Gynecologic
Endocrinology

Gynecologic Endocrinology

FOURTH EDITION

Edited by

JAY J. GOLD, M.D., F.A.C.P.

*Clinical Professor of Medicine
and Adjunct Professor of Obstetrics and Gynecology
University of Illinois College of Medicine
Chicago, Illinois*

and

JOHN B. JOSIMOVICH, M.D.

*Professor and Vice-Chairman
Department of Obstetrics and Gynecology
and Professor, Department of Pathology
UMDNJ–New Jersey Medical School
Newark, New Jersey*

PLENUM MEDICAL BOOK COMPANY • NEW YORK AND LONDON

Library of Congress Cataloging in Publication Data

Gynecologic endocrinology.

Includes bibliographies and index.
1. Endocrine gynecology. I. Gold, Jay J. II. Josimovich, John B., 1931–   .
[DNLM: 1. Endocrine Diseases. 2. Endocrine Glands — physiology.3. Genital Diseases,
Female. WP 505 G997]
RG159.G96   1986   618.1   86-22666
ISBN 0-306-42189-5

© 1987 Plenum Publishing Corporation
233 Spring Street, New York, N.Y. 10013

Plenum Medical Book Company is an imprint of Plenum Publishing Corporation

Printed in the United States of America

To our
wives, children, and grandchildren,
and to our office staffs

Contributors

A.A. ACOSTA, M.D.

Professor, Department of Obstetrics and Gynecology, Eastern Virginia Medical School, Norfolk, Virginia 23507

ROBERT N. ALSEVER, M.D.

Division of Endocrinology, Southern Colorado Clinic, Pueblo, Colorado 81004; and Clinical Associate Professor, Department of Medicine, University of Colorado Health Sciences Center, Denver, Colorado 80220

WILLIAM C. ANDREWS, M.D.

Professor, Department of Obstetrics and Gynecology, Eastern Virginia Medical School, Norfolk, Virginia 23507

DAVID F. ARCHER, M.D.

Associate Professor, Department of Obstetrics and Gynecology, University of Pittsburgh School of Medicine; and Department of Obstetrics and Gynecology, Magee-Womens Hospital, Pittsburgh, Pennsylvania 15213

JANICE M. BAHR, PH.D.

Professor, Department of Animal Sciences, University of Illinois, Urbana, Illinois 61801

WADI A. BARDAWIL, M.D.

Professor, Departments of Pathology and Obstetrics and Gynecology, University of Illinois, Chicago, Illinois 60612

OLGA M. BLAIR, M.D.

Associate Professor, Department of Pathology, St. Louis University School of Medicine, St. Louis, Missouri 63104

SANDRA ANN CARSON, M.D.

Assistant Professor and Attending Physician, Department of Obstetrics and Gynecology, Michael Reese Hospital and Medical Center, University of Chicago, Chicago, Illinois 60616

FRANK E. CHANG, M.D.

Clinical Instructor and Fellow in Reproductive Endocrinology, Department of Obstetrics and Gynecology, Ohio State University Hospitals, Columbus, Ohio 43210

M. YUSOFF DAWOOD, M.D., CH.B., M.MED, M.R.C.O.G.

Professor, Department of Obstetrics and Gynecology, Director, Division of Reproductive Endocrinology, University of Illinois College of Medicine, Chicago, Illinois 60612

WAYNE DECKER, M.D., F.A.C.S.

Executive Director, Fertility Research Foundation, New York, New York 10021

EUGENE R. DESOMBRE, PH.D.

Professor, Ben May Laboratory for Cancer Research, The University of Chicago, Chicago, Illinois 60637

CHARLES H. EMERSON, M.D.

Professor, Department of Medicine, Division of Endocrinology and Metabolism, University of Massachusetts School of Medicine, Worcester, Massachusetts 01605

CELSO-RAMON GARCIA, M.D.

Professor, Division of Human Reproduction, Department of Obstetrics and Gynecology, Hospital and Medical School of the University of Pennsylvania, Philadelphia, Pennsylvania 19104

J. GARCIA, M.D.

Director, Women's Hospital Fertility Center and IVF Program, Greater Baltimore Medical Center, Towson, Maryland 21204

JOHN G. GRUHN, M.D.

Associate Professor, Department of Pathology, Northwestern University School of Medicine, Chicago, Illinois 60611

DAVID L. HEALY, M.D., PH.D., M.R.A.C.O.G.

Lecturer, Department of Obstetrics and Gynaecology, Monash University, Queen Victoria Medical Center, Melbourne, Australia

ARTHUR L. HERBST, M.D.

Professor and Chairman, Department of Obstetrics and Gynecology, The University of Chicago, Chicago, Illinois 60637

JOHN A. HOLT, PH.D.

Associate Professor, Department of Obstetrics and Gynecology, The University of Chicago, Chicago, Illinois 60637

RAPHAEL JEWELEWICZ, M.D.

Associate Professor and Chief, Department of Obstetrics and Gynecology, Columbia University, College of Physicians and Surgeons, New York, New York 10032

JOHN B. JOSIMOVICH, M.D.

Professor and Vice-Chairman, Department of Obstetrics and Gynecology, and Professor, Department of Pathology, UMDNJ–New Jersey Medical School, Newark, New Jersey 07103

MOON H. KIM, M.D.

Professor and Director of Reproductive Endocrinology, Department of Obstetrics and Gynecology, Ohio State University Hospitals, Columbus, Ohio 43210

MARVIN A. KIRSCHNER, M.D.

Professor, Department of Medicine, New Jersey Medical School; and Newark Beth Israel Medical Center, Newark, New Jersey 07112

DAVID L. KLEINBERG, M.D.

Professor, Department of Medicine, New York University Medical Center; and Chief, Department of Endocrinology, Veterans Administration Medical Center, New York, New York 10016

BERTRAM LEVIN, M.D.

Professor and Chairman, Department of Diagnostic Radiology, Michael Reese Hospital and Medical Center; and Department of Radiology, Pritzker School of Medicine, University of Chicago, Chicago, Illinois 60618

EDWARD L. MARUT, M.D.

Director, In vitro Fertilization–Embryo Transfer Program, Division of Reproductive Endocrinology, Michael Reese Hospital and Medical Center; and Assistant Professor, Department of Obstetrics and Gynecology, Pritzker School of Medicine–University of Chicago, Chicago, Illinois 60616

S. J. MUASHER, M.D.

Department of Obstetrics and Gynecology, Eastern Virginia Medical School, Norfolk, Virginia 23507

JOHN R. MUSICH, M.D.

Chairman, Department of Obstetrics and Gynecology, William Beaumont Hospital, Royal Oak, Michigan 48072; and Department of Obstetrics and Gynecology, Wayne State University School of Medicine, Detroit, Michigan 48201

ROBERT S. NEUWIRTH, M.D.

Associate Professor, Department of Obstetrics and Gynecology, Columbia University College of Physicians and Surgeons; and Director, Department of Obstetrics and Gynecology, St. Luke's/Roosevelt Hospital, New York, New York 10025

MARIA I. NEW, M.D.

Professor and Chairman, Department of Pediatrics, Chief, Division of Pediatric Endocrinology, Acting Associate Program Director, Pediatric Clinical Research Center, The New York Hospital–Cornell Medical Center, New York, New York 10021

FRANCISCO I. REYES, M.D.

Professor and Director, Division of Reproductive Endocrinology, Department of Obstetrics and Gynecology, State University of New York, Downstate Medical Center, Brooklyn, New York 11203

GEORGE S. RICHARDSON, M.D.

Associate Professor of Surgery, Department of Gynecology, Harvard Medical School at the Massachusetts General and Vincent Memorial Hospitals, Boston, Massachusetts 02114

Z. ROSENWAKS, M.D.

Department of Obstetrics and Gynecology, Eastern Virginia Medical School, Norfolk, Virginia 23507

ANTONIO SCOMMEGNA, M.D.

Professor and Chairman, Department of Obstetrics and Gynecology, Michael Reese Hospital and Medical Center, University of Chicago, Chicago, Illinois 60616

BARBARA SHORTLE, M.D., PH.D.

Fellow in Reproductive Endocrinology, Department of Obstetrics and Gynecology, Columbia University, College of Physicians and Surgeons, New York, New York 10032

JOE LEIGH SIMPSON, M.D.

Professor and Chairman, Department of Obstetrics and Gynecology, University of Tennessee, Memphis, Memphis, Tennessee 38163

W.N. SPELLACY, M.D.

Professor and Chairman, Department of Obstetrics and Gynecology, University of Illinois College of Medicine, Chicago, Illinois 60612

EMIL STEINBERGER, M.D.

Texas Institute for Reproductive Medicine and Endocrinology; and Clinical Professor, Department of Internal Medicine, University of Texas Medical School at Houston, Houston, Texas 77002

JOHN C. M. TSIBRIS, PH.D.

Associate Professor, Department of Obstetrics and Gynecology, and Department of Physiology and Biophysics, University of Illinois at Chicago, Chicago, Illinois 60612

GERSON WEISS, M.D.

Professor and Chairman, Department of Obstetrics and Gynecology, University of Medicine and Dentistry of New Jersey–New Jersey Medical School, Newark, New Jersey 07103

CHARLES R. WIRA, PH.D.

Professor, Department of Physiology, Dartmouth Medical School, Hanover, New Hampshire 03756

Foreword

It has been exactly five years since I was privileged to write the foreword for the previous edition of this distinguished book on gynecologic endocrinology. Reproductive endocrinology has been established as a separate respected area in the general field of endocrinology, as well as in obstetrics and gynecology. Years ago the reproductive endocrinologist took long periods of time to answer questions, since most of the studies done then used bioassay methods. These studies were hastened by the work of Berson and Yalow with their development of the radioimmunoassay. They were later awarded the Nobel Prize for this work, since it unlocked many avenues of investigation in the field of endocrinology. It is now possible to measure small quantities of hormones in various biological tissues. Since that time high-pressure liquid chromatography and mass spectrometry have unlocked further secrets in this field with their capability of measuring ever smaller quantities of substances as well as their metabolites. Giant strides have been made in other diagnostic methods that interface with gynecologic endocrinology, notably in the field of radiology in the arena of tomography and CAT scans, and now nuclear magnetic resonance.

Progress will be pushed still further, and this fourth edition again identifies the leading edge of knowledge. Such new areas embrace the physiology of relaxin, the ontogeny of sexual differentiation, diagnostic procedures on the cervix, functional dysmenorrhea and anorexia nervosa, idiopathic edema, and the misunderstood premenstrual tension syndrome. Additional topics include the endocrinologic control of steroid receptors of the reproductive tract and breast malignancies, the management of diabetes mellitus during pregnancy, and several of our newest clinical arenas, including in vitro fertilization and control of the female immune system in the nonpregnant and pregnant states.

This is a large addition to an already very complete book. The authors of chapters in these areas are all scientists who have had personal experience in them and are considered experts. I continue to marvel at the progress of endocrinology in its never-ending search for additional truth, all of which ultimately relates back to superior clinical care for the patient. It is more and more difficult to mount serious investigative programs in this area as federal funding has diminished. The contributors to this book are individuals who will continue to lead investigations of the endocrine system and whose findings will translate from the laboratory workbench to clinical investigation, eventually becoming part of almost routine care for the practitioner of medicine. We are most indebted to Drs. Gold and Josimovich and the other contributors to this text, who have continued to make it a book of excellence.

Frederick P. Zuspan

Chairman, Department of Obstetrics and Gynecology
Ohio State University
Columbus, Ohio 43210

Preface

In this fourth edition of *Gynecologic Endocrinology,* it is a pleasure to be with our new publisher, Plenum Publishing Corporation. It is difficult to surpass prior excellence, but this edition boasts a multitude of outstanding new contributors as well as many of our old friends.

Unlike other books in the field, this one is purposely multiauthored to encompass a wide range of current expertise and a diversity of information. This approach will enable the sophisticated student and expert alike to cull the most important information without having to depend on didactic and often short-lived criteria or dicta.

This new edition includes information that has surpassed our best expectations for accomplishment in the field since the last edition. Endorphins and enkephalins, along with the bioamines and other regulatory CNS substances, assume additional prominence in CNS control. The diagnostic and therapeutic use of releasing hormones is becoming more commonplace, as is an improvement in delivery systems. Currently pulsatile pumps are being used, but eventually analogues may take their place in certain circumstances. Already the manufacturers of these factors and hormones are using advanced genetic techniques. In addition, the advent of monoclonal antibodies promises to simplify and improve the specificity of immunoassays in laboratories. The understanding of receptors has now been extended to intracellular postreceptor activities that may be blocked or enhanced in creating or treating disease processes. In vitro fertilization is now almost commonplace, with an explosion of in vitro fertilization centers around the world. Its original indications are now being broadened. In some areas of the country, surrogate parenting is being encouraged, and the time for ovarian transplants may not be too far off.

With so much already learned, it is hard to fathom what new areas remain for exploration, but they are many, and the surface of our learning has hardly been sanded, much less scratched. After reading the chapters in this book, the reader cannot help but be enthusiastic over prospects for future progress.

Jay J. Gold
John B. Josimovich

Skokie and Newark

Preface to the First Edition

There are several books available that are devoted to special phases of gynecologic endocrinology, and there are several endocrine texts that devote a few chapters to gynecologic endocrinology, but there is no book that adequately and completely compiles the latest information by knowledgeable authors into one text that can be used by physicians who are interested in this field.

This text was undertaken to fill the currently existing void. The field of gynecologic endocrinology has grown like Jack's legendary beanstalk. The contributions that have been made in this field over recent years and that have generated its growth as a specific field of endeavor are to be found in so many publications that any neophyte or interested sophisticate would be faced with a mammoth task of organization. What better way is there to solve this problem and ease the task for the progressive student than to go to the experts in each of the important subdivisions? In this manner these experts may pass on their knowledge, acquired through research, organized reading and interest, teaching, and experience. Adherence to this concept has produced a unified text that glows en masse from the brilliance generated by its contributors.

I am indebted to Dr. J. P. Greenhill for his generous remarks in the Foreword, and to my wife who has been secretary, critic, and a constant source of encouragement.

Jay J. Gold

Chicago, Illinois

Contents

IV. ENDOCRINE DISORDERS IN THE FEMALE

V. INFERTILITY AND ITS FUTURE

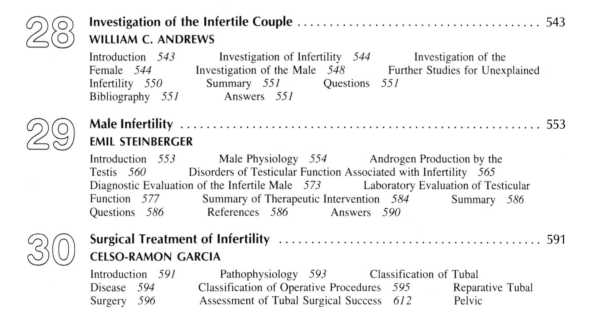

VI. NEW FRONTIERS IN GYNECOLOGIC ENDROCRINOLOGY

Gynecologic Endocrinology

FOURTH EDITION

Basic Anatomy and Physiology

1

Historical Introduction to Gonadal Regulation of the Uterus and the Menses

JOHN G. GRUHN

This chapter presents a selective historically oriented survey of the development of concepts from which modern gynecologic endocrinology arose. Current literature rarely permits consideration of how the basic facts and concepts developed and seldom provides historical perspective.

The uterus and the menses were recognized several millennia before the ovary was identified. The Sumerian birth goddess Nintu is shaped like a uterus, and the Egyptian hieroglyph Ankh depicted on the birth goddess Taurt resembles a uterus. The earliest known anatomic drawing of the uterus is from a ninth century manuscript copy of Soranus's *Gynecology*. Soranus, who practiced during the reigns of Trajan and Hadrian (98–138 A.D.), represents ancient obstetric and gynecologic practice at its apogee. Until the fourteenth century, it was widely believed that the human uterus was multichambered and could wander about the body, causing hysteria.

Discovery of the ovary is attributed to Herophilus

JOHN G. GRUHN • Department of Pathology, Northwestern University School of Medicine, Chicago, Illinois 60611.

of Chalcedon, an anatomist of the Alexandrian school of the fourth century B.C. and an originator of gross dissection. He is regarded as a father of scientific anatomy by the medical historian Karl Sudhoff. The lost original text of Herophilus is known to us because Galen copied from it into his *De Semine*. Kühn's translation from Galen uses the term *female testicle*. The anatomic analogy of the ovary and testicle was recognized long before their true function was suspected and before the term ovary came into use.

According to Aristotle (384–322 B.C.), the leading biologist of antiquity, seed produced in the male ducts developed in the soil of the menstrual coagulum of the female. Male seed provided form, motion, and soul for the child; female soil provided matter and body. Seed and soil combined to produce an egg that was the product of conception. The male testicles served as weights to keep the ducts straight. Aristotle also knew that farmers spayed animals to produce fatter animals; this eliminated the estrous cycle and the sex drive. Scientists failed to grasp the implication of this phenomenon until the 1870s.

Soranus also provided the earliest detailed gross

description of the ovaries, which he called didymi (literally twins). Temkin's 1956 translation notes "female seed seems not to be drawn on in generation since it is excreted externally."

Scrutiny of Vesalius's *De Fabrica* of 1543 reveals that the artist drew an epididymis on the "female testicle." Vesalius's book was the first to depict follicles in the "female testicle." He probably also saw the corpus luteum.

Fallopius, who thought the tubes vented noxious fumes from the uterus, wrote in 1562 that "anatomists assert . . . seed is made in the *testicles* of females. . . . But I have never seen seed."

Fabricius applied the name *ovarium* to the ovary of the hen in 1621 but did not apply the term to the human ovary. His *De Formatu Foetu* (1604) includes what is believed to be the first illustration of corpora lutea (from a sow).

Although Jan Swammerdam, Jan van Horne, and Niels Stenson conceived the idea that the "female testicle" is functionally comparable to the ovary of the bird, George Corner emphatically concluded that Regner de Graaf's detailed experimental observations published in 1672 established the concept that it is truly an ovary. An English translation of de Graaf's work by Jocelyn and Setchell appears in Supplement 17 of the *Journal of Reproduction and Fertility* in 1972. De Graaf mistook the entire follicle as an ovum, an error corrected by Carl von Baer, who first identified the true mammalian ovum in 1827. It was Albrecht von Haller (1708–1777), the greatest physiologist of his age, who designated the ovarian follicle as the graafian follicle. The term "female testicle" lingered long after de Graaf; it appears throughout Letter XXXVIII in Book III of Giovanni Baptista Morgagni's classic *De Sedibus et Causis Morborum* of 1761, which included "all of the common tumors" of the ovary.

Marcello Malpighi, generally considered the founder of microscopic anatomy, coined the term corpus luteum for the structure, which had previously been described by others. One of his descriptions appears in a letter written in 1681. Malpighi thought the follicle was derived from the corpus luteum.

Hippocrates, Aristotle, Galen, and Pliny assumed menstrual bleeding to be a cleansing or detoxifying process. In Leviticus the menstruating woman is considered unclean regarding the sexual activity and preparation of certain foods. Menses is the Latin term for month. In popular folklore the moon regulated the tides of women as well as the tides of the sea. As late as 1898, the physicist

Svante Arrhenius mistakenly believed he had demonstrated a mathematical correlation of lunar and menstrual cycles.

In 1775 Percival Pott removed both ovaries from a young woman for the correction of herniae. He noted that her menses ceased and her breasts shrank. Nineteen years later, in his doctoral thesis, John Davidge concluded: "Menstruation is attributable to a peculiar condition of the ovaries serving as a source of excitement to the vessels of the womb."

In 1797 Haighton recognized that coition induces ovulation in the rabbit. This appears to be the first description of induced ovulation.

The concept of internal secretion, proposed by Claude Bernard in 1855, would not be clearly applied to the ovary until 1900. During the 1850s, oophorectomy became a relatively common operation. By 1858 Karl Ludwig's famous *Lehrbuch der Physiologie* found loss of ovaries in humans to result in cessation of menses and shrinkage of the uterus.

Edward Pflüger, the leading German physiologist of his time, provided the first integrated theory of menstruation in 1863. He proposed that neural influences from distended follicles reflexly dilate pelvic and uterine vessels, causing engorgement, endometrial proliferation, and uterine bleeding.

During the 1870s the medical journals reported that a single episode of uterine bleeding lasting a few days occurred several days after oophorectomy. The phenomenon seemed inexplicable until the work of Allen in 1927–1928.

In 1873 Albert Peuch provided the first medical description of castrate atrophy of the sow uterus. The first published illustration of castrate atrophy of the sow uterus was provided by the distinguished gynecologist Alfred Hegar in 1878. Within two decades, the prevention of uterine atrophy in the castrate by experimental ovarian transplants would be utilized to establish the ovary as an organ of internal secretion.

In 1875 Oscar Hertwig, working with sea urchin eggs, established the principle that fertilization consists of the union of male and female nuclei. Herman Fol was the first to observe a starfish sperm cell actually fertilize a starfish ovum under his microscope in 1877. The discovery of the significance of fertilization ranks on a par with the discovery of the circulation in the seventeenth century.

Charles Brown-Sequard claimed he could obtain aqueous extracts from testicles (1889) and from ovaries (1890), with which he could rejuvenate men and women. Unfortunately, his extracts proved scientifically worthless. By 1895 Edward Schäfer, the leading physiologist in England, made the concept of internal secretion respectable in medicine, but he dismissed the theory of an endocrine function for the gonads for lack of experimental proof.

In 1895 Robert Tuttle Morris, a New York surgeon, pioneered the first successful human ovarian transplants, but his work was largely ignored at the time.

In 1896 G. T. Beatson reported that castration alleviated symptoms and signs of several patients with metastatic breast carcinoma.

In 1896 Emil Knauer, a young gynecologist in Vienna in Chrobek's department, removed ovaries from rabbits, grafted portions back, and demonstrated that ovarian grafts prevented castrate atrophy. Not until his monograph in 1900 did he refer to "internal secretion." He served in the chair of Obstetrics and Gynecology at Graz, Austria, from 1903 until 1934 and lived to use estrogenic hormone in his clinic. In 1898 Joseph Halban transplanted ovarian grafts subcutaneously into oophorectomized newborn guinea pigs in which uteri and tubes then developed normally. In 1900 he concluded: "We must assume . . . a substance . . . produced by the ovary . . . taken into the blood is able to exercise . . . influence upon the genital organs."

By 1900 Knauer and Halban had clearly demolished the theory proposed by Pflüger and proved the existence of an internal secretion from the ovary. It would take three additional decades of work to establish the existence of two ovarian hormones.

Between 1863 and 1898, five distinguished investigators—Pflüger, Waldeyer, Sobotta, Beard, and Prenant—studied the anatomy and function of the corpus luteum. In 1898 Louis-Auguste Prenant of Nancy was first to suggest: "there can be no doubt from a study of its histological appearance that it [the corpus luteum] acts . . . as a gland of internal secretion, releasing . . . products into the bloodstream." Prenant never attempted to test his thesis experimentally.

In 1900 Gustave Born of Breslau stimulated two of his former students to test his hypothesis that its function must be the protection of the early embryo. Working independently, Ludwig Fraenkel and Vilhelm Magnus demonstrated that spaying pregnant rabbits or cauterizing their corpora lutea caused resorption of embryos. By 1901 Fraenkel claimed the ovary had two functions: to provide ova and to facilitate their implantation in the uterus.

Magnus also noted that removal of the corpora lutea did not induce uterine atrophy, leading him to suspect that the ovarian stroma produces another substance, which maintains the uterus. Magnus was among the earliest investigators to predict the existence of two ovarian hormones.

The term hormone was suggested by Hardy and Vesey. It is derived from ὁρμάω (hormao), a Greek verb, meaning to excite or to arouse. Professor Starling used this term in his Croonian Lecture on the *Chemical Correlation of the Functions of the Body* in 1905.

By 1906 Francis Marshall, a foremost pioneer in the reproductive physiology of animals, could write:

> The ovary [provides] an internal secretion . . . elaborated by . . . follicular cells or . . . the stroma. This secretion . . . induces menstruation and heat. After ovulation . . . the corpus luteum is formed, and . . . provides a further secretion . . . essential for . . . attachment and development of the embryo in . . . pregnancy."

By 1910 the existence of gonadal hormones was no longer doubted. Between 1911 and 1918 four investigators were able to extract ovarian hormones with lipid solvents.

In 1907 and 1908 Leo Loeb, an American, demonstrated that a foreign body could induce a decidual reaction in the endometrium of nonpregnant guinea pigs or rabbits only if the corpus luteum was present. Between 1909 and 1910 P. Ancel and P. Bouin in France published the first illustrations from animals of what is now known to be progestational endometrium and proved this change to be related to the corpus luteum. At this time, the occurrence and significance of progestational or secretory change in the human endometrium was just beginning to be recognized.

The occurrence of normal cyclic changes in the human endometrium was completely unknown until they were clearly illustrated by two young assistants at the First University Women's Clinic in Vienna—Fritz Hitschmann and Ludwig Adler—whose classic paper, *The Structure of the Endometrium in the Sexually Mature Woman*, was published in the *Monatschrift für Geburtshilfe und Gynäkologie* in 1908. To appreciate the significance of their contribution we must review some background data. Recamier, a Parisian, introduced the curette in 1850, pathologists began to use the microscope in the mid-1800s, and essentially modern histologic technology was available during the late 1870s. After the development of anesthesia and the concept of asepsis during the late 1800s, essentially modern abdominal surgery developed. Surgical and histopathologic techniques were essentially tools. The development of the German University system with specialized gynecologic clinics and pathologic institutes brought together the clinical material, the investigative attitudes, and the appropriate tools and methods to explore problems.

Recamier's studies marked the beginning of histologic research on the endometrium. In his review of menstrual cyclic changes in the uterus, Novak wrote, "the earliest studies on the anatomy of the menstruating uterus were made by Kundrat and Engelmann," who reported studies on the uteri of cadavers in 1873. Novak credited Möricke as the first investigator who "avoided the use of dead material by studying scrapings from women in various stages of the menstrual cycle" in 1882. Möricke concluded that the endometrium remains intact during the cycle. Until Hitschmann and Adler's work, it was generally believed that the endometrium does not change significantly between menstrual periods. The normal secretory phase was widely misinterpreted as "endometritis glandularis hypertrophica."

Four excerpts and paraphrases are cited to permit the reader to judge the significance of Hitschmann and Adler's contribution.

1. This cycle develops in various phases, which are so characteristic that the chronologic relationship of the endometrium to menstruation can be determined with certainty, often to the exact day.
2. The menstrual bleeding itself is merely the last phase of the cyclical development of the endometrium, the removal of the previously decidualized endometrium, for the introduction of a new cycle in preparation for the acceptance of a fertilized egg.
3. Distinction between menstruation and other types of bleeding can be accomplished by microscopic study of endometrium.
4. Having demonstrated the cyclic variation of the endometrium, Hitschmann and Adler questioned whether the ovary went through corresponding cyclic changes.

Between 1911 and 1913, using the histologic changes of the endometrium as a baseline, Robert Meyer and his co-worker Carl Ruge, Jr., described the corresponding changes in the corups luteum from its formation to its ultimate fate. It was then possible to determine the stage of development of the corpus luteum from its histologic appearance.

Between 1909 and 1915, Robert Schröder also correlated human endometrial and ovarian changes in a series of papers. It was Schröder who first pointed out the difference between the basal and functional layers of the endometrium, who systematized the cyclic stages, and who first used the terms proliferative and secretory endometrium. The concepts of Hitschmann and Adler, of Meyer, and of Schröder are now an integral part of the data base that pathologists use daily to "date the endometrium." The standard current reference in English on *Dating the Endometrium* by Noyes, Hertig, and Rock appeared in 1950. Meyer, Schröder, and co-workers explained human menstruation based on morphologic studies of human endometrial and ovarian changes before it was possible to measure hormones. Morphologic studies led Meyer and Schröder to the concept that menstruation is the result of breakdown of progestational endometrium due to degeneration of the corpus luteum, which Meyer summarized in his famous dictum: "*Ohne ovulation, keine menstruation.*"

Robert Schröder is also credited with establishing endometrial hyperplasia as a clinicopathologic entity in 1914–1915, stressing that hyperplasia was the result of the persistent action of estrogen. In 1954 he provided a perspective on this work in English in the *American Journal of Obstetrics and Gynecology* (Endometrial hyperplasia in relation to genital function).

Endometrial biopsy still provides an activity assay, a bioassay that provides a pictorial display of the end result of hormonal action on the endometrial target tissue.

In 1910 Harvey Cushing together with Crowe and Homans provided the first unequivocal experimental demonstration of a relationship between the anterior pituitary and the ovary. They demonstrated that experimental hypophysectomy or clamping the pituitary stalk causes atrophy of the ovaries and the uterus. Similar studies were reported by Paulesco in 1907 and by Bell in 1917.

Additional early studies of the pituitary and of gonadotropic activity are summarized as follows:

1543   Vesalius
Described "Glandula pituitam cerebri excipiens."
1742   Lieutaud
Described the "pituitary portal vascular system."

1760 DeHaen
Described amenorrhea in patient with pituitary tumor.

1898 Compte
Found the pituitary to increase in size during pregnancy

1907 Tandler, Grosz
Found that in humans the pituitary enlarges after oophorectomy or orchiectomy.

1909 Erdheim, Stumme
Discovered that anterior pituitary lobe enlarges during pregnancy; "pregnancy cells" seen microscopically

1912 Aschner
Developed experimental transbuccal hypophysectomy; described genital hypoplasia as consequence of hypophysectomy; credited Engel, a pupil of Rokitansky, with awareness of this relationship

Between 1911 and 1915, four independent investigators (Henry Iscovesco, 1912; Ottfried Fellner, 1912–1913; Edmund Herrmann, 1915; and Robert Frank, 1915) successfully extracted ovarian hormones with lipid solvents, but their early work was initially largely ignored until Allen and Doisy called attention to it in 1923. Only Iscovesco attempted to use his extracts in patients in his practice.

In 1917 Charles R. Stockard and George Papanicolaou demonstrated in the guinea pig that the histologic cyclic changes that occur in the reproductive tract during the estrus cycle also occur in the vaginal mucosa and can be detected by cytologic examination of vaginal smears. Lataste's similar earlier studies in 1886 and 1887 were neither generally known nor used. It soon became obvious that Stockard and Papanicolaou's research provided a simple, rapid, accurate, reproducible, reliable method for studying the estrus or the menstrual cycle. The time of rupture of the follicle could be determined in small mammals almost within an hour. Before this simple procedure, it had been cumbersome and difficult to study the inconspicuous estrous cycles of the guinea pig, mouse, rat, and rabbit, which do not menstruate. The vaginal cytologic technique was promptly used by many investigators to facilitate major advances in reproductive biology. It was applied to the rat by Long and Evans whose *The Oestrus Cycle in the Rat and Its Associated Phenomena* was published in 1922.

The Papanicolaou technique also facilitated the discovery of "an ovarian hormone." Arthur Hertig wrote, "And so the tiny flame kindled by Stockard and Papanicolaou in 1917 was fanned into a blaze in 1923 . . . by Edgar Allen and Edward A. Doisy."

Edgar Allen (1892–1943) had used the Papanicolaou technique to study the estrous cycle of the mouse, and by 1922 he had demonstrated findings similar to those previously noted in the guinea pig by Stockard and Papanicolaou and in the rat by Long and Evans. During these studies, Allen noted that large mature ovarian follicles were usually present at the peak of the vaginal cytologic findings. He collected follicular fluid from sow's ovaries, injected the fluid into spayed mice and rats, demonstrated precisely that characteristic cytologic changes occur rapidly in the vaginal cells, and observed that typical estrous behavior promptly followed the cytologic changes.

Edward Doisy, born in 1893, became professor of biochemistry at Washington University in 1923. He became acquainted with Allen through the faculty baseball team. They first discussed collaboration as Doisy drove Allen home from school in his Model T Ford. They outlined the biochemical steps of their initial partial purification in their landmark 1923 paper. Potency accompanied the lipid solvent. They did not find the substance in either corpora lutea or commercial ovarian extracts and suggested that it was produced in follicles, was probably produced in all ovaries as ova mature, was not species specific, and was probably common to all female animals.

Their 1923 report was entitled, An Ovarian Hormone: Preliminary Report on Its Localization, Extraction and Partial Purification, and Action in Test Animals. They erroneously concluded there was only one ovarian hormone and that it was produced in the follicles.

In 1923 A. S. Parkes, another outstanding pioneer in reproductive biology, initially made an odd error. He mixed up a group of mice and mistakenly irradiated female mice thinking they were males. His first important discovery was to recognize that the irradiated ovaries in which all follicles were destroyed could produce enough estrogenic hormone to maintain uterine cyclic changes and estrus behavior. He provided the first objective proof that estrogenic hormone production was not limited to the follicles. Parkes was also involved in the naming of the hormone. Many terms were in use, including feminin, folliculin, menformin, progynon, and thelykinin. Doisy had suggested the term theelin (*thelys*, for "female" in Greek), but this term was protected by a university patent and could not be used generically. Parkes and Bellerby provided the name oestrin in 1926.

Early efforts to purify estrogenic hormone from ovarian or placental sources were often frustrated because of the presence of extraneous material in the tissue sources, but a series of surprising findings in urine soon permitted further progress. In 1926 S. Loewe and F. Lange found estrogenic substance in human urine. In 1927 Selmar Aschheim detected large amounts of estrogen in urine from pregnant women.

The use of urine, a watery source of the hormone, free from the extraneous materials from tissue sources, vastly simplified the task of the biochemists. Between 1929 and 1930, four groups of investiagtors independently obtained pure crystalline estrogenic hormone, and Doisy and Allen in the United States and Butenandt in Germany independently proposed the chemical formula $C_{18}H_{22}O_2$.

1929–1930   Doisy, Veler, and Thayer
St. Louis

1929   Butenandt
Göttingen

1930   Dingenmanse, deJonge, Kober, and Laquer
Amsterdam

1930   D'Amour and Gustavson
Denver

By 1930, Marrian demonstrated that a more potent substance is present in stale than in fresh urine. Later it would be learned that estrogen is excreted in conjugated form in fresh urine but is hydrolyzed in stale urine.

In 1932 the first International Conference on Standardization of Sex Hormones in London reached agreement on a standard for estrogen. At that meeting the terminology of estrone, estradiol and estriol was officially adopted. By 1938 E. C. Dodds and colleagues reported the first synthetic estrogen, stilbestrol. Problems of estrogen-related carcinogenesis and diethylstilbestrol (DES) syndromes soon emerged into prominence but are beyond the scope of this chapter.

Landmark studies on gonadotropins between 1921 and 1941 may be summarized as follows:

1921   Evans and Long
These workers studied intraperitoneal anterior pituitary extracts on the estrus cycle of rats.

1924   Evans
Alkaline extracts or ox pituitary inhibit estrous cycle and cause luteinization of follicles in the rat (*Note:* Ox pituitary is rich in LH; horse pituitary is rich in FSH.)

1926–1927   Smith, Engle
Two independent groups discovered a gonadotropic factor.

1926–1927   Zondek and Aschheim
Smith's technique of hypophysectomy provided a breakthrough for studies of pituitary trophic hormones. Hypo-

physectomized animals soon became a standard for the study of the number of gonadotropins and how they affected the ovary.

Smith's group demonstrated that hypophysectomized immature animals do not mature sexually.

They demonstrated that implantation of macerated pituitary induces precocious sexual maturity in immature rats and mice. Such implants may increase weight of immature mouse ovaries by a factor of 10 or 20. Later, in 1930, they proved that pituitary injections into hypophysectomized rats restored lost sexual function. Their work with hypophysectomized rats helped dispel criticism that the 1927 experiments were due to an effect on the pituitary of the experimental animals in that study.

Zondek's group demonstrated that extracts of anterior pituitary produce precocious puberty in immature mice.

1928   Fee and Parkes
Pituitary removal (by a crude partial decerebration) within 45 min after mating prevents ovulation.

1928   Zondek and Aschheim
The urine of pregnant women produces a gonadotropic effect similar to the action of pituitary gonadotropin. This became the basis for the famous Aschheim–Zondek urine pregnancy test.

1928   Zondek and Aschheim
There are two distinct gonadotropic hormones. Prolan A (later known as FSH) controls follicle maturation, the production of oestrone, and the estral reaction. Prolan B (later known as LH) controls luteinization.

1928–1929   Evans and Simpson
Gonadotropins are produced by pituitary basophils.

1929   Stricker and Gruter
Lactation was induced in ovariectomized pseudopregnant rabbits by administration of anterior pituitary extracts. This observation is the first experimental demonstration of a hypophyseal lactogenic substance.

1930   Collip
Extrahypophyseal origin of choriogonadotropin in early pregnancy urine was confirmed.

1931   Fevold, Hisaw, and Leonard; Hill and Parkes
Evidence that two different pituitary hormones influence the ovarian cycle was presented.

1932   Allen and Wiles
1933   Selye, Collip, and Thompson
Hypophysectomy was shown to inhibit lactation.

1933   Riddle, Bates, and Dykshorn
Prolactin was prepared, identified, and assayed as a hormone of the anterior pituitary.

1934   Fevold and Hisaw
Description of separation of FSH from LH was made.

1936   Evans, Korpi, Pencharz, and Wonder
Isolation of ICSH (later recognized as identical to LH) was accomplished.

1936   Marshall
"the internal rhythm is brought into relation with . . . other external phenomena . . . acting extraceptively through the nervous system and probably through the hypothalamus upon the anterior pituitary and thence upon . . . the ovary . . . . The primary periodicity is a function of the gonad, the anterior pituitary acting as a regulator. . . ." (The Croonian Lecture)

1938   Third Conference on Standardization of Sex Hormones
Agreement was reached on standardization of chorionic gonadotropin, mare serum gonadotropin, and prolactin. (Agreement on pituitary gonadotropins was not reached until after World War II.)

1940   Li, Simpson, and Evans
Preparation and physicochemical studies of interstitial cell stimulating hormone (ICSH) were accomplished.

Note: The terms FSH and LH are derived from the work of Evans's group.

In 1928 George Corner and Willard Allen studied adult rabbits ovariectomized after mating to evaluate the role of the corpus luteum. In 1929 they concluded:

> The evidence is now complete that in the rabbit the corpus luteum is an organ of internal secretion which has for one of its functions the production of a special state of the uterine mucosa (progestational proliferation). . . . The function of the proliferated endometrium is to . . . protect the free blastocysts and to make possible their implantation.

With the assistance of the lipid chemist, Walter Bloor, they obtained crude oily extracts of corpora lutea. Corner is credited with the discovery of the hormonal action of progesterone in 1929.

By 1931–1932, three groups of investigators working independently obtained almost pure crystalline material of high progestational activity: Fels and Slotta in Breslau, Fevold and Hisaw in Wisconsin, and W. Allen in Rochester.

By 1934 four groups of investigators were able to isolate crystalline progesterone from the corpus luteum and determine its structure: Allen and Wintersteiner in the United States, Butenandt and Westphal in Danzig, Germany, Hartmann and Wettstein in Switzerland, and Slotta, Ruschig, and Fels in Breslau, Germany. Wintersteiner worked with 75 mg crystals, Butenandt et al. had only 20 mg crystals obtained from the corpora lutea of 50,000 guinea pigs to determine the structure.

Fevold and Hisaw had used the term corporin for the hormone which obviously emphasized its source. Butenandt called the material luteosterone, which combined its source and its steroid nature.

Corner preferred the term progestin, which emphasized its biologic function. Parkes and Marrian were able to arrange a compromise in 1935, and the name progesterone was born "in a place of refreshment near the Imperial Hotel in Russell Square" in London at the time of The Second International Conference on The Standardization of Sex Hormones. Soon thereafter on August 16, 1935, Allen, Butenandt, Corner, and Slotta published a note in *Science* that resolved the nomenclature of corpus luteum hormone.

In 1920 Corner began to use the rhesus monkey for experimental studies because the cycle of the rhesus monkey closely resembles the human cycle. The monkey proved to be an ideal model to study the menstrual cycle ever since.

In 1923 Corner described anovulatory menstruation in the rhesus monkey and called attention to the previous work of Heape in 1897 and of van Herwerden in 1906. Between 1923 and 1927, George Corner, Willard Allen, and Carl Hartman each provided clear experimental proof that anovulatory cyclic bleeding occurs in rhesus monkeys. Novak appears to have described an early but inconclusive case in a woman in 1927. In 1932 Mazer and Ziserman claimed they had provided the first detailed report of this phenomenon in women in a paper entitled "Pseudomenstruation in the Human Female."

During 1927–1928, Edgar Allen noted that bilateral oophorectomy of rhesus monkeys was followed by uterine bleeding within a few days. His studies led him to propose an estrogen deprivation hypothesis in 1928 to explain menstruation. This hypothesis sharply contrasted with the Meyer-Schröder concept. Between 1928 and 1939, a host of investigators, including Allen, Corner, Engle, Greep, Hisaw, Pincus, Shelesnyak, Smith and Smith, and Zahl and Zuckerman, reported extensive experimental studies of menstruation. In 1939 George Corner summarized the data available at that time in "The Ovarian Hormones and Experimental Menstruation" in the *American Journal of Obstetrics and Gynecology*. By this time it was clear that both estrogen and progesterone must be considered in any working hypothesis. Corner provided a synthesis of the demonstrable experimental effects of estrogen and progesterone and the histomorphologic studies of the ovaries and the gonads.

During this time, the key role of the spiral coiled arteries of the endometrium in menstruation were elucidated by George Bartelmez at the University of Chicago between 1931 and 1941. His former associate John E. Markee also provided an elegant experimental method of observing menstruation in vivo by studies of endometrium transplanted into the anterior chamber of the eye of monkeys conducted between 1932 and 1946.

Limitations of space preclude historical review of topics such as ovarian steroidogenesis, radioimmunoassay (RIA) of hormones, feedback mechanisms, hypothalamic-releasing hormones, hormone receptors, and studies of the localization of hormones in tissues. Several of these topics are considered historically in subsequent chapters in this book. This introductory chapter has surveyed the elemental facets—the anatomic subunits and the hormones—that regulate the menstrual and the sexual rhythm. Once this basic information became available, attempts to use hormones and to manipulate the system inevitably followed rapidly. Short summarized the significance of the development of the contraceptive pill: ''No other scientific discovery in the field of reproduction has had greater impact on the general well-being of mankind.'' The body of this book reflects the exponential explosive progress of gynecologic endocrinology which has occurred during the past few decades.

A detailed bibliography may be obtained from the author by the interested reader.

2

The Neuroendocrine System

JANICE M. BAHR

INTRODUCTION

Neuroendocrinology is the study of the interaction between the nervous and endocrine systems. The premier site of this interaction is that of the hypothalamus and pituitary. The hypothalamus acts as a central station where neural and hormonal messages arising from internal and external stimuli are decoded and the appropriate message sent to the anterior pituitary. The Moore–Price theory, published in 1930, suggested a reciprocal influence between the gonads and the pituitary. The pituitary elaborated a gonad-stimulating hormone. In turn the gonads were thought to produce hormones that suppress the pituitary in a negative manner. This interaction was described as a seesaw, or a push–pull effect. The results of these experiments suggested that the anterior pituitary is the master gland that controls the gonads, adrenal cortex, and thyroid. This concept persisted until the late 1940s.

However, other researchers during this era, among them F. H. A. Marshall, the famous English physiologist, noted that external factors, such as day length, affect the breeding cycles of rabbits. Data published from several laboratories then demonstrated that localized electrical stimuli to precise regions of the hypothalamus alter function of the

ovary. Another key experiment that aided in tumbling the pituitary from its pedestal as the master gland was the blockade of the preovulatory luteinizing hormone (LH) surge by neural blocking drugs. These findings suggested that a neurogenic stimulus causes release of pituitary hormones. Moreover, anesthetizing rats at 1400 hr in proestrus but not at other times blocked the LH surge, suggesting a 24-hr rhythmicity in the control of LH. These initial studies laid the foundation for the study of neuroendocrinology, which has expanded into an extensive and fruitful field of investigation.[1,2]

Regardless of the degree to which the hormonal and neural systems are interlocked, the problem remained how neural signals were translated into action by the pituitary gland. The anterior pituitary gland is not innervated. The neural signal reaching the hypothalamus must therefore be translated into hormonal signal. Neurons in the hypothalamus produce neurohormones that are secreted into the capillary plexus and transported *via* a portal system to the anterior pituitary. The suggestion that neurons possess secretory functions was first proposed by Ernst Scharrer in 1928. The chemical nature of these neurohormones vary, ranging from biogenic amines to small peptides. The release of these neurohormones is regulated by the feedback of hormones from target tissues such as the thyroid, adrenal cortex, gonads, as well as by the higher levels of the brain.

JANICE M. BAHR • Department of Animal Sciences, University of Illinois, Urbana, Illinois 61801.

HISTORICAL BACKGROUND

Before discussing some of the details of the hypothalamic–hypophyseal relationships, a brief historical review is presented to show how these relationships were discovered and how they are investigated.

Electrolytic Lesions

One of the early approaches used in examining the relationship between the hypothalamus and the anterior pituitary was to place electrolytic lesions in discrete areas of the hypothalamus and determine which end-organ gland (e.g., thyroid, gonads) would be most obviously affected by these lesions. Such mapping has led to the postulate that specific and reasonably discrete regions of the hypothalamus are primarily concerned with the elaboration of releasing factors, which control the release of a specific pituitary hormone.

Deafferentation

Another approach widely used in neuroendocrinology is deafferentation. This technique involves inserting an appropriately fine cutting tool called a Halász knife, through the top of the skull and cutting the nerve tracks leading into the hypothalamus from its anterior to posterior aspect. It is also possible to cut completely around the hypothalamus, creating a hypothalamic island that has no nerve connections to the rest of the central nervous system (CNS). This technique permits the study of the relationship of the hypothalamus to the rest of the CNS.

Implantation of Hormones

The technique of implanting minute quantities of hormone (steroid or protein) into either the hypothalamus or the anterior pituitary makes it possible to distinguish between hypothalamic control centers and feedback control directly at the level of the anterior pituitary. This research has shown that, for most of the hormones studied, feedback may be exerted on both the hypothalamus and the pituitary, although the major feedback center appears to be the hypothalamus.

Adrenergic and Cholinergic Drugs

The use of cholinergic, adrenergic, and other drugs or tranquilizers to block the neural pathways

(primarily α sites) to and in the hypothalamus has also aided in elucidating the importance of hypothalamic control of the anterior pituitary. One of the most critical experiments in neuroendocrinology was performed by Sawyer and Everett in 1960.[1,2] These workers found that rats or mice anesthetized with pentobarbital (Nembutal) at a specific stage of the estrous cycle do not ovulate because the mechanism responsible for the release of gonadotropins has been blocked.[1] Similarly α-site-blocking drugs such as phenoxybenzamine (Dibenzyline) can be shown to block LH release in monkeys, a mechanism that may function in women as well. Neurotic or psychotic women who are given large doses of tranquilizers such as reserpine or chlorpromazine may have breast enlargement and start lactating. This effect is attributed to the action of the drugs on the hypothalamus, which normally produces a prolactin-inhibiting factor (PIF). Since this factor is inhibited by the drugs, prolactin (PRL) is released; in conjunction with other hormones, the PRL action leads to lactation.

Stalk Section

It is also possible to cut the stalk connecting the hypothalamus and the pituitary gland (Fig. 2-1). If this is done, the portal system, which normally carries the releasing factors to the anterior pituitary, is interrupted. The releasing factors cannot reach the pituitary gland and the glands controlled by the anterior pituitary degenerate either partially or completely.[3] The dependence of the pituitary gland on hypothalamic control can also be shown by removing the pituitary gland from its normal location and transplanting it to other sites, such as the kidney capsule or the anterior chamber of the eye.[4] If this is done, the pituitary gland releases very low levels of its hormones, with the exception of prolactin. However, the pituitary can be made to function again if releasing factors are infused into it.

Extraction of Releasing and Inhibiting Factors

The most convincing demonstration of the existence of releasing factors involves the chemical extraction of these factors from hypothalamic fragments.[5,6] Hypothalami of all large domestic animals and primates have yielded sufficiently high quantities of the various releasing factors to permit testing on human beings. Injections of such purified extracts into the carotid artery of experimental animals clearly showed that (1) there are separate releasing factors for growth hormone (GH), thy-

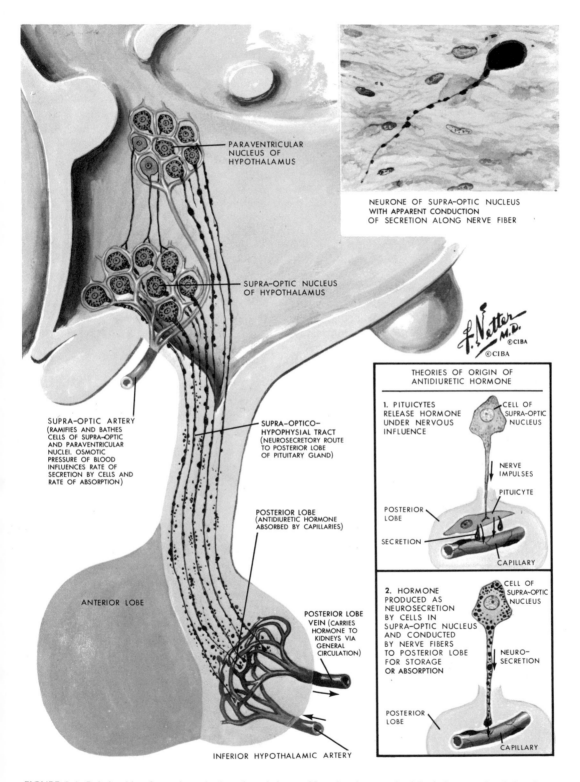

PARAVENTRICULAR NUCLEUS OF HYPOTHALAMUS

NEURONE OF SUPRA-OPTIC NUCLEUS WITH APPARENT CONDUCTION OF SECRETION ALONG NERVE FIBER

SUPRA-OPTIC NUCLEUS OF HYPOTHALAMUS

SUPRA-OPTIC ARTERY (RAMIFIES AND BATHES CELLS OF SUPRA-OPTIC AND PARAVENTRICULAR NUCLEI. OSMOTIC PRESSURE OF BLOOD INFLUENCES RATE OF SECRETION BY CELLS AND RATE OF ABSORPTION)

SUPRA-OPTICO-HYPOPHYSIAL TRACT (NEUROSECRETORY ROUTE TO POSTERIOR LOBE OF PITUITARY GLAND)

POSTERIOR LOBE (ANTIDIURETIC HORMONE ABSORBED BY CAPILLARIES)

ANTERIOR LOBE

POSTERIOR LOBE VEIN (CARRIES HORMONE TO KIDNEYS VIA GENERAL CIRCULATION)

INFERIOR HYPOTHALAMIC ARTERY

THEORIES OF ORIGIN OF ANTIDIURETIC HORMONE

1. PITUICYTES RELEASE HORMONE UNDER NERVOUS INFLUENCE

CELL OF SUPRA-OPTIC NUCLEUS

NERVE IMPULSES

PITUICYTE

POSTERIOR LOBE

SECRETION

CAPILLARY

2. HORMONE PRODUCED AS NEUROSECRETION BY CELLS IN SUPRA-OPTIC NUCLEUS AND CONDUCTED BY NERVE FIBERS TO POSTERIOR LOBE FOR STORAGE OR ABSORPTION

CELL OF SUPRA-OPTIC NUCLEUS

NEURO-SECRETION

POSTERIOR LOBE

CAPILLARY

FIGURE 2-1. Relationship of neurohypophysis to hypothalamus. Note that the posterior lobe is innervated and that the neurohypophyseal hormones originate in the hypothalamic nuclei.[2a] (Compare with Fig. 2-2.)

roid-stimulating hormone (TSH), and adrenocorti-cotropin (ACTH); (2) the same factor releases both follicle-stimulating hormone (FSH) and LH; and (3) PIF prevents the release of PRL. These extracts can also be added to pituitary gland organ cultures, where in the case of releasing factors, the amounts of hormone released into the culture medium can be greatly increased as compared with cultures to which extracts of brain tissue have not been added. In vitro studies have also shown that releasing factors not only cause the release of pituitary hormones but also significantly increase the rate of their synthesis.

In summary, to demonstrate clearly the existence of releasing factors and inhibiting factors for the anterior pituitary hormones, five criteria must be met:

1. Elimination of hypothalamic influences as through lesions of specific areas of the hypothalamus, should decrease or increase the release of the anterior pituitary hormone being studied. This method destroys cell bodies that produce specific releasing and inhibiting factors.
2. Releasing and inhibiting factors should be extractable from hypothalamic tissue.
3. Releasing and inhibiting factors must alter the synthesis and/or release of the anterior pituitary hormones using an assay that has been proved not to respond to nonspecific stimuli.
4. Releasing and inhibiting factors should be effective in vivo when applied directly to the anterior pituitary. Care must be taken that the administered factors do not reach the hypothalamus.
5. Releasing and inhibiting factors should be detectable in hypophyseal portal blood.

Moreover, changes in the concentration of these factors in the portal blood must result in concomitant changes in secretion of the anterior pituitary hormones.

Immunochemistry

Immunocytochemistry has been an excellent tool to identify the specific cell bodies that produce releasing and inhibiting factors. Antibodies specific to the releasing and inhibiting factors are conjugated to a chemical that will either fluoresce or produce a color when reacted with an appropriate substrate. This method is especially valuable spe-cifically, since the chemical structures of releasing and inhibiting factors have been elucidated and monoclonal antibodies can be generated against them. Monoclonal antibodies conjugated with an appropriate substance are reacted with thin slices of the hypothalamus and bind to cells that synthesize the specific releasing and inhibiting factors. Results from these studies have collaborated earlier findings.

Push–Pull Cannula

Finally, the push–pull cannula, a technique developed during the 1960s, has again become popular. The cannula consists of two needles, one fitted inside the other, permitting a fluid to be pumped into a localized area of the brain and be withdrawn through the outer needle. This approach used in experimental animals enables fluid to be sampled directly from specific hypothalamic regions and correlate concentrations of releasing and inhibiting factors with specific physiological conditions of the animal.[7]

POSTERIOR PITUITARY OR NEUROHYPOPHYSIS

The posterior pituitary or neurohypophysis, as indicated by its name, is a downgrowth of the ventral diencephalon and retains neural connections.[8] The supraoptic and paraventricular nerve bodies, located in the hypothalamus, send nerve tracts through the infundibulum terminating in the neural lobe (Fig. 2-1). Fenestrated capillaries, similar to those seen in other endocrine glands, surround the neural lobe. These capillaries transport the antidiuretic hormone (ADH) and oxytocin (OT) to their target organs as well as transport hormones between the anterior pituitary and neurohyphysis. The ADH is synthesized by both the supraoptic and paraventricular neurons, whereas OT is produced by only the supraoptic neurons. The posterior pituitary is a storage site for these two hormones.

During the late 1880s, the neurohypophysis was believed to be rudimentary. However, the observation that patients with diabetes insipidus lacked a functional neurohypophysis suggested that this tissue has an endocrine role. Later, the two nonapeptides, ADH and OT, were isolated. The biologic activity of these hormones depends on the presence of the carboxy-terminal amide group. Three other peptides, thyroid-releasing factor, substance

P, and growth-hormone inhibiting hormone, have also been found in the neurohypophysis.

The hormones of the neurohypophysis are synthesized as prohormones in cell bodies located in the supraoptic and paraventricular areas of the brain.[9] These hormones, bound to neurophysin, are transported in membrane-bound vesicles to the nerve terminals in the neurohypophysis. In response to a nerve stimulus, the hormone bound to the neurophysin is secreted. The neurons that produce ADH and OT are controlled by cholinergic and noradrenergic neurotransmitters as well as several octopeptides.[10] The fact that acetylcholine (ACh) releases ADH and OT explains the antidiuretic effects of tobacco smoking.

Antidiuretic Hormone

Since ADH is the principal hormone that regulates water diuresis by the kidney, it is logical that the most important regulator of ADH secretion is plasma osmolarity.[11] The secretion of ADH increases rapidly with increased plasma osmolarity. By contrast, water loading decreases ADH secretion. This regulation of ADH operates through a hypothalamic osmoreceptor neuron system. The effective circulating blood volume is only a secondary regulator of ADH. Approximately 10–25% reduction of blood volume is required to cause an increase in the release of ADH. Other substances, such as angiotensin II and endogenous opiates, can regulate ADH secretion as well.

Oxytocin

The second neurohypophyseal hormone, OT, controls milk letdown.[11] When an infant begins to nurse, there is approximately a half-minute delay before milk is available. Milk letdown depends on a reflex. Suckling initiates a neurogenic reflex by stimulating the nerves in the nipple. This stimulus travels *via* the spinal cord to the midbrain and finally to the hypothalamus, where OT is released. In turn, OT causes contraction of the myoepithelial cells in the mammary gland, and milk is expelled. A neural lesion of the paraventricular and supraoptic nuclei or neural stimuli such as pain or fright block OT release and milk letdown. In some women, the crying of a hungry baby can cause OT release and milk letdown. Oxytocin can also be released during sexual excitement and orgasm, resulting in milk letdown in lactating women.

The other action of OT is its involvement in labor. Actually, the first action of OT recognized was its ability to stimulate uterine contractions. Currently OT is used to induce labor and manage obstetric hemorrhage. Despite the widespread use of OT, its precise role in labor is questionable. For example, labor is normal in women who have diabetes insipidus. The fetal neural lobe does contain OT which may initiate labor. Once labor is started, maternal OT is secreted in spurts. As a result, a positive feedback is initiated with uterine contractions, leading to further release of OT.

NORMAL PHYSIOLOGY OF THE ANTERIOR PITUITARY AND MEDIAN EMINENCE

Anterior Pituitary

The pituitary gland consists of two separate glands: the posterior pituitary or neurohypophysis and the adenohypophysis.[12] The adenohypophysis, derived from the epithelial substrate (Rathke's pouch), consists of three parts: the pars tuberalis, pars intermedia, and pars anterior. The pars tuberalis is a thin layer of tissue that adheres to the median eminence and infundibulum. The pars intermedia is a thin layer of tissue adherent to the neurophypophysis separated from the pars anterior by the hypophyseal cleft. The pars anterior, more commonly called the anterior pituitary, is the lobular portion anterior and ventral to the hypophyseal cleft. The cells of the pars tuberalis may produce small amounts of TSH and LH. The pars intermedia, rudimentary in humans, comprises approximately 0.8% of the total weight of the pituitary gland.

The anterior pituitary, which produces six protein hormones, consists of different cell types (Fig. 2-2). Originally, three cell types—acidophils, basophils, and chromophobes—were identified on the basis of staining characteristics after histologic fixation of sectioned tissue. Later it was found that these unique cell types produce specific hormones. The acidophils (40% of the cells) produce GH and PRL, whereas the basophils (10% of the cells) are the cellular source for LH, FSH, TSH, and ACTH. Pituitary tumors, which produce abundant amounts of PRL, are rich sources of acidophils. By contrast, castration results in a hypertrophy of basophils, sometimes referred to as "castration cells." Immunocytochemistry studies, using specific antibodies against the various pituitary hormones, as well as electron microscopy have further documented the

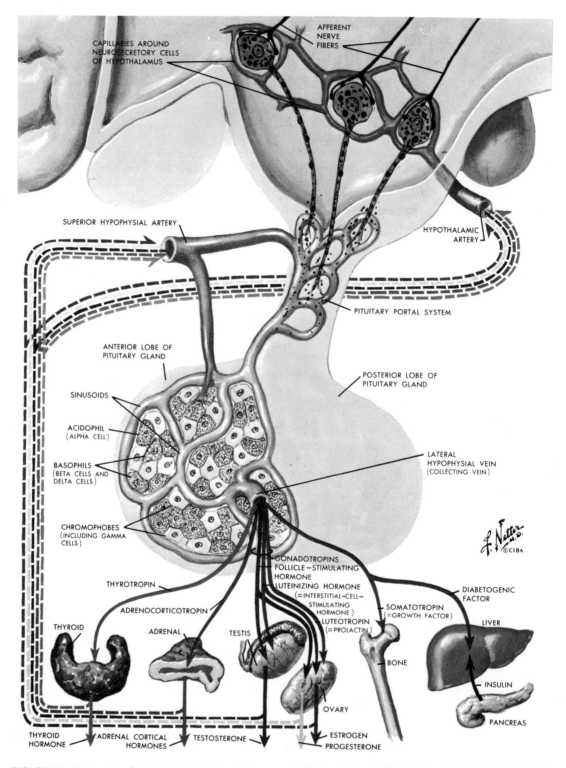

FIGURE 2-2. Relationship of adenohypophysis to hypothalamus and to the target glands. Note that the anterior lobe is linked to the hypothalamus via the portal system.[2a] (Compare with Fig. 2-1.)

cellular source of pituitary hormones. Five cell types have been identified: somatotrop (GH), mammotrop (PRL), thyrotrop (TSH), gonadotrop (FSH, LH), and corticotrop (ACTH, lipotropin hormone).

Median Eminence

An understanding of the regulation of the anterior pituitary gland by the hypothalamus requires an anatomic description of the neural and vascular connections between the hypothalamus and anterior pituitary.[13] The median eminence, the infundibulum of the hypothalamus, consists of neural, vascular, and epithelial components. The neural part has densely packed nerve endings from which all cell bodies arise in the ventral hypothalamus. There are two classes of neurons, the peptidergic and bioaminergic. The peptidergic neurons, as indicated by the name, produce small peptides called releasing and inhibiting factors or hormones. The bioaminergic neurons elaborate amines such as dopamine and norepinephrine. The median eminence is also the passageway for axons from the paraventriculohypophyseal and supraopticohypophyseal tracts, which terminate in the neurohypophysis.

The vascular component of the median eminence, called the hypophyseal portal system, is critical for the functioning of the anterior pituitary. It is the site of the capillary plexus, where the peptides and other neural transmitters secreted by cell bodies in the hypothalamus enter the blood and are transported to the anterior pituitary.[14] The median eminence receives blood from the superior hypophyseal stalk branch of the internal carotid. This capillary plexus is drained by the long portal veins into the pituitary sinusoids. The lower portion of the median eminence is supplied by blood from the inferior hypophyseal artery, which is drained by the short portal vessels into the pituitary. There is also evidence that blood flows from the pituitary to the medium eminence *via* the short portal vessels, which drain the anterior pituitary and neurohypophysis. An intimate vascular connection exists between the posterior and anterior pituitary. Apparently the unique anatomic structure provides the basis for the hormonal control exerted by the posterior pituitary over the anterior pituitary.[15]

Anterior Pituitary Hormones

The anterior pituitary secretes six major hormones: LH, FSH, TSH, GH, PRL, and ACTH. The anterior pituitary also secretes β-lipotropin (β-LPH). The biologic actions of these hormones are discussed in greater detail later. These hormones are large proteins, ranging in molecular weight from approximately 25,000 to 30,000. The hormones LH, FSH, and TSH are glycoproteins consisting of α- and β-subunits. The β-subunit confers specificity upon the hormone and differs in amino acid sequence among the three hormones. By contrast, the α-subunits are very similar. Both subunits are required for biologic activity of the hormones. The carbohydrate moieties of these hormones are important in regard to biologic activity and are altered by different physiologic conditions such as the presence or absence of gonads, photoperiod, and age, to name just a few.

The regulation of the secretion of anterior pituitary hormones has been an area of intense investigation dating back to the 1950s. Research during this period indicated that secretions from the neuronal elements of the hypothalamus regulate the secretions of the anterior pituitary. These neuronal products are transported to the anterior pituitary by the portal system, the vascular link between the hypothalamus and the anterior pituitary. Also during the 1950s, it was suggested that these neuronal products are small peptides. It was hypothesized that there would be a releasing and inhibiting hormone for each pituitary hormone. In other words, each hormone would have dual control. The search for the releasing and inhibiting factors created a challenge. After approximately 10 years of intense research, A. V. Schally and R. Guillemin, working independently isolated a tripeptide from tons of sheep and pig hypothalami identified as thyroid-releasing hormone (TRH). Besides releasing TSH, this small peptide is a potent releaser of PRL and in some cases of ACTH and GH. Schally and Guillemin were awarded the Nobel Prize in 1977 for their outstanding research.[5,16,17]

Shortly after the isolation of TRH, gonadotropin-releasing hormone (GnRH), a 10-amino acid polypeptide, was isolated. This releasing hormone stimulates release of both LH and FSH.[15,18] Differential release of this gonadotropin is due to subtle regulation by ovarian steroids and inhibin, a gonadal nonsteroidal substance, at the level of the pituitary. To date, no hypothalamic factor has been found that releases FSH specifically.

Somatostatin (growth hormone-inhibiting hormone, GHIF), a 14-amino acid that inhibits secretion of GH and TSH was next isolated from hypothalamic tissue. Shortly after this discovery, somatostatin was localized in the glands of the gastrointestinal (GI) tract, where it inhibits hormonal secretion by the GI tract and the pancreas as well as other GI actions. In 1982, a growth hormone-releasing hormone (GHRH) and corticotropic releasing hormone (CRH), consisting of approximately 41 amino acids, were isolated. Interestingly, the existence of a CRH was hypothesized during the 1950s but eluded researchers for approximately 30 years.[19-21]

The control of PRL, as judged from experiments in which the pituitary was transplanted to the kidney capsule, is primarily inhibitory. Therefore, a search for a PIF was undertaken. Data from a number of laboratories indicated that dopamine is the PIF.[22] Besides inhibiting PRL, dopamine can block release of LH, TSH, and in some cases GH. The remaining releasing and inhibiting factors, if they exist, have not yet been identified.

Neurotransmitters and Control of the Anterior Pituitary

Besides releasing and inhibiting hormones, the anterior pituitary is controlled by a number of neurotransmitters. There are dopaminergic neurons in the arcuate nucleus of the hypothalamus and median eminence. Numerous noradrenergic and serotonergic pathways, arising outside the hypothalamus, project to the hypothalamus.[23-25] The presence of choline acetyltransferase, an enzyme marker of ACh synthesis, in the hypothalamus and median eminence, suggests that the anterior pituitary may be under cholinergic control. High concentrations of γ-aminobutyric acid (GABA) in the hypothalamus and median eminence has also linked this neurotransmitter with pituitary control.

Regulation of the Anterior Pituitary by Other Neuropeptides

In addition to the releasing and inhibiting hormones and factors (not yet identified) and neurotransmitters, a number of other neuropeptides regulate the anterior pituitary. A partial list of these neuropeptides distributed in the hypothalamus and other brain regions includes substance P, neurotensin, vasoactive intestinal peptide, gastrin, cholecytokinin, met-enkephalin, leu-enkephalin, and β-endorphin.[26-30] Substance P, neurotensin, and vasoactive intestinal peptide increase PRL and GH release. There is increasing evidence that the met-enkephalin and leu-enkephalin, endogenous opiates, which are pentapeptides, regulate secretion of anterior pituitary hormones either directly or indirectly.

Role of External Stimuli

The secretion of pituitary hormones is regulated by small peptides and neurotransmitters produced by neurons in the hypothalamus and other regions of the brain. The release of these peptides and neurotransmitters is controlled by the feedback action of hormones from target organs. These hormones act at the level of the hypothalamus and in many cases, on the pituitary as well, where they modulate the response to neuropeptides from the hypothalamus. For example, the presence of certain levels of estrogen in the peripheral circulation will alter the response of the pituitary to GnRH. However, the body does not act as a self-contained unit. External stimuli such as photoperiod (length of day), odor, stress, and social interaction also modify the secretion of pituitary hormones, specifically those involved with reproduction. These external stimuli detected by the senses alter the production of neurotransmitters and neuropeptides by the brain. In turn, these substances modulate the secretion of releasing and inhibiting hormones and factors by the hypothalamus.

While numerous examples are available, only several are cited due to lack of space. In a large number of species, the effect of light on reproduction has been studied. The estrous cycle of the white laboratory rat is dependent on a daily exposure of light and darkness. Rats exposed to continuous light display constant estrus. The cyclic release of gonadotropins that occurs every 4–5 days is blunted. Instead, there is only a tonic release of gonadotropins, which causes the development of large follicles that produce high levels of estrogen but do not ovulate.

The role of odor in the regulation of reproduction is gaining importance. For years, it was known that female mice, previously housed in individual cages, when exposed to males, or even to male urine, will have synchronized estrous cycles.[31] A similar phenomenon appears to operate in humans.[32] For example, women who live together as roommates in dormitories have been found to have synchronized menstrual cycles. Recent studies indicate that in a group of women, one acts as the synchronizer. This effect of odor on the neuroendocrine system is brought about by pheromones. These chemical substances, detected by olfactory neurons, are present in various bodily secretions such as urine, perspiration, and saliva.

Other factors, such as stress, social interaction, and fear, alter pituitary function *via* the production of neurotransmitters and other neuropeptides. For example, pain can cause release of endorphins in the CNS. These endorphins bind to opiate receptors in the hypothalamus resulting in the release of PRL and GH and the suppression of TSH and gonadotropin release.

In summary, the few examples cited demonstrate how stimuli in our everyday environment alter the secretion of hormones by the pituitary gland. Moreover, these examples as well as other information presented document that the hypothalamus is the integrator for the neuroendocrine system.

PATHOPHYSIOLOGY

Malfunctioning of the neuroendocrine system can occur at the level of the hypothalamus and/or pituitary (see Chapter 15).[33-36] Disordered hypothalamic control of the anterior pituitary results in decreased secretion of the pituitary hormones, with the exception of PRL, which increases. Disorders of the hypothalamic–pituitary unit can occur at various levels. At the level of the brain, by activation of the stress response, suppression of normal gonadotropin secretion and GH secretion can result. There can also be defects in the neural input into the tuberhypophyseal system. This disturbance is manifested, for example, by loss of circadian rhythms and precocious puberty. Destruction of the stalk or interference with the hypophyseal portal system by surgical stalk section, tumors of the stalk region, and some inflammatory diseases blocks the communication pathway between the hypothalamus and pituitary. As a result, hypothalamic peptides and neurotransmitters that control the pituitary do not reach it. The pituitary itself can be the site of the defect. The pituitary can be destroyed by tumors or infarct. Tumors are classified according to their staining characteristics. Tumors of the chromophobes destroy normal pituitary tissue and cause hypopituitarism. In approximately 70% of cases, PRL secretion increases due to a decrease in PIF. Infarct occurs more frequently in pregnant women. During pregnancy, the pituitary enlarges and the blood supply to the pituitary is vulnerable. An episode of shock, such as postpartum uterine hemorrhage, can result in an infarcted pituitary and postpartum necrosis. One of the causes of hyperpituitarism is acidophil cell tumor. Elevated GH secretion causes gigantism in children and acromegaly in adults. The latter condition results in enlargement of hands and feet, protrusion of the lower jaw, coarse facial features, and increased body hair. Another hyperpituitary condition, due to small ACTH-secreting tumors and hyperplastic adrenals, is Cushing's disease. Removal of adrenals results in a rapid growth of these ACTH tumors. In turn, the elevated ACTH secretion and lipoprotein-related peptides cause hyperpigmentation of the skin. The growth of the tumor causes pressure in the sellar region and other neurologic signs.

RELEASING HORMONES AND THEIR USE IN THERAPY

The discovery of the hypothalamic releasing and inhibiting hormones that regulate the synthesis and secretion of pituitary hormones presented a tremendous potential for endocrine therapy.[37,38] Knowledge of the precise sequence of these hypothalamic peptides has facilitated their synthesis. Moreover, the replacement of one or several amino acids with other amino acids produces potent agonists and antagonists. As a result, an ample supply of these peptides can be used to alter pituitary function. Moreover, treatment with these releasing and inhibiting hormones causes no immunologic response that occurs when a hormone from a different species is given. Specific uses of the releasing and inhibiting hormones in therapy follow.

Gonadotropin releasing hormone, which releases LH and FSH, is used to induce spermatogenesis and testosterone production in men who do not produce adequate amounts of gonadotropins. Similar treatments are used in women to induce ovulation. This approach, giving GNRH in pulsatile fashion, has been effective in causing ovulation which resulted in pregnancy. This releasing factor is also employed as a diagnostic to assess disorders of the hypothalamus. Responses to synthetic GnRH will aid in the diagnosis of a wide range of endocrine diseases and syndromes. Several of these disorders are male and female infertility, panhypopituitarism, pituitary tumors, as well as other reproductive disorders, such as anorexia nervosa. The availability of potent antagonists of GnRH has suggested their use as a contraceptive. Oral administration of GnRH antagonists has blocked ovulation in rats. No data are available on the usefulness of these antagonists in humans.

The isolation of GHRF and GHIF suggested major breakthroughs for the control of GH secretion. However, to date GHRF and GHIF have only been tested in animals.

The knowledge that the inhibiting factor for PRL is dopamine has made possible the treatment of hyperprolactemia due to pituitary tumors. Hyperprolactinemia is usually associated with suppressed LH and FSH and a lack of normal menstrual cycles and ovulation. Derivatives of bromocriptine, a potent antagonist of dopamine, binds to dopamine receptors in the pituitary and decreases prolactin secretion. Normalization of LH and FSH levels occurs, and normal menstrual cycles are established.

The use of releasing and inhibiting hormones in treating endocrine disease is still in its infancy. During the next several years, the availability of these hormones for human use should increase markedly. Before these hormones can be marketed for human use, extensive testing in animal models and clinical trials in humans must be completed.

SUMMARY

Neuroendocrinology is the study of the neural and endocrine systems. The hypothalamus is the integrator for these two systems. It is at this site that neural messages are translated into chemical signals through the production of releasing and inhibiting hormones and factors. These small peptides are transported to the anterior pituitary *via* the hypophyseal portal system.

Until the 1950s, the anterior pituitary was considered a master gland that functions independently of the hypothalamus. However, through the keen observations of scientists at that time and the use of unique approaches, it was shown that the anterior pituitary was under the direct control of the hypothalamus. Techniques employed to study the hypothalamic control of the pituitary were electrolytic lesions, deafferentation, implantation of hormones, adrenergic and cholinergic drugs, stalk section, extraction of releasing and inhibiting factors from the hypothalamus, immunocytochemistry, and push–pull cannula.

The posterior pituitary or neurohypophysis is neural tissue, which is directly attached to the hypothalamus. ADH and OT produced by the supraoptic and paraventricular nuclei in the hypothalamus are stored in the posterior pituitary. These two octapeptides regulate water diuresis and milk letdown and labor.

By contrast, the anterior pituitary does not have neural connection with the hypothalamus. Instead, hypothalamic hormones are transported to the anterior pituitary *via* the hypophyseal portal system. The anterior pituitary consists of several different cell types called chromophobes, acidophils, and basophils, and cell function is established by immunocytochemistry. The acidophils synthesize and secrete PRL and GH, whereas the basophils are the source of FSH, LH, TSH, and ACTH. The production of these hormones is under the control of hypothalamic releasing and inhibiting hormones as well as the negative and positive feedback of hormones from the gonads, thyroid, and adrenal cortex. While the presence of a releasing and inhibiting hormone has been hypothesized for each pituitary hormone, only a gonadotropin-releasing hormone, thyroid-releasing hormone, growth hormone releasing and inhibiting hormones, corticotropin-releasing hormone, and prolactin-inhibiting hormone have been identified. The anterior pituitary is also controlled indirectly by other chemicals such as neurotransmitters, enkephalins, endorphins, and intestinal peptides, which alter the release of releasing and inhibiting hormones by the hypothalamus. External stimuli, such as light, stress, and social interactions, also modify secretion of pituitary hormones.

Disorders of the neuroendocrine system can occur at the level of the hypothalamus or pituitary, or both. In general, these disorders result in decreased secretion of the pituitary hormones, with the exception of prolactin, which increases.

The discovery of releasing and inhibiting hormones provides an excellent potential for clinical management and diagnosis of neuroendocrine diseases. To date, synthetic compounds of prolactin inhibiting hormone and gonadotropin-releasing hormone are available for clinical use.

QUESTIONS

1. Why is regulation of the anterior pituitary by the hypothalamus important?

2. How is the anterior pituitary regulated by the hypothalamus?

3. Why is the isolation and structural identification of releasing and inhibiting hormones important?

REFERENCES

1. Sawyer CH: Neuroendocrine regulation: The peptide neuron, introduction and historical background, in *Central Regulation of the Endocrine System*. New York, Plenum, 1978, pp 3–8*
2. Everett JW: Central neural control of reproductive functions of the adenohypophysis. *Physiol Rev* 44:373–431, 1964*
2a. Netter FN: *The CIBA Collection of Medical Illustrations: Nervous System* (Supplement to Vol. I). Summit, NJ, CIBA Pharmaceutical Company, 1957, pp 155–156
3. Adams JH, Daniel PM, Pritchard MD: Transection of the pituitary stalk in man. Anatomical changes in the pituitary gland. *J Neurol Neurosurg Psychiatry* 29:545–555, 1966
4. Everett JW, Nikitovich-Winer M: Physiology of the pituitary gland as affected by transplantation or stalk section, in Nalbandov, AV (ed): *Advances in Neuroendocrinology*. Urbana, University of Illinois Press, 1963, pp 289–313*
5. Guillemin R: Peptides in the brain: The new endocrinology of the neuron. *Science* 202:390–402, 1978
6. Knigge KM, Joseph SA, Hoffmann, GE, et al: Organization of LRF and SRIF neurons in the endocrine hypothalamus, in Reichlin S, Baldessarini RJ, et al (eds): *The Hypothalamus*, New York, Raven, 1978, pp 49–67*
7. Levine JE, Ramirez VD: 1980. In vivo release of luteinizing hormone-releasing hormone estimated with push–pull cannulae from the mediobasal hypothalamus of ovariectomized steroid-primed rats. *Endocrinology* 107:1782–1790
8. Reichlin S: *The Neurohypophysis*. New York, Plenum 1984*
9. Brownstein MJ, Russell JT, Gainer H: Synthesis, transport and release of posterior pituitary hormones. *Science* 207:373–378, 1980
10. Dierickx K, Vandesande R: Immunocytochemical demonstration of separate vasopressin–neurophysin and oxytocin–neurophysin neurons in the human hypothalamus. *Cell Tissue Res* 196:203–212, 1979
11. Pickering BT: Neurophypophysial hormones—Comparative aspects, in Jeffcoate SL, Hutchinson JSM (eds): *The Endocrine Hypothalamus*. London, Academic, 1978, pp 213–227*
12. Green JD, Harris GW: Neurovascular link between neurohypophysis and adenohypophysis. *J Endocrinol* 5:136–146, 1947
13. Harris GW: Neural control of the pituitary gland. *Physiol Rev* 28:139–179, 1948*
14. Krieger DT, Liotta AS: Pituitary hormones in brain: Where, how, and why? *Science* 205:366–372, 1979*
15. Peters LL, Hoefer, MT, Ben-Jonathan N: The posterior pituitary regulation of anterior pituitary prolactin secretion. *Science* 213:659–663, 1981
16. Schally AV: Aspects of hypothalamic regulation of the pituitary gland. Its implications for the control of reproductive processes. *Science* 202:18–20, 1981
17. Vale W, Rivier C, Brown M: Regulatory peptides of the hypothalamus. *Ann Rev Physiol* 39:473–527, 1977*
18. Knobil E: The neuroendocrine control of the menstrual cycle *Recent Prog Hormone Res* 36:53–88, 1980*
19. Krieger DT, Zimmerman EA: The nature of CRF and its relationship to vasopressin, in Martini L, Besser GM (eds): *Clinical Neuroendocrinology*. New York, Academic, 1978, pp 364–391*
20. Krulich L, Dhariwal AP: Stimulatory and inhibitory effects of purified hypothalamic extracts on growth hormone release from rat pituitary in vitro. *Endocrinology* 83:783–790, 1968
21. Pecile A, Olgiati VR: Control of growth hormone secretion, in Jeffcoate SL, Hutchinson JSM (eds): *The Endocrine Hypothalamus*. New York, Academic, 1978, pp 362–385*
22. Ben-Jonathan N, Oliver N, Weiner HJ, et al: Dopamine in hypophysial portal plasma of the rat during the estrous cycle and throughout pregnancy. *Endocrinology* 100:452–458, 1972
23. Adler EH, Johnson MD, Lynch CO, et al: Evidence that norepinephrine and epinephrine systems mediate the stimulatory effects of ovarian hormones on luteinizing hormone and luteinizing hormone releasing hormone. *Endocrinology* 113:1431–1438, 1983
24. Bloom FE: Contrasting principles of synaptic physiology: Peptidergic and non-peptidergic neurons, in Fuxe K, Hokfelt T, Luft R (eds): *Central Regulation of the Endocrine System*. New York, Plenum, 1979, pp 173–187*
25. Ganong WF: Neurotransmitters involved in ACTH secretion of catecholamines. *Ann NY Acad. Sci* 297:509–517, 1977
26. Dupont A, Cusan L: Evidence for a role of endorphins in the control of prolactin secretion, in Collu R, Barbeau A, Ducharme JR (eds); *Central Nervous System Effects of Hypothalamic Hormones*. New York, Raven, 1978, pp 283–300*
27. Goldstein A: Opioid peptides (endorphins) in pituitary and brain. *Science* 193:1081–1086, 1976
28. Kosterlitz HW: Endogenous opioid peptides: Historical aspects, in Hughes J (ed): *Centrally Acting Peptides*. Baltimore, University Park Press, 1978, p. 157
29. Malick JB, Robert MS: *Endorphins: Chemistry, Physiology, Pharmacology, and Clinical Relevance*. New York, Dekker, 1982*
30. Pearse AGE: Diffuse neuroendocrine system: Peptides common to brain and intestine and their relationship to the APUD concept, in Hughes J (ed): *Centrally Acting Peptides*. University Park Press, Baltimore, 1978, p 49
31. Aron C: Mechanisms of control of the reproduction function of olfactory stimuli in female animals. *Physiol Rev* 59(2):229–284, 1979
32. McClintock M: Pheromonal regulation of the ovarian cycle: Enhancement, suppression, and synchrony, in Vandenbergh JG (ed): *Pheromones and Reproduction in Mammals*. New York, Academic 1983, pp 113–149*
33. Daughaday WH, Cryer PE, Jacobs LS: The role of the hypothalamus in the pathogenesis of pituitary tumors, in Kohler PO, Ross GT (eds): *Diagnosis and Treatment of Pituitary Tumors*. Amsterdam and New York, Excerpta Medica, 1973, pp 26–34*
34. Perryman RL, Thorner MO: Clinical applications of the understanding of prolactin secretion, in Bhatnagar AS (ed): *The Anterior Pituitary Gland*. New York, Raven, 1983, pp 377–392*
35. Plum F, Van Uitert R: Nonendocrine diseases and disorder of the hypothalamus, in Reichlin S, Baldessarini RJ, Martin JB (eds): *The Hypothalamus*, Vol 56. New York, Raven, 1978, pp 415–473*
36. Rees LH: Human adrenocorticotropin and lipotropin (MSH) in health and disease, in Martini L, Besser GM (eds): *Clinical Neuroendocrinology*. New York, Academic, 1978, pp 402–404*

*Review article/chapter.

37. Frohman LA: Newer understanding of human hypothalamic–pituitary disease obtained through the use of synthetic hypothalamic hormones, in Reichlin S, Baldessarini RJ, Martin JB *The Hypothalamus*, Vol 56. New York, Raven, 1978, pp 387–413*

38. Yen SSC: The human menstrual cycle (integrative function of the hypothalamic–pituitary–ovarian–endometrial axis), in Yen SSC, Jaffe RB (eds): *Reproductive Endocrinology, Physiology, Pathophysiology, and Clinical Management.* Philadelphia, Saunders, 1978, pp 126–151*

ANSWERS

1. The hypothalamus acts as a transducer and as integrator for the anterior pituitary. Neural signals come from various parts of the body (internal stimuli) and from outside the body (external stimuli) to the hypothalamus. These neural signals are converted into a chemical signal (hormonal) and transported to the anterior pituitary, where the synthesis and secretion of anterior pituitary hormones are modulated.

2. The hypothalamus produces neurohormones which are secreted by nerve terminals into the capillary plexus in the median eminence. These hormones are then transported to the anterior pituitary by the hypophyseal portal system. The neurohormones are releasing and inhibiting factors (polypeptides), neurotransmitters (e.g., norepinephrine, dopamine, GABA), and neuropeptides (e.g., endorphins, enkephalins, vasoactive intestinal peptide).

3. First, knowledge of the presence of these hormones aids in understanding how the hypothalamus regulates the anterior pituitary. Second, elucidation of the structural identification of these hormones permits their synthesis and chemical modification. Third, these hormones have a tremendous potential for clinical use. They can be employed therapeutically to test pituitary function and to modify and regulate the pituitary.

3

Placental Endocrinology

DAVID L. HEALY

INTRODUCTION

The placenta is a temporary fetomaternal organ that sustains the growth and nutrition of the developing conceptus. Human beings have a villous hemochorial placenta in which trophoblast is in direct contact with maternal blood (Fig. 3-1). Syncytiotrophoblast is the outer layer of trophoblast, which is in direct contact with this blood; it derives from the cytotrophoblast, which is most prominent in early pregnancy (Fig. 3-2).

Clinical placental endocrinology has developed from and is based on physiologic studies. Several concepts currently seem vital to the obstetric usefulness of hormonal assays. The first of these is the biologic significance of the various placental hormones and substances measured in the maternal blood or urine. Hormonal effect and bioavailability is a function of the metabolic clearance rate, the avidity and number of carrier protein binding sites, the metabolic conjugates formed from the hormone, the biologic versus the immunologic activity of a measured substance, and the affinity and capacity of hormonal receptors. These factors are well illustrated by estriol, where only approximately 5% of the total estriol measured in the maternal circula-

tion is free bioactive steroid, for which there are few, if any, cytosol receptors in the uterus in late pregnancy (see section on Estrogen Function).

The second clinical concept is the predictive value of fetoplacental function tests. Chard and Klopper[1] have highlighted this analytic approach, defining predictive value as an index of the proportion of all patients with abnormal levels of the hormone being measured who also have the clinical abnormality. Predictive value is the information the obstetrician wants from a test. A predictive value of 25% or more would obviously be useful and human placental lactogen (hPL) measurement has been shown to have predictive value as a routine screening test for fetal health.[2] Unfortunately, this type of analysis has yet to be applied to other placental hormones. Estriol, human chorionic gonadotropin (hCG), schwangerschaft protein (SP_1), as well as hPL, are all secreted in large amounts from the placenta without known feedback-control mechanisms. These hormones either exist in excessive concentrations for their known actions or have no proven physiologic effect. The placenta therefore behaves, in engineering terms, like a free-running system with none of the negative feedback control that characterizes ovarian–pituitary hormone secretion. Unlike the gonads, the fetoplacental unit secretes much endocrine ''noise'' but relatively little ''signal'' to produce measurable biologic effects. Thus, pregnancies with very low estrogen forma-

DAVID L. HEALY • Department of Obstetrics and Gynaecology, Monash University, Queen Victoria Medical Centre, Melbourne, Australia.

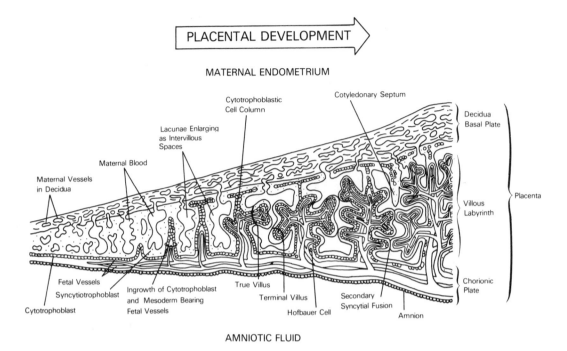

FIGURE 3-1. Schematic representation of the ontogeny of the human placenta (Adapted from Williams and Warwick.[248])

tion due to placental sulfatase deficiency or undetectable hPL levels develop perfectly satisfactorily with normal fetal growth.[3,4] Either these "hormones" have, in fact, no function unique to human pregnancy, or they are secreted in such excess that even trivial concentrations exert a satisfactory physiologic result on the fetus and the mother.

In one sense, these disturbing clinical experiments of nature do not matter if the clinician is using assays such as estriol and hPL solely as an index of trophoblast activity. Note that primate experiments have examined placental function in vivo completely separated from the fetus after the operation of fetectomy.[5] This model is important, as it showed that not only was progesterone secretion maintained while estrogen secretion fell but that these afetal pregnancies still labored at the usual gestational time and delivered their placentas normally. This extraordinary fact indicates that the fetus is not obligatory to primate labor and that the endocrine control of human parturition may lie elsewhere. One possibility is the interaction of the fetal

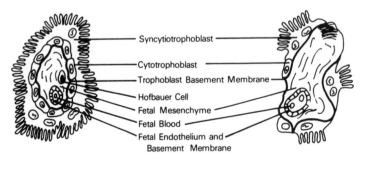

FIGURE 3-2. Diagram of a transverse section through a terminal villus of an early (left) and term (right) pregnancy. Note the prominent brush border of syncytiotrophoblast. Cytotrophoblast cells become infrequent with placental maturity and increasing fibrinoid deposits occur by term gestation (top right).

TABLE 3-1. Periplacental Peptides

Tissue	Peptide	Abbreviation
Syncytiotrophoblast	Chorionic gonadotropin	hCG
	Placental lactogen	hPL
	Corticotropin	ACTH
	β-Endorphin	β-END
	β-Lipotropin	β-LPH
	α-Melanocyte-stimulating hormone	α-MSH
	Nerve growth factor	NGF
Cytotrophoblast-placenta	Luteinizing hormone-releasing hormone	LHRH
	Thyrotropin-releasing hormone	TRH
	Somatostatin	SRIF
	Corticotropin-releasing factor	CRF
Cytotrophoblast-chorion laeve	Renin	REN
	Prolactin receptors	PRL-R
Decidua	Prolactin	PRL
	Relaxin	RLX
	Pregnancy associated plasma protein A	PAPP-A
	Ornithine decarboxylase	ODC
	Oxytocin receptors	OXY-R

membranes, the amniochorion, with the endometrial decidua.[6] These tissues are major sources of prostaglandins and represent the interface of the fetal and maternal systems. It is becoming apparent that abnormalities of this decidua–fetal membrane duality may affect pregnancy health: The amniochorion must now be regarded as major endocrine tissues of obstetric relevance.

A final concept that may direct future clinical placental endocrinology is the reported identification of many brain peptides in the placenta (Table 3-1). Small, neurotransmitter-size peptides appear to be localized in cytotrophoblast, whereas larger proteins are formed in the syncytiotrophoblast. The hypothesis is that secretion of substances like hCG is controlled by placental luteinizing-hormone releasing hormone (LHRH).[7] There is no proof of this

TABLE 3-2. Minimal Criteria for Putative Placental Hormones

Bioassay identification
Immunoassay or chromatographic identification
Accumulation during culture
Radiolabel incorporation
Specific mRNA (messenger ribonucleic acid) identified
Biochemical structure determined
Local receptors identified
Local function established

suggestion at this time. Indeed, mere immunohistochemical localization is but the first of a number of criteria to be satisfied before one could accept such an intriguing hypothesis as fact (Table 3.2).

The challenge of this chapter is to review placental hormones from a clinical viewpoint and to suggest future directions for obstetric endocrinology.

PLACENTAL STEROID HORMONES

Progesterone

Progesterone was purified from the corpus luteum by Corner and Allen in 1929[8] and was soon shown to be essential for the establishment of human pregnancy. In 1937, Venning and Browne[9] demonstrated that the placenta also synthetizes progesterone, which was found to metabolize to pregnanediol glucuronide, later excreted in urine. In a third classic report, Van Wagenen and Newton[5] described the endocrine effects of fetectomy in rhesus monkeys: Fetectomy left the placenta in situ, but progesterone secretion continued normally. This experiment proved that all placental progesterone precursors come from the mother and/or placenta, but not the fetus. It also implied that progesterone measurement would be useless as a test of fetal, as opposed to placental, function. Finally, in

1945, in one of the earliest human studies using steroidal isotopes, Bloch administered deuterium-labeled cholesterol to a pregnant woman and showed radiolabeled pregnanediol in her urine. This was the first demonstration that maternal cholesterol was the physiologic substrate for placental progesterone production.[10]

Origin, Synthesis, and Control

Progesterone is vital for human pregnancy: There are no obstetric situations wherein placental progesterone production is markedly low in which pregnancy continues. That the progesterone receptor antagonist, RU 486, will terminate pregnancy without altering plasma levels or actions of circulating estrogens gives further support to this keystone role of progesterone to human gestation.[11]

Figure 3-3 depicts major steroidal intermediates in placental progesterone synthesis. Most mammalian cells can synthesize cholesterol from acetyl coenzyme A. However, these condensation reactions are inefficient in the placenta. Sybulski and Venning[12] most clearly showed this when they perfused placentae with radiolabeled acetate but could not retrieve progesterone, although pregnenolone was rapidly converted to progesterone. When taken with Bloch's earlier reports, this work suggested that enzyme 20α-hydroxylase, the cholesterol side-chain cleavage enzyme, and 3β-hydroxysteroid dehydrogenase isomerase are rich in trophoblast and convert maternal cholesterol to progesterone.

Daily progesterone production reaches 75 mg at mid-gestation and 250 mg in term placenta.[13,14] This compares with 20 mg from the dominant corpus luteum. The cholesterol needed to synthesize such a large amount of progesterone in late pregnancy represents up to one-third of the daily maternal cholesterol production. Maternal cholesterol is esterified and transported by low-density lipoprotein (LDL) to bind to high-affinity receptors on trophoblast cells, where it is internalized. The complex is then hydrolyzed to release amino acids and cholesterol for progesterone synthesis.

Control of progesterone secretion from the placenta is poorly understood compared with the ovary. Corpus luteum progesterone production is governed by (1) luteinizing hormone (LH), and perhaps prolactin (PRL), presented in a pulsatile mode,[15] and (2) LDL as a cholesterol source.[16] Absence of LH or LDL markedly reduces luteal progesterone secretion. Corpus luteal progesterone secretion is

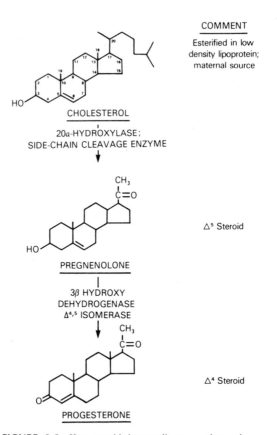

COMMENT

Esterified in low density lipoprotein; maternal source

CHOLESTEROL

20α-HYDROXYLASE;
SIDE-CHAIN CLEAVAGE ENZYME

Δ^5 Steroid

PREGNENOLONE

3β HYDROXY DEHYDROGENASE
$\Delta^{4,5}$ ISOMERASE

Δ^4 Steroid

PROGESTERONE

FIGURE 3-3. Key steroid intermediates to placental progesterone synthesis. Approximately 85% of the progesterone substrate comes from preformed cholesterol bound to low-density lipoprotein, which is hydrolyzed after entering the trophoblast cell. The 20α-hydroxylase enzyme is located in mitochondria, while the isomerase enzyme is found in the endoplasmic reticulum.

pulsatile: This pattern presumably reflects episodic stimulation by circulating gonadotropins.[17] By analogy, control of placental progesterone production might therefore be regulated at three sites: (1) supply of LDL, (2) 20α-hydroxylase and the cholesterol side-chain cleavage enzyme, and (3) 3α-hydroxysteroid dehydrogenase isomerase activity. The cholesterol side-chain cleavage enzyme is rate limiting for progesterone synthesis in the corpus luteum, where it is stimulated by LH. No such tropic hormone has been shown for placental progesterone synthesis. Indeed, the rate-limiting step in placental progesterone synthesis might be the number of LDL receptors on trophoblast. Certainly, hCG seems without effect on 20α-hydroxylase and cholesterol side-chain cleavage and did not alter progesterone secretion from human placenta either in vitro or in vivo.[18,19] Gonadotropin-releasing hormone has been identified in human cytotrophoblast but reported to inhibit, not stimulate, progesterone secretion.[20] Unlike their effects on adrenal steroidogenesis, ACTH (corticotropin) and the synthetic glucocorticoid, betamethasone, have no action on placental progesterone secretion.[21]

Progesterone is also produced by amnion, chorion, and endometrial decidua.[22,23] Many obstetricians believe that the amniochorion, or fetal membranes, are degenerated placental tissues of no endocrine significance. Nothing could be further from the truth. These tissues at the interface of the mother and fetus are now known to be major sources of prostaglandins, prolactin, and other progestogen-associated hormones. At this time, the ontogeny of these tissues, their capacity to synthesize progesterone, and the regulatory mechanisms governing production are unknown. Amniochorionic progesterone may contribute to prostaglandin release by these membranes. One such mechanism leading to labor may be that rising dehydroepiandrosterone sulfate (DHEAS) concentrations in amniotic fluid inhibit the isomerase enzyme and progesterone production in amniochorion.[24]

Other recent data suggest that the fetus might contribute in a direct way to progesterone secretion.

Challis and associates[25] examined women at 34 weeks gestation who had received synthetic glucocorticoids; their peripheral progesterone values were found to be decreased by about 20%. These workers suggested that the fetus synthesizes pregnenolone sulfate, which passes to the placenta as a progesterone substrate. Moreover, cortisol has been shown to inhibit the conversion of pregnenelone to progesterone during superfusion of human placental tissue.[26]

Maternal and Fetal Concentration

It is not known whether early placental progesterone secretion is pulsatile, nor are the contributions of the placenta and corpus luteum to circulating progesterone levels in the first trimester of pregnancy clearly defined. It has been deduced from 17-hydroxyprogesterone concentrations that up to 90% of plasma progesterone comes from the corpus luteum in the first 4 weeks of pregnancy, since the 17α-hydroxylase enzyme, which converts progesterone to 17-hydroxyprogesterone, is absent from the placenta.[27] Total plasma progesterone concentrations (25–75 ng/ml) typically fall from 4 to 8 weeks gestation as corpus luteum demise proceeds. Thereafter, plasma progesterone levels steadily rise as pregnancy advances, broadly reflecting the increase in placental mass (Fig. 3-4).

The concentration of progesterone in placental

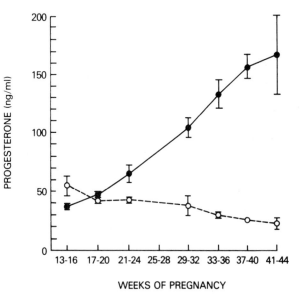

FIGURE 3-4. Progesterone concentrations in maternal plasma (●) and amniotic fluid (○) from the same subjects. Values represent mean ±SE. (From Johansson and Johansson.[249])

tissue is approximately 10^{-5} M. This level remains constant throughout pregnancy. Maternal plasma progesterone concentrations typically reach 200 ng/ml at term, when amniotic fluid levels are usually about 30 ng/ml.[28] Retroplacental blood progesterone values average 850 ng/ml at term gestation.[21] Noteworthy is the fact that circulating progesterone levels in the fetus are higher than in the mother: Umbilical venous and arterial values average 720 and 440 ng/ml, respectively, at term. This large venoarterial difference implies fetal uptake. Indeed, up to one-third of the progesterone produced daily by the placenta is metabolized by the fetus.

Metabolism in Mother and Fetus

The fate of progesterone in pregnancy was most directly studied by Pearlman in 1957,[14] who injected tritiated progesterone into the maternal circulation. Many reduced steroids resulted, including pregnanolone, 5α-pregnane-3,20-dione and 3α-hydroxy-5α-pregnane 20-one. These reactions occur in liver, which helps clear progesterone from plasma with a rapid half-life of 10–15 min. Significant amounts of progesterone are also stored in adipose tissue. All metabolic products are conjugated with glucuronic acid in the liver and kidneys and are excreted in urine and feces.

Pregnanediol glucuronide (3α,20-pregnanediol) is the major metabolite of progesterone in urine. It represents about 30% of a progesterone injection, and up to 100 mg/day is excreted in urine in late pregnancy.[9] Measurement of pregnanediol excretion is the only progesterone metabolite that has been evaluated by obstetricians as a test of pregnancy health, but unfortunately pregnanediol estimations have provided no help to clinicians in assessing fetal health. This is not surprising, given the physiology of this placental steroid as described above. In one strict sense, pregnanediol measurements are truly a placental function test, but this has no obstetric significance. Indeed, even after fetal death or experimental primate fetectomy, placental progesterone secretion continues unchanged.[29,30]

Fetal metabolism of progesterone is extensive and differs in several ways from that in the mother. First, tritiated progesterone perfused directly into the fetus accumulates in the liver. Here, reduction occurs not only at the 5β-, 3α-, and 20α-positions, as in the mother, but also at the 6β-, 14α-, and 15α-positions.[31] The metabolite 15α-hydroxyprogesterone seems to be uniquely formed by the fetus and may be a useful test of fetal liver function.

Second, radiolabeled progesterone accumulates in the fetal adrenal glands, where it is a major substrate for cortisol and mineralocorticoid synthesis.[32] This is an important fate for placental progesterone since the isomerase enzyme necessary for cortisol biosynthesis from pregnenolone is absent from the burgeoning fetal zone of the adrenal. Accordingly, performed $\triangle_4$-steroids like progesterone must be provided if increasing cortisol synthesis by the fetus is to proceed (Fig. 3.3).[33]

Third, the fetal gonad metabolizes placental progesterone. Progesterone is a major substrate for fetal testosterone synthesis.[34] The fetal ovary can also reduce progesterone to various androgens but lacks the aromatase enzyme necessary for estrogen formation.[35,36]

Function

Wherever progesterone is to act, it is widely appreciated that the free or unbound fraction of this hormone diffuses through cell membranes to bind to specific cytoplasmic receptors. Placental transport mechanisms are thus unnecessary for steroids to enter the fetal circulation. The cytoplasmic receptors in target cells are acidic proteins, lacking lipid or carbohydraate moieties. After hormone binding, each receptor is transformed into a DNA-binding form that attaches to specific chromatin acceptor sites. Modulation of gene transcription follows, resulting in synthesis, or the inhibition of synthesis, of specific proteins, which express the particular end point(s) characteristic of the actions of progesterone on that target cell.

The progesterone receptor is best characterized for chick oviduct. It is a dimer; the subunits have molecular weights of 80,000 and 110,000 daltons. Each component can bind progesterone separately.[37] Progesterone binds to the complete receptor with high affinity ($K_D = 1$ nm), but the resultant complex dissociates rapidly. Progesterone also binds with similar affinity to transcortin or corticosteroid binding globulin. Note that the concentration of transcortin binding sites in endometrium usually exceeds that of the conventional progesterone receptor. A synthetic 19-nor-progesterone, R 5020, is useful as a progestogen laboratory probe, since it dissociates more slowly from the receptor than progesterone and has minimal binding to corticosteroid binding globulin.[38]

Estradiol, cortisol, and testosterone exhibit negligible affinity for the progesterone receptor.

It is now clear that the progesterone cytoplasmic receptor is one protein synthesized by the action of estrogen on the endometrial epithelial cells in the proliferative phase. Progesterone receptors appear in these cells even early in the proliferative phase, long before progesterone secretion by the corpus luteum. A preovulatory increase in progesterone receptors reaches a concentration of about 3.0 pmoles/mg DNA, mainly due to a rise in the level of the cytoplasmic receptor. Approximately 12,000 progesterone receptors per endometrial cell have been identified at mid-cycle. As serum progesterone increases after ovulation, endometrial cytoplasmic progesterone sites decrease, whereas nuclear sites increase markedly. These observations are consistent with translocation. Nuclear progesterone receptors peak at 1 pmole/mg DNA on about day 20 of the human menstrual cycle. Like the estradiol receptor, the total number of progesterone receptors falls progressively during the luteal phase. Apparently, this is due to "down-regulation," or negative feedback effects of progesterone on its own receptors.[39] Progesterone may increase endometrial inactiviation of estradiol through the stimulation of 17β-estradiol dehydrogenase; this mechanism decreases the ratio of nuclear estradiol to estrone and decreases the synthesis of endometrial DNA.[40]

Progesterone receptor physiology during human pregnancy is still poorly understood. In the rat, the number of progesterone receptors in the cytosol of whole uterus is low at the start of pregnancy and steadily increases up to 30,000 receptors per cell just before birth.[41] Such receptor availability should permit an enhanced biologic response to circulating progesterone. In primates, progesterone acts through its endometrial receptor to increase fivefold the ratio of endometrial nuclear estrone : estradiol binding.[42] Presumably this helps nidation proceed.

A second function of the endometrial progesterone receptor is to facilitate the synthesis of several endometrial proteins such as prolactin; progestagen-associated-endometrial protein (PEP), or α-uteroprotein; and inhibitors of plasminogen activators.[6,43] These actions also seem to promote implantation.

In sheep, an acute increase in fetal cortisol levels in late gestation stimulates placental 17α-hydroxylase activity, acutely decreasing placental pro-

gesterone secretion and directly inducing labor.[44] Progesterone blocks myometrial contractility by increasing calcium binding to the sarcoplasmic reticulum and myometrial cell membrane.[45] Human labor has never been proved to begin from a similar sudden drop in progesterone production. In two prospective series of normal term primigravid patients, only some women showed decreases in plasma progesterone levels before labor, and these decreases were gradual and not acute.[46,47] In the latter study, mean plasma progesterone concentrations were 169 ng/ml at 36 weeks and 103 ng/ml in labor. Progesterone values 1 week before labor were equivalent to those measured during labor. Other studies have failed to show even this modest relationship. Note that no study has yet compared primate periplacental or amniochorionic progesterone concentrations or its receptor physiology before and during birth. And it is surely here, and not in peripheral blood, that progesterone exerts its physiologic role.

A fifth and final function of progesterone may be as an aid in preventing immunologic rejection of the fetus by the mother. Progesterone appears to inhibit the transformation of monocytes to macrophages.[48] Progesterone also seems to inhibit phytohemagglutinin- (PHA)-stimulated activation of human T lymphocytes in vitro.[49] However, the presence of progesterone receptors has not been formally proven in monocytes or in the various subsets of T lymphocytes from pregnant subjects.

Clinical Importance

Progesterone or pregnanediol measurements are rarely of clinical obstetric usefulness. Pregnanediol excretion is a poor predictor of abortion: 80% of women with low values spontaneously restore these to normal and continue their pregnancies.[50] In subjects with threatened abortion and low serum progesterone levels, only 60% eventually aborted.

In late pregnancy, perhaps one indication to measure progesterone values or pregnanediol excretion is in the patient with very low estriol levels. Normal progesterone/pregnanediol concentrations would support the diagnosis of a specific defect in estriol synthesis, such as placental sulfatase deficiency, rendering estrogen excretion an unreliable index of fetal health.

Rarely is there any clinical indication for progesterone administration in pregnant patients. Certainly, several double-blind controlled trials in pregnant women with past histories of recurrent spontaneous abortion have shown that progestagens are without value in preventing future abortion.[50,51] The not uncommon practice of prescribing progesterone suppositories or injections for 6–8 weeks to patients with luteal phase defects to supplement allegedly reduced luteal progesterone production has also not stood the test of double-blind controlled trials. Clinicians wishing to prescribe such therapy should first have demonstrated, in the conceptual cycle, that a real deficiency of progesterone exists.

This practice of prescribing progesterone to in-fertile women in early pregnancy has reached epidemic proportions in many in vitro fertilization (IVF) programs. Progesterone deficiency has never been shown to be the cause of the failure of transferred embryos to implant in the uterus. The fact that major IVF units have never used exogenous progesterone indicates that such therapy is quite unnecessary.[52]

An unconfirmed report of a double-blind, placebo-controlled trial showed prevention of premature labor in high-risk patients who received 250 mg 17α-hydroxyprogesterone caproate per week.[53]

Synthetic progestagens are teratogenic. Admin-

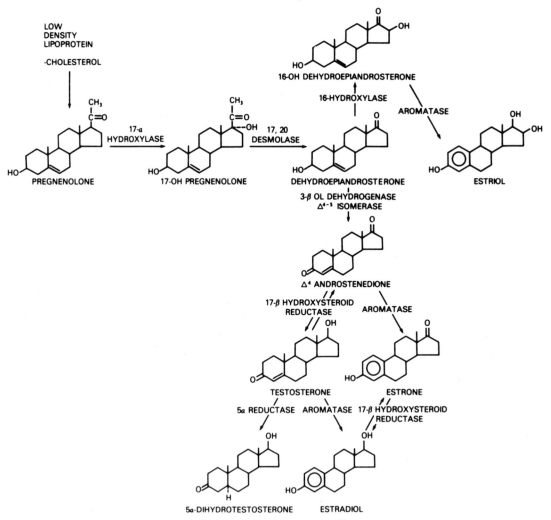

FIGURE 3-5. Principal intermediate structures in the synthesis of estrogens. Note that enzymes 17α-hydroxylase and 17,20-desmolase (horizontal arrows) are effectively absent from the human placenta but that the activities of the △4,5-isomerase, 17β-hydroxysteroid reductase and aromatase enzymes are intense.

istration of these steroids in early pregnancy is associated with an increased incidence of cardiovascular malformations and of hypospadias.[54] We believe that all these agents are contraindicated in pregnancy. Progesterone can be administered as a 50–100-mg IM injection, a rectal suppository, or even orally, although absorption is variable. Nevertheless, we believe it is only rarely clinically indicated: A true deficiency of progesterone should be established before exogenous progesterone is prescribed.

Estrogens

Estrogens are 18-carbon steroids with one aromatic ring containing double bonds between carbon atoms and one hydroxyl group on C-4 (Fig. 3-5). Estriol and estradiol were isolated from women in 1930 and 1936, respectively, and shown to be major human estrogens.[55,56] Estrogens were initially measured by the Kober reaction,[57] which analyzes their property of producing a yellow color in sulfuric acid, which turns pink in water. Brown[58,59] first developed estrogen assays sufficiently sensitive for aiding obstetric practice. His method involved the use of acid to hydrolyze estrogen conjugates from pregnancy urine. Free estrogens were then extracted, purified, and read by a spectrophotometric Kober reaction. Further advances came with estradiol measurements in nonpregnant women using double-isotope and later radioimmunoassay (RIA) techniques in extracted or unextracted plasma.[60]

Until 1964, it was considered axiomatic that the placenta completely synthesizes estrogens. Diczfalusy[31] then provided data that the fetus was vital for estrogen synthesis. He showed that the fetus and the placenta together form a fetoplacental unit that provides complementary enzymes vital for estriol synthesis. This insight has since dominated obstetric endocrinology.

Origin, Synthesis, and Control

In 1955, Brown reported that women produce 50–100 mg estriol and 15–20 mg estradiol daily at term gestation.[58,59] Zondek and Goldberg[61] then demonstrated urinary estriol measurements to be low in cases of fetal distress or death. In 1961, Frandsen and Stakemann[62] showed that urinary estriol excretion is also low in women carrying anencephalic fetuses and that these infants have small adrenal glands. Anencephalic fetuses were later found to have low plasma levels of the androgens DHEAS and 16-hydroxy-DHEAS, which are major products of the fetal adrenal glands.[63] Ryan[64] had previously shown that the placenta aromatized androgens to estrogens.

We are still unclear as to which factors regulate estriol synthesis by the fetoplacental unit. Estriol production throughout pregnancy is not apparently controlled by a feedback control mechanism between estrogen and pituitary–adrenal function. The placenta is certainly not rate limiting to estriol synthesis, as intra-amniotic injection of 100–200 mg DHEAS to normal women is followed by augmented estrogen secretion.[65]

About 90% of the estriol excreted by the mother derives from the fetal precursors at 20 weeks gestation.[66] It is now clear that DHEAS is the major substrate for placental estrogen production (Fig. 3-6). DHEAS is 16-hydroxylated in the fetal liver, and it is 16-hydroxy-DHEAS which is cleared by placental sulfatase and aromatase to produce estriol. At term, similar processes in the maternal adrenals and liver account for 10–15% of estriol precursor synthesis.[24]

What factors control fetal DHEAS secretion? Corticotropin (ACTH) is one obvious candidate as ACTH stimulates DHEAS secretion from the adult adrenal gland. ACTH (10^{-8}–10^{-9} M) will also stimulate DHEAS production from human fetal adrenal gland cells in vitro.[67] However, ACTH does not stimulate mitosis or DNA synthesis by these cells, unlike a related fetal pituitary peptide, α-melanocyte-stimulating hormone (α-MSH).[68] This implies that α-MSH, and not ACTH, stimulates the extraordinary growth of the fetal adrenal.

Other evidence indicates that ACTH is not the sole regulator of DHEAS secretion. Dexamethasone treatment suppresses fetal cortisol secretion by 90% but decreases DHEAS levels by only 60%.[69] Moreover, other peptides—chorionic gonadotropin (hCG); growth hormone (hGH); α-MSH; prolactin (PRL); angiotensin; and epidermal growth factor (EGF), or urogastrone—have all been reported to stimulate DHEAS secretion.[70–72] PRL is the most appealing of these putative fetal adrenal hormones. Fetal serum PRL concentrations rise as gestation proceeds,[73] and PRL increases DHEAS secretion not only in the fetus but in the adult as well.[74] Note, however, that chronic bromocriptine administration to a pregnant subject decreases fetal serum PRL levels but does not lower estriol excretion.[75]

Grumbach and associates[76] termed this second,

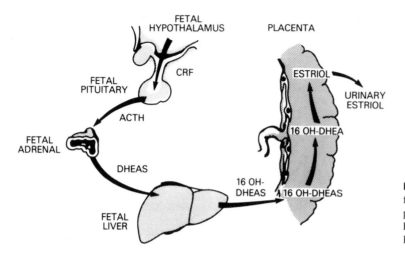

FIGURE 3-6. Predominant pathway for estriol synthesis. (Adapted with permission from Liggins in Human Reproductive Physiology, 1975, Blackwell).

non-ACTH, substance cortical androgen-stimulating hormone. It has been recently isolated as a 69,000-dalton peptide.[77] Although this factor was thought to be of pituitary origin, we recently reported that fetal primate thymectomy decreased adrenal gland size and DHEAS levels.[17] A thymic peptide might also stimulate fetal DHEAS secretion.

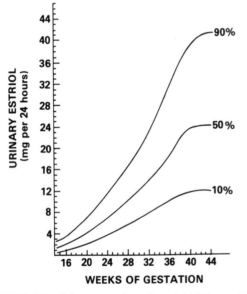

FIGURE 3-7. Urinary excretion of estriol-16-glucuronide throughout pregnancy. The upper and lower dotted lines represent the 90% and 10% confidence limits, respectively. (From Beischer et al.[250])

Maternal and Fetal Concentrations

It is vital to the proper understanding of the obstetric value of estrogen measurements that the physiologic variability in estrogen excretion be appreciated. For example, plasma estrone and estradiol concentrations increase from 6 weeks of pregnancy, but levels at term gestation range from 2 to 30 ng/ml and 12 to 90 ng/ml, respectively.[78] This wide range precludes the usefulness of these estrogens to obstetric practice. By contrast, estriol excretion increases 1000-fold during pregnancy (Fig. 3-7). Estriol concentrations also increase from typical mean concentrations of 39 nmoles/liter at 35 weeks to 56 nmoles/liter at 37 weeks of pregnancy.[78] These features, plus its predominantly fetal origin, have made estriol of particular interest to obstetricians as a fetoplacental function test. Fetal estriol levels are much higher than in the mother. Mean term estriol concentrations were 336 nmoles/liter in the umbilical vein and 367 nmoles/liter in the umbilical artery in one report.[79]

Estriol measurements in plasma, urine, or, more recently, saliva, all show coefficients of variation of 14–18% from one day to the next and of 30–34% from one women to the next at the same gestation.[80] These variations have clinical importance. It follows that a decrease in estriol of approximately 30%, or twice the coefficient of variation, must occur in a patient before a fall can properly be regarded as obstetrically significant. This is a major impediment to the clinical usefulness of estriol assays regardless of whether plasma or urinary measurements are used.

Mean term concentrations of maternal DHEAS and

16-hydroxy-DHEAS are 1.6 and 0.6 μmoles/liter, respectively.[81] Although these maternal androgens can be aromatized to estrone, estradiol, and estriol by the placenta, they seem to be poorly utilized. Mean fetal arterial DHEAS and 16-hydroxy-DHEAS concentrations are 5.0 and 10.5 μmoles/liter, respectively: mean umbilical vein 16-hydroxy-DHEAS values are 8.9 μmoles/liter, reflecting placental clearance of this steroid to form estriol.[81,82]

The half-life of DHEAS at term pregnancy is only 3h compared with 8–11 hr in nonpregnant women.[83] Exogenous DHEAS (50–200 mg IV) is rapidly (<1 hr) converted to estradiol (29%) but only slowly (5 hr) appears as estriol (17%).[84,85] These conversions occur even if the fetus is dead: Exogenous DHEAS injection is useless as a test of fetal health.[86]

A surge in fetal cortisol secretion induces a marked increase in estrogen excretion in sheep before labor begins and, in 1974, Turnbull and colleagues[47] reported in women that circulating levels of unconjugated estradiol also rose sharply before labor occurred. However, this finding was not confirmed in later studies.[87] Estradiol concentrations also do not increase before the onset of premature labor.[88] Estrogens do not appear to stimulate human labor.

Amniotic fluid also contains various estrogens. Estriol-16-glucosiduronate and estriol-3-sulfate-16-glucosiduronate are the major estrogens in this fluid. Free or unconjugated estriol rapidly diffuses into maternal tissue across the amniochorion and is not found in amniotic fluid.

Free steroids were also recently identified in saliva. Saliva estriol concentrations correlate with plasma unconjugated estriol levels. The day-to-day coefficient of variation of saliva estriol is 16.5%, which is comparable to plasma or urinary estimates, during pregnancy. Mean saliva estriol values are 7.0 nmoles/liter at term. These properties plus the ease of providing 50-μl repetitive samples suggest that saliva estriol might replace measurement of plasma estriol in assessing fetoplacental function.

Metabolism in Placenta, Mother, and Fetus

Circulating fetal androgens and estrogens are biologically inactive. This is because sulfation of steroids in the 3-position by the fetal liver and kidney inhibits bioactivity (Fig. 3-3). The fetal liver further hydroxylates DHEAS at the 15- and 16-positions to form 15-OH-DHEAS (Fig. 3-6). This capacity for 15-hydroxylation is seen only in fetal

life.[89] Estriol and estetrol are formed in the placenta due to its high content of sulfatase and aromatase enzymes.

Estriol then diffuses in the maternal circulation. Only 17% of circulating estriol is free or unbound to sex steroid-binding globulin or other carrier proteins.[90] Placental aromatase also prevents abnormal amounts of potent maternal androgens such as testosterone from masculinizing a female fetus.

Circulating estrogens are reconjugated with glucuronic acid in the maternal liver and excreted in bile and urine. The major biliary estrogen is estriol-3-sulfate-16-glucosiduronate: It is hydrolyzed by small-bowel bacteria to estriol-3-glucosiduronate which is then reabsorbed.[91] One-third of fetoplacental steroids enter bile by this route.[92] The kidney excretes not only estriol-16-glucosiduronate but free estriol as well. These metabolic pathways indicate that measurement of free or unconjugated estriol in plasma, urine or saliva is the most sensitive marker of fetoplacental estrogen synthesis.

Function

We still understand very little about the action of estriol during human pregnancy. In contrast to many studies measuring circulating estrogens, receptor technologies have infrequently been applied to human pregnancy tissues. Functional studies of estriol effects, in contrast to estradiol and estrone, are even fewer. The following questions arise: What is the precise role of estriol in human pregnancy? Does estriol merely represent endocrinologic noise from the fetoplacental unit or does it indicate a signal of major physiologic impact?

It is accepted that free or unbound estrogens diffuse through cell membranes to bind to specific cytoplasmic receptors. These receptors are acidic proteins without lipid or carbohydrate moieties. After estrogen binding, each receptor is transformed into a DNA-binding form that attaches to specific chromatin acceptor sites. Modulation of gene transcription follows, resulting in synthesis, or the inhibition of synthesis, of specific proteins in various pregnancy tissues.

The estradiol receptor from calf uterus may be the only estradiol binding site purified to homogeneity.[93] This receptor is a single polypeptide chain with a molecular weight of 70,000. It binds estradiol with high affinity (K_D = 0.1 nm), whereas estrone and estriol display approximately one-tenth this binding affinity. Glucocorticoids and progesterone have no affinity to the estradiol receptor.

As far as I am aware, no primate estradiol or estriol receptor has been isolated, purified, and characterized.

Estradiol receptors have been assessed throughout the menstrual cycle after dated endometrial biopsies in normal women.[94] The total cell content of estradiol receptor is high in the proliferative phase (2.0 pmoles/mg DNA), consistent with estrogen induction of this cytoplasmic receptor. Toward mid-cycle, the number of nuclear estradiol receptors doubles from 0.4 to 0.9 pmoles/mg DNA, in accord with translocation of the estradiol–receptor complex from the cytoplasm. At ovulation, there are approximately 8000 estradiol receptors per endometrial cell. After ovulation, the total concentration of estradiol receptor steadily falls throughout the luteal phase to a level (0.7 pmoles/mg DNA) below that seen in the follicular phase. Cytoplasmic receptor sites decrease early in the luteal phase, whereas nuclear receptors decline later. This loss of receptors for estradiol may be due to progesterone interference with replenishment of the cytoplasmic estradiol receptors, which is resynthesized early in the next menstrual cycle.[95]

This same mechanism probably operates during pregnancy. The total number of cytosol plus nuclear estrogen receptors was only 0.4 pmoles/mg DNA in pregnant subjects: Estrogen receptors were found only in the nucleus, 60% of which were occupied by estrogen.[96] These data suggest that the estrogen receptor is maximally saturated and that translocation to the nucleus occurs early in pregnancy. They further imply that no further biologic effect will result from the massive increases of estriol produced during the second and third trimesters.

The topography of estrogen receptors in the upper versus lower uterine segment, endometrium and amniochorion is not known. Rat studies show that estriol is short acting, while estradiol is a long-acting estrogen and that the reason for this is that estriol–receptor complexes are rapidly cleared.[97] Of course, estriol concentrations in human pregnancy are high and sustained and, in this circumstance, estriol is as potent as estradiol in promoting estrogen–nuclear receptor retention and uterine growth.[98] All estrogens seem to promote vascular permeability, mitosis and, in the uterus, synthesis of many proteins, including myometrial receptors for oxytocin and endometrial receptors for progesterone.[6] In addition, estrogen receptors have been reported in human uterine arteries.[99] This is clinically relevant as estriol has been reported to be the major estrogen increasing uteroplacental blood flow.[100]

Clinical Importance

Nearly 30 years after the first clinically useful estrogen assays, obstetricians still disagree as to whether these investigations are useful. This is a sad indictment of obstetric endocrinology. In one of the very few controlled prospective studies of the value of estrogen measurements in obstetrics, no clinical benefit from these tests was found.[101] Other obstetricians believe that estrogen assays do provide one index, albeit imprecise, of fetal health and that this information is worth having for clinical decision making. Support for this attitude comes from Beischer's study[102] of 6361 consecutive patients in whom 24-hr urinary estriol assays were performed in all pregnancies at 30 and 36 weeks gestation. In this routine screening program, estriol values below the 10th percentile were defined as abnormally low. Patients with one or more occasions of low estriol excretion had a perinatal mortality of 6.8% compared with a rate of 1.3% among those with normal estriol levels. Patients with low estriol excretion were hospitalized for bed rest and further evaluation.

The only purpose of estriol assays in obstetrics is to measure estrogen production by the fetoplacental unit. A 24-hr urinary assay, by summating excretion over the day, provides a more relevant index of estrogen production than does a single blood sample drawn for total or free estriol concentrations. However, we do acknowledge that 24-hr urine samples are inconvenient to collect, store, and handle. Nonfetoplacental causes for low estriol excretion are shown in Table 3-3. An incomplete urinary collection is the most common cause of "low estriol." Ampicillin and neomycin inhibit bacterial hydrolysis of estriol-3-sulfate-16-glucosiduronate; and a real reduction in plasma and urinary estriol results. Note that this mechanism is different from that of the urinary antiseptic, mandelamine, which liberates formaldehyde during the acid hydrolysis of estrogen conjugates and destroys all phenolic steroids. Phenolphthaline and other laxatives inhibit acid hydrolysis and also produce falsely low estimates. High-dose glucocorticoids, administered to the mother to prevent hyaline membrane disease in her premature infant, will lower urinary estriol excretion. Cortisol, at 100 mg/day for 2 days, or dexamethasone 6 mg/day for 2 days has been shown to

TABLE 3-3. Nonfetoplacental Causes of Low Urinary Estriol Excretion

Incomplete 24-hr collection
Exogenous glucocorticoids
   Dexamethasone
   Betamethasone
Antibiotics
   Ampicillin
   Neomycin
Urinary antiseptics
   Mandelamine
Laxatives
   Phenophthalein
Maternal disease
   Hepatic
   Renal

cross the placenta and suppress fetal ACTH and DHEAS secretion.[71] Finally, severe maternal liver or renal disease will reduce estriol conjugation and excretion.

Placental sulfatase deficiency is an enzyme defect that produces low urinary estriol excretion. It was initially described by France and Liggins in 1969.[103] Although initially thought to be rare, contemporary studies suggest that it is probably the commonest cause of estrogen excretion consistently below 3.0 mg/24 hr when fetal death or abnormality has been excluded. Placental sulfatase deficiency has an incidence of up to 1 : 800 when an obstetric population is screened by estriol assays.[4,104]

Many cases of incomplete or partial sulfatase deficiency are probably undiagnosed. Sulfatase deficiency is an X-linked recessive fetal disease: Only males manifest the condition. Sulfatase is absent not only in the placenta but also in fetal skin of severely affected males who usually develop ichthyosis, which has an incidence of 1 : 6000. Placental sulfatase deficiency should be suspected when urinary estriol excretion is persistently below 3.0 mg/24 hr in the absence of fetal death of anencephaly.[104]

Note that estriol levels are low but not zero, pregnanediol excretion is normal and amniotic fluid DHEAS concentrations are extremely high in this disorder. Exogenous DHEAS (100 mg IV) does not increase estrogen excretion, but dehydroepiandrosterone (DHEA) (100 mg IV) administration elevates estradiol levels four- to fourfold.[105] Mean urinary 16-hydroxy-DHEAS concentrations in affected pregnancies were 9.1 mg/24 hr (range 1.9–41.9) compared with 0.4 mg/24 hr (range 0–11.5) in normal pregnancies.[4] Such suspected cases of sulfatase deficiency must be confirmed after delivery by placental analysis: this is important not only for the infant's risk of ichthyosis but for future pregnancies as well. Measuring 7-[^{3}H]-DHEAS conversion, placental sulfatase activity was 194 ± 147 (mean ± SD) pmoles/mg protein per min in affected tissue compared with 2940 ± 184 pmoles/mg protein per min in normal placentae.[106]

The pregnancies typically show normal fetal growth and no fetal distress. Although prolonged pregnancy, an unripe cervix, and nonprogressive labor are alleged to characterize these patients, this is probably not true but merely reflects the few diagnosed cases. Sulfatase-deficient pregnancies can certainly deliver vaginally.[107]

Placental sulfatase deficiency is also an important clinical physiologic experiment of nature. Despite extremely low estrogen levels, maternal and fetal growth are normal. No fetal mortality or morbidity has ever been reported in this disorder. Estrogens appear permissive but certainly not fundamental to human fetal health and development.

A dynamic test of estrogen production, injecting DHEAS (50 mg IV), and measuring estradiol generation, has not been found useful.[108,109] Normal estradiol formation could occur even if the fetus were moribund: The insensitivity of this test was predictable from a knowledge of placental physiology. Estetrol (15α-hydroxyestriol) is formed from estradiol only by the fetal liver.[89] Maternal estetrol measurements were therefore a logical fetal function test and investigations found estetrol concentrations commonly but not always predicted fetal death: Estetrol seems no more clinically useful that estriol analyses.[110]

Although the estriol : estradiol shift occurs early in pregnancy, estrogen measurements are not useful for predicting spontaneous abortion. In one group of patients with threatened abortion, 23% of those with low estrogen levels delivered at term, whereas 21% of women with normal estrogen excretion aborted.[111]

Therapy with estrogens in pregnancy has been a sad chapter in obstetric endocrinology. Diethylstilbestrol (DES), a potent synthetic nonsteroidal estrogen was prescribed to 4–6 million pregnant women between 1945 and 1955 in an attempt to prevent recurrent abortion, premature labor, preeclampsia, and intrauterine death.[112] Eighty percent of female fetuses exposed to this compound at a time of mullerian duct differentiation developed vaginal adenosis and about 1 : 3000 of these females later acquired clear cell vaginal adenocarcinoma at a median age of 19 years.[113] Manifold other lesions—vaginal ridges, cervical ridges, hoods, pseudopolyps, uterine malformations, and synechiae, and in males, epididymal cysts and oligospermia—have been the legacy of the prescription of this estrogen without adequate controlled trials.[114]

Estriol excretion during the third trimester has been used to evaluate fetal health in every obstetric complication. As detailed earlier, controlled trials have been few and the estriol test, be it of urine or plasma, conjugated or free, is not predictive of acute obstetric complications. Low estriol values in preeclampsia, suspected intrauterine growth retardation (IUGR), and prolonged pregnancy are variously associated with increased perinatal mortality.[115–117] Low estriol excretion presumably reflects chronic fetoplacental insufficiency, but note that such fetal stress does not seem to result in secretion of fetal pituitary ACTH, which would be expected to elevate adrenal DHEAS secretion and thus raise—not lower—estrogen production. Unless glucose control is excellent, estriol measurements have no clear benefit on managing diabetic pregnancy.[118,119] Estriol estimations are valueless for predicting fetal death in rhesus isoimmunization.[120]

In all these complications, the value of estriol assays over other fetal function tests has rarely been proven. Urinary estrogen excretion was found inferior to placental lactogen (hPL) measurements as predictive of placental insufficiency in a recent study.[121] In all pregnancy complications, enough individual exceptions occur for the wise obstetrician to use other fetal assessments in addition to estriol assays to establish fetal well-being.

Most clinicians admit patients with low estriol excretion to hospital for further antenatal assessment. Many accept that bed rest alone improves estriol excretion.[122] The decision is typically between induction of labor and aiming for further intrauterine growth. An unconfirmed report found that intravenous therapy improved estriol excretion and presumably fetal outcome.[123]

Androgens and Corticosteroids

We have already reviewed the pivotal role of the fetal androgen dehydroepiandrosterone and its sulfate in placental estriol synthesis. There are no data to prove that the human placenta synthesizes androgens de novo. There is also no evidence that the placenta synthesizes glucocorticoids. Whereas several investigators have isolated cortisol, cortisone, aldosterone, and other corticosteroids from this tissue, the interpretation of these findings is impossible because the placenta contains appreciable amounts of maternal and fetal blood, both of which contain corticosteroids. The fetal adrenal is capable of synthesizing corticosteroids from placental progesterone, and these will also contribute to the amounts found in the placenta. Placental tissue incubated with progesterone does not form corticosteroids, consistent with the absence of the enzymes 17α-hydroxylase and 17,20-desmolase from this organ.

Previous experience with glucocorticoid therapy during human pregnancy for maternal disease (systemic lupus erythematosus, rheumatoid arthritis, Crohn's enteritis) is based mainly on the use of cortisone, hydrocortisone, prednisone, or prednisolone. These steroids, although given at pharmacologic doses, have very little effect on the fetus; birth weight of infants born to mothers treated with these steroids is either not affected or mildly decreased.[124] The cortisol production rate in most of these newborns is normal. The lack of fetal effects with these steroids is due mainly to their limited transplacental passage, which relates to their capacity to bind to maternal cortisol binding globulin and/or to their metabolism by placental enzymes.[125] In contrast to these glucorcorticoids, dexamethasone, even at the equivalent of maternal replacement doses (approximately 15 μg/kg per day), has marked effects on the fetal adrenal gland. Dexamethasone suppresses fetal adrenal function and fetal growth and at pharmacologic doses (80–160 μg/kg per day) caused fetal death.[126] Transplacental passage of dexamethasone has also been documented in women receiving dexamethasone in the last trimester of pregnancy for prevention of respiratory distress syndrome.[127]

Using this property, dexamethasone at 0.25 mg every 6 hr was prescribed from 10 to 40 weeks gestation to suppress adrenal androgen secretion and intrauterine masculinization of the genitals in a female fetus believed to have the 21-hydroxylase-deficient form of congenital adrenal hyperplasia.[128] This exciting case report indicates this form of fetal therapy as an alternative to neonatal surgical correction and indicates a new direction in obstetric endocrinology.

Total and unbound or free maternal plasma cortisol levels rise in pregnancy due to increases in cortisol binding globulin concentrations.[129] Glucocorticoid receptors are present in the placenta, chorion laeve and myometrium, but only chorion laeve tissue markedly produces cortisol from cortisone, which is a physiologically inactive glucocorticoid.[130] This paracrine production of cortisol affirms the functional significance of the human amniochorion and may promote immunological acceptance of the fetal allograft.

PLACENTAL PROTEIN HORMONES

Placental Lactogen

Human placental lactogen or chorionic somatomammotropin (hPL, hCS), a peptide secreted by the syncytiotrophoblast throughout gestation, was first clearly defined by Josimovich and MacLaren in 1962.[131] Their material showed considerable potency as a lactogenic factor in pigeon crop-sac assays and in promoting lactogenesis in rabbit mammary gland. Two groups found only 3% growth hormone (GH)-like activity in specific bioassays in rats such as the tibial length.[132,133] Because of its 80% amino acid identity with hGH, the term chorionic somatomammotropin was also suggested.[134] We shall use the term placental lactogen (hPL) in this chapter.

Structure

hPL is a single-chain polypeptide of 191 amino acids with two disulfide bonds and a molecular weight of 21,600. This sequence is 80% homologous with hGH but only 13% identical with prolactin (PRL).[135,136] The gene for hPL has been cloned, and the genes for hPL and hGH are located on chromosome 17 in close linkage.[138] By contrast, the PRL gene is found on chromosome 6.[138] As 92% of the nucleotides are homologous between hPL and hGH, Niall and colleagues[139] proposed that hPL arose in an evolutionary sense from a common ancestral molecule of hPL, hGH, and PRL by duplication of the hGH gene.

Origin, Synthesis, and Control

hPL synthesis by syncytiotrophoblast was proved by immunofluorescence localization and in vitro placental culture.[140,141] Placental production of hPL increases steadily with placental weight as pregnancy develops (Fig. 3-8). At term, the daily production rate of hPL is extraordinary: between 1 and 3 g/day is typically synthesized in late pregnancy.[142] At the end of pregnancy, hPL represents 10% of the proteins synthesized by placental polyribosomes.

Control of hPL synthesis is still poorly understood. This is remarkable, given the ease of obtaining placenta and the availability of stable hPL bioassays and radioimmunoassays. As for other placental hormones, there is little evidence that feedback control systems regulate hPL secretion. hPL release has been considered autonomous or governed by uteroplacental blood flow rather than by chemical messengers.[143,144] Insulin, at 10^{-10} M, has been reported to increase hPL secretion in vitro, but this finding awaits confirmation.[145] Dopamine has been shown to inhibit hPL release at pharmacologic concentrations (10^{-3} M)[146] whereas prostaglandins, cAMP, somatostatin, thyrotropin-releasing hormone, and arginine have all had unconfirmed reports of effects on hPL secretion.

Clinical hPL studies have also been contradictory. Autonomy of hPL secretion in vivo was suggested by absence of plasma hPL changes in women following induced rises and falls in serum glucose or amino acids.[140] By contrast, prolonged second-

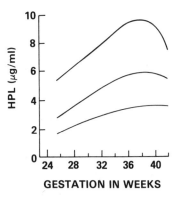

FIGURE 3-8. Normal range for hPL in maternal blood from 20 to 42 weeks gestation in 200 individuals, showing the mean ± 2 SD. (From Chard and Klopper.[1])

trimester fasting has been reported to elevate maternal hPL concentrations markedly.[147]

Maternal and Fetal Concentrations

hPL is detectable in maternal blood (7–10 ng/ml) 20–40 days after fertilization. Figure 3-8 shows that the increase closely follows placental mass and DNA content. Accordingly, concentrations of up to 40 µg/ml have been detected in multiple pregnancies. Maternal hPL levels show no nyctohemeral rhythm.[142]

Urine contains little hPL. Josimovich[148] found an urinary excretion of only 0.5 mg/day at term gestation. Fetal blood concentrations of hPL decline from 50 to 150 ng/ml at mid-gestation to 20–40 ng/ml at term.[149] The ratio of maternal to fetal hPL at delivery is therefore normally approximately 500 : 1, which surely reflects trophoblast being in direct contact with maternal blood (Fig. 3-2). By contrast to the fetus, amniotic fluid hPL concentrations are quite high, averaging 150 ng/ml at term.[150] This high concentration presumably reflects diffusion of hPL from chorion laeve into amniotic fluid and the slow degradation of proteins in this medium, since Chez and colleagues demonstrated slow diffusion in vitro.[151]

Metabolism

After removal of the placenta, hPL disappears from the maternal circulation rapidly according to a multicomponent logarithmic curve. The major portion of the hormone disappears, with a half-life of 12–30 min[152] (See review by Pavlou et al.[153]). The mean metabolic turnover rate was calculated to be 173 liters/day. The sites of metabolism of the hormone are unknown but are presumed to be similar to those responsible for degradation of hGH. Thus, liver and kidney are probably the major sites for hPL degradation, although adipose tissue may also be important.[154]

Function

Twenty years after its discovery and despite much effort from many investigators, the physiologic action of hPL is still unclear. Three factors are relevant here. First, several early human investigations reporting various metabolic actions of hPL used preparations that, in retrospect, were probably less somatotropic dimers or polymers.[133] Second, it is now certain that hPL, hGH, and PRL bind with varying affinity to both lactogenic and growth-promoting receptors, and this compounds the difficulty of determining a specific hPL action. Furthermore, there is considerable species-to-species variability in these three hormones,[155] and heterologous studies are difficult to relate to human physiology. Finally, recent reports show that up to 1 : 3000 human pregnancies have undetectable hPL levels in maternal blood.[3,156] Lactation, glucose tolerance tests, and, more importantly, fetal growth were quite normal in these affected pregnancies.[157,158] It is difficult to dismiss these several reports and their endocrine impact. It would seem that hPL has, at best, only a permissive and subsidiary role in human fetomaternal metabolism and that any or all of its functions can be satisfactorally performed by PRL, hGH, or other substances. Indeed, hPL may have no endocrine role whatsoever in human pregnancy, merely reflecting placental mass and being released in an open-ended, nonregulated fashion.[159]

In the human, Beck and Daughaday[152] found overnight infusion of hPL to increase insulin release in response to a glucose load, but to worsen glucose tolerance. Grumbach and colleagues[160] treated hypopituitary dwarfs with hPL doses 100–200 times the minimal effective dose of hGH and also found poorer glucose tolerance and increased free fatty acid mobilization, leading to the view that hPL serves to provide maternal glucose to the fetus. Unfortunately, this putative homeostatic mechanism has not been confirmed. Only small increases of hPL follow insulin-induced hypoglycemia, compared with large elevations in hGH,[161] while glucose ingestion produces no change in hPL concentrations.[162] Estrogens are at least equally likely as hPL to be the cause of the impaired carbohydrate metabolism of pregnancy even though the weak somatotropic effect of hPL may further increase insulin needs in late pregnancy.

It is remarkable that hPL has only 3% of growth hormone-like activity in various bioassays despite being 80% homologous to the hGH amino acid sequence. This fact, and the relatively low fetal hPL levels, mitigate against hPL exerting a growth-promoting action upon the fetus. There are some data that placental lactogen will stimulate somatomedin C (IGF I) and multiplication-stimulating activity (IGF II) So, release in various species (Handwerger (personal communication), but there is no proof of any somatotropic action in human fetal development.

Although hPL does have lactogenic activity in various bioassays, administration of hPL to non-pregnant subjects fails to induce lactation.[163] Moreover, maternal PRL concentrations increase by an order of the magnitude during pregnancy and could equally prepare the breasts for lactation and is the major stimulus for puerperal lactation.[164a] Nevertheless, Beck[164] showed that hPL can induce histologic changes consistent with lactogenesis in rhesus monkeys and it seems, on balance, that hPL and PRL both contribute to preparing the mammary gland for lactation.

Clinical Importance

Regardless of its uncertain physiologic actions, it is possible clinically to use hPL measurements as a placental function test. Routine screening with hPL sampling of an entire obstetric population has reported that hPL was an effective predictor of poor fetal outcome.[2]

hPL concentrations below 4.0 µg/ml after the thirtieth week indicated a fetal mortality of 24% in hypertensive pregnancy.[165] It is also evident that a combination of low maternal estrogen excretion and serum hPL measurement is highly predictive of definite intrauterine growth retardation.[132] Figure 3-9 shows hPL concentrations in an early series of 21 toxemic patients (7 with persisting essential hypertension, 9 with preeclampsia existing for greater than 1 week before blood sampling, 2 diabetic pa-

tients whose condition was complicated by vascular hypertension, 2 patients suffering from chronic glomerulonephritis with secondary hypertension, and 1 with allergic vasculitis causing decreased renal function and hypertension). In addition, Figure 3.9 gives the hPL values for five patients with idiopathic intrauterine growth retardation as judged by the delivery of babies varying between 1450 and 1930 g after 36 weeks gestation: It can be seen that 14 of the 21 hypertensive mothers had low serum hPL values. In contrast to the finding of Spellacy and colleagues,[166] however, Josimovich[132] found no prognostic value as to imminent (within 1 week) fetal demise, regardless of whether the hPL levels were in the normal or low range during the last trimester, although four of five babies born with severe fetal distress were associated with maternal hPL values that fell below the 50th percentile. Mothers of all five of the idiopathic dysmature babies—one was depressed at birth, and one died just before birth—had hPL concentrations that fell below the normal limits of 4 µg/ml, a finding consistent with earlier reports.

hPL concentrations have also been determined in a prospective study of 2733 patients with clinical evidence of fetal risk.[167] The results were reported or not reported in a randomized manner to the obstetrician. In the reported group, the perinatal mortality was 3.4%, compared with 15% in the unreported group. This study was important, as it indicated the usefulness in a controlled clinical trial of hPL measurements in identifying fetal risk.

hPL levels are high in multiple, diabetic, and rhesus-immunized pregnancies and tend to be low in threatened abortion and molar pregnancy. However, the predictive value is low in the individual patient and the determinations are only obstetrically useful in the well-controlled pregnant diabetic.

Chorionic Gonadotropin

Structure

Human chorionic gonadotropin (hCG) is a glycoprotein of 30% carbohydrate and a molecular weight of 36,700.[168] The peptide portion consists of an α- and β-subunit dissociable by hypertonic urea solutions. The α-subunit has 92 amino acids and a molecular weight of 14,500 and is essentially identical to the α-subunit of follicle-stimulating hormone (FSH), LH, and thyrotropin (TSH). The β-subunit contains 145 amino acids and has a mo-

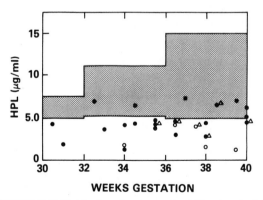

FIGURE 3-9. Distribution of representative hPL values in 21 mothers with preeclampsia and/or hypertension (●) and in 5 women carrying a fetus with fetal intrauterine growth retardation (IUGR) (○) in comparison with levels found in 95% of normal pregnant women (shaded area). Daggers represent eventual fetal death; asterisks, severe neonatal asphyxia.

lecular weight of 22,200. The hCG β-subunit is 80% identical to the β-subunit of LH but has a unique peptide of 30 amino acids at the C-terminal: It is this sequence which confers the specific biologic activity of hCG. The β-subunit is attached to five carbohydrate residues containing sialic acid at serine amino acids 121, 127, 132 and 138 of the C-terminal.[169]

Origin, Synthesis, and Control

Proof of the placental origin of hCG was first demonstrated in the culture of chorionic villi by Jones and colleagues.[170] Later immunofluorescent studies localized hCG production to syncytiotrophoblast.[171]

Recent studies show that both α- and β-subunits of hCG derived from separate and larger precursors, which are cleared by membrane-bound peptidases.[172] The subunits have separate genes that probably lie on the same chromosome. Synthesis of the β-subunit is rate limiting to the production of circulating hCG, whereas the α-subunit is secreted in excess.

Regulation of hCG secretion is still not clearly understood. Like LH secretion, recent studies show that hCG is released into the circulation in an episodic manner with pulses of hCG identified every 2 hr.[173]

Placenta has also been shown to synthesize a LHRH, which appears identical to hypothalamic LHRH.[7] These investigators also reported that placental LHRH was localized by immunohistochemistry to the cytotrophoblast and stimulated hCG secretion by syncytiotrophoblast.[174,175] This paracrine control mechanism would then be in a sense analogous to hypothalamic LHRH control of pituitary LH secretion, delivering a "pulse" of LHRH to release hCG every 2 hours. Physiologic studies to confirm this hypothesis have been contradictory. Although intravenous LHRH administration to pregnant monkeys has been claimed to increase circulating chorionic gonadotropin concentrations,[176] we were unable to confirm these results at various stages of pregnancy in rhesus monkeys.[177] Without in vivo supportive data, the role of LHRH in hCG regulation remains unproved.

Progesterone has been shown to inhibit hCG synthesis by placenta in vitro.[178] Whereas on the one hand this suggests a negative feedback control mechanism between hCG and corpus luteum progesterone secretion, it does not explain why placental progesterone does not constantly inhibit hCG production.

While physiologic control of hCG synthesis and release remains unknown, several pharmacologic actions have been identified. hCG secretion in vitro from normal placenta has been reported increased by dibutyryl cAMP[179] and pimozide,[180] while hCG release by choriocarcinoma cell lines has been claimed after epidermal growth factor or dopamine exposure.[180,181]

hCG has also been proved to originate from a wide variety of nonplacental tissues, both normal and neoplastic. These include not only trophoblast tumors but neoplasms of the ovary, testis, lung, stomach, and adrenal as well as normal adult and fetal liver and kidney.[182,183] The latter findings support a role for hCG in regulating fetal steroidogenesis: The interested reader is referred to a recent monograph for a more complete discussion of ectopic hCG production.[184]

Maternal and Fetal Concentrations

Although hCG has not been detected in culture media from 4- to 8-cell human embryos,[185] the hormone has been reported to be secreted by the blastocyst.[186] Maternal plasma contains detectable hCG within 2 days of embryo transfer or natural implantation and plasma hCG concentrations thereafter double every 2 days over the first 8–10 weeks of pregnancy. The early placenta secretes up to 100,000 IU of hCG daily. At approximately 10 weeks gestation, when the maximum maternal levels of hCG are obtained, plasma values range from 160 to 200 mIU/ml. During the second trimester, the well-known drop in hCG concentration occurs to about 10 mIU/ml, which remains essentially unchanged until delivery. Note that considerable hCG is nevertheless still secreted in late human pregnancy. Normal placental tissue also secretes free α-subunit whose levels exceed that of intact hCG after 8 weeks gestation, and free β-subunit for the first 16 weeks of pregnancy.[187]

hCG does cross the placenta and enters the fetal circulation to reach peak plasma concentrations at 8–12 weeks gestation.[188] Concentrations of 500 mIU/ml are not uncommon at this time. As there is no secretion of LH by the differentiating fetal pituitary at this gestation, hCG appears to be the major stimulus for testosterone secretion from the fetal Leydig cell. Anencephalic male fetuses produce little or no FSH or LH, but their genitalia differentiate normally.

Metabolism

hCG is cleared remarkably slowly from maternal plasma and disappears from the circulation according to a multicomponent logarithmic curve. The first phase has been estimated at 11 hr and the half-life of the second component at 23 hr.[189] The presence of N-acetylneuraminic (sialic) acid at the end of the carbohydrate residues appears to confer the primary resistance to metabolic clearance.[190] Like hPL, hCG is metabolized predominantly by the liver and kidney.

Function

Progesterone secretion from the corpus luteum of the fertile menstrual cycle becomes markedly enhanced concurrent with the appearance of hCG during implantation.[191] During this "rescue" of the corpus luteum by episodic exposure to hCG, luteal cell binding of hCG typically reaches 8–14 fmoles/mg protein.[192] Maintaining progesterone secretion by the corpus luteum for the first 6–7 weeks of pregnancy is a critical role for hCG. Note that at 8–10 weeks gestation, when hCG concentrations are highest, a significant reduction in hCG binding to 1–3 fmoles/mg protein to luteal tissue is observed.[193] At this time, the luteoplacental shift occurs and autonomy of the conceptus is established. Such hCG downregulation of corpus luteum progesterone secretion appears to involve two cellular events due to the presence of high and unremitting hCG exposure. The first event is a refractoriness of the adenylate cyclase enzyme within the luteal cell membrane and is associated with a loss of hCG receptors by internalization. The second lesion is a subsequent decrease in cAMP and progesterone formation.[194]

hCG appears to be the primary stimulus to the fetal Leydig cell to synthesize and secrete testosterone.[188] This action occurs before fetal pituitary LH secretion is established and is maximal from 11 to 17 weeks gestation. Fetal testosterone is vital for differentiation of the male genital tract. Receptors for hCG have been demonstrated in the fetal human testis at 16–20 weeks gestation and these binding sites respond in vitro to hCG at concentrations found in fetal plasma by testosterone secretion.[195]

Immunosuppressive properties have also been attributed to hCG.[196] It now seems clear that most, if not all the immunosuppressive activity of the hCG preparations used in these studies was due to other moieties. Early pregnancy factor is one such immunosuppressive embryonic protein that has been found in some hCG preparations.[197]

Clinical Importance

The diagnostic usefulness of hCG assay as a pregnancy test is clearly established: Bioassay, measuring ovarian hyperemia or hypertrophy, has a sensitivity of 1 IU of hCG/ml of urine or 400 mIU/ml of blood and can detect pregnancy 14 days after a missed period but fail to indicate an ectopic pregnancy associated with low production of hCG. Immunologic pregnancy tests, using Latex or hemagglutination inhibition were cheaper but had similar sensitivity. Radioimmunoassay for the β-subunit[198] or radioreceptorassay[199] have improved sensitivity, measuring 5–10 mIU/ml serum and can diagnosis pregnancy 6 days after conception. This is clinically useful in follow-up of trophoblastic disease.

Same-day β-subunit hCG assays, when combined with ultrasonography to examine for an intrauterine gestation sac, have proved of great help in the diagnosis and management of suspected ectopic pregnancy. Lundstrom et al.[200] reported on 64 patients with ectopic pregnancy who all had a positive hCG assay and in whom use of the assay led to earlier diagnosis and fewer ruptured ectopic pregnancies. In another study, 100 consecutive patients of reproductive age with acute pelvic pain were examined by a rapid hCG β-subunit RIA.[201] Twenty-four women had measureable β-subunit, and 22 of these had a pregnancy including 10 ectopic pregnancies: 76 gave negative results and only three had evidence of pregnancy.

The therapeutic use of hCG as a surrogate LH in managing chronic anovulation is established. Patients with spontaneous defects in positive feedback at mid-cycle and failure of an endogenous LH surge, hypogonadotropic patients receiving exogenous gonadotropin or patients on in vitro fertilization programs commonly receive hCG to induce ovulation. Pulsatile gonadotropin-releasing hormone regimens will reduce the need for hCG administration in most infertile patients with chronic anovulation.[202]

The prospect of fertility regulation in women by active immunization against the β-subunit of hCG was reported in 1976 by Talwar et al.[203] Difficulties in establishing immunogenicity and efficacy against hCG have appeared despite an intense effort by several laboratories to develop a suitable vaccine. The reader is referred to a monograph for a detailed analysis of the status of anti-hCG fertility regulation.[184]

OTHER PLACENTAL PROTEINS

Schwangerschaftsprotein 1

This is one of several proteins of placental origin identified during the past decade that are present in relatively high concentration but that have, as yet, no proven physiologic role.

SP_1 or $SP_{1\beta}$ is a 90,000-dalton β_1-globulin containing 30% carbohydrate that has been localized to syncytiotrophoblast.[204] SP_1, like hCG, has a long half-life of 22 hr in the maternal circulation and rises steadily as pregnancy advances (similar to hPL) to reach plasma concentrations of approximately 150 μg/ml at term gestation.[205] This compares with peak hPL levels of 7 μg/ml.

SP_1 has been detected within 2–3 days after implantation.[206] In late pregnancy, SP_1 radioimmunoassay has been applied to screening an entire obstetric population and low concentrations found predictive of general fetal risk.[207] It has been reported that SP_1 values are low in 60% of women who bear a growth-retarded infant, but the predictive value of a single abnormal SP_1 result in pregnancy is unknown.[208]

Pregnancy-Associated Plasma Protein A

Halbert's group isolated PAPP-A[209] and showed it to be an α_2-macroglobulin of 800,000 daltons. Bischof[210] later showed that PAPP-A is a dimer, with each monomer in turn being composed of two polypeptide chains of 200,000 daltons. Although originally believed to originate in the cytotrophoblast,[204] recent data indicate that PAPP-A is synthesized by maternal endometrial decidua[211] and merely localized to the placenta.

Maternal PAPP-A concentrations rise steadily until 30 weeks gestation and then rise more steeply up to and into labor.[212] If confirmed, this unique profile may be highly useful as a fetoplacental function test. Unlike hPL and SP_1, PAPP-A concentrations are not clearly related to placental mass. Moreover, PAPP-A levels are not reduced in pregnancies complicated by fetal growth retardation and seem elevated in the prodromal phase of preeclampsia.[213] PAPP-A has been found low in pregnancies destined for spontaneous miscarriage, be

these following natural conception or in vitro fertilization.[214] Clearly, confirmation of these results is awaited.

The function of PAPP-A is unknown. Various unsupported studies suggest that PAPP-A has immunosuppressive properties: In particular, it appears to inhibit complement activation.[215] This may relate to its elevation in preeclampsia and premature labor, where it may interact with another placental protein, PP5, as an antithrombin.

Hypothalamic Peptides

There appears to be localization of several hypothalamic–pituitary peptides within the placenta and amniochorion. Table 3.1 lists the variety of peptides localized to the various periplacental tissues. Note that pituitary peptides are localized by immunohistochemical studies to the syncytiotrophoblast, whereas the smaller hypothalamic–neurotransmitter peptides have been predominantly identified in cytotrophoblast. Note also that placental synthesis of these more recent peptides has certainly not been proven and usually only the immunoassayable presence and accumulation of the peptide has been shown with term placental extracts. Table 3.2 lists seven prerequisite criteria for such putative placental hormones. Paracrine regulation by cytotrophoblast-releasing factors of syncytiotrophoblast hormone release may occur in the human placenta but is certainly not proved at this time. As an example of this uncertainty, TRH has been identified in cytotrophoblast, but this appears to be chromatographically distinct from synthetic TRH.[216] Moreover, no TRH receptors have been found in syncytiotrophoblast and TSH-like activity certainly resides in highly purified and reconstituted synthetic α- and β-subunits of hCG.[217] Placental TRH seems to have no function.

PERIPLACENTAL HORMONES

Prostaglandins

Intrauterine prostaglandins mainly derive from arachidonic acid, originating predominantly from the essential fatty acid linoleic acid (Fig. 3-10). Arachidonic acid is a polyunsaturated 20-carbon atom chair with four double bonds and no nitrogen atoms. Arachidonic acid is liberated from cell membrane phospholipids by the enzyme phos-

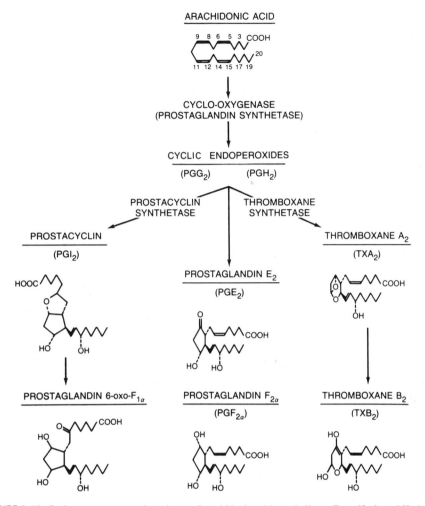

FIGURE 3-10. Cyclooxygenase cascade pathway of arachidonic acid metabolism. (From Healy and Hodgen.[251]

pholipase A_2, in response to many physical and hormonal stimuli. In the best-studied pathway, arachidonic acid is oxygenated rapidly by the enzyme prostaglandin synthetase, or cyclo-oxygenase, to form a family of prostaglandins that each contains only two double bonds.

The initial intermediates generated are two endoperoxides, PGG_2 and PGH_2. Both substances are pivotal in liberating at least three groups of prostanoids (Fig. 3.10). Prostaglandins PGF_2 and PGE_2 are among those most studied because of their potency at contracting the myometrium.[218] PGF_2 and thromboxane A_2 (TXA_2) are potent vasoconstrictors; conversely, PGE_2 and prostacyclin (PGI_2)

cause vasodilation.[219] PGI_2 also dissociates platelets, while TXA_2 aggregates platelets; both prostanoids are rapidly metabolized to form more stable products, including 6-oxo-PGF_1 and thromboxane B_2, respectively.

In placental endocrinology, prostacyclin (PGI_2) has attracted special interest, since its pharmacologic properties—vasodilation, platelet disaggregation, and increased renin release—are the converse of what is observed in patients with preeclampsia.[220] PGI_2 does not contract the human uterus.[221] PGI_2 is unique among placental hormones in being synthesized and released from all periplacental tissues—trophoblast, amnion, chorion laeve, decidua, umbilical cord, and myometrium.[222] Target tissues for placental PGI_2 are uncertain, but PGI_2 receptors have been demonstrated in platelets to be membrane bound and do demonstrate downregulation in the presence of high prostaglandin concentrations.[223]

Physiologic functions and the clinical importance of PGI_2 are still uncertain. The ability of trophoblast to invade endometrial vessels at implantation may depend on PGI_2 synthesis, which prevents immobilization by platelet aggregates.[224] Umbilical cord vessels produce more PGI_2 than do adult blood vessels, and this synthesis may be important in establishing the normal low resistance of the placental and fetal circulations.[225]

Several groups have now shown a deficiency of PGI_2 in preeclampsia,[226] and anecdotal case reports describe a decrease in blood pressure after intravenous PGI_2 administration to patients with severe preeclampsia.[227] Exciting though these reports are, the precise involvement of placental PGI_2 and other prostanoids in normal pregnancy physiology and to obstetric complications must await future study.

Decidual Prolactin

Although synthesized by maternal decidua, and not by the placenta, PRL is relevant to placental endocrinology as it is the most thoroughly studied of the newer periplacental proteins. Decidual PRL does provide the currently best model of cybernetic or paracrine hormone action in pregnancy tissues.

Origin, Synthesis, and Control

Application of the PRL radioimmunoassay to human pregnancy found amniotic fluid PRL concentrations of up to 4000 ng/ml or 100-fold higher than measured in maternal blood.[228] Where was amniotic fluid PRL coming from? Not the fetus and little from the maternal circulation, it seemed, as radiolabeled PRL injected into the fetal rhesus monkey did not reach amniotic fluid while passage of radiolabeled PRL was slow in transit from mother to amniotic fluid.[229]

Decidual synthesis of PRL was first proved by Riddick's group.[230] From and since that time, decidual PRL has been confirmed not only by radioimmunoassay but also by bioassay, radiolabel incorporation, identification of its primary amino acid sequence, and detection of its specific messenger RNA (mRNA) to be identical to pituitary PRL.[231–233]

Bromocriptine and dopamine inhibit, while estradiol and TRH potently stimulate, pituitary PRL release. All these modulators have no effect on decidual PRL secretion. Whereas this finding suggests that differing control mechanisms govern decidual and pituitary PRL release, calcium and progesterone appear capable of stimulating both pituitary and decidual PRL secretion.[234]

Surely progesterone stimulation of decidual PRL secretion acts *via* the decidual progesterone receptor, which is itself estrogen dependent. Such an estrogen–progesterone interdependance is really very similar to the estrogen–progesterone synergy previously demonstrated to stimulate pituitary PRL secretion.[235,236] This stimulatory mechanism thus seems common to both sites of PRL release in women. In addition to progesterone, the placenta seems to secrete a peptide, still incompletely purified, which also stimulates decidual PRL release.[237]

Two inhibitors of decidual PRL have been reported. Arachidonic acid, which is found in high concentration in amniochorion, inhibits decidual PRL secretion, although PGF_2 and indomethacin are without effect.[238] A decidual peptide, which is not PRL, of 38,000–45,000 mw has also been recently reported to inhibit decidual PRL release.[239] The precise physiologic role of these steroidal, nonsteroidal, and protein modulators of endometrial PRL secretion is uncertain. Progesterone, acting on an estrogen-primed endometrium, seems currently most likely to be the major stimulus to decidual PRL release.

Contribution to Maternal and Amniotic Fluid Compartments

Decidual PRL is the major source of PRL in amniotic fluid. Bromocriptine administration to pregnant women lowers maternal and fetal serum PRL values, but amniotic fluid PRL levels remain undisturbed.[75] There is a high correlation between decidual and amniotic fluid PRL concentrations and PRL localization and transport across the amniochorion has been formally demonstrated.[240,241] Amniotic fluid PRL is very slowly metabolized, and this surely contributes to the high concentrations observed in this medium.[229] By contrast, decidual PRL does not appear to enter the maternal circulation and does not contribute to the elevation of plasma PRL in human pregnancy.

Functions and Clinical Importance

A mandatory prerequisite for any biologic action of decidual PRL would be the demonstration of PRL receptors, since interaction with receptors is assumed to be the first step in the mechanism of action of protein hormones. We have identified such receptors in human chorion laeve.[155] The binding affinity (0.47×10^9 liters/mole) and capacity (175 fmole/mg) for lactogenic hormones in this tissue is similar to that described for PRL receptors in liver and mammary gland. Some patients in our study were found to have small amounts of receptor appearing within placental preparations, in keeping with the identical origin of the chorion laeve and chorion frondosum. No PRL binding was identified in decidua, amnion, or umbilical cord in our study. However, Leontic et al.[242] suggested the presence of PRL receptors in human amnion after studying water transport before and after in vitro exposure of amnion to an antibody directed toward a partially purified rabbit PRL receptor. A schema for the origin and entry of PRL into human amniotic fluid is shown in Fig. 3.11.

A major function of PRL in lower vertebrates is to conserve water and electrolyte balance, and PRL decreases the diffusional flow of water when applied to the human amnion.[242] We have shown that a PRL receptor defect is present in the chorion of women with chronic polyhydramnios, be that of an idiopathic or secondary nature.[235,243] The PRL receptor defect may cause the development of chronic polyhydramnios. Furthermore, studies in the pregnant rhesus monkey show that amniotic prolactin

levels markedly affect amniotic fluid volume, and protect the fetal extracellular fluid compartment vis a vis changes in amniotic fluid osmolality.[244,245]

A second function for the chorionic PRL receptor may be to modulate prostaglandin synthesis. It is known that PRL stimulates PGE and $PGF_{2\alpha}$ secretion from rat granulosal cells at low concentrations, while inhibiting prostoglandin formation at high concentrations.[246] A similar mechanism may operate between decidual PRL and chorionic prostaglandins during human pregnancy.

A third function for decidual PRL may be to stimulate fetal pulmonary surfactant formation. Certainly PRL receptors exist in fetal rhesus monkey and human fetal lung[243,247]; PRL stimulates phosphatidylcholine generation in human lung explants when added with cortisol and/or insulin.[247] There is some evidence that amniotic fluid can pass into the tracheobronchial tree and the concentration of tracheobronchial PRL correlates both with amniotic fluid PRL and lung surfactant values. This potential role for PRL from amniotic fluid and decidua, as well as from the fetal pituitary, awaits physiologic investigation in primates, since in lower species the direct effect of PRL on surfactant generation has been contradictory.[247]

SUMMARY

The obstetric value of placental steroidal and protein products has been largely empirical because the physiology of these substances is still not well understood. The human placenta appears to secrete products such as estriol, human placental lactogen, chorionic gonadotropin, and SP_1 without known feedback-control mechanisms.

Pregnancies with very low or absent circulating estriol levels due to placental sulfatase deficiency or genetic absence of human placental lactogen clinically develop normally, indicating that either little endocrine "signal" is necessary for the biologic effects of these substances or that they may have no unique action in human gestation.

The amniochorion, or fetal membranes, produce progesterone, cortisol, placental lactogen, prostaglandins, and bind prolactin. These tissues appear to be major endocrine organs providing a broad and dynamic interface between maternal endometrium and fetal tissues.

Paracrine or cybernetic endocrine communications may also exist between cytotrophoblast and

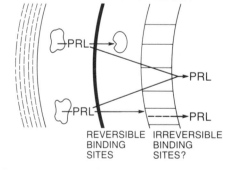

FIGURE 3-11. Paracrine interactions between PRL secretion by decidualized endometrium, PRL binding by fetal chorion laeve and the entry of PRL into amniotic fluid. (From Healy and Hodgen.[251])

syncytiotrophoblast by release of several neuro-transmitter size peptides by the former to regulate protein secretion by the latter tissue.

The role of prostacyclin, various pregnancy-associated plasma proteins and prolactin in such diverse obstetric complications as preeclampsia, placental abruption and polyhydramnios is provocative but awaits further clinical research. Estriol and human placental lactogen measurements are of limited but proven benefit in obstetric management when combined with biophysical estimates of fetal health.

QUESTIONS

1. Progesterone

    a. secretion from the human corpus luteum declines to that seen in the normal menstrual cycle once placental production becomes established.

    b. is synthesized by the placenta from cholesterol.

    c. enhances myometrial contractility.

    d. all of the above.

2. Estriol

    a. is synthesized by the placenta from precursors, which depend primarily on fetal adrenal conversion of 17-hydroxyprogesterone sulfate to dehydroepiandrosterone sulfate and fetal 16α-hydroxylation of the latter.

    b. (maternal serum estriol) and its conjugates may serve as a measure of fetal health in late pregnancy.

    c. is the most potent estrogen produced in late pregnancy.

    d. a and b.

3. Decidual prolactin production may

    a. contribute the majority of amniotic fluid prolactin.

    b. be suppressed by bromocryptine.

    c. maintain fetal serum prolactin levels.

    d. contribute most maternal serum prolactin.

4. Placental lactogen (chorionic somatomammotropin)

    a. is essential for successful continuation of human pregnancy to term.

    b. contributes to the insulin resistance in late pregnancy.

    c. is useful, when measured in the maternal serum, as a day-to-day measure of fetal health.

    d. None of the above.

REFERENCES

1. Chard T, Klopper A: *Placental Function Tests.* New York, Springer-Verlag, 1982
2. Grudzindkas JG, Gordon YB, Wadsworth J, et al: Is placental function testing worthwhile? An update on placental lactogen. *Aust NZ J Obstet Gynaecol* 21:103–1055, 1981
3. Hubert C, Descombey D, Mondon F, et al: Plasma human chorionic somatomammotropin deficiency in a normal pregnancy is the consequence of low concentration of messenger RNA coding for human chorionic somatomammotropin. *Am J Obstet Gynecol* 147:676–678, 1983
4. Taylor NF, Shackleton CHL: Gas chromatographic steroid analysis for diagnosis of placental sulfatase deficiency: A study of nine patients. J Clin Endocrinol Metab 49:78–86, 1979
5. Van Wagenen G, Newton WH: Pregnancy in the monkey after removal of the fetus. *Surg Gynecol Obstet* 77:539–552, 1943
6. Healy DL, Hodgen GD: The endocrinology of human endometrium. *Obstet Gynecol Surv* 38:509–530, 1983
7. Siler-Khodr TM, Khodr, GS: Extrahypothalamic luteinizing hormone-releasing factor (LRF): Release of immunoreactive LRF in vitro. *Fertil Steril* 32:294–296, 1979
8. Corner GW, Allen WM: Physiology of the corpus luteum. II. Production of a special uterine reaction (progestational proliferation) by extracts of the corpus luteum. *Am J Physiol* 88:326–339, 1929
9. Venning EM, Browne JSL: Urinary excretion of sodium pregnanediol glucuronidate in the menstrual cycle (an excretion product of progesterone). *Am J Physiol* 119:417, 1937
10. Bloch K: The biological conversion of cholesterol to pregnanediol. *J Biol Chem* 157:661–666, 1945
11. Healy DL, Chrousos GP, Schulte HM, et al: Pituitary and adrenal responses to the anti-progesterone and antiglucocorticoid steroid RU 486 in primates. *J Clin Endocrinol Metab* 57:863–865, 1983
12. Sybulski S, Venning EH: The possibility of corticosteroid production by human and rat placental tissue under in vitro conditions. *Can J Biochem Physiol* 39:203–214, 1961
13. Bengtsson LPH, Ejarque PM: Production rate of progesterone in the last month of human pregnancy. *Acta Obstet Gynecol Scand* 43:49–57, 1964
14. Pearlman WH: [16-^{3}H] Progesterone metabolism in advanced pregnancy and in oophorectomized-hysterectomized women. *Biochem J* 67:1–5, 1957
15. Yen SSC, Tsai CC, Naftolin F, et al: Pulsatile patterns of gonadotropin release in subjects with and without ovarian function. *J Clin Endocrinol Metab* 34:671–675, 1972
16. Tureck RW, Strauss JF: Progesterone synthesis by luteinised human granulosa cells in culture: The role of de Novo sterol synthesis and lipoprotein-carried sterol. *J Clin Endocrinol Metab* 54:367–369, 1982
17. Healy DL, Schenken RS, Lynch A, et al: Pulsatile progesterone secretion: Its relevance to clinical evaluation of corpus luteum function. *Fertil Steril* 41:114–119, 1984

18. Macome JC, Bischoff, K, Uma Bai R, et al: Factors influencing placental steroidogenesis in vitro. *Steroids* 20:469–485, 1972

19. Runnebaum B, Holzmann K, Bierwirith Y, et al: Effect of HCG on plasma progesterone during the lueal phase of the menstrual cycle and during pregnancy. *Acta Endocrinol* 69:739–746, 1972

20. Wilson EA, Jawad MJ: Luteinising hormone-releasing hormone suppression of human placental progesterone production. *Fertil Steril* 33:91–93, 1980

21. Tulchinsky D, Okada DM: Hormones in human pregnancy. IV. Plasma progesterone. *Am J Obstet Gynecol* 121:293–299, 1975

22. Gibb W, Lavoie JC, Roux J: In vitro conversion of pregnenolone to progesterone by term human fetal membranes. *Am J Obstet Gynecol* 136:631–634, 1980

23. Mitchell B, Cruikshank B, McLean D, et al: Local modulation of progesterone production in human fetal membranes. *J Clin Endocrinol Metab* 55:1237–1239, 1982

24. Siiteri PK, Seron-Ferre M: Fetoplacental unit and parturition in primates, in Novy MJ, Resko JA (eds): *Fetal Endocrinology*. New York, Academic, 1982, pp 1–34

25. Challis J, Patrick J, Richardson B, et al: Loss of diurnal rhythm in plasma estrone, estradiol and estriol in women treated with synthetic glucocorticoids at 34 to 35 weeks gestation. *Am J Obstet Gynecol* 139:338–343, 1981

26. Fraser RC, Delisle FE, Siiteri PK: Progesterone synthesis by superfused human placental minces and inhibition by cortisol. Society for Gynecological Investigation, 27th Annual Meeting, March 19–22, Denver, Colorado, 1980, Abst. 28

27. Yoshimi T, Strott CA, Marshall JR, et al: Corpus luteum function in early pregnancy. *J Clin Endocrinol* 29:225–231, 1969

28. Wiest WG: Estimation progesterone in biological tissues and fluids from pregnant women by double isotope derivative assay. *Steroids* 10:279–290, 1967

29. Coyle MG, Greig M, Walker J: Blood-progesterone and urinary pregnanediol and oestrogens in fetal death from severe pre-eclampsia. *Lancet* 2:275–277, 1962

30. Tullner WW, Hodgen GD: Effects of fetectomy on plasma estrogens and progesterone in monkeys (Macaca mulatta). *Steroids* 24:887–897, 1974

31. Diczfalusy E: Endocrine functions of the human feto-placental units. *Fed Proc* 23:791–804, 1964

32. Solomon S, Fuchs F: Progesterone and related neutral steroids, in Fuchs F, Klopper A (eds): *Endocrinology of Pregnancy*. New York, Harper & Row, 1971, pp 66–91

33. Huhtaniemi I: Studies on steroidogenesis and its regulation in human fetal adrenal and testis. *J Steroid Biochem* 8:491–497, 1977

34. Acevedo HF, Axelrod IR, Shikawa E, et al: Studies in fetal metabolism. II. Metabolism of progesterone-4^{14}C and pregnenolone-7^{3}H in human fetal testes. *J Clin Endocrinol Metab* 23:885–892, 1963

35. Bloch E: Metabolism of 4-^{14}C progesterone by human fetal testes and ovaries. *Endocrinology* 74:833–845, 1964

36. Jaffe R, Pion R, Eriksson G, et al: Studies on the aromatisation of neutral steroids in pregnant women. IV. Lack of oestrogen formation from progesterone. *Acta Endocrinol* 48:413–422, 1965

37. Grody WW, Schrader WT, O'Malley BW: Activation, transformation, and subunit structure of steroid hormone receptors. *Endocr Rev* 3:141–163, 1982

38. Raynaud JP: A tag for the progestin receptor, in McGuire WG, Raynaud JP, Baulieu EE (eds): *Progesterone Receptors in Normal and Neoplastic Tissue*. New York: Raven, 1977, pp 9–43

39. Walters MR, Clark JH: Relationship between the quantity of progesterone receptor and the antagonism of estrogen-induced uterotropic response. *Endocrinology* 105:382–386, 1979

40. Tseng L, Gurpide E: Effects of progestins on estradiol receptor levels in human endometrium. *J Clin Endocrinol Metab* 41:402–404, 1975

41. Logeat F, Vu Hai MT, Sartor P, et al: Uterine progesterone receptors during pregnancy, in Kimball KA (ed): *The Endometrium*. New York, SP Medical and Scientific Books, 1980, pp 127–145

42. Kreitmann-Gimbal B, Bayard F, Hodgen GD: Changing ratios of nuclear estrone to estradiol binding in endometrium at implantation: Regulation by chorionic gonadotropin and progesterone during rescue of the primate corpus luteum. *J Clin Endocrinol Metab* 52:133–137, 1981

43. Joshi SG: Progestin-regulated proteins of the human endometrium. *Semin Reprod Endocrinol* 1:211–236, 1983

44. Thorburn GD, Challis JRG: Endocrine control of parturition. *Physiol Rev* 59:863–918, 1979

45. Csapo AL: The "seesaw" theory of parturition. *CIBA Found Symp* 47:159–170, 1977

46. Csapo AL, Knobil E, Van Der Molen HJ, et al: Peripheral plasma progesterone levels during human pregnancy and labor. *Am J Obstet Gynecol* 110:630–632, 1971

47. Turnbull AC, Patten PT, Flint APF, et al: Significant fall in progesterone and rise in oestradiol levels in human peripheral plasma before the onset of labor. *Lancet* 1:101–104, 1974

48. Tansey TR, Padykula HA: Cellular responses to experimental inhibition of collagen degradation in the post partum rat uterus. *Anat Rec* 191:287–309, 1979

49. Clemens LE, Siiteri PK, Stites DP: Mechanisms of immunosuppression of progesterone on maternal lymphocyte activation during pregnancy. *J Immunol* 122:1978–1985, 1979

50. Shearman RP, Garrett WJ: Double-blind study of effect of 17-hydroxy progesterone caproate on abortion rate. *Br Med J* 1:292–295, 1963

51. Klopper A, MacNaughton MD: Hormones in recurrent abortion. *J Obstet Gynaecol Br Commonw* 72:1022–1028, 1965

52. Trounson AO, Leeton JF, Wood C, et al: Pregnancies in the human by fertilisation in vitro and embryo transfer in the controlled ovulatory cycle. *Science* 212:681–682, 1981

53. Johnson JWG, Austin KL, Jones GS, et al: Efficacy of 17α-hydroxyprogesterone caproate in the prevention of premature labor. *N Engl J Med* 293:675–680, 1975

54. Heinonen OP, Slone D, Shapiro S: Progestagens and pregnancy, in O.P. Heinonen, et al. (eds): *Birth Defects and Drugs in Pregnancy*. Littleton, MA, Publishing Sciences Group, 1977, pp 126–158

55. MacCorquodale DW, Thayer SA, Doisy EA: The isolation of the principal estrogenic substance of liquor folliculi. *J Biol Chem* 115:435–448, 1936

56. Marrian GF: The chemistry of oestrin. IV. The chemical nature of crystalline preparations. *Biochem J* 24:1021–1030, 1930

57. Kober S: Eine kolormetrische Bestimmung des Brunshormons (Menformon). *Biochem Zulschr* 239:209–212, 1931

58. Brown JB: A chemical method for the determination of oestriol, oestrone and oestradiol in human urine. *Biochem J* 60:185–193, 1955

59. Brown JB: Urinary excretion of oestrogens during the menstrual cycle. *Lancet* 1:320–323, 1955

60. Baird DT, Horton R, Longcope C: Steroid dynamics under steady state conditions. *Recent Prog Horm Res* 25:611–648, 1969

61. Zondek B, Goldberg S: Placental function and foetal death. (1) Urinary gonadotrophin tetration test in early pregnancy. (2) Urinary estradiol excretion test in advanced pregnancy. *J Obstet Gynaecol Br Commonw* 64:1–9, 1957

62. Frandsen VA, Stakemann G: The site of production of oestrogenic hormones in human pregnancy. *Acta Endocrinol* 38:383–391, 1961

63. Easterling WE, Simmer H, Dignam WJ, et al: Neutral C$_{19}$-steroids and steroid sulfates in human pregnancy. *Steroids* 8:157–178, 1966

64. Ryan KJ: Hormones of the placenta *Am J Obstet Gynecol* 84:1695–1713, 1962

65. Crystle CD, Dubin NH, Grannis GF, et al: Investigation of estrogen precursor availability in the regulation of estrogen synthesis in normal human pregnancy. *Obstet Gynecol* 42:718–724, 1973

66. Siiteri PK, MacDonald PC: Placental estrogen biosynthesis during human pregnancy. *J Clin Endocrinol Metab* 26:751–761, 1966

67. Tilders FJH, Parker C, Barnea A, et al: The major immunoreactive α-Melanocyte-stimulating hormone (α-MSH)-like substance found in human fetal pituitary tissue is not MSH but may be Desacetyl α-MSH (Adrenocorticotropin 1–13 NH$_2$). *J Clin Endocrinol Metab* 52:319–324, 1981

68. Rudman D, Hollins BM, Lewis NC: Effects of melanotropic peptides on fetal adrenal gland. *J Clin Invest* 65:822–828, 1980

69. Jaffe RB, Seron-Ferre M, Crickard K, et al: Regulation, and function of the primate fetal adrenal gland and gonad. *Recent Prog Horm Res* 37:41–103, 1981

70. Branchaud CT, Goodyer CG, Hall C, et al: Steroidogenic activity of hACTH and related peptides on the human neocortex and fetal adrenal cortex in organ culture. *Steroids* 31:557–572, 1978

71. Brown JB, Beischer NA, Smith MA: Excretion of urinary oestrogens in pregnant patients with cortisone and its analogues. *J Obstet Gynaecol Br Commonw* 75:819–828, 1968

72. Fujada K, Faiman C, Reyes FI, et al: The control of steroidogenesis by human fetal adrenal cells in tissue culture. I. Response to adrenocorticotropin. *J Clin Endocrinol Metab* 53:34–48, 1981

73. Clements JA, Reyes FI, Winter JSD, et al: Studies on human sexual development. III. Fetal pituitary and serum and amniotic fluid concentration of LH, HCG, and FSH. *J Clin Endocrinol Metab* 42:9–16, 1976

74. Healy DL: Human prolactin physiology. Doctoral Thesis, Monash University, 1978

75. Bigazzi M, Ronga R, Lancranjan I, et al: A pregnancy in an acromegalic woman during bromocriptine treatment: Effects on growth hormone and prolactin in the maternal, fetal and amniotic compartments. *J Clin Endocrinol Metab* 48:9–12, 1979

76. Grumbach MM, Richards GE, Conte FA, et al: Adrenal androgens, in James VHT, Serio M, Gusisti G, Martini L

(eds): *The Endocrine Function of the Human Adrenal Cortex*. New York, Academic, 1978, pp 64–97

77. Parker LN, Lifrak ET, Odell WD: A 60,000 molecular weight human pituitary glycopeptide stimulates adrenal androgen secretion. *Endocrinology* 113:2092–2096, 1983

78. Buster JE, Abraham GE: The applications of steroid hormone radioimmunoassay to clinical obstetrics. *Obstet Gynecol* 46:489–499, 1975

79. Shutt DA, Smith ID, Shearman RP: Oestrone, oestradiol-17 and oestriol levels in human foetal plasma during gestation and at term. *J Endocrinol* 60:30–33, 1974

80. Klopper A, Wilson G, Cooke I: Studies on the variability of urinary oestriol and pregnanediol output during pregnancy. *J Endocrinol* 43:295–300, 1969

81. Laatikainen T, Pelkonen J, Apter D, et al: Fetal and maternal serum levels of steroid sulphates, unconjugated steroids, and prolactin at term pregnancy and in early spontaneous labor. *J Clin Endocrinol Metab* 50:489–494, 1980

82. Tulchinsky D, Osathanondh R, Belisle S, et al: Plasma estrone, estradiol, estriol and their precursors in pregnancies with anencephalic fetuses. *J Clin Endocrinol Metab* 45:1100–1103, 1977

83. Belisle S, Osathanondh R, Tulchinsky D: The effect of constant infusion of unlabeled dehydroepiandrosterone sulfate on maternal plasma androgens and estrogens. *J Clin Endocrinol Metab* 45:544–550, 1977

84. Kauppila A, Ylikorkala O: Stable prolactin level after enhanced estradiol production following dehydroepiandrosterone sulphate. *Am J Obstet Gynecol* 138:271–272, 1980

85. Madden JD, Gant NF, MacDonald PC: Study of the kinetics of conversion of maternal plasma dehydroepiandrosterone sulfate to 16-hydroxy dehydroepiandrosterone sulfate estradiol, and estriol. *Am J Obstet Gynecol* 132:392–395, 1978

86. Korda AR, Challis JJ, Anderson ABM, et al: Assessment of placental function in normal and pathological pregnancies by estimation of plasma oestradiol levels after injection of dehydroepiandrosteorone sulphate. *Br J Obstet Gynaecol* 82:656–661, 1975

87. Mathur RS, Landgrebe S, Williamson HO: Progesterone, 17α-hydroxyprogesterone, estradiol, and estriol in late pregnancy and labor. *Am J Obstet Gynecol* 136:25–27, 1980

88. Cousins LM, Hobel CJ, Chang RJ, et al: Serum progesterone and estradiol-17 levels in premature and term labor. *Am J Obstet Gynecol* 127:612–615, 1977

89. Gurpide E, Schwers J, Welch MT, et al: Fetal and maternal metabolism of estradiol during pregnancy. *J Clin Endocrinol Metab* 26:1355–1365, 1966

90. Tulchinsky D: Placental secretion of unconjugated estrone, estradiol and estriol into the maternal and the fetal circulation. *J Clin Endocrinol Metab* 36:1079–1087, 1973

91. Levitz M, Katz J: Enterohepatic metabolism of estriol-3-sulphate 16-glucosiduronate in women. *J Clin Endocrinol Metab* 28:862–868, 1968

92. Adlercruetz H: Hepatic metabolism of estrogens in health and disease. *N Engl J Med* 290:1081–1083, 1974

93. Puca GA, Medici N, Molinari AM, et al: Estrogen receptor of calf uterus: An easy and fast purification procedure. *J Steroid Biochem* 12:105–113, 1980

94. Bayard F, Damilano S, Robel P, et al: Cytoplasmic and nuclear estradiol and progesterone receptors in human endometrium. *J Clin Endocrinol Metab* 46:635–648, 1978

95. Hsueh AJW, Peck EJ, Clark JH: Progesterone antagonism

of the oestrogen receptor and estrogen-induced uterine growth. *Nature (Lond)* 254:337–339, 1975

96. Giannopoulos G, Goldberg P, Shea TB, et al: Unoccupied and occupied estrogen receptors in myometrial cytosol and nuclei from non-pregnant and pregnant women. *J Clin Endocrinol Metab* 51:702–705, 1980

97. Clark JH, Paszko Z, Peck EJ: Nuclear binding and retention of the receptor–estrogen complex: Relation to the agonistic and antagonistic properties of estriol. *Endocrinology* 100:91–96, 1977

98. Martucci C, Fishman J: Direction of estradiol metabolism as a control of its hormonal action—luteotrophic activity of estradiol metabolites. *Endocrinology* 101:1709–1715, 1977

99. Lantta M, Karkkainen J, Lehtovirta P: Progesterone and estradiol receptors in the cytosol of the human uterine artery. *Am J Obstet Gynecol* 147:627–633, 1983

100. Resnick R, Killam AP, Battaglia FC, et al: The stimulation of uterine blood flow by various estrogens. *Endocrinology* 94:1192–1196, 1974

101. Duenhoelter JH, Whalley PJ, MacDonald PC: An analysis of the utility of plasma immunoreactive estrogen measurements in determining delivery time of gravidas with a fetus considered at high risk. *Am J Obstet Gynecol* 125:889–898, 1976

102. Beischer NA: Low oestriol excretion: Incidence, significance and treatment in an obstetric population. *Med J Aust* 2:379–380, 1975

103. France JT, Liggins GC: Placental sulfatase deficiency. *J Clin Endocrinol Metab* 29:138–141, 1969

104. Oakey RE: Placental sulphatase deficiency: Antepartum differential diagnosis from foetal adrenal hyperplasia. *Clin Endocrinol (Oxf)* 9:81–88, 1978

105. France JT, Seddon RJ, Liggins GC: A study of a pregnancy with low estrogen production due to placental sulfatase deficiency. *J Clin Endocrinol Metab* 36:1–9, 1973

106. Marton I, Oakey RE: 3β-hydroxysteroid dehydrogenase-isomerase activity in placentae from pregnancies complicated by steroid sulphatase deficiency. *J Steroid Biochem* 13:475–479, 1980

107. Reti LL, Kelsey GP, Stewart CR: Vaginal delivery in placentae sulphatase deficiency. Two case reports with some unusual features. *Br J Obstet Gynaecol* 89:1054–1055, 1982

108. Pupkin MJ, Nagey DA, Schomberg DW, et al: The dehydroepiandrosterone loading test. III. A possible placental function test. *Am J Obstet Gynecol* 134:281–288, 1979

109. Tulchinsky D, Osathamondh R, Finn A: Dehydroepiandrosterone loading in diagnosis of complicated pregnancy. *N Engl J Med* 294:517–521, 1976

110. Tulchinsky D, Frigoletto FD, Ryan KJ, Plasma estetrol as an index of fetal well-being. *J Clin Endocrinol Metab* 40:560–567, 1975

111. Jouppila P, Huhtaniemi I, Tapanainen J: Early pregnancy failure: Study by ultrasonic and clinical methods. *Obstet Gynecol* 55:42–47, 1979

112. Noller KL, Fish CR: Diethylstilboestrol usage: Its interesting past, important present and questionable future. *Med Clin North Am* 58:5793–5810, 1974

113. Herbst AL, Ulfelder H, Poskener DC: Adenocarcinoma of the vagina. *N Engl J Med* 284:878–880, 1971

114. Kaufman RH, Binder GL, Gray PM, et al: Upper genital tract changes associated with exposure in utero to diethylstilbestrol. *Am J Obstet Gynecol* 128:51–59, 1977

115. Beischer NA, Brown JB: Current status of estrogen assays in obstetrics and gynecology. Part 2: estrogen assays in late pregnancy. *Obstet Gynecol Surv* 27:303–343, 1972

116. MacLeod SC, Mitton DM, Avery CR: Relationship between elevated blood pressure and urinary estriols during pregnancy. *Am J Obstet Gynecol* 109:375–382, 1971

117. Gorwill RH, Sarda IR: Hormonal studies in pregnancy. II. Unconjugated estriol in maternal peripheral vein, cord vein and cord artery serum at delivery in pregnancies complicated by intrauterine growth retardation. *Am J Obstet Gynecol* 127:17–25, 1977

118. Distler W, Gabbe SG, Freeman RK, et al: Estriol in pregnancy. V. Unconjugated and total plasma estriol in the management of pregnant diabetic patients. *Am J Obstet Gynecol* 130:424–431, 1978

119. Whittle MJ, Anderson D, Lowensohn RI, et al: Estriol in pregnancy. VI. Experience with unconjugated plasma estriol assays and antepartum fetal heart rate testing in diabetic pregnancies. *Am J Obstet Gynecol* 135:764–772, 1979

120. Klopper A, Stephenson R: The excretion of pregnanediol and of oestriol in pregnancy complicated by Rh immunisation. *J Obstet Gynaecol Br Commonw* 73:982–985, 1966

121. MacDonald DJ, Scott JM, Gemmell RS, et al: A prospective study of three biochemical fetoplacental tests: Serum human placental lactogen, pregnancy-specific-glycoprotein, and urinary estrogens and their relationship to placental insufficiency. *Am J Obstet Gynecol* 147:430–436, 1983

122. Beischer NA, Drew JH, Kenny JM: The effect of rest and intravenous infusion of hypertonic dextrose on subnormal estriol excretion in pregnancy. *Clin Perinatol* 1:253–261, 1974

123. Chang A, Abell D, Beischer NA, et al: Trial of intravenous therapy in women with low urinary estriol excretion. *Am J Obstet Gynecol* 127:793–797, 1977

124. Warrell DW, Taylor R: Outcome for the foetus of mothers receiving prednisolone during pregnancy. *Lancet* 1:117–118, 1968

125. Murphy BEP, Clark SJ, Donald IR, et al: Conversion of maternal cortisol to cortisone during placental transfer to the human fetus. *Am J Obstet Gynecol* 118:538–541, 1974

126. Novy MJ, Walsh SW: Dexamethasone and estradiol treatment in pregnant rhesus macaques: Effects on gestational length, maternal plasma hormones, and fetal growth. *Am J Obstet Gynecol* 145:920–931, 1983

127. Funkhouser JD, Peevy KJ, Mockridge PB, et al: Distribution of dexamethasone between mother and fetus after maternal administration. *Pediatr Res* 12:1053–1056, 1978

128. Evans MI, Chorousos GP, Mann DL, et al: Abnormal genital masculinization in congenital adrenal hyperplasia (CAH): Attempted prevention by adrenocortical suppression in utero. Society for Gynaecological Investigation, Washington, DC, 1983, 497

129. Simmer HH, Frankland MV, Greipel M: Unbound unconjugated cortisol in umbilical cord and corresponding maternal plasma. Materno-fetal gradient: Comparison of methods. *Gynecol Invest* 5:199–221, 1974

130. Murphy BEP: Chorionic membrane as an extra-adrenal source of foetal cortisol in human amniotic fluid. *Nature (Lond)* 266:179–180, 1977

131. Josimovich JB, MacLaren J: Presence in the human placenta and term serum of a highly lactogenic substance immunologically related to pituitary growth hormone. *Endocrinology* 71:209–220, 1962

132. Josimovich JB: Hormonal physiology of pregnancy, in Gold JJ, Josimovich JB (eds): *Gynecologic Endo-*

crinology, 3rd ed. Hagerstown, MD, Harper & Row, 1980, pp 147–174

133. Li CH: On the characterization of human chorionic somatomammotrophin. *Ann Sclavo* 12:651–666, 1970

134. Li CH, Grumbach MM, Kaplan SL, et al: Human chorionic somatomammotropin (HCS): Proposed terminology for designation of a placental hormone. *Experientia* 24:1188–1196, 1968

135. Li CH, Dixon JS, Chung D: Primary structure of human chorionic somatomammotropin (HCS) molecule. *Science* 173:56–58, 1971

136. Shome B, Parlow AF: Human pituitary prolactin (hPRL). The entire linear amino acid sequence. *J Clin Endocrinol Metab* 45:1112–1115, 1977

137. Shine J, Seeburg PH, Martial JA, et al: Construction and analysis of recombinant DNA for HCS. *Nature (Lond)* 270:494–499, 1977

138. Owerbach D, Rutter WJ, Cooke NE, et al: The prolactin gene is located on chromosome 6 in humans. *Science* 212:815–816, 1981

139. Niall HD, Hogan ML, Sawer R, et al: Sequence of pituitary and placental lactogenic and growth hormones: Evolution from a primordial peptide by gene reduplication. *Proc Natl Acad Sci USA* 68:866–873, 1971

140. Grumbach MM, Kaplan SL: Placental origin and purification of chorionic growth hormone-prolactin and its immunoassay in pregnancy. *Trans NY Acad Sci* 27:167–188, 1964

141. Sciarra JJ, Kpalen SL, Grumbach MM: Localization of anti-human growth hormone serum within the human placenta: Evidence for a human chorionic "growth hormone—prolactin." *Nature (Lond)* 199:1005–1007, 1963

142. Beck P, Parker ML, Daughaday WH: Radioimmunologic measurement of human placental lactogen in plasma by a double antibody method during normal and diabetic pregnancies. *J Clin Endocrinol Metab* 25:1457–1467, 1965

143. Chard T: Human placental lactogen, in Martini L, James VHT (eds): *Endocrinology,* vol 4. London, Academic, 1983, pp 167–192

144. Spellacy WN, Tech ES, Buhi WC, et al: Value of human chorionic somatomammotropin in managing high-risk pregnancies. *Am J Obstet Gynecol* 109:588–592, 1971

145. Hochberg Z, Perlman R, Brandes JM, et al: Insulin regulates placental lactogen and estradiol secretion by cultured human term trophoblast. *J Clin Endocrinol Metab* 57:1311–1313, 1983

146. Macaron C, Famuyiwa O, Singh SP: In vitro effect of Dopamine and Pimozide on human chorionic somatomammotropin (HCS) secretion. *J Clin Endocrinol Metab* 47:168–170, 1978

147. Tyson JE, Austin KH, Favenholt JW: Prolonged nutritional deprivation in pregnancy: Change in human chorionic somatomammotropin and growth hormone secretion. *Am J Obstet Gynecol* 109:1080–1086, 1971

148. Josimovich JB: The human placental lactogen, in Astwood EB, Cassidy CE (eds): *Clinical Endocrinology.* New York, Grune & Stratton, 1968, p. 658

149. Novy MJ, Aubert ML, Kaplan SL, et al: Regulation of placental growth and chorionic somatomammotropin in the rhesus monkey. *Am J Obstet Gynecol* 140:552–562, 1981

150. Niven PAR, Ward RTH, Chard T: Human placental lactogen levels in amniotic fluid in rhesus isoimmunisation. *J Obstet Gynaecol Br Commonw* 81:988–990, 1974

151. Chez RA, Josimovich JB, Schultz S: The transfer of human placental lactogen across isolated amnion-chorion. *Gynecol Invest* 1:312–318, 1970

152. Beck P, Daughaday WH: Human placental lactogen: Studies of its acute metabolic effects and disposition in normal man. *J Clin Invest* 46:103–110, 1967

153. Pavlou C, Chard T, Letchworth AT: Circulating levels of human chorionic somatomammotrophin in late pregnancy: Disappearance from the circulation after delivery, during labour, and circadian variation. *J Obstet Gynaecol Br Commonw* 79:629–637, 1972

154. Singer W, Desjardins P, Friesen HG: Human placental lactogen. An index of placental function. *Obstet Gynaecol* 36:222–227, 1970

155. Herington AC, Graham J, Healy DL: The presence of lactogen receptors in human chorion laeve. *J Clin Endocrinol Metab* 51:1466–1468, 1980

156. Sideri M, de Virgilis G, Guidobono F, et al: Immunologically undetectable human placental lactogen in a normal pregnancy. Case report. *Br J Obstet Gynaecol* 90:771–773, 1983

157. Borody JB, Carlton MA: Isolated defect in human placental lactogen synthesis in a normal pregnancy. Case report. *Br J Obstet Gynaecol* 88:447–449, 1981

158. Nielsen PV, Pedersen H, Kampmann EM: Absence of human placental lactogen in an otherwise uneventful pregnancy. *Am J Obstet Gynecol* 135:322–326, 1979

159. Gordon YB, Chard T: The specific proteins of the human placenta: Some new hypotheses, in Klopper A, Chard T (eds): *Placental Proteins.* Berlin, Springer-Verlag, 1979, pp 1–21

160. Grumbach MM, Kaplan SL, Sciarra JJ, et al: Chorionic growth hormone prolactin: Secretion, disposition, biologic activity in man and postulated function in the "growth hormone" of the second half of pregnancy. *Ann NY Acad Sci* 148:501–531, 1968

161. Brinsmead MW, Bancroft BJ, Thorburn GD, et al: Fetal and maternal ovine placental lactogen during hyperglycaemia, hypoglycaemia and fasting. *J Endocrinol* 90:337–343, 1981

162. Pavlou C, Chard T, London J, et al: Circulating levels of HPL in late pregnancy effect of glucose loading, smoking and exercise. *Eur J Obstet Gynecol Reprod Biol* 3:45–50, 1973

163. Josimovich JB, Stock RJ, Tobon H: Effects of primate placental lactogen upon lactation, in Josimovich JB, Reynolds M, Cobo E (eds): *Lactogenic Hormones, Fetal Nutrition and Lactation.* New York, Wiley, 1974, pp 335–350

164. Beck P: Lactogenic activity of human chorionic somatomammotropin in rhesus monkeys. *Proc Soc Exp Biol Med* 140:183–187, 1972

164a. Healy DL, Burger HG: Review: Human prolactin. Recent advances in physiology and therapy. *Aust NZ J Obstet Gynaecol* 17:61–78, 1977

165. Teoh ES, Spellacy WN, Buhi WC: Human chorionic somatomammotrophin (HCS): A new index of placental function. *J Obstet Gynaecol Br Commonw* 78:673–685, 1971

166. Spellacy WN, Gohen WD, Carlson HL: Human placental lactogen levels as a measure of placental function. *Am J Obstet Gynecol* 97:560–570, 1967

167. Spellacy WN, Buhi WC, Birk SA: The effectiveness of human placental lactogen as an adjunct in decreasing perinatal deaths. *Am J Obstet Gynecol* 121:835–840, 1975

168. Birken S, Fetherstron J, Desmond J, et al: Partial amino acid sequence of the preprotein form of the sub-unit of HCG and identification of the site of subsequent proteolytic cleavage. *Biochem Biophys Res Commun* 85:1247–1253, 1978

169. Kessler MJ, Reddy NS, Shah RH, et al: Structure of N-glycosidic carbohydrate units of HCG. *J Biol Chem* 254:7901–7909, 1979

170. Jones GES, Grey CO, Gey MK: Hormone production by placental cells maintained in continuous culture. *Bull John Hopkins Hosp* 72:26–38, 1943

171. Thiede HA, Choate JW: Chorionic gonadotropin localization in the human placenta by immunofluorescent staining. II. Demonstration of HCG in the trophoblast and amnion epithelium of immature and mature placentae. *Obstet Gynecol* 22:433–443, 1963

172. Birken S, Canfield RE: In S Segal (ed): Chorionic Gonadotropin. New York, Plenum, 1980, pp 65–83

173. Owens O'd M, Ryan KJ, Tulchinsky D: Episodic secretion of human chorionic gonadotropin in early pregnancy. *J Clin Endocrinol Metab* 53:1307–1309, 1981

174. Khodr GS, Siler-Khodr T: Localisation of luteinizing hormone-releasing factor in the human placenta. *Fertil Steril* 29:523–526, 1978

175. Khodr GS, Siler-Khodr T: The effect of luteinizing hormone-releasing factor on human chorionic gonadotropin secretion. *Fertil Steril* 30:301–304, 1978

176. Siler-Khodr T, Khodr GS: Production and activity of placental releasing hormones, in Novy MJ, Resko JA (eds): *Fetal Endocrinology*, New York, Academic, 1981, pp 183–210

177. Healy DL, Hodgen GD: Does luteinizing hormone-releasing hormone really stimulate HCG secretion? (Submitted for publication, 1984)

178. Wilson EA, Jawad MJ, Dickson LR: Suppression of human chorionic gonadotropin by progestational steroids. *Am J Obstet Gynecol* 138:708–713, 1980

179. Hussa RO, Pattillo RA, Ruckert ACF, et al: Effects of butyrate and debutyryl cyclic AMP on hCG-secreting trophoblastic and non-trophoblastic cells. *J Clin Endocrinol Metab* 46:69–76, 1978

180. Macaron C, Kynel M, Famuyiw O, et al: In vitro effect of dopamine and pimozide on human chorionic gonadotropin secretion. *Am J Obstet Gynecol* 135:499–502, 1979

181. Benveniste R, Speeg KV, Carpenter G, et al: Epidermal growth factor stimulates secretion of human chorionic gonadotropin by cultured human choriocarcinoma cells. *J Clin Endocrinol Metab* 46:169–172, 1978

182. Fusco FD, Rosen SW: Gonadotropin-producing carcinomas of the lung. *N Engl J Med* 275:507–515, 1966

183. McGregor WG, Kuhn RW, Jaffe RB: Biologically active chorionic gonadotropin: Synthesis by the human fetus. *Science* 22:306–308, 1983

184. Jones WR: *Immunological Fertility Regulation*. Melbourne, Blackwell, 1982

185. Shutt DA, Lopata A: The secretion of hormones during the culture of human preimplantation embryos with corona cells. *Fertil Steril* 35:413–416, 1981

186. Landesman R, Coutinho EM, Saxena BB: Detection of human chorionic gonadotropin in blood of regularly bleeding women using copper intrauterine contraceptive devices. *Fertil Steril* 27:1062–1066, 1976

187. Harrison RF, O'Moore RR, McSweeney J: Maternal plasma hCG in early human pregnancy. *Br J Obstet Gynaecol* 87:705–711, 1980

188. Clements JA, Reyes FI, Winter JSD, et al: Studies on human sexual development. III. Fetal pituitary and serum and amniotic fluid concentrations of LH, CG and FSH. *J Clin Endocrinol Metab* 42:9–19, 1976

189. Yen SSC, Llerena O, Little B, et al: Disappearance rates of endogenous luteinizing hormone and chorionic gonadotropin in man. *J Clin Endocrinol Metab* 28:1763–1767, 1968

190. Van Hall EV, Vaitukaitis JL, Ross GT: Effects of progressive desialyation on the rate of disappearance of immunoreactive (hCG) from plasma in rats. *Endocrinology* 89:11–15, 1971

191. Hodgen GD, Ross GT, Turner CK, et al: Pregnancy diagnosis by a haemagglutination inhibition test for urinary macaque chorionic gonadotropin (mCG). *J Clin Endocrinol Metab* 38:927–928, 1974

192. Bolton RA, Coulam CB, Ryan RJ: Specific binding of human chorionic gonadotropin to human corpora lutea in the menstrual cycle. *Obstet Gynecol* 56:336–338, 1980

193. Rajaniemi HJ, Ronnberg L, Kauppila A, et al: Luteinizing hormone receptors in human ovarian follicles and corpora lutea during menstrual cycle and pregnancy. *J Clin Endocrinol Metab* 52:307–313, 1981

194. Catt KJ, Harwood JP, Clayton RN, et al: Regulation of peptide hormone receptors and gonadal steroidogenesis. *Recent Prog Horm Res* 36:557–622, 1980

195. Huhtaniemi IT, Korenbrot CC, Jaffe RB: hCG binding and stimulation of testosterone biosynthesis in the human fetal testis. *J Clin Endocrinol Metab* 44:963–967, 1977

196. Kay MD, Jones WR: Effect of human chorionic gonadotropin on in vitro lymphocyte transformation. *Am J Obstet Gynecol* 109:1029–1033, 1971

197. Morton H, Rolfe B, Caranagh A: Early pregnancy factor: Biology and clinical significance, in Grudzinskas JE, Feisner B, Seppale M (eds): *Placental Proteins*. Sydney, Academic, 1982, pp 391–406

198. Vaitukaitis JL, Braunstein GD, Ross GT: A radioimmunoassay which specifically measures human chorionic gonadotropin in the presence of human luteinizing hormone. *Am J Obstet Gynecol* 113:751–758, 1972

199. Saxena BB, Hasan SH, Hadur R, et al: Radioreceptor assay of human chorionic gonadotropin: Detection of early pregnancy. *Science* 184:973–975, 1974

200. Lundstrom V, Bremme K, Eneroth P, et al: Serum beta-human chorionic gonadotrophin levels in the early diagnosis of ectopic pregnancy. *Acta Obstet Gynecol Scand* 58:231–233, 1979

201. Seppala M, Tontti K, Ranta T, et al: Use of a rapid hCG beta-subunit radioimmunoassay in acute gynaecological emergencies. *Lancet* 1:165–166, 1980

202. Hurley DM, Brian R, Burger HG: Ovulation induction with subcutaneous pulsatile gonadotropin-releasing hormone: Singleton pregnancies in patients with previous multiple pregnancies after gonadotropin therapy. *Fertil Steril* 40:575–579, 1983

203. Talwar GP, Sharma NC, Dubey SK, et al: Isoimmunization against human chorionic gonadotropin with conjugate of processed β-subunit of the hormone and tetanus toxoid. *Proc Natl Acad Sci USA* 73:218–223, 1976

204. Lin TM, Halbert SP: Placental localization of human pregnancy-associated plasma proteins. *Science* 193:1249–1252, 1976

205. Klopper A, Buchan P, Wilson G: The plasma half-life of

placental hormones. *Br J Obstet Gynaecol* 85:738–747, 1978

206. Grudzinskas JG, Gordon YB, Jeffrey D, et al: Specific sensitive determination of pregnancy-specific β-glycoprotein by radioimmunoassay: A new pregnancy test. *Lancet* 1:333–335, 1977

207. Gordon YB, Grudzinskas JG, Lewis JD, et al: Circulating levels of pregnancy specific β-glycoprotein and human placental lactogen in the third trimester of pregnancy and their relationship to parity, birthweight and placental weight. *Br J Obstet Gynaecol* 84:642–647, 1977

208. Chapman MG, Jones WR: Pregnancy specific-1 glycoprotein (SP-1) in normal and abnormal pregnancy. *Aust NZ J Obstet Gynaecol* 18:172–175, 1978

209. Lin TM, Halbert SP, Kiefer D, et al: Characterization of four human pregnancy-associated plasma proteins. *Am J Obstet Gynecol* 118:223–236, 1974

210. Bischof P: Purification and characterization of pregnancy associated plasma protein-A. *Arch Gynecol* 227:315–326, 1979

211. Duberg S, Bischoff P, Schindler AM: In vitro production of PAPP-A, in Grudzinskas A, Chard T, Seppala M (eds): *International Conference on Placental Proteins*. London, Blackwell, 1981, p 6

212. Smith R, Bischof P, Hughes G, et al: Studies on pregnancy-associated plasma protein A in the third trimester of pregnancy. *Br J Obstet Gynaecol* 86:882–887, 1979

213. Toop K, Klopper A: Effect of anticoagulants on the measurement of pregnancy-associated plasma protein-A (PAPP-A). *Br J Obstet Gynaecol* 50:150–155, 1983

214. Sinosich MJ, Smith DH, Grudzinskas JG, et al: The prediction of pregnancy failure by measurement of pregnancy-associated plasma protein A (PAPP-A) following in vitro fertilisation and embryo transfer. *Fertil Steril* 40:539–541, 1983

215. Bischof P: Pregnancy associated plasma protein-A: An inhibitor of the complement system. *Placenta* 2:29–34, 1981

216. Youngblood WW, Humm J, Lipton MA, et al: Thyrotropin-releasing hormone-like bioactivity in placenta: Evidence for the existence of substances other than pyroglu-His-Pro-NH_2 (TRH) capable of stimulating pituitary thyrotropin release. *Endocrinology* 106:541–546, 1980.

217. Nisula BD, Tahadouros GS, Carayon P: Primary and secondary biologic activities intrinsic to the human chorionic gonadotropin molecule, in Segal SJ (eds): *Chorionic Gonadotropin*. New York, Plenum, 1980, pp 17–35

218. Karim SMM: Action of prostaglandin in the pregnant woman. *Ann NY Acad Sci* 180:483–498, 1971

219. Armstrong JM, Lattimer N, Moncade S, et al: Comparison of the vasodepressor effects of prostacyclin and 6-oxo-prostaglandin F_1 with those of prostaglandin E_2 in rats and rabbits. *Br J Pharmacol* 62:125–130, 1978

220. Miyamori I, Fitzgerald GA, Brown MJ, et al: Prostacyclin stimulates the renin angiotensin system in man. *J Clin Endocrinol Metab* 49:943–944, 1979

221. Omini C, Folco GC, Pasargiklian R, et al: Prostacyclin (PGI_2) in the pregnant human uterus. *Prostaglandins* 17:113–120, 1979

222. Bamford DS, Jogee M, Williams KI: Prostacyclin formation by the pregnant human myometrium. *Br J Obstet Gynaecol* 87:215–218, 1980

223. Siegl AM, Smith JB, Silver MJ, et al: Selective binding

site for [^{3}H]prostacyclin on platelets. *J Clin Invest* 63:215–220, 1979

224. Rakoczi I, Tihanyi K, Falkay G, et al: Prostacyclin production in trophoblast, in Lewis PJ, Moncada S, O'Grady J (eds): *Prostacyclin in Pregnancy*. York, Raven, 1983, pp 15–25

225. Remuzzi G, Misani R, Muratore D, et al: Prostacyclin and human foetal circulation. *Prostaglandins* 18:341–348, 1979

226. Downing I, Shepard GL, Lewis PJ: Reduced prostacyclin production in pre-eclampsia. *Lancet* 2:1374, 1980

227. Lewis PJ: Does prostacyclin deficiency play a role in pre-eclampsia?, in Lewis PJ, Moncade S, O'Grady J (eds): *Prostacyclin in Pregnancy*. New York, Raven, 1983, pp 215–220

228. Tyson JE, Hwang P, Guyda H, et al: Studies of prolactin secretion in human pregnancy. *Am J Obstet Gynecol* 113:14–20, 1972

229. Josimovich JB, Weiss G, Hutchinson DL: Sources and disposition of pituitary prolactin in maternal circulation, amniotic fluid, fetus and placenta in the pregnant rhesus monkey. *Endocrinology* 94:1364–1371, 1974

230. Maslar IA, Riddick DH: Prolactin production by human endometrium during the normal menstrual cycle. *Am J Obstet Gynecol* 135:751–754, 1979

231. Clements J, Whitfield P, Cooke N, et al: Expression of the prolactin gene in human decidua-chorion. *Endocrinology* 112:1133–1134, 1983

232. Golander A, Hurley T, Barrett J, et al: Prolactin synthesis by human chorion-deciduial tissue: A possible source of prolactin in the amniotic fluid. *Science* 202:311–313, 1978

233. Healy DL, Kimpton WG, Muller HK, et al: The synthesis of immunoreactive prolactin by decidua-chorion. *Br J Obstet Gynaecol* 86:307–313, 1979

234. Daly DC, Maslar IA, Riddick DH: Term decidua response to estradiol and progesterone. *Am J Obstet Gynecol* 145:679–683, 1983

235. Healy DL, Herington AC, O'Herlihy C: Chronic idiopathic polyhydramnios: Evidence for a defect in the chorion laeve receptor for lactogenic hormones. *J Clin Endocrinol Metab* 56:520–523, 1983

236. Williams RF, Barker DL, Cowan BD, et al: Hyperprolactinemia in monkeys: Induction by an estrogen–progesterone synergy. *Steroids* 38:321–331, 1981

237. Handwerger S, Barry S, Markett E, et al: Stimulation of the synthesis and release of decidual prolactin by a placental polypeptide. *Endocrinology* 112:1370–1374, 1983

238. Handwerger S, Barry S, Barrett J, et al: Inhibition of the synthesis and secretion of decidual prolactin by arachidonic acid. *Endocrinology* 109:2016–2021, 1981

239. Markoff E, Howell S, Handwerger S: Inhibition of decidual prolactin release by a decidual peptide. *J Clin Endocrinol Metab* 57:1282–1286, 1983

240. Healy DL, Muller HK, Burger HG: Immunofluorescence shows localisation of prolactin to human amnion. *Nature (Lond)* 265:642–643, 1977

241. Riddick DH, Maslar IA: The transport of prolactin by human fetal membranes. *J Clin Endocrinol Metab* 52:220–224, 1981

242. Leontic EA, Schrueter JJ, Andreassen B, et al: Further evidence for the role of prolactin on human fetoplacental osmoregulation. *Am J Obstet Gynecol* 133:435–438, 1979

243. Healy DL: The clinical significance of endometrial PRL. *Aust NZ J Obstet Gynecol* 24:111–115, 1984
244. Josimovich JB, Merisko K, Boccella L, et al: Binding of prolactin by fetal rhesus cell membrane fractions. *Endocrinology* 100:557–563, 1977
245. Josimovich JB, Merisko K, Boccella L: Amniotic prolactin control over amniotic and fetal extracellular fluid water and electrolytes in the rhesus monkey. *Endocrinology* 100:564–570, 1977
246. Knazek RA, Christy RJ, Watson KC, et al: Prolactin modifies follicle-stimulating hormone-induced prostaglandin synthesis by the rat granulsa cell. *Endocrinology* 109:1566–1572, 1981
247. Mendelson CR, Johnston JM, MacDonald PC, et al: Multihormonal regulation of surfactant synthesis by human fetal lung *in vitro*. *J Clin Endocrinol Metab* 53:307–317, 1981
248. Williams L, Warwick L, (eds): *Gray's Anatomy*, 36th ed, Philadelphia, Saunders, 1980, p. 125 (fig. 2.39)
249. Johansson ED, and Johansson LE: Progesterone levels in amniotic fluid and plasma for women, I. Levels during normal pregnancy. *Acta Obstet Gynecol Scand* 40:339–344, 1971
250. Beischer NA, Brown JB, Smith MA, Townsend L: Studies in prolonged pregnancy. II. Clinical research and urinary estriol excretion in prolonged pregnancy. *Amer J Obstet Gynecol* 103:483–488, 1969
251. Healy DL, Hodgen GD: The endocrinology of human endometrium. *Obstet Gynecol Survey* 38:509–530, 1983

ANSWERS

1. a

2. d

3. a

4. b

Hormonal Physiology

4

Hormonal Physiology of the Ovary and Adrenal Cortex

GEORGE S. RICHARDSON

INTRODUCTION

The central mission of the ovary is to provide fertilizable ova, but it also has a complicated secondary agenda, made possible by the fact that it secretes steroidal and possibly nonsteroidal hormones: (1) the long-term project, beginning in intrauterine life and extending through puberty, of developing the genital organs and the secondary sex characteristics; (2) the preparation, during each cycle, of the genital tract for reception of sperm and the transport and implantation of the fertilized ovum; (3) the nurture of the oocyte and the provision of factors necessary for controlling meiotic division; and (4) participation in the refined dialogue with pituitary and hypothalamus that makes possible the specifically human phenomenon of single ovulation.

The mission of the adrenal cortex is to help maintain metabolic needs and water–electrolyte homeostasis in times of stress to the body and, to a lesser extent, to provide such support even in normal, nonstress circumstances.

GEORGE S. RICHARDSON • Department of Gynecology, Harvard Medical School at the Massachusetts General and Vincent Memorial Hospitals, Boston, Massachusetts 02114.

STEROIDOGENESIS IN OVARY AND ADRENAL

The principal hormonal secretions of the ovary are estradiol, produced by the follicular apparatus in amounts of up to 500 μg/day, and progesterone, produced by the corpus luteum in amounts of 25–30 mg/day. As Ryan[1] has emphasized, all steroid hormones are synthesized by pathways that all steroidogenic tissues have in common. These tissues—the adrenal gland, ovary, testis, and placenta—are characterized by more or less complete blocks at certain reactions so that the compound before the block constitutes the major secretory product of the gland. Specifically, the adrenal gland is capable of all the reactions shown in Figure 4-3. Little or no aromatization (reactions 5 and 6) takes place in the adrenal, however, and only a portion of the gland, the zona glomerulosa, carries out reaction 9. The normal ovary does not carry out reactions 5, 7, 8, and 9. In order to produce testosterone, the testis only requires the reactions shown in the upper half of Figure 4-3 and does not require reactions 5, 6, 7, 8, or 9. The placenta is incapable of all the reactions beyond reaction 1, except for reactions 5 and 6. This is another way of saying that it can produce progesterone but requires androgenic precursors in order to produce estrogen. The general importance of the biosynthetic sequence is such that it is well to examine it in some detail.[2]

Steroid Structure

The basic steroid skeleton (cholestane) is shown in Figure 4-1. The carbons are numbered 1–27 and the rings labeled A, B, C, and D. It must be noted that in a diagram such as this the constituent carbon atoms are located at the junctions and ends of straight lines. This convention is also adopted in diagramming the rather complicated steps in the formation of cholesterol from acetate. The 27-carbon structure shown is that of cholestane. The number of carbons in the molecule is conventionally denoted by a subscript: cholestane is a C_{27} compound. The carbon atom in position 27 is denoted C-27. As successive carbons are removed in order, beginning at C-27, the remaining skeleton is referred to by a name that is used as the base of systematic nomenclature: C_{27} is cholane; C_{21}, pregnane; C_{19}, androstane; C_{18}, estrane; and C_{17}, gonane. Side chains or groups that project backward from the plane of the diagram are referred to as being in the α-position and are shown as being attached by dashed lines. Those that project forward are in the β-position and are connected by heavy lines. The rings of the molecule are not planes like the ring of benzene but have the "chair" conformation as shown on the right in Figure 4-1. Figure 4-1 also illustrates the rather larger change in molecular shape that results when the substituent at C-5 is shifted from the α- to the β-position: In the α-position, it is on the side of the molecule opposite C-19, and the ring fusion is referred to as A,B-*trans*. In the β-position it is on the same side as C-19, and the conformation is A,B-*cis*. Aromatization of ring A to form a ring of the benzene-type changes the A ring conformation from that of a chair to a flat structure. The shift of a single hydroxyl (-OH) group from an α- to a β-position can make an almost all-or-none difference in biologic activity: estradiol-17β and testosterone (also 17β) are active, while estradiol-17α and epitestosterone (also 17α) are inactive. A hydroxyl group attached to a benzene ring is neither α nor β, but in the plane of the molecule. It readily loses a proton (H^+) to the medium: Estrogens are polar because they are weak acids. Such hydroxyl groups are referred to as phenolic (phenol equals hydroxybenzene).

Pregnenolone is the parent steroid in hormone biosynthesis. Its systematic name is 3β-hydroxy-pregn-5-en-20-one. The double bond at C-5, C-6 is commonly referred to as Δ^5; compounds with this configuration are biologically inactive relative to the Δ^4 compounds, which have the double bond at C-4, C-5.

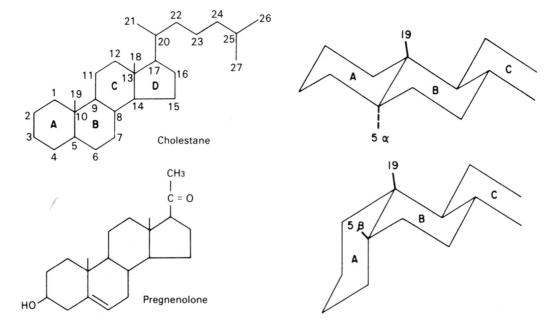

FIGURE 4-1. Structure of steroid hormones.

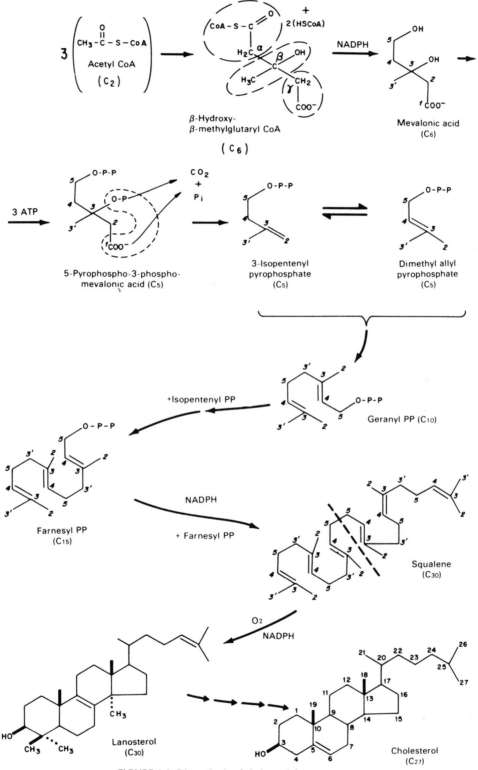

FIGURE 4-2. Biosynthesis of cholesterol from acetate.

From Acetate to Cholesterol

The steps in the biosynthesis of cholesterol are shown in Figure 4-2. The drawings are not stereochemically accurate but are arranged to make it easier to see how the isoprenoid units contribute to the final structure. The numbering scheme of mevalonic acid is carried through into squalene for the same reason. Three molecules of acetic acid, activated by being chemically bonded to coenzyme A (CoA), are condensed to form β-hydroxy-β-methylglutaryl CoA. This compound is reduced in turn by reactions requiring reduced nicotinamide adenine dinucleotide phosphate (NADPH) to mevalonic acid, a 6-carbon compound (C_6). The enzyme that accomplishes this, hydroxymethylglutaryl reductase (HMG CoA reductase), is rate-limiting for the biosynthetic sequence from acetate. The amount of this enzyme decreases in the presence of cholesterol in the form of low-density lipoprotein (LDL)[3]. Mevalonic acid is phosphorylated in three steps by adenosine triphosphate (ATP) and is decarboxylated to yield isopentenyl pyrophosphate, which exists in equilibrium with dimethyl allyl pyrophosphate. The two C_5 compounds now condense to form geranyl pyrophosphate (C_{10}). The attachment of an additional molecule of isopentenyl pyrophosphate forms the compound farnesyl pyrophosphate (C_{15}). Two molecules of this compound now condense in a head-to-tail fashion to form squalene, a compound originally found in shark oil but now known to be present in many mammalian tissues. An attack by molecular oxygen at one end of the molecule in the presence of NADPH sets off a series of interactions that lead to the formation of carbon–carbon bonds and the production of lanosterol (C_{30}). This sterol is the largest molecule in the series. In a sense, everything that follows is the breakdown of what has just been built. Although ATP energy is required in the steps already described, it is no longer needed for the steps that follows.

From Cholesterol to Pregnenolone

Specific uptake of lipoprotein cholesterol in the form of LDL is the principal means by which the adrenal glands, luteinized ovaries, and placenta acquire substrate for steroidogenesis.[3] The steps between cholesterol (C_{27}) and pregnenolone (C_{21}) are illustrated at the top of Figure 4-3. At least three enzymes are involved in splitting off the side chain of cholesterol to yield isocaproic aldehyde and progesterone: 20α-hydroxylase, 22-hydroxylase, and 20,22-desmolase. These enzymes are located in the mitochondria and require NADPH and molecular oxygen. The 20α-hydroxylation of cholesterol is the rate-limiting reaction and is consequently a control point at which luteinizing hormone (LH) acts in the ovary and ACTH in the adrenal. It is not the sole point of LH action, however. LH (and hCG) increase the number of specific binding sites for LDL. LH may also make possible the cleavage of C_{20} compounds to form C_{19} compounds, and there is evidence that LH affects the cleavage of cholesterol esters to form free cholesterol. It must be remembered that most of the work concerning LH action has been done on the corpus luteum, which contains a large amount of stored cholesterol.

From Pregnenolone to the Corticoids, Androgens, and Estrogens

The generally accepted sequence as shown in Figure 4-3 consists of 10 steps performed by a number of enzymes that is greater than 10 because of the existence of isozymes. Some intermediate compounds exist or are hypothesized; these are considered later. It should be noted that the absence of reaction 1 (3 β-hydroxysteroid dehydrogenase deficiency) deletes all the compounds below the second row and makes dehydroepiandrosterone (DHEA) (and its sulfate) the end product of biosynthesis. Similarly, deletion of reaction 2 (17-hydroxylase deficiency) eliminates all the compounds to the right of the first column and down through the next-to-bottom row. Corticosterone, but not cortisol, is formed, and the sex steroids, with the exception of progesterone, are absent, whereas aldosterone, at the end of the chain, is still formed. Deletion of reaction 3 (desmolase deficiency) eliminates the major androgens and estrogens, whereas the absence of reactions 5 and 6 (aromatase deficiency) leaves androgens, but not estrogens, as end products. Deficiency of reaction 7 (21-hydroxylase deficiency) is the biochemical defect underlying the most common form of the adrenogenital syndrome: Glucocorticoids and mineralocorticoids are produced inefficiently and the sex steroids become the major end products. In this condition, reaction 8 (11-hydroxylation) is unaffected, and some of the excess 17-hydroxyprogesterone is metabolized by hydroxylation at C-11 to form 21-deoxycortisol, while androstenedione is metabolized to 11β-hydroxyandrostenedione (not shown in Fig. 4-3). The absence of reaction 8 (11-hydroxylase deficiency)

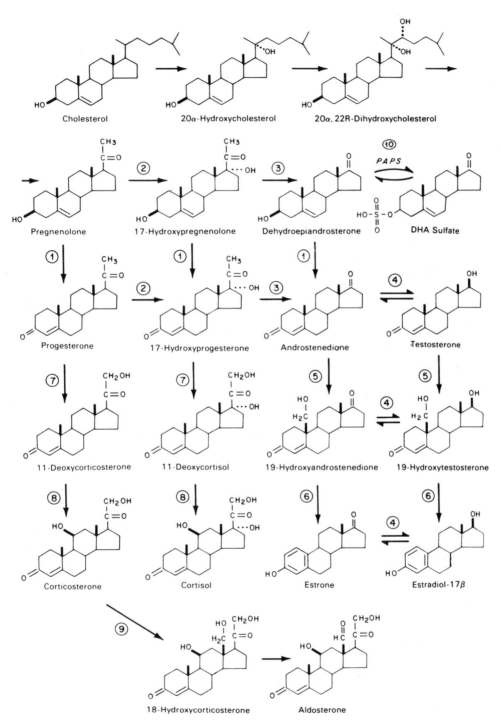

FIGURE 4-3. Steroidogenesis from cholesterol.

is the defect underlying the second most common form of congenital adrenal hyperplasia: The sex steroids and a mineralocorticoid, 11-deoxycorticosterone, are still produced, but cortisol and aldosterone are not. It must be remembered in all this that different isoenzymes may carry out the same reaction, so that the deletion of a single one of them will not produce the complete block that might be anticipated from the schema.

Further study of the schema shows that in some instances several different pathways can lead to the same end product. The androgens and estrogens, for example, can be formed by a Δ^5-pathway that postpones reaction 1 until dehydroepiandrosterone is formed. Cortisol is in fact formed in part in the adrenal gland by a Δ^5 pathway that bypasses progesterone and proceeds by way of 17-hydroxyprogestrone. There is less flexibility, however, in the pathways to aldosterone on the one hand and to cortisol on the other. These are kept separated by the fact that a compound that is already hydroxylated at C-21 (11-deoxycorticosterone, corticosterone, aldosterone) cannot be a substrate for reaction 2 (17-hydroxylation). Furthermore, in the bovine, at least, the glomerulosa layer of the adrenal cortex, where aldosterone is formed, lacks 17-hydroxylase activity. In the adrenal glands, hydroxylation at C-21 (reaction 8) precludes loss of the side chain to form androgens and estrogens (reaction 3). When 11β-hydroxylated compounds that lack a 21-hydroxyl are formed, as in conditions of deficient 21-hydroxylation, the resulting compounds are no longer substrates for 21-hydroxylation.[4]

Reaction 1: Δ^5-3β-ol to Δ^4-3-Ketone

The currently proposed official name for this microsomal enzyme does not distinguish the two steps that must occur in this conversion: the dehydrogenase step that gives rise to the 3-ketone and the isomerase step that changes the Δ^5 to Δ^4. The two activities do seem to go together during purification of the enzyme system.[5] Other evidence suggests that the dehydrogenase step is rate limiting. It is not known whether there are different isoenzymes for C_{21} and C_{19} substrates. It has been pointed out that the reaction works as a generating system for reduced nicotinamide adenine dinucleotide (NADH). A transhydrogenase, also located in the microsomal compartment of the cell, then transfers the hydrogen from NADH to nicotinamide adenine dinucleotide phosphate (NADP), forming NADPH, the cofactor required for most of the subsequent reactions.

This is the first steroidogenic reaction to have been detected histochemically. NADH made available by reaction 1 was detected by the reduction of tetrazolium to the colored compound formazan, a reaction carried out by dihydrolipoamide reductase, present in the tissue. On the basis of this staining reaction, the theca of the ovarian follicle, but not the granulosa, was long considered the main site of follicular steroidogenesis. Recent evidence from experiments on the adrenal glands of rats indicates that ACTH directly stimulates the synthesis of this enzyme.[6]

Reaction 2: 17-Hydroxylation

Hydroxylation of C_{21} steroids at the 17-position is an essential step before side-chain cleavage to form C_{19} steroids. A ketone must be present at C-20; 20α-dihydroprogesterone cannot undergo side-chain cleavage. The enzyme is located in the microsomal fraction of the cell. The side chain is β-oriented, so that the hydroxyl group has to be α-oriented: it seems unnecessary, therefore, to include the α in referring to 17-hydroxypregnenolone or 17-hydroxyprogesterone. The same enzyme probably serves both precursors, pregnenolone being more rapidly hydroxylated than progesterone. This reaction can precede reaction 1 in the pathway leading to cortisol. In the adrenal gland, the enzyme system for this reaction is present in the zona fasciculata and zona reticularis but not in the zona glomerulosa. The adult rat adrenal synthesizes only corticosterone, but not the 17-hydroxylated glucocorticoids cortisol and cortisone. The young rat adrenal can make cortisol, and 17-hydroxylation occurs in the adrenals of both age groups as an intermediate step in androgen formation.

Reaction 3: C_{21} to C_{19} Steroids

The side-chain cleavage of C_{21} steroids by the 17,20-desmolase results in the formation of C_{19} steroids that are weak androgens: 17-hydroxypregnenolone becomes dehydroepiandrosterone (DHEA), and 17-hydroxyprogesterone becomes androstenedione. The enzyme (steroid 17–20 carbon–carbon lyase, commonly called desmolase) operates in close associate with the 17-hydroxylase. The hydroxylase, and not the desmolase, is rate limiting with respect to side-chain cleavage.

Reaction 4: 17β-Hydroxysteroid Dehydrogenases

This oxidoreduction is the only freely reversible reaction shown in Figure 4-3. The enzymes are soluble and use either NAD or NADP, with a preference for the former. On the whole, equilibrium is in the direction of the more potent steroids, testosterone and estradiol, which have the 17β-hydroxyl, rather than the less potent 17-ketosteroids, androstenedione and estrone. The NADH:NAD ratio in target tissues determines whether the more active or the less active steroid preponderates locally.

Reactions 5 and 6: 19-Hydroxylation and Aromatization

These reactions have been studied in great detail in placental tissue. In both the ovary and the placenta, the reactions take place in the microsomes and require NADPH and molecular oxygen. Androstenedione is converted to 19-hydroxyandrostenedione and then, *via* a second hydroxylation at C-19, to 19-aldoandrostenedione. A third hydroxylation at C-2 results in the spontaneous loss of C-19 as formic acid, with dehydrogenation to form a double bond at C-1.[7] Note that the aromatic (phenolic) A ring is common to all estrogenic steroids.

Reactions 7–9: Formation of Corticoids and Aldosterone

These reactions of 21-, 11-, and 18-hydroxylases are not found in normal ovarian tissue; however, 11-hydroxylation has been claimed for polycystic ovaries,[8] and both cortisol-secreting[9] and aldosterone-secreting[10] tumors of the ovary have been reported.

Reaction 7: 21-Hydroxylation

Like the 17-hydroxylating and 19-hydroxylating enzymes, this adrenal enzyme is also located in the microsomes and requires NADPH and molecular oxygen. It was the first of the steroid-oxygenating enzyme systems to be thoroughly studied, beginning with the pioneering work of Ryan and Engel.[11] Its clinical importance in relationship to the adrenogenital syndrome has already been noted. The adrenal enzymes for the 21-hydroxylation of progesterone and 17-hydroxyprogesterone may be different.[4] In any event, the 21-hydroxylation of progesterone to form 11-deoxycorticosterone occurs primarily in the zona glomerulosa and leads to al-

dosterone formation, while the 21-hydroxylation of 17-hydroxyprogesterone to form 11-deoxycortisol occurs in the zona fasciculata and zona reticularis. The Δ^5 compound 17-hydroxypregnenolone can be 21-hydroxylated to form 17,21-dihydroxypregnenolone, another possible pathway to the formation of 11-deoxycortisol that is not shown in Figure 4-3. Hydroxylation at C-21 seems to be a prerogative of the adrenal gland, but it has also been reported as occurring in polycystic ovaries.

Reaction 8: 11β-Hydroxylation

With this step and with reaction 9 we return to the mitochondria for other oxygenations involving NADPH and molecular oxygen. The 21-hydroxysteroids 11-deoxycorticosterone and 11-deoxycortisol are the normal substrates, but there may be different enzymes for each. The 11-hydroxylation of 17-hydroxyprogesterone to form 21-deoxycortisol (not shown in Fig. 4-3) is a reaction that becomes evident in states of deficient 21-hydroxylation.[4] Under some circumstances, androstenedione may be metabolized to form 11β-hydroxyandrostenedione. It is likely that another enzyme is involved in the 11β-hydroxylation of C_{21} compounds without the 21-hydroxyl, and that still another is involved in the 11β-hydroxylation of C_{19} compounds. The reaction of 11β-hydroxylation is the finishing touch to steroid biosynthesis in the sense that 11β-hydroxysteroids are no longer substrates for 21-hydroxylation.

Reaction 9: 18-Hydroxylation

The formation of aldosterone is carried out in the mitochondria of the adrenal zona glomerulosa.[12] It is not surprising to find that 18-hydroxylation involves NADPH and molecular oxygen, like the other oxygenations we have seen. It might seem logical to suppose that aldosterone is formed by hydroxylating the C-18 methyl group to form 18-hydroxycorticosterone and then dehydrogenating to form the aldehyde. In actuality, 18-hydroxycorticosterone is not a precursor but a by-product, with the reaction proceeding *via* a geminal diol at C-18.

Reaction 10: Sulfurylation and Sulfatase Activity

Human adrenal and ovarian tissue is capable of sulfurylating DHEA and estradiol. The enzyme 3β-hydroxysteroid sulfotransferase in the case of

DHEA, or estrone sulfotransferase in the case of estrone, transfers the sulfate group from 3'-phosphoadenylyl phosphosulfate (PAPS) to the hydroxyl group at C-3. It is essential for the human placenta to be able to hydrolyze DHEA sulfate, an important precursor in placental steroidogenesis. This is not true of the ovary, which has only small amounts of the required enzyme, sulfatase.

Hydroxylation Reactions: The Oxygenases

Oxidation means the removal of electrons, as occurs when atoms of hydrogen are removed to form a double bond or to convert a hydroxyl function to a ketone. Such reactions are usually reversible, their direction depending on whether cofactor is available in the reduced or the oxidized state. Reaction 4 is an example.

Oxygenation, on the other hand, takes molecular oxygen and attaches it to the steroid as a hydroxyl function. Examples of such reactions are cholesterol side-chain cleavage and reactions 2, 3, 5, 6, 7, and 8. All these reactions require NADPH and molecular oxygen. Three of these, cholesterol side-chain cleavage and reactions 8 and 9, take place in the mitochondria. The rest are associated with the microsomes. All the reactions involve cytochrome P450, a hemoprotein whose action is inhibited by carbon monoxide (CO). The term comes from the fact that CO evokes a change in absorbance that is maximal at 450 nm. Activity is restored even in the presence of CO on exposure to light at the same wavelength. The mitochondrial cholesterol side-chain-cleaving enzyme system consists of the P450 hemoprotein, an iron–sulfur (Fe_2–S_2) protein (adrenodoxin in the adrenal, testodoxin in the testis), and a flavoprotein containing flavine adenine dinucleotide (FAD), and NADP (H).[13] Electrons are passed from NADPH to FAD to the iron–sulfur protein and finally to the metalloenzyme complex that takes up molecular oxygen and attaches it to the steroid. The overall reaction is as follows:

$$\text{Steroid H} + \text{donor} \cdot H_2 + O_2 \rightarrow \text{steroid OH} + \text{donor} + H_2O$$

where "donor" represents the P450 system.

P450 is located in mitochondria characterized by cristae with a uniquely vesicular appearance. At least four substrate-specific P450 hemoproteins are associated with (1) cholesterol side-chain cleavage ($P450_{scc}$), (2) cholesterol sulfate side-chain cleav-

age, (3) 11β-hydroxylation ($P450_{11\beta}$), and (4) 18-hydroxylation.[4]

Evidence from several sources suggests that (3) and (4) may be the same enzyme.[14] They are not distinguishable by immunochemical and histochemical techniques; they are affected in parallel fashion in congenital adrenal hyperplasia; they respond in parallel fashion in normal humans in response to adrenocorticotropic hormone (ACTH) stimulation and metyrapone blockage and in selectively bred rats a single gene seems to regulate both enzymes.

The microsomal P450 enzyme systems are associated with smooth endoplasmic reticulum. They differ from the mitochondrial system described above in several respects: (1) there is no nonheme iron–sulfur protein, (2) cytochrome b_5 may be involved in the electron transfer, (3) the microsomal flavoproteins are immunologically distinct, and (4) a phospholipid(phosphatidyl)choline may be an obligatory component.[4]

Adrenal Steroidogenesis

It must not be supposed that Figure 4-3 is a representation of adrenal physiology. While the adrenal gland is the most completely versatile steroidogenic organ, it also has some limitations.[13,15] The gland can and does synthesize cholesterol from acetate but, like the corpus luteum, it prefers to use circulating cholesterol rather than the ATP-wasting "scratch recipe." Cholesterol sulfate is present in plasma, but it crosses membranes poorly and is not an important precursor. The adenal cell, like other steroidogenic cells as well as fibroblasts, has a cell-surface receptor that specifically binds the apoprotein component of LDL and contributes the exogenous cholesterol. The precursor cholesterol in the adrenal cell comes from three sources: (1) from outside, by way of the LDL receptor; (2) from hydrolysis of stored cholesterol esters; and (3) from acetyl CoA, as in Figure 4-2. Acute ACTH stimulation depletes the ester cholesterol, and continued stimulation increases the amount of LDL receptor at the cell surface. When circulating LDL is deficient, or the stimulus is strong and continued, synthesis from acetyl CoA is called into play.[16]

The pathways to cortisol and to aldosterone are segregated in different zones. The adult adrenal gland can form 3β-hydroxysteroid sulfates of pregnenolone, 17-hydroxypregnenolone, and DHEA. In addition, it can and does use a separate biosynthetic pathway for the sulfated compounds: pregnenolone sulfate, 17α-hydroxypregnenolone sulfate, and dehydroepiandrosterone sulfate (DHEAS).[17] This pathway is most important in the fetal adrenal.[18]

The major adrenal androgen is DHEA, which, with its sulfate and some androstenedione, is secreted in significant amounts at pubertal adrenarche. Estrogens are not formed in the normal adrenal gland but arise as a result of peripheral aromatization of androgens.[15]

Adrenal Structure and the Regulation of Adrenal Androgen Biosynthesis: Adrenarche and "Adrenopause"

About 80% of the fetal adrenal cortex consists of an inner zone, called the fetal zone, which is not present in the adult. The outer 20% is the definitive zone, which will give rise to the three layers of the adult, consisting, from within outward, of the zona reticularis (by volume 7% of the cortex, putative site of androgen synthesis, but also a site of glucocorticoid synthesis), the zone fasciculata (73% of the cortex, the major site of glucocorticoid synthesis), and the zone glomerulosa (20% of the cortex, the site of aldosterone biosynthesis). The fetal zone has a relative deficiency of Δ^5-3β-hydroxysteroid dehydrogenase (reaction 1 in Fig. 4-3) but is rich in sulfurylating enzyme. A glance at Figure 4-3 shows that under these conditions DHEA and DHEAS become the major end products, especially when large quantities of pregnenolone formed by the placenta are presented to the fetal adrenal as substrate.[19] The fetal zone involutes after delivery, and in infants 1 to 2 years old constitutes less than 20% of the cortex.[20] The adult zona reticularis first appears between ages 3 and 7, and it has been noted that the percentage of subjects with a continuous reticular zone parallels the adrenarchal rise in the serum concentration of DHEAS.[21] The level of free DHEA in serum has been documented in children from the neonatal period through 15 years of age. In both girls and boys, a fall to low levels during the first year of life is followed by a progressive rise first detectable between ages 6 and 7.[20] This change is accompanied by responses to the administration of ACTH consistent with decreased levels of Δ^5-hydroxysteroid dehydrogenase (reaction 1, Fig. 4-3) and increased levels of 17-hydroxylase and desmolase (reactions 2 and 3), both tending to increase the production of androgen.[22] These in vivo observations confirm the results of in vitro incubations of whole adrenal glands.[22] While it appears that the fetal zone and the zona reticularis are the sites of androgen production, and histochemical observations are consistent with this, direct proof is lacking. The functional zonation of the gland may indeed be the result of local circulation and the pooling of steroid products that favor some reactions regionally while inhibiting others.[23]

Throughout childhood, the plasma cortisol concentration and the cortisol secretory rate remain constant.[21] What changes is the adrenal response to ACTH. If this change is due to involution of the fetal zone, and later, to proliferation of a biochemically similar zona reticularis, what mediates the involution and the proliferation? Is there an "adrenarchal factor"[22] that causes the zona reticularis to proliferate? Does a pituitary adrenal androgen stimulating hormone (AASH) exist, as has often been suggested? Evidence for the existence of such a hormone, a glycopeptide of molecular weight 60,000, has been presented.[24] While ACTH stimulates the production of both cortisol and DHEA by adrenal cells in vitro, this putative AASH stimulates production of androgen alone.

The phenomenon in men and women of age 40 and older of falling levels of urinary 17-ketosteroid, a reflection of falling levels of serum DHEA and DHEAS, has been called "adrenopause." Like adrenarche, stress and recovery from stress, and a number of pathologic states, "adrenopause" also poses the problem of the dissociation between the control of the secretion of androgen and that of cortisol.

The Mechanism of Action of Tropic Hormones in Steroidogenesis

Mechanisms worked out for ACTH are in all probability applicable in a general way as well to LH in its action on the corpus luteum. In both instances the tropic hormone stimulates steroidogenesis by increasing the rate of cleavage of the side chain of cholesterol to form pregnenolone. The tropic stimuli increase aldosterone formation and aromatization also, however, as shown in Table 4-1.

ACTH binds with high affinity and specificity to receptor sites on the plasma membrane that are coupled with adenyl cyclase. Binding in vitro is associated with activation of the cyclase and formation of

TABLE 4-1. Tropic Stimuli in Steroidogenesis: Cells and Reactions Affected[a,b]

Tropic stimulus	Cell	Reaction affected
ACTH	Adrenal fasciculata and reticularis	Cholesterol side-chain cleavage
Angiotensin II	Adrenal glomerulosa	Cholesterol side-chain cleavage
ACTH	Adrenal glomerulosa	Cholesterol side-chain cleavage
Serotonin	Adrenal glomerulosa	Cholesterol side-chain cleavage
Increased K^+	Adrenal glomerulosa	Cholesterol side-chain cleavage
Severely decreased Na^+	Adrenal glomerulosa	Cholesterol side-chain cleavage
Na^+ deficiency	Adrenal glomerulosa	18-Hydroxylation
K^+ uptake	Adrenal glomerulosa	18-Hydroxylation
hCG (?)	Adrenal fetal zone	Cholesterol (sulfate?) to pregnenolone sulfate
LH (hCG)	Leydig	Cholesterol side-chain cleavage
FSH	Sertoli	Aromatization
LH (hCG)	Theca, luteinized granulosa	Cholesterol side-chain cleavage
FSH	Follicular granulosa	Aromatization

[a]ACTH, adrenocorticopic hormone; hCG, human chorionic gonadotropin; LH, luteinizing hormone; FSH, follicle-stimulating hormone.
[b]From Richardson.[2]

intracellular cyclic adenosine monophosphate (cAMP). cAMP binds to a specific intracellular receptor protein associated with a protein kinase:

$$ATP + a\ protein \rightarrow ADP + a\ phosphoprotein$$

Similar cAMP-dependent protein kinases have been demonstrated in a number of tissues as well as the adrenal. Their activation consists of dissociation of the catalytic subunit (C) from the receptor subunit (R):

$$\underset{(inactive)}{R \cdot C} + cAMP \rightarrow R \cdot cAMP + \underset{(active)}{C}$$

Although cAMP-dependent protein kinase has been purified from bovine adrenal cortex, and many protein substrates for it exist within the adrenal cortical cell, only the first of six criteria for the mediation of the cAMP effect by protein phosphorylation seems to have been established.[25] These criteria require that (1) the cell type involved should contain a cAMP-dependent protein kinase, (2) protein that bears a functional relationship to a cAMP-mediated process should be phosphorylated in vitro, (3) in vitro phosphorylation should lead to modified function, (4) stoichiometric correlation should exist between in vitro phosphorylation and modified function, (5) phosphorylation in vivo should be demonstrable in response to cAMP. So far, in fact, only phosphorylase kinase, glycogen synthetase, and triglyceride lipase have been shown to fill all but the fifth criterion.[26]

Whereas steroid hormones act on cells by an effect on the genome involving the transcription of new message, messenger ribonucleic acid (mRNA), ACTH is fully active when gene transcription is blocked by actinomycin D. Even when new protein formation is blocked by cycloheximide, ACTH can stimulate the formation of cAMP and of intracellular free cholesterol. The observed effects under these conditions fit the phosphorylation hypothesis: In the absence of protein synthesis, there can still be an increase in the activation state (phosphorylation) of existing proteins such as adenylate cyclase, cAMP-dependent protein kinase, cholesterol esterase, and cholesterol synthetase.[13] In the presence of cycloheximide, free cholesterol accumulates and is translocated by a heat-stable carrier protein to the mitochondria, but steroidogenesis does not occur. It has been demonstrated that the synthesis of a labile protein is required, the function of which is unknown. Evidence has been presented that this protein enables the mitochondrial free cholesterol to bind to cytochrome $P450_{scc}$.[13]

A version of the mechanism of ACTH action that is also applicable to the mechanism of action of LH and hCG is found in Figure 4-4, which also illustrates the regulatory mechanism involving the LDL receptor. At the top left, ACTH interacts with the receptor component of the adenyl cyclase complex at the cell surface (plasma membrane). The cyclase is activated, and cAMP (adenosine 3,5'-monophosphate) is produced within the cell. cAMP activates (+) the protein kinase, which in turn activates cho-

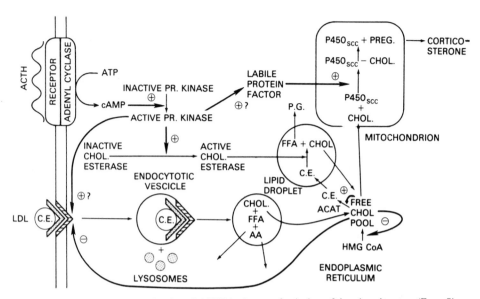

FIGURE 4-4. Proposed mechanism of action of ACTH in the zona fasciculata of the adrenal cortex. (From Simpson.[13])

lesterol esterase, converting cholesterol ester (CE) in the lipid droplet into free fatty acid (FFA) and free cholesterol (CHOL). Prostaglandin (PG) is also released from its conjugated form. The resultant increase in the free cholesterol pool has a negative effect ($-$) on de novo synthesis of cholesterol from acetate by inhibition at the level of β-hydroxy-β-methyl glutaryl coenzyme A (HMG CoA) and a negative effect on the number of LDL receptors at the cell membrane (long bottom arrow). The free cholesterol in the pool enters the mitochondrion (upper right) presumably bound to heat-stable carrier protein (not shown). If for any reason the level of the pool of free cholesterol rises, cholesterol acyl transferase (ACAT) is stimulated ($+$), resulting in more esterification and more CE contributed to the lipid droplet. The lipid droplet also receives cholesterol from the plasma by the LDL receptor mechanism. The coated pit at the cell surface ($>>$, lower left) that receives the LDL particle invaginates to form an endocytotic vesicle. Lysosomal enzymes break down the surface apoprotein of the LDL particle into amino acids (AA), while the CE in the core is broken down to FFA and CHOL, which is added to the pool.

The active protein kinase is shown as stimulating ($+$) the labile protein factor. Actually, this is new protein synthesis, and the arrow should show the kinase stimulating ribosomal translation. The newly formed labile protein enters the mitochondrion, where it stimulates ($+$) the binding of intra-

mitochondrial cholesterol to P450 associated with cleavage of the cholesterol side chain ($P450_{scc}$). The product, pregnenolone, leaves the mitochondrion to undergo reactions 1 and 7; reenters for reaction 8, which is carried out by mitochondrial $P450_{11\beta}$; and exits as the ultimate glucocorticoid (for the rat), corticosterone.

Calcium is required for hormonal stimulation of steroidogenesis, in the adrenal gland and in the ovary, both for ACTH or LH stimulation of adenylate cyclase and for stimulation of the subsequent steps by cAMP.[25,27] The ability of calcium to cause clustering and phase separation of membrane phospholipids could be part of the hypothesized role of ACTH in cholesterol binding and translocation at the inner mitochondrial membrane.[13] Where calcium is involved in hormone action participation of the calcium-binding transmitter protein calmodulin is to be expected, and a role for calmodulin in corticosteroidogenesis has in fact been established.[28]

Regulation of Aldosterone Biosynthesis

The biosynthesis of aldosterone in the adrenal zona glomerulosa is under multifactorial control: It is stimulated by ACTH, angiotensin II, serotonin, increased levels of potassium ion, and decreased levels of sodium ion.[12,29] ACTH may have a permissive role for the other stimuli. The situation is complicated by the fact that sodium depletion acts both directly and by stimulating the secretion of angiotensin II. Its action and that of potassium may be exerted at steps between progesterone and aldosterone, while angiotensin II and serotonin may both act by a mechanism similar to that shown in Figure 4-4.

Steroidogenesis in the Ovarian Follicle: The Two-Cell Theory

The most striking feature of the follicle from the point of view of steroidogenesis is the separation of theca from granulosa by a basement lamina. On the basis of histochemical observations the theca was long thought to be the major site of steroidogenesis in the mature follicle. Like cells of the adrenal cortex, the Leydig cells of the testis, and the cells of the corpus luteum, these cells have morphologic features, as seen electron microscopically, associated with steroid secretion: an abundance of smooth endoplasmic reticulum, spherical mitochondria with tubular cristae, lipid droplets, and conspicuous Golgi apparatus.[30] By contrast, the granulosa cells have the appearance of protein-synthesizing cells with abundant rough endoplasmic reticulum.[31] A tremendous amount of effort has been devoted to elucidating the respective roles in steroidogenesis of the two cell types, beginning with the ingenious experiments on rats conducted by Falck (see also Ref. 32), who in 1959 introduced fragments of theca, granulosa, and vagina into the anterior chamber of the eye and reported that estrogenic changes in the vagina occurred only when both granulosa and theca were present. The careful experiments of Ryan and co-workers[33] confirmed the synergism of the two cell types in the synthesis of both progesterone and estrogen from acetate in vitro.[33] Dorrington made the important discovery that follicle-stimulating hormone (FSH) stimulates rat granulosa cells in vitro to aromatize. In these experiments, added testosterone in the medium was required as precursor in order for detectable amounts of estradiol to be formed.

Subsequent experiments by Tsang et al.[34,35] with human theca and granulosa cells in vitro pointed to a clear difference of function of the two compartments. Theca, but not granulosa, was found to synthesize androgen (androstenedione). The effective tropic stimulus was hCG (equivalent to LH); FSH was ineffective. Conversely, granulosa, but not theca, was capable of aromatizing androstenedione provided in the medium, the granulosa cells of large follicles exhibiting the greatest activity. The production of estradiol was proportional to the concentration of androstenedione. Others have reported a granulosal aromatase activity 700 times as great as thecal aromatase in human preovulatory follicles.[36] Curiously, aromatase activity in vitro is stimulated by the presence of an androgen that cannot be used as a precursor, 5α-dihydrotestosterone.[37]

The tidy concept that emerges from these experiments is that in vivo the theca carries out most of the steroidogenesis characteristic of the follicular phase, except for the production of estradiol, which is carried out in the granulosa from precursor (androstenedione, testosterone) provided by the theca. Furthermore, many workers have been tempted to speculate that the granulosa simply does not have the full array of steroidogenic enzymes and that, like the placenta, it is capable of progesterone synthesis (when luteinized), and of aromatization, but not capable of the steps between (reactions 2 and 3) that provide precursor androgens. Many studies by Ryan and co-workers, however, have failed to demonstrate any real enzyme deficiency on the part of the granulosa. This work culminates in a detailed comparison of the capacity of three compartments (granulosa, theca, and stroma) to produce progesterone, androgens (androstenedione, testosterone, 5α-dihydrotestosterone) and estrogens (estrone, estradiol).[36] Human follicular tissue was incubated for a 48-hr period, and the production of these steroids was measured by radioimmunoassay (RIA). Small (1–8-mm) and large (>8-mm) follicles, healthy and atretic, were compared in four phases of the menstrual cycle: early, mid-, and late follicular and luteal.

The most striking overall result was that all three compartments were capable of producing all six steroids. Both granulosa and theca from atretic follicles, however, produced normal or increased amounts of androgens, but no estrogens, and very little progesterone. Their healthy counterparts produced increasing amounts of progesterone and estrogen as the follicular phase advanced, the production and the increase exhibited by tissue from large follicles being much greater than that from small ones. Even stromal tissue produced increasing amounts of progesterone. On the whole, the performance of this compartment was qualitatively similar to, but quantitatively very much less than, that of the theca of small follicles, some of which probably were present in the stromal samples. Steroid production by tissue from follicles of the luteal phase was generally low. In the experiments, the incubations were carried out in the presence of serum, which could have provided a small amount of steroid precursor, and steroid conjugates were not measured. In addition, the granulosal preparations were suspensions of dispersed cells, while the others consisted of tissue fragments, so that a quantitative comparison of granulosa with theca and stroma was not possible.

In a further extension of these experiments,[39] tissue from the different compartments was cocultured in an effort to determine whether there was cellular synergism in steroidogenesis. It was concluded that peak secretion of estrogen by the follicle required the synergism of both theca and granulosa.

The compartments are defined by in vivo conditions wherein the cells have a close and special relationship. In vitro they are not so related, and every cell has equal access to the artificial environment provided. In vivo, during the follicular phase, the environment of the thecal cells is that of the systemic plasma, while the environment of the granulosa cells is that of the follicular fluid. Measurements on this fluid show gonadotropin levels that are lower than those of plasma (FSH at about 60% and LH about 30% of plasma levels in the late follicular phase[40]). By contrast, as follicular size and number of granulosa cells increase, estradiol concentrations go from 50 to 1700 ng/ml (1000 times the level in preovulatory plasma) and progesterone concentrations from 40 to 90 ng/ml (4 times the level of mid-luteal plasma), while the concentration ratio of androgen : estrogen falls progressively to <1. In all probability, the specialized microenvironment of the follicle is the one that is optimal for the oocyte.

In vivo experiments that can differentiate the functions of theca and granulosa are difficult to devise because of the element of uncontrolled trauma that is necessarily involved. One experimental design is to remove the granulosa by aspiration and to observe the effect on steroid concentrations in the ovarian venous effluent. When this experiment was first attempted in monkeys, it was concluded that the theca, not the granulosa, was the main secreting element; repetition of this experiment with greater care, however, gave the opposite result.[41] Within 15 min of removing the granulosa cells from the dominant follicle, ovarian vein concentrations of progesterone, estradiol, and androstenedione had fallen to less than 30% of their previous levels. The difference in results from those of the earlier experiment was explained by venous stasis induced by the method of blood sampling in the latter.

The main function of the compartmental separation between theca and granulosa in the follicular phase appears to be to hold the steroidogenic capacity of the granulosa in check. Steroids are not made by the scratch recipe from acetate but from precursor cholesterol in the form of LDL.[3,42] LDL cholesterol cannot cross the basement membrane and therefore is not available to the granulosa before ovulation.[43]

GERM CELL AND OOCYTE

At 3 weeks of intrauterine life, the germ cells first become recognizable. They enter the primordia of the gonads as these begin to form at 4–5 weeks. Their numbers increase by mitosis to a population peak of 7 million at 5 months. This level falls to 2 million at birth and to 0.3 million at puberty.[44] Since only about 400–500 ovulations occur during reproductive life, more than 99% of these cells are lost, most or all of them through the process of follicular atresia. The primary oocyte is a diploid cell with a full postsynthetic complement of DNA. Meiotic changes begin in nuclei of these cells by 3 months of fetal life; the process stops at the diplotene stage, equivalent to G_2 of somatic cells. Meiosis resumes whenever ovulation occurs, from 15 to 45 years later, when the primary oocyte divides by separation of homologous sets of chromosomes (reduction division) into the first polar body (haploid) and the secondary oocyte (haploid), which remains at a stage equivalent to G_1 of somatic cells. Only when a sperm enters does the secondary oocyte divide, without chromosomal reduction, into the second polar body (haploid) and the mature ovum (haploid). The latter, containing 25% of the DNA of the primary oocyte, goes on to form the female pronucleus, which fuses with the male pronucleus to form the zygote.

FOLLICULOGENESIS

Identifiable follicles first appear in the ovary after 4 months gestation (see Fig. 4-5). FSH, first detectable in fetal serum at 12 weeks and peaking at 5 months, is undoubtedly involved. The appearance at 7 months of fully functioning follicles and the beginning of significant estrogen secretion by the fetal ovary coincides with an increased rate of growth of the fetal uterus. The continued growth of the ovary in the years up to menarche is shown in Figure 4-6. Again, an increased rate of uterine growth coincides with the appearance of antral follicles. It is generally believed that most of the increase in ovarian weight represents interstitial

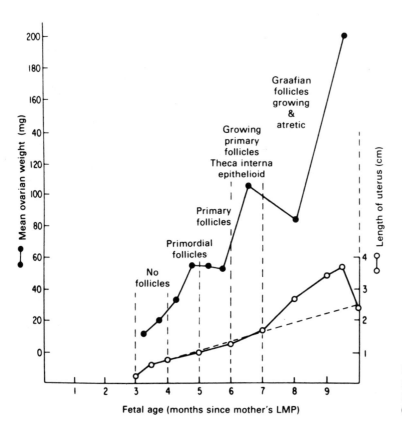

FIGURE 4-5. The ovary during fetal life. Growth and development correlated with growth of the fetal uterus. (From Ross and Vande Wiele.[119])

tissue contributed by follicles that have undergone atresia. The premenarcheal ovary is a polycystic ovary with a smooth surface free of ovulatory scars, and indeed its structure and hormonal milieu may be quite similar to that of some of the polycystic ovarian syndromes of adults.[45,46] In Figure 4-7 progressive follicular growth is displayed on the left side of the ovary, the successive stages being illustrated from the hilus upward. Most of the follicles in the normal ovary are primordial follicles only 50 μm in diameter, consisting of an oocyte and a single layer of flattened granulosa cells surrounded by a basement membrane. The first step in the transition from the primordial to the primary follicle (Fig. 4-7, lower left) is the increase in the size of the oocyte from 50 to 100 μm in diameter, a process completed when the follicle is only 150 μm in diameter. At the same time, the oocyte becomes surrounded by the zona pellucida, a layer rich in mucopolysaccharide. This structure has three functions: At the time of fertilization, it (1) binds to sperm specifically according to species, (2) blocks the entry of more sperm after fertilization, and (3) protects the early embryo on its

travels before implantation.[47] The zona is not a solid shell around the oocyte, since microvilli from the oocyte penetrate it for a short distance, whereas processes from the granulosa cells extend all the way through to make contact with the oocyte.[44] The granulosa cells now proliferate, forming multiple layers of cells joined by gap junctions that permit direct transmission of small molecules, such as cAMP, between cells.[48] At this point, the follicle has reached a diameter of ~200 μm. The entire process of follicular growth thus far has occurred independently of gonadotropin stimulation. It has been suggested that epithelial growth factor (EGF) may be involved. The granulosa cells have now acquired receptors for FSH and are ready for their next stage of growth.

Unlike the transition from primordial to primary follicles, the transition from the solid mature primary follicle ("growing follicle" in Fig. 4-7, lower left) to the antrum-containing secondary follicle ("maturing follicle" in Fig. 4-7) depends on gonadotropin, chiefly FSH, while estrogen also has a quasicatalytic role. LH and its equivalent, hCG, do not stimulate ovarian growth or secretion

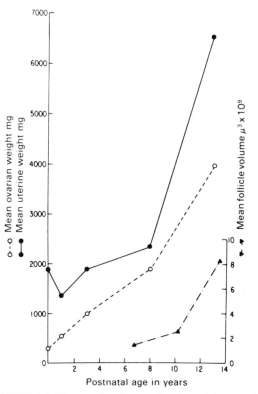

FIGURE 4-6. The prepubertal ovary. Ovarian weight and volume of the largest nonatretic follicle correlated with growth of the uterus. (From Ross and Vande Wiele.[119])

in the absence of FSH, explaining the absence of pseudoprecocious puberty in girls with hCG-secreting tumors.[49,50] The granulosa cells secrete the glycosaminoglycans (mucopolysaccharides) that fill the antrum and the interstitial spaces, with chondroitin sulfuric acid preponderating in the antral fluid and hyaluronic acid in the corona–cumulus complex that surrounds the oocyte (upper left inset, Fig. 3-7). Steroids are present at higher concentrations in this fluid than in plasma, and proteins and gonadotropins are present at lower concentrations.[31,40] The androgen to estrogen ratio is high in follicles destined for atresia and low in preovulatory follicles. Granulosa cells continue to multiply as the follicle grows, doubling in number for every 2 mm of growth until the follicle reaches 1 cm in diameter, and continuing to increase slowly thereafter.[51]

Does Figure 4-7 give a plausible picture of the distribution of follicles in a normal ovary? In humans, single ovulation means that there is only one dominant follicle (labeled ''Graafian follicle'')

in each cycle. It should not coexist with a corpus luteum (see Fig. 4-7) because follicular maturation is arrested during the luteal phase. Folliculogenesis in the luteal phase does indeed resume in monkeys if the corpus luteum is excised, but suppression is maintained if the corpus luteum is replaced by a progesterone-releasing silastic implant.[52] Administration of hCG will also suppress folliculogenesis after luteectomy, acting by maintaining progesterone secretion in the remaining ovarian tissue.[53] Indeed, the next follicle is recruited from whichever ovary secretes the least amount of progesterone at this time. Whatever the reason, the explanation is not insensitivity of the follicles to gonadotropin during that phase of the cycle, since in primates ovulation can be induced even in the midluteal phase by gonadotropin administration.[54] Indeed, the sensitivity of the follicular granulosa to stimulation by FSH increases as the luteal phase proceeds.[55] The size distribution and growth rate (as measured by thymidine labeling) of preantral follicles remains the same in monkeys in both the follicular and the luteal phase.[56,57] The number of antral (secondary) follicles remains constant from the late follicular through the luteal phase, but most of them are atretic; the best developed nonatretic follicle is 4 mm in diameter at the onset of menstruation.[55]

The requirements of human in vitro fertilization have led to new knowledge about the follicular environment that is associated with mature, fertilizable oocytes. These are summarized in the discussion of the putative oocyte maturation inhibitor. The cumulus cells that surround the oocyte at the time of ovulation (Fig. 4-7, insert upper left) become separated from each other by interstitial mucus as maturation proceeds. These cells secrete androgen, estrogen, and progesterone; with maturation, testosterone secretion continues, estradiol secretion increases 2 times, and progesterone secretion increases 3 times.[58]

ESTROGEN AND HORMONE RECEPTORS IN FOLLICULOGENESIS

In 1940, Pencharz and Williams independently demonstrated that estrogen administration will maintain ovarian weight and ovarian responsiveness to gonadotropins in hypophysectomized rats.[30] Twenty years later, Bradbury found that putting 0.5–1.0 mg estradiol crystals on one ovary of a rat caused a unilateral increase of weight and

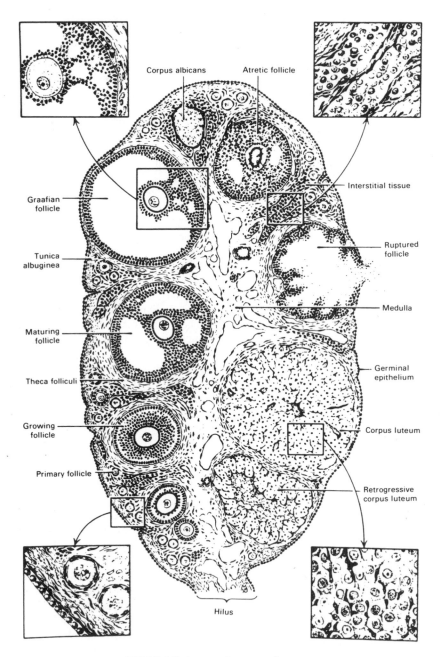

Corpus albicans

Atretic follicle

Graafian
follicle

Tunica
albuginea

Maturing
follicle

Theca folliculi

Growing
follicle

Primary follicle

Interstitial tissue

Ruptured
follicle

Medulla

Germinal
epithelium

Corpus luteum

Retrogressive
corpus luteum

Hilus

FIGURE 4-7. A composite mammalian ovary.

gonadotropin responsiveness.[59] Our current understanding of the mechanisms involved has not yet been extended to humans and primates but remains dependent on research on the hypophysectomized immature female rat (HIFR), which has continued in a steady stream.[60-62] The level of receptor is a good measure of the sensitivity of a tissue to hormone, and in HIFR estrogen administration not only stimulates granulosal proliferation (increase in cellular DNA and uptake of labeled thymidine) but a short-term (4-day) increase in the amount of estradiol receptor per cell as well. In both rats[63] and humans,[64] FSH alone is inactive in stimulating folliculogenesis, and, as noted before, LH is inactive in stimulating follicles that have not already responded to FSH.[49,50]

After priming with estradiol, however, the ovaries of HIFR are responsive to FSH, and the level of receptor rises again,[65] slowly if estrogen administration is stopped but rapidly if it is continued.[62] LH receptor, previously undetectable, appears for the first time and rises steeply when FSH administration follows estrogen priming.[62] Small amounts of LH (hCG) are necessary for continued follicular development, and in intact rats progesterone has been found to increase the sensitivity of the growing follicle to these low levels of LH.[66]

Conversely, LH (hCG) has a negative effect on follicular development induced in HIFR by estrogen alone. It promotes androgen production which leads to cessation of follicular growth and atresia.[67,68] This phenomenon may help explain physiologic atresia and may bear a distant relationship to the polycystic ovarian syndrome, with its high LH:FSH ratio.

SELECTION OF THE PREOVULATORY (DOMINANT) FOLLICLE

By day 5-7 of the menstrual cycle in primates, the dominant follicle gives evidence of its presence by a higher concentration of estradiol in the venous effluent of the ovary that bears it than in that of the opposite side.[52] By day 7, also, higher levels of LH receptor in the dominant follicle than in other follicles can be demonstrated by the injection of fluorescein-labeled hCG and scanning of microscopic sections. By day 8-10, the other follicles are no longer responsive to FSH or hCG, an effect possibly caused by the putative follicle regulatory protein. The dominant follicle that will provide the single

ovulation characteristic of humans is the one with the highest antral concentration of estrogen and the lowest androgen to estrogen ratio, and its granulosa cells contain the most aromatase.[36] How does the dominant follicle get ahead of the others? The follicle with the most estrogen is also the one that is most sensitive to FSH and LH. FSH levels fall before they rise again at the time of the midcycle surge; at these lower levels, the most sensitive follicle has an advantage. The secretion of a follicle regulatory protein would make that advantage decisive.

The dominant follicle and its reincarnation, the corpus luteum, exert their primacy for all but the first 5 days of the menstrual cycle, during which recruitment of follicles and selection of the dominant one occurs. It has been calculated that it takes about 25 days for follicular development from the earliest antral phase to ovulation.[55] If the dominant follicle or the corpus luteum is destroyed, however, ovulation occurs in half that interval of time, implying that half-prepared antral follicles are always available. Cautery of the dominant follicle in the rhesus on the tenth day of the cycle was followed by ovulation 12.4 ($\pm$ 0.9 SEM) days later, and after removal of the corpus luteum it occurred 12.8 ($\pm$ 0.9 SEM) days later.[52] The slightly elevated levels of FSH present during menstruation (intercycle FSH elevation) have been considered a necessary stimulus to the recruitment of a cohort of follicles, one of which will become dominant.[69] Research in primates, however, suggests that although the intercycle elevation may be desirable for optimal development of the corpus luteum later on, it is not obligatory for follicular recruitment, selection of the dominant follicle, and ovulation.[70]

OVULATION

A sustained secretion of estrogen for some 60 hr, together with the production over a period of 12 hr of progesterone by preovulatory follicles, is essential in inducing the onset of the FSH-LH surge.[71,72] Ovulation occurs 34-35 hr after onset of the surge and 10-12 hr after the peak.[73] Follicle rupture is not simply a bursting of the wall under increased hydrostatic pressure. The pressure does not in fact increase with increased follicular volume. Instead, the follicle becomes more distensible, perhaps under the influence of progesterone. Pressure recordings obtained by transducer in the follicles of rabbits do show contractile activity, however, which is increased by the administration of hCG or prostaglandin $F_{2\alpha}'$.[74] The theca adjacent to the basement lamina contains myosin, as demonstrated by immunofluorescence studies, and electron microscopic examination shows contractile elements similar to those of smooth muscle.[75] Adrenergic nerve fibers are demonstrable in the ovary, the function of which may be more concerned with the maintenance of a constant follicular pressure rather than with contraction. Sectioning of these nerves in rabbits does not prevent ovulation from occurring normally. Proteolysis at the site of follicle rupture (the stigma) is manifested on electron microscopy by "melting" of the collagen network. An increased amount of plasminogen activator, but not collagenase, is detectable locally.[76] In addition, a direct affect of LH on lysosomal activity has been suggested.

The protaglandins clearly play a key role in ovulation.[74] In rats and rabbits, ovarian production of PGE and PGF peaks at ovulation. LH stimulates ovarian prostaglandin synthesis (curiously, a GnRH analogue is capable of doing the same).[77] Indomethacin, a drug that blocks prostaglandin synthesis, also blocks hMG-hCG-induced ovulation in monkeys; administration of $PGF_{2\alpha}$ is capable of overriding the block.[74]

The vascular and biochemical events at the site of ovulation are comparable to the events at the onset of inflammation. The similarities and differences between the two processes have been extensively reviewed.[78]

FORMATION, MAINTENANCE, AND LYSIS OF THE CORPUS LUTEUM

Formation of the corpus luteum is marked by luteinization of the remaining granulosa cells, which now accumulate lipid and take on the appearance of steroidogenic cells. The basement membrane (lamina propria) that separated this epithelium from its stroma breaks down, and there is an invasion of blood vessels and lymphatics. As in the growth of cancers, an angiogenic factor secreted by the luteinizing cells may be involved.[79,80] Ultimately there will be a distinctive vascular architecture, with a central vein draining the mass. The theca interna contributes smaller and darker theca luteal (or paraluteal) cells to the luteal cells formed from the granulosa.[81] Lipid-rich K (for ketosteroid) cells appear in this tissue; at first thought to be steroidogenic, these are now considered macrophages. Capillary invasion of the granulosa begins on day 2, reaching the center of the mass by day 4. The secretory peak is reached by day 8. Thereafter, regression of vessels and fatty degeneration or simple atrophy of cells begins. The history of the corpus luteum is classically divided into four phases: (1) proliferation and hyperemia, (2) vascularization, (3) maturity or bloom, and (4) regression. It takes 7–10 months for the retrogressive corpus luteum to become a corpus albicans, a grossly white-appearing, collagen-rich scar, shown at the top of Figure 4-7.

Levels of receptor-binding LH (hCG) are high in human ovaries in the periovulatory period, then decline slightly, followed by an increase to a peak on days 22–23 of the menstrual cycle, followed by a slow decline thereafter to undetectable levels after day 27.[82,83] Early work on induction of ovulation by hMG administration followed by hLH (human LH) in humans indicated that daily administration of hLH was required for maintenance of luteal function.[84] A luteal life span of almost 15 days was achieved, but it could not be further extended by continued administration of hLH. While these experiments suggest that the human corpus luteum requires a luteotropic factor and that the luteotropic factor is LH, other recent experiments in rhesus monkeys suggest that gonadotropins are not luteotropic.[85] Daily administration of a potent inhibitory LHRH analogue starting the first day after ovulation lowered serum LH and FSH levels markedly without affecting luteal life span, secretion of estrogen or progesterone, or secretory responsiveness to hCG.

What causes the demise of the cyclic corpus luteum (luteolysis)? The level of LH receptors falls as the corpus luteum ages; curiously, in monkeys at least, androgen secretion persists after progesterone secretion has decreased.[86] The administration of estradiol in the mid-luteal phase in monkeys decreases progesterone secretion and shortens luteal life span.[87] The contributors of these observations have noted that there is normally a mid-luteal plateau in estradiol secretion, which is of sufficient magnitude to be the physiologic mediator of luteolysis. Their supposition that estrogen acts by lowering LH secretion assumes that LH is luteotropic. The ultimate step in luteolysis appears to be brought about by prostaglandin $F_{2\alpha}$.[88]

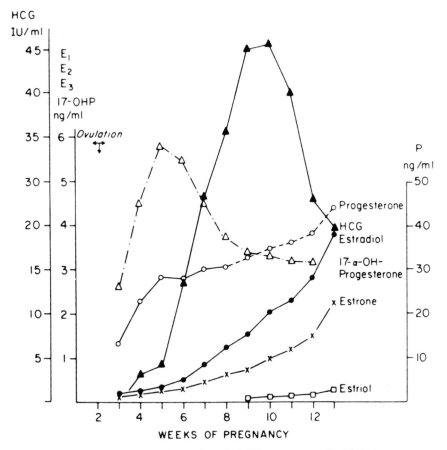

FIGURE 4-8. Mean plasma values of human chorionic gonadotropin (hCG), progesterone (P), 17α-hydroxyprogesterone (17-OHP), and unconjugated estrone (EI), estradiol (E2), and estriol (E3) of 10 normal patients followed weekly from the third to thirteenth week of pregnancy. ↓ , Presumed time of ovulation. (From Tulchinsky and Hobel.[91])

What saves the corpus luteum in the event of pregnancy (corpus luteum rescue)? In monkeys, implantation occurs, and monkey chorionic gonadotropin is detectable in serum as early as days 8–9 of pregnancy.[89] If LH cannot maintain the corpus luteum, CG clearly can: Its administration during the early luteal phase brings about a persistent secretion of progesterone, and appropriate dosage can mimic the responses of early pregnancy.[89]

In humans, as illustrated in Figure 4-8, the corpus luteum of pregnancy is already ceasing to function despite a continuing increase in the level of hCG.[90,91] The open triangles in Figure 4-8 represent secretion of 17-hydroxyprogesterone by the corpus luteum (the placenta cannot synthesize 17-hydroxysteroids), whereas the open circles represent the sum of progesterone secretion by the corpus luteum and placenta combined. Luteal secretion peaks at 4–5 weeks, but by 7–8 weeks it is no longer important to maintain pregnancy: The luteoplacental transition has been accomplished. Even though the corpus luteum of pregnancy appears completely spent at this early stage, it is nonetheless potentially functional in special circumstances, as shown in experiments on postpartum monkeys whose corpora lutea were able to respond to administered hCG with increased progesterone secretion.[92]

LUTEINIZATION INHIBITOR AND STIMULATOR[93]

Granulosa cells obtained from large preovulatory porcine follicles will undergo luteinization spontaneously in tissue culture. Cells from small, immature follicles can be induced to undergo luteinization, chemically demonstrable by an increase in LH/hCG receptor and progesterone production, in response to the addition of FSH to the medium (insulin, cortisol, thyroxine, and serum must also be present). Fluid from small follicles contains material that inhibits this response [luteinization inhibitor (LI)], whereas fluid from large follicles contains material that stimulates it [luteinization stimulator (LS)]. Inhibitory material with a molecular weight less than 1000 has been demonstrated in human follicular fluid, especially the fluid obtained from immature follicles.[94] The inhibition appears to be mediated at the level of adenylate cyclase.

FOLLICLE REGULATORY PROTEIN

Is the dominant follicle simply the follicle that wins, or is it indeed dominant over other follicles? It was observed by DiZerega and Hodgen[95] that hMG (FSH-LH) treatment stimulated follicular growth in monkeys during the early to mid-follicular phase (days 1–6), in the luteal phase, in mid-pregnancy, postabortion, and postpartum. The same treatment in the late follicular phase (days 8–10), however, did not increase the production of estradiol, did not prevent single ovulation by the dominant follicle, did not increase the number of follicles (quiescent opposite ovary at laparotomy on day 12), and did not prevent a normal luteal phase from ensuing. The data suggested that the dominant follicle might actually be secreting a substance that inhibited the response of other follicles to gonadotropin. Subsequently, a heat- and trypsin-labile material unique to the dominant follicle was purified from human ovarian venous blood[96] and human follicular fluid[97] that inhibited the follicular response of hypophysectomized, estrogen-primed immature female rats to hMG. Active material was also obtainable from the media used for the culture of human granulosa cells,[98] and the studies were extended to porcine follicular fluid and porcine granulosa cells, where a substance of similar properties was found to inhibit the induction of LH/hCG re-

ceptor by FSH in a dose-related manner, without affecting the binding of FSH,[99] and to inhibit aromatase activity.[100] Administration of the material from porcine follicular fluid to monkeys for the first 14 days of the menstrual cycle blocked ovulation in two of five animals and prolonged the follicular phase, lowering estrogen secretion and resulting in an inadequate luteal phase in the other three.[101] Studies of human follicular fluid aspirated in conjunction with a program of in vitro fertilization[100] showed a direct proportionality in unstimulated cycles between levels of the inhibitor, of estrogen, and of inhibin in the fluid, and an inverse relationship to the concentration of progesterone. The material, protein of 12,500–16,000 daltons with isoelectric points of pH 4.5 and 6.5, is a larger molecule than inhibin and does not suppress gonadotropin secretion. Its mechanism of action is unclear.

OOCYTE MATURATION INHIBITOR

Within 30–48 hr before ovulation the human oocyte completes meiotic maturation that had been prepared for years earlier with nuclear changes that had stopped at the diplotene stage. It was recently discovered that follicular fluid contains a substance that, when added to immature porcine oocytes incubated in appropriate medium, inhibits maturation in a dose-related manner.[93] This assay has been used to demonstrate a progressive fall in OMI in human follicular fluid as the follicle matures. A study using material obtained from patients undergoing in vitro fertilization and embryo transfer[102] has found that the follicular environment associated with mature fertilizable oocytes is characterized by a fluid volume of 2–4.5 ml, a high progesterone to estrogen ratio (1.58), a low androstenedione to estrogen ratio (0.3), and a low level of OMI (1 unit/ml). OMI is a small molecule (2000 daltons); efforts at purification show heterogeneity with two to three molecular species present. In vitro studies with porcine material indicate that OMI is secreted by granulosa cells, production being greatest by granulosa cells from small follicles and least by cells from large ones.

INHIBIN (INHIBIN F, FOLLICULOSTATIN, GONADOSTATIN)

A substance has been demonstrated in human follicular fluid that inhibits the production of FSH by rat pituitary cells in vitro in a dose-dependent manner.[93] The lowest levels are found in atretic follicles and in follicles of the luteal phase (most of which are not functional), with the amount increasing as follicles mature, being maximal in preovulatory fluids. In vitro studies on human material show that granulosa cells secrete the substance. Measurement in serum has not been successful in the absence of a sensitive radioimmunoassay, so that it is not possible at present to document the physiological role, if any, of this substance in primates.

Administration of steroid hormone-free (charcoal-extracted) porcine follicular fluid, however, to primates for 5–7 days early in the menstrual cycle[103] delays preparation of the dominant follicle for a corresponding number of days. Channing[93] hypothesized that inhibin F acts as a signal to the hypothalamic–pituitary axis that registers the total number of unripe follicles in the ovary. Inhibin F thus could account for the reduced gonadotropin secretion of childhood and its increase at puberty (with FSH preponderant) as continuing atresia lowers the number of follicles to some critical level, and also for the preponderance of FSH over LH in the high gonadotropin levels occurring when the store of follicles is exhausted at the menopause. The low levels of inhibin F in follicular fluid from polycystic ovaries[104] have been interpreted to explain the preponderance of LH over FSH in that syndrome. Unfortunately, progress in the purification of inhibin F has not kept step with physiologic observations, let alone speculation.

PROLACTIN

Prolactin is a hormone with multiple functions throughout the phylogenetic series but no definite function in humans aside from its role in lactation. It is of interest in relationship to ovarian function because of its definite luteotropic role in some species and because of its association with amenorrhea and infertility with or without galactorrhea. There is no evidence for a luteotropic role of prolactin in humans, but in monkeys an association has been observed between lactation and persistence of the corpus luteum of pregnancy.[105] In addition, monkeys made hyperprolactinemic by hypothalamic lesions have corpora lutea that fail to regress completely after functioning normally for an appropriate span of time, but do regress when prolactin is suppressed by bromocriptine.[106]

The association of hyperprolactinemia and infertility has led to research that has revealed a number of negative effects of prolactin. The concentration of the hormone in the human ovarian follicular fluid is inversely related to the concentration of progesterone and, when prolactin is added in vitro to the medium of preovulatory granulosa cells, the production of progesterone is inhibited in a dose-related manner over the range 20–100 ng/ml. Patients with amenorrhea, galactorrhea, and hyperprolactinemia have been found unresponsive to the administration of human menopausal gonadotropin.[107] These observations were confirmed by experiments with human follicular tissue fragments in vitro: Prolactin not only blocked the secretion of progesterone and estradiol but blocked the stimulatory action of hCG as well.[108] In vitro ovulation by perfused rabbit ovaries is prevented by adding prolactin to the medium.[109] Curiously, study of the fluid of follicles prepared for the harvesting of ova for in vitro fertilization showed that the best results were obtained from those with the highest concentrations of prolactin.[110]

GONADOTROPIN-RELEASING HORMONE

Pharmacologic doses of GnRH analogues are capable of producing luteolysis in normal women and, as with prolactin, research has demonstrated a number of direct inhibitory effects of these substances on the ovary. Most of the experiments have been carried out on rats: Receptors of GnRH have been found in the ovary,[111,112] GnRH agonists block granulosal steroidogenesis in vitro,[113,114] and GnRH itself in vitro inhibits basal and LH-stimulated cAMP accumulation and progesterone secretion by luteal cells.[115] These results have been confirmed by experiments on human granulosa cells in vitro that demonstrate inhibition of progesterone secretion by an agonistic analogue of GnRH in a dose-related manner, beginning at 10^{-10} M concentration.[116] An antagonistic analogue reversed the effect, suggesting competition for a receptor at the cell surfaces. The effect was not observable, however, until the cells had been cultured in the presence of agonist for at least 96 hr. It has been speculated that GnRH-like peptides are normally secreted in the ovary by atretic follicles under the influence of low levels of LH, and the name "gonadocrinin" has been coined for these putative ovarian hormones.[117]

RELAXIN

Discovered by Hisaw 55 years ago as the agent responsible for relaxing the guinea pig symphysis preparatory to parturition, relaxin has been completely characterized chemically in several mammalian species and measured in the circulation by radioimmunoassay.[118] Its function, however, remains unknown. It is a polypeptide molecule of 6000 daltons that strongly resembles insulin and its related compounds, the somatomedins and other growth factors—in vitro it potentiates the action of insulin by increasing the binding of insulin to its receptor. Occasionally detectable by RIA in the serum of nonpregnant women during the luteal phase, relaxin is a hormone of pregnancy that normally becomes detectable by postconception day 14. Administration of hCG to women from day 8–10 of the luteal phase induces relaxin secretion; earlier injection, on day 2–3, is ineffective. The site of its production is the corpus luteum, which as a result must be classified as a polypeptide-secreting as well as a steroidogenic organ (see Chapter 5).

QUESTIONS

1. In the ovary, which of the enzymatic reactions listed below take place?

   a. 3 β-ol steroid dehydrogenase
   b. 18 β-hydroxylase
   c. 20, 22 desmolase
   d. a and c

2. In the adrenal cortex, which of the enzymatic activities listed below take place?

   a. 3 β-ol steroid dehydrogenase
   b. 21 β-hydroxylase
   c. 11 β-hydroxylase
   d. All of the above

3. Which of the following statements appear true?

   a. ACTH stimulates cAMP production in the adrenal cortex.
   b. ACTH stimulates activation of an adrenocortical protein kinase, which, in turn, stimulates a cholesterol esterase.
   c. LH inhibits cAMP production in the ovary.
   d. a and b

4. Aldosterone production in the adrenal cortex is

   a. stimulated by ACTH.
   b. stimulated by reduced serum K$^+$ levels.
   c. inhibited by angiotensin II.
   d. all of the above.

REFERENCES

1. Ryan KJ: The endocrine and neuroendrocine control of reproduction, in Reid, DE, Ryan, KJ, Bernirschke K (eds): *Principles and Management of Human Reproduction.* Philadelphia, Saunders, 1972, pp 1–133
2. Richardson GS: Steroidogenesis, in Sciarra JJ (ed): *Gynecology and Obstetrics,* Vol 5. Hagerstown, MD, Harper & Row, 1984, pp 1–17
3. Gwynne JT, Strauss JF: The role of lipoproteins in steroidogenesis and cholesterol metabolism in steroidogenic glands. *Endocr Rev* 3:299–329, 1982
4. Finkelstein M, Shaefer JM: Inborn errors of steroid biosynthesis. *Physiol Rev* 59:353–406, 1979
5. Ford HC, Engel LL: Purification and properties of the 5-3 beta-hydroxysteroid dehydrogenase-isomerase system of sheep adrenal cortical microsomes. *J Biol Chem* 249:1363–1368, 1974
6. Rybak SM, Ramachandran J: Mechanism of introduction of 5-3 beta-hydroxysteroid dehydrogenase-isomerase activity in rat adrenocortical cells by corticotropin. *Endocrinology* 111:427–433, 1982
7. Goto J, Fishman J: Participation of a nonenzymatic transformation in the biosynthesis of estrogens from androgens. *Science* 195:80–81, 1977
8. Maschler I, Salzberg M, Finkelstein M: 11 beta-Hydroxylase with affinity to C-21 deoxysteroids from ovaries of patients with polycystic ovary syndrome. *J Clin Endocrinol Metab* 41:999–1002, 1975
9. Marieb NJ, Spangler S, Kashgarian MD, et al: Cushing's syndrome secondary to ectopic cortisol production by an ovarian carcinoma. *J Clin Endocrinol Metab* 57:737–740, 1983
10. Todesco S, Terribile V, Borsatti A, et al: Primary aldosteronism due to a malignant ovarian tumor. *J Clin Endocrinol Metab* 41:809–819, 1975
11. Ryan KJ, Engel LL: Hydroxylation of steroids at carbon 21. *J Biol Chem* 225:103–114, 1957
12. Makin HLJ: *Biochemistry of Steroid Hormones.* Oxford, Blackwell, 1975
13. Simpson ER: Cholesterol side chain cleavage, cytochrome P450, and the control of steroidogenesis. *Mol Cell Endocrinol* 13:213–227, 1979
14. Sonino N, Levine LS, Vecsei P, et al: Parallelism of 11 beta- and 18-hydroxylation demonstrated by urinary free hormones in man. *J Clin Endocrinol Metab* 51:557–560, 1980
15. Nelson DH: *The Adrenal Cortex: Physiological Function and Disease,* Philadelphia, Saunders, 1980
16. Brown MS, Kovanen PT, Goldstein JL: Receptor-mediated uptake of lipoprotein-cholesterol and its utilization for steroid synthesis in the adrenal cortex. *Recent Prog Horm Res* 35:215–257, 1979
17. Bernstein S, Solomon S: *Chemical and Biological Aspects of Steroid Conjugation.* New York, Springer-Verlag, 1970
18. Ryan KJ, Tulchinsky D: *Maternal–Fetal Endocrinology.* Philadelphia, Saunders, 1977
19. Peterson RE: Cortisol, in Fuchs F, Klopper A (eds): *Endo-*

crinology of Pregnancy, 2nd ed. Hagerstown, MD, Harper & Row, 1977, pp 157–176

20. DePeretti E, Forest MG: Unconjugated dehydroepiandrosterone plasma levels in normal subjects from birth to adolescence in human: The use of a sensitive radioimmunoassay. *J Clin Endocrinol Metab* 43:982–991, 1976

21. Schiebinger RJ, Albertson BD, Cassoria FC, et al: The developmental changes in plasma adrenal androgens during infancy and adrenarche are associated with changing activities of adrenal microsomal 17-hydroxylase and 17,20-desmolase. *J Clin Invest* 67:1177–1182, 1981

22. Rich BH, Rosenfield RL, Lucky AW, et al: Adrenarche: Changing adrenal response to adrenocorticotropin. *J Clin Endocrinol Metab* 52:1129–1136, 1981

23. Hornsby PJ, Aldern KA: Steroidogenic enzyme activities in cultured human definitive zone adrenocortical cells: Comparison with bovine adrenocortical cells and resultant differences in adrenal androgen biosynthesis. *J Clin Endocrinol Metab* 58:121–127, 1984

24. Parker LN, Lifrak ET, Odell WD: A 60,000 molecular weight human pituitary glycopeptide stimulates adrenal androgen secretion. *Endocrinology* 113:2092–2096, 1983

25. Gill GN: ACTH regulation of the adrenal cortex. *Pharmacol Ther* 2:313, 1976

26. Walsh DA, Ashby CD: Protein kinases: Aspects of their regulation and diversity. *Recent Prog Horm Res* 29:329–359, 1973

27. Veldhuis JD, Klase PA: Mechanisms by which calcium ions regulate the steroidogenic actions of luteinizing hormone in silated ovarian cells in vitro. *Endocrinology* 111:1–6, 1982

28. Carsia RV, Moyle WR, Wolff DJ, et al: Acute inhibition of corticosteroidogenesis by inhibitors of calmodulin action. *Endocrinology* 111:1456–1461, 1982

29. Schulster D, Burnstein S, Cooke BA: *Molecular Endocrinology of the Steroid Hormones*. London, Wiley, 1976

30. Ferenczy A, Richart RM: *Female Reproductive System: Dynamics of Scan and Transmission Electron Microscopy.* New York, Wiley, 1974

31. McNatty KP: Cyclic changes in antral fluid hormone concentrations in humans, in Lipsett MB, Ross GT (eds): *Clinics in Endocrinology and Metabolism*, Vol 7, No 3. Philadelphia, Saunders, 1978, pp 577–600

32. Richardson GS: *Ovarian Physiology*. Boston, Little Brown, 1967

33. Ryan KJ: Ovarian function and gynecologic endocrinopathies. *Int J Gynecol Obstet* 8:608–612, 1970

34. Tsang BK, Armstrong DT, Whitfield JF: Steroid biosynthesis by isolated human ovarian follicular cells in vitro. *J Clin Endocrinol Metab* 51:1407–1411, 1980

35. Tsang BK, Moon YS, Simpson CW, et al: Androgen biosynthesis in human follicles: Cellular source, gonadotropic control and adenosine 3′,5′-monophosphate mediation. *J Clin Endocrinol Metab* 438:153–158, 1979

36. Hillier SG, Reichert LE, Van Hall EV: Control of preovulatory follicular estrogen biosynthesis in human ovary. *J Clin Endocrinol Metab* 52:847–846, 1981

37. Hillier SG, De Zwart FA: Evidence that granulosa cell aromatase induction/activation by follicle-stimulating hormone is an androgen receptor-regulated process in vitro. *Endocrinology* 109:1303–1305, 1981

38. McNatty KP, Makris A, DeGrazia C, et al: The production of progesterone, androgens, and estrogens by granulosa cells, thecal tissue, and stromal tissue from human

ovaries in vitro. *J Clin Endocrinol Metab* 49:687–699, 1979

39. McNatty KP, Makris A, DeGrazia C, et al: Steroidogenesis by recombined follicular cells from the human ovary in vitro. *J Clin Endocrinol Metab* 51:1286–1292, 1980

40. McNatty KP, Hunter WM, MacNeilly AS, et al: Changes in the concentration of pituitary and steroid hormones in the follicular fluid of human Graafian follicles throughout the menstrual cycle. *J Endocrinol* 64:555–571, 1975

41. Marut EL, Huang SC, and Hodgen GD: Distinguishing the steroidogenic roles of granulosa and theca cells of the dominant ovarian follicle and corpus luteum. *J Clin Endocrinol Metab* 57:925–930, 1983

42. Carr BR, Sadler RK, Rochelle DB, et al: Plasma lipoprotein regulation of progesterone biosynthesis by human corpus luteum tissue in organ culture. *J Clin Endocrinol Metab* 52:875–881, 1981

43. Tureck RW, Mastroianni L Jr, Blasco L, Strauss JF: Inhibition of human granulosa cell progesterone secretion by a gonadotropin-releasing agonist. *J Clin Endocrinol Metab* 54:1078–1080, 1982

44. Baker TG: Primordial germ cells; oogenesis and ovulation, in Austin CR, Short RV (eds): *Reproduction in Mammals*. Cambridge, Cambridge University Press, 1972

45. Merrill JA: Morphology of the prepubertal ovary: Relationship to polycystic ovary syndrome. *South Med J* 56:225, 1963

46. Peters H, McNatty KP: *The Ovary. A Correlation of Structure and Function in Mammals.* Berkeley and Los Angeles, University of California Press, 1980, p 108

47. East IJ, Keenan AM, Larson SM, et al: Scintigraphy of normal mouse ovaries with monoclonal antibodies to ZP-2, the major zona pellucida protein. *Science* 225:938–941, 1984

48. Erickson GF: Normal ovarian function. *Clin Obstet Gynecol* 21:31–52, 1978

49. Bode HH, Bercu BB, Beitins IZ, et al: Intracranial hCG secreting tumor in a prepubertal girl. *Pediatr Res* 10:336, 1976

50. Sklar CA, Conte FA, Kaplan SL, et al: Human chorionic gonadotropin-secreting pineal tumor: Relation to pathogenesis and sex limitation of sexual precocity. *J Clin Endocrinol Metab* 53:656–660, 1981

51. McNatty KP, Smith DM, Makris A, et al: The microenvironment of the human andral follicle: Interrelationships among the steroid levels in antral fluid, the population of granulosa cells, and the status of the oocyte in vivo and in vitro. *J Clin Endocrinol Metab* 49:851–860, 1979

52. DiZerega GS, Hodgen GD: Folliculogenesis in the primate ovarian cycle. *Endocr Rev* 2:27–49, 1981

53. DiZerega GS, Hodgen GD: The intraovarian progesterone gradient: A spatial and temporal regulator of folliculogenesis in the primate ovarian cycle. *J Clin Endocrinol Metab* 54:495–499, 1982

54. DiZerega GS, Hodgen GD: Cessation of folliculogenesis during the primate luteal phase. *J Clin Endocrinol Metab* 51:158–160, 1980

55. McNatty KP, Hillier SG, Can den Boogaard AMJ, et al: Follicular development during the luteal phase of the human menstrual cycle. *J Clin Endocrinol Metab* 56:1022–1031, 1983

56. Zeleznik AF, Wildt L, Schuler HM: Characterization of ovarian folliculogenesis during the luteal phase of the menstrual cycle in rhesus monkeys using ^{3}H-thymidine autoradiography. *Endocrinology* 107:982–988, 1980

57. Koehring MJ: Cyclic changes in ovarian morphology during the menstrual cycle in Macaca mulatta. *Am J Anat* 126:73–101, 1969

58. Laufer N, DeCherney AH, Haseltine FP, et al: Steroid secretion by the human egg–corona–cumulus complex in culture. *J Clin Endocrinol Metab* 58:1153–1157, 1984

59. Bradbury, JT: Direct action of estrogen on the ovary of the immature rat. *Endocrinology* 68:115–120, 1961

60. Goldenberg RL, Reiter EO, and Ross GT: Follicle response to exogenous gonadotropins: An estrogen-mediated phenomenon. *Fertil Steril* 24:121–125, 1973

61. Goldenberg RL, Vaitukaitis JL, Ross GT: Estrogen and FSH interactions on follicle growth in rats. *Endocrinology* 90:1492–1498, 1972

62. Richard JS: Hormonal control of ovarian follicular development: A 1978 perspective. *Recent Prog Horm Res* 35:343–373, 1979

63. Lostroh AJ, Johnson RE: Amounts of interstitial cell-stimulating hormone and follicle-stimulating hormone required for follicular development, uterine growth and ovulation in the hypophysectomized rat. *Endocrinology* 79:991–996, 1966

64. Jewelewicz R, Warren M, Dyrenfurth I, et al: Physiological studies with purified human pituitary FSH. *J Clin Endocrinol Metab* 32:688–691, 1971

65. Richards JS, Midgley AR Jr: Protein hormone action: A key to understanding ovarian and follicular luteal cell development. *Biol Reprod* 14:82–94, 1976

66. Richards JS, Bogovich K: Effects of hCG and progesterone on follicular development in the immature rat. *J Clin Endocrinol Metab* 111:1429–1438, 1982

67. Louvet JP, Harman SM, Ross GT: Effects of hCG, hICSH and hFSH on ovarian weights in estrogen-primed hypophysectomized immature rats. *Endocrinology* 96:1179–1186, 1975

68. Louvet JP, Harman SM, Ross GT: Evidence for a role of androgens in follicular maturation. *Endocrinology* 97:366–372, 1975

69. Ross GT, Cargille CM, Lipsett MB, et al: Pituitary and gonadal hormones in women during spontaneous and induced ovulatory cycles. *Recent Prog Horm Res* 26:1–62, 1970

70. DiZerega GS, Nixon WE, Hodgen GD: Intercycle serum follicle-stimulating hormone elevations: Significance in recruitment and selection of the dominant follicle and assessment of corpus luteum normalcy. *J Clin Endocrinol Metab* 50:1046–1048, 1980

71. Hoff JD, Quigley ME, Yen SSC: Hormonal dynamics at midcycle: A reevaluation. *J Clin Endocrinol Metab* 57:792–796, 1983

72. Liu JH, Yen SSC: Induction of midcycle gonadotropin surge by ovarian steroids in women: A critical evaluation. *J Clin Endocrinol Metab* 57:797–802, 1983

73. WHO Task Force: Temporal relationships between ovulation and defined changes in the concentration of plasma estradiol-17 beta, luteinizing hormone, follicle-stimulating hormone, and progesterone. *Am J Obstet Gynecol* 183:383–895, 1980

74. LeMaire WJ, Clar MR, March JM: Biochemical mechanism of ovulation, in Hafez ESE (ed) *Human Ovulation*. Amsterdam, Elsevier/North-Holland, 1979, pp 159–175

75. Owman C, Sjoberg NO, Wallach EE, et al: Neuromuscular mechanisms of ovulation, in Hafez ESE (ed): *Human Ovulation*. Amsterdam, Elsevier/North-Holland, 1979, pp 57–100

76. Strickland S, Beers WH: Studies on the role of plasminogen activator in ovulation. *J Biol Chem* 21:5694–5702, 1976

77. Clark MR: Stimulation of progesterone and prostaglandin E accumulation by LHRH and LHRH analogs in rat granulosa cells. *Endocrinology* 110:146–152, 1982

78. Espey LL: Ovulation as an inflammatory reaction: A hypothesis. *Biol Reprod* 22:73–106, 1980

79. Gospodarowicz D, Thakral KK: Production of a corpus luteum angiogenic factor responsible for proliferation of capillaries and neovascularization of corpus luteum. *Proc Natl Acad Sci USA* 75:847–851, 1978

80. Koos RD, LeMaire WJ: Evidence for an angiogenic factor from rat follicles, in Greenwald, GS, Terranova PF (eds): *Factors Regulating Ovarian Function*. New York, Raven, 1983, pp 191–195

81 Zuckerman S, Weir BJ: *The Ovary* (3 vols). New York, Academic, 1977

82. Wardlaw S, Lauersen NH, Saxena BB: The LH–hCG receptor of the human ovary at various stages of the menstrual cycle. *Acta Endocrinol (Copenh)* 79:568–576, 1975

83. McNeilly AS, Sharpe RM, Fraser HM, et al: Changes in the binding of hCG/LH, FSH, and prolactin to human corpora lutea during the menstrual cycle and pregnancy. *J Endocrinol* 87:315–325, 1980

84. Van de Wiele RL, Bogumil J, Dyrenfurth I, et al: Mechanisms regulating the menstrual cycle in women. *Recent Prog Horm Res* 26:65–104, 1970

85. Balmaceda JP, Borghi MR, Coy DH, et al: Suppression of postovulatory gonadotropin levels does not affect corpus luteum function in rhesus monkeys. *J Clin Endocrinol Metab* 57:866–868, 1983

86. Knobil E: On the regulation of the primate corpus luteum. *Biol Reprod* 8:246, 1973

87. Schoonmaker JN, Bergman KS, Steiner RA, et al: Estradiol-induced luteal regression in the rhesus monkey: Evidence for an extraovarian site of action. *Endocrinology* 110:1708–1715, 1982

88. Sotrel L, Helvacioslu A, Dowers S, et al: Mechanisms of luteolysis: Effect of estradiol and prostaglandin $F_{2\alpha}$ on corpus luteum LH/hCG receptors and cyclic nucleotides in the rhesus monkey. *Am J Obstet Gynecol* 139:134–140, 1981

89. Ottobre JS, Stouffer, RL: Persistent versus transient stimulation of the macaque corpus luteum during prolonged exposure to human chorionic gonadotropin: A function of age of the corpus luteum. *Endocrinology* 114:2175–2182, 1984

90. Yoshimi T, Strott CA, Marshall JR, et al: Corpus luteum function in early pregnancy. *J Clin Endocrinol Metab* 29:225–230, 1969

91. Tulchinsky D, Hobel CJ: Plasma hCG, estrone, estradiol, estriol, progesterone and 17 alpha-hydroxyprogesterone in human pregnancy. III. Early normal pregnancy. *Am J Obstet Gynecol* 117:884–893, 1973

92. Thau S, Seidman LS, Brook J, et al: Human chorionic gonadotropin maintains plasma progesterone at pregnancy levels in rhesus monkeys. *Endocrinology* 101:704–707, 1981

93. Channing CP, Anderson LD, Hoover DJ, et al: The role of nonsteroidal regulators in control of oocyte and follicular maturation. *Recent Prog Horm Res* 38:331–408, 1982

94. Hillensjo T, Chari S, Nilsson L, et al: Inhibition of progesterone secretion in cultured human granulosa cells by a

low molecular weight fraction of human follicular fluid. *J Clin Endocrinol Metab* 56:835–838, 1983

95. Dizerega GS, Hodge GD: The primate ovarian cycle: Suppression of hMG induced follicular growth. *J Clin Endocrinol Metab* 50:819–825, 1980
96. Dizerega GS, Goebelsmann U, Nakamura RM: Identification of protein(s) secreted by the preovulatory ovary with suppress follicle response to gonadotropins. *J Clin Endocrinol Metab* 54:1091–1096, 1982
97. Dizerega GS, Marrs RP, Roche PC, et al: Identification of protein(s) in pooled human follicular fluid which suppress follicular response to gonadodotropins. *J Clin Endocrinol Metab* 56:35–41, 1983
98. Dizerega GS, Marrs RP, Campeau JD, et al: Human granulosa cell secretion of protein(s) which suppress follicular response to gonadotropins. *J Clin Endocrinol Metab* 56:147–155, 1983
99. Montz FJ, Vjita EL, Campeau JD, et al: Inhibition of LH/hCG binding to porcine granulosa cells by a follicular fluid protein(s). *Am J Obstet Gynecol* 148:436–441, 1984
100. Dizerega GS, Campeau JD, Lobo RA, et al: Activity of a human follicular fluid protein(s) during normal and stimulated ovarian cycles. *J Clin Endocrinol Metab* 57:838–846, 1983
101. Dizerega GS, Wilks JF: Inhibition of the primate ovarian cycle by a porcine follicular fluid protein. *Fertil Steril* 41:635–638, 1984
102. Channing CP, Liu CQ, Jones GS, et al: Decline of follicular oocyte maturation inhibitor coincident with maturation and achievement of fertilizability of oocytes recovered at midcycle of gonadotropin-treated women. *Proc Natl Acad Sci USA* 80:4184–4188, 1983
103. Dizerega GS, Turner CK, Stougger RL, et al: Suppression of FSH dependent folliculogenesis during the primate ovarian cycle. *J Clin Endocrinol Metab* 52:451–456, 1981
104. Tanabe K, Gagliano P, Channing CP, et al: Levels of inhibin F activity and steroids in human follicular fluid from normal women and women with polycystic ovarina disease. *J Clin Endocrinol Metab* 57:24–31, 1982
105. Weiss G, Dierschke DJ, Karsh FJ, et al: The influence of lactation on function in the rhesus monkey. *Endocrinology* 93:954–959, 1973
106. Richardson DW, Goldsmith LT, Pohl CR, et al: The role of prolactin in the regulation of the primate corpus luteum. *J Clin Endocrinol Metab* 60:501–504, 1985
107. Mroueh AM, Siler Khodr TM: Ovarian refractoriness to gonadotropins in cases of inappropriate lactation: Restoration of ovarian function with bromocryptine. *J Clin Endocrinol Metab* 43:1398–1401, 1976
108. Demura M, Ono M, Demura H: Prolactin directly inhibits basal as well as gonadotropin-stimulated secretion of progesterone and 17 beta-estradiol in the human ovary. *J Clin Endocrinol Metab* 54:1246–1250, 1982

109. Hamada Y, Schlaff S, Kobayashi Y, et al: Inhibitory effect of prolactin on ovulation in the in vitro perfused rabbit ovary. *Nature (Lond)* 285:161–163, 1980
110. Laufer N, Botero-Ruiz W, DeCherney AH, et al: Gonadotropin and prolactin levels in follicular fluid in human ova successfully fertilized in vitro. *J Clin Endocrinol Metab* 58:430–434, 1984
111. Clayton RN, Harwood JP, Catt KJ: Gonadotropin-releasing hormone analogue binds to luteal cells and inhibits progesterone production. *Nature (Lond)* 280:90, 1979
112. Reeves JJ, Sequin C, Lefebre FA, et al: Similar luteinizing hormone releasing hormone binding sites in rat anterior pituitary and ovary. *Proc Natl Acad Sci USA* 77:5567, 1980
113. Behrman HR, Preston SL, Hall AK: Cellular mechanism of antigonadotropic action of LHRH in the corpus luteum. *Endocrinology* 107:656–664. 1980
114. Magoffin DA, Reynolds DS, Erickson GF: Director inhibitory effect of GnRH on androgen secretion by ovarian interstitial cells. *Endocrinology* 109:661–663, 1981
115. Hsueh AJW, Wang C, Erickson CF: Direct inhibitory effect of gonadotropin-releasing hormone on follicle stimulating hormone induction of luteinizing hormone receptor and aromatase activity in rat granulosa cells. *Endocrinology* 106:1697–1705, 1980
116. Turek RW, Mastroianni L Jr, Blasco L, et al: Inhibition of human granulosa cell progesterone secretion by a gonadotropin-releasing agonist. *J Clin Endocrinol Metab* 54:1078–1080, 1982
117. Ying SY, Guillemin R: Gonadocrinins: Peptides in ovarian follicular fluids stimulating the secretion of pituitary gonadotropins. *Proceedings of the Sixty-Second Annual Meeting of the Endocrine Society, Washington DC*, 1979 p 158, abst
118. Weiss G: Relaxin. *Annu Rev Physiol* 46:43–52, 1984
119. Ross GT, Vande Wiele RL: The ovaries, in Williams RH (ed.): *Textbook of Endocrinology*, 5th Ed. Philadelphia, Saunders, 1974

ANSWERS

1. d

2. d

3. d

4. a

5

Physiology of Relaxin

GERSON WEISS

INTRODUCTION

During the 1920s, Hisaw[1] determined that there are three active principles in the ovary, which he named theelin, folliculin, and relaxin. Theelin has since been renamed estrogen, and folliculin has been renamed progesterone. The third substance, a water-soluble factor that could cause interpubic ligament formation in estrogen-primed guinea pigs, thus "relaxing" the pelvis, was named relaxin, a name maintained to the present. Research in the physiology of relaxin has been hampered by the fact that, until recently, technology to characterize, purify, and measure relaxin in humans was not available. During the 1950s, clinical studies were performed using impure, relaxin-containing extracts of pregnant sow ovaries containing variable and sometimes minimal amounts of relaxin. Since the preparations varied, the study results varied and results could not be repeated. During the 1970s the structure of relaxin was determined and sensitive radioimmunoassays (RIAs) were developed, permitting reproducible physiologic studies.

GERSON WEISS • Department of Obstetrics and Gynecology, University of Medicine and Dentistry of New Jersey–New Jersey Medical School, Newark, New Jersey 07103.

STRUCTURE

Relaxin is a basic peptide hormone weighing approximately 6000 daltons. The hormone consists of two dissimilar peptide chains linked by disulfide bridges. There is significant structural homology to insulin, the somatomedins, and nerve growth factor. While relaxin and insulin have almost identical three-dimentional structure, they do not share biologic activity.[2] There is less than 25% amino acid homology between relaxin and insulin. Unlike insulin, the amino acid sequence of relaxin is poorly conserved across species lines.[3] The known relaxin structures—those in pig, rat, human, and shark—have less than 50% amino acid homology.[4]

SPECIES SPECIFICITY

While relaxin is detectable in the circulation of mammals during pregnancy, the secretory patterns vary widely. The major source of circulating relaxin is the corpus luteum in rats, pigs, cows, and primates. The endometrium produces relaxin in the guinea pig, and the placenta is the major source of relaxin in the pregnant mare.

Relaxin-mediated interpubic ligament formation is important for parturition in the mouse and guinea pig but not in the rat or primate. Relaxin is obligatory for cervical ripening and dilation in the pig and rat.[5] There is no clear analogy for this in women.

MEASUREMENT OF RELAXIN

The classic bioassay for relaxin is the guinea pig pubic symphysis palpation assay. This assay is based on the induction of pubic symphysis relaxation by relaxin in estrogen primed guinea pigs. The scoring involves subjective manipulation of the pubic symphysis. This is the most specific bioassay. Several laboratories use the mouse pubic symphysis direct-measurement assay. This less expensive assay is not as specific as the guinea pig assay. Relaxins from various species do not necessarily show parallel activity in a given assay, suggesting different potencies.[6]

Relaxin inhibits myometrial contractions in all mammals studied. This inhibition has been used as a bioassay. There is as yet no species specific radioimminoassay for human relaxin. However, human relaxin cross-reacts significantly with several anti-porcine relaxin antibodies. This has been used as the basis for a currently used radioimmunoassay for human relaxin.

SOURCES OF RELAXIN IN THE HUMAN FEMALE

The corpus luteum of pregnancy is the major source of relaxin in human pregnancy.[7] This organ accounts for all the measurable circulating relaxin. Luteectomy in pregnancy results in a prompt fall in circulating relaxin.[8] Relaxin is present in high (μg/g) tissue concentrations in the corpus luteum of pregnancy.[9] Relaxin is also found in the corpus luteum of the nonpregnant state, but in concentrations one to two orders of magnitude lower than in the corpus luteum of pregnancy.

Relaxin has been found in low (ng/g) concentrations in placenta, myometrium, and decidua. Low concentrations have also been noted in other tissues during pregnancy. It is not as yet clear whether decidual and placental relaxin is a luteal product in the blood of these other tissues and/or membrane-bound on the cells of these tissues. It is possible that low concentrations of relaxin are produced locally. This is an important point to differentiate since human pregnancy can be maintained after the mid-first trimester in the absence of the corpus luteum. If relaxin is only luteal then it is difficult to see how it

could have a significant role in later pregnancy. If it is produced locally then it may have a major role in pregnancy maintenance even in the absence of the corpus luteum.[6]

RELAXIN IN THE NONPREGNANT STATE

Relaxin is occasionally detected in the circulation in the luteal phase of nonpregnant women. It has also been found in breast cyst fluid of nonpregnant women. Thomas et al.[10] detected relaxin in the peritoneal fluid during the mid-luteal phase in nonpregnant women; they postulated that relaxin may have uterine activity even before it is found in the circulation during early pregnancy, by direct uterine transport from peritoneal fluid. Acute treatment with gonadotropin-releasing hormone (GnRH) can increase levels of circulating relaxin in nonpregnant luteal-phase women. Quagliarello et al.[11] showed that human chorionic gonadotropin (hCG) given on days 8–10 of the luteal phase is capable of inducing relaxin secretion. Although this treatment produces an abrupt rise in serum progesterone concentrations, relaxin does not become detectable for 2–6 days afterwards. Levels of serum progesterone fall, while relaxin levels rise, suggesting different control mechanisms of the hormones even though their secretion is stimulated by the same exogenous stimulus.

The timing of the hCG injections is critical to relaxin secretion. When the hCG injections were given on days 2–3 of the luteal phase, no relaxin secretion was detectable. In studies in which hCG was used to induce ovulation after human menopausal gonadotropin was given to mature a follicle, relaxin was undetected in the luteal phase. However, if these women conceived during the treatment cycle, then relaxin was detected at the time of the missed menses. This is presumably due to endogenous luteal stimulation from the blastocyst. Since hCG stimulus was given in all these experiments but the response was variable, it appears that appropriate ovarian conditions are necessary for relaxin secretion. Constant doses of hCG are not capable of maintaining relaxin secretion in the nonpregnant state for more than 2 weeks.

RELAXIN AND PREGNANCY

Relaxin is detectable in serum by the time of the missed menses. Levels rapidly rise and concentra-

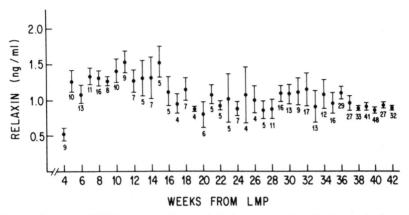

FIGURE 5-1. Relaxin levels (mean ±SEM) in women with normal singleton pregnancies. Numbers under data points indicate the number of women sampled during that week of pregnancy. Reprinted with permission from the American College of Obstetricians and Gynecologists (Obstetrics and Gynecology, 59: 167–170, 1982).

tions in both serum and the corpus luteum are highest in the first trimester of pregnancy. By the end of the first trimester of pregnancy, the serum levels have fallen by approximately 20%. Concentrations then remain stable throughout pregnancy (Fig. 5-1). There appears to be no diurnal variation in serum relaxin concentrations. There is no prelabor elevation in serum relaxin in women, as there is in pigs and rodents. Labor does not elevate relaxin. Levels fall after delivery and are undetectable within a few days. hCG can increase relaxin secretion from the postpartum corpus luteum. Nursing does not prolong relaxin secretion, suggesting that prolactin is not luteotropic in the puerperium.

The human pregnancy corpus luteum, rescued by hCG in the late luteal phase of pregnancy cycles, is present and active throughout pregnancy. It secretes progesterone throughout pregnancy. Progesterone, however, cannot be used as a luteal marker in pregnancy, since most circulating progesterone in human pregnancy is placental in origin. Since virtually all circulating relaxin is derived from the corpus luteum, it can serve a number of luteal functions throughout pregnancy. Oxytocin, or prostaglandins E_2 and $F_{2\alpha}$ in doses adequate to produce labor, do not affect relaxin levels in serum. These agents are thus not acutely luteolytic in human pregnancy.

Relaxin concentrations in serum seem related to the amount of luteal tissue present in an individual. When multiple corpora lutea are present, as in multiple pregnancies, there is a tendency for higher circulating relaxin concentrations to be present. Relaxin concentrations are normal in toxemic pregnancy but tend to be low in both postmature pregnancies and women in premature labor.

ROLE OF RELAXIN IN WOMEN

The physiology of relaxin in women has not been well understood since the hormone has only recently been measurable and no human hormone is as yet available for study.

Human relaxin decreases the amplitude of spontaneous human myometrial contractions in vitro.[12] Progesterone, which alone has little effect on this system, synergizes with relaxin in this action. Doses of relaxin and progesterone, which are ineffective independent together inhibit myometrial contraction amplitude.[13] Since relaxin and progesterone are both luteal products, and the corpus luteum is necessary for maintenance of early pregnancy, it is likely that these hormones act in concert physiologically in the maintenance of human pregnancy. In fact, the secretion pattern of relaxin, its human myometrial actions, and the necessity of the corpus luteum in maintaining early human pregnancy suggest that the major actions of relaxin in women occur at the beginning of pregnancy.

A mechanism of action of relaxin on myometrial activity has been suggested by Nishikori et al.[14] These workers showed that myosin light-chain kinase activity, myosin light-chain phosphorylation, and calcium activated ATPase activity were decreased by relaxin.

While relaxin is responsible for cervical softening, ripening, and dilatation in several subprimate species, there is no evidence that relaxin is physiologically involved in human cervical ripening. However, several groups have used pharmacologic doses of porcine relaxin to aid in cervical ripening and advancement of the Bishop score in women.[15]

Other actions of relaxin seen in experimental animals have not been as yet looked for in women. In rodents, the mammary gland is a target organ for relaxin. Uterine weight, glycogen, and nitrogen content were increased by relaxin in experimental animals.[5] In rats, relaxin increases the binding of insulin to its receptor and increases glucose uptake in adipocytes. This suggests a role for relaxin is making cells more sensitive to the effects of insulin, countering the diabetogenic effects of pregnancy.

RELAXIN IN THE MALE

Relaxin has not been found in the circulation in men. Relaxin is present, however, in seminal plasma in concentrations one to two orders of magnitude higher than contained in pregnancy serum. Relaxin is produced in the prostate. It is found in high concentrations in the seminal plasma of men with congenital absence of the vas deferens and seminal vesicles. Relaxin is present in higher concentrations in the first part of the ejaculate. Relaxin affects sperm motility and attenuates the loss of motility seen over time in washed human sperm. Relaxin augments the penetration of sperm into cervical mucus. Relaxin antisera immobilize human sperm but this action can be blocked by excess relaxin.[16] Antibodies to insulin, also found in seminal plasma, do not affect sperm motility. These data suggest that relaxin may have an important role in sperm motility and penetration of sperm into the female reproductive tract. Relaxin, an exocrine male secretion, and an endocrine female hormone may thus facilitate fertility.

FUTURE TRENDS

The previous decade saw major advances in understanding the chemistry of relaxin. Sensitive radioimmunoassays permitted descriptions of the secretion patterns of relaxin in several species. It is likely that technical advances in the near future will provide significant quantities of human relaxin as well as monoclonal antibodies to various relaxins. These tools will clarify the physiologic roles of relaxin, elucidate its mechanisms of action, and en-

able testing of human relaxin as a potentially useful pharmacologic agent.

SUMMARY

Relaxin is a peptide product of the pregnancy corpus luteum. The stimulus for relaxin secretion is chorionic gonadotropin. Relaxin is detectable in serum throughout pregnancy, but its greatest concentration is in the first trimester. The physiologic action of relaxin in human pregnancy has not been determined. It is known, however, that relaxin inhibits myometrial contractions and may affect cervical ripening. Relaxin is also present in semen plasma; relaxin augments sperm motility.

ACKNOWLEDGMENT. This work was supported in part by grant HD 12395 from the National Institutes of Health.

QUESTIONS

1. To what substances is relaxin structurally related?

2. What is the secretion pattern of relaxin during human pregnancy?

3. What are some actions of relaxin?

4. What are some sources of relaxin?

REFERENCES

 1. Hisaw FL: Experimental relaxation of the pubic ligament of the guinea pig. *Proc Soc Exp Biol Med* 23:661–663, 1928
 2. Steinetz BG, Schwabe C, Weiss G (eds): Relaxin: Structure, function and evolution. *Ann NY Acad Sci* 380, 1982
 3. John MJ, Borjesson BW, Walsh JR, et al: Limited sequence homology between porcine and rat relaxins: Implications for physiological studies. *Endocrinology* 108:726–729, 1981
 4. Hudson P, Haley J, John M, et al: Structure of a genomic clone encoding biologically active human relaxin. *Nature (Lond)* 301:628–631, 1983
 5. Schwabe C, Steinetz BG, Weiss G, et al: Relaxin. *Recent Prog Horm Res* 34:123–211, 1978.*
 6. Bigazzi M, Greenwood FC, Gasparri F (eds): *Biology of Relaxin and Its Role in the Human. International Congress Series No. 610.* Excerpta Medica, Amsterdam
 7. Weiss G, O'Byrne EM, Steinetz BG: Relaxin: A product of the human corpus luteum of pregnancy. *Science* 194:948–949, 1976
 8. Weiss G, Byrne EM, Hochman JH, et al: Secretion of progesterone and relaxin by the human corpus luteum at midpregnancy and at term. *Obstet Gynecol* 50:679–681, 1977

*Review article or chapter.

9. O'Byrne EM, Flitcraft JF, Sawyer WI, et al: Relaxin bioactivity and immunoactivity in the human corpora lutea. *Endocrinology* 102:1641–1644, 1978

10. Thomas K, Loumaye E, Donnez J: Immunoreactive relaxin in the peritoneal fluid during spontaneous menstrual cycle in women. *Ann NY Acad Sci* 380:126–130, 1982

11. Quagliarello J, Goldsmith L, Steinetz B, et al: Induction of relaxin secretion in nonpregnant women by human chorionic gonadotropin. *J Clin Endocrinol Metab* 51:74–77, 1980

11a. Szlachter BN, Quagliarello J, Jewelewicz R, et al: Relaxin in normal and pathogenic pregnancies. *Obstet Gynecol* 59:167–170, 1982

12. Szlachter N, O'Byrne EM, Goldsmith L, et al: Myometrial-inhibiting activity of relaxin containing extracts of human corpora lutea of pregnancy. *Am J Obstet Gynecol* 136:584–586, 1980

13. Sarosi P, Schmidt CL, Essig M, et al: The effect of relaxin and progesterone on rat uterine contractions. *Am J Obstet Gynecol* 145:402–405, 1983

14. Nishikori K, Weisbrodt NW, Sherwood OD, et al: Relaxin alters rat uterine myosin light chain phosphorylation and related enzymatic activities. *Endocrinology* 111:1743–1745, 1982.

15. MacLennan AH, Green RC, Bryant-Greenwood GD: Ripening of the human cervix and induction of labor with purified porcine relaxin. *Lancet* 1:220–223, 1980

16. Sarosi P, Schoenfeld C, Berman J, et al: Effect of anti-relaxin antiserum on sperm motility in vitro. *Endocrinology* 112:1860–1861, 1983

ANSWERS

1. Relaxin is structurally related to insulin, the somatomedins, and nerve growth factor.

2. Relaxin is present in serum from the time of the missed period. It is highest in first trimester then declines by 20% and is stable throughout the duration of the pregnancy.

3. Relaxin inhibits myometrial contractions, causes ripening of the pregnant cervix at term, and augments sperm motility.

4. The corpus luteum of pregnancy is the major source of circulating relaxin in women. Relaxin may also be produced by decidua. In the male there is evidence that the prostate produces relaxin.

Normal Growth and Development of the Female

RAPHAEL JEWELEWICZ and BARBARA SHORTLE

INTRODUCTION

Growth and development is a continuous process that begins at the moment of conception, accelerates during the antenatal period, continues rapidly during infancy and then through childhood and puberty. During puberty, the secondary sexual characteristics appear and mature, the adolescent growth spurt takes place, fertility is attained, and significant physical, psychological, and behavioral changes occur, transforming the child into an adult.

Although the mechanisms that control the onset of puberty in humans are complex and not completely understood, development of specific and sensitive hormone assays during the past two decades have made possible studies in human subjects that provide new insight into the dynamics and interrelationships of the various hormones that regulate hypothalamic, pituitary, and gonadal function from early fetal life to adulthood. This chapter traces the development of neuroendocrine function in relationship to growth and sexual maturation of the female.

RAPHAEL JEWELEWICZ and BARBARA SHORTLE • Department of Obstetrics and Gynecology, Columbia University, College of Physicians and Surgeons, New York, New York 10032.

DEVELOPMENT OF THE SEXUALLY UNDIFFERENTIATED EMBRYO

After penetration of the oocyte by sperm, the fertilized ovum undergoes mitosis, yielding two blastomeres with a diploid amount of DNA in their nuclei. Mitotic division of blastomeres continues until the blastocyst stage is reached. This important entity has two cellular compartments: (1) the trophoblast, which eventually gives rise to the chorion (placenta); and (2) the internal embryoblast, which gives rise to the yolk sac, amniotic sac, and embryo. From a new study of 417 preimplantation embryos in an in vitro fertilization program, Edwards et al.[1] found that many embryos are in the two-cell stage by 28 hr, the four-cell stage by 43 hr, and the eight-cell stage by 54 hr after insemination, respectively. The mean doubling time of cells is 15.82 hr. The blastocyst begins to form 4–5 days after fertilization. Table 6-1 calculates mean midstage times.

Immediately after implantation, a series of cellular migrations and alterations begin in the embryo that are essential for the normal differentiation of the organism. At 2 weeks of age, the conceptus consists of a two-layered trophoblast surrounding a mass of primary mesoderm. Within the mesoderm, there are two cavities, that is, the primitive amniotic

TABLE 6-1. Estimates of Time (in Hours) from
Insemination to Attain Specified Stages of Development[a]

Cell stage	Estimate of midpoint of cleavage stages (±SE)	Upper 95% point of distribution[c]
2-cell	33.2 ± 1.3	47
4-cell	49.0 ± 1.3	63
8-cell	64.8 ± 1.8	84
16-cell	80.7 ± 2.4	106
Morula[b]	96.8 ± 4.9	115
Early blastocyst	112.7 ± 2.9	130

[a]From Edwards et al.[1]

[b]Estimates for the 2-, 4-, 8-, and 16-cell stages were obtained from the
exponential growth curves; those for morula and early blastocyst, by
direct computation.

[c]These figures give the estimated time from insemination by which 95%
of the embryos will have attained the specified stage.

cavity and the cavity of the yolk sac. The embryo
lies as a two-layered disc between these two cavities. A number of invaginations appear in the primary mesoderm, merging and forming the first
coelomic cavity. At the same time, part of the primary mesoderm at the posterior end of the embryo
condenses to form the body stalk that will connect
the embryo and the placenta. At this stage, the anterior and posterior ends of the embryo can be distinguished. During the third week, ectodermal cells
near the midline of the posterior half of the embryonic disc divide rapidly, forming a linear structure,
which is the primitive streak. From this streak, the
cells migrate out between the ectodermal and endo-
dermal layers, forming a trilaminar embryo. The
embryonic disc, which was initially round, elon-
gates. A portion of the ectoderm thickens to form
the neural plate and the edges of the neural plate
bend dorsally to form the neural folds. The mesoderm along the neural folds thickens and undergoes
segmentation to form the somites of the body. The
embryo folds on itself, that is, the head and tail ends
bend toward each other, with the yolk sac gradually
pinched off from the gut but remaining connected
by the yolk stalk. Swellings called blood islands
appear in the primary mesoderm around the yolk
sac and give rise to the vascular system. While the
neural folds join to form the neural tube, cells from
their lateral margins form the neural crest from
which cells migrate ventrally to form the sympathetic ganglia. Other cells migrate from the neural crest to form the adrenal medulla. By 3½ weeks,
the human embryo has a cylindrical body attached
to the yolk sac at midpoint. The neural groove is

closed, the neural crests are apparent, pharyngeal
pouches are forming, and the thyroid diverticulum
is present. The lung and liver buds are also present,
the heart tubes fuse and begin to pulsate, and the
embryonic coelom is lined with mesoderm. Within
the following few weeks all the organ systems proceed to develop rapidly. At 4 weeks, the mesonephric tubules (also known as wolffian ducts) are
rapidly differentiating and projecting into the coelom on either side as a ridge beside the mesentery.
The most caudal portion of these ducts develop into
the metanephros and eventually become the kidney
and ureter. Alongside the mesonephros, another
pair of ducts develop independently, the para-
mesonephric or mullerian ducts which, in the
female, will become the fallopian tubes, uterus and
upper two-thirds of the vagina. Over the mesonephros there is a fold of peritoneum that becomes
fibrous in its caudal end and forms the inguinal
ligament of the mesonephros, while its upper portion becomes the round ligament of the uterus. This
is the anatomic state in the sexually undifferentiated
embryo around the sixth to seventh week after nidation. A timetable of events is presented in Table
6-2.

Sex is determined at the time of fertilization, but
the embryonic gonads play an essential role in the
sexual differentiation of the fetus. By castrating
rabbit fetuses prior to sexual differentiation, Jost[2]
showed in a series of classical experiments that all
the newborns were phenotypic females irrespective
of the genetic sex. Except for the absence of
gonads, the fetuses had normal female external and
internal genitalia. These studies established that
male-type differentiation requires fetal testicular
activity, while female-type differentiation may be
independent of hormonal influence and does not
require endocrine activity of the ovary. There is
considerable clinical evidence in humans confirming Jost's observations. Thus, in the absence of
functioning embryonic testes and whether or not
ovaries are present, the embryo will develop into a
phenotypic female.

DEVELOPMENT OF THE FEMALE FETUS

External Genitalia

The external genitalia develop in connection with
the genital tubercle, a conical prominence caudal to
the umbilical cord that appears around the fifth

TABLE 6-2. Timetable and Staging of Human Prenatal Development[a]

Period	Age[b] (days)	Length (mm)	External characteristics
Embryonal			
Blastogenesis	0–2	0.2	Unicellular (fertilized oocyte)
	2–4	0.2	Blastomeric (16–20 blastomeres, morula)
	4–6	0.4	Blastodermic (blastocyst)
			Bilaminar embryo stage (round-shaped embryonic disc)
	6–15	0.1	Bilaminar plate
			Primary yolk sac
		0.2–0.4	Secondary yolk sac
			Trilaminar embryo stage (pear-shaped embryonic disc)
	15–17	0.4–1.0	With primitive streak
	17–20	1.0–2.0	With notochordal process
Early organogenesis			Early somite stage (shoe-sole-shaped embryo)
	20–21	1.5–2.0	Completely open neural groove
	21–26	1.5–4.0	Neural tube closing, both ends open
	26–30	3–5	One or both neuropores closed
			Stage of limb development (C-shaped embryo)
	28–32	4–6	Bud of proximal extremity
	31–35	5–8	Buds of proximal and distal extremities
	35–38	7–10	Proximal extremity, two segments
	37–42	8–12	Proximal and distal extremity, two segments
	42–44	10–14	Digital rays, foot plates
	44–51	13–21	Digital tubercles
	51–53	19–24	Digits, toe tubercles; late embryonal stage (embryo with differentiated extremities including fingers and toes)
	52–56	22–25	Eyes open
	56–60	27–35	Fusing eyelids
Fetal	60–182+	31–200	Fetus with fused eyelids
Perinatal	170–266+	201–350	Third-trimester fetus (newborn with open eyes)

[a]Adopted partly from Jirásek.[74]
[b]Age from conception.

week. About 6–7 weeks the tubercle becomes clearly defined as a phallus, but the specific external genitalia of either sex are not formed until the tenth week. The cloacal membrane is an epithelial structure in the ventral portion of the embryo, caudal to the genital tubercle. The embryonic cloaca is divided into two sinuses by a urogenital fold that will become part of the perineum. The cloacal membrane will split so that the anal part will connect with the rectum, the ventral part will be incorporated with the lower part of the bladder to form the urethra, and the dorsal part will join with the caudal end of the fused mullerian ducts to form the vagina.

On either side of the cloaca there are swellings that later develop into the genital folds, which extend to join the genital tubercle. The genital folds become the labia minora, while the genital tubercle becomes the clitoris. The labia majora develop from swellings at the outer side of the genital folds (Fig. 6-1).

Uterus, Fallopian Tubes, and Vagina

The cephalad portion of the mullerian ducts becomes the fallopian tubes which open to the peritoneal cavity. The caudal portions of the mullerian ducts fuse to form the uterus, cervix, and upper two-thirds of the vagina. Concomitantly, an invagination of the inferior part of the cloaca is converted into the lower one-third of the vagina.

The uterus, cervix, and upper vagina are at first solid and later become septate. The cervix is the first part of the genital system to lose its longitudinal septum, then the vagina, and at 4–5 months, the uterus loses its septum. Failure of these septae to

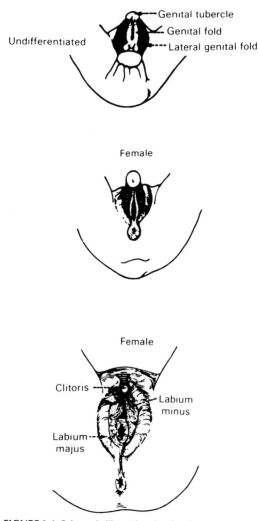

Undifferentiated

Genital tubercle
Genital fold
Lateral genital fold

Female

Female

Clitoris

Labium
minus

Labium
majus

FIGURE 6-1. Schematic illustration showing the development of the external genitalia from the undifferentiated state. (From Kistner.[75])

disappear results in congenital anomalies of the genital tract.

Ovaries

Ten days after fertilization, the primordial germ cells appear in the yolk sac as large cells with clear cytoplasm. They stain deeply with an alkaline phosphatase reaction and are readily distinguishable histochemically from the other cells. On the twelfth day, they migrate to the hindgut: 3 days later, they have migrated by ameboid movements into the

mesonephric folds. Concomitantly, a genital ridge appears over the ventral part of the mesonephros on each side. Initially it consists of mesenchyme alone, but soon cordlike protrusions of cells move in to form the sex cords. Later (at 4–5 weeks), the germ cells move from the genital ridges into the sex cords to form the cortex of the gonad. At the embryonic age of 6 weeks, the sex cords break up into separate clumps of cells. By the eighth week, if the gonad is to become an ovary, the sex cells seem to organize the mensenchymal elements of the gonad.

Differentiation of the ovary begins about the twelfth week, when oocytes begin to appear. Basically three types of follicles develop during the fetal period, i.e., primordial, preantral and antral (Fig. 6-2). By the sixteenth week, primordial follicles appear, also called resting follicles, containing one large primitive ovum (oogonium) surrounded by smaller, moderately differentiated cells that become granulosa cells. Less well-differentiated stromal cells become theca cells, and completely nondescript elements remain in the connective tissue. The stroma thickens at the periphery to form a capsulelike tunica albuginea and the fetal germinal epithelium thins out to a single layer of cuboidal epithelium covering the adult ovary. The oogonia undergo extensive mitotic activity, so that by the age of 20–21 weeks their number reaches a maximum of about 7 million. Thereafter, mitosis ceases and no further ova are produced for the rest of the individual's life.

A number of preantral follicles are found between medulla and cortex by 24 weeks. In these follicles the oocyte is larger, with a number of layers of granulosa cells surrounding it. A theca layer and zona pellucida are also present.

The third type of follicle, known as the graafian or antral follicle, appears no earlier than 26 weeks of gestation.[3] This consists of a mature oocyte, layers of granulosa cells, a theca layer outside the basement membrane, and a fluid-filled cavity.

A corpus luteum was recently reported in a 36-week fetus who succumbed to the respiratory distress syndrome.[4] This is probably the first time such an occurrence has been observed at this gestational age.

The ovaries continue to increase in size until term.[5] At birth, the oogonia have begun the first meiotic division and are called primary oocytes. They remain dormant in prophase until ovulation occurs many years later. At birth there are about 1 million oocytes in the ovaries, but the number has

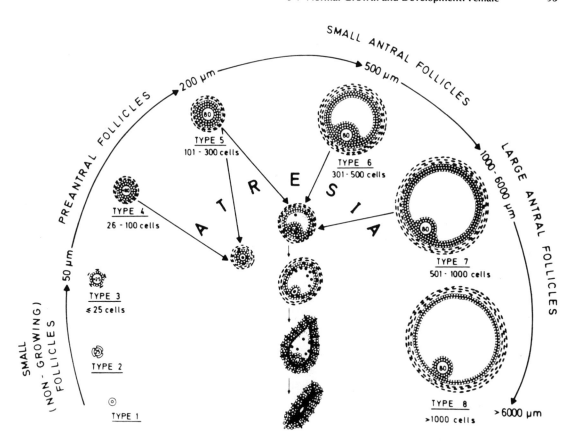

FIGURE 6-2. Classification of follicles in the human ovary. (From Peters et al.[37])

declined to approximately half a million by the time of puberty.[6–8] Indeed some ova begin to undergo the process of atresia starting at 20–21 weeks gestation, which continues until ovarian failure at menopause.

Aside from its function of producing oocytes during the antenatal period, the fetal ovary becomes capable of synthesizing hormones.[9] Aromatization is possible at 10 weeks,[10] and androgen formation at 12–18 weeks.[11] Reyes et al,[12] detected a low concentration of E_2-17-β-OH (estradiol) (0.5 pg/mg) in fetal ovaries at 10–22 weeks gestation. Steroidogenesis is limited, however, up to 22 weeks due to a deficiency of gonadotropin receptors.[13]

The enzyme 3β-hydroxysteroid dehydrogenase appears in granulosa cells at the beginning of the fourth month of gestation, and increases thereafter.[14] The ovaries have been found to synthesize progesterone at 20–22 weeks.[15]

NEUROENDOCRINE FUNCTION IN THE FETUS

In the human fetus of both sexes, the fetal gonad is affected by two gonadotropins, placental chorionic gonadotropin (hCG) early in gestation, and follicle-stimulating hormone (FSH) and luteinizing hormone (LH) secreted by the fetal pituitary later in gestation. Unlike the testis, the fetal ovary is only minimally affected by hCG, its growth and intrauterine function being more dependent on the pituitary gonadotropins.[16] The pituitary content of gonadotropins, particularly FSH, is much higher in female fetuses than in male, and secretion of gonadotropins begins earlier in females than in males.[17,18]

In order of appearance, gonadotropin-releasing hormone (GnRH) is present in human fetal brain by 5½ weeks gestation. By 8–10 weeks, the hypo-

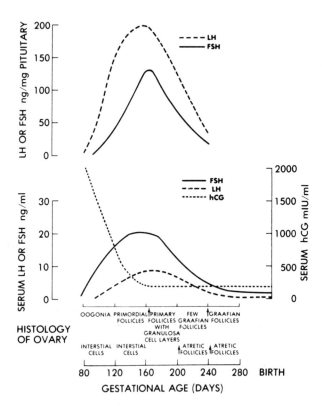

FIGURE 6-3. Pattern of serum LH, FSH, hCG, and pituitary LH and FSH in the female human fetus during gestation is correlated with the developmental histology of the fetal ovary. (From Kaplan and Grumbach.[21])

thalamus contains significant concentrations of immunoreactive GnRH (0.5–5 pg/mg).[19]

The development of the fetal central nervous system (CNS), particularly the hypothalamic–pituitary–portal systems, correlates well with gonadotropin synthesis and secretion. Gonadotrophs are present in fetal pituitary by 10½–13 weeks, with a rapid rise in number by 25 weeks.[20] FSH is present in fetal pituitary by 68 days and peaks at mid-gestation (140–160 days). Peak levels of LH are attained earlier (105–139 days), its concentration being greater than that of FSH throughout most of the gestational period.[21] It appears that the α-subunit is synthesized first at 10 weeks, with the β-subunit not being present until 15 weeks.[22]

In terms of fetal plasma levels, peak levels of gonadotropins are attained between 14 and 24 weeks gestation, with levels equivalent to those of castrated adults.[23] This corresponds to the phase of maximal follicular development in the fetal ovary.[24] Following this phase there is a decrement of FSH and LH until term, when levels are undetectable (Fig. 6-3).

Gonadotropins are essential for fetal ovarian fol-

licular growth. This was shown using anencephalic fetuses as a model to study the effect of pituitary formation on gonadal development.[25,26] These fetuses have only about 2% of the normal amount of gonadotropins, with the pituitary gland being very small. The ovaries in turn are small, with follicular development not progressing beyond the preantral stage.[18]

The rise in gonadotropins early in gestation may be due to unrestrained stimulation by GnRH of the fetal pituitary. The decrement late in gestation may be due to inhibitory feedback mechanisms, with progressively greater sensitivity of the hypothalamus to levels of circulating sex steroids, although they be low.

INTRAUTERINE FETAL GROWTH

During intrauterine life, the fetus grows by cellular multiplication, with excessive linear growth rates. As can be seen in Figure 6-4, peak velocities of 10–11 cm/month occur at 4–5 month gestation, followed by a gradual decline in rate during the

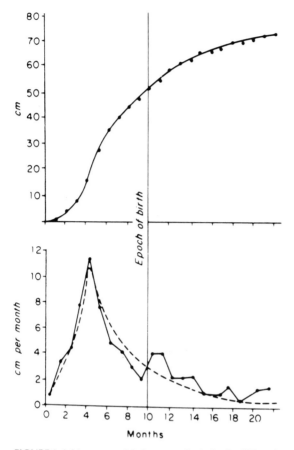

FIGURE 6-4. Linear growth in lunar months during fetal life and in the first postnatal year. The slowing of late fetal growth rate is compatible with the concept of constraints to growth by the uterus and is followed postnatally by a brief period of accelerated catch-up growth. (From Felig et al.[27])

femur growth rate begins at 3.15 mm/week and slowly declines to 1.55 mm/week toward 40 weeks gestation (Fig. 6-5). As shown, the calculation of gestational age of fetal FL is accurate up to 24 weeks, before normal biologic variation causes widening of the growth curve limits. After 22 weeks gestation, there is a linear relationship between FL and BPD, with a normal ratio of 79.8%[30] (Fig. 6-6). This ratio provides a quality-control check on FL and BPD measurements and can be used in the diagnosis of microcephaly, hydrocephalus, and short-limbed dwarfism.

THE NEWBORN PERIOD

In the newborn girl, umbilical cord blood contains the following levels of sex steroids: estrone (900–4000 ng/dl), estradiol (200–1600 ng/dl), estriol (1200–15,000 ng/dl), and progesterone (12,000–50,000 ng/dl).[31] However, peripheral blood concentrations are 50 times lower than umbilical cord blood. By 5 days of age, estradiol levels are <1.4 ng/dl and progesterone <200 ng/dl,[31] with undetectable hCG levels.

As noted, during the first week of life estrogen blood levels fall rapidly, rising again in the second week and continuing to rise during the first year of life.[32] Although the increase in estradiol correlates with the large number of graafian follicles in the ovary, part of the estradiol may be of adrenal origin. Plasma testosterone levels are similar to those of the mother (or normal adult female), but after 1 week they fall and remain low (0.04 ng/dl) until puberty.[33] Pituitary FSH and LH output is negligible at birth, but during the first week of life circulating gonadotropin levels increase secondary to withdrawal of placental steroids, continuing upward until 3 months of age, when they are considerably higher than in prepubertal children, with FSH levels higher in females than in males.[33]

INFANCY AND CHILDHOOD

After this peak of infant FSH and LH at 3 months, there is a decline, with a nadir at 3–4 years of age.[34] The hypothalamic–pituitary–gonadal relationship becomes established by 2 years of age. From infancy through childhood, small but measurable amounts of FSH and LH are secreted,[35] and

third trimester, leveling off to approximately 2 cm/month.[27] Fetal weight doubles during the last 8 weeks gestation due to the formation of increasing amounts of adipose tissue. At birth, females have a slightly smaller head circumference than that of males, weighing an average of 150 g less; body length is shorter by 0.9 cm.[28] However, bone age is 2 weeks ahead of that in males, and by 1 year this difference has increased to 8 weeks.

Assessment of intrauterine growth can be made by ultrasonographic evaluation of fetal femur length (FL) or by biparietal diameter (BPD). In particular, evaluating FL from 14 weeks until term, O'Brien and Queenan[29] describe an asymptotic curve similar to that for BPD. Calculated fetal

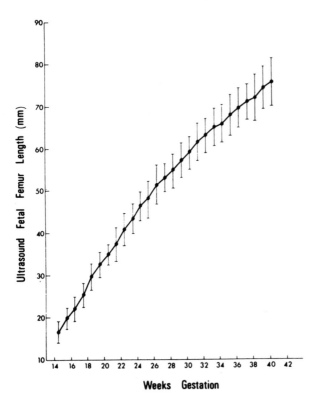

FIGURE 6-5. Graph of the mean ultrasound femur length ±2 SD for each week of gestation from 11 weeks to term. (From O'Brien and Queenan.[29])

circulating gonadotropin levels remain steady until the onset of puberty (Fig. 6-7).

Follicular growth and atresia occur at all ages. During childhood, the ovary is not quiescent, as was shown in studies conducted on children who died in accidents.[36,37] Small follicles exist in the outer cortex of the ovary, representing about 97% of all follicles present,[36] constituting the group from which all growing follicles emerge. During this period, the ovary grows in size secondary to an increase in stroma and in number of fluid-filled follicles as well. All follicles that have entered the growth phase before ovulation occurs become atretic. Hence, in childhood follicular growth and atresia are ongoing processes, with the result that the ovary is by no means a dormant organ, as was previously believed.

Between the ages of 4–8 years there are low serum levels of gonadotropins and sex steroids. It is interesting that compared with female infants, older girls are less responsive to GnRH in terms of FSH secretion.[38,39] In contradistinction, prepubertal rhesus monkeys are capable of estrogen production[40] and can be caused to ovulate by administration of human menopausal gonadotropins (hMG) and hCG.[41]

Agonadal children have been found to have high levels of serum and urinary gonadotropins.[42] It may be inferred that in normal girls there is some mechanism whereby gonadotropin secretion is sup-

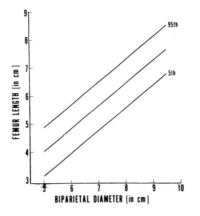

FIGURE 6-6. Ninety percent confidence interval of the relationship between femur length and BPD from 23 to 49 weeks gestation ($R = 0.85$; $p < 0.0001$). (From Hohler and Quetel.[30])

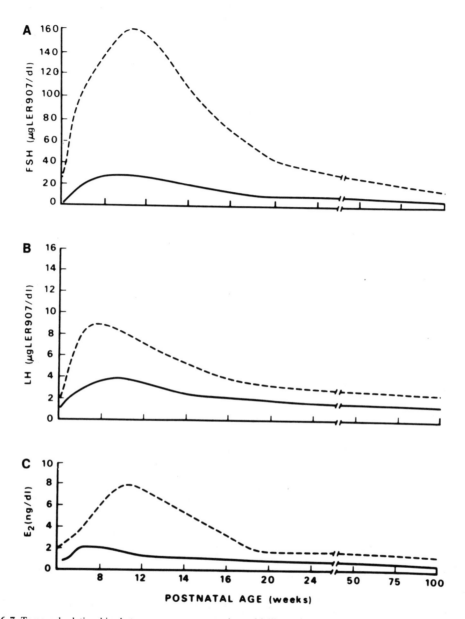

FIGURE 6-7. Temporal relationships between serum concentrations of follicle-stimulating hormone (A), luteinizing hormone (B), and estradiol (C) in girls during infancy. (———) Median concentration at each age; (– – –) upper normal limit. (From Winter et al.[31])

pressed. However, there is no indication of pre-pubertal estrogen secretion in normal girls.

PERIPUBERTAL HORMONAL CHANGES

The initiation of puberty is brought about by maturation of the hypothalamic–pituitary complex and the input of the CNS that integrates a variety of intrinsic and extrinsic stimuli. This hypothalamic–pituitary complex was named the gonadostat by Grumbach and, as currently understood, it develops in two stages:

First, the negative feedback mechanism is operative early in childhood, probably from mid- to late fetal life. The threshold of sensitivity of the

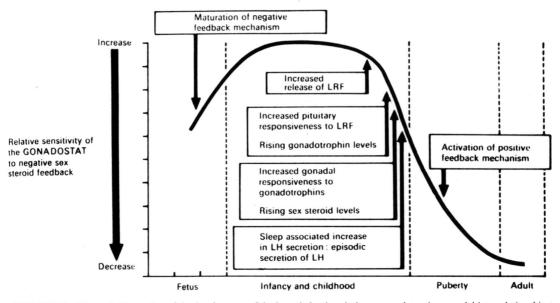

FIGURE 6-8. Schematic illustration of the development of the hypothalamic–pituitary–gonadotropin–gonadal interrelationship to the onset of puberty. (From Grumbach et al.[16])

gonadostat is very high and extremely sensitive to the suppressive effect of small amounts of circulating gonadal steroids. The circulating concentration of estrogens and gonadotropins is correspondingly low. With the onset of puberty, the hypothalamic gonadostat becomes progressively less sensitive to the suppressive effect of the gonadal steroids and more gonadotropins are secreted from the pituitary. Grumbach et al.[16] showed that the hypothalamic gonadostat in prepubertal children is 6–15 times more sensitive to circulating estrogens than after puberty. There is no evidence of episodic LH secretion in children before puberty, but beginning in early puberty intermittent LH secretion is observed only during sleep.[43] This is characterized by widely fluctuating plasma LH concentrations. There is, most probably, a maturation phenomenon related to changes in the central nervous system that affects pulsatile release of GnRH and possibly participates in the prepubertal increase in pituitary response to GnRH[44] (Fig. 6-8).

Second, the second stage of pubertal development is maturation and activation of the positive feedback effect of estrogens that occurs in girls about mid- to late puberty.[45] The progressive maturation of the hypothalamic–pituitary gonadal axis and increasing secretion of gonadotropins and gonadal steroids occur simultaneously with the development stages described by Tanner and correlate better with bone age than with chronologic age[16] (Fig. 6-9).

NEUROENDOCRINE DEVELOPMENT DURING PUBERTY

To reiterate, the pituitary response to GnRH is minimal in prepubertal children and is enhanced at the onset of puberty.[46] This increase in pituitary sensitivity may be secondary to either increased secretion of GnRH or increased secretion of estrogen. In humans estrogen appears to play a special role in pituitary maturation and pituitary response to hypothalamic stimulation.[47] An interesting sex difference has been noticed in the pituitary response to exogenous GnRH. Prepubertal and pubertal girls release significantly more FSH than do boys at all stages of sexual maturation, suggesting that the pituitary gonadotropes of prepubertal girls are more sensitive to GnRH than those of boys.[35]

Prolactin secretion shows a pattern similar to gonadotropin secretion in females. Serum prolactin is elevated at birth, decreases to low levels during the first week of life and remains low during childhood. In a study of 80 girls between the ages of 8–15 years, a twofold rise in prolactin levels was

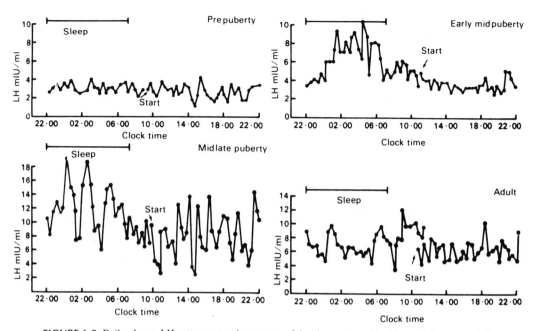

FIGURE 6-9. Daily plasma LH patterns at various stages of development in girls. (From Weitzman et al.[76])

found to occur, with a statistically significant rise between 14–15 years of age, paralleling a rise in serum estrogen levels. These data suggest that increased prolactin secretion occurs in late puberty.[48–50]

An increase in adrenal activity takes place in the latter half of childhood, preceding the onset of puberty; this phase of development is termed adrenarche. The earliest changes begin around the age of 6 years, when there is an increase in secretion of dehydroepiandrosterone (DHEA), dehydroepiandrosterone sulfate (DHEAS), and Δ^4-androstenedione.[51] The prepubertal concentration of plasma testosterone is the same in boys (6.62 ± 2.46 ng%) as in girls (6.8 ± 2.48 ng%) and is of adrenal origin.[52] Ducharme et al.[53] found a certain sequence in the secretion of adrenal steroids during puberty. Plasma DHEA increases first from the age of 6, followed by an increase in Δ^4-androstenedione from age 8 to 10. Testosterone and estrogens increase at the time of onset of puberty. The prepubertal development of adrenal steroidogenesis is not under direct ACTH or gonadotropin control.[54] Maturation of the adrenal may be related to maturation of the gonadostat. DHEA and Δ^4-androstenedione may act directly on the hypothalamus, or *via* conversion to estrogens. Circumstantial support for this theory comes from clinical investigation. It has been observed that children with gonadal dysgenesis, but normal adrenarche have nyctohumoral rhythms of plasma LH, while children with adrenal insufficiency have delayed puberty.[55] In addition, agonadal children show an increase in 17-ketosteroid (17-KS) excretion after being given estrogen, and children with precocious adrenarche show increased levels of estradiol.[56] Androgens of adrenal origin may affect maturation of the hypothalamus and therefore the timing of puberty. A summary of events from conception to puberty is found in Figure 6-10.

GROWTH AND SEXUAL MATURATION DURING PUBERTY

The Adolescent Growth Spurt

At adolescence, maturation of the gonads is accompanied by acceleration of somatic growth, development of the secondary sex characteristics, and attainment of reproductive capacity. The growth curve for a child runs steeply in early life, after which it gradually levels off. Around the time of puberty, it suddenly becomes steep again; this acceleration of growth is termed the adolescent spurt. (Figs. 6-11 and 6-12). Adolescent girls may reach

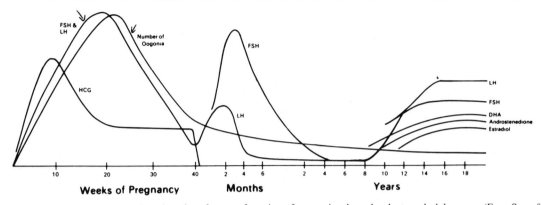

FIGURE 6-10. Gonadotropin levels and number of oocytes from time of conception through puberty and adolescence. (From Speroff et al.[77])

their maximal growth rate any time between the tenth and fourteenth birthday. The mean age of reaching peak height velocity in girls studied by Marshall and Tanner in England was 12.14 ± 0.14 years, with a standard deviation of 0.88 years.[57] The adolescent spurt does not begin at the same time in all parts of the body. The trunk reaches its maximal growth rate about 6 months after the legs. Growth of the feet accelerates first, about 4 months before the lower legs; thus, the feet may become temporarily disproportionately large in some children. The pelvic outlet is wider at birth in girls than in boys and, as a result of growth at puberty, girls' hips become wider in relationship to their shoulders.[58]

Development of Secondary Sex Characteristics and Reproductive Organs

An increase in the number of superficial cells in the vaginal smear heralds the approach of puberty. This indication of estrogenic activity can be detected before any other signs of sexual development and provides a practical and simple test when a child's developmental status is in question.

The vagina begins to lengthen before the secondary sex characteristics appear and continues to do so until shortly after menarche. Prepubertal growth of the uterus is due mainly to growth of the myometrium. The endometrium develops concomitantly with the secondary sex characteristics.[58]

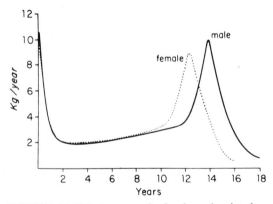

FIGURE 6-11. Velocity curves for females and males show gradual increases in rates of weight gain from 2 years until adolescence. (From Felig et al.[27])

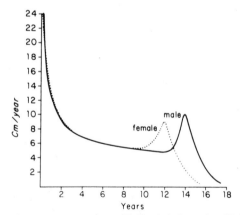

FIGURE 6-12. Velocity curves for length (<2 years) and height (2–18 years) for females and males show deceleration of growth rate from infancy until the onset of adolescence. (From Felig et al.[27])

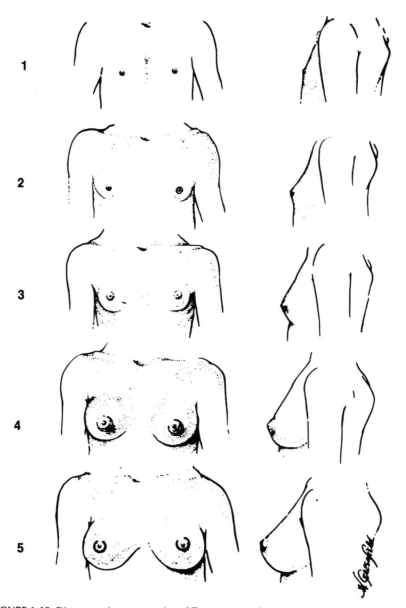

FIGURE 6-13. Diagrammatic representation of Tanner stages of breast development. (From Williams.[64])

Breast Development (Thelarche)

On the basis of appearance, adolescent breast development can be divided into five stages[59] (see Fig. 6-13):

Stage 1   This is the infantile stage, which persists from infancy until changes of puberty begin.

Stage 2   The breast and papilla are elevated in a small mound, and the diameter of the areola increases; this is the first indication of pubertal changes in the breast.

Stage 3   The breast and areola are further enlarged and have the appearance of a small adult breast with a continuous round contour.

Stage 4   The areola and papilla further enlarge

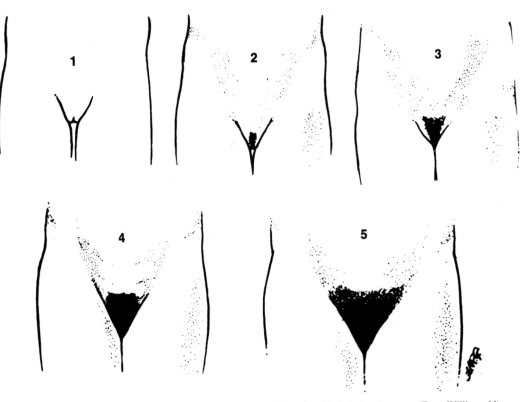

FIGURE 6-14. Diagrammatic representation of Tanner stages of female pubic hair development. (From Williams.[64])

to form a secondary mound above the contour of the remaining breast.

Stage 5   The typical adult breast has a smoothed round contour; The secondary mound seen in stage 4 has disappeared.

The process of breast development from stage 2 to 5 takes an average 4 years, but the duration and stages of breast development vary greatly between individuals. In some girls, stage 5 is never reached, with stage 4 persisting until the first pregnancy or even beyond. In others, stage 4 is very short, or inapparent. The vast majority of girls achieve adult breast size between the ages of 11–19.[60]

Pubic Hair Development (Pubarche)

Pubic hair growth can also be described in five stages (Fig. 6-14):

Stage 1   This is the infantile stage, in which there is no true pubic hair.

Stage 2   Sparse growth of long slightly pigmented hair appears first on either the labia majora or mons pubis.

Stage 3   An increase in the amount of hair spreads sparsely over the mons pubis; it is considerably darker, coarser, and more curly than in stage 2.

Stage 4   The hair is adult in character but covers a smaller area than in most adults.

Stage 5   The hair is distributed in an inverse triangular pattern, with some spread to the medial surface of the thighs, characteristic of an adult female.

Axillary hair appears concomitantly with pubic hair. The adult distribution of hair is usually attained between 12–17 years of age.

The range of ages at which pubic hair growth begins is very similar to that for the beginning of breast development, but in a given individual pubic hair growth and breast development do not necessarily begin at the same time. There is usually some breast development before pubic hair appears and sometimes the breast may progress to stage 4 without pubic hair growth. On the other hand, in some girls pubic hair appears before there is any breast development.[58]

Cutaneous Gland Development

Axillary and pubic apocrine glands begin to function at approximately the same time that pubic and axillary hair appear. While examining young girls, a change in odor of the axillary and pubic areas is an early clinical indication of pubertal changes. The sebaceous glands and merocrine sweat gland of the general body also become more active at about the same time.[58]

Menarche

Menarche is the onset of menses. There are great variations in the age at which menarche occurs in different populations and countries, and even between social groups. Girls in the higher socioeconomic classes tend to have earlier menarche than do girls in the lower classes.[58] Lifestyle too is very important. Children who are not athletically active have an earlier menarche,[61] as have blind children, who presumably have a more sedentary lifestyle.[62]

In the United States the mean age at menarche is 12.65 years, with a standard deviation of 1.17 years.[63] In England the average age is 13.0 years, with a standard deviation of approximately 1 year.[57] Accordingly, a range of 9–16 years constitutes the period during which the onset of menses might be regarded as normal; it should be considered abnormal when menses appear before the age of 9 or are delayed beyond age 16.[64] Different mean ages of menarche have been reported in different races, but it is difficult to distinguish between the effect of race itself and that of differences in nutrition, climate, culture, and other factors. Within the same race, a significant relationship was found between menarche and mean temperature, and menarche was usually later at higher than at lower altitudes and in rural than in urban communities.[65]

During the past 100 years, the mean age at menarche in Europe, North America, and some other countries has become progressively earlier at a rate of 3–4 months per decade. This trend is continuing in many countries, but there are signs that it may be leveling off.[66]

The mean age at onset of menarche precedes the mean age of regular menses by about 14 months;

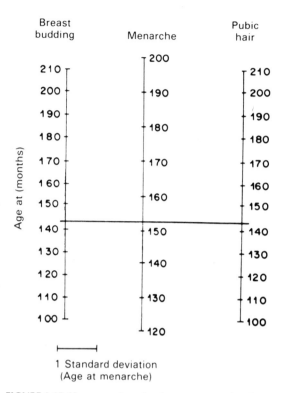

FIGURE 6-15. Nomogram for estimating age at menarche when the age of appearance of breast budding and pubic hair is known. (From Zacharias et al.[63])

painful menses are noted at a mean interval of 10 months later. Zacharias et al.[67] constructed a nomogram based on the ages at which breast budding, pubic hair, and menarche appear, from which it is possible to predict the age of menarche when the age of breast budding and appearance of pubic hair is known (Fig. 6-15).

Frish[70] hypothesized that weight, or more precisely total body fat, plays a critical role in the onset of menses.[68,69] Menarche is associated with attainment of an average critical body weight of about 47 kg. The average critical weight represents a critical body composition of fat, as a percentage of total body weight, which is attained at varying weights and heights within a population. About 17% of body composition as fat is probably needed for menarche to occur and about 22% for the onset and maintenance of regular ovulatory cycles. Frish and McArthur[71] have constructed a weight for height graph from which the expected time of menarche can be predicted when the height and weight are known (Fig. 6-16). This graph can be used for

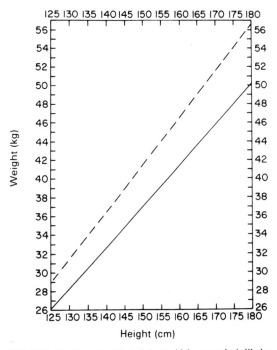

FIGURE 6-16. The weight for height at which menarche is likely to occur (solid line) and at which ovulatory cycles are likely to be maintained (broken line). (From Frish and McArthur.[68])

clinical evaluation of primary amenorrhea. It should be pointed out, however, that although this is an interesting hypothesis, it has not been universally accepted and has been criticized because its conclusions were drawn from derived rather than observed data.

An interesting study that clarifies the above discussion was conducted by Warren.[72] Onset of menarche was studied in career-oriented girls subjected to a severe energy drain versus a control group in which the career goal was of a sedentary nature (ballet dancers vs. music students) Menarche was considerably delayed in the dancer group, occurring at a mean of 15.4 years vs. 12.6 years for the control group. The dancers' body weight and calculated body fat were considerably less than controls ($p < 0.05$). In two-thirds of dancers, sexual development and onset of menarche correlated with a drop in exercise secondary to injury, causing forced rest of 2 months duration. Weight gain was minimal or absent during this period. Return of the amenorrheic state occurred in 11 of 13 dancers with resumption of exercise. It was concluded that energy drain may have a modulatory effect on the hypothalamic–pituitary set point at puberty, and in com-

bination with low body weight may prolong the prepubertal state.

Aside from menarche, other parameters were studied. Pubarche was found to occur at a normal age. This is not surprising, since pubarche is related to androgen secretion, and high testosterone levels have been reported in female runners.[73] Breast development was also remarkably delayed in all dancers, however. All girls (100%) showed no development or slight, at 13 years of age, and 75% were at Tanner stage 3 at menarche. Thus, thelarche occurred significantly later than for normal children,[57,63] in which 62% have reached Tanner stage 4 at menarche.

SUMMARY

Growth and development of the female, like that in any living organism, is a complex process that begins at the moment of fertilization. The early embryonic development is similar for both sexes until the eighth week, when the fetal gonads (testes) become active. In the absence of functioning embryonic testes, the embryo develops into a female. Growth and function of the embryonic ovary is affected by the pituitary gonadotropins. During infancy and childhood, secretion of gonadotropins and gonadal steroids is low. At adolescence, maturation of the hypothalamic–pituitary complex occurs. The gonadostat becomes progressively less sensitive to the suppressive effect of estrogens, with the result that more gonadotropins are secreted that induce follicular maturation, increased estrogen production, and acceleration of somatic growth and development. The secondary sex characteristics appear and reproductive capacity is reached, transforming the child into an adult female. Maturation of the adrenals, adrenarche, has an important role in the process of puberty. Finally, somatic changes and attainment of a certain weight and body composition are critical factors in the onset and maintenance of menses. All these factors are closely integrated and interdependent.

QUESTIONS

1. What is the most common cause of congenital anomalies of the genital tract in women?

2. What initiates puberty?

3. What are the major changes during puberty?

REFERENCES

1. Edwards RG, Purdy JM, Steptoe PC, et al: The growth of human preimplantation embryos in vitro. *Am J Obstet Gynecol* 141:408–416, 1981

2. Jost A, Vigier E, Crepin J, et al: Studies on sex differentiation in mammals. *Recent Prog Horm Res* 29:1–41, 1973

3. Pryse-Davies J, Dewhurst, CJ: The development of the ovary and uterus in the foetus, newborn and infant: A morphological and enzyme histo-chemical study. *J Pathol* 103:5–25, 1971

4. Miles PA, Penney LL: Corpus luteum formation in the fetus. *Obstet Gynecol* 61:525–529, 1983

5. Siiteri PK, Wilson JO: Testosterone formation and metabolism during male sexual differentiation in the human embryo. *J Clin Endocrinol Metab* 38:113–125, 1974

6. Federman DD: *Abnormal Sexual Development.* Philadelphia, Saunders, 1967

7. Page EW, Villee CA, Villee DB: *Human Reproduction.* Philadelphia, Saunders, 1972

8. Reid DE, Ryan KJ, Benirschke K: *Principles and Management of Human Reproduction.* Philadelphia, Saunders, 1972

9. Lemprecht SA, Zor H, Tsafriri A, et al: Action of prostoglandin E_2 and of luteinizing hormone on ovarian adenylate cyclase, protein kinase and ornithine decarboxylase activity during post-natal development and maturity in the rat. *J Endocrinol* 57:217–233, 1973

10. George FW, Wilson JD: Conversion of androgen to estrogen by the human fetal ovary. *J Clin Endocrinol Metab* 47:550–555, 1978

11. Payne AH, Jaffe RB: Androgen formation from pregnenolone sulfate by the human fetal ovary. *J Clin Endocrinol Metab* 39:300–304, 1974

12. Reyes FI, Winter JSD, Faiman C: Studies on human sexual development I. fetal gonadal and adrenal sex steroids. *J Clin Endocrinol Metab* 37:74–78, 1973

13. Wilson EA, Jawad MJ: The effect of trophic agents on fetal ovarian steroidogenesis in organ culture. *Fertil Steril* 32:73–79, 1979

14. Goldman AS, Yakovac WC, Bongiovanni AM: Development of activity of 3β-OH-steroid dehydrogenase in human fetal tissues and in two anencephalic newborns. *J Clin Endocrinol* 26:14–22, 1965

15. Jungmann RA, Schweppe JS: Biosynthesis of sterols and steroids from acetate-^{14}C by human fetal ovaries. *J Clin Endocrinol Metab* 28:1599–1604, 1968

16. Grumbach MM, Roth JC, Kaplan SL, et al: Hypothalamic–pituitary regulation of puberty. Evidence and concepts derived from clinical research, in Grumbach MM, Grave GD, Mayer FE (eds): *The Control of the Onset of Puberty.* New York, Wiley, 1974, p 115*

17. Siler-Khodr TM, Morgenstern LL, Greenwood FC: Hormone synthesis and release from human fetal adenohypophysis in-vitro. *J Clin Endocrinol Metab* 39:891–905, 1974

18. Grumbach MM, Kaplan SL: Ontogenesis of growth hormone, insulin, prolactin and gonadotropin secretion in the human fetus, in Gross KW, Nathanielsz P (eds): *Advances in Foetal and Neonatal Physiology.* New York, Cambridge University Press, 1973, p 462*

19. Winters AJ, Eskay RL, Porter JC: Correlation and distribution of TRH and LRH in the human fetal brain. *J Clin Endocrinol Metab* 39:960–963, 1974

20. Baker BL, Jaffe RB: The genesis of cell types in the adenohypophysis of the human fetus as observed with immunocytochemistry. *Am J Anat* 143:137–161, 1975

21. Kaplan SL, Grumbach MM: The ontogenesis of human foetal hormones. II. Luteinizing hormones (LH) and follicle stimulating hormones (FSH). *Acta Endocrinol (Copenh)* 81:808–829, 1976

22. Bugnon C, Bloch B, Fellman D: Cytoimmunological study of the ontogenesis of the gonadotropic hypothalamopituitary axis in the human fetus. *J Steroid Biochem* 8:565–577, 1977

23. Grumbach MM, Kaplan SL: Fetal pituitary hormones and the maturation of the CNS regulation of anterior pituitary function, in Gluck L (ed): *Modern Perinatal Medicine.* Chicago, Yearbook, 1974, pp 247–256*

24. Reyes FI, Boroditsky RS, Winter JSD, et al: Studies on human sexual development. II. Fetal and maternal serum gonadotropin and sex steroid concentration. *J Clin Endocrinol Metab* 38:612–617, 1974

25. Ross GT: Gonadotropins and preantral follicular maturation in women. *Fertil Steril* 25:522–543, 1974

26. Ch'in KY: The endocrine glands of anencephalic foetuses. A quantitative and morphological study of 15 cases. *Chinese Med J [Suppl]* 2:63–90, 1938

27. Felig P, Baxter JD, Broadus AE, et al: *Endocrinology and Metabolism.* New York, McGraw-Hill, 1981

28. Smith DW: *Major Problems in Clinical Pediatrics.* Vol 15: *Growth and Its Disorders.* Philadelphia, Saunders, 1977

29. O'Brien GD, Queenan JT: Growth of the ultrasound fetal femur length during normal pregnancy. Part I. *Am J Obstet Gynecol* 141:833–837, 1981

30. Hohler CW, Quetel TA: Comparison of ultrasound femur length and biparietal diameter in later pregnancy, *Am J Obstet Gynecol* 141:759–762, 1981

31. Winter JS, Faiman C, Reyes FI, et al: Gonadotropins and steroid hormones in the blood and urine of prepubertal girls and other primates. *Clin Endocrinol Metab* 7(3):513–530, 1978

32. Bidlingmaier F, Versmold H, Knorr D: Plasma estrogens in newborns and infants, in Forest MG, Bertrand J (eds): *Colloque international sur l'endocrinologie sexuelle de la periode perinatal,* Vol. 32. Paris, INSERM, 1974, pp 299–314

33. Forest MG, Sizonenko PC, Cathiard AM, et al: Hypophysealgonadal function in humans during the first year of life. *J Clin Invest* 53:819–828, 1974

34. Winter JSD, Faiman C, Hobson WC, et al: Pituitary–gonadal relations in infancy: 1. Patterns of serum gonadotropin concentrations from birth to four years of age in man and chimpanzee. *J Clin Endocrinol Metab* 40:545–551, 1975

35. Grumbach MM: Onset of puberty, in Bernberg SR (ed): *Puberty—Biologic and Psychological Components.* London, Stenfert Kroese B.V., 1975, p 2*

36. Block E: Quantitative morphological investigations of the follicular system in women. *Acta Anat* 16:108–123, 1952

37. Peters H, Himelstein-Braw R, Faber M: The normal development of the ovary in childhood *Acta Endocrinol (Copenh)* 82:617–630, 1976

38. Garnier PE, Chaussain J-L, Binet E, et al: Effect of synthetic LH-RH in the release of gonadotropin in children and adolescents. VI. Relations to age, sex and puberty. *Acta Endocrinol (Copenh)* 77:422–434, 1974

39. Dickerman Z, Prager-Lewin R, Laron Z: Response of plas-

*Review article or chapter.

ma LH and FSH to synthetic LH-RH in children at various pubertal stages. *Am J Dis Child* 130:634–638, 1976

40. Lemons TA, Foster DL, Jaffe RB: Aromatization by the immature rhesus monkey ovary. *Endocrinology* 94:1181–1184, 1974

41. Weiss G, Rifkin I, Atkinson LE: Induction of ovulation in premenarchal rhesus monkeys with human gonadotropins *Biol Reprod* 14:401–404, 1976

42. Conte F, Grumbach MM, Kaplan SL: Variations in plasma LH and FSH with age in 35 patients with XO gonadal dysgenesis. *Pediatr Res* 6:353, 1972

43. Judd HL, Parker DC, Yen SSC: Sleep–wake patterns of LH and T release in prepubertal boys. *J Clin Endocrinol Metab* 44:865–869, 1977

44. Boyar RJ, Finkelstein H, Roffwarg H, et al: Synchronization of augmented luteinizing-hormone secretion with sleep during puberty. *N Engl J Med* 287:582–586, 1972

45. Reiter ED, Kulin HE, Hamwood SM: The absence of positive feedback between estrogens and luteinizing hormone in sexually immature girls. *Pediatr Res* 8:740–745, 1974

46. Job JC, Garnier PE, Chaussain JL, et al: elevation of serum gonadotropins (LH and FSH) after releasing hormone (LH-RH) injection in normal children and in patients with disorders of puberty. *J Clin Endocrinol Metab* 35:473–476, 1972

47. Odell WD: The role of the gonads in sexual maturation, in Grumbach MM, Grave GD, Mayer FE (eds): *The Control of the Onset of Puberty.* New York, Wiley, 1974, p 313*

48. Aubert MI, Grumbach MM, Kaplan SL: The ontogenesis of human fetal hormones. III. Prolactin. *J Clin Invest* 56:155–164, 1975

49. Ehara Y, Yen SSC, Siler TM: Serum prolactin levels during puberty. *Am J Obstet Gynecol* 121:995, 1975

50. Guyda HJ, Friesen HG: Serum prolactin levels in humans from birth to adult life. *Pediatr Res* 7:534–540, 1973*

51. Sizonenko PC: Endocrine laboratory findings in pubertal disturbances. *Clin Endocrinol Metab* 4(1):173–206, 1975

52. Forest MG, Saez JM, Sann L, et al: La Function gonadique chez le nourrisson et l'enfant. Notions physiopathélogique et exploration. *Arch Fr Pediatr* 31:587–617, 1974

53. Ducharme JR, Forest MG, DePeretti E, et al: Plasma adrenal and gonadal sex steroids in human pubertal development. *J Clin Endocrinol Metab* 42:468–476, 1976

54. Forest MG, DePeretti M, Bertrand J: Hypothalamic–pituitary–gonadal relationship in man from birth to puberty. *Clin Endocrinol* 5:551–569, 1976*

55. Boyar RM, Finkelstein JW, Roffwarg H, et al: Twenty-four hour luteinizing hormone and follicle-stimulating hormone secretory patterns in gonadal dysgenesis. *J Clin Endocrinol Metab* 37:521–525, 1973

56. Warne GL, Carter JN, Faiman C, et al: Hormonal changes in girls with precocious adrenarche. A possible role for estradiol and prolactin. *J Pediatr* 92:743–747, 1978

57. Marshall WA, Tanner JM: Variations in patterns of pubertal changes in girls. *Arch Dis Child* 44:291–303, 1969

58. Marshall WA: Growth and sexual maturation in normal puberty. *Clin Endocrinol Metab* 4(1):3–25, 1975*

59. Tanner JM: *Growth at Adolescence,* 2nd ed. Blackwell, Oxford, 1962

60. Barnes HV: Physical growth and development during puberty. *Med Clin North Am* 59(6):1305–1317, 1975*

61. Malina RM, Harper AB, Averit HH, et al: Age at menarche in athletes and non-athletes. *Med Sci Sports* 5:11–13, 1973

62. Zacharias L, Wurtman RJ: Blindness: Its relation to age of menarche. *Science* 144:1154–1155, 1964

63. Zacharias L, Wurtman RJ, Schatzoff M: Sexual maturation in contemporary American girls. *Am J Obstet Gynecol* 108:833–846, 1970

64. Williams, RH: Disorders of sex differentiation, in Williams RH (ed): *Textbook of Endocrinology,* 6th ed. Philadelphia, Saunders, 1981, pp 422–505;

65. Roberts DF: Race, genetics and growth. *J Biosoc Sci [Suppl.]* 1:43–67, 1969

66. Tanner JM: Trend towards earlier menarche in London, Oslo, Copenhagen, The Netherlands and Hungary. *Nature (Lond)* 243:95–96, 1973

67. Zacharias L, Wurtman RJ: Age at menarche, genetic and environmental influences. *N Engl J Med* 280:868–875, 1969

68. Frish RE, McArthur JW: Menstrual cycles: Fatness as a determinant of minimum weight for height necessary for their maintenance or onset. *Science* 185:949–951, 1974

69. Frish RE, Revelle R: Height and weight at menarche and a hypothesis of menarche. *Arch Dis Child* 46:695–701, 1971

70. Frish RE: Critical weight at menarche, initiation of the adolescent growth spurt, and control of puberty, in Grumbach MM, Grave GG, Mayer FE (eds): *The Control of Onset of Puberty.* New York, Wiley, 1974, pp 178–179

71. Billewicz WZ, Fellows HM, Hytten CA: Comments on the critical metabolic mass and the age of menarch. *Ann Human Biol* 3:363–374, 1976

72. Warren MP: The effect of exercise on pubertal progression and reproductive function in girls. *J Clin Endocrinol Metab* 51:1150–1157, 1980

73. Dale E, Gerlach DH, Wilhite AL: Menstrual dysfunction in distance runners. *Obstet Gynecol* 54:47, 1979

74. Jirásek JE: Prenatal development: Growth and Development, in: Sciarra JJ, Dilts PV, Gerbie AB (eds): *Gynecology and Obstetrics.* Philadelphia, Harper and Row, 1985, vol 2, pp 1–12

75. Kistner RW: *Gynecology Principles and Practices,* 2nd ed, Chicago, Yearbook Medical Publishers, 1971, p 18

76. Weitzman et al.: *Recent Progress in Hormone Research,* Vol 31, 1975, p 399

77. Speroff L, Glass RH, Kase JG: *Clinical Gynecologic EEndocrinology and Infertility,* 2nd ed, Baltimore, Williams and Wilkins, 1978, p 65

ANSWERS

1. The female genital organs develop by fusion of the mullerian ducts. The upper part of the mullerian ducts becomes the fallopian tubes, while its lower part forms the uterus, cervix, and upper two-thirds of the vagina. The uterus, cervix, and upper vagina are at first solid and later become septate. Later, the septae disappear; failure of the septae to disappear results in congenital anomalies of the genital tract.

2. Initiation of puberty is caused by maturation of the hypothalamic–pituitary complex. It develops in two stages. First, during early childhood until the onset of puberty, the negative feedback mechanism is the overriding component. As a result, the circulating levels of estrogens and gonadotropins is low. Second, with the onset of puberty, the positive feedback effect of estrogens takes place. With maturation of the hypothalamic–pituitary–ovarian axis, there is an increase in secretion of gonadotropins and gonadal steroids, eventually resulting in appropriate physical development and menarche.

3. Around the time of puberty, with the increase in estrogen levels a significant acceleration of growth occurs, the adolescent spurt, along with typical changes in breast development (the five Tanner stages) and pubic hair. Axillary and pubic apocrine glands begin to function. The last stage is onset of menses–menarche.

7

Thyroid Function and Disease in the Female

CHARLES H. EMERSON

INTRODUCTION AND HISTORICAL BACKGROUND

The thyroid has attracted the interest of observers for centuries. Goiter in women is depicted in artwork from the ancient Egyptians, the Aztecs, and many other cultures. In 1656, Warton suggested that the gland was more prominent in women because its role was to round out and beautify the neck.[1] Gull's report in 1874 "On a cretinoid state supervening in adult life in women," was one of the first descriptions which drew attention to similarities between myxedema and cretinism. A few years later, Ord provided the first comprehensive description of myxedema.[1] Its title emphasized the point that this disease was seen predominantly in women. It is now clear that women are more susceptible than men to all the common thyroid diseases including autoimmune disorders (Graves' disease, Hashimoto's thyroiditis), simple goiter, and thyroid neoplasia. Moreover, some of the most important clinical features of thyroid dysfunction

are due to the effects of thyroid hormone on female reproductive tissues and, some thyroid diseases are secondary to an abnormality of a female reproductive organ. Finally, many thyroid problems are seen exclusively in women because they are related to pregnancy. It is not therefore surprising that thyroid disorders are frequently encountered in the practice of obstetrics and gynecology. In order to understand these disorders, an understanding of normal thyroid physiology is important.

THYROID PHYSIOLOGY

Iodine and Thyroid Hormone Formation

The thyroid produces two hormones: thyroxine (T4) and 3,5,3'-triiodothyronine (T3). These have profound effects on almost every tissue of the body. The gland weighs approximately 20 g and consists of two lobes that adhere to the lateral aspects of the trachea. The lobes are joined by the isthmus, which crosses the trachea just above the sternal notch. The basic unit of the thyroid gland is the follicle. This consists of a group of epithelial cells surrounding a central pool of thyroglobulin-rich colloid. Thyroglobulin is a protein with a molecular weight of

CHARLES H. EMERSON • Department of Medicine, Division of Endocrinology and Metabolism, University of Massachusetts School of Medicine, Worcester, Massachusetts 01605.

660,000. It contains covalently linked T4 and T3. This arrangement permits the thyroid to store relatively large amounts of hormone.[2]

Thyroid hormone synthesis can be divided into several discrete steps.[3] These consist of (1) transport of circulating iodide into the thyroid against a concentration gradient (the iodide trap), (2) organification of iodide followed by generation of monoiodotyrosine (MIT) and diiodotyrosine (DIT) residues linked to thyroglobulin, (3) coupling of these residues to form thyroglobulin-associated T3 or T4, and (4) limited digestion to release T4 and T3 for secretion. It is apparent from this scheme that iodide is essential for thyroid hormone production. Two major factors influence iodide uptake and organification. The first of these is the plasma concentration of iodide. During iodide deficiency, the plasma iodide concentration falls. The thyroid has the ability to compensate by trapping and organifying a much greater percentage of the circulating iodide. In iodide excess, plasma iodide levels are increased and the thyroid compensates by decreasing the transport of iodide into the gland. This process is called iodide autoregulation and is an intrinsic property of the thyroid.[4] The pituitary hormone thyrotropin, thyroid-stimulating hormone (TSH), also regulates thyroid iodide uptake. TSH is essential for normal iodide uptake and organification. If TSH secretion is excessive, the uptake and organification of circulating iodide are increased. Other thyroid stimulators besides TSH, such as the thyroid-stimulating immunoglobulins of Graves' disease and thyroid-stimulating substance(s) produced by trophoblastic tumors, also increase iodide uptake.

Structure, Transport, and Metabolic "Activation" of Thyroid Hormone

Figure 7-1 presents the structure of the thyroid hormones T4 and T3. It can be seen that T4 contains two iodine atoms linked to the outer aromatic ring and two linked to the inner ring. T3 is identical to T4 except there is only a single iodine atom in the outer ring. Figure 7-1 also shows the structure of 3,3′,5′-T3 or reverse T3 (rT3). Its structure is similar to that of T3 except that a single iodine atom is linked to the inner rather than the outer ring. The thyroid is the only tissue in the body capable, under normal circumstances, of producing T4. After secretion, more than 99% of the circulating T4 is bound to three serum proteins. These are thyroxine-binding globulin (TBG), thyroxine-binding prealbumin (TBPA), and albumin.[5] The distribution of circulating T4 among these proteins in normal subjects is approximately 60, 30, and 10% for TBG, TBPA, and albumin, respectively. However, it is the concentration of unbound or free T4 in the circulation that actually reflects thyroid status. Thus, in making the diagnosis of hyper- or hypothyroidism, the concentration of free T4 must be assessed.

In contrast to T4, only about 20% of the circulating T3 comes from thyroid secretion. The remaining T3 is generated in "peripheral" tissues by the action of enzymes known as outer ring deiodinases. These enzymes convert T4 to T3. The same tissues also contain inner-ring deiodinase enzymes that convert T4 to reverse T3. Reverse T3 displays little or no hormonal activity. These enzymatic steps are depicted in Figure 7-1, which emphasizes the point that T4, secreted from the thyroid, can either be

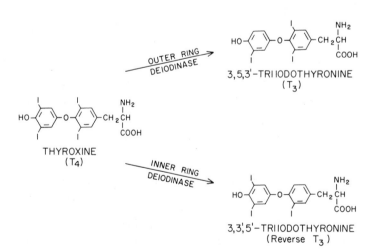

FIGURE 7-1. Metabolism of thyroxine (T4) after secretion by the thyroid. T4 must be converted to triiodothyronine (T3) by enzymatic removal of the outer ring iodine before it becomes hormonally active. Removal of the inner ring iodine by another enzyme produces reverse T3, which is hormonally inactive. The metabolism of T4 in maternal and fetal circulations is probably strikingly different.

converted to its metabolically active form, T3, or inactivated to form rT3. The reactions are physiologically regulated. Starvation and severe illness of any kind decrease the peripheral conversion of T4 to T3.[6] Therefore, in anorexia nervosa or severe illness the plasma concentration of T3 is low. This is currently regarded, however, as a physiologic response, not a state of true hypothyroidism. Many drugs and hormones also decrease the peripheral conversion of T4 to T3. These include propranolol, prednisone, and other glucocorticoid steroids, X-ray contrast agents such as iopanoic acid, and the cardiac agent amiodarone.[7]

Thyroid Hormone Actions: T4 vs. T3

Like the steroid hormones, many of the most important effects of thyroid hormone are mediated at the cell nucleus. Brain, pituitary, heart, lung, liver, kidney, and uterus contain high-affinity, limited-capacity nuclear receptors for T3.[8] In some of these tissues, the thyroid hormone response is proportional to the number of receptors occupied by T3. T4 binds poorly to nuclear receptors and probably must be converted to T3 to be hormonally active. However, it is misleading to think of T3 as metabolically active and T4 as an inactive. This is because the cell nucleus has two sources of T3: circulating T3 and T3 generated from circulating T4 after it is taken up by the cell and converted to T3. Some tissues, such as liver and kidney, derive almost all their nuclear T3 from circulating T3. Other tissues, such as brain, obtain the major portion of nuclear T3 from circulating T4. Thus, plasma T3 concentrations reflect the thyroid status of organs such as liver, while plasma T4 may be a more reliable index of thyroid status in the brain.[9] The fetus is of interest in this regard, since plasma T4 concentrations during the last trimester are near the normal adult range, whereas plasma T3 levels are almost undetectable. T3 interacts at the nuclear level with the linker portion of DNA to initiate a process that ultimately results in enzyme synthesis. In some cases, this can be related to one of the classic effects of thyroid hormone. For example, it is postulated that thyroid hormones increase tissue respiration, and therefore the basal metabolic rate (BMR), by stimulating the synthesis of plasma membrane Na-K-ATPase.[10] So many effects of thyroid hormone have been described that a complete review of them is beyond the scope of this chapter. Those that are particularly important will become apparent in the discussion of hyper- and hypothyroidism.

The Hypothalamic–Pituitary–Thyroid Axis

Thyroid hormone secretion is almost completely under the control of pituitary TSH. TSH stimulates all phases of thyroid hormone production from iodide uptake to T4 and T3 secretion. In TSH deficiency, thyroid function is severely compromised. TSH secretion, in turn, is dependent on the hypothalamic peptide thyrotropin-releasing hormone (TRH). TRH is the smallest of the hypothalamic releasing factors and contains only three amino acids. It is found in high concentrations in the most basal part of the hypothalamus, the median eminence. From there it is carried to the TSH-secreting cells, called thyrotrophs, by the pituitary portal circulation. TRH is a potent stimulus for TSH secretion in humans and animals. By contrast, thyroid hormones inhibit TSH secretion. TRH and thyroid hormone interact so as to maintain TSH secretion at a normal rate.[11] For example, even mild thyroid hormone deficiency enhances the TSH secretory response to TRH. But when the pituitary is exposed to small excesses of thyroid hormone, the TSH response to TRH is markedly suppressed.[11] Therefore, the negative feedback effect of thyroid hormone on TSH secretion can largely be explained by the ability of thyroid hormone to antagonize the response of the pituitary thyrotrophs to endogenous TRH. The TSH response to TRH is augmented in women as compared with men.[12] This effect is related to the estrogen and androgen status of women. In women who are receiving oral contraceptives the TSH response to TRH is enhanced.[13] In humans testosterone decreases the TSH response to TRH.[14]

THYROID FUNCTION TESTS

The clinical goals of thyroid function tests are twofold. The first is to determine whether the patient is producing a normal amount of thyroid hormone. The second is to determine the nature of thyroid enlargement and to rule out a malignant process. Thyroid cancer is usually associated with normal production of thyroid hormone. Therefore, the chances of a thyroid malignancy are much less if hyper- or hypothyroidism is detected. Thyroid function tests can be divided into several categories: (1) tests that measure or provide an index of serum thyroid hormone concentrations, (2) tests that assess the hypothalamic-pituitary axis, (3) tests that evaluate thyroid anatomy and physiology, and (4) miscellaneous tests.

Tests that Measure Serum Thyroid Hormone Hormones

These tests include the serum T4, the T3 resin uptake (T3 RU), the free thyroxine index (FTI), and the serum T3. The serum T4 concentration is currently measured by radioimmunoassay (RIA). In practice, it is a measurement of the protein bound fraction, since more than 99.9% of the T4 in serum is bound to TBG, TBPA, or albumin. If the serum TBG is normal, the serum T4 is usually an accurate index of thyroid status. When serum TBG is increased or decreased, the T4 is changed in a similar direction. However, the patient is still euthyroid because the free T4 concentration, which determines thyroid status, is normal. Serum TBG concentrations are elevated in pregnant women or those taking estrogen-containing medications. In these patients, the serum T4 should be high normal or mildly elevated. The T3 resin uptake test (T3 RU) should be ordered at the same time as the T4. This test can be used to determine whether the T4 is abnormal because of true thyroid disease or because the serum TBG concentration is outside the range of normal. The nomenclature for the T3 RU is misleading, since this test is not a measure of the serum T3 concentration. Instead, it provides an index of the amount of TBG in serum that is not saturated with T4. Accordingly, the T3 RU is dependent on both the serum T4 and TBG concentrations. While this seems complex, the interpretation of the T3 RU and the serum T4 is relatively simple and can be summarized as follows: In hyperthyroidism the serum T4 and T3 RU are both increased; in hypothyroidism these tests tend to be decreased. By contrast, when the serum T4 is increased because of an increase in serum TBG, the T3 RU is low; when the serum T4 is low because the serum TBG is decreased, the T3 RU is elevated. The free thyroxine index (FTI) or T_7 is a derived expression that takes advantage of this situation. The FTI is calculated by multiplying the T3 RU by the T4. The FTI is increased in hyperthyroidism and decreased in hypothyroidism because in these situations both the T4 and the T3 RU is either elevated (hyperthyroidism) or depressed (hypothyroidism). The FTI is usually normal in women taking estrogen-containing medications because the increase in the T4 is compensated for by a decrease in the T3 RU. However, if the TBG concentration is extremely high or low, the FTI will be somewhat outside the range of normal, even though the patient is euthyroid. This problem should be suspected if there is a marked disparity between the results of the serum T4 and T3 RU. In this situation, other studies are required to establish or rule out thyroid dysfunction. Finally, it must be noted that the T4, T3 RU, and FTI may give misleading results in patients who are very ill,[15] in patients receiving certain drugs, or in rare patients with unusual serum T4-binding proteins.[16]

Measurement of the serum T3 concentration by RIA is an important thyroid function test in the diagnosis of hyperthyroidism. Because the serum T3 is low in many conditions besides hypothyroidism, this test has no place in the workup of suspected hypothyroidism. Like T4, more than 99% of circulating T3 is bound to TBG. The serum T3 is therefore modestly elevated in pregnant women or in those taking estrogen. In some patients with hyperthyroidism, the production rate of T3 is high, whereas that of T4 is much closer to normal. In these cases, called "T3 toxicosis," the FTI is normal, but the serum T3 concentration is elevated. In "T3 toxicosis," a serum T3 measurement is required to make the diagnosis of hyperthyroidism.

Tests of the Hypothalamic–Pituitary–Thyroid Axis

These tests take advantage of the fact that the hypothalamic–pituitary axis is very sensitive to changes in circulating thyroid hormones. The useful tests in this category are the serum TSH and the TSH response to the administration of TRH. A high serum TSH and normal T4 is a very early sign of thyroid failure. This combination is frequently observed after treatment of Graves' disease with radioactive iodine (RAI) or surgery, in early Hashimoto's thyroiditis, and in patients receiving the antithyroid drug lithium. The serum TSH provides both sensitive and specific information. With the exception of rare patients who have TSH-secreting pituitary tumors, a serum TSH value of greater than 20 μU/ml is diagnostic of primary hypothyroidism. Peripheral resistance to the metabolic actions of thyroid hormone is also associated with elevated serum TSH levels, but values are usually well below 20 μU/ml in these unusual patients.[17]

The TRH test is useful in the diagnosis of hyperthyroidism. It should be employed in cases where clinical features suggest hyperthyroidism, but other thyroid function tests are borderline. After placing an intravenous line for TRH administration and blood collection, a basal blood sample is obtained. Following this, 400 μg of synthetic TRH is administered as a bolus. Blood is collected 15, 30, 60, and 90 min after TRH administration and TSH is measured in all samples. In normal subjects, the basal TSH is usually less than 6 μU/ml. After TRH, the serum TSH increases by at least 3 μU/ml. Peak TSH levels usually occur about 30 min after TRH. In primary hypothyroidism, the basal TSH is elevated and the TSH response is exaggerated. In most forms of hyperthyroidism, the basal TSH is low or undetectable and the TSH shows little or no change after TRH. Hyperthyroidism is very unlikely if the serum TSH increases by more than 3 μU/ml after TRH. However, failure of TSH to rise after TRH does not firmly establish the diagnosis of hyperthyroidism. This is also seen in some severely ill patients, in patients taking the antiarrhythmic drug amiodarone, and in acute psychiatric conditions. Theoretically, the TRH test should also be useful to distinguish between hypothyroidism that results from hypothalamic TRH deficiency (hypothalamic hypothyroidism) and hypothyroidism secondary to pituitary disease. Unfortunately, in clinical studies the TRH test does not clearly distinguish between patients with hypothalamic and pituitary disease.[18]

Tests of Thyroid Anatomy and Physiology

The major tests in this category are the 24-hr thyroid iodine uptake and the thyroid scan. These tests involve the administration of RAI and should not be performed in pregnant women. The 24-hr thyroid iodine uptake test is performed by administering tracer amounts of RAI. The thyroid is scanned 24 hr later, and the percentage of the administered iodine concentrated by the thyroid is calculated. In normal individuals residing in the United States the 24 hr iodine uptake ranges from about 12 to 30%. Very low values will be obtained if the patient has been exposed to large amounts of iodine. Iodine exposure can come from many sources. Some, but not all are dietary. For example, vaginal douching with polyvinyl–pyrrolidone–iodine markedly lowers the 24-hr iodine uptake.[19] In addition, iodine-containing medications and radiographic contrast agents are a well-recognized source of pharmacologic doses of iodine. The 24-hr iodine uptake is useful in the differential diagnosis of hyperthyroidism. This test may be low, normal, or high in different forms of hyperthyroidism. The

24-hr iodine test is also performed before RAI treatment of hyperthyroidism to calculate the treatment dose. Despite previous use, the 24-hr radioactive iodine uptake is of little value in determining whether a patient has hypothyroidism or hyperthyroidism.

The thyroid scan is used to determine the size and shape of the gland and assess the function of enlarged regions. Technetium 99-, ^{123}I, and ^{131}I have been used as thyroid scanning agents. The use of ^{131}I is discouraged, particularly in young patients, because of the radiation exposure. Although ^{99m}Tc scans require less time than ^{123}I, they do not provide the best information, since ^{123}I discriminates better than ^{99m}Tc between normal thyroid tissue and thyroid cancer. In fact, some thyroid carcinomas concentrate ^{99m}Tc very well, whereas this is rarely the case for ^{123}I.

Miscellaneous Tests

Three other very useful thyroid function tests are measurement of serum antibodies to thyroid tissue (anti-thyroid antibody test), measurement of the serum thyroglobulin, and needle biopsy of the thyroid. One of the hallmarks of autoimmune thyroid diseases is the presence of circulating antibodies directed against different cellular components of the thyroid gland. Sensitive tests are now available to measure antibodies directed against two of these components, namely, thyroglobulin and thyroid microsomes. Moderately or strongly positive tests for antithyroglobulin and antimicrosomal antibodies should be considered a marker for autoimmune thyroid diseases (Graves' disease, Hashimoto's thyroiditis). The titer of these antibodies does not reflect the severity of thyroid dysfunction. For example, it is not unusual to find patients with early Hashimoto's thyroiditis who are euthyroid but have antimicrosomal antibody titers of 1 : 25,000. The tests for anti-thyroid antibodies are not completely specific for autoimmune thyroid diseases. Low titers of anti-thyroglobulin and anti-microsomal antibodies are sometimes seen in subacute thyroiditis, multinodular goiter, and thyroid cancer.[20]

In normal subjects, small amounts of thyroglobulin are secreted by the thyroid. In patients with simple goiter or thyroid cancer, much larger quantities of thyroglobulin leak into the circulation. Therefore, the serum thyroglobulin cannot be used to distinguish between benign and malignant thyroid disease. Rather, it is used as a marker that thyroid tissue is present. In patients with thyroid cancer, who have had total ablation of thyroid tissue, the development of metastatic disease can be detected by the presence of thyroglobulin in serum.[2,21] Fine-needle aspiration biopsy is becoming widely used to evaluate the malignant potential of hypofunctioning thyroid nodules.[22,23] The test is safe and relatively painless. Experience is necessary in order to obtain an adequate sample and the test must be read by a pathologist who is thoroughly familiar with thyroid cytology.

THYROID PATHOPHYSIOLOGY

Susceptibility to Thyroid Disease in Women

Simple goiter, thyroid nodules, hyperthyroidism, and hypothyroidism are far more prevalent in women than in men.[24] The female to male ratio of simple goiter is about 8 : 1. Mild iodine deficiency may be an important basis for this increased susceptibility of women to goiter. Women are vulnerable to iodine deficiency during pregnancy and possibly during each menstrual cycle because the renal iodide clearance is increased.[25,26] Iodine deficiency need not be associated with hypothyroidism in order to induce thyroid enlargement. Experimental studies indicate that TSH has a greater effect on thyroid growth in the iodine-deficient as compared with the iodine-sufficient animal.[27] Another factor that might explain the propensity of women to develop goiter is that during pregnancy they may be exposed to thyroid-stimulating substances of placental origin.[28–30]

The female to male ratio in Graves' disease and Hashimoto's thyroiditis is in some series more than 6 : 1.[31,32] The preponderance of these autoimmune diseases in women is in accord with the finding that women have a predilection to almost all autoimmune diseases. The basis for this susceptibility has not been established. One theory is that the absence of the Y chromosome, which carries protective histocompatability antigens, makes women more susceptible to autoimmune disease.[33] Differences in the production of estrogen and androgen between men and women may influence the expression of autoimmune disease as well.[34]

Hyperthyroidism

Differential Diagnosis

Hyperthyroidism is a condition in which thyroid hormone production is greater than required to maintain the euthyroid state. This definition takes into consideration the rare syndrome of peripheral resistance to the metabolic actions of thyroid hormone. In this syndrome the production rate of thyroid hormone is high in order to maintain the euthyroid state.[17] The diagnosis of hyperthyroidism begins with the finding of clinical features of thyroid hormone excess. Thyroid function tests that confirm the diagnosis are a high serum FTI and T3 and lack of a TSH response to TRH administration. Hyperthyroidism has many etiologies. The most common cause in women is Graves' disease. This autoimmune disorder is associated with the production of antibodies to the TSH receptor. These antibodies were previously called the long-acting thyroid stimulator (LATS) and are currently referred to as thyroid-stimulating immunoglobulins (TSI). TSI produces many, if not all, of the metabolic effects of TSH. As a result of their action, the thyroid becomes diffusely enlarged and secretes large amounts of T4 and T3. A diffuse goiter can be appreciated by palpation or by thyroid scan, and the iodine uptake is markedly elevated. Patients with Graves' disease frequently have circulating antibodies to thyroglobulin and to thyroid microsomes. The thyroid is infiltrated with lymphocytes, and there is evidence that, over the course of many years, the autoimmune process may produce hypothyroidism. Ophthalmopathy is one of the extrathyroid hallmarks of Graves' disease that helps establish the diagnosis.[35] Graves' ophthalmopathy is probably a manifestation of the autoimmune process. Pathologically, the extraocular muscles are swollen, and there is infiltration of the retrobulbar space with lymphocytes and protein-rich fluid. This produces varying degrees of proptosis. More severe forms of ophthalmopathy are characterized by diplopia, exposure keratitis due to inability to close the eyelids, and loss of visual acuity due to compression of the optic nerve. Almost all patients with Graves' disease have ophthalmopathy, but many have few clinical signs. Fortunately, severe ophthalmopathy is rare and symptomology is usually limited to a sensation of discomfort in the eyes. There is a high incidence of other autoimmune diseases in Graves' disease, particularly myasthenia gravis, pernicious anemia, idiopathic thrombocytopenic purpura, and vitiligo.

Toxic multinodular goiter is the second most common form of hyperthyroidism. This disease develops in some patients with long-standing simple or multinodular goiter. Consequently, toxic multinodular goiter is more frequent in elderly patients. Toxic solitary nodule is a variant of toxic multinodular goiter. This lesion may be seen in younger women. It is almost never malignant. The diagnosis of toxic multinodular goiter and toxic solitary nodule is based on the presence of nodular thyroid enlargement, as detected by physical examination and thyroid scan. Hyperthyroidism in toxic multinodular goiter and toxic solitary nodule results from unregulated release of thyroid hormone from the nodular lesions. If the nodules are small, the amount of thyroid hormone released is also small and feedback inhibition of TSH maintains serum thyroid hormone in the near-normal range. Exposure to pharmacologic amounts of iodine will greatly increase the amount of thyroid hormone produced by these nodules and can convert a euthyroid patient to one with thyrotoxicosis.[36] Iodine-induced hyperthyroidism is slow in onset and typically persists for some time after the period of iodine exposure.

The term "destructive" hyperthyroidism can be applied to a group of syndromes whose course is quite different from Graves' disease, toxic multinodular goiter, or toxic adenoma.[37] Graves' disease and nodular thyroid disease are characterized by sustained hyperproduction of thyroid hormone. The onset is often insidious. By contrast, destructive hyperthyroidism is characterized by the abrupt onset of hyperthyroid symptoms. This is because, in destructive hyperthyroidism, a major portion of the hormone stored in the thyroid is released in a rapid and uncontrolled fashion. Since thyroid hormone synthesis is not increased, the duration of hyperthyroidism is brief. In addition, because of TSH suppression during the hyperthyroid period, and because of damage to the gland by the destructive process, a period of hypothyroidism often persists for several weeks or months before normal function is resumed. Surprisingly, destructive hyperthyroidism is usually not a cause of permanent hypothyroidism. The major forms of destructive hyperthyroidism are subacute thyroiditis, painless thyroiditis, and postpartum thyroiditis. In subacute thyroiditis, the thyroid becomes tender and painful. Pain is sometimes referred to the ear, jaw, and even the chest. Most cases of subacute thyroiditis are thought to result from viral infections.[38] Painless thyroiditis (spontaneously resolving thyroiditis, lymphocytic thyroiditis, hyperthyroiditis) is similar to subacute thyroiditis in that there is a rather sudden onset of hyperthyroidism.[39] However, pain and thyroid tenderness are absent. The cause of painless thyroiditis is unknown. Postpartum thyroiditis is a fascinating entity that probably has more than one underlying cause (see the section on pregnancy).

Destructive hyperthyroidism should be suspected in patients with hyperthyroidism of abrupt onset and in those with thyroid pain and tenderness. A very low 24-hr RAI uptake is strong support for the diagnosis.

The remaining causes of hyperthyroidism are very rare. These include TSH-producing pituitary tumors, isolated pituitary resistance to the feedback effects of thyroid hormone, and factitious hyperthyroidism. This can be caused by surreptitious ingestion of T4 (Synthyroid, Levothyroid), T3 (Cytomel) or T4/T3 mixtures (desiccated thyroid, Proloid, Euthroid). In factitious hyperthyroidism, the serum thyroid hormone levels reflect what the patient is ingesting. The diagnosis requires a high index of suspicion and should be suspected when there is no goiter and the 24-hr RAI uptake is depressed. Unexplained atrial fibrillation is common in these patients.

Ovarian teratomas (struma ovarii) are a very rare cause of hyperthyroidism.[40,41] These tumors sometimes contain thyroid tissue. These patients may be clinically hyperthyroid with elevated serum T4 and/or T3 concentrations. They have no goiter and the 24-hr RAI uptake is depressed. A whole-body scan showing uptake of RAI in the ovarian tumor is necessary to document this diagnosis.[40,41]

Clinical Features

The clinical features of hyperthyroidism are due to direct effects of thyroid hormone on many organs, including those of the reproductive system.[42,43] Table 7-1 lists the most prominent signs and symptoms of hyperthyroidism. The heat intolerance, increased sweating, and warm skin are probably secondary to increased tissue oxygen consumption and thermogenesis produced by thyroid hormone. Tachycardia is at least partially a reflex response to the increase in basal metabolic rate (BMR), but thyroid hormone also directly influences cardiac tissue. This results in increased contractility and probably accounts for the high incidence of atrial fibrillation in hyperthyroidism. Proximal muscle weakness is common in established hyperthyroidism and is the major manifestation of thyrotoxic myopathy. Dyspnea, a frequent complaint in severe hyperthyroidism, is in part due to intercostal muscle weakness. Thyroid hormone is more catabolic for muscle than for fat tissue, which is why thyroid hormone is not useful in the treatment of obesity.[44] Most of the eye manifestations of hyperthyroidism are confined to those with Graves' disease. Thyroid hormone excess does

TABLE 7-1. Clinical Features of Hyperthyroidism

Symptoms	Signs
Hypomenorrhea	Diaphoresis
Amenorrhea	Warm skin
Heat intolerance	Stare
Nervousness	Emotional lability
Increased appetite	Hyperkinetic movements
Weight loss	Tremor
Hyperdefecation	Tachycardia

cause upper eyelid retraction, producing lid lag and stare. These clinical signs resolve when the patient becomes euthyroid. By contrast, the clinical features of Graves' opthalmopathy do not necessarily improve with anti-thyroid drug treatment.

Hyperthyroidism and the Female Reproductive System

In hyperthyroid women, menses occur at normal intervals, but flow is scanty.[45,46] Hypomenorrhea becomes more pronounced as the severity of hyperthyroidism increases. In most patients, however, the cycles are ovulatory, as shown by endometrial biopsy, urine pregnanediol measurement, and a rise in plasma progesterone following the mid-cycle surge in LH and FSH.[45,46] In patients with severe hyperthyroidism, secondary amenorrhea may develop. These patients lack mid-cycle FSH and LH peaks, and their plasma progesterone concentrations remain constantly low, confirming anovulation.[46,47] Hyperthyroid women usually resume normal menstrual periods when treated with antithyroid drugs. The pathogenesis of the hypomenorrhea and amenorrhea of hyperthyroidism is unclear. As shown in Figure 7-2, plasma LH and FSH concentrations in hyperthyroid women are elevated throughout the menstrual cycle as compared with those of controls, except at the time of the mid-cycle peak.[46] The mean peak of the mid-cycle LH surge is slightly lower than in euthyroid women, while the peak of the mid-cycle FSH surge is similar. Plasma estrogens (estradiol 17 β-estrone) have been reported to be elevated throughout the menstrual cycle in some studies[46] and in the normal range in other studies.[48] Even in this latter study, however, there was a decline in the plasma esterone and estradiol concentrations with treatment of hyperthyroidism. Plasma progesterone[47] concentra-

tions are normal unless the patient develops amenorrhea. Serum androstenedione has been reported to be normal in women with hyperthyroidism,[48,49] but the androstenedione production rate is increased in some women.[48] Plasma testosterone concentrations are consistently elevated when measured in hyperthyroid subjects.[48,50−55]

Hyperthyroidism is associated with an almost threefold increase in plasma sex hormone binding globulin (SHBG) concentrations. Thyroid hormone appears to increase directly the production of SHBG.[56,57] The increase in SHBG probably accounts for the increase in plasma testosterone and may partially account for increased plasma estradiol concentrations. Although an early study suggested that the conversion of testosterone to estradiol and of androstenedione to estrone was increased in hyperthyroidism, this finding was not confirmed by a more recent study.[48,49] Akande and Anderson[58] hypothesized that the increase in SHBG associated with hyperthyroidism leads to diminished free estradiol. This in turn decreases the negative feedback effect of estradiol on LH, accounting for high plasma LH concentrations during most of the menstrual cycle and a decrease in the positive feedback effect of estrogen at mid-cycle. This decrease in positive feedback accounts for the fact that the mid-cycle LH surge is decreased and, if the defect is severe enough, the LH surge is lost altogether. This theory would account for anovulation, absence of progesterone production during the luteal phase, and amenorrhea. The LH response to LHRH is increased in some hyperthyroid women, even if they do not have menstrual disturbances.[59,60] This fits with the concept that negative feedback on gonadotropin secretion is decreased in hyperthyroidism.

T3 receptors have been identified in the rat uterus,[61] and thyroid hormone alters the effects of estrogen on uterine growth.[62] Thyroid hormone also appears to effect the activity of 5α-reductase pathways for steroid metabolism.[63] The clinical significance of these effects is not clear. The increase in SHBG synthesis produced by thyroid hormone may be particularly significant under unusual circumstances. For example, a patient with thyrotoxicosis, an ovarian hilus cell tumor, and markedly elevated serum testosterone was noted to lack virilization. It was postulated that the high levels of SHBG that resulted from hyperthyroidism protected this patient from the effects of the testosterone produced by the ovarian tumor.[64] Because thyroid hormone

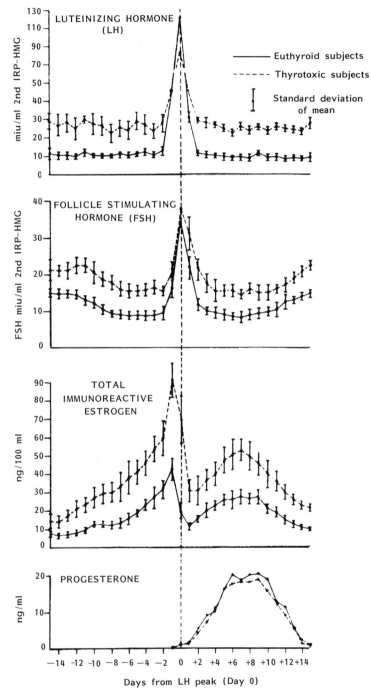

FIGURE 7-2. Circulating levels of gonadotropins, estrogens, and progesterone in hyperthyroid women. The relationship of this hormonal profile to hypomenorrhea, the characteristic menstrual pattern of hyperthyroidism, is unclear. (From Akende and Hockaday[46].)

increases SHBG, it has been used to blunt androgen effects in hirsute women.[57] This treatment is experimental, however, and more studies are needed before it can be recommended.

Hypothyroidism

Differential Diagnosis

In the United States autoimmune thyroid diseases account for most cases of hyperthyroidism. Hypothyroidism is common in many patients with Graves' disease, regardless of treatment. This complication results not only from treatments such as RAI or surgery but also from the underlying autoimmune thyroiditis.[65] Hypothyroidism is the major complication of Hashimoto's thyroiditis (chronic lymphocytic thyroiditis, struma lymphomatosa). This disorder is characterized by lymphocytic infiltration of the thyroid with the formation of germinal centers, one of the manifestations of a cell-mediated immune process directed against the thyroid. Another is the presence of circulating antibodies to thyroglobulin and thyroid microsomes. Titers of these antibodies are usually higher than seen in Graves' disease. Most patients with Hashimoto's thyroiditis present with a small goiter that is usually firm and may be finely nodular. In some cases, physical examination suggests only a solitary nodule. More often, thyroid enlargement is diffuse. Many patients with autoimmune thyroid failure never have a palpable goiter; In these patients thyroid atrophy is probably more characteristic.

Although many drugs have antithyroid properties, lithium carbonate is the only agent in wide use. In as many as 10% of patients who receive lithium carbonate for more than 1 year, hypothyroidism develops.[66] Hypothyroidism is also caused by inherited defects in thyroid hormone synthesis, but these disorders are very rare.

Clinical Features

Table 7-2 lists some of the prominent signs and symptoms of hypothyroidism. It must be emphasized that even when patients are found to have moderately severe hypothyroidism by laboratory criteria, these features may be subtle; many ''classic'' signs or symptoms are often absent. Thyroid function tests should be obtained even if the index of suspicion for hypothyroidism is low. Constitutional symptoms are common in hypothyroidism.[67,68] These include cold intolerance, lassitude, constipation, and hypersomnolence. Although

TABLE 7-2. Clinical Features of Hypothyroidism

Symptoms	Signs
Menorrhagia	Constipation
Galactorrhea[a]	Muscle cramps
Dry, puffy skin	Paresthesias
Periorbital edema	Rheumatic complaints
Cold intolerance	Bradycardia
Lethargy	Growth retardation

[a]Rare, resolves with thyroid hormone treatment.

some weight gain occurs, hypothyroidism is rarely the cause of massive obesity. As many as 85% of patients with hypothyroidism have changes in the skin and subcutaneous tissue. The skin is dry, cool, pale, and coarse, and the subcutaneous tissue is infiltrated with protein-rich fluid. The facies of a patient with moderately severe hypothyroidism, before and after treatment, are shown in Figure 7-3.

In hypothyroidism the clearance of albumin and other proteins from the interstitial space is decreased.[69] This is the basis of the nonpitting edema (myxedema) and accounts for a wide variety of clinical manifestations. These include periorbital edema, swelling of the skeletal muscles including the tongue, and myxedematous effusions into the pericardial, pleural, and peritoneal cavities. In long-standing hypothyroidism, the skin has a yellowish hue as the result of carotene deposition. The hair and scalp are thin and dry. Patchy hair loss is a late sign of hypothyroidism. Some patients with Hashimoto's thyroiditis have oval, well-circumscribed areas of hair loss (alopecia areata). This lesion is not due to hypothyroidism but rather to an associated autoimmune disorder.

Bradycardia is the most prominent cardiovascular manifestation of hypothyroidism. The electrocardiogram (ECG) shows decreased voltage with flat T waves. The finding of pleural and pericardial effusions may lead to an erroneous diagnosis of congestive heart failure. Pulmonary symptoms are uncommon in hypothyroidism unless the advanced condition leads to myxedema; in these patients, central hypoventilation is a life-threatening clinical problem. The most prominent gastrointestinal symptoms are constipation and vague abdominal discomfort. In advanced myxedema paralytic ileus sometimes develops. Symptoms related to bladder dysfunction are unusual. In myxedema coma, urinary retention sometimes occurs. Musculoskeletal symptoms are frequent in hypothyroidism and usu-

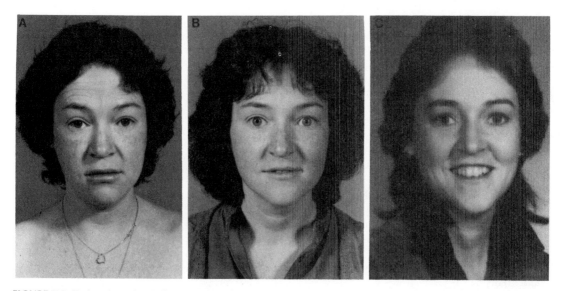

FIGURE 7-3. Facies of a patient before treatment of hypothyroidism (left). The same patient is shown 2 months (middle) and 16 months (right) after thyroid hormone replacement. Note the improvement in the sallow, lethargic appearance. (Courtesy of Dr. M. Safran.)

ally consist of muscle stiffness or cramps. Arthralgias and synovial thickening have been described, but significant joint effusions are unusual. Neurologic abnormalities include paresthesias of the distal extremities, ataxia, and psychosis. Paresthesias may be due to compression of small sensory nerves. Large nerves are sometimes compressed by swollen tendon sheaths leading to entrapment neuropathies such as the carpel tunnel syndrome. Hypothyroidism is one of the major causes of growth failure in the adolescent. Pubertal development is also affected. Hypothyroidism should always be ruled out in girls with growth failure, abnormal pubertal development, and galactorrhea.

Certain laboratory findings suggest the diagnosis of hypothyroidism. Because lipid abnormalities are frequent, hypothyroidism must be ruled out in all patients with hypercholesterolemia or hypertriglyceridemia. The CPK is often increased, and the SGOT and LDH may be modestly elevated. The elevation of CPK is largely due to the MM isoenzyme. Many hypothyroid patients have a mild anemia; iron deficiency is frequently associated with anemia. This is probably the result of menorrhagia. The incidence of pernicious anemia is increased in Hashimoto's thyroiditis. The possibility of vitamin B_{12} deficiency must therefore be considered in hypothyroid patients who are anemic.

Hypothyroidism and the Female Reproductive System

The menstrual abnormalities of hypothyroidism are, in a sense, the opposite of those that occur in hyperthyroidism. Whereas hyperthyroidism is characterized by hypomenorrhea, hypothyroid patients tend to have menorrhagia. Metropathia hemorrhagia is characteristic of patients with more long-standing hypothyroidism. This term was used by Albright to describe periods of amenorrhea interrupted, on a random basis, by endometrial oozing or hemorrhage.[45,70] In a few patients, prolonged amenorrhea occurs. Menstrual disturbances are associated with a high incidence of anovulation. Goldsmith et al.[45] found that 7 of 10 patients with "definite clinical and laboratory evidence of myxedema" were anovulatory; most of these patients had menorrhagia. These and other data clearly establish that fertility is decreased in hypothyroidism. Indeed, until recently the occurrence of pregnancy in a hypothyroid woman was considered unusual.[71-73] Before 1980, less than 50 cases of pregnancy had been reported. However, the notion that hypothyroidism presents a major barrier to conception may be incorrect. For example, Montoro et al.[74] recently documented 11 pregnancies in 9 women who had unequivocal laboratory evidence of hypothyroidism. All these patients were seen during a 5-year period at the same large medical center. Both the degree and the duration of hypothyroidism probably influence fertility. Many of the patients in Montoro's series had moderately severe hypothyroxinemia, but in some cases hypothyroidism had resulted because thyroid hormone had not been taken on a regular basis.

Thyroid hormone is effective in restoring normal ovulatory menstrual cycles in hypothyroid women. In the past these results led to its widespread use to treat patients with infertility and habitual abortion.[73] Thyroid hormone treatment was justified on the grounds that hypothyroidism could not be ruled out by the thyroid function tests then available. As laboratory tests for hypothyroidism are now far more sensitive and specific, there is no longer a rationale for treating infertile women with thyroid hormone unless laboratory tests show evidence of hypothyroidism.

There is remarkably little information concerning the secretion, clearance, and metabolism of reproductive hormones in hypothyroid patients. As would be expected, the plasma concentration of SHBG is decreased.[57] This accounts, in part, for the fact that plasma testosterone and total immunoreactive estrogen concentrations are decreased.[75] In anovulatory women, plasma LH and FSH concentrations are decreased, and the FSH/LH ratio is modestly elevated. This is in contrast with the plasma FSH and LH values seen in hyperthyroidism.[46]

Since hypothyroidism decreases reproductive function in the adult it is paradoxical that, in long-standing juvenile hypothyroidism, clinical features suggestive of sexual precocity may develop.[76,77] These features include enlargement of the breasts, precocious menstruation, hypertrophy of the labia minora, and estrogenization of the vaginal mucosa. The effects of hypothyroidism on somatic and sexual maturation are in some ways quite different. In juvenile hypothyroidism the bone age is retarded. By contrast, compared with euthyroid patients with the same bone age (but a lower chronologic age), the plasma gonadotropin concentrations are elevated and there is more advanced maturation of the breasts and reproductive organs.[78] Some of the features of juvenile hypothyroidism go beyond advanced sexual maturation and suggest a disturbance in reproductive hormone dynamics. As demonstrated in Figure 7-4, several studies show that cystic ovaries are not unusual in juvenile hypothyroidism.[79,80] Galactorrhea is also not uncommon. Galactorrhea is also rarely a feature of adult hypothyroidism; in these patients, it is abolished by thyroid hormone treatment.[81-83] However, most adult patients with galactorrhea had received estrogens or had recently been pregnant.

Goiter and Thyroid Nodule

Pathophysiologically, a goiter can be thought of as resulting from a primary or secondary process. Primary goiters are the result of benign or malignant neoplasms of the thyroid gland. In these patients thyroid enlargement is asymmetric, and one or more nodules may be present. Secondary goiters are due to stimulation of the thyroid by external factors (thyrostimulatory goiter) or to invasion of the thyroid by a foreign process (thyroinvasive goiter).

Thyrostimulatory goiters are caused by many factors. One of the most important of these is TSH. In many forms of primary hypothyroidism, the thyroid retains the capacity to respond to the growth-promoting effects of TSH. Since plasma TSH is uniformly elevated, thyrostimulatory goiter inevitably develops. TSH-dependent thyrostimulatory goiters occur in iodine deficiency, when antithyroid drugs are administered, in congenital defects of thyroid hormone synthesis, and in acquired thyroid diseases such as Hashimoto's thyroiditis. In the United States, Hashimoto's thyroiditis is by far the most common cause of TSH-dependent thyrostimulatory goiter. Iodine-deficiency goiter is currently considered rare in the United States because many processed foods contain iodine. Small goiters develop in some patients who are receiving lithium carbonate. This drug has antithyroid effects; plasma TSH concentrations are frequently mildly elevated during its administration.[66] Congenital defects of thyroid hormone synthesis are uncommon. They become apparent in neonatal life, infancy, or early childhood. Goiters occur in patients with TSH-secreting pituitary tumors, but these lesions are very rare.

Thyrostimulatory goiters are also caused by the thyroid-stimulating immunoglobulins of Graves' disease, by growth hormone, and by substances related to chorionic gonadotropin.[28-30] Thyroid-stimulating immunoglobulins are the major reason for goiter in Graves' disease. These autoantibodies bind to the TSH receptor and produce almost all the effects of TSH itself. In acromegaly, the thyroid is one of the many organs that enlarge under the influence of growth hormone. (The goiter associated with hyperproduction of chorionic gonadotropin and related substances is discussed in the section on

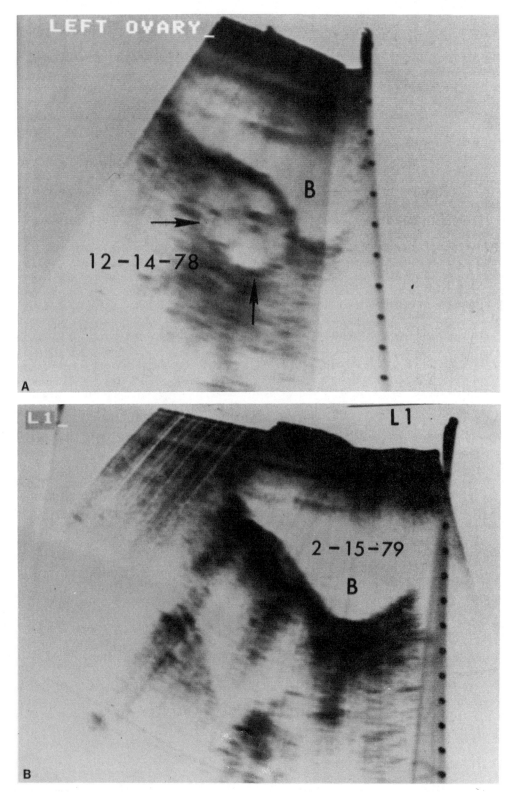

FIGURE 7-4. Regression of a multicystic ovary with thyroid hormone treatment in a patient with juvenile hypothyroidism. The ovarian ultrasound images before treatment (A) and after treatment (B) are shown. Hypothyroidism should be considered in prepubescent or early pubescent girls with cystic ovaries. (From Riddlesberger et al.[80])

the thyroid in pregnancy.) Thyrostimulatory goiters are usually diffuse, since the entire gland is stimulated. After prolonged stimulation there is a tendency for nodule formation to occur. The 24-hr RAI uptake is frequently elevated in thyrostimulatory goiter.

Simple goiter is one of the most common forms of goiter. Its pathogenesis is unclear. One hypothesis is that these goiters begin with very mild hypothyroidism leading to TSH-dependent thyrostimulatory goiter. Later, nodule formation occurs. Most patients with simple goiter are euthyroid and the 24-hr RAI uptake is normal. In the late stage, hyperthyroidism (toxic multinodular goiter) may develop. Thyroid enlargement occurs when any of a wide variety of processes invade the thyroid (thyroinvasive goiter), including neoplasms, infections, and granulomas. These goiters are characteristically asymmetric and often contain one or more nodules. In Hashimoto's thyroiditis, lymphocytic invasion of the thyroid occurs in varying degrees. In some cases, this is so focal that only a solitary nodule can be palpated. Hashimoto's thyroiditis is therefore an example of both thyrostimulatory and thyroinvasive goiter. The process that is most evident in a given case will determine the degree to which thyroid enlargement is diffuse or focal.

The most useful tests in the evaluation of goiter and thyroid nodules are the FTI, the thyroid scan, and thyroid needle biopsy. Thyroid malignancy is unlikely if the patient is hyperthyroid or hypothyroid or if the thyroid scan shows that the enlarged region concentrates iodine more avidly than surrounding tissue. The chances of thyroid cancer are increased if the patient has been treated in childhood or infancy with radiation. Rapid thyroid enlargement is also cause for concern. It may be due, however, to a benign process, such as bleeding into a cyst. If the enlarged region concentrates iodine poorly, needle biopsy is required to guide the decision for or against thyroid surgery. Although thyroid surgery is the only procedure that will completely rule out thyroid cancer, this operation is only indicated in carefully selected patients, as most goiters and thyroid nodules are benign.

MANAGEMENT OF THYROID DISEASES

Graves' Disease

The initial goal in the management of Graves' disease is to restore serum thyroid hormone levels to normal. This can be achieved with the antithyroid drugs propylthiouracil (PTU), methimazole, or carbimazole. Propranolol is also useful in this phase, since it blunts many of the effects of excess thyroid hormone. When antithyroid drugs are prescribed, the patient should be made aware of their possible side effects and instructed to discontinue medication immediately if signs or symptoms of agranulocytosis develop. As control of thyrotoxicosis is achieved, the dose of antithyroid drug is reduced and propranolol can be discontinued. There is no rationale for continuing propranolol when the patient is euthyroid. Three forms of therapy have been used in the long-term management of Graves' disease: (1) continued treatment with antithyroid drugs, (2) subtotal resection of the thyroid gland, and (3) RAI. Each treatment has its benefits, but none is ideal. Unlike surgery or RAI, antithyroid drugs do not cause permanent hypothyroidism. However, they do not cure the underlying disease and must be taken indefinitely unless a remission occurs. The chance of remission after 1 year of treatment ranges from approximately 15 to 50%.[84] Antithyroid drugs may produce agranulocytosis. However, since RAI or thyroid surgery often involves the use of antithyroid drugs, this potential problem is associated with almost all the treatment protocols for Graves' disease. Surgery offers prompt control of hyperthyroidism and eliminates the need for continued therapy with antithyroid drugs. Its disadvantages are the morbidity and mortality associated with general anesthesia, injury to the recurrent laryngeal nerves, and hypoparathyroidism. These complications are minimized if the patient is euthyroid at the time of surgery and if the procedure is performed by an experienced thyroid surgeon. Preoperative treatment with propranolol alone is not favored unless unusual circumstances are present. Propranolol has no effect on the high serum thyroid hormone levels.

RAI is as effective as surgery in ablating thyroid tissue, and its use avoids surgical complications. In many patients, it is advisable to achieve euthyroidism before RAI. In uncontrolled hyperthyroidism, RAI may precipitate thyroid storm. The disadvantage of RAI is that its therapeutic effects are delayed for several months. Some patients require a second treatment with RAI.

When RAI was first introduced, it was used only in women beyond the child-bearing period. There was concern that this treatment would increase the risk of neoplasia and damage ovarian germ cells. RAI is now used in young women with Graves' disease, but these concerns have not been completely resolved.[85] While there is little question that RAI is the treatment of choice for older patients, some endocrinologists avoid using this therapy in young women. Like surgery, RAI increases the tendency to develop hypothyroidism in later years.

Toxic Multinodular Goiter, Toxic Solitary Nodule

Since remission is unlikely, ablative therapy is the usual method of treating toxic multinodular goiter. But since this disorder tends to occur in older persons, RAI is usually the treatment of choice. Older patients are likely to have associated medical problems and may not tolerate the increase in thyroid hormones that tends to occur during the first 2 weeks after RAI treatment. Therefore, most patients with toxic multinodular goiter should be treated first with antithyroid drugs. RAI is administered after they become euthyroid. Antithyroid drugs must be stopped for at least 3 days before RAI and can be resumed 1 week after the treatment dose is administered.

Toxic solitary nodules occur in young as well as older patients. Ablative therapy is indicated if the patient is clearly hyperthyroid by clinical and laboratory criteria. RAI has been recommended on the grounds that this lesion is almost always benign and, in contrast to patients with Graves' disease, is less likely to cause hypothyroidism. However, relatively large doses of RAI are required to treat large toxic nodules. Theoretically, this could increase the incidence of carcinoma in surrounding normal tissue.[86] In addition, a recent report indicates that hypothyroidism may occur after this treatment.[87] Some authorities therefore prefer surgery rather than RAI to treat younger patients with toxic solitary nodule.[88] The morbidity and mortality associated with surgery for toxic solitary nodule is somewhat less than for Graves' disease, since unilateral rather than bilateral thyroid resection is required.

Hypothyroidism

The treatment of choice for hypothyroidism is L-thyroxine. T3 is not recommended because it does not restore serum T4 levels to normal and produces unstable serum T3 concentrations. Dessicated thyroid, a mixture of T4 and T3, is also not recommended because the hormone content of different preparations is not standardized. The usual replacement dose of T4 is 0.15–0.20 mg/day. In patients over the age of 60, T4 requirements are 0.10–0.15

mg, while some young patients require more than 0.20 mg/day.[89,90] When treatment of hypothyroidism is begun, 0.025–0.05 mg/day of T4 should be administered. This is especially important when there is cardiovascular disease, or when hypothyroidism is severe or of long duration. In these patients thyroid hormone replacement is gradually increased on a weekly or biweekly basis. This minimizes the possibility of angina or myocardial infarction. In addition, a recent report suggests that abrupt replacement of thyroid hormone in young patients may induce pseudotumor cerebri.[91]

When the dose of T4 is about 0.1 mg/day in older patients, and 0.15 mg/day in young patients, it should be maintained for 6 weeks. At this time, FTI and TSH are measured. If TSH is still elevated, the dose of T4 can be increased by 0.025 mg/day and the patient tested again at 6 weeks. When full replacement is achieved, serum TSH should be normal and the FTI in the normal range or slightly elevated. The treatment of pituitary hypothyroidism should follow guidelines similar to those employed for primary hypothyroidism. However, serum TSH cannot be used as a guide for full replacement. Instead, enough T4 should be administered to restore the FTI to normal. If ACTH deficiency is present, it is mandatory that the patient receive adrenal glucocorticoid replacement before thyroid hormone treatment is begun.

THE THYROID IN PREGNANCY AND THE POSTPARTUM

Maternal Thyroid Physiology

Many thyroid function tests change during pregnancy, but the production rate of T4 is actually quite stable. An early observation was that the BMR was elevated, largely the result of added fetal demands for oxygen, not a change in thyroid status.[92] The percentage 24 hr iodine uptake is also increased.[26,93] The plasma iodide is decreased because of transfer of iodide to the fetus and a decreased renal threshold for iodide excretion. In response to the fall in plasma iodide, the thyroid increases the percentage of circulating iodide that is trapped and organified (iodide autoregulation). The actual amount of iodide concentrated by the thyroid is similar, however, in pregnant and nonpregnant women.[93]

As a result of estrogen production by the fetal placental unit, serum TBG concentrations rise during pregnancy. There is a concomitant rise in serum

T4, T3, and rT3 levels, which peak at about 18 weeks gestation.[94-99] The increase in these hormones is almost entirely due to a change in the TBG bound fraction. Free T4 concentrations may change slightly, but the data on this point have been contradictory.[99] A recent longitudinal study found free T4 slightly elevated in early pregnancy and declined thereafter.[99] These changes were attributed to changes in T4 secretion rate. However, an older study could find no difference in the T4 turnover rate in age matched pregnant and nonpregnant women.[100] Plasma TSH levels are in the normal range during pregnancy. TSH levels tend to increase very slightly from the seventh week of gestation until term.[99] Several TSH-like substances in the placenta have been described.[30] The effect of these substances on thyroid function in normal pregnancy, if any, has not been defined. One or more of these substances are probably important in the hyperthyroidism of hydatidiform mole.

Fertility is not completely impaired in hypothyroidism. Therefore the possibility of this disorder cannot be discounted simply because the patient is pregnant. Early diagnosis and treatment are important because of the adverse effects of maternal hypothyroidism on fetal viability and development. The extent of this problem is difficult to gauge. Using clinical and laboratory criteria to establish the diagnosis of hypothyroidism, Greenman et al.[101] observed a poor outcome in six of seven pregnancies involving untreated hypothyroid women. There was one spontaneous abortion at 12 weeks and one stillborn infant at 38 weeks. Developmental defects were noted in the remaining four infants. By contrast, Montoro et al.[74] noted one stillbirth and one abnormally developed infant in nine pregnancies involving untreated or partially treated hypothyroid women. Other studies have attempted to examine the relationship between maternal hypothyroidism and fetal status. Unfortunately in many cases a low serum T4, protein-bound iodine (PBI), or butanol extractable iodine (BEI) was used as the only criteria for the diagnosis of hypothyroidism. However, fetal–placental dysfunction, regardless of cause, will be associated with decreased estrogen production. As a result, the normal rise in plasma TBG and T4 associated with pregnancy will be blunted or absent.

Current thyroid function tests can accurately diagnose primary hypothyroidism in pregnancy. As in nonpregnant women, the FTI is low and the TSH elevated. The FTI and TSH should be performed in women with goiter, a history of thyroid disease, or symptoms suggestive of hypothyroidism. If hypothyroidism is confirmed, administration of 0.1–0.15 mg/day L-thyroxine should be instituted. In contrast, to the case in nonpregnant women, the goal is to restore the patient to the euthyroid state as quickly as possible. The FTI and TSH should be monitored during the remainder of pregnancy and the dose of T4 adjusted to maintain the FTI in normal range.

Maternal and Neonatal Hyperthyroidism

The diagnosis of hyperthyroidism is made in about 1 in 500 pregnancies.[102] Untreated hyperthyroidism is associated with premature labor, low birth weight, and a slight increase in neonatal mortality.[102] Maternal death can also occur,[103] but the relative risk of this complication is unknown. The basis for fetal complications in untreated hyperthyroidism is not clear. Almost no thyroid hormone crosses the placenta in euthyroid women.[104] However, when supraphysiologic doses of T4 and T3 are administered to experimental animals, the fetal pituitary–thyroid axis is suppressed,[105] indicating that maternal thyroid hormone has entered the fetal circulation. Therefore, uncontrolled maternal hyperthyroidism may be complicated by fetal hyperthyroidism.

The options for treatment of hyperthyroidism in pregnant women are limited.[92] Radioactive iodine is absolutely contraindicated because of fetal radiation exposure.[106] Fetal hypothyroidism has been reported when RAI was inadvertently administered as early as the thirteenth week of gestation.[107] Other radiation-related sequelae are also theoretically possible. Stable iodine, such as SSKI or Lugol's solution, is contraindicated except if there is an immediate threat to the mother's life or in special circumstances (discussed below). Stable iodine is a potent inhibitor of thyroid hormone secretion in the fetus. Therefore, neonatal goiters are associated with the maternal administration of iodine. Some of these goiters have been large enough to cause asphyxiation.[108]

The antithyroid drugs are the most widely used form of therapy for pregnant women with hyperthyroidism.[109-114] Some authorities recommend propylthiouracil (PTU) in preference to methimazole or carbimazole because the use of methimazole has been associated with the scalp lesion aplasia cutis in newborns.[112] Methimazole also may cross the placenta more readily than PTU.[115] Nevertheless, fetal hypothyroidism and fetal goiter are of concern in PTU-treated patients. Antithyroid drugs cause these problems if excess amounts reach the fetus. The mechanism is the same as seen in animal studies. Antithyroid drugs induce fetal hypothyroidism, serum TSH levels become elevated, and goiter develops. PTU-induced hypothyroidism is not the only cause of neonatal goiter. Maternal thyroid-stimulating immunoglobulins also cross the placenta.[116,117] It is clear that some cases of neonatal goiter are due to TSI, particularly when there is associated neonatal hyperthyroidism. Despite these concerns, most infants of mothers who received antithyroid drugs during pregnancy are euthyroid and do not have goiter. In some of the infants who were hypothyroxinemic at birth, maternal T4 levels were also low, suggesting excessive treatment with antithyroid drugs.[118] However in other studies the correlation between maternal T4 concentrations at term and neonatal T4 levels is poor.[113,114]

Current recommendations are that PTU be administered in as low a dose as possible. It is reasonable to begin with 150 mg bid. This dose should be tapered, ideally to $\leq$ 100 mg/day. Serum T4 concentrations should be monitored approximately once a month. The goal is to maintain the maternal T4 or FTI in the range that is high normal or borderline elevated for pregnancy. There is no rationale for adding replacement doses of thyroid hormone in an effort to prevent PTU-induced fetal hypothyroidism. This treatment interferes with the ability to use maternal thyroid hormone concentrations as a guide to PTU dosage. With close follow-up evaluation, most patients with Graves' disease can be managed on low doses of PTU, and in some cases the drug can be discontinued altogether, as Graves' disease tends to go into remission during the second and third trimesters. Long-term studies, although limited, suggest that in utero exposure to PTU does not have an adverse effect on physical or intellectual development.[119]

Subtotal thyroidectomy is one of the methods of treating Graves' disease. In pregnant women this therapy is probably best reserved for those who have had adverse reactions to antithyroid drugs. Surgery should be avoided during the first trimester. Before surgery, an effort should be made to render the patient as euthyroid as possible. In place of antithyroid drugs, which cannot be used because of previous adverse reactions, a saturated solution of potassium iodide, 3 drops twice daily, can be administered. Larger doses should be avoided. They are more likely to be associated with hyper-

sensitivity reactions and have no added antithyroid activity.[120] The use of SSKI in this situation is justified because it protects the mother during the perioperative period. However, iodide treatment should not be extended beyond 10 days. Fortunately, most iodide-induced neonatal goiters have been associated with prolonged maternal ingestion of iodide. Preoperative treatment with propranolol is also advisable, since many patients with Graves' disease do not become completely euthyroid during iodide treatment.[120] Propranolol is not a drug of choice in pregnant women with Graves' disease, and its use should be restricted to special circumstances. Whereas some reports suggest that propranolol causes intrauterine growth retardation (IUGR), fetal bradycardia, neonatal hypoglycemia, and other problems, these difficulties have not been encountered in all studies.[121-123]

Occasionally, hyperthyroidism and goiter develop in infants of mothers with Graves' disease. Symptoms characteristically occur several days or weeks after delivery. Neonatal thyrotoxicosis is caused by the transplacental passage of TSI. Symptoms resolve as the titer of circulating TSI in the infant's circulation declines. The incidence of neonatal thyrotoxicosis in neonates born of women with Graves' disease ranges from 0 to 12% in different series.[112,113] Neonatal thyrotoxicosis is apt to develop if maternal titers of TSI are high.[117]

The differential diagnosis of hyperthyroidism in pregnancy includes not only Graves' disease but also hydatiform mole.[120] This tumor is the source of thyroid-stimulating substances that produce typical thyrostimulatory hyperthyroidism (goiter, high RAI uptake). It has been suggested that human chorionic gonadotropin itself is responsible for the hyperthyroidism of hydatidiform mole, but there is also evidence against this theory.[125,126] Hyperthyroidism may be present in more than 50% of patients with hydatiform mole.[124,127] Evacuation of the hydatidiform mole results in prompt resolution of the clinical and laboratory features of hyperthyroidism.[124]

It has recently been reported that the serum T4, T3 RU, and FTI are elevated in a high percentage of patients with severe hyperemesis gravidarum.[129] The serum T3 and the TSH response to TRH were measured in some of these patients. In many the T3 was elevated, and the TSH response to TRH was flat. These patients would therefore be considered to have hyperthyroidism by conventional laboratory criteria. However, the nature of their thyroid disturbance is unclear. No goiter was present, and

thyroid function tests became normal when hyperemesis gravidarum was treated by conventional
means. Some signs and symptoms of hyperthyroidism were present, but they were nonspecific. Similar abnormalities in thyroid function
tests have been noted in acutely psychotic patients.[130,131] Since some of the features of hyperemesis gravidarum suggest a psychic disturbance, it
is likely that these patients share a common mechanism with respect to their thyroid disturbance. The
pathogenesis of this problem is completely unclear.

Maternal Thyroid Enlargement

Thyroid enlargement is said to be characteristic
of pregnancy. However, there are few controlled
studies of this phenomenon. Crooks et al.[132] noted
that the incidence of goiter was increased in pregnancy among women from Scotland, while this was
not the case in Iceland, a region where the dietary
content of iodine is high. The tendency to goiter in
pregnancy seems to be related to relative iodine
deficiency. Thyroid stimulators of placental origin
also may play a role, but this is speculative. Despite
this role for iodine deficiency, the administration of
stable iodine to pregnant women is contraindicated,
as this treatment produces large fetal goiters.

Postpartum Thyroid Dysfunction

Because autoimmune diseases tend to be exacer-
bated after delivery, women are vulnerable to thyroid dysfunction during the postpartum period.

Postpartum thyroid dysfunction occurs in patients
who are in remission from Graves' disease,
Hashimoto's thyroiditis, and painless thyroiditis.[133–136] The evolution of postpartum thyroid
dysfunction is depicted in Figure 7-5. The hyperthyroidism of Graves' disease is characterized by
high RAI uptake and increased synthesis of thyroid
hormone. In Hashimoto's, gradual onset of hypothyroidism is the rule. Patients with a history of
these disorders may experience a typical exacerbation of the underlying disease or destructive hyperthyroidism may develop. Why typical features of
the underlying disease develop in some patients
while destructive hyperthyroidism develops in others is not clear. Perhaps destructive hyperthyroidism is a manifestation of a very sudden and intense
autoimmune process. The hallmarks of destructive
hyperthyroidism are abrupt onset of symptoms, a
self-limited course, and a low RAI uptake. Subjects
with a history of painless thyroiditis (spontaneously
resolving thyroiditis, lymphocytic thyroiditis), one
of the causes of destructive hyperthyroidism, are
susceptible to the development of a relapse after
delivery.[136] Figure 7-5 also depicts the different
courses that may occur after the development of
postpartum thyroid dysfunction. In typical Graves'
disease, recovery is likely, but in some cases the
disease persists. Most of those patients in whom
destructive hyperthyroidism develops will recover
—often after an intervening period of hypothyroidism. A few patients, usually those with underlying
Hashimoto's thyroiditis, do not regain thyroid
function after the development of hypothyroidism.

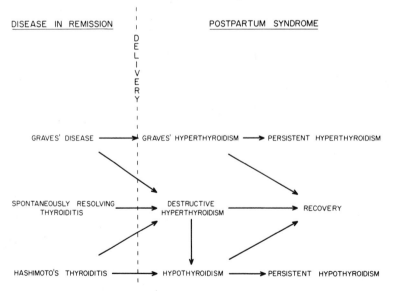

FIGURE 7-5. Evolution and natural
history of postpartum thyroid dysfunction. Autoimmune thyroid diseases tend to go into remission during
pregnancy. Several months after delivery, relapse is not unusual, and the
clinical features may be atypical.

The diagnosis of postpartum thyroid dysfunction requires a high index of suspicion. Goiter is frequently absent, and thyroid pain and tenderness are unusual. In some cases, the period of hyperthyroidism is so brief that it may be missed. Laboratory features can also be atypical. In hypothyroid subjects, the FTI is low but, because the recent hyperthyroidism may cause the TSH to be suppressed; this can lead to an erroneous impression of pituitary hypothyroidism. However, if the hypothyroidism persists, TSH secretion will increase. The treatment of postpartum thyroid dysfunction depends on the clinical and laboratory features. Antithyroid drugs are not indicated for destructive hyperthyroidism, but a short course of propranolol may prove beneficial. Antithyroid drugs are useful if severe Graves' hyperthyroidism develops. Sub-replacement doses of L-thyroxine are indicated for symptomatic patients with postpartum hypothyroidism. Full replacement should be avoided until it becomes clear that normal thyroid function will not resume.

Fetal Thyroid Physiology

The fetal thyroid can be recognized as early as the fourth week of gestation, but its size remains stable for the next 6 weeks. Around the tenth week, the rate of growth accelerates, microfollicles devoid of colloid are present, and small amounts of noniodinated thyroglobulin are synthesized.[137] By the eleventh week, the thyroid is able to concentrate iodine and incorporate it into thyroxine, monoiodotyrosine (MIT), and diiodotyrosine (DIT). Shortly thereafter, T4 can be detected in the fetal circulation.[138-142] The ontogenic pattern of each iodothyronine in the fetal circulation differs. In comparison with maternal plasma, fetal plasma T4 is low until the twentieth week of gestation, when it begins to rise steadily. Around the thirty-sixth week, maternal levels are reached, and at term fetal plasma T4 exceeds maternal plasma T4. T3 is undetectable in fetal plasma at 30 weeks gestation. At term, fetal serum T3 concentration is 50 ng/dl, a value at least threefold lower than that of maternal serum.[142] By contrast, rT3 levels in fetal serum are higher than in maternal serum from the third trimester until term. The lack of correlation between the concentration of various iodothyronines in maternal and fetal plasma reflects the fact that little intact T4, T3, or rT3 is transferred across the placenta. Most of the T4 and T3 in the fetal circulation appears to come from fetal sources. It has recently been found that the human placenta contains potent deiodinase activity.[143] T4 is converted to rT3 rather than to T3. T3 itself is very actively deiodinated by placenta inner-ring deiodinase. It may be that the relatively low levels of T3 in fetal plasma are attributable to rapid degradation of T3 in the placenta and to a low production rate of T3 from T4 by the fetoplacental unit. Placental deiodination of T4 to rT3 may account for the relatively high levels of rT3 in fetal plasma.

In contrast to T4 and T3, a significant portion of the rT3 in the fetal circulation and amniotic fluid of some species appears to come from maternal sources. In rats maternal thyroidectomy reduces fetal serum rT3 levels.[144] Amniotic fluid rT3 concentrations are even more dependent on maternal thyroid function than is fetal serum rT3. In rats maternal thyroidectomy reduces amniotic fluid rT3 to levels found in combined maternal–fetal hypothyroidism.[144] The influence of maternal thyroid status on fetal serum and amniotic fluid rT3 may be due to an ability of the placenta and fetal membranes to convert maternal T4 to rT3. The rT3 generated in these tissues then enters fetal compartments. Enzymatic deiodination of T4 and T3 may also be one reason, in addition to permeability, that transplacental movement of intact T4 and T3 is poor. These concepts have recently been reviewed.[145]

The fetus, at least during the last trimester, appears to be euthyroid with respect to plasma T4 concentrations and to be ''hypothyroid'' with respect to plasma T3 concentrations. It seems likely that tissue requirements for T4 and T3 may differ between intra and extrauterine life. For example, thyroid hormone is of critical importance for brain maturation.[141] The relatively high concentration of T4 in comparison with T3 in fetal serum is probably appropriate for the demands of the brain, since other studies indicate that the brain derives its nuclear T3 largely from circulating T4, not from circulating T3.[9] By contrast, the requirements of the fetus for thermogenesis are less than those of extrauterine life. Few estimates have been made of the relative roles of circulating T4 and T3 in thermogenesis, but it seems likely that circulating T3, rather than circulating T4, is of major importance. After delivery, plasma T3 concentrations surge,[142] probably essential for the maintenance of body temperature as the fetus moves from an insulated to an exposed environment.

Fetal Hypothyroidism

Neonatal screening for congenital hypothyroidism is now performed in most regions of the United States, Canada, and Western Europe. The incidence of congenital hypothyroidism is approximately 1 in 5000 births.[146] Screening for hypothyroidism is one of the most cost-effective programs of this type. Untreated congenital hypothyroidism results in severe mental retardation; the cost of caring for these patients far exceeds the cost of screening programs. Congenital hypothyroidism is usually due to thyroid agenesis or is associated with the development of ectopic, hypoplastic tissue. Pituitary hypothyroidism and congenital defects of thyroid hormone synthesis are unusual. Most infants with congenital hypothyroidism have euthyroid mothers, but on rare occasions women with autoimmune thyroiditis will give birth to hypothyroid children. There is little the obstetrician can do to prevent or even detect congenital hypothyroidism in utero. Measurement of amniotic fluid rT3 levels have not been shown to predict fetal hypothyroidism and may actually be more a measure of maternal thyroid status.[144,147]

Despite these difficulties, the obstetric history should include questions regarding prior thyroid disease or delivery of hypothyroid infants. Endocrine consultation is advisable if the latter history is positive and an FTI and TSH should be performed in the neonate. It must be stressed that the normal range for the FTI in the newborn is higher than in the adult. If the normal range for the adult FTI is used, some cases of congenital hypothyroidism will be missed.

SUMMARY

Treatment of thyroid diseases is not central to the practice of obstetrics and gynecology. However, the ability to recognize these disorders and an understanding of the principles of treatment are important for several reasons. Graves' disease, the most common cause of hyperthyroidism, is far more prevalent in women than in men. This is also true for Hashimoto's thyroiditis, the most frequent cause of hypothyroidism. Fertility is decreased in both hyperthyroidism and hypothyroidism; each of these conditions is associated with its own spectrum of menstrual disturbances. Hypomenorrhea is characteristic of hyperthyroidism, whereas menorrhagia is a feature of hypothyroidism. Amenorrhea is a late occurrence in both disorders. Although these and other clinical features should alert the clinician to the possibility of a thyroid disturbance, laboratory studies must support the diagnosis. The primary tests used for the diagnosis of hypothyroidism are the FTI and the serum concentration of TSH. The FTI and the serum T3 concentration are the major tests used in the diagnosis of hyperthyroidism. As these and other thyroid-function tests are now quite sensitive and specific, there is no need to use thyroid hormone to treat infertility, menstrual disturbances, or recurrent abortions if thyroid-function tests indicate that the patient is euthyroid.

An understanding of maternal–fetal thyroid physiology is essential in the management of pregnant women with hypothyroidism or hyperthyroidism. TSH and thyroid hormones are not transferred across the placenta; the fetal and maternal hypothalamic–pituitary–thyroid axis are therefore relatively independent. Maternal hypothyroidism and hyperthyroidism have an adverse effect on fetal survival and development. Diagnosis of maternal hypothyroidism and restoration of the serum FTI to normal should be achieved as early as possible during gestation. Serum T4 and T3 are elevated in pregnancy because of the estrogen-induced increase in serum TBG. The FTI is normal. Despite the fact that the antithyroid drugs cross the placenta the treatment of choice for maternal hyperthyroidism is PTU. The does of PTU should be as low as possible and designed to maintain the maternal FTI in the high normal range. Thyroid function must be monitored frequently during pregnancy and, because of the tendency for Graves' disease to remit during the second and third trimesters, it is often possible to discontinue PTU.

Women with subclinical Graves' disease, Hashimoto's thyroiditis, and painless thyroiditis are susceptible to the development of a relapse of their underlying disease about 3 months after delivery. Some patients experience transient hyperthyroidism followed by hypothyroidism. Postpartum thyroid dysfunction is not rare. The diagnosis requires a high index of suspicion because goiter is often absent and the clinical and laboratory features change from week to week. Thyroid function may be disturbed in hyperemesis gravidarum, but antithyroid drugs are usually not indicated. Hydatidiform mole and ovarian teratomas are unusual causes of hyperthyroidism in women.

ACKNOWLEDGMENT. This work was supported in part by National Institutes of Health & Research grant AM 27850.

QUESTIONS

1. Of the following thyroid function tests, the only reliable test in the diagnosis of hypothyroidism is

    a. The serum T3 concentration.
    b. a high titer of serum anti-microsomal antibodies.
    c. the 24-hr RAI uptake.
    d. the serum T3 RU.
    e. the FTI.

2. In women who are pregnant or taking estrogens,

    a. the T4 is normal, the T3 RU is high, and the FTI is low.
    b. The T4 is high, the T3 RU is low, and the FTI is normal.
    c. the T4 is high, the T3 RU is high, and the FTI is normal.
    d. the T4 is high, the T3 RU is low, and the FTI is elevated.

3. Clinical features associated with hyperthyroidism are

    a. menorrhagia.
    b. galactorrhea.
    c. hypomenorrhea.
    d. growth retardation.
    e. muscle cramps.

4. The most common cause of hyperthyroidism in women is

    a. Graves' disease.
    b. hydatidiform mole.
    c. toxic multinodular goiter.
    d. ovarian teratoma.
    e. facticious ingestion of thyroid hormone.

5. Are there well-established indications for the use of thyroid hormone in women without thyroid enlargement who have normal values for serum TSH and FTI?

6. The optimal method of treating pregnant women with hyperthyroidism is

    a. stable iodides for rapid control followed by propylthiouracil (PTU).
    b. high-dose PTU with added thyroid hormone to avoid maternal hypothyroidism.
    c. PTU in the first trimester followed by radioactive iodine in mid-gestation.
    d. low-dose PTU.
    e. methimazole with propranolol.

7. Does increased sex hormone binding globulin (SHBG) synthesis alter plasma testosterone and estrogen concentrations in hyperthyroidism?

REFERENCES

1. Werner SC: Historical resume, in Werner SC, Ingbar SH (eds): *The Thyroid: A Fundamental and Clinical Text.* Hagerstown, MD, Harper & Row, 1978, pp. 3–6.
2. Van Herle AJ, Vassart G, Dumont JE: Control of thyroglobulin synthesis and secretion. *N Engl J Med* 301:239–248, 1979.
3. Degroot LJ, Niepomniszcze H: Biosynthesis of thyroid hormone: Basic and clinical aspects. *Metabolism* 26:665–718, 1977.
4. Ingbar SH: Autoregulation of the thyroid: The response to iodide excess and depletion. *Mayo Clin Proc* 47:814–823, 1972.
5. Robbins J, Cheng SY, Gershengorn MC, et al: Thyroxine transport proteins of plasma. *Recent Prog Horm Res* 34:477–519, 1978.
6. Schimmel M, Utiger RD: Thyroidal and peripheral production of thyroid hormones. *Ann Intern Med* 87:760–768, 1977.
7. Cavalieri RR, Pitt-Rivers R: The effects of drugs on the distribution and metabolism of thyroid hormones. *Pharmacol Rev* 33:55–80, 1981.
8. Oppenheimer JH, Schwartz HL, Surks MI, et al: Nuclear receptors and the initiation of thyroid hormone action. *Recent Prog Horm Res* 32:529–565, 1976.
9. Larsen PR, Silva JE, Kaplan MM: Relationships between circulating and intracellular thyroid hormones: Physiological and clinical implications. *Endocr Rev* 2:87–102, 1981.
10. Edelman IS: Thyroid thermogenesis. *N Engl J Med* 290:1303–1308, 1974.
11. Utiger RD: Tests of the hypothalamic–pituitary–thyroid axis, in Werner SC, Ingbar SH (eds): *The Thyroid: A Fundamental and Clinical Text.* Hagerstown, MD, Harper & Row, 1978, pp 367–374.
12. Synder PJ, Utiger RD: Response to thyrotropin releasing hormone (TRH) in normal man. *J Clin Endocrinol Metab* 34:380–385, 1972.
13. Ramey JN, Burrow GN, Polackwich RJ, et al: The effect of oral contraceptive steroids on the response of thyroid stimulating hormone to thyrotropin-releasing hormone. *J Clin Endocrinol Metab* 40:712–714, 1975.
14. Morley JE: Neuroendocrine control of thyrotropin secretion. *Endocr Rev* 2:396–436, 1981.
15. Wartofsky L, Burman KD: Alterations in thyroid function in patients with systemic illness: The euthyroid sick syndrome. *Endocr Rev* 3:164–217, 1982.
16. Rajatanavin R, Braverman LE: Euthyroid hyperthyroxinemia. *J Endocrinol Invest* 6:493–505, 1984.
17. Refetoff S, Salazar A, Smith TJ, et al: The consequences of inappropriate treatment because of failure to recognize the syndrome of pituitary and peripheral tissue resistance to thyroid hormone. *Metabolism* 32:822–834, 1983.
18. Synder PJ, Jacobs LS, Rabello MM, et al: Diagnostic value of thyrotrophin-releasing hormone in pituitary and hypothalamic disease. *Ann Intern Med* 81:751–757, 1974.
19. Safran M, Braverman L: Effect of chronic douching with polyvinyl-pyrrolidone-iodine on iodine absorption and thyroid function. *Obstet Gynecol* 60:35–40, 1982.
20. Abreau CM, Vagenakis AG, Roti E, et al: Clinical evalua-

tion of a hemagglutination method for microsomal and thyroglobulin antibodies in autoimmune thyroid disease. *Ann Clin Lab Sci* 7:73–78, 1977.

21. Schneider AB, Bekerman C, Favus M, et al: Continuing occurrence of thyroid nodules after head and neck irradiation—Relation to plasma thyroglobulin concentration. *Ann Intern Med* 94:176–180, 1981.

22. Gershengorn MD, McClung MR, Chu EW, et al: Fine needle aspiration cytology in the preoperative diagnosis of thyroid nodules. *Ann Intern Med* 87:265–269, 1977.

23. Miller JM, Hamburger JI, Kini S: Diagnosis of thyroid nodules. *JAMA* 241:481–484, 1979.

24. Tunbridge WMG, Evered DC, Hall R, et al: The spectrum of thyroid disease in a community: The Wickham survey. *Clin Endocrinol (Oxf)* 7:481–493, 1977.

25. Noble MJD, Rowlands S: Utilization of radioiodide during pregnancy. *J Obstet Gynaecol Br Commonw* 60:892–894, 1953.

26. Aboul-Khair SA, Crooks J, Turnbull AC, et al: The physiological changes in thyroid function during pregnancy. *Clin Sci* 27:195–207, 1964.

27. Bray GA: Increased sensitivity of the thyroid in iodine depleted rats to the goitrogenic effects of thyrotropin. *J Clin Invest* 47:1640–1647, 1968.

28. Harada A, Hershman JM, Reed AW, et al: Comparison of thyroid hormone concentrations in the sera of pregnant women. *J Clin Endocrinol Metab* 48:793–797, 1979.

29. Taliadouros GS, Canfield RE, Nisula BS: Thyroid-stimulating activity of chorionic gonadotropin and luteinizing hormone. *J Clin Endocrinol Metab* 51:855–860, 1978.

30. Everett RB, MacDonald, PC: Endocrinology of the placenta, in Creger WP, Coggins CH, Hancock EW (eds): *Annual Review of Medicine*. Palo Alto, CA, Annual Reviews, Inc., pp. 484–485, 1979.

31. Furszyfer J, Kurland LT, McConahey WM, et al: Graves' disease in Olmstead county, Minnesota, 1935 through 1967. *Mayo Clin Proc* 45:636–644, 1970.

32. Mogensen EF: The epidemiology of thyrotoxicosis in Denmark. *Acta Med Scand* 208:183–186, 1980.

33. Adams DD, Knight JG: H gene theory of inherited autoimmune disease. *Lancet* 1:396–398, 1980.

34. Rocklin RE, Kitzmiller JL, Kaye MD: Immunobiology of the maternal–fetal relationship, in Creger WP, Coggins CH, Hancock EW (eds): *Annual Review of Medicine*. Palo Alto, CA, Annual Reviews, Inc., 1979, pp 386–387.

35. Werner SC: The eye changes of Graves' disease. *Mayo Clin Proc* 47:969–974, 1972.

36. Vagenakis AG, Wang C, Burger A, et al: Iodine-induced thyrotoxicosis in Boston. *N Engl J Med* 287:523–527, 1972.

37. Amino N, Tanizawa O, Mori H, et al: Aggravation of thyrotoxicosis in early pregnancy and after delivery in Graves' disease. *J Clin Endocrinol Metab* 55:108–112, 1982.

38. Hamburger JI: Subacute thyroiditis: Diagnostic difficulties and simple treatment. *J Nuc Med* 15:81–89, 1974.

39. Nikolai TF, Brosseau J, Kettrick MA, et al: Lymphocytic thyroiditis with spontaneously resolving hyperthyroidism (silent thyroiditis). *Arch Intern Med* 140:478–482, 1980.

40. Emge LA: Functional and growth characteristics of struma ovarii. *Am J Obstet Gynecol* 40:738–750, 1940.

41. Kempers RD, Dockerty MB, Hoffman DL, et al: Struma ovarii: Ascitic, hyperthyroid and asymptomatic syndromes. *Ann Intern Med* 72:883–893, 1970.

42. Crooks J, Murray IPC, Wayne EJ: Statistical methods applied to the clinical diagnosis of thyrotoxicosis. *Q J Med* 28:211–234, 1969.

43. Gorman CA: Unusual manifestations of Graves' disease. *Mayo Clin Proc* 47:926–933, 1972.

44. Rivlin RS: Therapy of obesity with hormones. *N Engl J Med* 292:26–29, 1975.

45. Goldsmith RE, Sturgis SH, Lerman J, et al: The menstrual pattern in thyroid disease. *J Clin Endocrinol Metab* 12:846–855, 1952.

46. Akande EO, Hockaday TDR: Plasma concentration of gonadotropins, oestrogen, progesterone in thyroxtoxic women. *Br J Obstet Gynecol* 82:541–555, 1975.

47. Akande EO: Plasma progesterone concentration in thyrotoxic women with menstrual disturbance. *Am J Obstet Gynecol* 122:887–889, 1975.

48. Ridgeway EC, Maloof F, Longcope C: Androgen and oestrogen dynamics in hyperthyroidism. *J Endocrinol* 95:105–115, 1982.

49. Southren AL, Olivo J, Gordon GG, et al: The conversion of androgens to estrogens in hyperthyroidism. *J Clin Endocrinol Metab* 38:207–214, 1974.

50. Crepy O, Dray F, Sabaoun J: Role des hormones thyroidiennes dans les interactions entre la testosterone et les proteines seriques. *CR Acad Sci D* 264:2651–2653, 1967.

51. Gordon G, Southren AL, Tochinoto S, et al: Effect of hyperthyroidism and hypothyroidism on the metabolism of testosterone and androstenedione in man. *J Clin Endocrinol Metab* 29:164–170, 1969.

52. Clark AF, Calandra RS, Bird CE: Binding of testosterone and 5 alpha-dihydrotestosterone to plasma proteins in humans. *Clin Biochem* 4:89–103, 1971.

53. Chopra IJ, Tulchinsky D: Status of estrogen–androgen balance in hyperthyroid men with Graves' disease. *J Clin Endocrinol Metab* 38:269–277, 1974.

54. Chopra IJ, Abraham GE, Chopra U, et al: Alterations in circulating oestradiol-17 beta in male patients with Graves' disease. *N Engl J Med* 286:124–129, 1972.

55. Ridgeway EC, Longcope C, Maloof F: Metabolic clearance and blood production rates of estradiol in hyperthyroidism. *J Clin Endocrinol Metab* 41:491–497, 1975.

56. Ruder H, Corvol P, Mahaoudeau JA, et al: Effects of induced hyperthyroidism on steroid metabolism in man. *J Clin Endocrinol Metab* 33:382–387, 1971.

57. Anderson DC: Sex-hormone-binding globulin. *Clin Endocrinol* 3:69–96, 1974.

58. Akdande EO, Anderson DC: Role of sex-hormone-binding globulin in hormonal changes and amenorrhea in thyrotoxic women. *Br J Obstet Gynaecol* 82:557–561, 1975.

59. Tanaka T, Tamai H, Matsuzka F, et al: Gonadotropin response to luteinizing hormone releasing hormone in hyperthyroid patients with menstrual disturbances. *Metabolism* 30:323–326, 1981.

60. Distiller LA, Sagel J, Morley JE: Assessment of pituitary gonadotropin reserve using luteinizing hormone-releasing hormone (LRH) in states of altered thyroid function. *J Clin Endocrinol Metab* 40:512–515, 1975.

61. Evans RW, Farwell AP, Braverman LE: Nuclear thyroid hormone receptor in rat uterus. *Endocrinology* 113:1459–1463, 1983.

62. Kirkland JL, Gardner RM, Mukku VR, et al: Hormonal control of uterine growth: The effect of hypothyroidism on estrogen-stimulated cell division. *Endocrinology* 108:2346–2351, 1981.

63. Hellman L, Baradlow HL, Zumoff B, et al: The influence of thyroid hormone on hydrocortisone production and metabolism. *J Clin Endocrinol Metab* 21:1231–1247, 1961.

64. Sutton GP, Lyles KW, Wilbe RH: Steroid secretion and testosterone binding in a woman with an ovarian hilus cell tumor and thyrotoxicosis. *Am J Obstet Gynecol* 141:535–538, 1981.

65. Wood LC, Ingbar SH: Hypothyroidism as a late sequela in patients with Graves' disease treated with antithyroid agents. *J Clin Invest* 64:1429–1436, 1979.

66. Emerson CH, Dyson WL, Utiger RD: Serum thyrotropin and thyroxine concentrations in patients receiving lithium carbonate. *J Clin Endocrinol Metab* 36:338–346, 1973.

67. Watanakunakorn C, Hodges RE, Evans TC: Myxedema. *Arch Intern Med* 116:183–190, 1965.

68. Blum M: Myxedema coma. *Am J Med Sci* 264:432–443, 1972.

69. Parving HH, Hansen JM, Nielson SL, et al: Mechanisms of edema formation in myxedema-increased protein extravasation and relatively slow lymphatic drainage. *N Engl J Med* 301:460–465, 1979.

70. Scott JC, Mussey E: Menstrual patterns in myxedema. *Am J Obstet Gynecol* 90:161–165, 1964.

71. Echt CR, Doss, JF: Myxedema in pregnancy. *Obstet Gynecol* 22:615–620, 1963.

72. Kennedy AL, Montgomery DAD: Hypothyroidism in pregnancy. *Br J Obstet Gynaecol* 85:225–230, 1978.

73. Potter JD: Hypothyroidism and reproductive failure. *Surg Gynecol Obstet* 50:251–255, 1980.

74. Montoto M, Collea JV, Fraiser D, et al: Successful outcome of pregnancy in women with hypothyroidism. *Ann Intern Med.* 94:31–34, 1981.

75. Akande EO: Plasma concentration of gonadotrophins, oestrogen and progesterone in hypothyroid women. *Br J Obstet Gynaecol* 82:552–556, 1975.

76. Van Wyk JJ, Grumbach MM: Syndrome of precocious menstruation and galactorrhea in juvenile hypothyrodism: An example of hormonal overlap in pituitary feedback. *J Pediatr* 57:416–435, 1960.

77. Costin G, Kershnar AK, Kogut MD, et al: Prolactin activity in juvenile hypothyroidism and precocious puberty. *Pediatrics* 50:881–889, 1972.

78. Barnes ND, Hayles AB, Ryan RJ: Sexual maturation in juvenile hypothyroidism. *Mayo Clin Proc* 48:849–856, 1973.

79. Lindsay AN, Voorhess ML, Macgillivray MH: Multicystic ovaries detected by sonography. *Am J Dis Child* 134:588–592, 1980.

80. Riddlesberger MM, Kuhn JP, Munschauer RW: The association of juvenile hypothyroidism and cystic ovaries. *Radiology* 139:77–80, 1981.

81. Bayliss PFC, van't Hoff W: Amenorrhea and galactorhoea associated with hypothyroidism. *Lancet* 2:1399–1400, 1969.

82. Edwards CRW, Forsyth IA, Besser GM: Amenorrhea, galactorrhea, and primary hypothyroidism with high circulating levels of prolactin. *Br Med J* 3:462–464, 1971.

83. Shahshahani MN, Wong ET: Primary hypothyroidism, amenorrhea, and galactorrhea. *Arch Intern Med* 138:1411–1412, 1978.

84. Wartofsky L: Low remission after therapy for Graves' disease. *JAMA* 226:1083–1088, 1973.

85. Emerson CH, Braverman LE: Thyroid irradiation—One view. *N Engl J Med* 303:217–219, 1980.

86. Gorman CA, Robertson JS: Radiation dose in the selection of 131-I or surgical treatment for toxic thyroid adenoma. *Ann Intern Med* 89:85–90, 1978.

87. Goldstein R, Hart IR: Follow-up of solitary autonomous thyroid nodules treated with 131-I. *N Engl J Med* 309:1473–1482, 1983.

88. Hamburger J: The autonomously functioning thyroid. *N Engl J Med* 309:1512–1513, 1983.

89. Stock JM, Surks MI, Oppenheimer JH: Replacement dosage of L-thyroxine in hypothyroidism. *N Engl J Med* 290:529–533, 1974.

90. Rosebaum RL: Levothyroxine replacement dose for primary hypothyroidism decreases with age. *Ann Intern Med* 96:53–55, 1982.

91. Van Dop C, Conte FA, Koch TK, et al: Pseudotumor cerebri associated with initiation of levothyroxine therapy for juvenile hypothyroidism. *N Engl J Med* 308:1076–1080, 1983.

92. Burrow GN: Hyperthyroidism during pregnancy. *N Engl J Med* 298:150–153, 1978.

93. Aboul-Khair SA, Crooks J, Turnbull AC, et al: The physiological changes in thyroid function during pregnancy. *Clin Sci* 27:195–207, 1964.

94. Osathanondh R, Tulchinsky D, Chopra IJ: Total and free thyroxine and triiodothryronine in normal and complicated pregnancy. *J Clin Endocrinol Metab* 42:98–104, 1976.

95. Parlow ME, Oddie TH, Fisher DA: Evaluation of serum triiodothyronine and adjusted triiodothyronine (free triiodothyronine index) in pregnancy. *Clin Chem* 23:490–492, 1977.

96. Harada A, Hershman JM, Reed AW, et al: Comparison of thyroid stimulators and thyroid hormone concentrations in the sera of pregnant women. *J Clin Endocrinol Metab* 48:793–797, 1979.

97. Yamaoto T, Amino N, Tanizawa O, et al: Longitudinal study of serum thyroid hormones, chorionic gonadotrophin and thyrotrophin during and after normal pregnancy. *Clin Endocrinol (Oxf)* 10:459–468, 1979.

98. Cooper E, Aickin CM, Burke CW: Serum concentrations of 3,3′,5′-triiodothyronine (reverse T3) in normal pregnancy. *Clin Chim Acta* 106:347–349, 1980.

99. Weeke J, Dybkjaer L, Granlie K, et al: A longitudinal study of serum TSH, and total and free iodothyronines during normal pregnancy. *Acta Endocrinol (Copenh)* 101:531–537, 1982.

100. Dowling JT, Appleton WG, Nicoloff JT: Thyroxine turnover in human pregnancy. *J Clin Endocrinol Metab* 27:1749–1750, 1967.

101. Greenman GW, Gabrielson MO, Howard-Flanders J, et al: Thyroid dysfunction in pregnancy. *N Engl J Med* 267:426–431, 1962.

102. Niswander KR, Gordon M, Berendes HW: *The Women and Their Pregnancies.* Philadelphia, Saunders, 1972, 1.246.

103. Sugrue D, Drury MI: Hyperthyroidism complicating pregnancy: Results of treatment by antithyroid drugs in 77 pregnancies. *Br J Obstet Gynaecol* 87:970–975, 1980.

104. Roti E, Gnudi A, Braverman LE: The placental transport, synthesis and metabolism of hormones and drugs which affect thyroid function. *Endocr Rev* 4:131–149, 1983.

105. Knobil E, Josimovich JP: Placental transfer of thyrotropin, thyroxine, triiodothyronine and insulin in the rat. *Ann NY Acad Sci* 75:895–904, 1959.

106. Green HG, Gareis FJ, Shepard TH, et al: Cretinism associated with maternal sodium iodide I-131 therapy during pregnancy. *Am J Dis Child* 122:247–249, 1971.

107. Russell KP, Rose H, Starr P: The effects of radioactive iodine on maternal and fetal thyroid function during pregnancy. *Surg Gynecol Obstet* 104:560–564, 1957.

108. Carswell F, Kerr MM, Hutchison JH: Congenital goitre and hypothyroidism produced by maternal ingestion of iodides. *Lancet* 1:1241–1243, 1970.

109. Herbst AL, Selenkow HA: Hyperthyroidism during pregnancy. *N Engl J Med* 273:627–633, 1965.

110. Talbert LM, Thomas CG Jr, Holt WA, et al: Hyperthyroidism during pregnancy. *Obstet Gynecol* 36:779–785, 1970.

111. Worley RJ, Crosby WM: Hyperthyroidism during pregnancy. *Am J Obstet Gynecol* 119:150–155, 1974.

112. Mujtaba Q, Burrow GN: Treatment of hyperthyroidism in pregnancy with propylthiouracil and methimazole. *Obstet Gynecol* 46:282–286, 1975.

113. Cheron RG, Kaplan MM, Larsen PR, et al: Neonatal thyroid function after propylthiouracil therapy for maternal Graves' disease. *N Engl J Med* 304:525–538, 1981.

114. Lamberg BA, Ikonen E, Teramo L, et al: Treatment of maternal hyperthyroidism with antithyroid agents and changes in thyrotrophin and thyroxine in the newborn. *Acta Endocrinol (Copenh)* 97:186–195, 1981.

115. Marchant B, Brownlie BEW, Hart DM, et al: The placental transfer of propylthiouracil, methimazole and carbimazole. *J Clin Endocrinol Metab* 45:1187–1193, 1977.

116. Dirmikis SM, Munro DS: Placental transmission of thyroid-stimulating immunoglobulins. *Br Med J* 2:665–666, 1975.

117. Zakarija M, McKenzie JM: Pregnancy-associated changes in the thyroid-stimulating antibody of Graves' disease and the relationship to neonatal hyperthyroidism. *J Clin Endocrinol Metab* 57:1036–1040, 1983.

118. Ibbertson HK, Seddon RJ, Croxson MS: Fetal hypothyroidism complicating medical treatment of thyrotoxicosis in pregnancy. *Clin Endocrinol* 4:521–523, 1975.

119. Burrow GN, Bartsocas C, Klatskin EH, et al: Children exposed in utero to propylthiouracil. *Am J Dis Child* 116:161–165, 1968.

120. Emerson CH, Anderson AJ, Howard WJ, et al: Serum thyroxine and triiodothyronine concentrations during iodide treatment of hyperthyroidism. *J Clin Endocrinol Metab* 40:33–36, 1975.

121. Veland K, McAnulty JH, Veland FR, et al: Cardiovascular diseases in pregnancy: Special consideration in the use of cardiovascular drugs. *Clin Obstet Gynecol* 24:809–823, 1981.

122. Eliahou HE, Silverberg DS, Reisin E, et al: Propranolol for the treatment of hypertension in pregnancy. *Br J Obstet Gynecol* 85:431–436, 1978.

123. Rubin PC: Beta-blockers in pregnancy. *N Engl J Med* 305:1323–1326, 1981.

124. Higgins HP, Hershman JM, Kenimer JG, et al: The thyrotoxicosis of hydatidiform mole. *Ann Intern Med* 83:307–311, 1975.

125. Kenimer JG, Hershaman JM, Higgins HP: The thyrotropin in hydatidiform moles in human chorionic gonadotrophin. *J Clin Endocrinol Metab* 40:480–489, 1975.

126. Amir SM, Sullivan RC, Ingbar SH: In vitro responses to crude and purified hCG in human thyroid membranes. *J Clin Endocrinol Metab* 51:51–58, 1980.

127. Galton VA, Ingbar SH, Jimenez-Fonseca J, et al: Alterations in thyroid hormone economy in patients with hydatidiform mole. *J Clin Invest* 50:1345, 1971.

128. Hershman JM, Higgins HP: Hydatidiform mole—A cause of clinical hyperthyroidism. *N Engl J Med* 284:573–577, 1971.

129. Bouillon R, Naesens M, Van Assche FA, et al: Thyroid function in patients with hyperemesis gravidarum. *Am J Obstet Gynecol* 143:922–926, 1982.

130. Spratt DI, Pont A, Miller MB, et al: Hyperthyroxinemia in patients with acute psychiatric disorders. *Am J Med* 73:41–48, 1982.

131. Morley JE, Shafer RB: Thyroid function screening in new psychiatric admissions. *Arch Intern Med* 142:591–593, 1982.

132. Crooks J, Tulloch MI, Turnbull AC, et al: Comparative incidence of goitre in pregnancy in Iceland and Scotland. *Lancet* 1:625–627, 1967.

133. Walfish PG, Ginsberg J: Postpartum thyroid disease. *Ann Intern Med* 88:128, 1978.

134. Amino N, Mori H, Iwatani Y, et al: High prevalence of transient post-partum thyrotoxicosis and hypothyroidism. *N Engl J Med* 306:849–852, 1982.

135. Amino N, Tanizawa O, Mori H, et al: Aggravation of thyrotoxicosis in early pregnancy and after delivery in Graves' disease. *J Clin Endocrinol Metab* 55:108–112, 1982.

136. Dahlberg PA, Jansson R: Different aetiologies in postpartum thyroiditis. *Acta Endocrinol (Copenh)* 104:195–200, 1983.

137. Olin P, Ekholm R, Almquist S: Biosynthesis of thyroglobulin related to the ultrastructure of the human fetal thyroid gland. *Endocrinology* 87:1000–1014, 1970.

138. Hodges RE, Evans TC, Bradbury JT, et al: The accumulation of radioactive iodine by human fetal thyroids. *J Clin Endocrinol Metab* 15:661–667, 1955.

139. Shepard TH: Onset of function in the human fetal thyroid: Biochemical and radioautographic studies from organ culture. *J Clin Endocrinol* 27:945–957, 1967.

140. Greenberg AH, Czernichow P, Reba RC, et al: Observations on the maturation of thyroid function in early fetal life. *J Clin Invest* 49:1790–1803, 1970.

141. Fisher DA, Dussault JH, Sack J, et al: Ontogenesis of hypothalamic–pituitary–thyroid function and metabolism in man, sheep, and rat, in Greep RO (ed): *Recent Progress in Hormone Research,* Vol 33. New York, Academic, p 59.

142. Fisher DA, Klein AH: Thyroid development and disorders of thyroid function in the newborn. *N Engl J Med* 304:702–712, 1981.

143. Roti E, Fang SL, Green K, et al: Human placenta is an active site of thyroxine and 3,3′,5-triiodothyronine tyrosyl ring deiodination. *J Clin Endocrinol Metab* 53:498–501, 1981.

144. El-Zaheri MM, Vagenakis AG, Hinerfeld L, et al: Maternal thyroid function is the major determinant of amniotic fluid 3,3′,5′-triiodothyronine in the rat. *J Clin Invest* 67:1126–1133, 1981.

145. Emerson CH, Braverman LE: Peripheral deiodination of thyroid hormones in placenta and fetal membranes. *Hormone Metab Res (Suppl)* 14:56–62, 1984.

146. Burrow GN, Dussault JH: *Neonatal Thyroid Screening.* New York, Raven, 1980.

ANSWERS

1. e

2. b

3. c

4. a

5. No

6. d

7. Yes

Diagnostic Procedures

8

Hormone Assays in Endocrine Systems

ROBERT N. ALSEVER

INTRODUCTION

A quarter of a century ago, the hormonal milieu surrounding our body systems was relatively simple and based on intuition and some selected bioassayable end points. With the development of improved radioimmunoassay (RIA) techniques, our knowledge and understanding of the endocrine system have mushroomed at an exponential rate, making it nearly impossible for physicians to keep pace with it. This chapter emphasizes hormonal assays and discusses their meaning as they might relate to gynecologic endocrinology.

Endocrine testing in any system requires certain concepts in order to obtain results that are accurate and meaningful. As a general rule, endocrine tests may be obtained in the basal state as random samples, and after stimulation-suppression testing. When a hormone is thought to be deficient, random or basal hormone levels will often be within the normal range. Therefore, when deficiency is considered, stimulation testing is necessary to docu-

---

ROBERT N. ALSEVER • Division of Endocrinology, Southern Colorado Clinic, Pueblo, Colorado 81004; and Department of Medicine, University of Colorado Health Sciences Center, Denver, Colorado 80220.

ment true deficiency. Suppression testing is indicated when hormone excess or overproduction is suspected. Stimulation testing will usually cloud the diagnostic milieu where overproduction is suspected and more often will confuse rather than aid the clinician (Table 8-1).

The magnificent armamentarium of the clinical laboratory now places the burden of wise choice on the clinical physician. Certain points are critical in choosing or interpreting any set of endocrine data. First, one needs a thorough understanding of the feedback loops involved with almost every hormone in the endocrine system. With the exception of gonadotropin control, most systems operate on a negative feedback loop. Maximal information from the hormone testing protocols will be obtained with feedback loops in mind. Second, circadian rhythms and wide fluctuations from minute to minute (pulsatility) frequently occur in hormone systems. Third, differences among men, women, children, and the elderly will frequently yield differing laboratory results.[1,2] In interpretation, these factors should be kept in mind. Several preceding chapters have detailed some of these differences, and some texts detail these as they apply to endocrine testing.[1]

It is the purpose of this chapter to provide an

TABLE 8-1. Evaluation of Endocrine Function

Hyperfunction suspected		
Basal	Suppression	Interpretation
Normal	Normal	Normal
Increased	Normal	Normal
Increased	Nonsuppressed	Hyperfunction

Hypofunction suspected		
Basal	Stimulation	Interpretation
Normal	Normal	Normal
Low	Normal	Normal
Low	Nonstimulated	Hypofunction

outline of test procedures that may be used in evaluating a patient with a gynecologic endocrine disorder. By its very nature, this chapter cannot be disease oriented, but must be test oriented. Where common, key disorders are delineated as they apply to endocrine testing. For the reader's convenience, selected hormone tests and their normal values are given in concise form in Table 8-2. Certain of these values may vary somewhat, depending on the method used and the reference laboratory. Finally, endocrine testing protocols have been similarly concisely outlined in Tables 8-3 through 8-9.

PROCEDURES FOR TESTING

With the exponential rise in the number of sophisticated endocrine studies, there has been a similar exponential rise in reference laboratories. Most tests are so specialized and so infrequently done that unreliable results will occur in laboratories performing them infrequently. Most reference laboratories are regionally located to give the clinician easy access to their services. Because accurate and reliable results are so critical to the diagnosis of endocrine disease in this decade, it is important to select a good reference laboratory. While one tends to be cost conscious in selecting a laboratory, one should be chosen on the basis of its reputation and reliability rather than its cost.

In order for a laboratory to perform tests properly, it is critical that it be provided with adequate information and samples. In order to assure this, the laboratory should be consulted on all unusual tests. Proper labeling and transportation of samples are as critical to valid results as is use of the proper test protocol. As an example, many 24-hr urines require the presence of a preservative. An improper preservative will result in total loss of the 24-hr urine, which may have been collected at a critical time. Routinely, urinary creatinines should be collected on all 24-hr urines to judge the adequacy of collection by the patient and to permit comparison of one set of assay values with another done on a different occasion.

In the testing protocols outlined in the tables, a basal level should be obtained before initiating the test. Second, when obtaining multiple test samples, it is important to obtain them through an indwelling needle to minimize trauma. Stress from multiple venipuncture may cause abnormal laboratory results.

HORMONE ASSAY PROCEDURES

The RIA was the serendipity child of Dr. Solomon Berson and Dr. Rosalyn Yalow during the late 1950s.[3] In an effort to observe the metabolism of radioactive insulin (RAI) in humans with and without diabetes, they found, surprisingly, that in diabetics treated with insulin, radioiodinated insulin had an extremely prolonged half-life in the serum. This prolongation in half-life was noted to be due to intravascular binding of insulin by insulin antibodies. Initial attempts to publish their discovery resulted in rejection from several leading scientific journals. Further experiments indicated that unlabeled insulin displaced the labeled insulin from the antibody. Berson and Yalow developed a purified antibody by immunizing guinea pigs against insulin; they published the first insulin assay in 1959. Crude bioassays, however, continued to be the rule until the late 1960s, when RIA of hormones in biologic fluids began to flourish. RIA during the past decade has enabled monumental advances in endocrinology and has had a revolutionary impact in our understanding of the endocrine system. For this work, Berson and Yalow received a Nobel Prize in 1977.

The RIA is based on the principle of competitive protein binding.[4] Using the RIA, a known amount of plasma into which an unknown amount of hormone or ligand (polypeptide, glycoprotein, or steroid hormone) is allowed to come into equilibrium with a known amount of isotopically labeled "tracer" hormone. To this mixture, a known amount of antibody directed against that hormone is added. This is allowed to come into equilibrium, and then either an antigammaglobulin raised

TABLE 8-2. Normal Adult Fasting Values[a]

Hormone	Units	Sex	Cycle	Value
ACTH	pg/ml			20–100
Androstenedione	ng/ml	Male		20–200
		Female		20–250
Compound S (11-desoxycortisol)	ng/dl			>120
Cortisol	mcg/dl		a.m.	10–25
			p.m.	5–12
Cortisol, urine[b]	mcg/24hr			20–100
DHEA-S	mcg/dl	Male		190–550
		Female		60–350
Dihydrotestosterone	ng/dl	Male		20–75
		Female		5–30
Estradiol, 17β	pg/ml	Male		10–50
		Female	Follicular	10–150
			Luteal	5–300
			Menopausal	0–25
Estrogen, urine[b]	mcg/24hr	Male		5–20
		Female	Follicular	5–25
			Luteal	25–80
			Menopausal	5–20
Estrone	pg/ml	Male		15–60
		Female		15–150
FSH	mIU/ml	Male		4–13
		Female	Follicular	4–17
			Midcycle	13–50
			Luteal	4–15
			Menopausal	30–200
Free testosterone	pg/ml	Male		80–200
		Female		2–9
Growth hormone	ng/dl	Male		<5
		Female		<8
17-hydroxycorticosteroids[b]	mg/24hr			4–11
17-hydroxypregnenolone[b]	ng/ml			0.3–3.5
17-hydroxyprogesterone[b]	ng/dl	Male		30–200
		Female	Follicular	20–80
			Luteal	80–300
			Menopausal	4–50
17-Ketosteroids[b]	mg/24hr	Male		8–20
		Female		6–15
17-ketogenic steroids[b]	mg/24hr	Male		5–23
		Female		3–15
LH	mIU/ml	Male		6–23
		Female	Follicular	5–30
			Midcycle	75–1000
			Luteal	3–40
			Menopausal	30–200
Pregnenolone	ng/ml			0.3–2
Progesterone	ng/dl	Male		12–30
		Female	Follicular	2–90
			Luteal	400–3000
			Menopausal	3–30
Prolactin	ng/ml			0–25
Reverse-T3	ng/dl			20–60
Somatomedin C	U/ml	Male		0.34–1.9
		Female		0.45–2.2
T4	mcg/dl			5–11.5
Thyroxine-binding globulin	mcg/ml			15–35
T3 uptake	percent			Varies
T3-RIA	ng/dl			80–190
Testosterone	ng/dl	Male		250–1200
		Female		20–70
TSH	μU/ml			0–6

[a]Results will vary slightly with different assay methods.
[b]Assumes urine creatinine 0.8–2.0 gm/24hr.

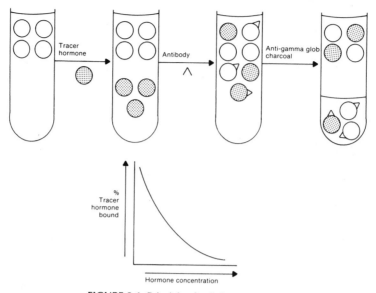

FIGURE 8-1. Principle of radioimmunoassay.

against the first antibody, or charcoal, ethanol or other precipitating agent is added to separate that hormone which is bound to the first antibody from that which is free or unbound. Other methods include solid-phase antibodies or antigens. Then, after centrifugation of this final sample, the supernatant contains the free hormone, both isotopically labeled and native, whereas in the precipitate, antibody bound to both native and isotopically labeled hormone is found. Since a known quantity of tracer hormone and a known quantity of antibody have been added and with competition by the tracer and native hormones for the antibody, the curve derived from the varying amount of native hormone will be a function of its concentration (Fig. 8-1). The more native hormone that is added to the system, the less isotopically labeled hormone will be bound to a known quantity of antibody. This results in a typical standard curve for competitive protein-binding assays which, although simplified, demonstrates the concept. When a sample with an unknown quantity of hormone is added to the system, the concentration of this native hormone can be determined utilizing this concept by computing the percentage of tracer hormone bound in the system at the end of the assay time.

TESTING PROTOCOLS

Growth Hormone

Growth hormone measurements in gynecologic endocrinology are rarely required. Short stature due to growth hormone deficiency is rare, and details regarding its evaluation can be found in most textbooks.[1] Other situations in which we frequently measure growth hormone include evaluation of acromegaly (some women with acromegaly may present with amenorrhea, hirsutism, or acne) or patients in whom we suspect pituitary neoplasm which may result in growth hormone deficiency in the adult. Testing protocols are shown in Table 8-3.[1,5,6] All tests for stimulation of growth hormone have been proven effective. Most consistent, independent of age, is stimulation of growth hormone by insulin-induced hypoglycemia. The response of growth hormone to all stimulatory tests diminishes with age. Sleep-induced growth hormone release rarely occurs above the age of 65.

In the diagnosis of acromegaly, measurement of somatomedin C is probably the most sensitive test. Somatomedin C is one of several growth factors that represent proteins synthesized within the liver in response to growth hormone. Somatomedin C levels are invariably elevated in cases of acromegaly, even when the serum growth hormone levels may appear to be normal. In cases with chronic liver disease, however, somatomedin C levels may be abnormally low (Table 8-2).

Thyrotropin-releasing hormone (TRH) normally does not increase growth hormone levels. Patients with acromegaly however frequently respond with a rise in growth hormone levels after administration of TRH. With the administration of glucose, patients with acromegaly may exhibit a paradoxical rise in growth hormone.

TABLE 8-3. Growth Hormone

	Growth hormone stimulation	
Test	Procedure	Normal response
Insulin hypoglycemia	0.1 U/kg regular insulin IV push; samples every fifteen minutes $\times$ 1 hr	Glucose falls greater than 50%; GH rises two to three-fold and achieves a level greater than 8 ng/ml
Sleep	Sample drawn 60–90 minutes after onset of sleep	GH greater than 7 ng/ml
Arginine	30 g i.v. over 30 min; samples every 30 min $\times$ 2 hr	GH rises three-fold and achieves a level greater than 8 ng/ml
L-Dopa	500 mg orally and samples at 40, 60, 90, and 120 min	GH rises to a level greater than 6 ng/ml
Exercise	Vigorous exercises $\times$ 15 min; samples 30, 40, and 60 min after exercise	GH rises to a level greater than 7 ng/ml

	Growth hormone suppression	
Test	Procedure	Normal response
Glucose	100 gm oral glucose. Samples $\frac{1}{2}$, 1, 2, 3, 4, and 5 hr to include glucose	GH falls to less than 2 ng/ml between $\frac{1}{2}$ and 2 hr

Stimulation-suppression testing of growth hormone is most useful in the follow up of growth hormone secreting pituitary tumors.

Growth hormone releasing factor, a 44-amino acid polypeptide hormone, has recently been synthesized and has biologic activity. It is likely that this will be measured in serum in the future and may be useful in therapy and in the diagnosis of states of abnormal growth hormone secretion.[7]

Prolactin

The importance of prolactin in gynecologic endocrinology has been bolstered by recent reports indicating that elevated levels are frequently found in pitiutary neoplasms[8,9] (Chapter 23). Until recently, the function of prolactin, other than its critical importance in breast development and milk secretion in lactating females, was only speculated upon. It now appears that prolactin may have minimal effects on salt and water metabolism, may inhibit myometrial response to oxytocin in several species, and appears to have a direct androgen-stimulating effect on the adrenal in the adult female.[9a] Stimulation tests of prolactin are shown in Table 8-4. No good suppression tests for prolactin exist at present. The most convenient and best standardized test for prolactin stimulation still remains thyrotropin-releasing hormone (protirelin)

administration. Patients with prolactin-secreting tumors usually exhibit little change in prolactin levels in response to TRH: This suggests autonomy.[1] The alert reader will note that this breaks one of the basic rules: When a hormone is suspected to be overproduced, suppression testing is the best test. Since there are no good suppression tests, stimulation testing represents our best available test to evaluate this system.

Transient elevations in basal prolactin levels usually represent physiologic secretory spikes of this hormone. When abnormally elevated, prolactin levels should be repeated to rule this out as a cause of spurious elevation. A number of drugs will falsely elevate the serum prolactin concentration. Dopamine antagonists that block dopamine receptors include phenothiazines, butyrophenones, and benzamides (metoclopramide).[1] Dopamine antagonists that deplete dopamine concentrations include reserpine and α-methyldopa. Other drugs that increase prolactin concentrations include oral contraceptive agents, isoniazid, cimetidine, and antidepressants. Stress, surgery, or psychological stress may increase serum prolactin secretion, as will hypothyroidism. Basal fasting serum prolactin levels greater than 300 ng/ml need not be repeated and suggest the presence of a pituitary tumor. Prolactin levels greater than 100 ng/ml are associated with a 50% risk of pituitary neoplasm.

TABLE 8-4. Evaluation of Pituitary Prolactin

Prolactin stimulation			Prolactin suppression
Test	Procedure	Normal response	No tests
Chlorpromazine	25 mg orally; samples at 60 and 90 min	Prolactin increases two to three-fold	
TRH (protirelin)	500 mcg given i.v. push; samples at 15 and 30 min	Prolactin increases three to five-fold	
Metoclopramide	10 mg given i.v. push; samples at 20 and 60 min	Prolactin increases five to ten-fold	

Alpha Subunit

Three glycoprotein pituitary hormones, TSH, LH, and FSH, and the placental hormone, HCG, share a common alpha subunit. The beta subunit is what gives the molecule its specificity, while the alpha subunit completes its molecular structure. Both intact glycoprotein molecules and free alpha subunit are secreted by the pituitary, placenta, and some HCG-producing tumors. Stimulation of the pituitary with TRH will yield increased levels of both TSH and alpha subunit. The clinical importance of the alpha subunit was not recognized until the initial report of Rosen et al.[9b] Since that time, measurement of the alpha subunit in the plasma of patients with suspected pituitary tumors has shown that some patients with amenorrhea or hypogonadism with normal levels of other pituitary hormones have tumors secreting increased amounts of the alpha subunit. In cases of suspected "nonsecreting" pituitary tumors, levels for the alpha subunit should be obtained, since it may provide evidence of a pituitary tumor that was not evident on routine studies and would provide a marker for follow-up of treatment regimens.[9c] Moreover, its use in the follow-up of patients with HCG-secreting tumors may prove to be more sensitive than the measurement of HCG, itself.

Antidiuretic Hormone

The two most common clinical situations in which antidiuretic hormone (ADH), or vasopressin, may be abnormal are diabetes insipidus and the syndrome of inappropriate ADH secretion (SIADH). Too often, the diagnosis of diabetes insipidus is based on the hospital measurement of the patient's urine output and oral intake. Unfortunately, this is not performed under standardized conditions, which would differentiate between psycho-genic water drinking and the patient with true deficiency of ADH. When hormone deficiency is suspected, stimulation testing provides the most reliable means of evaluation.

Stimulation testing of ADH is performed most simply by utilizing water deprivation according to the method of Miller.[10] If psychogenic water drinking is suspected, longer periods of deprivation may be needed. Fluid restriction should begin at 6:00 a.m., unless psychogenic water drinking is suspected (when earlier restriction is needed). At the onset of the test, the patient should void and be weighed, and a sample obtained for urine osmolality. Urine collections for the determination of osmolality and body weights are done at hourly intervals thereafter. When the urinary osmolality plateaus so that the change in two consecutive urines is less than 30 mOsm, a serum osmolality and serum ADH are obtained and the patient is weighed and given 5 units of aqueous vasopressin subcutaneously. Exactly 1 hr later, a final urine specimen is obtained for osmolality determination. In normal subjects with normal renal function, the maximum urine osmolality before vasopressin administration should be greater than the serum osmolality. The serum osmolality should be less than 300 mOsm with an appropriate antidiuretic hormone concentration for the osmolality achieved (Table 8-10).[11] The urine should be concentrated to greater than 500 mOsm, and there should be little or no increase in urine osmolality after vasopressin (less than 5% of the previous specimen).

Where SIADH is suspected, confirmation of the inappropriate secretion of this hormone may be confirmed by simultaneous measurement of serum ADH levels and serum osmolality (Table 8-5). While waiting for the return of these results, however, the diagnosis may be made (assuming there is no renal disease and Addison's disease) by demonstrating that the urine osmolality is inappropriately

TABLE 8-5. Plasma AVP Levels

Plasma AVP (pg/ml)	Plasma osmolality (mOsm/kg)
<1.5	270–280
<2.5	280–285
1–5	285–290
2–7	290–295
4–12	295–300

concentrated as compared with the simultaneously obtained serum osmolality, and the urinary sodium is greater than 10 in the absence of diuretics. Water loading is not needed to confirm this diagnosis. SIADH has been reported to occur after psychological stress with no evidence of neoplasm or other significant disorder. In addition, it is a common concomitant of stress during aging when release of ADH is excessive. A number of drugs will interfere with ADH levels and water metabolism; they include clofibrate, carbamazine, diphenylhydantoin, chlorpropramide, corticosteroids, tolbutamide, and declomycin.[1]

Hypothalamic–Pituitary–Adrenal Axis

The hypothalamic–pituitary–adrenal axis (HPA) operates in a negative feedback loop. The hypothalamus and pituitary are sensitive to minute changes in the circulating serum cortisol level. No other adrenal steroids produce significant alterations in this system other than cortisol. Normal basal ACTH Levels are noted in Table 8-1. There are no standardized testing protocols using stimulation and suppression studies with the measurement of ACTH only. As a consequence, we rely on urinary and serum steroids together with ACTH, which have been demonstrated to accurately reflect alterations in the HPA.

For the sake of simplicity, it can be stated that the adrenal synthesizes three classes of hormones: sex steroids (zona reticularis, zona fasciculata), glucocorticoids (zona reticularis, zona fasciculata), and mineralocorticoids (zona glomerulosa). All adrenal steroids are derived from the parent compound, cholesterol, and steroid synthesis proceeds from the common precursor, Δ^5-pregnenolone (Fig. 8-2) through specific and well-documented hydroxylation steps to result in their respective products.

Recognition of these hydroxylations has resulted in our ability to diagnose multiple adrenal enzyme deficiencies important in evaluating patients with

gynecologic problems. Specific defects and their clinical and biochemical characteristics may be found outlined in detail elsewhere.[1] Suffice it to say that those most commonly seen include 21-hydroxylase deficiency with androgenization and salt losing; 11-hydroxylase deficiency with masculinization and hypertension; and 17-hydroxylase deficiency with lack of secondary sexual characteristics, as well as hypertension, and amenorrhea. A review of Figure 8-2 with a specific hydroxylase deficiency in mind demonstrates which end products might be expected to be elevated in these cases.

Adrenal Androgens and Estrogens

It is clear that the adrenal androgens and estrogens have a minor role in sexual differentiation and maturation. They are critical for the maintenance of secondary sex characteristics, which is evident in the patient with adrenal insufficiency. Conversely, premature adrenarche in a prepubertal female or male will result in pubic hair and occasional axillary hair development, without other secondary sex characteristics. Further description of sex steroids will be covered in the section on the hypothalamic–pituitary–gonadal axis. The masculinizing effects of adrenal androgens are usually seen when these hormones are produced in excess, as with adrenal enzyme deficiencies (partial or complete), adrenal carcinoma, Cushing's syndrome, and adrenal adenomas. Compared with testosterone, however, the androgenicity of adrenal steroids is rather small. Most potent are androstenedione, androsterone, and dehydroepiandrosterone. Although testosterone is produced in part by the adrenal gland, adrenal-derived testosterone amounts to less than 5% of the contribution to the total daily 17-ketosteroid production rate.

Adrenal androgens are most commonly measured in the urine. Perhaps the most commonly requested measurement of adrenal androgen metabolites in the urine are the urinary 17-ketosteroids (Table 8-1). Measurement of these compounds is a simple procedure (see Fig. 8-3). Compounds included in 17-ketosteroid measurements are androstenedione, dehydroepiandrosterone, androsterone, etiocholanolone, androstanedione, as well as their sulfates, glucuronides, and 11-hydroxylated derivatives. Testosterone is not a 17-ketosteroid, since testosterone has a hydroxyl group rather than a ketone at the C-17 position. Metabolic breakdown products of testosterone contribute to less than 5% of ketosteroid production.[1]

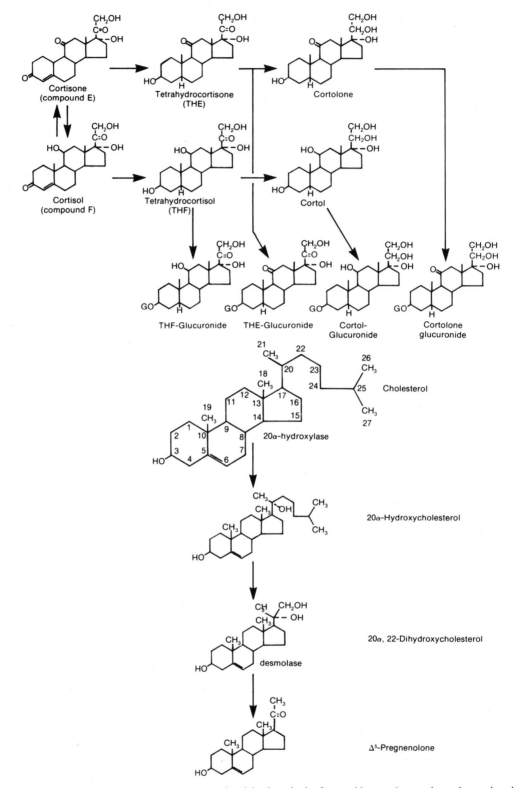

FIGURE 8-2. Steroid biosynthetic pathways. – – –→ , only minimal synthesis after age 11 years; *, may also undergo adrenal 11-hydroxylation and appear as 11-hydroxy and 11-keto 17-ketosteroids.

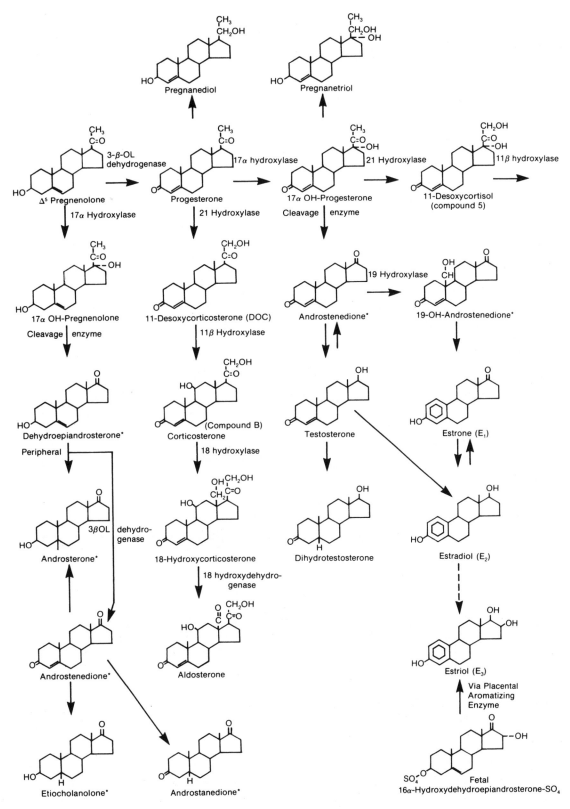

FIGURE 8-2. (*Continued*)

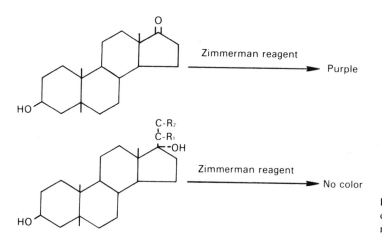

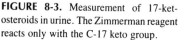

FIGURE 8-3. Measurement of 17-ketosteroids in urine. The Zimmerman reagent reacts only with the C-17 keto group.

17-Ketosteroid excretion increases with age throughout puberty. It plateaus at age 30–40 and then gradually declines. As a rule of thumb, children excrete approximately 1 mg of ketosteroids per year of age until puberty.[1] Most obese patients will fall within a normal range for 17-ketosteroids, or slightly above. Patients with adrenal carcinomas are said to have the highest levels of 17-ketosteroids. As a general rule in the hirsute woman, elevated levels of 17-ketosteroids reflect an adrenal source for androgenicity, rather than an ovarian source.

Dehydroepiandrosterone sulfate now is a commonly measured 17-ketosteroid, measured in the serum rather than in the urine. Extraordinarily high levels are reported in adrenal carcinoma.

Adrenal Glucocorticoids

Two commonly used methods for the determination of urinary glucocorticoids are currently employed. These include urinary 17-hydroxycorticosteroids and urinary 17-ketogenic steroids. A number of drugs will interfere with the determination of urinary 17-hydroxycorticosteroids, including chloral hydrate, chlordiazepoxide, chloromycetin, chlorpromazine, digitalis, meprobamate, paraldehyde, quinidine, and spironolactone.[12] In addition, urinary glucose may cause a falsely low result and, as might be expected, bilirubin ill cause interference, since this is a colorometric reaction that depends on the color yellow. Urinary 17-hydroxycorticosteroids primarily measure 11-desoxycortisol (compound S), cortisol (compound F),

cortisone (compound E), and tetrahydrocortisone and tetrahydrocortisol. It is estimated that this method measures roughly 50% of total daily cortisol production.

Measurement of urinary 17-ketogenic steroids is considered by many to be a simpler and more reliable method. 17-Ketogenic steroids bear no relationship to 17-ketosteroids. The term merely refers to the method of measurement (Fig. 8-4). It measures the following steroids: 11-desoxycortisol, cortisol, cortisone, tetrahydrocortisone, tetrahydrocortisol, cortolones, and pregnanetriol. Many authorities believe that 17-hydroxypregnenolone, 17-hydroxyprogesterone, and progesterone are not 17-ketogenic steriods.

Probably more discriminating than any other test for Cushing's disease is the measurement of urinary free cortisol.[1,13] All tests that measure urinary steroids may be increased in patients with depression, or who are under stress, and may be decreased in patients who are taking diphenylhydantoin or in those with renal disease or liver disease. Moreover, it is virtually impossible to do meaningful suppression–stimulation studies in patients with these disorders, making the diagnosis of Cushing's disease in these states extremely difficult.

Measurement of glucocorticoids in serum and plasma has been the method of choice for a number of years. With the advent of RIA, accuracy and specificity for cortisol has been dramatically improved. Single samples or two samples taken in the morning and in the evening have little diagnostic value for the determination of diurnal variation

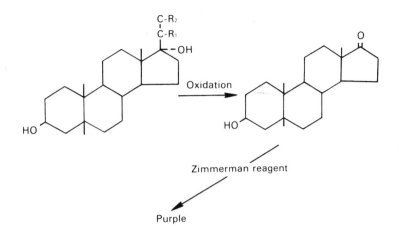

FIGURE 8-4. Measurement of 17-ketogenic steroids in urine.

(Table 8-1). That is, failure to demonstrate diurnal variation on two cortisol samples is insufficient evidence to warrant further investigation. If one wishes to prove loss of diurnal variation, serum cortisols should ideally be obtained every 2–4 hours in a 24-hr study to yield meaningful information. Abolition of the circadian rhythm of cortisol is seen in patients with liver disease and in patients undergoing time-zone shift (jet lag) but is not influenced by depression or changes with light and dark in human subjects.

Stimulation of the adrenal gland may be accomplished by direct stimulation with ACTH or by indirect stimulation of the hypothalamic pituitary end of the loop. Currently, there are five commonly used stimulation studies (Tables 8-6 and 8-7): (1) a rapid ACTH stimulation test, an excellent screening procedure that can be performed as an outpatient in the office in an hour's time; (2)

prolonged ACTH stimulation, which can be done as an outpatient over 4–5 days or in a hospital setting (this is used as a confirmatory test or only when Addison's disease is highly suspect); (3) the standard metyrapone test; (4) rapid metyrapone test, which can be conveniently done as an outpatient but not infrequently produces nausea and vomiting, which may invalidate the test; and (5) insulin hypoglycemia, which is an especially useful method if other hormones need to be measured (e.g., growth hormone, prolactin).[6] It is expected that at some time within the next 5 years, corticotropin releasing factor, a 41-amino acid polypeptide hormone that causes release of ACTH, β-endorphin, and melanotropin will be available as a rapid stimulation test as well.

The oral metyrapone test is commonly employed that involves integrity of both ends of the hypothalamic pituitary axis. Metyrapone acts as an

TABLE 8-6. Cortisol Stimulation

Test	Procedure	Result
Rapid cortrosyn (screening)	Serum cortisol, then 250 mg; cortrosyn i.v. or i.m. push; serum cortisol 30 and 60 min following injection	Cortisol should increase at least 7 mcg/dl to a value of greater than 18 mcg/dl
Prolonged cortrosyn (confirmatory)	Daily 24-hr urine for 17-hydroxycorticosteroids and creatinine beginning at 8:00 a.m. and daily 4:00 p.m. serum cortisol × four days; day 2 begin daily 4-hr infusion of 500 mcg Cortrosyn i.v.	Serum cortisol will increase to greater than 30 mcg/dl and 17-hydroxycorticosteroids to 30-40 mg/24hr

TABLE 8-7. Evaluation of Pituitary ACTH

ACTH stimulation		
Test	Procedure	Normal response
Insulin	0.1 U/kg regular insulin i.v. push; samples every 15 min × one hour	Glucose falls greater than 50%; cortisol rises at least 10 mcg/dl to a value greater than 20 mcg/dl
Standard metyrapone	Begin daily 24-hr urine for 17-ketogenic steroids at 8:00 a.m. × 3 days; at beginning of second 24-hr urine, 750 mg metyrapone is given orally every four hours × six doses	A two-and-a-half- to three-fold increase in 17-ketogenic steroids on day 2 or 3
Overnight metyrapone	At midnight give 30 mg/kg metyrapone orally; draw samples for cortisol and Compound S[a] (metyrapone) at 8:00 a.m.	Serum cortisol less than 8 mg/dl and Compound S greater than 8 mcg/dl

ACTH suppression		
Test	Procedure	Normal response
Overnight dexamethasone	At 11:00 p.m., 1.0 mg dexamethasone and 5 mg Valium; serum cortisol at 8:00 a.m.	8:00 a.m. serum cortisol less than 5 mcg/dl
Standard dexamethasone	Begin 24-hr urine for 17-hydroxycorticosteroids and creatinine daily × 5 days at 8:00 a.m.; on days 2 and 3 dexamethasone 0.5 mg. p.o. every six hours beginning at 8:00 a.m.; days 4 and 5 dexamethasone 2 mg. p.o. every six hours beginning at 8:00 a.m.	17-hydroxycorticosteroids fall to less than 4 mg/24hr on 2 mg dose
Outpatient dexamethasone	Day 1 at 8:00 a.m. begin dexamethasone 0.5 mg orally every 6 hr; obtain serum cortisol at 4:00 p.m. on day 2; day 3 change at 8:00 a.m. to 2 mg dexamethasone orally every 6 hr; day 4 at 4:00 p.m. obtain serum cortisol	Serum cortisol on day 2 less than 5 mcg/dl; on day 4 less than 10 mcg/dl

[a] 11-desoxycortisol

enzyme inhibitor at the 11-hydroxylation step (and probably 18-hydroxylation as well); it results in a fall in the serum cortisol, a rise in the 11-desoxycortisol, and consequently a rise in corticotropin-releasing factor and ACTH. This rise in ACTH further increases adrenal steroid output that can be measured as 17-ketogenic steroids (not 17-hydroxycorticosteroids). Failure of this mechanism to operate (i.e., failure of urinary steroids to increase) would suggest a lesion at the level of the hypothalamus, pituitary, or adrenal. Having proved that the adrenal functions normally in response to exogenous ACTH, one could then state that the lesion lay in the region of the hypothalamus and pituitary.

The reader will note that 17-ketosteroids were not included in all tests of stimulation mentioned thus far. No standardized stimulation test exists for 17-ketosteroids. However, most clinicians believed that hirsute women who exhibit a marked rise in 17-ketosteroids after the administration of ACTH may represent a variant or a mild 21- or 11-hydroxylase deficiency. Clinically, many of these patients respond to adrenal suppression.

Suppression testing of the adrenal can be done only by suppressing the hypothalamic pituitary loop of the axis. The drug of choice for suppression testing is dexamethasone, a synthetic cortisol analogue that is recognized by the pituitary and hypothalamus as cortisol. It is preferred over the

TABLE 8-8. Use of the Standard Dexamethasone Suppression Test

| | Urinary 17-ketogenic steroids or 17-hydroxycorticosteroids | | |
	Dexamethasone (2 mg)	Dexamethasone (8 mg)	ACTH level
Normal	Suppressed	Suppressed	Normal
Cushing's disease	Greater than 50% suppression	Suppressed	Normal, high
Adrenal adenoma	No suppression	No suppression	Low
Ectopic ACTH	No suppression	No suppression	Often high

other drugs because its half-life is significantly longer and because its metabolites constitute only a minute fraction of the total steroid excretion in the urine. Basically, the following three protocols are available for adrenal suppression (Table 8-8):

1. *Overnight dexamethasone suppression test:* This represents an excellent outpatient screening study. Patients with obesity suppress; those with suspect Cushing's do not. It is now currently most commonly employed in the diagnosis of psychiatric depressive illness. Patients with depressive illnesses exhibit lack of suppression in samples taken 9 and 17 hr after the administration of an overnight dexamethasone dose. If done properly, and the patient is not depressed, the test has a false-negative rate of less than 10% of patients with Cushing's syndrome. Diphenylhydantoin increases the metabolism of dexamethasone and may result in lack of suppression. Oral contraceptive agents increase cortisol-binding globulin and may give falsely elevated results in patients who suppress normally.

2. *Standard dexamethasone suppression study:* This protocol is more burdensome than the rapid screening study and may require hospitalization. The same abnormalities may cause abnormal results in this testing protocol.

3. *Prolonged dexamethasone suppression test:* The use of serum cortisols is a recent addition to our diagnostic armamentarium.[15] It has the drawback of being a new test and lack of large experience, but it looks like an excellent alternative. Abnormal results should be viewed with caution, however, since highly stressed patients in a home setting may yield abnormal results.

Typically, the standard dexamethasone suppression study is used to separate patients with normal adrenal function from those with Cushing's disease, Cushing's syndrome due to adrenal adenoma, or ectopic ACTH. Typical responses are shown in Table 8-7. These values may be compared to those values obtained after ACTH stimulation. While this test is generally accurate, there are many reports of Cushing's syndrome due to pituitary disease or adrenal adenoma, undergoing periods of remission, during which testing may be entirely normal. Patients who are highly suspect should undergo repeat testing. Moreover, some patients with Cushing's disease may fail to suppress, in the manner characteristic of an adrenal adenoma. Ectopic ACTH production has been reported in patients with pancreatic carcinoma, pheochromocytoma, neurogenic sarcoma, oat cell carcinoma of the lung, endometrial carcinoma, and thymoma.

In 1984, ovine corticotropin-releasing factor was isolated, synthesized, and tested in patients with Cushing's syndrome. It appears to be a rapid and useful test to differentiate pituitary Cushing's disease from Cushing's syndrome due to ectopic ACTH, adrenal adenomas and adrenal carcinomas. The neurotransmitter is given intravenously; samples for ACTH are obtained before and after injection. Patients with Cushing's disease from pituitary origin should respond with a substantial increase in their ACTH levels while those with nonpituitary etiology respond with little or no rise in their serum ACTH levels. At present the numbers of patients studied are small and some overlap will be expected so that the specificity of the test will likely be as good as the dexamethasone suppression test. Its primary advantage will be that it is rapid and can be done as an outpatient. Further studies will be required to determine its clinical value.[15a,15b]

Hypothalamic–Pituitary–Gonadal Axis

Testing of the hypothalamic–pituitary–gonadal (HPG) axis is perhaps the most difficult of all endocrine systems in which to perform meaningful tests.

Factors making this difficult include the knowledge that sex steroids and gonadotropins not only change from minute to minute but also may exhibit pulsatility in the adult female, as well as significant changes during the varying stages of puberty. Moreover, tests in prepubertal children are difficult to interpret.[16–18] The lack of foolproof stimulation–suppression testing of this axis adds further to the difficulty. For these reasons, only those tests that tell us the net effect of the HPG axis on a given patient remain our best procedures. These include such clinical tests as chromosomal analysis, vaginal cytology, general physical and pelvic examinations, the patient's history and evaluation of growth and development, and alterations in the menstrual cycle. Clinical tests are well covered in previous chapters; this section concerns itself primarily with laboratory testing.

The ovaries have the ability to synthesize both estrogen and androgen in the prenatal period, as well as in adulthood. With the exception of the 11β-hydroxylase enzyme that they lack, the ovaries are able to synthesize androgen from cholesterol and contain the same enzyme systems as the adrenal gland.[1] The ovarian follicle is the major source of estrogen in the female and is under the stimulating control of pituitary FSH. The corpus luteum is the major source of progesterone and its metabolite pregnanediol. Although we recognize that the menstrual cycle involves both positive and negative feedback at the pituitary hypothalamic level by estrogen and possibly androgen, the details are not yet clear. While the ovaries have the capability of synthesizing androgen, the major site of androgen production is the adrenal. Thus, during puberty, breast development (ovarian) and hair growth (adrenal) may not be simultaneous.

Testing of the patient in the basal state will frequently yield maximal information regarding the HPG axis. For instance, an amenorrheic woman with low serum estradiol, high LH and FSH and failure to exhibit withdrawal bleeding after progesterone, obviously has evidence of ovarian disease. Conversely, a woman with low FSH and LH levels and low estradiol levels has functional or structural disease at the level of the hypothalamus and pituitary, provided there is adequate evidence that the uterus is capable of responding to estrogen. A woman with a high luteinizing hormone (LH) level combined with a slightly elevated serum testosterone level with normal menstrual cycling may actually have no disease, but rather, a mid-cycle LH surge and a mild slight increase in testosterone, which accompanies it. In a patient with amenorrhea, however, it may represent polycystic ovary syndrome or pregnancy, since human chorionic gonadotropin (hCG) crossreacts with LH in all RIAs for LH. Finally, a serum testosterone of 20 µg/dl in an 8-year-old girl would be considered abnormal, while in a female in stage III puberty it would be considered normal.

In small children, serum LH and FSH values may be within the normal adult range until the age of 2–4, when they fall to quite low levels. During stage II puberty and thereafter, serum gonadotropins may reach normal adult levels.[16,17] In the postmenopausal state, there is a marked increase in serum LH and FSH levels into a range seen with ovulation. Over the ensuing decades, these levels may gradually fall to levels that are only slightly elevated.

Ovarian products commonly measured include estrogens, progesterone, 17-hydroxyprogesterone, and testosterone (Table 8-1). While the 24-hr urine still remains a reasonable way to measure total estrogens, this is being rapidly replaced by serum determinations of estrogens. Estradiol-17β is the major estrogen in females and is consequently the common estrogen measured in serum and urine. Prepubertal females have levels of 17β-estradiol and progestogens similar to the menopausal adult.

Testosterone is secreted in much lower amounts in females than in males throughout life. However, during the first 3 months of life, a high proportion of testosterone is free, i.e., not bound to sex hormone-binding globulins (SHBG). These values then return to normal, prepubertal ranges. In the adult female, free testosterone remains the active available form of testosterone. Testosterone decreases its own binding globulin and consequently, in many women with hirsutism or acne, total testosterone may be within the normal range. Ideally, free testosterone should be measured in all women with signs of excessive androgenization. Recent development of assays for serum free testosterone alleviates the binding problems and provides more accurate diagnosis in women with excessive androgen production (Table 8-1).

Stimulation testing of LH basically involves only two agents—clomiphene citrate and luteinizing hormone releasing hormone (LHRH) or gonadorelin (Table 8-9).

The use of clomiphene as a test of hypothalamic–pituitary integrity in females is difficult. In pre-

TABLE 8-9. Evaluation of Pituitary Luteinizing Hormone

Luteinizing hormone stimulation		
Test	Procedure	Normal response
Clomiphene (female)	100 mg orally daily × 5 days	Rise in LH by day 5–9, similar to midcycle surge
Clomiphene (male)	100 mg orally daily × 1 week	Rise in LH by 25–300% at end of 1 week
LHRH (gonadorelin)	100 mcg i.v. push or s.q.; samples at 15, 30, 45, and 60 min	LH should rise to a value greater than 24 and double the baseline in males and in females

Luteinizing hormone suppression		
Test	Procedure	Normal response
Estrogen	Ethinyl estradiol	Not standardized
Testosterone	Testosterone proprionate	Not standardized

pubertal females during early puberty, clomiphene may suppress gonadotropin[18] and may even prevent ovulation. In the adult patient with amenorrhea, clomiphene administration may be started at any time provided pregnancy has been excluded. In some normal menstruating females, clomiphene may block the LH surge and hence, ovulation. Failure to demonstrate a rise in LH or FSH may not document the presence of hypothalamic–pituitary disease.

LHRH (gonadorelin) has been shown to stimulate both LH and FSH secretion in children as well as adults. Changes in FSH, however, are smaller; as a consequence, they are rarely measured during testing protocols. In patients with pituitary disease, one would expect to find low serum levels of gonadotropins, low estrogens, and a poor response to LHRH. By contrast, patients with hypothalamic disease will exhibit, as a general rule, normal or enhanced and prolonged response to LHRH (e.g., chronic illness, anorexia nervosa). Unfortunately, clear-cut separation may not always hold true, and interpretation of results must be with caution.[6]

Stimulation testing at the level of the ovaries can be carried out in conjunction with clomiphene administration, provided adequate hypothalamic–pituitary function is present. However, no standards regarding estrogen and testosterone secretion are available for stimulation testing. Primary stimulation of the ovaries is carried out using hCG, which is rarely used as a diagnostic tool.

Suppression testing of the HPG axis generally falls within the same categories noted above. Since

we do not understand the mechanism by which puberty is triggered and the subsequent development of the "gonadostat" as well as the feedback systems involved in normal menstrual cycling, suppression testing is somewhat difficult. While ethinyl estradiol is frequently used to suppress the ovaries, as well as simple oral contraceptive steroids, no standards exist for suppression studies with either agent.[1] Others have attempted to use dexamethasone suppression to help diagnose the source of androgen excess. This has been carried out in a manner similar to the standard dexamethasone suppression test. Frequently, changes in testosterone or 17-ketosteroid levels are used as an endpoint of suppression.

It should be clear that the most reliable test of the HPG axis that we currently have are those obtained in the basal state. Stimulation testing with LHRH may prove a valuable tool in certain cases.

Hypothalamic–Pituitary–Thyroid Axis

Testing of the hypothalamic–pituitary axis (HPT) is based on the concept that it operates on a negative feedback loop. Thyrotropin releasing hormone (TRH) is secreted by the hypothalamus; it effects release of thyroid stimulating hormone (TSH) into the peripheral circulation. The binding of TSH to the thyroid receptor increases the iodine uptake, hormone synthesis and proteolysis of preformed hormone in thyroglobulin. In addition, it effects release of thyroid hormone into the peripheral circulation. Thyroid hormone is basically stored in two forms: thyroxine (T4) and tri-iodothyronine (T3). These two hormones are stored in a 3 : 4 ratio, respectively, and when released into the circulation, their ratio is 10 : 1 and the ratio of total distribution is 60 : 1. Of the circulating T3 levels, 70–90% are derived by peripheral degradation of T4. Alternate or additional degradatory pathways include further reduction to reverse T3 and diiodothyronine (T2). Circulating levels of T4 and T3 act at both the hypothalamus and pituitary to inhibit further TSH release. TRH and TSH are not turned on again until the level of thyroid hormone falls below a setpoint of the hypothalamus. At that point, the cycle begins again.

Like many other hormones, when T4 and T3 circulate in the peripheral blood, they are bound to specific binding proteins. For instance, T4 is 99.96% bound to thyroxine-binding globulins, so what is measured in the blood is a direct reflection of the protein binding under normal circumstances. The amount that remains free, regardless of the amount that is bound, remains constant in normal circumstances. T3 is also protein bound. In pregnancy and with estrogen or oral contraceptive treatment, thyroxine values are usually elevated, since estrogen induces synthesis of thyroxine-binding globulin. However, the amount that remains free in the circulation and has biologic activity remains normal. Conversely, when serum proteins are low, secondary to chronic liver disease, congenital low thyroxine-binding globulin, nephrotic syndrome, or protein-losing enteropathies, the amount of thyroxine-binding protein is low. Consequently, the amount of total T4 is also low, but the amount circulating free and biologically active remains the same. Any measurement of T4 or T3 alone is invalid and must be accompanied by a measure of protein binding.

The resin triiodothyronine uptake (RT3U) is designed to give an indirect estimate of thyroxine-binding globulin. Unfortunately, many people consider this a thyroid function test. This concept is in error, since RT3U gives no information regarding the amount of circulating thyroid hormone. Under normal circumstances, when serum proteins are low resulting in a low T4, the RT3U will be elevated. Conversely, when serum thyroxine-binding proteins are elevated owing to pregnancy, oral contraceptives, or estrogen therapy, the RT3U will be low.

Utilizing a product of the T4 and RT3U or TBG, one may calculate a free thyroxine index. The free thyroxine index (FT4I) represents a T4 value that has been corrected for protein-binding abnormalities. This calculation must be performed on all patients in whom T4 or T3 concentration is being measured to determine the state of the patient's thyroid function. To confuse the issue, the free thyroxine index has a number of "catchy" pseudonyms coined by various commercial manufacturers for use: T7, T12, T4N, ETR, and TI.

Thyroxine values are shown in Table 8-1. In children, the values are somewhat higher than seen in adults. T3 by RIA is proportionally increased in T3 toxicosis, treated hyperthyroidism, iodine deficiency, goiter and early thyroid failure. Conversely, it is decreased in the early newborn, old age, protein-calorie malnutrition, starvation, and severe illness. Reverse-T3 (rT3) levels are shown in Table 8-1. It is rarely required for measurement, except in special circumstances.

A syndrome recently described may result in abnormal thyroid function tests which appear in many seriously ill patients. The so-called "euthyroid sick" syndrome patients are frequently found to have low T4, free thyroxine index, and T3 by RIA levels, but normal or increased T3 levels and frequently normal T4 levels by equilibrium dialysis (free T4).[19] Their response to TRH is usually normal, and the syndrome is characterized by decreased production and increased metabolic clearance of T4, as well as shunting of T4 production from T3 to rT3, an inactive thyroid hormone. These patients have normal serum TSH. This syndrome is thought to represent a biologic adaptation to illness and is usually not treated.

Serum TSH is a glycoprotein synthesized by the anterior pituitary whose alpha chain is identical to that of LH and FSH. Normal values are shown in Table 8-1, which are very slightly increased in women and in the elderly. Moreover, it is estimated that 4% of the elderly are indeed hypothyroid.[2] The TSH and T4 are commonly used in combination in newborn screening for hypothyroidism, estimated to occur in 1 in 4000 births. Timing of sampling for TSH and T4 is critical, since TSH levels rise immediately after birth and T4 levels may fall. Moreover, in premature infants, there may be subnormal TSH and T4 values, suggesting hypothalamic hypothyroidism, but probably representing a "euthyroid sick" syndrome.

With the improved array of thyroid function tests, stimulation and suppression testing of the thyroid is rarely needed (Figs. 8-5 and 8-6). Thyroid

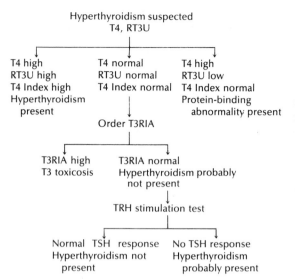

Hyperthyroidism suspected
T4, RT3U

T4 high	T4 normal	T4 high
RT3U high	RT3U normal	RT3U low
T4 Index high	T4 Index normal	T4 Index normal
Hyperthyroidism present		Protein-binding abnormality present

Order T3RIA

T3RIA high
T3 toxicosis

T3RIA normal
Hyperthyroidism probably
not present

TRH stimulation test

Normal TSH response
Hyperthyroidism not
present

No TSH response
Hyperthyroidism
probably present

FIGURE 8-5. Evaluation of hyperthyroidism by algorithm.

suppression studies still remain useful (Table 8-10), although they are rarely needed. The availability of TRH should decrease the use of suppression studies.

TRH stimulation (Table 8-9) is now available to all clinicians. It depends on the integrity of the pituitary for normal stimulation. The test is most commonly employed in the situation in which hypothyroidism is demonstrated by a low free thyroxine index and is thought to be pituitary or hypothalamic in origin by the finding of a low serum TSH.

Some have found it useful in the diagnosis of autonomous thyroid nodules and in subclinical hypothyroidism (Fig. 8-5). Failure to demonstrate a rise in TSH after the administration of TRH can indicate one of six possibilities: (1) hypothalamic hypothyroidism, (2) suppression of the pituitary by excessive thyroid hormone levels or concentrates, (3) normal result or laboratory error, (4) depression, (5) drug interference, or (6) aging.

Unfortunately, ^{131}I is still used as a diagnostic tool. Many clinicians are unaware that routine scanning and uptake doses of radioactive iodine may deliver 50–200 rad to the thyroid gland. Moreover, the ^{131}I uptake is an extremely poor thyroid function test, except to tell the clinician how the thyroid handles iodine. Hypothyroid patients may have elevated ^{131}I uptakes and hyperthyroid persons may have normal ^{131}I uptakes. For this reason, ^{131}I uptakes should rarely be used, unless treatment with radioactive iodine is contemplated, *or* unless the diagnosis of thyroiditis with hyperthyroidism is being considered. If scanning is desired, ^{123}I or Tc^{99m} scanning yields information regarding thyroid morphology and nodule evaluation with an extremely low level of radiation to the thyroid.

Pancreas

The islet cells of the human pancreas synthesize and secrete multiple hormones, three of which are insulin, glucagon, and somatostatin. For the purpose of this section, we may quickly dispense with glucagon and somatostatin as not playing a signifi-

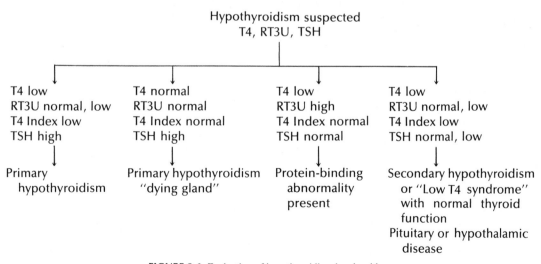

Hypothyroidism suspected
T4, RT3U, TSH

T4 low	T4 normal	T4 low	T4 low
RT3U normal, low	RT3U normal	RT3U high	RT3U normal, low
T4 Index low	T4 Index normal	T4 Index normal	T4 Index low
TSH high	TSH high	TSH normal	TSH normal, low

Primary
hypothyroidism

Primary hypothyroidism
"dying gland"

Protein-binding
abnormality
present

Secondary hypothyroidism
or "Low T4 syndrome"
with normal thyroid
function
Pituitary or hypothalamic
disease

FIGURE 8-6. Evaluation of hypothyroidism by algorithm.

TABLE 8-10. Evaluation of Pituitary TSH

	TSH stimulation	
Test	Procedure	Normal response
TRH (protirelin)	500 mcg given i.v. push; samples at 30 and 60 min	Increment in TSH 5–25 μU/ml above baseline at 30 min, followed by a rapid fall
	TSH suppression	
Test	Procedure	Normal response
T3	Baseline ^{131}I uptake at 24 hr; then 50 mcg T3 orally bid × seven days; obtain second ^{131}I uptake at 24 hr on day 7	^{131}I uptake falls to less than 50% of baseline and less than 30% 24-hr uptake
T4	Baseline ^{131}I uptake at 24 hr; then 3 mg T4 orally as single dose; seven days after T4 second ^{131}I uptake at 24 hr	^{131}I uptake falls to less than 50% of baseline

cant role in gynecologic endocrinology. However, we are all aware of the implications of diabetes during pregnancy, and this is covered in detail in Chapter 26. While diabetes mellitus is frequently sought as a possible cause for amenorrhea in otherwise healthy women, diabetes not clinically obvious (subclinical, latent or chemical) is almost never the cause of amenorrhea. In order to produce significant amenorrhea, one must have major biochemical alterations resulting from insulin deficiency (i.e., ketosis, gluconeogenesis from protein precursors that result in protein-calorie malnutrition and weight loss).

Many believe that the glucose tolerance test has reached the precise pinnacle of clinical diagnosis. It is the growing opinion of many diabetologists that glucose tolerance is rarely, if ever, indicated in clinical medicine. Many consider a single fasting blood glucose sufficient. A fasting glucose concentration should be obtained after a 12-hr overnight fast. Current criteria indicate that most individuals have normal whole blood glucose of 60–95 mg/dl and plasma or serum glucoses of 70–115 mg/dl. However, in order to make a diagnosis of diabetes mellitus, the fasting serum or plasma glucose must be greater than 130 mg/dl.[20] To obtain the popular 2-hr postprandial blood glucose, the subject should not be ill, under any significant stress, or taking any medications that may deteriorate glucose tolerance. If at all possible, this test should be performed on an outpatient basis. Finally, the subject should be ingesting at least 150 g of carbohydrate daily for 3 days before the test. After

an overnight 12-hr fast, the patient should be instructed to eat a high-carbohydrate breakfast consisting of 100 g of carbohydrate. A convenient meal would be two slices of toast, a cup of milk, a cup of orange juice, and 3/4 cup of cereal with a small amount of sugar (a meal consisting of approximately 75 g of carbohydrate). A 2-hr postprandial blood sugar is then obtained exactly 2 hr after the last bite of meal was consumed. In normal subjects, this plasma glucose value should be less than 140 mg/dl. However, to make a diagnosis of diabetes mellitus, this value should be more than 160 mg/dl.[20] Some investigators believe that a 10-mg/dl increment should be added for every decade over 50 (we would accept a 2-hr postprandial glucose of 200 mg/dl in an 80-year-old person before diagnosing diabetes).

In the pregnant woman, the usual normal criteria cannot be applied for glucose tolerance testing. The reader is referred to Chapter 26 for normal values.

Reactive hypoglycemia is an overdiagnosed "nondisease." It is never a cause for gynecologic problems. Suffice it to say that normal blood glucose levels may be extraordinarily low without

TABLE 8-11. Normal Serum Glucose Values After 100 g Oral Glucose

	Fasting	1 hr	1½ hr	2 hr	3 hr	4 hr	5 hr
Upper limit	110	185	165	140	130	110	110
Lower limit	60	60	50	45	35	45	60

symptoms of reactive hypoglycemia (Table 8-11).[21,22]

FUTURE OF HORMONE ASSAY IN ENDOCRINOLOGY

Improved techniques in hormone assays will not only increase our understanding of endocrinology in the future but make measurement of previously unheard or poorly understood hormones and neurotransmitters commonplace. Spillover of hormonal assay techniques can already be seen in the proliferation of information about infectious disease and therapeutic drug monitoring. Its spillover into other areas of medicine will become more evident.[23]

Enzyme-labeled immunoassays (EMIT, ELISA), are already replacing classic RIA. On the basis of competitive and noncompetitive protein-binding assays, they eliminate the hazard of radioactive materials by using colorometric methods with solid-phase bound enzymes. These are currently available for some thyroid hormone assays and numerous drug assays. Their application to more drug assays will be common in the future.[7]

Perhaps the most promising advancement in hormone assays is the development of monoclonal antibodies, providing a major advance in the field.[24] Monoclonal antibody production requires specialized techniques: obtaining antibodies from culture cell lines obtained by hybridization of non-secretory myeloma cells with lymphoid cells from a hyperimmunized animal with selection of stable clones that secrete the desired antibody. Monoclonal antibodies are currently being used commercially in the assay of prostatic alkaline phosphatase, carcinoembryonic antigen, α-fetoprotein, and pregnancy testing. They will improve sensitivity and specificity of assays such as parathyroid hormone. Current problems with parathyroid hormone occur because of antibodies against various antigenic sites on the molecule. Monoclonal antibodies will increase our ability to use the PTH assay accurately to differentiate between primary hyperparathyroidism and malignant disease. Monoclonal antibodies are also being used in some laboratories to evaluate growth hormone and insulin dynamics, to evaluate mullerian-inhibiting substance in fetal endocrinology, and in the search for ''inhibin'' for FSH feedback. Their future use will include quantitative measurement of insulin receptors, TSH re-

ceptors, and estrogen receptors. They will be extremely useful in understanding autoimmune disease and in improving our abilities in treatment, as we are now seeing in terms of insulin-dependent diabetes mellitus. Finally, they will help us define and characterize new molecules.

We will see increasing use of radioreceptor assays in which receptors are used as binding agents in radioligand assays. Radioreceptor assays are closer to true biologic assays than RIA because the receptor or binding agent is part of the normal biologic process: a receptor rather than an antibody. Current application of radioreceptor assays can be seen in the development of the assay for thyroid-stimulating immunoglobulins in the diagnosis and treatment of Graves' disease.

Finally, we see rapid proliferation in our understanding and localization of hypothalamic and brain neurotransmitters, such as corticotropin-releasing factor, growth hormone-releasing factor, LHRH, and TRH, which will be able to be measured in serum, enhancing our ability in diagnosis. Moreover, these agents have potential in treatment of certain endocrine disease.

SUMMARY

Knowledge of negative feedback systems, stimulation of hypofunctioning states and suppression of hyperfunctioning states remains the backbone of endocrine testing. Our hormone assays are only as good as the clinician who orders them and does them correctly, and the reference lab who performs them. Tests of growth hormone secretory dynamics for diagnosis of excessive growth hormone secretion are best measured using somatomedin C. Prolactin stimulation tests are currently our only means of evaluating prolactin secretory dynamics, other than measurement in the basal state, and frequently can be used to diagnose status or activity of a pituitary neoplasm. Because of fluctuation in ACTH levels and serum cortisols, the 24-hr excretion rate of steroids still remains one of our best diagnostic tests of adrenal function. These tests include 17-ketosteroids, which measure androgen production, and 17-hydroxycorticosteroids and 17-ketogenic steroids, which measure cortisol and/or its by-products. The standard test of suppression of the hypothalamic–pituitary–adrenal axis remains the dexamethasone suppression test, although certain rapid screening tests are available. ACTH stimulation using synthetic ACTH, metyrapone stimulation, and insulin hypoglycemia represent the three best tests for defining hypothalamic-adrenal insufficiency. The hypothalamic–pituitary–gonadal area is the most difficult to evaluate. Currently, tests taken in the basal state accompanied by historical information and physical examination, represent the mainstay of diagnosis. Stimulation testing with LHRH is useful in some cases of hypothalamic–pituitary disease. The array of thyroid function tests now available permit the clinician to diagnose with accuracy the presence of hyper- or hypothyroidism in most patients.

The clinician should be aware of a number of disease and psychological states that will alter the endocrine system, hence endocrine results. In addition, a large number of drugs also alter endocrine testing as well.

Radioimmunoassay and its offshoots using noncompetitive protein-binding and radioreceptor assays will continue to increase our knowledge of the endocrine system and the availability of endocrine tests.

QUESTIONS

1. Is the 17-ketosteroid measurement a good test of adrenal function?

2. What factors other than Cushing's syndrome may produce an abnormal overnight dexamethasone suppression test?

3. If repeat LH levels are 300 mIU/ml on several occasions in a patient with amenorrhea, what would be the possibilities?

4. A patient with nephrotic syndrome has a T4 of 2.0, TBG of 12, a low free thyroxine index, and a TSH of 2. What is the diagnosis?

5. Metyrapone testing on a female with weight loss and amenorrhea shows no increased urinary 17-ketogenic steroids. Does this patient have Addison's disease?

REFERENCES

1. Alsever RN, Gotlin RW: *Handbook of Endocrine Tests in Adults and Children,* 2nd ed. Chicago, Yearbook Medical, 1978*

*Review article/chapter.

2. Nasr H: Endocrine disorders in the elderly. *Med Clin North Am* 67:481, 1983*
3. Yalow R: Radioimmunoassay. *Science* 200:1236, 1978
4. Odell WD, Franchimont P: *Principles of Competitive Protein-Binding Assays.* New York, Wiley, 1983*
5. Greenwood FC, Landon J, Stamp TCB: The plasma sugar, free fatty acid, cortisol and growth hormone response to insulin I. In control subjects. *J Clin Invest* 45:429, 1966
6. Lufkin EG, Kao PC, O'Fallon WM, et al: Combined testing of anterior pituitary gland with insulin, thyrotropin-releasing hormone and luteinizing-hormone releasing hormone. *Am J Med* 75:383, 1983
7. Hershman J: Advancing in tandem: Clinical endocrinology and clinical chemistry. *Clin. Chem.* 29:237, 1983*
8. Kleinberg DL, Noel GL, Frantz AG: Galactorrhea: A study of 235 cases including 48 with pituitary tumors. *N Engl J Med* 295:659, 1977
9. Robinson AG, Nelson PB: Prolactinoma in women: Current therapies. *Ann Intern Med* 99:115, 1983*
9a. Vermeulen A, Say E, Rubens R: Effect of prolactin on plasma DEA(s) levels. *J Clin Endocrinol Metab* 44:1222, 1977
9b. Rosen SW, Weintraub BW: Ectopic production of the isolated alpha subunit of the glycoprotein hormones. *N Eng J Med* 290:1441, 1974
9c. Ridgeway EC, Klibanski A, Landenson PW, et al.: Pure alpha secreting pituitary adenomas. *N Eng J Med* 304:1254, 1981
10. Miller M, Moses AM, Streeten DH: Recognition of partial defects in antidiuretic hormone secretion. *Ann Intern Med* 73:721, 1970
11. Hays RM: Antidiuretic hormone. *N Engl J Med* 295:659, 1977
12. Constanton NV, Kakat HF: Drug-induced modifications of laboratory tests—Revised 1973. *Am J Hosp Pharm* 30:24, 1973*
13. Weiss ER, Rayyis SS, Nelson DH, et al: Evaluation of stimulation and suppression tests in the etiological diagnosis of Cushing's syndrome. *Ann Intern Med* 71:941, 1969
14. Carroll BJ, Schroeder K, Mukhopadhyay S: Plasma dexamethasone concentrations and cortisol suppression response in patients with endogenous depression. *Clin Endocrinol Metab* 51:433, 1980
15. Ashcraft MW, VanHerle AJ, Vener SL, et al: Serum cortisol levels in Cushing's syndrome after low- and high-dose dexamethasone supression. *Ann Intern Med* 97:21, 1982
15a. Chrousos, GP, Schultz HM, Oldfield EH, et al: The corticotropin-releasing factor stimulation test: An aid in the evaluation of patients with Cushing's syndrome. *N Engl J Med* 310:622, 1984
15b. Muller OA, Stalla GK, Werder K: Corticotropin releasing factor: A new tool for the differential diagnosis of Cushing's syndrome. *J Clin Endocrinol Metab* 57:227, 1983
16. Winter JSD, Faiman C: Pituitary gonadal relations in male children and adolescents. *Pediatr Res* 6:126, 1972
17. Winter JSD, Faiman C: Pituitary gonadal relationships in female children and adolescents. *Pediatr Res* 7:948, 1973
18. Kulin HE, Grumbach MM, Kaplan SL: Gonadal–hypothalamic interaction in prepubertal and pubertal man: Effect of clomiphene citrate on urinary follicle-stimulating hormone and luteinizing hormone and plasma testosterone. *Pediatr Res* 6:162, 1972
19. Wartofsky L, Burman KD: Alterations in thyroid function in patients with systemic illness: The "euthyroid sick" syndrome. *Endocrinol Rev* 3:164, 1982*

20. Harris M, Cahill G, and members of NIH Diabetes Data Group Workshop: A draft classification of diabetes mellitus and other categories of glucose tolerance. *Diabetes* 28:1039, 1979

21. Merrimee TJ, Tyson JE: Hypoglycemia in man. Pathologic and physiologic variants. *Diabetes* 26:161, 1977

22. Hofeldt FD, Dippe S, Forsham PH: Diagnosis and classification of reactive hypoglycemia based on hormonal changes in response to oral and intravenous glucose. *Am J Clin Nutr* 25:1193, 1972

23. Klee G: Strategies for communicating the values and limitations for endocrine tests. *Clin Lab Med* 2(4):803, 1982

24. Eisenbarth GS, Jackson RA: Application of monoclonal antibody techniques to endocrinology. *Endocr Rev* 3:26, 1982

ANSWERS

1. No. Many cases of Cushing's syndrome will have normal or low levels of 17-ketosteroids. In cases of adrenal hypofunction, urinary ketosteroids are still inadequate to diagnose hypofunction. The clinician should resort to stimulation testing of 17-hydroxycorticosteroids or ketogenic steroids. To evaluate adrenal cortisol production in an excess state, basal 17-hydroxycorticosteroids, 17-ketogenic steroids, or urine free cortisol should be obtained.

2. Oral contraceptive agents, stress, diphenylhydantoin, phenobarbitol, and depression.

3. LH-secreting pituitary tumor, pregnancy, molar pregnancy, or excessive androgen production.

4. The patient may have "euthyroid sick" syndrome, especially if this is accompanied by renal failure or recent onset of illness. More than likely, the patient has low T4 binding secondary to loss of thyroxine-binding globulin through the kidneys.

5. This test has merely demonstrated lack of response in the hypothalamic–pituitary axis. To demonstrate whether this is a problem in the pituitary gland or in the adrenal gland, a prolonged ACTH stimulation test must be done. If the adrenal demonstrates responsiveness, the patient has a defect at the level of the hypothalamus and pituitary, and the clinician should proceed to an insulin tolerance test. If no responsiveness to prolonged ACTH is demonstrated, the patient has Addison's disease.

9

Hormonal Cytopathology of the Vagina

OLGA M. BLAIR

INTRODUCTION

Evaluation of the hormonal status of women by the use of vaginal smears remains one of the most practical, reliable, and economical tests available. Pouchet[1] in 1847 was the first to correlate the cyclic changes in human and animal ovaries and the cyclic changes in cellular material of unstained vaginal secretions. Stockard and Papanicolaou[2] reported the examination of the vaginal fluid and its cellular component in the guinea pig. Later Papanicolaou[3-5] and others[6-10] have made significant contributions to the understanding of the clinical uses of hormonal vaginal cytology. Understanding the advantages and limitations of the hormonal assessment by means of vaginal cellular responses helps show that the study of vaginal cytology can be of optimal clinical value. This chapter reviews the hormonal patterns of cellular response under various physiologic and pathologic conditions.

OLGA M. BLAIR • Department of Pathology, St. Louis University School of Medicine, St. Louis, Missouri 63104.

CYTOLOGIC TECHNIQUES

Methods of Collection

In order to obtain cytologic hormonal studies that are accurate and reliable, it is of paramount importance that the following procedure be done. The patient should be instructed to avoid intercourse for at least 48 hr before the test and not to use a vaginal douche for 24 hr before obtaining the specimen.[8,10] The material is to be collected from the upper third of the lateral wall of the vagina, avoiding contamination with cervical material[9,11,12] and excessive pressure.[13] If the examination is repeated, ideally the same area is to be sampled. The materials are smeared quickly on one-end frosted slides. Prescored V-C-E smears also can be used for hormonal assessment.[14] The smears are fixed immediately, preferably in 95% alcohol, but a spray fixative can be used with good results. The smears are then submitted to the laboratory together with a completed statement of the clinical data. The importance of good communication between the clinician and the cytopathologist in this area cannot be overemphasized.

TABLE 9-1. "Pap" Staining Technique

1. 95% ethanol	8–10 dips
2. 50% ethanol	8–10 dips
3. Tap water	8–10 dips
4. Harris hematoxylin	2 min
5. Running tap water until water is clear	
6. 0.5% HCl/70% ethanol	2–3 dips
7. Tap water	2 changes
8. 1.5% NH$_4$OH/70% ethanol	1–3 dips
9. Tap water	8–10 dips
10. 70% ethanol	8–10 dips
11. 80% ethanol	8–10 dips
12. 95% ethanol	8–10 dips
13. OG-6	1 min
14–15. 95% ethanol (two changes)	10 dips each
16. EA-50	1–2 min
17–18. 95% ethanol (two changes)	10 dips each
19–20. 100% ethanol (two changes)	10 dips each
21–23. Xylene	8–10 dips each

Coverslip with permount.
All staining times must be constantly adjusted as they are used and new stain is added.

Staining Procedures

The smears are stained by the Papanicolaou (Pap) method[15,16] with some modifications, as shown in Table 9-1.

The Schorr staining method[17,18] is also used with excellent results, as shown in Table 9-2. The supravital stain used by Rakoff[19] to stain wet smears provides a rapid staining procedure (see Table 9-3).

Phase-contrast microscopy provides a rapid office procedure, as described by Wied.[20,21] Castellanos and co-workers[22,24] introduced the

TABLE 9-2. Schorr's Staining Technique

Stain S3 (method)	
50% ethyl alcohol	1 dl
Biebrich Scarlet	0.5 g
Orange G	0.25 g
Fast Green FCF	0.075 g
Phosphotungstic acid	0.5 g
Glacial acetic acid	1.0 ml

Method
Wet smears are fixed in 95% ethyl alcohol (1–2 min).
Stain is placed in solution S3 for 1–2 min
Dehydrate in 70%, 95% and absolute alcohol.
Clean in xylene and mount.
Superficial cells are stained brilliant orange-red.
Intermediate and parabasal cells are stained in shades of green according to degree of maturation.

TABLE 9-3. Rakoff's Staining Technique

Collection of the specimen: cotton-tip applicator
Stain

Light green 5% aqueous solution	83 ml
Eosin Y, 1% aqueous solution	17 ml

Method
1. Add 3 drops of stain solution to 2 ml saline.
2. Immerse and agitate cotton-tip applicator into the solution.
3. Place 1 drop of the solution on a slide, coverslip, and examine under the microscope.

cytologic examination of the urinary sediment for hormonal assessment, which has proved useful in the hormonal assessment of various endocrinopathies.

The Cell Population on Vaginal Smears

The expected cell components observed on vaginal smears, as seen with the Papanicolaou stain,[3,16,25] are as follows

Superficial Cell. The superficial cells are those located closer to the surface of the stratified squamous epithelium and overlie the intermediate cells. The superficial cell nucleus is dark, and small (less than 6 μm) and is referred to as pyknotic. The cytoplasm of this cell is thin, large, and acidophilic (Fig. 9-1).

Intermediate Cell. On histologic preparation the intermediate cell is situated between the superficial cell above and the parabasal cell below. On Pap stains, the cell nucleus is round or oval and vesicular; the cytoplasm is pale blue or blue-green and infrequently acidophilic.

Parabasal Cell. This cell is located between the intermediate cell layer above and the smaller basal cells below. The cell nucleus is round or oval with discrete nuclear membrane and a regular chromatin pattern. The cytoplasm is often round and dense, the density being its hallmark. More often, their cytoplasm stains pink or blue, and less frequently, pink-orange. Parabasal cells are seen in those situations in which the epithelium has not properly matured or there is inflammation.

Basal Cell. This cell type is situated close to the basement membrane below and the parabasal cells above and do not exfoliate under normal condi-

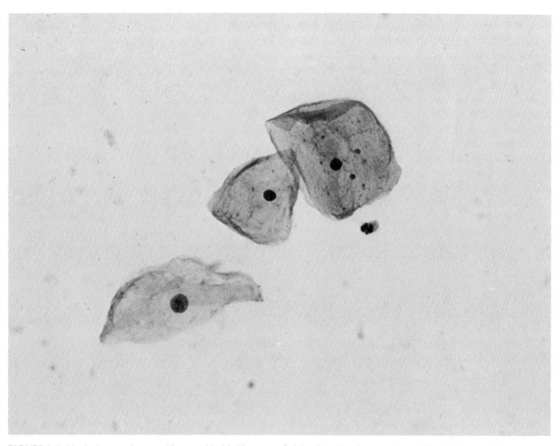

FIGURE 9-1. Vaginal smear from an 18-year-old girl. Note superficial cells and an intermediate cell in the foreground. Note lipid intracytoplasmic granules in one of the superficial cells. Pap stain ×312.

tions. They may be difficult to recognize in substandard or poor preparations. Occasionally they may be recovered from patients with cervical erosions.[26]

Anucleated Superficial Cells. This cell originates in the skin, and it is seen as a contaminant; in some cases, however, it may be "related to hyperkeratosis and leukoplasia."[26] The anucleated superficial cell has a delicate pink cytoplasm, their nucleus is either not seen, or it may leave a shadowy space. Intracytoplasmic nuclear chromatin granules may be seen.

Microorganisms and Inflammatory Responses

Vaginal smears taken at a time when there is excessive growth of Doederlein bacilli may show (1) cytolysis[28] due to enzymatic action charac-

terized by cytoplasmic cell loss so that only free nuclei are found. In conditions of cytolysis or severe inflammation, the smears would be unsatisfactory for hormonal evaluation.[10,26] The presence of severe inflammation in vaginal smears, regardless of the organism involved (e.g., coccoid bacteria, *Trichomonas, Candida*) may alter the normal ratio of the vaginal epithelial cells in the smear and thus may lead to an erroneous cytohormonal reading.[10,26] In any of the above situations, the smears should be repeated following the appropriate treatment.

Recommendations for Cytohormonal Assessments

The reliability of the cytohormonal evaluation of the female patients will depend on the adherence to a consistent methodology in obtaining, staining and interpretation and final reporting in a manner that indicates effective communication between the cytopathologist and the clinician.[29-31] The following recommendations are pertinent. It is the responsibility of the clinician to provide all clinical data. The patient should be instructed to avoid intercourse, drug treatment, douches, and so forth before she is tested. The smears are to be obtained from the upper third of the lateral wall of the vagina. Serial daily smears are also indicated if endocrinopathies are suspected or if the time of ovulation is to be determined. A cytohormonal reading should not be issued if there is inflammation, cytolysis, or contamination with cervical material or if the smears are not properly fixed (air dried smears). Any unsatisfactory report should be followed by a repeat of the smears in keeping with the report recommendation.

CYTOLOGY UNDER PHYSIOLOGIC CONDITIONS

Birth to Menarche

The vaginal cellular patterns from birth to menarche have been studied.[10,22,23,26,32-34] At birth, the smear patterns reflect the effects of the mother's hormones, so there is an intermediate cell pattern. In subsequent weeks, the smear will show an atrophic, parabasal type pattern with fluctuations to an intermediate cell pattern. This pattern will remain unchanged until the perimenarchal period. At this time, superficial cells, indicating the production of sex hormones, will reappear. However, the reappearance of a pattern of proliferation-maturation will happen in an irregular fashion reflecting the functional variabilities of the onset of the menarche.

The Menstrual Cycle

The vaginal smears during the normal menstrual cycle will reflect the various sex hormones acting during the cycle. During the proliferative phase of the cycle until ovulation, the smears will show a progressive increase in the numbers of mature superficial cells as manifested in the maturation index. At the time of ovulation, the cell pattern in the smear will indicate predominance of superficial cells in keeping with the peak of estrogen production at that time. During the second half of the cycle

and after the production of progesterone, the smears will exhibit a progressive intermediate cell pattern with the appearance of crowding folded intermediate cells (Fig. 9-1) and with an abundance of glycogen contributed by the intermediate cells. Doederlein bacilli will appear in increasing numbers, and leukocytosis will occur. The menstrual smear characteristically contains blood, endometrial cells, and endometrial fragments, some in various stages of degeneration. Histiocytes appear toward the end of the menstrual phase. Throughout menstruation, the squamous epithelial cells are of the intermediate type. In the anovulatory cycles the smears will show no progesterone effect, since there is failure of corpus luteum formation. The cellular pattern in the vaginal smears will be dependent on the estrogenic activity of the follicles and will fluctuate from one patient to another.

ASSESSMENT OF HORMONAL EFFECTS

Estrogen-Related Patterns

Estrogen and, more specifically, estradiol[36-38] have been found to correlate well with the maturation of the vaginal epithelium as seen in histologic sections and in vaginal smears. These studies include determinations of the in situ estrogen concentration by radioimmunoassay (RIA).[39] The vaginal epithelium appears to be more sensitive to the effects of estrogens than the endometrium.[40] The vaginal epithelium response to estrogens is that of proliferation and maturation expressed in the vaginal smear cell pattern by the predominance of superficial cells.[40-43] The superficial cell intracytoplasmic granules first reported by Nieburgs[44] and observed by others[45,46] represents a cellular manifestation of the estrogenic effects. These perinuclear cytoplasmic granules are of varying sizes and stain either light-yellow or blue with the Pap stain. In an attempt to facilitate a numerical expression that will convey to the clinician the degree of epithelial maturation, a number of indices are used to report hormonal patterns in smears. Nylkicek in 1951[47] described for the first time, the maturation index (MI). Since then, a number of cellular indices are available for reporting.[10,45-52] An estimation of the hormonal status of the woman will be more accurate if a baseline or initial smear is counted and expressed in any of the following indices.

Eosinophilic Index

This index represents a count of 100 pink-stained superficial cells. It is based on the assumption that mature squamous cells will stain deep pink; however, this reaction is dependent to some degree on the pH of the vagina, which in turn may be influenced by inflammation. Therefore, inflammatory reactions may interfere with the reliability of the results.

Karyopyknotic Index

The KI is expressed in the percentage of superficial cells with pyknotic nuclei. At least 200 cells, or preferably 300 cells per smear are counted. The results of the KI is of clinical value before the menarche, the first half of the normal menstrual cycle, anovulation, after the menopause, and in those patients with feminizing tumors.[43] Pitfalls in interpretation result in those patients with inflammation, multihormonal administration, and the use of digitalis.

Maturation Index

The MI is a percentage of the number of squamous cells in the smear. At least 200, and preferably 300, cells are counted. The report is issued totaling the percentages and issued left to right: parabasal, intermediate, and superficial cells. The MI is a most accurate predictor of estrogen effects and is useful in the hormonal assessment of postmenopausal patients.

Maturation Value

The MV also is a count of 200 normal squamous cells on different fields in the smear; it includes a count of various types of squamous cells in the smear. Each cell type is given a preassigned value as follows:

Superficial eosinophil cell (1.0)
Superficial cyanophilic cell (0.8)
Large intermediate cell (0.5)
Small intermediate cell (0.5)
Parabasal cell (0.0)

The percentage of each cell type is multiplied by its given value, the totals are added, and the final figure without a decimal is the maturation value. A smear with adequate maturation will have an MV from 6 to 10; in one with atrophy, the MV is 0.

DeLaguna et al.,[50] Meisels,[51] and more recently Jensen et al.[52] showed this index to be highly sensitive for diagnostic and investigative purposes and of practical value for data processing in the evaluation of a large patient population.

If a woman is undergoing digitalis therapy and she necessitates hormonal assessment by vaginal smears, she should be taken off digitalis before the Pap smear is obtained, since it is known that digitalis is associated with a superficial cell pattern, yielding an erroneous hormonal assessment.[53,54]

Progesterone-Related Patterns

Progesterone[55,56] induces the regression of the pattern of maturation of the stratified squamous epithelium from a matured superficial cell pattern to one of intermediate cell preponderance. This is seen in the smears as a tendency of the cells to appear crowded and folded. Three indices are used in estimating progesterone effect: the navicular cell index, the crowded cell index, and the folded cell index. The navicular cell index applies to the percentage of navicular cells in the smear. The crowded cell index gives the percentage of crowded cells (four or five or more cells cluttered together) versus the isolated cells.

Similarly, the folded cell index indicates the percentage of cells with folded cytoplasmic borders in proportions to the percentage of flat cells in the smear. The results of these two indices are of value when serial smears are evaluated rather than one single examination.

Androgen-Related Patterns

It is controversial as to whether there is a definite androgenic pattern in smears.[58,59] Pundel[59] described a vacuolated intermediate or parabasal cell, glycogen-laden, and with a large pale nucleus. Rakoff[19] disputed the reliability of these cells as an indicator of androgenicity, since those cells may also be seen in estrogen deficiency or in low progesterone effects. On the other hand, it has been shown that when androgens are administered to a woman whose vaginal epithelium is atrophic,[43] the atrophic pattern is reverted to one of incomplete maturation. Conversely, when androgens are given to women with estrogenic patterns, the result is that of intermediate cell proliferation. Wachtel[43] suggested that cytology plays a role in the control of androgenic therapy by establishing the smallest doses that will produce a change from atrophic to one of intermediate cell proliferation "within a given time."

CYTOLOGY OF PREGNANCY AND ABORTION

In 1925, Papanicolaou[60] first reported the cellular patterns associated with pregnancy in the guinea pig when he described the predominant cell pattern of navicular cells and thought navicular cells were a feature of the first trimester of pregnancy. Since then, studies of smear cell patterns during pregnancy in humans[61-67] have further proved the value of cytology as a predictive measure of the outcome of normal pregnancy and its complications.[68-76,78-84]

Cell Patterns in Pregnancy

Smears from women with normal uncomplicated pregnancy are characterized by a continuous predominance of intermediate cells and navicular cell change reflecting the vaginal epithelial changes related to production of estrogen progesterone by the corpus luteum and by the placenta.[61] Navicular cells appear during the early weeks, and the numbers increase all through the first trimester. Since these cells are glycogen rich, the growth of the Doederlein bacilli will lead to cytolysis with loss of cell cytoplasm similar to that seen in Fig. 9-2. Since intermediate cells and navicular cells also may be seen in conditions of estrogenic imbalance and of androgenic stimulation, the diagnosis of pregnancy based on cytology alone may not be entirely accurate, unless a comparison is made of the smear patterns after estrogen therapy. After administration of

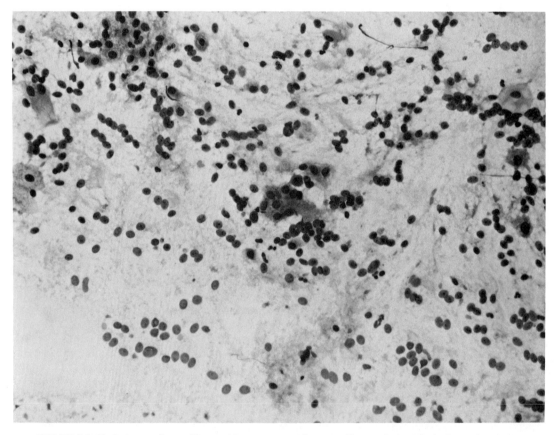

FIGURE 9-2. Vaginal smear from a 56-year-old postmenopausal woman. Note marked cytolysis. Pap stain ×312.

estrogens, smears from pregnant women will show no change in the cell pattern.[63] Smears obtained from the anterior fornix,[65] the cervix,[66] or from the upper third of the lateral wall of the vagina[67] have been employed with similar results.

Lichtfus in 1959[69] introduced the practical use of cytology in the pregnancy at term and pointing out its usefulness in detecting whether the patient is before term, at term, or post-term. The before-term smear shows intermediate and navicular cells; at term, the navicular cells decrease, and superficial cells are seen, whereas the post-term smear is characterized by the appearance of basal cells. Pundel[62,68] similarly found a 90% accuracy in the smear pattern as a predictor of the at-term patient; however, others have disclaimed it.[65,67,70,71] Abrams[70] showed that "serial lateral wall smears failed to reveal specific cellular alternatives that might enable the prediction of the date of delivery."

Postnatal smears frequently show an atrophic pattern characterized by numerous parabasal cells with features of intermediate and navicular cells. Papanicolaou[68] gave those cells the name "postpartum cells." It is generally believed that an atrophic pattern of various degree will persist for 3–4 months after delivery unless estrogens have been administered. Estrogens will induce a normal pattern or at least normal-appearing parabasal cells earlier than 4 months postdelivery.

Cellular Patterns of Abortion

Premature Rupture of Membranes

The cytologic diagnosis of premature rupture of the membranes depends on the demonstration of vernix caseosa cells. These cells are polygonal anucleated squames with a delicate grayish-white cytoplasm that sometimes stains slightly red with the Pap stain. Often, the vernix caseosa cells contain intracytoplasmic lipid that can be demonstrated by the Nile blue stain; this stain is reliable if done in smears obtained after the thirty-second week of gestation, since cells from the skin sebaceous glands will be formed by then. However, Gall[79] showed the presence of vernix caseosa cells as early as 25 weeks gestation. Averette[74] reported 97% accuracy in the diagnosis of premature rupture of membranes (PRM) with the use of a rapid staining technique using 0.25% pinacyanole chloride. The technique is as follows:

1. Collect vaginal material with gloved finger.
2. Smear immediately on slide.
3. Fix immediately in 95% ethyl alcohol.
4. Cover the smear with staining solution: 0.25% solution of pinacyanole chloride in 50% methyl alcohol. Stain for 20 sec.
5. Wash with tap water.
6. Examine under microscope, low power.

Results

The polygonal translucent vernix caseosa cells will be further characterized by the absence of perinuclear halos, and their cytoplasm will show delicate intracytoplasmic lines, best seen at high power.

Bercovici and co-workers evaluated the vaginal smears[77] and other hormonal parameters[78] in women with PRM and observed good correlation between the vaginal and urinary sediment, cytologic findings, and the plasma RIA levels for progesterone. In two-thirds of patients, he found the vaginal smears to have a "washed-out" appearance with "weak staining" of the cells and marked reduction or disappearance of the vaginal flora, features his group considered useful in establishing the diagnosis of PRM.

McLennan and McLennan[82] evaluated vaginal wall smears from 200 pregnant women considered at high risk. The smears were evaluated for KI, scoring of navicular cells, and cell wrinkling and clumping; it was found that the vaginal smear patterns predicted the outcome of the pregnancies in 54%, but only in 32% of those who actually aborted. Furthermore, they reemphasized their previous findings[73] that "colpocytograms are not reliable predictors of the pregnancy outcome in individual patients."

The cytologic diagnosis of missed abortion and fetal death may be difficult, since the cellular pattern of parabasal cells of postpartum type may be inconsistently present. Pundel[62] indicated, and others agree,[68] that in the absence of inflammation, vaginal smears made of large parabasal and intermediate cells, unchanged for at least 4 days, indicate fetal death. Furthermore, Pundel[68] restated that "during pregnancy, the smears for hormonal evaluation always must be collected from the lateral vaginal wall, not from the ectocervix" and that "the appearance of morphologically normal parabasal cells during pregnancy must be regarded as an 'alarm'."

A predictive diagnosis of fetal death can be made by daily administration of oral estrogen with a smear, then showing numerous superficial cells indicating fetal death.

In all types of abortion, the smears contain blood. In inevitable abortion, and in incomplete abortion, the smears may contain endometrial cells. In incomplete abortion, in addition, one often encounters endocervical cells and occasional syncytiotrophoblasts. The presence of decidual cells in early abortion may lead to a false atypical cytology.[75,76]

THE MENOPAUSE

Vaginal smears play an important role in the assessment of menopausal patients, and particularly in those patients who require estrogen therapy.[84-99] The cytologic findings in menopausal patients may show a wide spectrum of changes ranging from persistent or elevated estrogenic pattern to one of complete atrophy. There is no given interval in years for complete atrophy to be manifested, since it will depend on the individual patient's complete cessation of ovarian function, a fact that varies as well. A vaginal smear consisting almost entirely of parabasal cells with low KI and low MV characterizes complete atrophy (Figs 9-3 and 9-4). Those smears will usually show a concomitant leukocytic response. Most frequently, however, the vaginal smear pattern is one of high estrogenic effect. Meissels[85] studied 7354 vaginal smears in 5920 menopausal cases, and the MV in 50% of those cases remained low (below 49); complete atrophy (MV = 0) was seen in 21% of patients. In the remaining 50%, moderate activity was present but below that seen with normal genital function, and these values remained unchanged for those patients. In 10%, the patients had high estrogenic values (MV = above 65). Morse[86] recently demonstrated that in menopausal patients, smears from the lateral wall of the vagina had a high KI and correlated with the degree of proliferation of the vaginal epithelium and with the plasma levels of estriol but not with the levels of estrone. Thus, these findings seem to support the concept that estriol is the biologically important estrogen here and indicated the importance of vaginal cytology in the menopausal patient. Other authors have also observed high levels of estriol[87] and estrogen[88] levels to correlate with the vaginal hormonal patterns. Benjamin[88] suggests that the KI and the MV are more useful in evaluating "estrogen deficiency than excess in the post-menopause."

Excessive estrogenic effect may result from sources other than the ovary.[26,27,31,43,92,93] The age group in which the menopause usually occurs is also the age group associated with other diseases such as diabetes, liver disease, and heart failure; in some of these patients, digitalis is administered. Stone[92] observed increased estrogen effect as reflected by KI and MV in the vaginal smears of patients under digitalis therapy. Variabilities in the estimation of the cytologic pattern of estrogenic effect may also result from excessive vaginitis.[93]

Vaginal hormonal cytology is of significant value in the postmenopausal woman undergoing any type of estrogen therapy,[94-98] particularly to estimate the appropriate dosage. However, Wied[99] indicated that in following estrogen therapy with cytology, vaginal smears may show severe cytolysis and resulting leukorrhea (Fig. 9-2) that may "mask an estrogenic effect." He suggested that, in those cases, a bacteriostatic drug is to be given 24 hr before obtaining the vaginal smear.

CYTOLOGY OF AMENORRHEA

The assessment of vaginal smears may play an important role in the evaluation and management of the patient with amenorrhea, and more specifically of those patients who have never ovulated.[9,17,27,31,40,100-105] Amenorrhea may be classified into two major groups: primary and secondary and/or according to the site of origin: uterine, ovarian, pituitary–adrenal, hypothalamic, and psychogenic.[13,100] The cytologic study of the amenorrheic patient and more specifically the patient suspected of having primary amenorrhea should include the obtaining of serial smears over a long interval of not less than 28–30 days. The results of cytology offer the greatest value when combined with a complete endocrinologic and in some cases genetic evaluation. We shall consider the cytologic results in the following subtypes of primary amenorrhea.

Amenorrhea of Uterine Origin

In patients with congenital absence of the uterus, the ovaries are physiologically normal. The patients ovulate but do not menstruate. Vaginal smears in these patients are cyclically normal,[100] a feature that will assist in excluding the diagnosis of testicular feminization syndrome. In patients with this disorder, there is a persistent ''proliferative'' (superficial cell) type smear and negative sex chromatin pattern.[9,19,43,100] Batrinos[100] and Efstratiades[102] showed that a superficial-type pattern correlates with breast development where estrogenic secretion is expected to exist.

Amenorrhea of Ovarian Origin

In patients with either absence of the ovaries, or with failure of ovarian function, the vaginal smears are characterized by an atrophic pattern.[9,19,27,40,43,100–104]

Gonadal Dysgenesis

Anatomically, gonadal dysgenesis refers to the absence of gonadal differentiation involving one or both gonads. Bilateral gonadal dysgenesis is most frequently found in patients with Turner's syndrome due to the absence of a sex chromosome (45,X). Less frequently, bilateral gonadal dysgenesis is present in phenotypic females with primary amenorrhea and either a 46,XX or a 46,XY karyotype, a condition known as ''pure gonadal dysgenesis.'' A third variety of gonadal dysgenesis is usually unilateral and is associated with sex chromosomal mosaicism (45,X/46,XY) in genetic males with ambiguous or female type external genitalia.

Turner's Syndrome

Patients with this disorder are phenotypic females with normal external genitalia, infantile uterus and fallopian tubes and bilaterally dysgenetic gonads represented by fibrous streaks. Short stature is present in almost all cases, and webbing of the

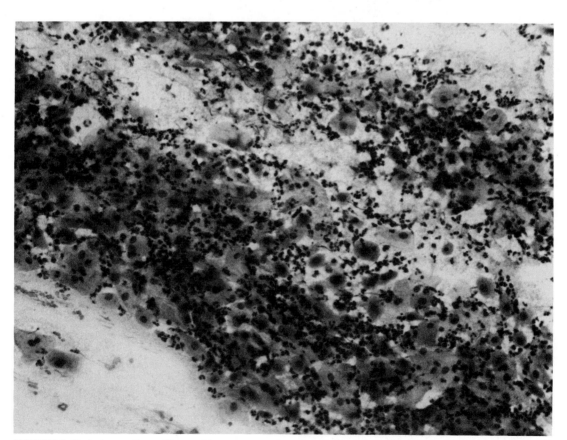

FIGURE 9-3. Vaginal smear from a 58-year-old postmenopausal woman. Observe the numerous large parabasal cells and the severe inflammatory reaction. Pap stain ×312.

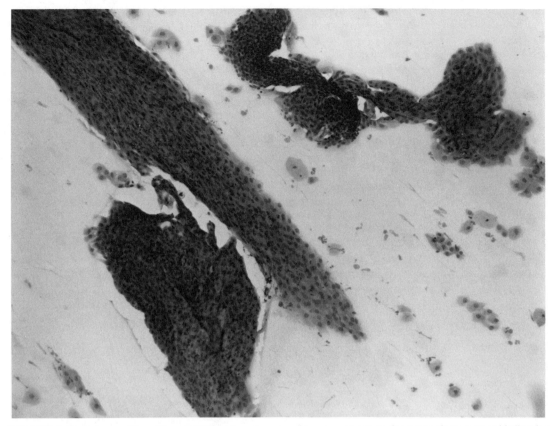

FIGURE 9-4. Vaginal smear from a 76-year-old 23-year postmenopausal woman. Note large fragments of squamous epithelium in a dried smear. Pap stain ×125.

neck occurs in about 35% of cases. Other congenital anomalies associated with this syndrome include a high incidence of coarctation of the aorta and renal anomalies, the former usually detected in the neonatal period.

Lack of estrogen stimulation results in absence or poor development of breasts, pubic and axillary hair, and infantile size of the internal genitalia, which are always female type. Menses are absent, and the vaginal smears accurately reflect the absence of estrogen effect, i.e., the smears resemble the atrophic pattern of post-menopausal women (Figs. 9-3 and 9-4). In those patients with a single X chromosome (45,X), Barr bodies are absent.

Pure Gonadal Dysgenesis

This relatively rare syndrome presents as a phenotypic female of normal or increased height who has absent or minimal breast development and female-type internal genitalia. There are no stig-

mata of Turner's syndrome. The karyotype is either 46,XX, or more frequently 46,XY. Therefore, the sex chromatin pattern can be either positive or negative. In either case, the vaginal smear accurately reflects severe estrogen deficiency and consistently shows an atrophic pattern. Patients with this syndrome plus a 46,XY karyotype have a high incidence of gonadal tumors, particularly gonadoblastoma.

Unilateral ("Mixed") Gonadal Dysgenesis

Unilateral gonadal dysgenesis is most frequently encountered in sex chromosomal mosaics, particularly 45,X/46,XY. In this group, genital ambiguity is common, although the internal genitalia are female type with a unilateral streak gonad and varying degrees of testicular differentiation of the contralateral gonad. However, about 25% of these patients have female external genitalia without ambiguity at birth. In this group without genital ambiguity, the vaginal smears are of the atrophic type because of the absence of estrogen stimulation. In fact, androgenic effects may be noticeable in some patients in whom clitoral hypertrophy develops at puberty.

Unilateral gonadal dysgenesis may also be associated with 45,X/46,XX sex chromosomal mosaicism: these are genetic and phenotypic females with normal or subnormal estrogen effect noticed in the vaginal smears. Usually, some degree of ovarian differentiation is present and phenotypically, some features of Turner's syndrome are likely to be present.

Stein–Leventhal Syndrome

The Stein–Leventhal syndrome occurs in young, somewhat obese females who show hirsutism, menstrual disorders, oligomenorrhea, or amenorrhea.[105,106] The pathology of the ovaries in these patients consists of bilateral enlargement, fibrosis of the ovarian capsule, multiple follicular cysts of various sizes and absence of corpora lutea. Stromal luteinization may be present. Cytologic findings do not contribute to a specific diagnosis since the smear may show an estrogenic pattern. In those patients who are treated by wedge resection of their ovaries,[106] a study of their vaginal smear is useful to determine the time of onset of normal ovarian function.

Ovarian Tumors

The vaginal smears from patients with estrogen producing cysts and tumors in the young age group are not diagnostic, specifically, since their vaginal smear pattern is one of nonspecific estrogenic effect. Johnston[107] observed a predominant intermediate cell pattern with MI of 0/78/22. It is difficult to diagnose androgen-producing tumors, including arrhenoblastomas, and functioning hilus cell tumors by cytologic examination. Their vaginal smears may be either proliferative, intermediate, or atrophic type, in keeping with the variabilities of the activities of androgenic hormones.

Amenorrhea of Pituitary–Adrenal and Hypothalamic Origin

The vaginal smears in amenorrhea associated with pituitary or hypothalamic dysfunction are of no diagnostic value. The cell patterns observed are of various degrees of atrophy. The amenorrhea of Chiari-Frommel syndrome resulting in inhibition of the gonadotropin hormones with elevated prolactin is clinically manifested by galactorrhea involution of the uterus and amenorrhea. These patients show a pattern of severe atrophy (Figs. 9-3 and 9-4).

EFFECT OF HORMONAL ADMINISTRATION AND CONTRACEPTION

Administration of Estrogens and Antiestrogens

Vaginal cytologic evaluation is of importance in the management of women who are undergoing or are about to be placed on therapy using estrogens.[10,40,43] The postmenopausal woman, and the young surgical castrate are among the clinical groups in which estrogens are often used; in both groups, vaginal cytology provides a convenient means of determining the estrogenic response of the vaginal epithelium as well as the effective dosage of the drug. Either the KI, the MI, or the MV is used to evaluate the estrogenic effects. In the postmenopausal patient, the vaginal smear patterns related to estrogen therapy will depend on the type of epithelial pattern for a specific patient at the time she is placed on estrogens. In those women who undergo complete vaginal epithelial atrophy, the responses to estrogens will be consistently observed and as reflected in their subsequent MI. On the other hand, for a patient who does not show complete vaginal epithelial atrophy, and who has either an intermediate or a superficial cell pattern, the estimation of the response to administered estrogens will be difficult and of limited value.[10] In addition, prolonged administration of estrogens in some patients may be associated with an overgrowth of Doederlein bacilli, which results in marked cytolysis (Fig. 9-2) necessitating a bacteriostatic agent before cytologic examination. Likewise, some women given prolonged estrogen therapy show variabilities in vaginal pattern, and some will only show a persistent life-long intermediate cell pattern.[10,43] Drugs that act as antiestrogens[108,109] are used in certain infertile patients in order to induce ovulation. Shirai[108] showed that Clomiphene citrate given to anovulatory patients has an effect on the vaginal smear pattern expressed by a lack of increase of cornified cells and low eosinophilic index after the seventh day of therapy. This finding suggests that the vaginal response "is a result of the anti-estrogenic effect of clomiphene citrate." By contrast, the administration of the cis-isomer of clomiphene citrate results in variable responses in the vaginal cell pattern.

Administration of Progestogens and Androgens

Progestogens are synthetic steroids that have an antiovulation effect. They are derivatives of either testosterone, 19-nortestosterone, 17 α-hydroxy-progesterone, or progesterone. The vaginal smear hormonal patterns in women treated with any of these drugs will depend on the progestogen–estrogen dosage for each drug, i.e., if progesterone or estrogen/progesterone combinations are given, the smears will show no cyclic pattern and the presence of navicular cells similar to that of endogenous progesterone effect. Wied[10] and others[55–57] indicate that the response to progestogens will depend on the preexisting cell pattern. In surgical castrates,[110] the administration of progesterone induces a pattern similar to that of the luteal phase of the cycle. Androgens, like progestogens, induce a vaginal cellular response dependent on the existing cell pattern before the administration of the drug.[10,11,38,58,59]

Administration of Contraceptive Drugs

The administration of contraceptive drugs, aside from possible atypical cellular patterns,[111] may be associated with a cytohormonal response[112,113] that is dependent on the formula and dosage of the particular contraceptive used. Sequential (oral or parenteral), long-acting oral or parenteral, and continuous progestogenic drugs do not induce pathognomonic cell patterns, but their vaginal smear responses depend on the concentrations of estrogens or progesterones. Reyniak et al.[112] evaluated the vaginal smear effects of combined and sequential therapy; he observed that the cytohormonal patterns were dependent on the timing of the drug administration in reference to the cycle, i.e., a high estrogenic effect at the beginning of the cycle when the estrogen alone was acting; the addition of progesterone resulted in cell folding and crowding when progesterone alone was acting.

HORMONAL PATTERNS OF MISCELLANEOUS CONDITIONS

An attempt has been made to demonstrate the possible applications of hormonal cytopathology in other clinical situations.[114–117] In reviewing the vaginal smears in 62 cases of endometriosis, Schmidt[114] found the smears to show a high KI, but he gave no absolute criteria for the specific diagnosis of endometriosis. Stoll[116] observed that hormonal vaginal cytology is useful in selecting those early postmenopausal patients with cancer of the breast who might undergo castration or hormonal therapy; he observed that those patients with changes in serial smear patterns during estrogen therapy had a higher rate of tumor regression. Moracci and Berlingieri[116] employed hormonal cytologic evaluation in seven young women who underwent reconstruction of their vagina because of congenital absence of the vagina. He was able to demonstrate the estrogenic effects of 1 mg estriol on smears taken from the artificial vagina. Tetracyclines, similar to digitalis,[26,27] may induce maturation expressed in an intermediate cell pattern on vaginal smears.

SUMMARY

Cytology has a very important role in the hormonal evaluation of women under physiologic conditions as well as in the evaluation of various endocrine disorders. The contribution of the technique is maximized if there is an effective interchange of data between clinicians and cytopathologists, particularly as it pertains to the cytopathologic technique employed, the method of reporting the hormonal readings, and subsequent follow-up management of the patient. Regarding the cytopathologic techniques, the following aspects are to be emphasized. The vaginal smears are to be obtained from the upper third of the lateral wall of the vagina and fixed immediately. Conditions that will render the test unsatisfactory, such as air drying, cytolysis, and excessive inflammatory changes, will necessitate a repeat smear. In all patients it is preferable to obtain a baseline smear in order to assess a certain pattern for that time. In the estimation of ovulation, and in endocrinopathies, the optimal hormonal pattern estimations result from serial smears. The discrepancies of hormonal readings seen in certain conditions may only be due to the individual hormonal responses, but they may also be due to the variations of the site from which the cytologic material is obtained. The usefulness of this technique as a diagnostic or predictive method will be enhanced if these considerations are met.

QUESTIONS

1. In order to assess the hormonal response of the vaginal epithelium, materials for Pap smears are collected from

a. the lower portion of the lateral wall of the vagina.

b. the mid-portion of the lateral wall of the vagina.

c. the upper third of the lateral wall of the vagina.

d. the anterior wall of the vagina.

e. the introitus

2. The estrogenic effect on the vaginal epithelium may be accurately predicted by the

a. folded cell index.

b. maturation index.

c. crowded cell index.

d. eosinophilic index.

e. maturation value.

3. A Pap smear is obtained from the vaginal wall in a pregnant woman. Parabasal cells are seen on the smear. Repeated Pap smears show an unchanged pattern. The cytologic findings are suggestive of

a. pregnancy at term.

b. incomplete abortion.

c. fetal death.

d. threatened abortion.

e. inevitable abortion.

REFERENCES

1. Pouchet FA: *Theorie positive de l'ovulation spontanée et de la fecondation des mammifères et de l'espèce humaine, basée sur l'observation de tante la serie animale.* Paris, Bailliere, 1847

2. Stockard CR, Papanicolaou GN: A rhythmical "heat period" in the guinea pig. *Science* 46:1176–1182, 1917

3. Papanicolaou GN: The sexual cycle in the human female as revealed by vaginal smears. *Am J Anat* 52(suppl):519–637, 1933*

4. Papanicolaou GN: Existence of a "post-menopause" sexual rhythm in women, as indicated by the study of vaginal smears. *Anat Rec* 55(suppl):71–72, 1933

5. Frankel L, Papanicolaou GN: Growth, desquamation and involution of the vaginal epithelium of fetuses and children with consideration of the related hormonal factors. *Am J Anat* 62:427–441, 1938

6. Rakoff AE: Gynecological endocrinology, in Meggs JV, Sturgis S (eds): *Progress in Gynecology,* Vol 2. New York, Grune & Stratton, 1950*

7. Pundel JP: *Les frottis vaginaux endocriniens.* Paris, Masson, 1952, Paris.

8. Wachtel E, Plester JA: Hormonal assessment by vaginal cytology. *J Obstet Gynaecol Br Emp* 61:155–161, 1954

9. Rakoff AE: The vaginal cytology of gynecologic endocrinopathies. *Acta Cytol* 5:153–167, 1961

10. Wied GL, Bibbo M: Evaluation of endocrinologic condition by exfoliative cytology, in Gold, JJ (ed): *Gynecologic*

11. Wied GL: Importance of the site from which vaginal cytologic smears are taken. *Am J Clin Pathol* 25:742–750, 1955

12. Soost HJ: Comparative studies on the degree of proliferation of the vaginal and ectocervical epithelium in the hormonal evaluation of a patient by means of exfoliative cytology. *Acta Cytol* 4:199–209, 1960

13. Rubio CA, Stormby N, Kock Y, et al: Studies on the distribution of abnormal cells in cytologic preparations. VI. Pressure exerted by the gynecologist during smearing. *Gynecol Oncol* 15:39–395, 1983

14. Meisels A: Superiority of the V-C-E smear. *Acta Cytol* 13:1–2, 1969

15. Papanicolaou GN: A new procedure for staining vaginal smears. *Science* 95:438–439, 1942

16. Papanicolaou GN, Trout HF: *Diagnosis of Uterine Cancer by the Vaginal Smear.* New York, Commonwealth Fund, 1943

17. Shorr E, Papanicolaou GN: Action of gonadotrophic hormones in amenorrhea as evaluated by vaginal smears. *Proc Soc Exp Biol Med* 41:629–636, 1939

18. Shorr E: New technique for staining vaginal smears. *Science* 94:545–546, 1941.

19. Rakoff AE: Hormonal cytology in gynecology. *Clin Obstet Gynecol* 4:1045–1061, 1961*

20. Wied GL: Techniques for collection and preparation of cytologic specimens. *Clin Obstet Gynecol* 4:1031–1044, 1961

21. Wied GL: Phase contrast microscopy in office technique for pre-screening of cytologic vaginal smears. *Am J Obstet Gynecol* 71:806–817, 1956

22. Castellanos HA, Sturgis SH: Urinary cytology in the endocrine evaluation of the normal female, in *Progress in Gynecology,* Vol IV. Grune & Stratton, New York, 1963, pp 98–120

23. Castellanos H, O'Marchae PJ, Yahia C, et al: Urethral cytology in the diagnosis of secondary amenorrhea. *JAMA* 187:631–636, 1964

24. Baraggino E, Dalla-Pria S, Pezzetta A, et al: The validity of the urocytogram compared to colpocytology in hormonal cytodiagnosis. *Clin Exp Obstet Gynecol* 7:57–61, 1980

25. Papanicolaou GN, Trout HF, Marchetti AA: *The Epithelia of Woman's Reproductive Organs.* New York, Commonwealth Fund, 1948

26. Frost JK: Gynecologic and obstetric clinical cytopathology, in Novak ER, Woodruff JD (eds): *Novak's Gynecologic and Obstetric Pathology.* Philadelphia, Saunders, 1979, pp 689–734

27. Koss LG (ed): *Diagnostic cytology and Its Histopathologic Bases,* Vol I, 3rd ed. Philadelphia, Lippincott, 1979

28. Bercovici B, Schechter A, Golau J: Cytolysis in normal and complicated pregnancy. *Am J Obstet Gynecol* 116:831–834, 1973

29. Symposium on Cytological Terminology: *Acta Cytol* 2:26, 1958

30. Wied GL: Terminology of cytologic reporting of endocrinologic conditions (editorial). *Acta Cytol* 8:383–384, 1964

31. Wied GL, Bibbo M: *Hormonal Cytology of the Female Genital Tract. Pathways to Conception.* Springfield, IL, Charles C Thomas, 1971*

32. Wied GL, Keebler CM: Vaginal cytology of female children. *Am NY Acad Sci* 142:646–653, 1967

33. Sonek M: Vaginal cytology in childhood and puberty. I.

*Review article/chapter.

Newborn through prepuberty. *J Repr. Med.* 2:39–56, 1969

34. Kaufman RH, Leeds LJ: Cervical and vaginal cytology in the child and adolescent. *Pediatr. Clin North Am* 19:547–557, 1972
35. Zinca V, Cirlan M: The reproduction of hormonal effect by macromolecular RNA. *Acta Cytol* 13:679–684, 1969
36. Punnonen R, Lukola A: High affinity binding of estrone, estradiol and estriol in human cervical myometrium and cervical and vaginal epithelium. *J Endocrinol Invest* 5:203–207, 1982
37. Schneider V, Friedrich E, Schlindler AE: Hormonal cytology: A correlation with plasma estradiol, measured with radioimmunoassay. *Acta Cytol* 21:37–39, 1977
38. Wied GL, Davis ME: Synergism antagonism of sex steroids as determined by the vaginal epithelial cells. *Ann NY Acad Sci* 83:207–216, 1959
39. Holderegger C, Keefer DS, Babler W, et al: Quantitative autoradiographic analysis of in situ estrogen concentration by individual cell types of mouse target organs: Dose-uptake studies. *Biol Reprod* 25:719–724, 1981
40. deNeef JC: *Clinical Endocrine Cytology.* New York, Harper & Row (Hoeber), 1965
41. Symposium on Administered Estrogens: *Acta Cytol.* 2:331–442, 1958
42. Symposium on Hormonal Cytology: *Acta Cytol* 12:87–127, 1968
43. Wachtel E: *Exfoliative Cytology in Gynaecological Practice.* Washington, DC, Butterworth, 1964, pp 55–144*
44. Nieburgs HE, Zucker HS: Cytoplasmic granules and estrogen effect. *Acta Cytol* 2:367–369, 1958
45. Maillet M, Charasini DJ, Cava E, et al: Significant hormonal changes in patterns of lipid granules in vaginal exfoliated cells. *Acta Cytol* 22:479–482, 1978
46. Lahiri T, Chowdhury JR: Lipid patterns in vaginal cells exfoliated from different physiologic conditions. *Acta Cytol* 25:572–577, 1981
47. Nylkicek O: Importance of vaginal cytograms for diagnosis and therapy in the deficiency of oestrogenic hormones. *Gynaecologia* 131:173–178, 1951
48. Symposium on the Cytologic Indices for Hormonal Assessment: *J Reprod Med* 2:1–12, 1969
49. Teter J: The use of selected cytologic indices for evaluation of estrogenicity of synthetic compounds. *Acta Cytol* 16:366–375, 1972
50. DeLaguna JG, Garcia G, Urrutia M, et al: Importancia de los signos R.S. y R.R. en el pronostico y tratamiento del carcinoma cervico-uterino. *Rev Inst Nac Canc (Mexico)* 1:331–349, 1958
51. Meisels A: Computed cytohormonal findings in 3,307 healthy women. *Acta Cytol* 9:328–333, 1965
52. Jensen MR, Kaplan BJ, Marrs RP, et al: Maturation value as an indicator of the serum estrogen concentration during treatment with gonadotropins. *Acta Cytol* 25:251–254, 1981
53. Britch CM, Azar HA: Estrogen effect in exfoliated vaginal cells following treatment with digitalis. A case report with experimental observations in mice. *Am J Obstet Gynecol* 85:989–993, 1963
54. Navab A, Koss LG, LaDue JS: Estrogen like activity of digitalis. Its effect on the squamous epithelium of the female genital tract. *JAMA* 194:30–32, 1965
55. Wied GL, Davis ME: Comparative activity of progestational agents on the human endometrium and vaginal

epithelium of surgical castrates. *Ann NY Acad Sci* 71:599–616, 1958
56. Symposium on the Effects of Progestational Agents: *Acta Cytol* 6:211–310, 1962
57. Heber, KR: The effect of progesterones on vaginal cytology, *Acta Cytol* 19:103–109, 1975
58. Symposium on Androgenic Effects on Vaginal Epithelial Cells: Acta Cytol 1:70–102, 1957
59. Pundel JP: Is there a physiological cell type which may be defined as androgenic cell type? *Acta Cytol* 1:82–86, 1957
60. Papanicolaou GN: The diagnosis of early human pregnancy by the vaginal smear method. *Proc Soc Exp Biol Med* 22:436, 1925
61. Pundel JP, Van Meensel F: *Gestation et cytologie vaginale.* Paris, Masson, 1951
62. Pundel JP: Vaginal cytology as prognostic method in pregnancy. *Acta Cytol* 3:231–234, 1959
63. Pundel JP: Effect of administered estrogens on the vaginal epithelium during pregnancy and the post-partum period. *Acta Cytol* 3:241–243, 1959
64. von Haam E: The cytology of pregnancy. *Acta Cytol* 5:320–329, 1961
65. Birtch PK: Hormonal cytology of pregnancy. *Clin Obstet Gynecol* 4:1062–1074, 1961*
66. Soule SD: The practical value of vaginal cytology in pregnancy. I. Cytological prediction of the fate of early pregnancy, *Acta Cytol.* 8:364–367, 1964
67. Hammond DO: A critical evaluation of the value of vaginal cytology for the determination of "biological term." *Acta Cytol* 9:340–343, 1965
68. Pundel JP: Symposium on Hormonal Cytology in Pregnancy: *J Reprod Med* 2:101–110, 1969
69. Lichtfuss CJP: Vaginal cytology at the end of pregnancy. Acta Cytol 3:247. 1959
70. Abrams RY, Abrams J: Vaginal cytology during the final weeks of pregnancy. *Acta Cytol* 6:359–364, 1962
71. Hindman WM, Schwalenberg RR, Efstatim TD: A study of vaginal smears in late pregnancy and pregnancy at term. *Acta Cytol* 6:365–369, 1962
72. Malek J, Kobilkova EC, Cehc E, et al: Vaginal cytologic patterns during the biological preparation for labor. *Acta Cytol* 11:444–448, 1967
73. McLennan MT, McLennan CE: Hormonal patterns in vaginal smears from puerperal women. *Acta Cytol* 19:431–433, 1975
74. Averette HE, Ferguson JH: Cytodiagnosis of ruptured fetal membranes. *Am J Obstet Gynecol* 87:226–230, 1963
75. Danos M, Halmquist ND: Cytologic evaluation of decidual cells: A report of two cases with false abnormal cytology. *Acta Cytol* 11:325–330, 1967
76. Holmquist ND, Danos M: The cytology of early abortion. *Acta Cytol* 11:262–266, 1967
77. Bercovici B, Diamant YZ: Vaginal cytology of premature rupture of membranes. *Obstet Gynecol* 39:861–865, 1972
78. Bercovici B, Yaffe H, Segal S: Vaginal and urinary cytology and blood hormone examinations in patients with premature rupture of membranes. *Acta Cytol* 24:208–211, 1980
79. Gall SA, Spellacy WN: Cytologic diagnosis of ruptured membranes. *Obstet Gynecol* 24:732–735, 1964
80. Bamford SB, Mitchell GW, Bardarwil WA, et al: Vaginal cytology of pregnant habitual aborters with skin homografts. *Acta Cytol* 11:257–261, 1967
81. Soszka S, Wisniewski L: Cytological evaluation of fetal

death and an attempt to determine the time of its occurrence. *Acta Cytol* 11:403–409, 1967

82. MeLennan MT, McClennan CE: Use of vaginal wall cytologic smears to predict abortion in high-risk pregnancies. *Am J Obstet Gynecol* 114:857–860, 1972

83. Bercovici B, Diamant Y, Polishuk WZ: A simplified evaluation of vaginal cytology in third trimester pregnancy complication. *Acta Cytol* 17:67–72, 1973

84. Wied GL: Climateric amenorrhea: A cytohormonal test for differential diagnosis. *Obstet Gynecol* 9:646–649, 1957

85. Meisels A: The menopause. A cytohormonal study. *Acta Cytol* 10:49–55, 1966

86. Morse AR, Hutton JD, Murray MAF, et al: Relation between the karyopyknotic index and plasma estrogen concentrations after the menopause. *Br J Obstet Gynaecol* 86:981–983, 1979

87. deWaard F, Pot H, Tonckens-Naninga NE, et al: Longitudinal studies on the phenomenon of post-menopausal estrogen production. *Acta Cytol* 16:273–278, 1972

88. Benjamin F, Duetsch S: Immunoreactive plasma estrogens and vaginal hormone cytology in post-menopausal women. *Int J Gynecol Obstet* 17:546–550, 1980

89. Papanicolaou GN, Shorr E: The action of ovarian follicular hormones in the menopause as indicated by vaginal smears. *Am J Obstet Gynecol* 31:806–831, 1936

90. Wied GL: The effect of physiological sex hormones on the vaginal epithelium of patients with inactive ovaries. *Acta Cytol* 1:75–76, 1957

91. Højgaard K, Henriksen HM, Højgaard JB, et al: Superficial eosinophilic squamous epithelial cells in vaginal smears from post-menopausal women. *Acta Obstet Gynecol Scand* 61:429–431, 1982

92. Stone DF, Sedlis A, Stone MI, et al: Estrogen-like effects in the vaginal smears of post menopausal women. *Acta Cytol* 5:349–352, 1967

93. Lin TJ, So-Bosita JL: Pitfalls in the interpretation of estrogenic effect in post-menopausal women. *Am J Obstet Gynecol* 114:929–931, 1972

94. Lin TJ, So-Bosita JL, Brar HK, et al: Clinical and cytologic responses of post-menopausal women to estrogen. *Obstet Gynecol* 41:97–107, 1973

95. Henzel MR, Moyer DL, Townsend D, et al: Quantitation of the estrogenic effects of mestranol on human endometrium and vaginal mucosa. *Am J Obstet Gynecol* 115:401–405, 1973

96. Bercovici B, Uretzki G, Palti Y: The effects of estrogen on cytology and vascularization of the vaginal epithelium of climateric women. *Am J Obstet Gynecol* 113:98–103, 1972

97. Hustin J, Van den Eynde JP: Cytologic evaluation of the effect of various estrogens given in post-menopause. *Acta Cytol* 21:225–228, 1977

98. Mattson LA, Cullberg G: Clinical evaluation of treatment with estriol vaginal cream versus suppository in post-menopausal women. *Acta Obstet Gynecol Scand* 62:397–401, 1983

99. Wied GL: The cytologic changes of the vaginal epithelial cells and the leukorrhea following estrogenic therapy. *Am J Obstet Gynecol* 70:51–58, 1955

100. Wachtel E: The cytology of amenorrhea. *Acta Cytol* 10:56–61, 1966

101. Batrinos, ML, Efstratiades MG: Vaginal cytology in primary amenorrhea. *Acta Cytol* 16:376–380, 1972

102. Efstratiades M, Panitsa-Faflia C, Batrinas M: Vaginal cytology in endocrinopathies. *Acta Cytol* 27:421–424, 1983

103. Boszle P, Sandor G, Laszlo J: Vaginal cytology and the human menopausal gonadotropin-test (HMG-cytohormonal test). Cases of gonadal dysgenesis. *Acta Cytol* 21:22–25, 1977

104. Teter, J, Boczkowski K: Cytohormonal pattern and histologic studies in cases of pure gonadal dysgenesis. *Acta Cytol* 11:449–455, 1967

105. Bamford SB, Mitchell GW, Bardawil WA, et al: Vaginal cytology in polycystic ovarian disease. *Acta Cytol* 9:322–327, 1965

106. Stein IF: The management of bilateral polycystic ovaries. *Fertil Steril* 6:189–205, 1955

107. Johnston WW, Goldstein WR, Montgomery MS: Clinicopathologic studies in feminizing tumors of the ovary. III. The role of genital cytology. *Acta Cytol* 15:334–338, 1971

108. Shirai E, Iizuka R, Notake Y: Clomiphene citrate and its effects upon ovulation and estrogen. *Fertil Steril* 23:331–338, 1972

109. Pandya G, Cohen MR: The effect of cis-isomer of clomiphene citrate (cis-Clomiphene) on cervical mucus and vaginal cytology. *J Reprod Med* 8:133–138, 1972

110. Wied GL, del Sal JR, Dargan AM: Progestational and androgenic substances tested on the highly proliferated vaginal epithelium of surgical castrates. I. Progestational substances. *Am J Obstet Gynecol* 75:98–111, 1958

111. Fuertes-de la Haba A, Pelegrina I, Bangdiwala IS, et al: Changing patterns in cervical cytology among oral and non-oral contraceptive users. *J Reprod Med* 10:3–10, 1973

112. Reyniak JV, Sedlis A, Stone D, et al: Cytohormonal findings in patients using various forms of contraception. *Acta Cytol* 13:315, 1969

113. Wied GL, Davis ME, Frank R, et al: Statistical evaluation of the effect of hormonal contraceptives cytological smear pattern. *Obstet Gynecol* 27:327–336, 1966

114. Schmidt ALC, Christiaans APL: The vaginal smear pattern in cases of endometriosis. *Acta Cytol* 9:247–250, 1965

115. Stoll BA: Vaginal cytology as an aid to hormone therapy in post-menopausal cancer of the breast. *Cancer* 20:1807–1813, 1967

116. Moracci E, Berlingieri D: Hormonal evaluation of vaginal smears from artificial vagina. *Acta Cytol* 17:131–134, 1973

ANSWERS

1. c

2. b

3. c

10

Cervical Mucus

JOHN C. M. TSIBRIS

INTRODUCTION

Cervical mucus is a gel-like material that fills the endocervical canal and controls the entry of spermatozoa and microorganisms into the upper genital tract. The functions of the cervical mucus are dependent on its physical properties and the presence of key enzymes and other proteins.

The structure–function and the rate of secretion of cervical mucus change during the menstrual cycle and apparently correlate with the normal fluctuations of sex hormones (estrogens, progesterone). This chapter presents some of the current knowledge about the physical properties, chemical composition, and applications to clinical practice of the hydrodynamic and other parameters of human cervical mucus. New findings on cervical mucus peroxidases will be also discussed along with their projected use in the study of reproduction.

A number of excellent reviews[1–7] describe the historical background, recent developments in basic studies, and diagnostic uses of human cervical mucus. The latter include the postcoital test, in vitro mucus penetration tests, and rheologic (flow) properties of cervical mucus, which are routinely used to evaluate infertile couples. With the increased in-

terest in artificial insemination and "test-tube" babies, the cervical mucus, an easily accessible secretion, could prove most useful in determining the optimal time for insemination, embryo transfer, and so on, thereby improving the outcome of these procedures.

PRODUCTION AND PHYSIOCHEMICAL PROPERTIES

Cervical mucus is produced in the crypts or in the complex folds of endocervical columnar epithelium. The columnar cells consist of nonciliated secretory cells and kinociliated cells.[3] Cervical mucus that collects in the posterior fornix of the vagina contains varying amounts of fluids from the endometrium, oviducts, ovarian follicle, and peritoneum, as well as cells and cellular debris from the epithelium of the upper reproductive tract, white blood cells, and microorganisms.

Before ovulation there is a large increase in the surface of the endocervical epithelium and increased secretion of clear mucus is observed (600 mg/day at mid-cycle compared with 20–60 mg/day at other times). The diameter of the cervical os increases from 1 to 3 mm.

Around the time of ovulation, the pH of endocervical mucus increases to 6.8–7.4, whereas in the mid-proliferative and mid-secretory phases it re-

JOHN C. M. TSIBRIS • Department of Obstetrics and Gynecology, and Department of Physiology and Biophysics, University of Illinois at Chicago, Chicago, Illinois 60612.

mains at 6.0–6.6. At the vaginal fornix, the pH remains around 4.6 throughout the cycle. The ejaculate raises the pH by 0.5–2.0 units in the posterior fornix of the vagina and the endocervical canal; the increased pH is maintained for 1–6 hr.[4,8]

Cervical mucus can be separated by centrifugation into an aqueous and a gel phase. The relative amounts of the two phases vary during the menstrual cycle.

Aqueous Phase

Although the cervical mucus is a heterogeneous mixture of secretions, the chemical composition of which changes during the cycle, a few general comments can be made:

- At mid-cycle cervical mucus contains 98% water (0.5% proteins) and 90% water at other times (2.5–3.0% proteins).[9]
- Soluble proteins in the mucus originate from serum and from secretions of the reproductive tract. The aqueous phase contains NaCl, calcium, and many other ions, but among the nondialyzable material, 30% is soluble proteins and 70% mucins. High estrogen levels decrease protein concentration in the cervical mucus whereas progesterone, in the presence of estrogens during the secretory phase, increases protein concentration. Prescribed estrogens and progestagens have the same effect as do the natural hormones.

Among the soluble proteins are albumin, transferrin, haptoglobulins, immunoglobulins IgG, IgA, and IgM,[2,10], α-amylase, alkaline phosphatase,[11] lactoferrin, peroxidases,[12] lysozymes, plasminogen activator, α_1-antitrypsin, and several other proteinase inhibitors. Estrogen administration decreases the apparent level of nonspecific proteinases in cervical mucus, whereas progestagens increase it.[2]

It was recently discovered that preovulatory cervical mucus contains relatively large amounts of prostaglandins (range: 1–5 ng/g wet mucus); by comparison, blood contains 10–100 pg/ml and sperm 100–500 μg/ml. The prostaglandin concentration decreases at mid-cycle;[13] their origin is unknown. Luteinizing hormone (LH) has been found in human cervical mucus, and its concentration shows a nadir at ovulation.[14] The pre- and postovulatory levels of mucus LH are two to three times higher than peak LH levels observed in serum (LH concentrations are expressed as mIU per g mucus or ml serum, respectively).

Gel Phase

The main components of this phase are cervical mucins, which are highly glycosylated sialoglycoproteins. Mucins are very large proteins (molecular weight range: $7–15 \times 10^6$). These cross-linked proteins form the structural frame of cervical mucus. In order to maintain the gel structure, both disulfide bonds and hydrophobic interactions are needed, because both 6 M guanidine hydrochloride and 10 mM dithiothreitol are necessary to solubilize the gel effectively.[15–17] The chemical composition of cervical mucins (after removal of nonmucin components of the gel phase) does not differ greatly from other mucin-type glycoproteins found in the respiratory or gastrointestinal tract.[18] Proteins constitute 20% and saccharides (neutral, sialylated, or sulfated) 80% of mucin by weight. The protein component of cervical mucins consists mainly of serine and threonine (38% of the total amino acids) and contains very few lysine, histidine, tyrosine, methionine (3% of total), or cysteine (3% of total residues); most of the cysteine residues are carboxymethylated. Cysteine, basic, and aromatic amino acids are probably concentrated in a "naked" (lacking glycosylated residues) segment of mucins; these segments are susceptible to proteolytic attack.[6] Oligosaccharides range in size from di- to decasaccharides and are therefore intermediate in size between ovine submaxillary mucins and the large, complex polysaccharides of bronchial and gastric mucins.

It is not clear whether the polysaccharide composition of human cervical mucins changes during the menstrual cycle; the structure of some oligosaccharides does change during the cycle. It appears that there are no significant differences in the carbohydrate components of mucins from women belonging to different blood groups within the ABO system.[6,17]

Although the sialic acid content of cervical mucins does not correlate with the rheologic properties of mucus, there is evidence that the ratio of L-fucose to sialic acid does correlate. Moreover, a sialyl transferase and a few fucosyl transferases have been identified in mucus,[6] but their role in regulating the physical properties of mucins or the possible regulation of these transferases by hormones remains unclear.

When the ionic strength or pH is varied in vitro,

there is no significant change on the viscoelasticity of mucus. Therefore, electrostatic interactions between charged groups in the gel phase are not deemed important. In vivo the changes in pH are not so large as to greatly modify the charge of the ionizable groups present.

Studies of mucin structure using various denaturing-chaotropic agents (e.g., phenol, calcium and lithium salts, urea and guanidinium salts) suggest[19] that noncovalent aggregation of mucins may be more extensive than covalent aggregation. Current methods, most of which are "destructive," do not permit detailed knowledge of the three-dimensional structure of cervical mucus, which, according to current hypotheses, is the main regulator of sperm penetration through the cervical canal.

Nuclear magnetic resonance (NMR), a very powerful nondestructive technique, had been used earlier by Odeblad[6,7] to gain some insight into the structure of cervical mucus. Odeblad and others used a variety of biophysical methods and have formulated models that describe how mucin chains are arranged in the gel phase of cervical mucus. The main points of our present understanding are as follows:

- The three-dimensional structure of cervical mucus is in a dynamic state which changes continuously and is under the control of estrogens and progestogens. Under the influence of estrogens alone (late proliferative phase), the mucus becomes watery and mucins are arranged in strings or micelles, with an approximate diameter of 0.5 µm, which stretch from the major endocervical crypts to the external os. These micelles allow the formation of "highways"[5] for sperm migration. This clear mucus was designated by Odeblad as E_S and is in a mixture with type E_L mucus, the latter having a less regular structure with spaces allowing the penetration but not rapid transport of spermatozoa. At ovulation, cervical mucus consists of 22% E_S, 75% E_L, and 3% type G mucus. Scanning electron microscopy (SEM) has been used extensively in the study of cervical mucus; despite the unavoidable distortion of SEM specimens from the natural, unperturbed state, impressive SEM photographs[20] show mid-cycle cervical "channels" with a diameter of 30–35 µm. In the early proliferative and secretory phases, the diameter of the mucin network openings decreases to 2–6 and 4–6 µm, respectively.

- After ovulation, and under the influence of rising progesterone, cervical mucus becomes relatively scanty, cloudy and sticky, thus prohibiting sperm penetration. This is the predominantly G state in the Odeblad nomenclature and contains 90% of the G-type mucus, a meshwork of cross-linked polypeptide strands. The presence of proteins that could anchor adjacent mucin strands together to give G mucus has been suggested by Gibbons.[21] However, no specific cross-linking proteins have been identified as yet in cervical mucus.

- Lee et al.[6,7] have used laser light scattering, a method causing negligible perturbations, and proposed that mucus is made of random-coiled rather than cross-linked macromolecules. During the luteal phase, the 10% decrease in water content would cause the mucus to become more compact and thus unpenetrable by spermatozoa.

- Wolf et al.[6,7] have proposed however that the increase in the degree of hydration at midcycle could account for the observed changes in the hydrodynamic properties of cervical mucus.

Since purified mucins contain very small numbers of amino acids with "cross-linkable" side chains (e.g., cysteine, tyrosine), one would suspect that mucins by themselves cannot form the observed complex network through covalent bonds, unless the "naked" segments are enriched in such residues and there is a "cross-linking" molecule. Additional studies of the interaction between soluble proteins and mucins are needed to clarify how the three-dimensional structure is held together. A mid-cycle decrease in the extent of the putative cross-linking between mucins and nonmucin proteins would account for most experimental observations.

SPERM PENETRATION OF CERVICAL MUCUS

Spermatozoa are able to penetrate the cervix only during the late proliferative and early secretory phases of the menstrual cycle, a span of approximately 6 days.[4] Important aspects of sperm migration have been elucidated from in vivo studies in animals and in women during artificial insemination or insemination followed by removal of the uterus and oviducts. Such studies showed that the percentage of motile sperm and the percentage of sperm with normal morphology are higher in cervical mucus than in semen.[22] Thus, the mucus seems to exclude most abnormal sperm; the mechanism of exclusion is not yet clear but mucus does not act as a simple filter since it does not collect abnormal sperm.

After sperm deposition in the vagina at midcycle, there is a rapid phase (1.5–3 min) in the transport of spermatozoa to the cervical canal and up to the internal os. Since the in vitro sperm velocity in preovulatory mucus reaches a maximum of 0.1–3 mm/min, the finding of sperm in the ampulla within 5 min of ejaculation suggests that its travel may be facilitated in some way. Small carbon particles of sperm size deposited in the vagina of animals have also been found to progress into the upper part of their uterus.

Spermatozoa can move in a linear fashion through the cervical mucus forming a stretch, like a military phalanx, along an ''invisible'' channel of cervical mucus that seems to give direction to sperm movement. The formation of phalanges is probably due to stretching of mucus, which acts as a ''superelastic material,''[7] rather than to proteolytic invasion of mucus by sperm. Channels located in the center of the cervical canal lead directly to the uterine cavity, whereas some sperm are diverted to the crypts.

It is estimated that one spermatozoon out of 2000 does penetrate the mucus, while the rest are destroyed by the hostile vaginal environment or are phagocytosed. The rapid migration of sperm, achieved presumably by the inherent mobility of the spermatozoa, is followed by the slower colonization of the cervical crypts as more spermatozoa leave the ejaculate. The sperm concentration in the cervical canal is maximal (100,000–200,000) for about 2 hr and steadily declines after 6 hr.[4]

The normal mid-cycle endocervix is a major storage depot for spermatozoa, and the most favorable environment for sperm survival within the whole reproductive tract[22] because it contains very few leukocytes, adequate nutrients and can wash out or dilute semen components clinging to the sperm. Proof of the favorable cervical environment for sperm survival is the finding[23] that sperm extracted from cervical mucus 56 hr after artificial insemination are able to undergo the acrosomal reaction and penetrate the zona pellucida in vitro; however, the fertilizing life span of human sperm is estimated at 48 hr.

ANTIBACTERIAL ACTIVITY OF CERVICAL MUCUS

A bactericidal role has been suggested for cervical mucosa and cervical mucus because the normal uterine cavity is sterile and only infrequently are bacteria found in the cervical canal.[24,25] In addition to the ''mechanical'' barrier to the passage of microorganisms, cervical mucus must also contain bacteriostatic substances since day 14 mucus[25] has higher in vitro inhibitory activity for growth of vaginal bacteria and fungi (e.g., *Micrococcus lysodeicticus, Staphylococcus aureus, Candida albicans*) than mucus from days 10, 18, or 22; at mid-cycle, leukocyte counts are also at their lowest. Mucus from women fitted with an intrauterine device (IUD) or on estrogen–progesterone contraceptives have similar antimicrobial capacity for *M. lysodeicticus*, whereas the latter group shows much reduced capacity for the other microorganisms tested in this study.[25] Resistance to ascending infection may be impaired during menstruation as a result of alteration in the cervical protective mechanisms. Odeblad had studied mid-cycle mucus from women with chronic or acute cervical inflammation and found its viscoelasticity and NMR parameters to resemble those of luteal phase mucus.

The cervix, which is the major site of immunologic activity in the female genital tract[2,26] exhibits well-developed antibacterial and phagocytic activities mediated by complement, lysozyme, lactoferrin, and opsonizing antibodies. At the same time, in some cases, local and systemically produced antibodies may prevent sperm motility and penetration of the cervical mucus by agglutination or other mechanisms. Thus, bacteria and viruses may cause infertility, although chronic cervicitis may not be an absolute factor, since cervicitis is found in pregnant women.[5] The results of the postcoital test would clarify whether it is necessary to treat the inflammation with antibiotics or other means.[5]

USE OF CERVICAL MUCUS IN CLINICAL TESTS OF INFERTILITY

The physical properties of cervical mucus are evaluated in the following two tests of the fertile period:

1. *Spinnbarkeit* (threadability or elasticity) of mucus reaches a maximum at mid-cycle and

is obtained by measuring the length of a mucus thread stretched between two glass plates.

2. *Ferning,* first observed by Papanicolaou, is the crystalline fernlike pattern obtained when mucus is dried on a microscope slide. Ferning increases at mid-cycle, is common to mucus from other parts of the body, and is due to the interaction of NaCl with E-type mucus.

Cervical etiology (factor) is suspected in 5–10% of all infertility cases. Two clinical tests are performed at mid-cycle to evaluate infertile couples: the postcoital test (PCT) and the in vitro mucus-penetration test.

The PCT or Sims-Huhner test involves the microscopic evaluation of cervical mucus and sperm, 2–4 hr after intercourse. A good PCT suggests that there is satisfactory estrogen stimulation of the cervix, adequate sperm number, and good sperm quality, good coital technique, and no significant antisperm immunity factors present in the woman's secretions. A poor or negative PCT test is meaningless in the presence of poor mucus, but in the presence of good mucus it indicates that further testing is warranted. The most common problem with the performance of the PCT is improper (not at mid-cycle) timing of mucus collection. A good method to predict ovulation by a few days might abrogate more than one-half the observed abnormal PCT.

The in vitro mucus penetration test is not performed as frequently as the PCT but provides complementary information and allows more flexibility than the PCT. It requires mid-cycle cervical mucus and fresh semen from the patient's husband or from a donor; the husband's semen may also be tested with mucus from another fertile woman. The penetration of the mucus and the fate of sperm entering the mucus are observed. The use in the test of flat capillary tubes permits photomicrography and sophisticated semen analysis that can also provide valuable research data.[5,26] A comprehensive account of the above clinical tests is given in chapter 27.

CERVICOVAGINAL PEROXIDASES AND PREDICTION OF THE TIME OF OVULATION

The cervix and cervical mucus are a key part of the mechanism that synchronizes the entry of sper-matozoa into the uterine cavity with the availability of the ovum. Since the cervical mucus is easily accessible by nontraumatic procedures, many methods use it to determine the fertile period of the menstrual cycle and specifically the time of ovulation. Methods that take advantage of changes in the rheologic properties of cervical mucus have already been mentioned. Fluctuations during the cycle in the chemical content of cervical mucus have also been explored, such as the mid-cycle increase in the concentration of glucose[5,11] or NaCl.[28] However, the mid-cycle concentrations of enzymes such as lysozyme, α-amylase, and alkaline phosphatase decline relative to their early proliferative and mid-secretory levels. None of these methods[11] has been widely accepted because they are not practical or have not been correlated with precise parameters of the time of ovulation, such as serum LH levels. In clinical practice, the basal body temperature, *Spinnbarkeit,* and ferning are routinely used despite their limitations.

Daily determinations of serum or urine LH, estradiol, serum progesterone, urine pregnanediol, or their metabolites (e.g., glucuronides) have proved useful but are not practical, fast, or economical.[11]

A peroxidase, extracted from cervical mucus (sampled at the external os), shows great promise as a predictor of ovulation.[12] The colorimetric assay uses H_2O_2 and a plant phenol, guaiacol as outlined in Figure 10-1. The copper-red color produced can be easily quantitated with the naked eye because of the large changes occurring in the peroxidase levels. Notice that 0.5 M $CaCl_2$ is used to extract this enzyme from cervical mucus. The color is stable for 5 min, although in the spectrophotometric assay[12] the rate of increase declines after the first minute or so.

In studies of human endometrium[29] designed to determine whether a correlation existed between guaiacol peroxidase (a known marker of estrogen dependence of rat uterine tissue) and estrogen receptors, we found that the peroxidase activity was localized mainly in the mucosa of the endocervical canal. Moreover, during the menstrual cycle, the specific activity of the peroxidase (activity units per g wet tissue) fluctuated and declined sharply before ovulation. In these hysterectomy specimens, the day of the cycle was determined by histologic examination of the endometrium.

In postmenopausal women, the peroxidase content of the cervical mucosa was only a small fraction of the premenopausal levels.

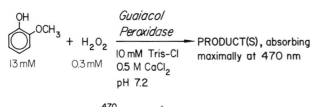

G-Px content : ΔA^{470} per min / g wet tissue

FIGURE 10-1. The guaiacol peroxidase (G-Px) assay. The enzyme is extracted from cervical mucus with Ca^{2+} and the rate of color development (maximum absorbance at 470 nm) is measured with a recording spectrophotometer. Because of the high Ca^{2+}, simple methods to measure protein are not applicable and the specific content is expressed per gram wet mucus. The structure of the product(s) is unknown; because of the possibility of autooxidation of guaiacol, the structure of the reaction products may not be stable after a few minutes.

Recent studies[30,31] with 40 ovulatory woman cycles (Fig. 10-2) showed that

- Cervical mucus contains very large concentrations of guaiacol peroxidase at all times except 3–5 days before and during ovulation.

- The preovulatory decline in peroxidase concentration is steep enough to be perceived by the naked eye.
- 1–2 days after ovulation the high peroxidase levels return, signaling the end of the fertile period.
- At the end of the ovulatory cycle, the peroxidase declines again.

Both cervical mucus and vaginal peroxidases always showed the 3–5-day drop in concentration regardless of the "regularity" of the ovulatory cycle, namely, whether the woman ovulated 3 days or 13 days after the end of menses.

In anovulatory cycles, either spontaneous or due to the use of oral contraceptives, the peroxidase levels increase right after the end of menses and stay high throughout the cycle. Similar peroxidase patterns are observed when vaginal "secretions," sampled with a "cotton swab" at the posterior fornix, are tested (data not shown).

Since blood was collected daily (Fig. 10-2), we were able to test for correlations between peroxidase and LH, estradiol, or progesterone levels. Statistically significant correlations were found[30] between estradiol and peroxidase (a negative correlation, only between days -7 to -1), and progesterone and peroxidase (a positive correlation between days 0 to $+12$); no correlation was found between LH and enzyme levels. Such correlations do not, of course, prove a cause–effect relationship but point to an association reminiscent of the estrogen/progesterone effects on the structure of cervical mucus.

Guaiacol peroxidase may regulate the cyclic changes observed in the rheologic and sperm penetration characteristics of cervical mucus (1) by being a structural component of the tight structure

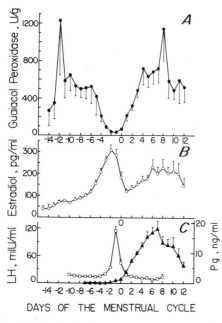

FIGURE 10-2. Guaiacol peroxidase content (A) of cervical mucus, serum estradiol; (B) of luteinizing hormone (LH) and progesterone (Pg); and (C) during the menstrual cycle. Each point is the mean value from 40 normal ovulatory woman cycles; the bar represents the SE. Note that the peroxidase data are plotted on a logarithmic scale. Serum estradiol, LH, and Pg were determined by radioimmunoassay. Day 0 is the LH + 1 day, the presumed day of ovulation. The rising Pg levels are the indication that ovulation did occur.

of the gel, and (2) by catalyzing some important reaction.

Peroxidases are a family of hemoproteins that, in the presence of H_2O_2 or hydroperoxides, catalyze the oxidation of a variety of substrates. Peroxidases are used routinely to iodinate proteins at tyrosine residues, and these reactions are most valuable in the preparation of ^{125}I-labeled tracers for radioimmunoassays and for other uses in clinical and basic research. In this context, it is interesting that after intravenous injections of ^{131}I-labeled iodide,[1] large amounts of tracer were concentrated in the cervical mucus, perhaps by peroxidase-catalyzed covalent binding to cervical proteins.

Peroxidases can also catalyze the cross-linking of proteins through tyrosine side chains, since tyrosine dimers have been isolated.[32,33] A peroxidase-catalyzed reaction is implicated in the mechanism to prevent polyspermy in sea urchin eggs[34] and again involves the cross-linking of proteins. Women who were given intravenous guaiacol[1] or guaifenesin orally (a guaiacol analogue and common antitussive)[35] showed an improvement in their cervical mucus, which in the guaifenesin study was also shown to improve their fertility. Since estrogen administration also improves the cervical mucus of infertile patients, two questions arise: What is the common feature between estrogens and guaiacol, and what is the natural substrate(s) of guaiacol peroxidase? Estrogens and guaiacol are phenols; therefore, this peroxidase may act on endogenous phenols, such as estrogens and estrogen metabolites, the catecholestrogens.[36] Our in vitro studies[29] had shown that 2-hydroxyestrogens are more potent inhibitors of guaiacol peroxidase than estrogens. It is possible that estrogens/catecholestrogens are "suicide" sustrates of guaiacol peroxidase. When peroxidase antibodies become available it can be determined whether the peroxidase is present but inactive in mid-cycle mucus. Since human cervical mucosa contains very small numbers of estrogen receptors,[37] it should not escape our attention that the regulation of cervical secretions by estrogens may not be exerted *via* the classic genomic route.

Since estrogen levels rise again at the mid-secretory phase (Fig. 10-2), progesterone must override the hypothetical in vivo inhibition of guaiacol peroxidase by estrogens. Another possibility is that the preovulatory peroxidase may have a different origin (e.g., from eosinophils) from the secretory peroxidase, or the secretory per-

oxidase may not be inhibited by estrogens. Further characterization is needed to classify the peroxidase(s) and possibly distinguish them from peroxidases in leukocytes or from other sources.

One of our volunteers contracted a severe yeast infection on day -8 and her cervical mucus peroxidase remained high throughout the cycle despite treatment that alleviated her symptoms. Interestingly, after treatment the peroxidase in her vaginal secretions (sampled at the posterior fornix) showed the mid-cycle "dip."

Freshly prepared seminal plasma inhibited guaiacol peroxidase from cervical mucosa.[29] This in vitro inhibition may be due to reducing agents or proteolytic enzymes in seminal plasma.

The peroxidase pattern shown in Figure 10-2 has been observed in all normal ovulatory cycles tested. After more testing is done it may prove that such pattern constitutes evidence that the cycle is normal and ovulation has occurred. Administration of Pergonal, to induce ovulation, caused an increase in serum estradiol, improved the cervical mucus, and showed a concomitant decrease in cervical mucus guaiacol peroxidase.[38]

SUMMARY

This chapter attempts to show the importance of cervical mucus in the reproductive process. Cervical mucus has unique properties that enable it to vary with hormonal stimuli altering its physical status and effects on sperm transport. It helps in evaluating fertility status and compatibility with semen and by measuring changes in peroxidase content that may be a predictor of ovulation timing with its many potential applications.

QUESTIONS

1. Cervical mucus becomes thin and watery when serum estrogen levels rise. What do you expect cervical mucus to be like in pregnancy? Explain your answer.

2. To achieve conception but prevent defective spermatozoa from fertilizing the egg, would thick cervical mucus be needed? Explain your answer.

REFERENCES

1. Weiss G: Effect of steroid hormones on cervical mucus, in Briggs MH (ed): *Advances in Steroid Biochemistry and Pharmacology,* Vol I. London, Academic, 1970, pp 137–162.*
2. Schumacher GFB: Humoral immune factors in the female reproductive tract and their changes during the cycle, in Dhindsa DS, Schumacher GFB (eds): *Immunological Aspects of Infertility and Fertility Regulation.* New York, Elsevier/North-Holland, 1980, pp 93–141.*
3. Hafez ESE: The cervix and sperm transport, in Hafez ESE (ed): *Human Reproduction. Conception and Contraception,* 2nd ed. Hagerstown, MD, Harper & Row, 1980, pp 221–252.*
4. Fordney-Settlage D: A review of cervical mucus and sperm interactions in humans. *Int J Fertil* 26:161–169, 1981.*
5. Joyce D, Vassilopoulos D: Sperm–mucus interaction and artificial insemination. *Clin Obstet Gynaecol* 8:587–610, 1981.*
6. Chantler E: Structure and function of cervical mucus, in Chantler EN, Elder JB, Elstein M (eds): *Mucus in Health and Disease*—II. New York, Plenum, 1982, pp 251–263.*
7. Elstein M: Cervical mucus: Its physiological role and clinical significance, in Chantler EN, Elder JB, Elstein M (eds): *Mucus in Health and Disease*—II. New York, Plenum, 1982, pp 301–318.*
8. Kroeks MVAM, Kremer J: The pH of the lower third of the genital tract, in Insler V, Bettendorf G (eds): *The Uterine Cervix in Reproduction.* Stuttgart, Thieme, 1977, pp 109–118.
9. Odeblad E: The functional structure of human cervical mucus. *Acta Obstet Gynecol Scand* 47(suppl 1):59–79, 1968.
10. Davis KP, Maciulla GJ, Yannane ME, et al: Cervical mucus immunoglobulins as an indicator of ovulation. *Fertil Steril* 62:388–392, 1983.
11. Moghissi KS: Prediction and detection of ovulation. *Fertil Steril* 34:89–98, 1980.*
12. Tsibris JCM, Thomason JL, Kunigk A, et al: Guaiacol peroxidase levels in human cervical mucus: A possible predictor of ovulation. *Contraception* 25:59–67, 1982.
13. Charbonnel B, Kremer M, Gerozissis K, et al: Human cervical mucus contains large amounts of prostaglandins. *Fertil Steril* 38:109–111, 1982.
14. Moreno-Escallon B, Chappel S, Blasco L: Luteinizing hormone in cervical mucus. *Fertil Steril* 37:536–541, 1982.
15. Wolf DP, Sokoloski JE, Litt M: Composition and function of human cervical mucus. *Biochim Biophys Acta* 630:545–558, 1980.
16. Yurewicz EC, Matsuura F, Moghissi KS: Structural characterization of neutral oligosaccharides of human midcycle mucins. *J Biol Chem* 257:2314–2322, 1982.
17. Carlstedt I, Lingren H, Sheehan JK, et al: Isolation and characterization of human cervical mucus glycoproteins. *Biochem J* 211:13–22, 1983.
18. Allen A: Mucus—A protective secretion of complexity. *Trends Biochem Sci* 9:169–173, 1983.*
19. Creeth JM: Constituents of mucus and their separation. *Br Med Bull* 34:17–24, 1978.*
20. Daunter B, Lutjen P: Cervical mucus, in Hafez ESE, Kenemans P (eds): *Atlas of Human Reproduction by Scanning Electron Microscopy.* Lancaster, England, MTP Press, 1982, pp 55–59.
21. Gibbons RA, Sellwood R: The macromolecular biochemistry of cervical secretions, in Blandau RJ, Moghissi K (eds): *The Biology of the Cervix.* Chicago, The University of Chicago Press, 1973, pp 251–265.
22. Hanson FW, Overstreet JW: The interaction of human spermatozoa with cervical mucus in vivo. *Am J Obstet Gynecol* 140:173–178, 1981.
23. Gould JE, Overstreet JW, Hanson FW: Assessment of human sperm function after aging in vitro. *Fertil Steril* 35:240, 1981. (abst)
24. Sparks RA, Puppier BGA, Watt PJ, et al: Bacteriological colonization of uterine cavity: Role of tailed intrauterine contraceptive device. *Br Med J* 282:1189–1191, 1981.
25. Zuckerman H, Kahana A, Carmel S: Antibacterial activity of human cervical mucus. *Gynecol Invest* 6:265–271, 1975.
26. Jones WR: Immunology of infertility. *Clin Obstet Gynecol* 8:611–638, 1981.*
27. Katz DF, Overstreet JW, Houson FW: A new quantitative test for sperm penetration in cervical mucus. *Fertil Steril* 33:179–186, 1980.
28. McSweeney DJ, Sbarra AJ: A new cervical mucus test for hormone appraisal. *Am J Obstet Gynecol* 88:705–709, 1964.
29. Tsibris JCM, Trujillo YP, Fernandez BB, et al: Distribution of guaiacol peroxidase in human endometrium and endocervical epithelium during the menstrual cycle. *J Clin Endocrinol Metab* 54:991–997, 1982.
30. Tsibris JCM, Langenberg PC, Khan-Dawood FS, et al: Cervicovaginal peroxidases: Sex hormone control and potential clinical uses. *Fertil Steril* 44:236–240, 1985.
31. Tsibris JCM, Virgin SD, Khan-Dawood FS, et al: Cervicovaginal peroxidases: Markers of the fertile period. *Obstet Gynecol* 67:316–320, 1986.
32. Bayse GS, Michaels AW, Morrison M: The peroxidase-catalyzed oxidation of tyrosine. *Biochim Biophys Acta* 284:34–42, 1972.
33. Aeschbach R, Amado R, Neukom H: Formation of dityrosine cross-links in proteins by oxidation of tyrosine residues. *Biochim Biophys Acta* 439:292–301, 1976.
34. Foerder CA, Shapiro BM: Release of ovoperoxidase from sea urchin eggs hardens the fertilization membrane with tyrosine cross-links. *Proc Natl Acad Sci USA* 74:4214–4218, 1977.
35. Check JH, Adelson HG, Wu CH: Improvement of cervical mucus with guaifenesin. *Fertil Steril* 37:707–708, 1982.
36. Merriam GR, Lipsett MB (eds): *Catechol Estrogens.* New York, Raven, 1983.*
37. Tsibris JC, Fort FL, Cantor B, et al: The uneven distribution of estrogen and progesterone receptors in human endometrium. *J Steroid Biochem* 14:997–1003, 1981.
38. Tsibris JCM, Thomason JL, Gold JJ, et al: Le mucus cervical et sa teneur en guaiacol péroxidase: un procédé possible pour prédire l'ovulation. *Contraception Fertil Sexual* 11:25–27, 1983.

*Review article/chapter.

ANSWERS

1. Whether or not progesterone is present seems to be more important for the structure of cervical mucus than estradiol concentration alone. In pregnancy you have high estrogen

and high progesterone concentrations and the mucus forms a thick plug of the cervical canal.

2. No. Thick mucus does not permit entry of either normal or defective spermatozoa. Normal mid-cycle mucus screens, by some unknown mechanism, the penetration of abnormal sperm. Even at mid-cycle, cervical mucus represents a tortuous path, and most abnormal sperm do not seem to make it through.

11

Endometrium

WADI A. BARDAWIL

"On this soft anvil all mankind was made"
John Wilmot, Earl of Rochester[1]

INTRODUCTION

John Wilmot's statement underscores the importance of the uterus, particularly the endometrium, as a vital tissue in human biology, for not only does mankind develop in this endometrium, but also lives up to 1–2% of the life-span within it.

This unique tissue characterized by its dynamic ability to change continuously does so with exquisite regularity, modulated by powerful sex hormones—estrogens and progesterone. These changes consist of growth (regeneration), differentiation (secretion), and destruction (menstruation). They occur cyclically, nearly once a month during the life of the human female from menarche to menopause and are referred to as the menstrual cycle.

During the management of the female patient, the gynecologist frequently needs to assess the condition of the endometrium. Because it is an endocrine target organ, this condition cannot be assessed without a histological examination in many in-

WADI A. BARDAWIL • Departments of Pathology and Obstetrics and Gynecology, University of Illinois, Chicago, Illinois 60612.

stances. No single serum test or battery of tests can conveniently substitute for a histopathological study of the endometrium. Thus, there is the need for understanding the morphology and function of the endometrium in normal and abnormal states, as well as for expertise in the procurement, handling, and preservation of this tissue for proper processing and interpretation.

In addition, the necessity of communicating in advance with the pathologist(s) to map diagnostic strategy needs to be underscored. This practice, as desirable as it may be, is infrequent but is becoming more readily used.

This chapter deals with some of the basic diagnostic principles concerning the endometrium as they relate to the normal and abnormal states. It is directed to the student of gynecological endocrinology and pathology.

HISTORICAL CONSIDERATIONS*

The origin of gynecological endocrinology dates back to nearly 150 years ago, when Claude Bernard, the father of endocrinology, promulgated the neurovascular–endocrine concept and when Jacques Récamier introduced curettage as a surgical procedure before the French Academy of Medicine

---

*See the special historical introductory chapter to this volume.

(which, historians relate, created furor among its members).

By the end of the last century, the ovaries were recognized as organs of internal secretion. Hitschmann and Adler[2] are credited with pioneer descriptions of cyclical variations of the endometrium in vivo. It was not until the isolation and characterization of estrogens by E. Allen and Doisy in 1923[3] and of progresterone by Corner and W. Allen in 1929[4] that a new era based on experimentation had begun. Thereafter, a large number of classic contributions to the anatomy and physiology of the endometrium were made, notably those of E. Allen,[5,6] W. M. Allen,[7] Bartelmez,[8-11] Daron,[12,13] Corner,[4,14,15] Hartmann,[16] Hertig,[17,18] Hisaw,[19] Phelps,[20,21] Ramsey,[22] Wislocki,[23] Velardo,[24-26] and Kasprow.[27]

Sometime after the pioneer work done on the endometrium by Hitschmann and Adler,[2] Schröeder,[28] and others, Rock and Bartlett[29] introduced quantitative interpretations of the endometrial changes during the menstrual cycle. These changes were modified by Hertig[17] and eventually culminated in the universally accepted criteria for dating of the endometrium by Noyes et al.[30]

NORMAL ENDOMETRIUM

The endometrium develops from the mesoderm within the mullerian duct system. Because of its responsiveness to estrogen and progesterone, it is considered an endocrine target organ, although the possibility of being an endocrine organ itself has not yet been settled. It has been claimed to secrete relaxin[31,32] and in tissue culture to produce prolactin.[33]

In viewing the cytohistoarchitecture of the uterus, one finds the endometrium firmly attached to the myometrium, forming with it the endomyometrial junction. On section, this is seen as a slightly irregular indented line of demarcation. In infancy and senility, this line of demarcation is less distinct.

Morphological Considerations

Conceptually, the following histologic description pertains to the endometrium in its basic state. The morphodynamics of this tissue, unless specified, are discussed under dating of the endometrium.

The endometrium is composed of epithelium and stroma or lamina propria. The epithelium forms glands (glandular) and covers the surface of the endometrium (surface). Both are lined by pseudostratified columnar or cuboidal cells supported by a basement membrane. The glandular epithelium orginates in the proximity of the myoendometrial junction, forms tubular glands, courses toward the surface following twisting paths, and ends in glandular ostia from which it continues with the surface epithelium. Whereas most of the glandular cells are of secretory type, some are ciliated. The surface epithelium has a greater but variable number of ciliated cells.

The stroma is populated by highly specialized connective tissue cells whose nuclei are round and oval with scanty cytoplasm that projects thin processes forming a fine anastomotic network with their neighbors. Here one observes delicate reticulum fibers surrounding stromal cells. Collagen appears rather scantily in the normal cycling endometrium.[34,35] The ground substance is abundant but is markedly influenced by the phase of the cycle.

Dispersed in the stroma are mast cells,[36] lymphocytes, and macrophages; during the late secretory phase, numerous neutrophilic leukocytes and decidual granulocytes (Körnchenzellen) are seen as well.[37,38] The normal endometrium varies in thickness from 0.1 to 0.8 cm or more. It is thin in infancy, during the early proliferative phase and in senility. It is thick in the secretory phase and in pregnancy.

The endometrium is topographically divided into two poorly defined zones, the basalis and the functionalis. The basalis is a thin layer of undifferentiated endometrium in contact with the myometrium. It is generally not modified by sex hormones during the menstrual cycle. However, a change may be appreciated under a greater stimulus, such as in pregnancy. The functionalis occupies the rest of the endometrium, usually the upper two-thirds or more. It owes its name to its responsiveness to the ovarian sex steroid hormones during the cycle. Late in the secretory phase, the functionalis is further subdivided into a superficial layer (or compacta), and a deeper layer (or spongiosa). The compacta is demarcated by a dense zone of predecidual cells, and the spongiosa by a richly glandular zone with little intervening stroma.

Arterial blood is supplied to the human endometrium by the radial–spiral arteries, branches of the myometrial arcuate arteries.[39] The radial–spiral arteries enter the endomyometrial junction, giving rise to subterminal branches, the basal or straight arteries, and the spiral arteries. The basal arteries terminate in a rich capillary network supplying blood to the basalis and the lower functionalis. These basal arteries are neither influenced by ovarian hormones nor modified by menstruation.[39,42] However, they contribute to the formation of a new functionalis after shedding of the menstrual endometrium.

The spiral arterioles continue their radial sinuous course in the endometrial stroma between glands, spiraling and branching, and forming an extensive subepithelial capillary network. The spiral arteries supply the upper two-thirds of the functionalis. They are influenced by estrogen and progesterone and are also involved in menses.[40]

The return venous circulation begins with the rich capillary system and venous plexuses from periglandular, subepithelial, and stromal vessels. The venous system from the functionalis and basalis, unlike the arterial supply, is accomplished by a single rather than a double vascular system. The venules of the human endometrium grow, mature, and degenerate with the menstrual cycle. It should be noted that regeneration of arterioles and venules after menses does not necessarily restore the vasculature to the original topography.[20]

There is a paucity of reports on the lymphatic circulation of the human endometrium. In nonpregnant and pregnant monkeys, lymphatics form an extensive network in the lower functionalis and basalis. The superficial functionalis is devoid of lymphatics[23]; Robbard et al.[41] reported on the distribution of lymphatics in the human uterus from material removed at autopsy, but gave no description of the endometrial lymphatics.

Some nerve fibers penetrate the endometrium along the basal arteries, others along the spiral arteries, for a short distance, into the functionalis.[42,43] The nerves terminate in free endings in the stroma.[44]

Physiological Considerations

In addition to sperm capacitation, the fundamental function of the endometrium is its preparation to provide optimal conditions for the nidation of the blastocyst. This feat is accomplished cyclically by the fine regulatory mechanism of the ovarian estrogens and progesterone and their reciprocal actions on the pituitary gland and its gonadotropins, follicle-stimulating hormone (FSH) and luteinizing hormone (LH) under the influence of hypothalamic releasing factors. FSH induces the ovarian follicle to secrete estrogens (estrogenic substances) and, in combination with LH, a low level of preovulatory progesterone. These gonadotropins amplify the theca interna anatomically and physiologically and induce the lutein cells to secrete progesterone. The adenohypophyseal gonadotropins in turn are inhibited by the ovarian hormones through a feedback mechanism *via* the hypothalamus.

The ovarian sex steroid hormones, with other possible unknown factors, regulate the cyclic activity of the endometrium in alternating phases of growth and regression. Keep in mind that to the physiologist, the periods of growth and regression of the endometrium do not necessarily correspond to the anatomic proliferative and secretory phases.

Period of Growth

The endometrial growth begins after menstruation and ends some 4 ± 2 days before the onset of menstruation.[45] At this time, regression begins irrespective of whether the cycle is ovulatory or anovulatory. The growth phase is biphasic, corresponding to the anatomic periods of proliferation and differentiation. The initial phase of endometrial growth is under the influence of estrogen. This hormone induces synthesis of RNA and DNA, causing proliferation of both epithelial and stromal cells. It enhances deposition of ground substance in the stroma through increased permeability and metabolic activity. The spiral arteries and veins respond to the estrogenic stimulus. They elongate disproportionately faster to the increase of thickness of the endometrium.[39] Adapting to the space limitations, these vessels twist, coil, and branch. In addition, it should be noted that several enzymes increase during this period: alkaline phosphatase (AKP), β-glucuronidase (BGU), glucose 6-phosphatase (G6Pase), and triphosphopyridine nucleotide diaphorase (TPNH).[46]

After ovulation, growth (differentiation) is under the influence of both estrogen and progesterone, with dominance of the latter. This combination of hormones inhibits cell proliferation, largely through repression of RNA and DNA synthesis for mitoses and evokes cell differentiation; the endometrial glands secrete materials rich in glycogen, proteins, lipids, and enzymes. There is an increase in acid phosphatase (ACP), succinic dehydrogenase (SDH), cytochrome oxidase (CO), malic dehydrogenase (MDH), and isocitric dehydrogenase

(CDH) activity. Part of the stroma transforms to predecidua.[46]

The predecidua provides a supporting rigid wall to the progesterone-induced branching spiral arterioles. After ovulation, estrogen exerts a greater influence on capillaries supplying the stroma, while progesterone influences the vessels around glands and under the epithelium.[45] Concomitant with the increased vascularity, there is increase in blood volume supplied to the endometrium. "The basic characteristic of the growth phase is a progressive increase in the volume of blood delivered to and circulating within the endometrial functionalis or nidation area."[21] If ovulation occurs, the volume of blood increases from the level that will not support the implanting conceptus to that which will support it. Here also rests the differences between ovulatory and anovulatory cycles.[21] Concomitant with increased blood volume there is enhanced vascular permeability and metabolic activity. Fluids, proteins, and solids are deposited in the ground substance and in the glandular secretions. The 22-day secretory endometrium contains greater total wet weight ($3.8\times$), increased water ($3.6\times$), and protein ($5.7\times$) compared with that of the 9-day proliferative endometrium.[47] The water content of the endometrium during the cycle approximately parallels the double-hump curve of the blood estrogen level.

The metabolic activity of the endometrium parallels the increase in vascular growth. It reaches the highest level in the 21–22-day secretory endometrium (nidation time) and remains high until regression sets on and secretory function ceases. Thus, it appears that the main function of the endometrium during the growth period is to prepare an anatomical and biochemical bed for nidation of the traveling fertilized egg that is already in the endometrial cavity in the form of a blastocyst.

Regression

Unless nidation of the blastocyst takes place and trophoblastic activity supports the corpus luteum, regressive changes ensue. Regression correlates with the rapid drop of estrogen and progesterone secretion from the regressing corpus luteum. The time when the amount of progesterone is inadequate to produce progestational changes may determine the onset of bleeding.[19]

It has been reported that the mechanism for bleeding rests on the rhythmic spastic contractions of the spiral arterioles, further aided by uterine contractions. The precise mechanism of menstruation, while not fully understood, is most probably multifactorial as follows:

1. *Role of the radial arteries:* Bartelmez[11] demonstrated frequent luminal constrictions of the radial arteries in the uterus throughout the cycle. Measurements of the overall diameter of sites of constriction seem to indicate that the radial arteries do not contract but become elongated; this stretching causes reduction in lumen and blood flow that is responsible for ischemia of the surface and bleeding.[48]

2. *Role of the spiral arterioles:* With the fall of estrogen primarily, but also of progesterone, the endometrium loses fluid (20–40%). With the fluid loss there is shrinkage of the endometrium, with consequent compression and collapse of the spiral arterioles and venules, resulting in ischemia, microinfarcts, and bleeding.[12,13] In addition, the fall in progesterone is responsible for degenerative changes of the spiral arteriolar wall.

3. *Role of the decidua:* The compacta, which had given support to the spiral arterioles, venules, and capillaries, degenerates and softens. Without this support, the frail, thin-walled vessels subjected to internal blood pressure, rupture. Softening of the decidua may result from a reduction in size of predecidual cells by the discharge of cytoplasmic organelles and materials and the effect of such discharged organelles and materials on neighbor cells and fibers. Some of the discharged organelles and materials may be released from decidual granulocytes: relaxin, fibrinolysins, and esterases capable of degrading reticulum fibers and ground substances. The bulk, however, derive from premenstrually chemotactically attracted neutrophils. As these cells phagocytize or break down, they release potent proteolytic lysosomal enzymes that contribute greatly to the menstrual phenomenon. The role of toxic oxygen radicals is a new concept emerging in inflammation; however, its relationship to menstruation requires further elucidation.

The stage is then set, and menstruation begins; the spiral arterioles rupture and thrombose, venules bleed, and the stroma and glands break down. In all, some of the functionalis mixed with blood is eliminated in 3–5 days.

As menstruation progresses, the degrading enzymes and anticoagulants are eliminated, the reparative forces enter into action. Under the influence of renewed estrogenic secretions, blood vessels grow again, and glandular epithelium proliferates. From its glandular ostia, surface epithelium regenerates covering raw areas. Polymorphonuclear cells are eliminated with the menstrual discharge. The new endometrium is now infiltrated with lymphocytes whose role is unknown. With the regression phase completed, a new cycle begins.

Dating of the Endometrium (Morphological Timing)

The normal menstrual cycle is customarily divided into two phases: proliferative (follicular) and secretory (progestational, progravid, or luteal).

The length of the menstrual cycle ranges from 25 to 35 days, occasionally longer. The variability largely depends on the proliferative phase because the secretory phase is of constant 14 days duration.

Evaluation of the endometrium should be made in relationship to the patient's basal temperature, hormone levels, and the histological findings. Timing of the endometrial biopsy is paramount in the infertile patient. For maximum information, biopsy should be taken, conditions permitting, within the first hours of the onset of menstruation. Otherwise, the biopsy should be taken several days after the temperature rise of a biphasic temperature chart. It would be a futile exercise to attempt a biopsy procedure in the infertile patient during the proliferative phase, unless it happens to be at bleeding time of an anovulatory cycle. The gynecological patient with diverse pathology, however, can be biopsied practically at any time as dictated by the patient's medical condition.

Dating of the endometrium as presented in this chapter is in keeping with the criteria established by Hertig,[17] Noyes et al.,[30] and Noyes and Haman[49] (Fig. 11-1).

In dating the endometrium, the pathologist relates findings to an idealized cycle of 28 days. The first day of the cycle and proliferative phase corresponds to the onset of menstruation. Ovulation time is arbitrarily assigned day 14 of the 28-day cycle irrespective of the length of the proliferative phase. This measure is necessary to relate the dating to the ideal 28-day cycle, since the secretory phase, from ovulation to onset of menstruation, is of constant 14-day duration.

Proliferative Endometrium

The proliferative endometrium cannot be dated on a daily basis. The best a pathologist can do is to estimate this phase as late menstrual–early proliferative, early, mid-, or late proliferative. All the changes described below should be interpreted as part of a continuum. That which the pathologist sees is an interrupted still picture of the process.

Late Menstrual–Early Proliferative Endometrium (Days 1–5)

This is the stage of the endometrium in restoration to its base state. One finds mixed features of the late menstrual and early proliferative changes. As the menstrual detritus is discharged and before completion of menstruation, the viable endometrium proliferates from the stratum basalis and lower functionalis. Mitoses are seen in both epithelium and stroma. At this time, the surface is incompletely epithelialized. Lymphocytes infiltrate the stroma (chronic physiologic endometritis). Polymorphonuclear leukocytes, plentiful during early menstruation, are only occasionally seen at this time.

Early Proliferative Endometrium (Days 5–8)

At this stage, proliferation of both glands and stroma proceeds. Mitoses are numerous. The endometrium thickens. The glands are tubular, straight, and sparse and their epithelium pseudostratified. The surface epithelium regenerates from the broken glandular ostia. The height of the surface epithelium is uneven and gets lower away from the glandular mouths. The stromal cells are of the "naked nucleus" type. Lymphocytic infiltrates may be seen (Fig. 11-2).

Mid-proliferative Endometrium (Days 8–11)

The mid-proliferative endometrium is characterized by increasing thickness. The glands are tortuous and more numerous as they grow at a faster rate than the stroma. The surface epithelium is uniform in height. The endometrial stroma becomes temporarily edematous, correlating with the first peak of blood estrogen level in the cycle (Fig. 11-3).

Late-Proliferative Endometrium (Days 11–14)

From days 11 to 14 of the cycle, the endometrium reaches maximal proliferation. The glands have be-

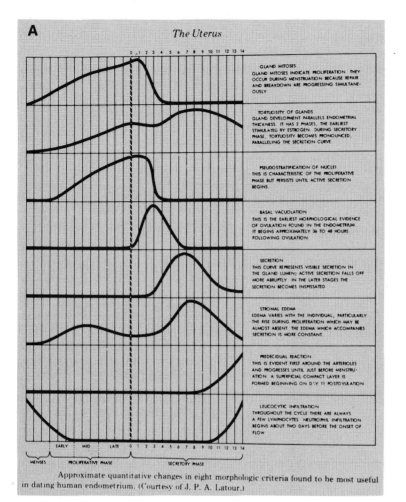

A   *The Uterus*

GLAND MITOSES
GLAND MITOSES INDICATE PROLIFERATION THEY OCCUR DURING MENSTRUATION BECAUSE REPAIR AND BREAKDOWN ARE PROGRESSING SIMULTANE-OUSLY

TORTUOSITY OF GLANDS
GLAND DEVELOPMENT PARALLELS ENDOMETRIAL THICKNESS IT HAS 2 PHASES, THE EARLIEST STIMULATED BY ESTROGEN. DURING SECRETORY PHASE, TORTUOSITY BECOMES PRONOUNCED, PARALLELING THE SECRETION CURVE

PSEUDOSTRATIFICATION OF NUCLEI
THIS IS CHARACTERISTIC OF THE PROLIFERATIVE PHASE BUT PERSISTS UNTIL ACTIVE SECRETION BEGINS.

BASAL VACUOLATION
THIS IS THE EARLIEST MORPHOLOGICAL EVIDENCE OF OVULATION FOUND IN THE ENDOMETRIUM. IT BEGINS APPROXIMATELY 36 TO 48 HOURS FOLLOWING OVULATION.

SECRETION
THIS CURVE REPRESENTS VISIBLE SECRETION IN THE GLAND LUMEN; ACTIVE SECRETION FALLS OFF MORE ABRUPTLY IN THE LATER STAGES THE SECRETION BECOMES INSPISSATED

STROMAL EDEMA
EDEMA VARIES WITH THE INDIVIDUAL, PARTICULARLY THE RISE DURING PROLIFERATION WHICH MAY BE ALMOST ABSENT THE EDEMA WHICH ACCOMPANIES SECRETION IS MORE CONSTANT

PREDECIDUAL REACTION
THIS IS EVIDENT FIRST AROUND THE ARTERIOLES AND PROGRESSES UNTIL JUST BEFORE MENSTRU-ATION A SUPERFICIAL COMPACT LAYER IS FORMED BEGINNING ON DAY 11 POSTOVULATION

LEUCOCYTIC INFILTRATION
THROUGHOUT THE CYCLE THERE ARE ALWAYS A FEW LYMPHOCYTES NEUTROPHIL INFILTRATION BEGINS ABOUT TWO DAYS BEFORE THE ONSET OF FLOW

EARLY   MID   LATE   0 1 2 3 4 5 6 7 8 9 10 11 12 13 14

MENSES   PROLIFERATIVE PHASE   SECRETORY PHASE

Approximate quantitative changes in eight morphologic criteria found to be most useful in dating human endometrium. (Courtesy of J. P. A. Latour.)

FIGURE 11-1. (A) Schematic representation of histologic changes of the endometrium during the menstrual cycle. (From Noyes et al.[30]) (B) Schematic representation of histologic and histochemical changes during the menstrual cycle. (From Dallenbach-Hellweg.[52]) Both A and B form morphological criteria important in dating the human endometrial cycle.

come very tortuous, so that many more glands are seen on sections. Mitoses are numerous exceeding at times the numbers seen in carcinomas of the endometrium. Curiously, many mitoses appear protruding into the lumen.[50] Mobilization of the dividing cells, as they enlarge, is possibly directed toward the site of lesser resistance. The stromal edema decreases. Mast cells, although seen throughout the proliferative phase, are more numerous in the late proliferative endometrium.[36] Occasional small irregular vacuoles of secretion containing glycogen may be seen at this stage in some glands of the upper functionalis. Low-level preovulatory progesterone is responsible for this phenomenon and should not be confused with the clearly defined vacuoles of the early secretory endometrium (Fig. 11-4).

Secretory Endometrium

After ovulation, the endometrium differentiates. This is expressed morphologically by characteristic fixation, dehydration, and staining artifacts of histopathological specimens, permitting the skillful pathologist to date the secretory endometrium from day to day with remarkable precision. It has been customary to date the secretory endometrium departing from ovulation time—day 14 and so on to day 28 or onset of menstruation. It has recently been recommended, however, that ovulation time be considered as day 0 and subsequent days as postovulatory (P.ov.) 1, 2, 3, and so on.

The morphological parameters of the secretory endometrium in sequence are (1) glandular secretion, its site of appearance, mobilization, and re-

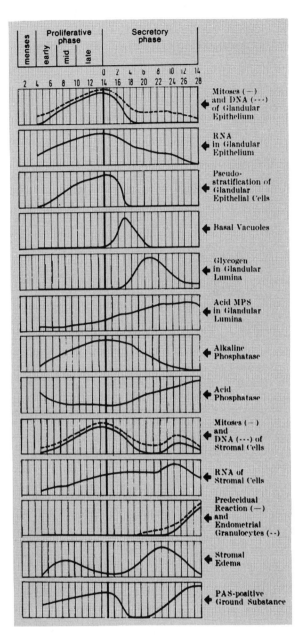

FIGURE 11-1. *(Continued)*

lease; (2) stromal edema, and (3) predecidual reaction. All these changes are localized in the functionalis. Secretory responses of the basalis may occur, however, in cases of progestational hyperplasia.

The first evidence of secretion appears on day 16 (P.ov. 2), as subnuclear vacuoles in the glandular cells. Not all cells in the same gland contain vacuoles, giving it a motheaten appearance. The nuclei of the vacuole-laden cells occupy an apical position. At day 17 (P.ov. 3), the subnuclear vacuoles increase, so that all cells of the gland have a uniform appearance. The nuclei in apical position form a monolayer. Thenceforth, pseudostratification of epithelium is lost. By day 18 (P.ov. 4), some vacuoles are mobilized to the cell apex, and still others

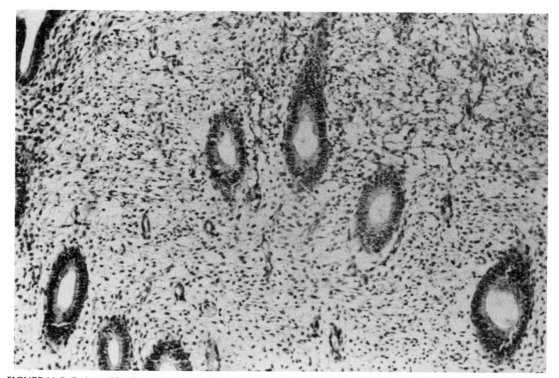

FIGURE 11-2. Early proliferative endometrium. Glands are sparse. Stromal cells are "naked nucleus" type. Some lymphocytes are seen in stroma. (X104)

are discharged into the lumen. The nuclei revert to the basal position. There is evidence that some cell organelles are discharged with the secretion.[95,96] On day 19 (P.ov. 5), much of the secretion has been already released. On day 20 (P.ov. 6), the glands appear secretorily exhausted. There is, however, electron microscopic evidence of continued secretion. On day 21 (P.ov. 7), the endometrial stroma becomes increasingly edematous reaching maximum by day 22 (P.ov. 8), increasing thickness of the endometrium to approximately 0.6–0.8 cm. The endometrium is then ideally conditioned for nidation. Should fertilization occur, the blastocyst would already be in the uterine cavity in the process of implantation; otherwise, edema subsides shortly thereafter. Day 23 (P.ov. 9) is characterized by prominence of the spiral arterioles brought about by predecidual changes of the perivascular stromal cells. These cells enlarge their cytoplasm and become amphophilic and distinct. New islands of predecidual reaction appear subepithelially by day 24 (P.ov. 10). The islands of predecidua enlarge and coalesce by day 25 (P.ov. 11). At this stage, the

glands dilate, increase their tortuosity affected by shrinkage of endometrium and loss of stromal fluid. This change correlates with the initiation of the decline in blood levels of estrogen and progesterone. The glandular epithelium is projected into the lumen giving to the gland a sawtoothed appearance. Some secretion accumulates in the lumen and stains more intensely acidophilic. By day 26 (P.ov. 12), all islands of predecidua coalesce forming a solid zone, the compacta layer, in the midst of which there are a few constricted glands. Beneath the compacta lies the spongiosa layer formed by numerous glands and a relatively scanty stroma. On day 27 (P.ov. 13), also called premenstrual endometrium, the compacta is infiltrated by myriads of neutrophilic leukocytes (actue physiologic endometritis). The predecidual cells under the effects of anoxia degenerate and stain faintly.

Hamperl[37] and Hellweg[38] pointed out that many of the alleged polymorphonuclear leukocytes infiltrating the predecidua are indeed a distinct predecidual cell whose shrunken cytoplasm contains phloxinophilic granules (decidual granulocytes,

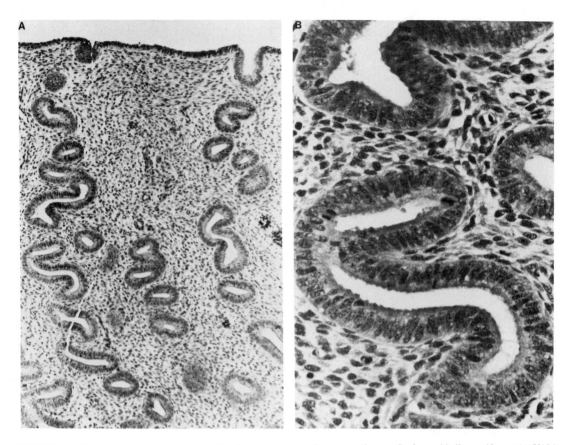

FIGURE 11-3. Mid-proliferative endometrium. Glands are numerous, mitoses conspicuous. Surface epithelium uniform. (A) (X104) (B) (X416)

Körnchenzellen). These granules contain relaxin, esterases, and acid phosphatase, which play an important lytic role in menstruation.[32,52] Late in the secretory phase, slight focal reactivation of secretion may be seen in some endometrial glands (Figs. 11-5 through 11-16).

Menstruation

On day 28 (P.ov. 14), the secretory phase has ended and menstruation ensues. The predecidual cells dissociate, small lakes of blood and fluids are formed throughout the compacta. Heavy infiltration of polymorphonuclear leukocytes with their proteolytic lysosomal enzymes contribute to the lysis of the stroma (Fig. 11-16). The endometrial glands break down. The first day of menstruation shows that the surface epithelium, although fractured and altered by anoxia, is still in place. By the second day, the surface epithelium may be lost,

together with some superficial endometrium. These changes progress on the third, fourth, and fifth days of the ensuing cycle, at which time signs of regeneration from the basalis and viable functionalis become evident.[53] Simultaneously, the cleaning-up process takes place. Cellular debris from necrotic polymorphonuclear leukocytes, and stromal cells trapped in the stroma during menstruation is eliminated by phagocytosis. Scavenger macrophages containing phagocytic vacuoles are frequently seen under or between epithelial cells. This phenomenon, described by Bartelmez,[8] in the menstrual endometrium of monkeys, is a useful diagnostic feature of menstruation (Fig. 11-17). Similar vacuoles can be seen, however, in destructive endometrial disease such as carcinoma, severe endometritis and rare cases of cystic and adenomatous hypoplasia. Again, with a renewed estrogen tide a new cycle is heralded.

Noyes[54] reported that responses of the endo-

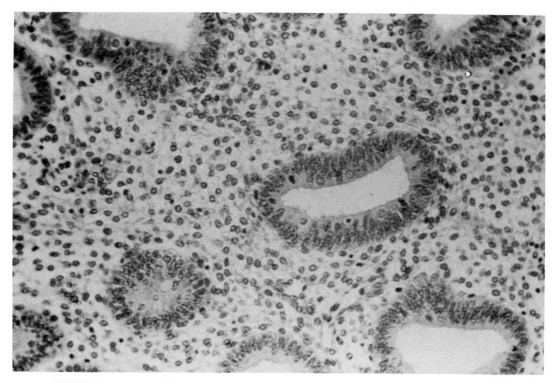

FIGURE 11-4. Late proliferative endometrium. Maximal pseudostratification. Mitoses at peak. (X260)

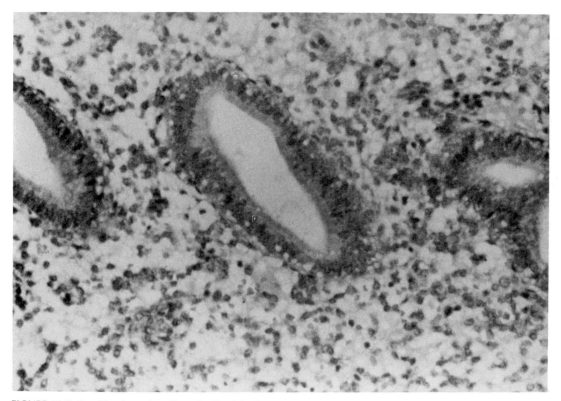

FIGURE 11-5. Day 16 endometrium (P.ov. 2). Glandular basal vacuoles are scattered, giving a motheaten appearance. (X416)

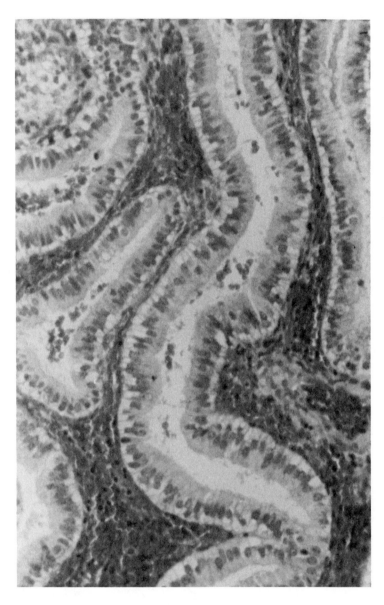

FIGURE 11-6. Day 17 endometrium (P. ov. 3). Basal vacuoles are uniformly present. (X416)

metrium are uniform throughout the mucosa. An exception should be made, however, of the lower uterine segment. Here the endometrium is akin to the basalis. As such, responses are minimal and not fully representative of the whole endometrium. For reliable dating, therefore, endometrial samples should be obtained from the fundus.[55] The date ascribed to the endometrium should be that of the most advanced aspect seen on the section.

Following the guidelines given above, accuracy and reliability of dating of the endometrium, within 2 days variability, are over 80%.[55] This figure was arrived at by reading biopsies and also by using other parameters, such as menses, presence, location, and state of development of the fertilized eggs, as well as changes in tubal mucosa.[55,56]

In summary, the proliferative endometrium is interpreted as early, mid-, or late proliferative. This is based on the presence of mitoses and estimation of the degree of proliferation. The secretory endometrium can be dated on a daily basis using secretion, edema, predecidua, and leukocytic infiltration as parameters. Substantial secretion begins at day 16 (P.ov. 2) and peaks at 17 (P.ov. 3) to 18 (P.ov.

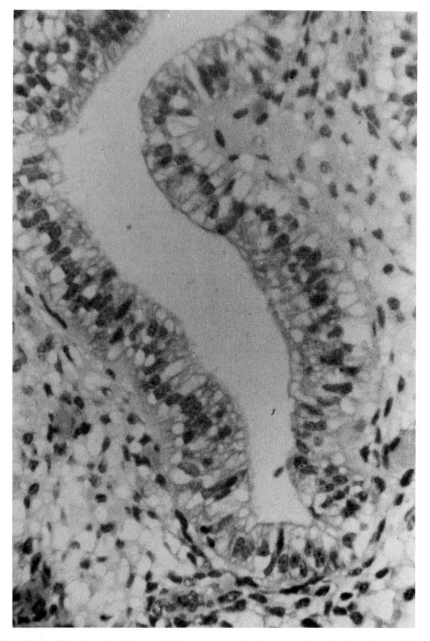

FIGURE 11-7. Day 18 endometrium (P. ov. 4). Secretory vacuoles in supranuclear and subnuclear position. (X416)

4). Edema is most conspicuous at day 22 (P.ov. 8). Predecidual reaction becomes apparent first at day 23 (P.ov. 9) and increases progressively until menses. Leukocytic infiltration is seen at day 27 (P.ov. 13). It is to be noted that the peaks of secretion, edema, and predecidual reaction do not overlap in the normal menstrual cycle.

Histochemical and Cellular Morphophysiological Considerations

Since the menstrual cycle is regulated primarily by estrogens and progesterone, receptor or binding sites for these hormones must be present in target cells. Indeed, receptor sites (R) have been demon-

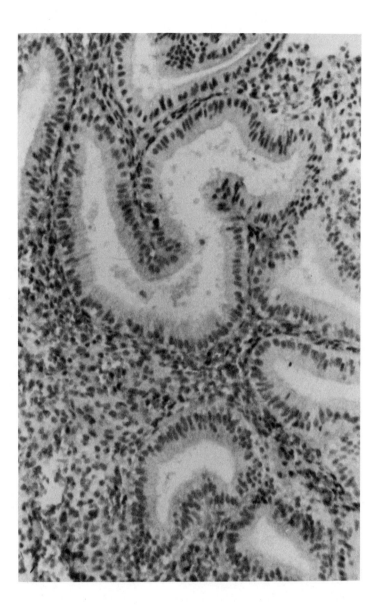

FIGURE 11-8. Day 19 endometrium (P. ov. 5). Most of the secretory vacuoles have been discharged into the lumen. Nuclei have reverted to basal position. (X260)

strated in the endometrium for estrone (E_1), estradiol (E_2), estriol (E_3), and progesterone (P) in cytosol and nuclear fractions of the cells.[57–59] The receptors are present, at variable concentrations, throughout the cycle irrespective of the cycle phase. Kreitmann-Gimbel et al.[60] demonstrated in monkeys constant ratios between E_1R and E_2R; e.g., 1 : 1, 1 : 0.75, and 1 : 2.5–3.5 in the proliferative phase, secretory phase, and pregnancy at time of implantation, respectively.[60] Tsibris et al.[59] reported the uneven distribution of E_2R and PR in the human endometrium. The concentration of cytoplasmic R is higher at the fundus and lower toward the low uterine segment, while the nuclear R maintain an inverse relationship, lower at fundus. Using rat monoclonal antibodies raised against MCF-7 human breast carcinoma high-affinity ER (estrophilin), Press and Greene, and Press et al.,[61–63] found specific nuclear localization of ER in epithelia and stromal cells by immunoperoxidase technique in all early, mid-, and late proliferative phase endometria. Staining of the basalis was surprisingly weak. Specific staining gets weaker as proliferation advances. Staining of mid- and late secretory endometrium is scanty, spotty, and limited to only occasional epithelial and stromal cells. By contrast, the

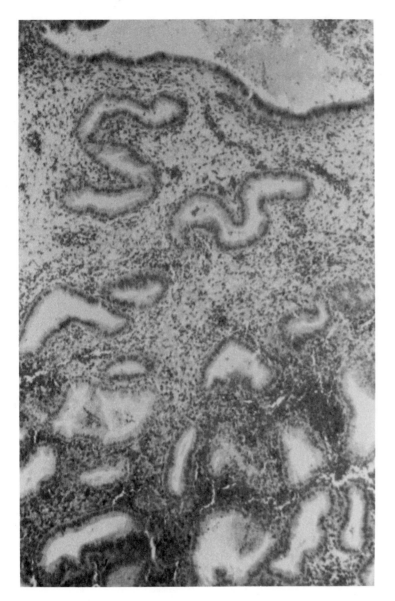

FIGURE 11-9. Day 20–21 endometrium (P. ov. 6–7). Glands are mostly secretorily exhausted, cells low cuboidal. Stromal edema manifest. (X104)

basalis during the secretory phase stains intensely. Postmenopausal endometria stain strongly in the nuclei of both epithelium and stroma. No cytoplasmic staining was observed in any of the endometria studied.

Prostaglandins

The possible role of prostaglandins has been added to the mechanism of menstruation. PGE and $PGF_{2\alpha}$ are produced by the endometrium. They are both at a low level during the proliferative and early secretory phase (100 ng/g tissue) increasing nearly five- to sevenfold beginning late in the secretory phase (500–700 ng/g tissue) for the $PGF_{2\alpha}$ and at onset of menstruation for PGE. These levels of prostaglandin synthesis in relationship to the cycle suggest a progesterone influence.[64]

Peroxidases, Immunoglobulins

Peroxidases have been localized in glandular epithelium and in granulocytes.[65] Guaiacol peroxidase was found at a very low level throughout the

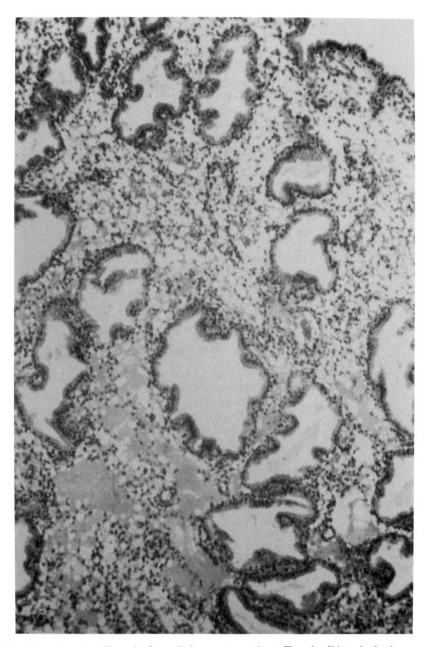

FIGURE 11-10. Day 22 endometrium (P. ov. 8). Stromal edema most prominent. The role of histamine has been proposed for this change. Glands are tortuous and dilated. (X260)

cycle in the fundal endometrium, contrasting sharply with the level of the enzyme in the low uterine segment and endocervical mucosa.[66] Immunoglobulins have been reported in the endometrium.

Histochemistry

Proliferative Endometrium

The proliferative endometrium is characterized by an increase in RNA, AKP, BGL, G6Pase, and

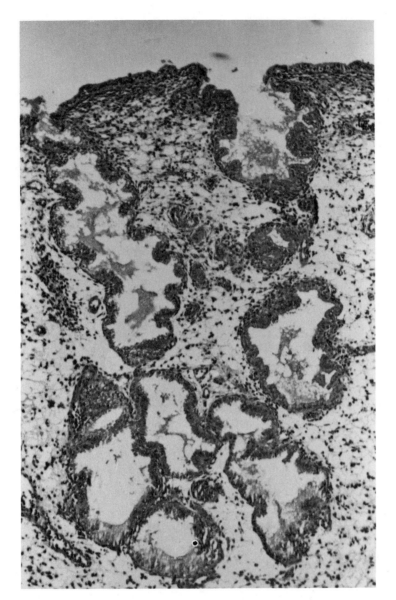

FIGURE 11-11. Day 23 endometrium (P. ov. 9). Incipient perivascular predecidual reaction gives prominence to the spiral arterioles. (X104)

NADPH (TPNH), whereas glycogen and glycoproteins are not significantly produced. Nonspecific esterases are seen in the proliferative as well as in the secretory phases (see Plate 11-1).

Secretory Endometrium

The secretory endometrium is characterized by production of glycogen, glycoproteins, proteins, and lipids; and also by increases in the following enzymes: acid phosphatase (ACP), glucose 6-phosphate dehydrogenase (G6PD), lactic dehydrogenase (LDH), succinic dehydrogenase (SDH), cytochrome oxidase (CO), malic dehydrogenase (MDH), and isocitric dehydrogenase (ICDH) (plate 11-1).

RNA

Estrogens induce cellular enrichment of ribosomes and RNA, and thus, higher protein synthesis for internal cell consumption and DNA synthesis

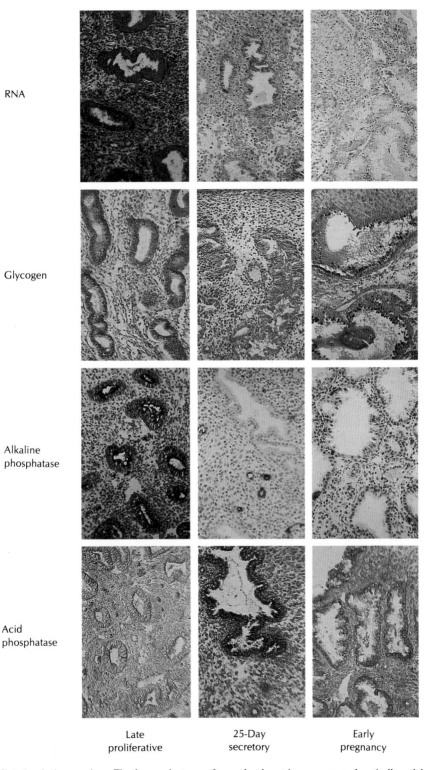

RNA

Glycogen

Alkaline
phosphatase

Acid
phosphatase

Late
proliferative

25-Day
secretory

Early
pregnancy

PLATE 11-1. Histochemical comparison. The three major types of normal endometrium are arranged vertically and the histochemical reactions, horizontally, for comparison of the several reactions in different stages of development. (From McKay et al.[46])

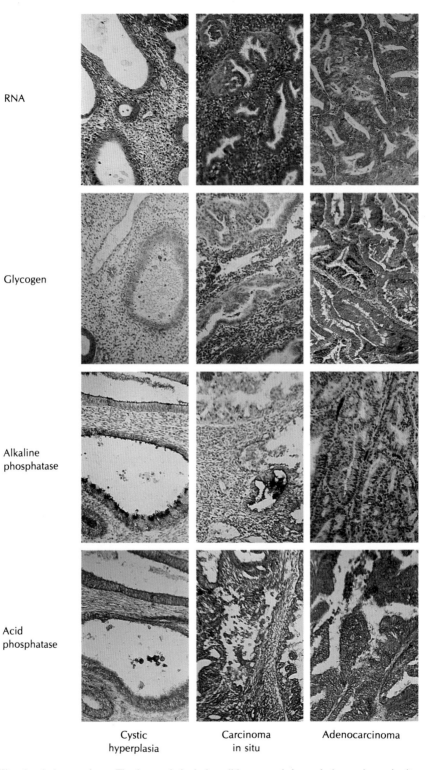

RNA

Glycogen

Alkaline
phosphatase

Acid
phosphatase

Cystic
hyperplasia

Carcinoma
in situ

Adenocarcinoma

PLATE 11-2. Histochemical comparison. The three pathological conditions—cystic hyperplasia, carcinoma in situ, and adenocarcinoma—are arranged vertically and the several histochemical reactions, horizontally, for comparison. (From McKay et al.[51])

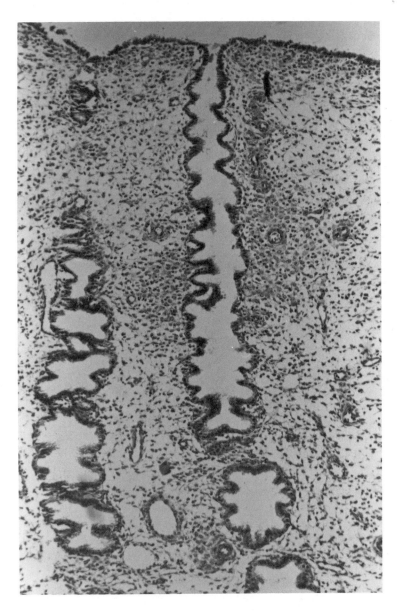

FIGURE 11-12. Day 24 endometrium (P. ov. 10). Note predecidual reaction increment around spiral arterioles. New islands of predecidua appear under surface epithelium. (X104)

for mitoses, both in vitro and in vivo. Progesterone interrupts RNA synthesis for cell replication while maintaining protein synthesis for secretion.[67] RNA, identified as ribonuclease-sensitive basophilia in the cytoplasm of both epithelial and stromal cells, is richest during the proliferative phase (see Plate 11-1A–C). It increases gradually with the progression of the cycle. After ovulation, basophilia is abated. In association with secretory activity the RNA granules clump and are secreted with the vacuoles of secretion into the glandular lumina. A possible related mechanism of this phenomenon may be the progesterone-induced acid phosphatase interference with estrogen receptors.[68]

Alkaline Phosphatase

Alkaline phosphatase is a membrane-bound enzyme (associated with membrane synthesis) present during the proliferative phase in the glandular and surface epithelium. AKP reaches a peak shortly after ovulation (2–3 days); then, as AKP is dis-

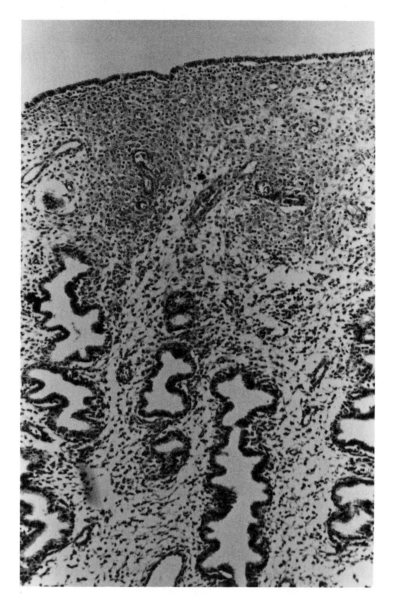

FIGURE 11-13. Day 25 endometrium (P. ov. 11). Islands of predecidua coalesce. Glands have sawtoothed appearance. (X104)

charged with the secretion, it fades rapidly as a cellular constituent. The stroma does not stain appreciably for AKP except for the endothelium, which stains at all times of the cycle (see Plate 11-1G–I).

β-Glucuronidase

BGL is an estrogen-dependent enzyme involved in the process of cell growth. Its activity is confined to the glands with only a low level in stroma and vessels; after ovulation its activity decreases very rapidly. Essentially, BGL parallels the AKP curve.

Glucose 6-Phosphatase

G6P is an enzyme involved in the metabolism of carbohydrates localized in the endoplasmic reticulum and nuclear membranes of glandular epithelial cells.[69] G6P becomes evident in the midproliferative endometrium, peaks at about ovulation, and decreases rapidly at about nidation time.

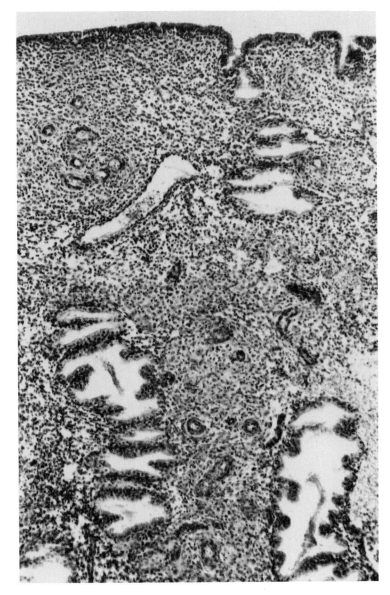

FIGURE 11-14. Day 26 endometrium (P. ov. 12). Formation of the compacta layer is complete. Some superficial glands are compressed. (X104)

Glucose 6-Phosphate Dehydrogenase

G6PD like G6P is also involved in the metabolism of carbohydrates and follows a similar curve. It differs in that the drop after day 22 follows a slower slope.

Lactic Dehydrogenase

LDH is a very important catalytic enzyme of the secretory phase involved in aerobic and anaerobic metabolism of carbohydrates through interconversion of lactate and pyruvate. It stains intensely in glands and vessels during the whole secretory phase. The stroma shows only trace amounts.

Succinic Dehydrogenase

This enzyme is localized in the glandular epithelium. It begins to rise at about mid-proliferative endometrium and plateaus and decreases at mid-secretory endometrium. The stroma shows only

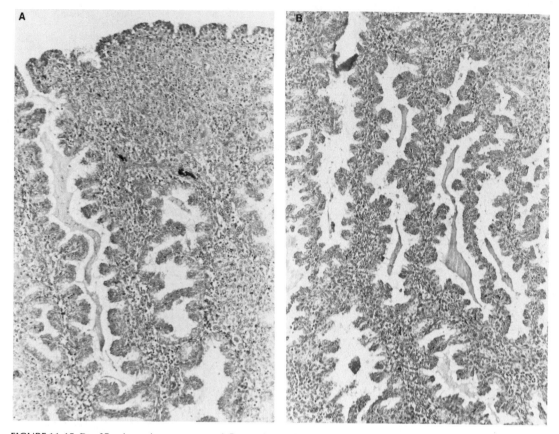

FIGURE 11-15. Day 27 endometrium, premenstrual (P. ov. 13). (A) Compacta layer is infiltrated by polymorphonuclear leukocytes. (X104) (B) Spongiosa layer. "Serrated" glands contain abundant inspissated secretion. (X104)

traces without meaningful variations. Isocitric (ICDH) and malic (MDH) dehydrogenases show a similar histochemical pattern, one of continuous progression from mid-proliferative endometrium with maximum staining in the secretory phase. Again, the staining is localized in the glands. Stromal staining is minimal.

Acid Phosphatase

This enzyme is demonstrated during the whole secretory phase in the glandular epithelium (see Plate 11-1J–L). The stroma does not stain conspicuously until late near-menstruation. However, some granules of stain can be observed on leukocytes infiltrating the stroma. Progesterone induces inactivation of nuclear estrogen receptor in the hamster uterus mediated by acid phosphatase.[68]

Triphosphopyridine Nucleotide Diaphorase

TPNH is localized intensely in the glandular epithelium during the proliferative phase and moderately during the secretory phase, and in the vasculature throughout the cycle. The stroma shows only traces.

Diphosphopyridine Nucleotide Diaphorase

DPNH shows an inverse type of localization to the TPNH. Staining of glands is moderate during proliferative endometrium and intense during the secretory phase, with traces of staining in the stroma.

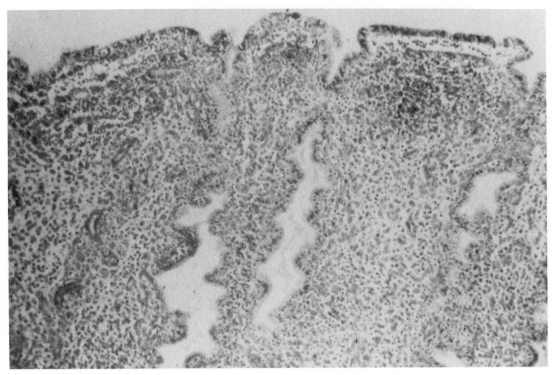

FIGURE 11-16. Day 1, menstrual endometrium (P.ov. 14). Focal stromal hemorrhages, dissolution of predecidua, more marked on left side. (X260)

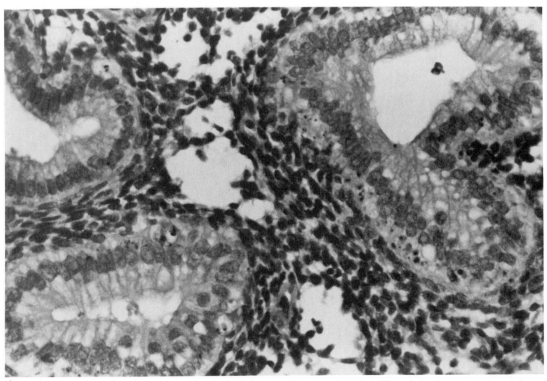

FIGURE 11-17. Menstrual endometrium. Note cell debris at base and between glandular cells, probably in phagocytic vacuoles. A mopping-up mechanism? (X416)

Nonspecific Esterases

Localization of NSE is variable in different endometria. Activity is localized in the cytoplasm of surface and glandular epithelium. The stain is uniform throughout the cytoplasm. Some luminal secretions reveal enzyme activity. Macrophages in the stroma stain intensely.

Glycogen and Glycoproteins

The glycogen content of the proliferative endometrium is meager. Some small granules may be seen in glandular epithelium before ovulation. After this, glycogen becomes abundant and follows the path of the secretory vacuoles, basal first, then apical, and finally luminal. In the stroma, predecidua and decidua contain abundant stainable glycogen (see Plate 11-1D–F). Glycoprotein (mucin) in the proliferative endometrium is scanty and limited to the basal membrane and to some of the glandular tips. During the secretory phase, glycoprotein is also scanty except at sites of maximal glycogen secretion. Mast cells scattered in the stroma stain intensely.

For more details on histochemistry, the reader is referred to the publications by Struemer and Stein,[70] McKay et al.,[46,51] Velardo and Rosa,[25,54] and Boutselis.[71]

Oxygen Uptake

After menstruation, the basal endometrium and remaining functionalis is poorly vascularized. Growth and metabolism proceed under hypoxic conditions; thus glycolysis may be anaerobic. Oxygen consumption of the proliferative endometrium is low, increasing slightly late in this phase. A shift to aerobic glycolysis occurs in the secretory endometrium when oxygen consumption may reach twice the level of that in the proliferative endometrium.[72,73]

Electron Microscopic Examination of the Endometrium

Transmission (TEM) and scanning electron microscopy (SEM) have not proved useful diagnostic tools of the normal or abnormal endometrium. Nevertheless, they have enhanced our knowledge of the basic structure and function of the mucosa. A succinct account of salient features not already apparent by light microscopy will be presented. For fur-

ther details, the reader is referred to the excellent reviews and contributions in the literature by Cavazos and Lucas,[74] Ferenczy and Richart,[75] and Wynn and Wooley.[76]

During the early proliferative phase, reflecting a low degree of activity related to regeneration and repair, the glandular cells of the endometrium demonstrate a paucity of ultrastructural elements. The nuclei are smooth and oval. The cytoplasmic organelles are scanty, simple, and small. Few glycogen granules may be seen in the cytoplasm. Parallel with the degree of proliferation, the nuclei turn gradually irregular. Euchromatin, reflecting active cell division (DNA replication), occupies most of the nucleus. The nucleolus becomes prominent. The cytoplasmic organelles increase in number, size and complexity. Glycogen granules are associated with undeveloped bundles of microtubules and microfilaments. Centrioles can be seen at the apex and remnants of spindle filaments around nuclei. The apical membrane is dense and microvilli subtle. The cells present lateral tight junctions. The Golgi apparatus is positioned supranuclearly. Abundant rough endoplasmic reticulum (RER) and smooth endoplasmic reticulum (SER) develop.

In the secretory endometrium more nuclear–RER interconnections are expressed morphologically by greater convolutions and indentations of the nuclear surface and physiologically by continued protein synthesis. A thick rim of heterochromatin concentrates at the nuclear periphery. The nucleolus develops a unique microchannel system,[77] and this nucleolar structure persists through the secretory phase. Giant mitochrondria may be seen in association with circumferential loops of endoplasmic reticulum, specifically at about ovulation time.[78,79] Large deposits of glycogen are observed at the base of the cells at this time, associated with well-developed microtubules and microfilaments (transport system). Large mitochondria with complex cristae concentrate apically. Later, at midsecretory phase, abundant glycogen appears in the apical cytoplasm in association with lysosomes. Reflecting secretory activity, homogeneous intercellular electron-dense material appears at the apex. Also, the apical membrane becomes irregular with projecting vacuoles containing glycogen and cell organelles. The microvilli enlarge and assume club shapes. Annular lamellae present in proliferative phase are no longer seen at this stage. Late in the secretory phase, the cells decrease in size, and again the cell organelles decrease in number, size, and complexity. Glycogen decreases significantly (regression). Lysosomes increase, reflecting enzymatic lytic activity (digestion).

In keeping with the light microscopic findings, the stromal cells from the stratum basalis do not change appreciably throughout the cycle.[74] The stromal cells are divided into two categories: the superficial and deep cells. The superficial cells are those under the glandular and surface epithelium and around vessels. These differ from the deep cells in their ability to better differentiate towards a fibroblastic appearance.

The stromal cells from day 5 to 10 of the cycle, like their epithelial counterpart, are simple. The cytoplasm is scanty; the organelles develop and gradually enrich the cytoplasm. The cell membrane is distinct, except at some areas of condensation, which are associated with intra- and extracellular deposits of collagen.

From day 15 on, the cells continue their differentiation toward a fibroblastic type. The cells develop blunt processes that appear separated from the rest of the cytoplasm by rows of microvesicles and filaments, probably resulting from mitotic activity. The fate of this structure is unknown. The Golgi apparatus is well developed and may contain tropocollagen fibers within vesicles that may be discharged in the intercellular space.

From day 20, the stromal cells reach maximum differentiation. Glycogen is synthesized in large amounts through the remainder of the secretory phase. On day 25, the cells show evidence of differentiation to predecidua cells. They become round or acquire polygonal shapes. In contrast with epithelial cells, the RER and SER are maximally developed at this stage. Cell-to-cell contacts are prominent in the decidua. Finally, autophagic lysosomes become numerous.

In interpreting the EM changes of the endometrium during the menstrual cycle, it is worthwhile paraphrasing the statements of Cavazos and Lucas. Governed by estrogens, the intracellular changes in the proliferative endometrium reflect the activity of five different intracellular systems: (1) the reproductive, genetic, and control system; (2) the protein synthesis and transport system; (3) the carbohydrate synthesis and transport system; (4) the secretory apparatus; and (5) the digestive system. During the secretory phase, modulated by progesterone, there is an increase in carbohydrate synthesis and transport system activity, as well as an increase in activity of the secretory apparatus. Protein synthesis is maintained but there is a marked decrease in both lysosomal and growth activity.[74]

Scanning Electron Microscopic Examination of Endometrium

Proliferative Phase

The surface of the endometrium is smooth with interspersed oval glandular ostia. These become larger and rolled as the cycle progresses.[75] At larger magnifications, two distinct types of cells are seen, ciliated and secretory, at an approximate ratio of 20 : 1. The size and number of microvilli appear to increase from the proliferative to the secretory phase.

Secretory Endometrium

The flat surface of the proliferative phase gives rise to a convoluted appearance with emergence of ridges and clefts obscuring glandular ostia. By the mid-secretory phase, the microvilli swell terminally with transported secretions, some of which may be seen at glandular mouths. At menstruation, the surface of the endometrium as expected turns shaggy. The ciliated cells decrease in number.

Endometrium in the Fetus, Infant, and Preadolescent

The fetal endometrium is hardly recognizable. It consists of a single layer of epithelium supported by a scanty indistinct stroma. Occasional glands may be seen. At birth, there may be more glands and evidence of maternal hormonal stimulation. Focal proliferation, secretion (Fig. 11-18), predecidual transformation, menstrual changes, and even decidual granulocytes have been reported.[80] A few days after birth, these changes disappear with the endometrium reverting to its primitive state. From that time on the endometrium develops very gradually, reaching maturity at menarche. This is uniquely the longest normal proliferative phase cycle in the life of the female. Readers interested in fetal and preadolescent endometrium are referred to the review article by Valdes–Dapena.[81]

The Endometrium during Senility

After menopause, the endometrium is reduced to its minimal expression. It resembles the stratum basalis. The glands are sparse and round. Secretion in the lumen is mucinous and frequently inspissated. Mitoses are rare. Upon atrophy, some glands dilate in what has been called cystic hyperplasia, in

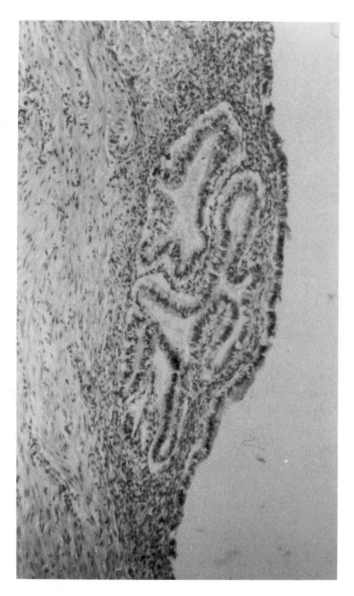

FIGURE 11-18. Endometrium from newborn infant at term (autopsy). Focus of secretory glands recapitulating day 17 of cycle. (X260) (From St. Margaret's Hospital, Boston, A-71-29.)

this case a misnomer, since it is the result of atrophy (Fig. 11-19).

Endometrium during Pregnancy

The endometrium that has nidated a blastocyst does not undergo regression. Instead, a state of intense physiological activity and anatomical differentiation persists at least until rescue of the corpus luteum by the placenta.

At implantation, and for a short time thereafter, support of the endometrial structure and function is derived from a surge of progesterone secretion from the corpus luteum stimulated by the early secretion of trophoblastic human chorionic gonadotropin (hCG) hormone. This is morphologically and biochemically evident by day 24 (2–3 days postimplantation).[82,83] After implantation, the volume of blood supplied to the endometrium expands rapidly,[21] especially at the implantation site.

The metabolic activity of the endometrium is augmented during pregnancy and follows the pattern of the secretory endometrium as evidenced by chemical determinations and histochemical studies.

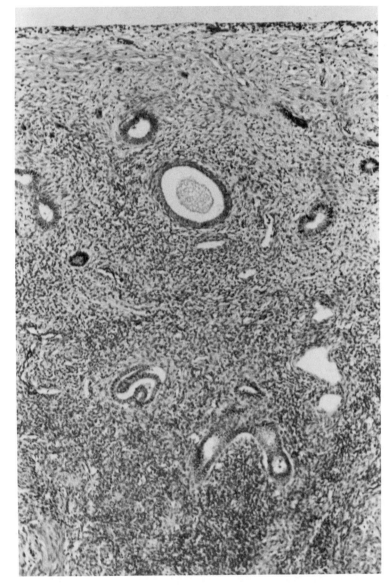

FIGURE 11-19. Senile atrophy, endometrium, full thickness. Glands are sparse and inactive. Stroma, spindle cells near surface, collagenized (X260)

A detailed description of the endometrium during pregnancy follows.

ENDOMETRIAL RESPONSES

The pattern of endometrial responses, and that of the menstrual cycle for that matter, can be modified by variations in the levels, ratios or sequence of estrogen and progesterone, as well as with certain pharmacologic products with either estrogenic or progesteronelike effects. The endometrial responses to such stimuli may be excessive or restrictive and are referred to here as hyperplasia or hypoplasia, respectively.

Endometrial Changes Effected Primarily by Progesterone

Progestational/Gestational Hyperplasia

Noyes et al.[30] demonstrated that in the normal menstrual cycle secretory vacuolization, stromal edema, and predecidual transformation occur se-

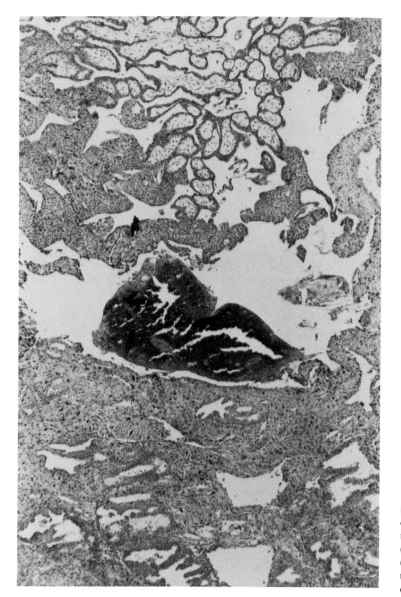

FIGURE 11-20. Implantation site, conceptus, 19 days estimated gestation age. Avascular chorionic villi (above), characteristic hematoma (middle) and endometrium with gestational hyperplasia (below). Numerous placental site giant cells. (X40)

quentially with peaks corresponding to days 17, 22, and 28 of the cycle, respectively. Although there may be slight overlapping of these changes, one is usually dominant at any one designated time. Should secretory vacuolization, stromal edema, and predecidual/decidua significantly overlap, this would indicate a state of heightened activity of the secretory phase endometrium known as progestational hyperplasia.[82] The prototype of progestational hyperplasia is the endometrium associated with normal pregnancy. Progestational hyperplasia

can also be seen in abnormal pregnancies, including ectopic pregnancy, in cases of synchronous multiple corpora lutea and exogenous progesterone administration.

Gestational Hyperplasia (Pregnancy). Gestational hyperplasia is a condition of heightened activity of the secretory phase endometrium induced by pregnancy. Hertig[82] indicated that subtle changes suggestive of pregnancy can be seen in the endometrium by day 21–22 of the cycle, and defini-

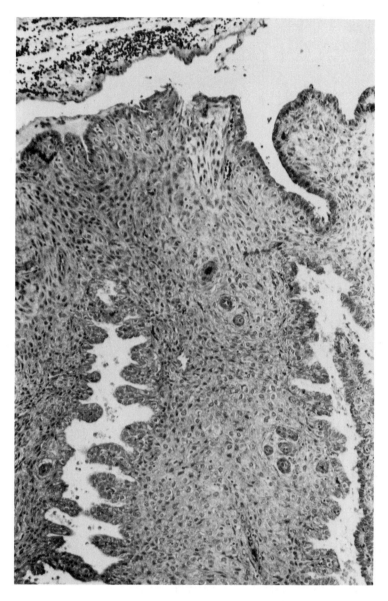

FIGURE 11-21. Same case shown in Figure 11-20, different site. Depicts well-formed decidua, serrated hypersecretory glands, and hypertrophic spiral arterioles. (X104)

tive changes by day 24–25. These changes progress rapidly until a fully developed decidua is formed.

Gestational hyperplasia of the endometrium is characterized by the presence of markedly twisted, serrated, hypersecretory glands and an edematous decidua that by day 28 of the cycle has formed a well-defined compacta layer (Figs. 11-20 through 11-22). The spiral arterioles are hypertrophic to a degree beyond that seen in the normal menstrual cycle; they are congested and lined by hyperplastic endothelium (Fig. 11-21).

Focal atypical epithelial changes (AEC) in some glands can be seen haphazardously distributed in the endometrium; these are better known as the "Arias-Stella" phenomenon,[84,85] (Fig. 11-23). AEC have also been described in the stroma and endocervical epithelium and, quite rarely, in the absence of pregnancy. The AEC is a hormone-dependent polyploidy associated with both normal and abnormal chorionic tissues. The AEC cells are large and protrude into the lumen. The nucleus is large and hyperchromatic.

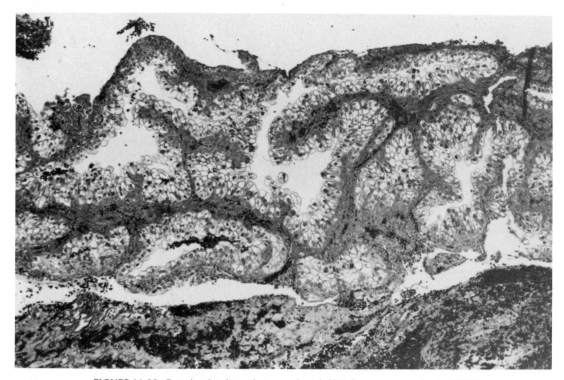

FIGURE 11-22. Gestational endometrium, postabortal. Note hypersecretory glands. (X416)

In curetted material from complications of pregnancy, the pathologist frequently finds trophoblast and other placental elements as absolute evidence of pregnancy, as well as fragments of the Nitabuch layer. At the meeting of the International Society of Gynecologic Pathologists in 1983, Mazur reported the presence of empty nuclei in glandular cells of endometrium associated with choriocarcinoma and hydatidiform moles. This interesting and as yet not understood phenomenon has been seen in our laboratory in material from abortions (Fig. 11-24).

At the implantation site, the decidua and myometrium may contain single or multinucleated giant cells called placental site giant cells (Fig. 11-25A). The nature of these cells has been the subject of considerable controversy. Recently, at least three types of cells have been distinguished by their antigenic localization. Some are positive for hCG and are presumably trophoblast. Others are periodic acid-Schiff (PAS) positive and are probably decidua. A third type positive for actin is suggestive of a myogenic origin (R. V. O'Toole, personal communication). Figure 11-25 depicts several placental site giant cells. One of these shows cytoplasmic cross-striations observed in our laboratory. This finding may have intriguing implications on the pathogenesis of heterologous components in sarcomas and carcinosarcomas of the uterus.

Ectopic Pregnancy. The nature of the endometrium in ectopic pregnancies depends on the quality of the conceptus. Many of the tubal pregnancies are pathological ova and/or are abortive and thus are frequently hormonally insufficient to stimulate a corpus luteum. In a study of 115 cases of ectopic pregnancies, Romney et al.[86] found 30% of endometria in a proliferative phase, 40% in secretory phase, 10% menstrual or regenerating, and 20% with good decidua formation.

At times, patients with ectopic pregnancy may expel a decidual cast that shows microscopic features of progestational hyperplasia without chorionic tissues. These findings may permit the pathologist to alert the clinician of the possibility of an unexpected ectopic pregnancy.

Exogenous Progesterone Administration. Postovulatory administration of progesterone may induce a mild progestational hyperplasia followed by breakthrough bleeding. The cycle may not be sig-

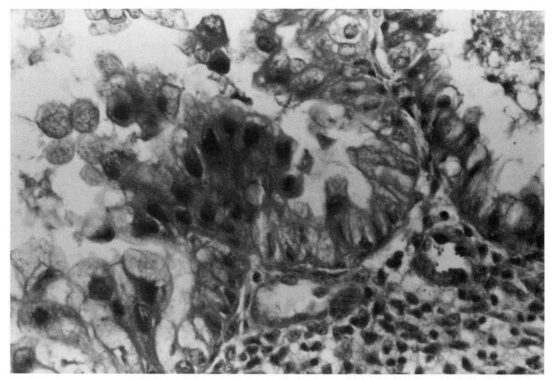

FIGURE 11-23. Gestational endometrium, postabortal. Note atypical epithelial change (AEC, Arias-Stella). (X416)

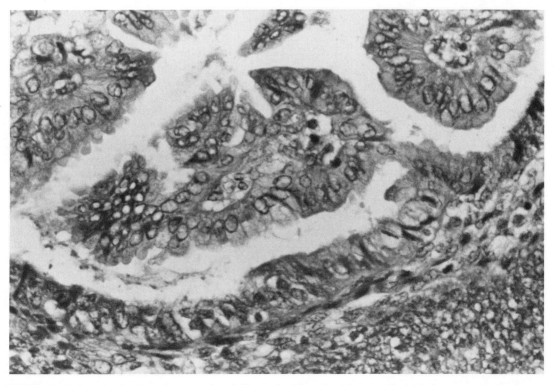

FIGURE 11-24. Gestational endometrium, post abortal. Shows glandular cells with ''empty'' nuclei. Case not previously reported. (X416)

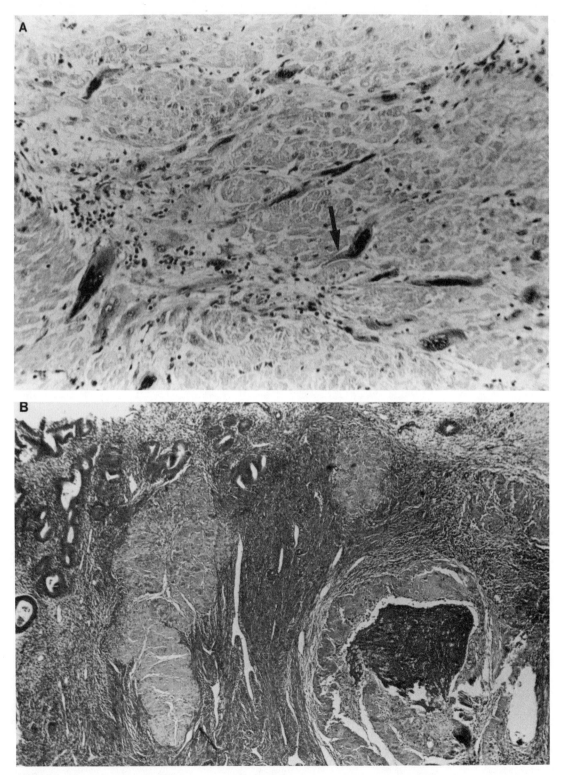

FIGURE 11-25. (A) Placental site giant cells. Cytoplasmic cross-striations are clearly seen in cell located paracentrally, right lower quadrant. These cells are probably the ones that, under proper oncogenic stimulus, may contribute to the heterologous sarcomatous elements of the uterus. See text description. (X416) Case not previously reported. (From St. Margaret's Hospital, Boston, S-58-111-B.) (B) Subinvolution placental site. Involution of decidua and gaping blood vessels (1 month postdelivery). (X104) (Ober and Grady.[155])

nificantly prolonged by progesterone. This is in contrast to the effect by hCG. Long-term progesterone administration may induce atrophy of the endometrium.

If progesterone is given during the proliferative phase, it may inhibit the development of both follicles and ovulation, causing arrest of the proliferative activity. Progesterone given at onset of menstruation may induce irregular shedding.[87] (To readers interested in the subjects of gestational hyperplasia, AEC, and uterine placental relationships refs. 83, 85, and 88 are recommended.)

Progestational Hypoplasia

Luteal-Phase Defect. This syndrome was recognized by Jones in patients whose common denominator was the presence of a deficient corpus luteum and/or an underdeveloped secretory endometrium.[89,90] The etiology of this syndrome is multifactorial. Some cases may reflect a disturbance in the hypothalamic–pituitary axis with hyperprolactinemia. In others the corpus luteum is either small, poorly developed and/or deficient in receptors for gonadotropins. In still others, the endometrium has an altered ratio of receptivity for E_1, E_2, and P. In this regard, Levy et al.[90a] found very low concentrations of E_2R (0.8 pmoles/mg DNA) and P_4R (1.3 pmoles/mg DNA) in luteal-phase defect endometria even lower than in the late secretory endometrium. Daly et al.[90b] correlate the above findings with the lack of, or deficient decidualization in, luteal-phase defect. This in turn accounts for the low prolactin secretion by such endometrium. Paradoxically, many patients with luteal phase defect show hyperprolactinemia.

Dietetic, genetic, and other factors have also been proposed. Whatever the cause, the corpus luteum secretes a low level of progesterone, which at the peak of the secretory phase may not exceed 3 mg/ml of plasma.[91–93]

Recently, it has been suggested that the deficient luteal phase may at times represent an anovulatory cycle in which a deficient corpus luteum may originate from luteinized unruptured follicles.[94] Aluteal cycles have been reported as severe forms of luteal-phase defects.[95]

A properly timed biopsy of the endometrium is perhaps the most efficient diagnostic procedure for luteal-phase defects.[96] A full-thickness biopsy from the uterine fundus should be taken within the first 6 hr of menstruation before the fine anatomical details of the endometrium become distorted (Her-

tig). If this is not possible, biopsy taken late in the late secretory phase would be a second choice.

The anatomical features of the defective luteal-phase endometrium are those of progestational hypoplasia. If menstruation had begun, menstrual changes would be seen in an underdeveloped endometrium such as day 22 or 23 secretory endometrium (Fig. 11-26). The decidua may be absent or insignificant. The glands may be sparse and rounded and contain scanty secretion. If menstruation had not as yet occurred, the endometrium would be markedly underdeveloped. To be significant in infertility, the luteal phase defect should be repetitive in several cycles. Thus, a biopsy should be taken in at least two cycles to establish the diagnosis.

Ablation of the Corpus Luteum. Removal of the corpus luteum will bring about regressive changes of the endometrium. If ablation is performed during the immediate postovulatory period, differentiation of the endometrium is inhibited. At more advanced stages of the secretory phase, regression and menstrual changes will follow. Removal of the corpus luteum in pregnancy during the first 4–6 weeks of gestation may lead to degeneration of the decidua and abortion. Rescue of the corpus luteum by the placenta takes approximately 7–10 days after progesterone secretion by the corpus luteum is under the influence of hCG hormone and without which progesterone secretion cannot be sustained at high levels. This usually takes place at some 5–7 weeks gestation when time placental progesterone reaches a level sufficient to support the endometrium.

Effects of Synthetic and other Exogenous Agents

Clomid (Clomiphene Citrate). This nonsteroidal, nonhormone compound is a member of the triarylethelene substances with estrogen–antiestrogen action. The antiestrogenic action is believed to be mediated at the level of the hypothalamic–pituitary axis, probably by lowering the threshold of the inhibiting influences of estrogens on the axis. This leads to the secretion of gonadotropins followed by induction of ovulation.

The antiestrogenic effect on the endometrium is evidenced by the regressive changes on the proliferative and hyperplastic endometria.[97–99] The estrogenic action of the drug is substantiated by the increased ovarian steroidogenesis and urinary estrogen excretion.

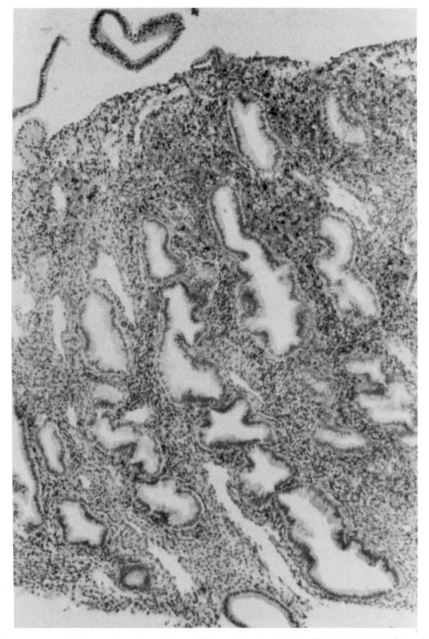

FIGURE 11-26. Luteal-phase defect, endometrium. Menstrual changes in upper portion. Underdeveloped endometrium corresponds to days 22 and 23. (X260) (From St. Margaret's Hospital, Boston, S-72-362.)

The endometrial responses to Clomid depend on the time of administration in the cycle and the endocrine dysfunction or background of the patient. Using Clomid as an ovulatory drug, Kistner obtained best results in patients whose endometria was in a proliferative phase at the time of treatment and poorer responses in patients with atrophic endometrium. When ovulation took place, subsequent biopsies revealed any of the following endometrial types: secretory, atypical secretory, or menstrual. A number of patients failed to ovulate and biopsies indicated either proliferative arrest or atrophic endometrium.[97]

Patients with cystic and adenomatous hyperplasia, anaplasia, or carcinoma in situ (CIS) treated with Clomid frequently reverted to a cycling endometrium, although some of those patients later returned to their original status. It should be noted, however, that nearly 50% of patients with cystic and adenomatous hyperplasia may spontaneously revert to normal cycles coincidentally with the first curettage.

Pergonal or Postmenopausal Gonadotropins. Pergonal is a concentrate of urinary postmenopausal gonadotropins containing 75 IU of both FSH and LH per ampule. It is used primarily as an ovulation inducer. Gonadotropins, whose actions are mediated by the ovary, do not directly modify the structure of the endometrium. If ovulation is induced, a normal menstrual cycle will follow.

Effect of Synthetic Progestagens–Estrogens. Most available progestagens derive from the 19-norsteroids (e.g., Norethynodyel, ethynodiol acetate) and are related to testosterone or 17α-acetoxyprogesterone (e.g., medroxyprogesterone, chloramadione) related to progesterone. The number of products is increasing rapidly.

These compounds are used, either in continuous or cyclical regimens, combined with estrogen primarily for the control of ovulation. They are also used for the treatment of a number of organic and dysfunctional gynecological disorders.

Estrogens are available in multiple forms. Some of the most commonly used are ethynyl estradiol, ethynyl estradiol-3 methyl ether (mestranol), and 17α-dihydroequilin (Premarin).

The effects of these drugs on the endometrium differ with (1) the potency of the compound and duration of treatment, (2) the day of the menstrual cycle when administered, (3) the receptivity of the target organs, (4) the pathological disorder of the recipient, and (5) how the patient metabolizes the drug, rendering products with either estrogenic or androgenic activity.

The pathologist can easily identify endometria influenced by progestational agents given singly or in combinations with estrogen. The identification of the exact type and dosage of drug used, however, requires great expertise.

The response to estrogens is a dose-related proliferation of the glands and stroma. The endometrium responds to progestagens in the form of glandular secretion and/or decidualization in this order in an endometrium properly primed with estrogen. Withdrawal bleeding may follow within a few days after interruption of the medication. A low

dosage progestagen given for several weeks may bring about breakthrough bleeding. With ab initio administration of high dosage of progestagens for long periods of time, the following sequence of events may be observed. First, the initial secretory activity is abolished and the endometrium remains in a state of arrested proliferation. This is followed by atrophy of glands in the midst of a markedly decidualized stroma, or secretory arrest. Finally, there is complete atrophy of glands and then of stroma. Different progestagens induce different morphological changes. With derivatives of 19-norsteroids, there is a greater decidualization. Electron microscopic examination shows that the nucleolar channel system does not appear and that the apical surface of the secretory glandular cell is smooth. There is also a preponderance of stroma over glandular ratio, and atrophy occurs more rapidly. While derivatives of progesterone primarily influence the glands, the stromal DNA increases as the ER and Golgi enlarge. Sometimes, a breakthrough decidual cast may be shed. Stromal hemorrhages may account for breakthrough bleeding. Long-term treatment may readily render endometrium refractory to further stimulus by progestagens. Atrophy of the stroma follows a prolonged decidualization.[52]

In 1966, Ober[100] summarized the morphology of the endometrium under progestagen or progestagen–estrogen (P/PS) influence in the following manner: 19-norsteroids in high to mid-dosage in continuous or cyclic combined regimens produce an endometrium with hyperinvoluted glands, conspicuous predecidual reaction, suppressed spiral arterioles, and a marked dilatation of venules. At a daily dosage of ≤ 2.0 mg (low) the glands are involuted and the spiral arterioles suppressed, but the decidual reaction is infrequent and weak and the venules are mildly, if at all, dilated. 19-Norsteroids at medium dosage given for 20 days without added estrogen render a late secretory endometrium with marked variation not only from site to site within the same endometrium, but from person to person as well.

17α-Acetoxyprogesterone derivatives at high and medium dosage given in a cyclic combined regimen with estrogen produces similar results to the 19-norsteroid but less intense. When given sequentially, it produces an early secretory endometrium resembling the normal endometrium but chronologically retarded by as much as 5 days. Predecidual response is minimal and dilation of venules is inconstant (approximately 20–25%).[100] Similar observations were reported using Mes-

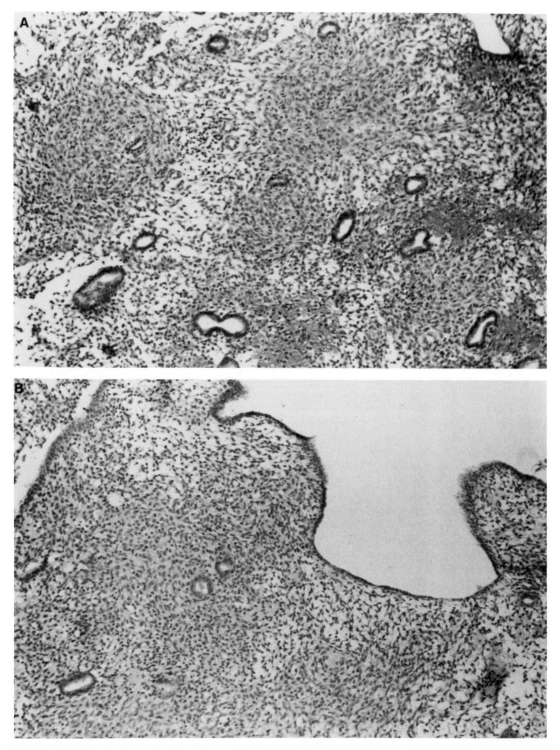

FIGURE 11-27. Long-term progestagen response, endometrium (Ovulen). (A) Patchy stromal decidualization, glands arrested and/or atrophic, and spiral arterioles are inconspicuous. (X104) (From University of Illinois, Chicago, S-84-1972.) (B) Irregularities of surface. (X104) (C) Discordant responses, decidualization of stroma, glandular arrest. Note dissolution of lower decidua, suggesting mechanism of decidual cast shedding. Breakthrough bleeding has occurred. (X104)

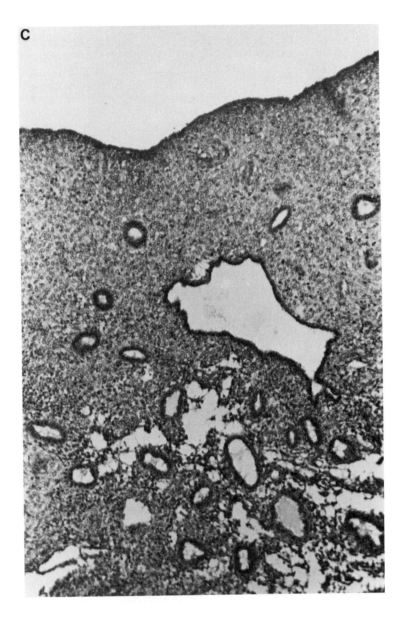

FIGURE 11-27. (*Continued*)

tranol, 80 μg/day × 20 with added chlormadinone 2 mg/day during the last 5 days of estrogen treatment.[101]

With nearly all combinations of P/PS regimens, the common denominator is the inhibition of the development of the spiral arterioles. This change probably accounts for the modification in morphology of the vascular and stromal elements of the endometrium.

Long-Term Combination Regimens. Again, with nearly all long-term combination regimens, the pro-

liferative phases are progressively shortened. As a consequence, the glands and stroma eventually develop poorly and irregularly. It appears that the endometrium needs a sufficient preparatory estrogenic stimulus of 14 days or longer for proper secretory differentiation. Since this does not happen in long-term combined regimens, the secretory endometrium that follows a poorly developed proliferative endometrium is itself equally poor.

The added effect of discordant glandular and stromal growth to the haphazardously distributed islands of predecidua give irregularity in thickness and surface to the endometrium (Fig. 11-27A,B). Irregularities of the surface are magnified by the polypoid excrescencies, cracks, and defective cilioneogenesis of the epithelium so neatly described by SEM.[102] Under the surface of the endometrium, one may observe congestion and stromal hemorrhages. These may be responsible for the breakthrough hemorrhages, which at times can be protracted requiring curettage of the endometrium (Fig. 11-27C).

Long-term sequential regimens will rarely produce atrophy of the endometrium. In fact, patients have been followed for years without untoward effects. With some frequency, however, the estrogenic effect prevails over the progestagen, inducing hyperplastic changes of the endometrium which are mild in approximately 50% and severe in 13%. Silverberg and Makowski[103] called attention to adenocarcinoma appearing in young women taking oral contraceptives. Figure 11-42A–D depicts one such case seen in our laboratories. (Additional information on the chemical changes, histochemistry, electron microscopy, and the mechanism of action of the progestagens on the endometrium, can be obtained from refs. 74, 102, 102a, 104–107.)

Endometrial Changes Primarily Effected by Estrogen

Anovulatory Cycle. The anovulatory cycle is a hypothalamic–pituitary axis controlled estrogenic-influenced monophasic cycle, resulting from failure of LH surge and consequent failure of ovulation. Anovulatory cycles can occur as isolated or repetitive events more commonly occurring at either menarche or menopause.

The length of the anovulatory cycle is governed by the duration and activity of the ovarian follicle before undergoing atresia. The cycles end by withdrawal bleeding shortly after the decline in estrogens.

Morphologically, the anovulatory cycle is recognized by the presence of a proliferative endometrium during the entire length of the cycle. Secretory activity is absent. Other parameters can aid in the diagnosis, such as the presence of keratinization in the vaginal cytology and a monophasic temperature chart.

The degree of proliferation of the endometrium reflects the degree of estrogenic levels. Thus, features of early, mid-, and late proliferative endometrium can be seen in different endometria.

Sedlis and Kim[108] reported a thick band of sub-epithelial collagen or basement membrane in a number of anovulatory endometria (17%). This inconstant feature, when clearly evidenced, can be of diagnostic value. Later in the anovulatory cycle, the endometrium differs from the normal late proliferative endometrium in some of its enzymatic patterns. For instance, the alkaline phosphatase disappears, while the acid phosphatase increases. This pattern is not seen in the normal proliferative endometrium.

The diagnosis of an anovulatory cycle can be best made in curettage material taken at the time of bleeding. The coexistence of "menstrual changes" with a proliferative endometrium establishes the diagnosis. The so-called "menstrual changes" in a proliferative endometrium differ from the normal menstrual endometrium. In the former there are thromboses of sinuses and venules associated with infarct necrosis. However, there may also be some dissociation of the tissues as well (Fig. 11-28).

Dallenbach-Hellweg[52] indicated that stromal granulocytes are not present in the anovulatory endometrium; thus, the lytic enzymes are not operable in the anovulatory bleeding. However, lytic enzymes can be derived from broken polymorphonuclear leukocytes present in the area of necrosis.

When the factors responsible for anovulation cease, the endometrium may revert to normal ovulatory cycles. On the other hand, when follicles enlarge and continue secreting estrogens for awhile longer, the endometrium may turn hyperplastic for at least as long as the excessive stimulus persists.

Endometrial Hyperplasia. Endometrial hyperplasia is a common abnormal proliferative condition resulting from long-standing estrogenic or estrogenic-like stimulus unopposed by progesterone. The disorder is disabling because of metrorrhagic tendencies and carries a high risk at cancer. The relationship of hyperplasia to estrogens is well documented, for it has been induced both experimentally[109–111] and clinically.[97]

The association between estrogen-producing lesions of the gonads, such as follicular cysts, polycystic ovaries, ovarian stromal hyperplasias and neoplasias, and hyperplasia of the endometrium is well known. Endometrial hyperplasia may also develop in some patients with adrenal gland disorders and liver disease. Digitalis, diethylstilbestrol (DES), and other nonsteroidal drugs may stimulate the endometrium in an estrogenlike manner.

The degree of hyperplasia may vary widely from

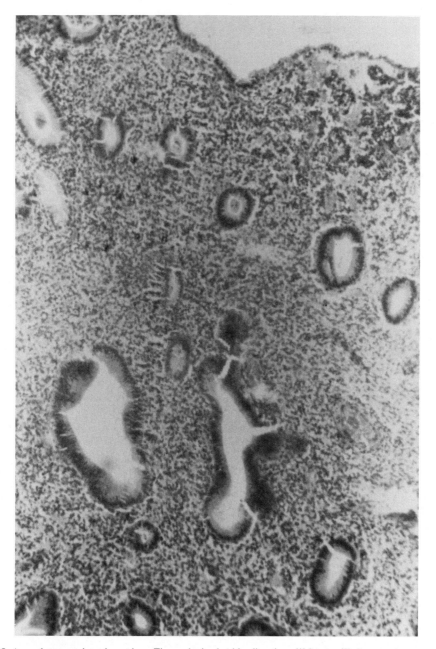

FIGURE 11-28. Anovulatory cycle endometrium. Tissue obtained at bleeding time. "Menstrual" changes seen upper right. Some hyperplastic changes of glands. (X260)

mild and focal to diffuse and severe. It can be so severe that it merges imperceptibly with carcinoma in a "continuum from hyperplasia to carcinoma."[112] A classification based on severity and anatomical patterns used by Hertig is as follows: (1) cystic hyperplasia, (2) cystic and/or adenomatous hyperplasia, (3) cystic and/or adenomatous hyperplasia with anaplasia (dysplasia), and (4) carcinoma in situ.

Unless otherwise specified, all hyperplasias share with the normal proliferative endometrium, histocytomorphometry, estrogen and progesterone receptor contents, histochemistry[51] (see Plate 11-2 following page 200), TEM, and SEM.[74,75]

Cystic Hyperplasia. Cystic hyperplasia represents a mild form or perhaps an initial step in the spectrum of hyperplasias. The glands are spherically dilated and lined by tall or cuboidal pseudostratified epithelium. The number of glands may be increased in proportion to the severity of the lesion. Mitoses are seen, but their numbers may not be significant factors. Although the endometrial stroma is usually mildly hyperplastic as well, the prominence of the dilated glands overshadows the stromal changes. Cystic hyperplasia is also known as cystic glandular hyperplasia. The mechanism for the cystic dilation is unknown. Histogenesis has been related to either obstruction of the glands or asynchronism between glandular and stromal growth.

The term of cystic hyperplasia is often applied to the cystic atrophic glands seen in postmenopausal patients who, preceding menopause, had either a series of anovulatory cycles or a mild cystic hyperplasia. A more appropriate name is regressive hyperplasia, given by Novak and Woodruff.[113]

Cystic and/or adenomatous hyperplasia. These terms are given to more severe and complex patterns of hyperplasias. The glands branch off at different levels like fingers or radiate from the main gland. Because of their tortuosity, the glands may appear as ''back to back.'' Some of the branches may pinch off of the main gland forming secondary glands (Figs. 11-29 through 31). One of these patterns designated by Gore as Hertig type consists of cystic gland(s) associated with numerous small ones clustered about the mother gland.[114,115] Hertig-type adenomatous hyperplasia was described in curettage material of patients who subsequently developed carcinoma.[116]

These crowded compact glands are similar to those that compelled Halban to his famous pronouncement, *Nicht ein Karzinom aber besser heraus* (not a carcinoma, but better out), and to Meyer's adenoma malignum.

Cystic and/or adenomatous hyperplasia with anaplasia (dysplasia) and carcinoma in situ. Cystic and/or adenomatous hyperplasia with anaplasia is a more complex pattern of hyperplasia with an added degree of dedifferentiation. The anaplastic glands may be irregular, pale, or acidophilic. The epithelial cells have irregular nuclei. On occasions, the anaplastic glands are distinctly acidophilic, tall and irregular. Their large nuclei have irregular membranes, dispersed fine granular chromatin and prominent nucleoli. Small papillary buds may be present and project into the lumen. These glands correspond to the classical Hertig-type adenocarcinoma in situ described by Hertig et al.[115–117] These glands are truly anaplastic, as they express a deranged histochemical pattern corresponding to the secretory rather than proliferative endometrium.[51] Other in situ forms corresponding to the different varieties of endometrial adenocarcinomas have also been recognized.[114,115] Abell listed six forms of adenocarcinoma in situ as follows: the classical Hertig type, cribriform, acanthoid (adenoacanthoma), secretory, papillary, and mesonephroid (clear cell)[118] (Figs. 11-32, 11-33).

Adenocarcinoma in situ of the endometrium is a controversial entity. The author has elected to describe this entity under hyperplasias in order to emphasize a conservative therapy. The difficulty in making a diagnosis of adenocarcinoma in situ is discussed by Abell.[118] In his study of 89 cases diagnosed by curettage, 17 demonstrated no atypicality following hysterectomy, and 11 others were already invasive. Kurman and Norris[119] indicated that the only reliable criterion of malignancy is invasion of the endometrial stroma. Adenocarcinoma in situ should not be confused with the occasional focus of secretory activity occasionally seen in hyperplastic endometria or with tubal metaplasia. Evidence of stromal invasion should disqualify the lesion from the in situ category.

Cystic and/or adenomatous hyperplasia of the endometrium and CIS correspond to some of the atypical hyperplasias type 2 and 3 of Campbell and Barter,[120] and to some of the moderate to severe adenomatous hyperplasias and carcinoma stage 0 of Gusberg and Kaplan[121] and Gusberg.[122]

Hyperplasias of the endometrium are common disabling metrorrhagic disorders that carry a significant risk of malignant progression or transformation. The protracted bleeding in these patients is due to thrombosis of endometrial sinuses and venules with microinfarcts (Fig. 11-29A) These lesions are fundamentally similar to those in cycling anovulatory bleeding but are more severe.

The frequency of malignant progression correlates well with the degree and complexity of the hyperplastic pattern. This is lower in patients with plain cystic hyperplasia and much greater in cystic and adenomatous hyperplasia with anaplasia. This has been demonstrated in retrospective studies[123,124] in prospective studies[121] and in studies of the uninvolved endometrium at hysterectomy of pa-

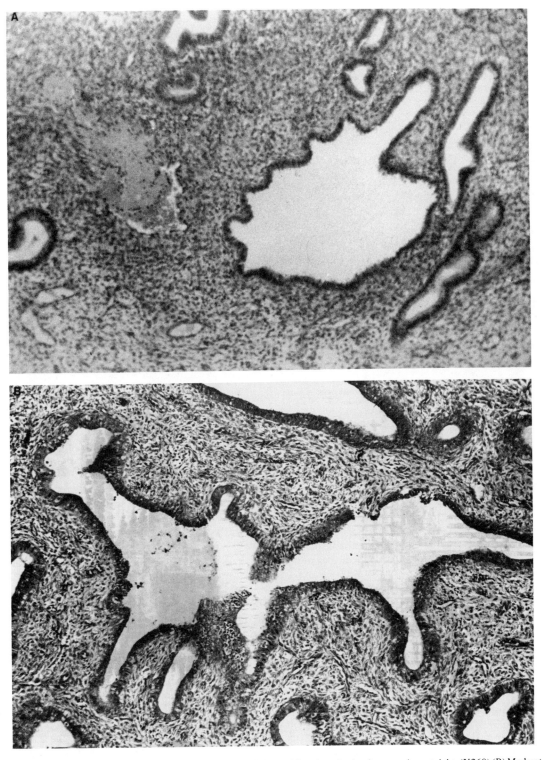

FIGURE 11-29. Cystic and adenomatous hyperplasia. (A) Mild case. Note thrombosis of venous sinus at right. (X260) (B) Moderate case. Note glandular fingerlike projections. (X104)

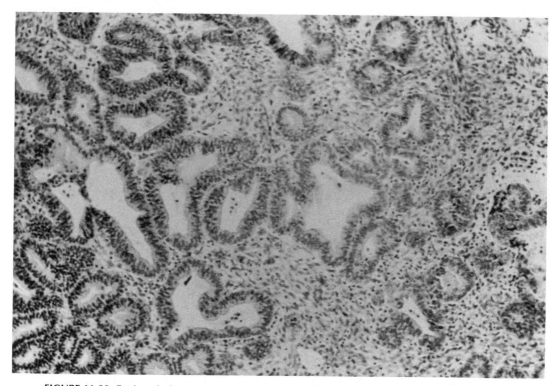

FIGURE 11-30. Cystic and adenomatous hyperplasia, severe. Glands are cystic, crowded, and irregular. (X260)

tients with carcinoma.[125] The association of adenocarcinoma to endometrial hyperplasia was found to be 15%, 24%, and 45% in hyperplasias type I, II, and III, respectively.[120]

Hyperplasia of endometrial stroma. Isolated hyperplasia of endometrial stroma is an extremely rare condition (Fig. 11-34). We have seen a case of marked stromal hyperplasia and sarcoma associated with osteoid formation in a 24-year-old obese patient receiving a high dose of Provera for sleep apnea (Fig. 11-42A–F). This patient developed, in association with the stromal change, a well-differentiated adenocarcinoma.

OTHER DYSFUNCTIONAL BLEEDING SYNDROMES

Asherman's Syndrome

In 1948, Asherman[126] described a syndrome of obstructive amenorrhea from cervical stenosis due to a previous trauma that he called amenorrhea traumatica. Resumption of menstruation, in these pa-

tients, followed corrective cervical dilatation and endometrial curettage.

The characteristic lesions in Asherman's syndrome are endometrial synechiae and, at times, hematometra. Synechiae result when healing and bridging takes place between two contacting opposite sides of the endometrium, having been previously destroyed by a vigorous curettage or by a severe inflammatory process. In either case, the basalis must also be affected for synechiae to be formed. The microscopic diagnosis can be made only when the bridging scar tissue and/or myometrium is included in the specimen and in the light of a good clinical history. Asherman's syndrome should become less common with the advent of the aspirate biopsy procedure (vabra) currently in vogue,

We had the opportunity to study a case at St. Margaret's Hospital, Boston, a possible variant of Asherman's syndrome with congenital connotations. The cross section of the uterus at the level of the internal os showed obstruction of the canal by endometrium whose glands gave a histological sievelike appearance.

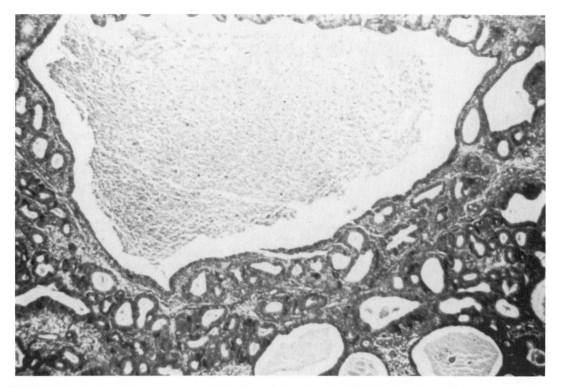

FIGURE 11-31. Cystic and adenomatous hyperplasia with anaplasia, severe. Probably already carcinoma. This case was associated with 1.0 cm thecoma in one ovary. (X260) (From St. Margaret's Hospital, Boston, S-69-605.)

Irregular Shedding

This dysfunctional uterine bleeding syndrome is clinically characterized by a prolonged menstruation (7–14 days or longer), elevated urinary pregnandiol excretion during menstruation, and an endometrium, which when sampled at an appropriate time, shows features of premenstrual, menstrual, and proliferative phase endometria[127] (Fig. 11-35).

The anatomical diagnosis is difficult to make without a clinical history and properly timed endometrial curettage. This should be done some 5–7 days after initiation of menses; otherwise, the endometrium may have an entirely normal appearance.

Irregular shedding has been associated with abnormal persistent progesterone stimulus of the endometrium at about the time of menstruation. In fact, it has been induced experimentally in normal women with progesterone administered at the onset of bleeding.[87] Among the clinical conditions responsible for persistent progesterone stimulus are persistently active corpus luteum, cystic or otherwise, multiple spontaneous or induced corpora lutea, retained placental tissues from abortions, and normal or ectopic pregnancies. Irregular shedding has also been observed in association with submucosal leiomyomas, polyps, and postabortal subinvolution of the placental site.[87,127]

Dallenbach-Hellweg[52] attributes tissue changes or lack thereof to progesterone influenced failure of relaxin release from granulocytes. The basic pathophysiological defect results from the asynchronous shedding and involution of the menstrual endometrium resulting in endometrial patches at variance with the phase. Thus, at 5 days into the menstrual period, premenstrual, menstrual, and proliferative endometria are observed, with the latter resulting from areas of earlier menstruation, involution, and regeneration. Some areas with inadequate involution may show characteristic star-shaped glands surrounded by shrunken stroma condensed around the glands. Eventually, the entire endometrium undergoes proliferation and the cycle proceeds as usual. Curettage in some of these patients may not only be diagnostic, but may render therapeutic benefits.

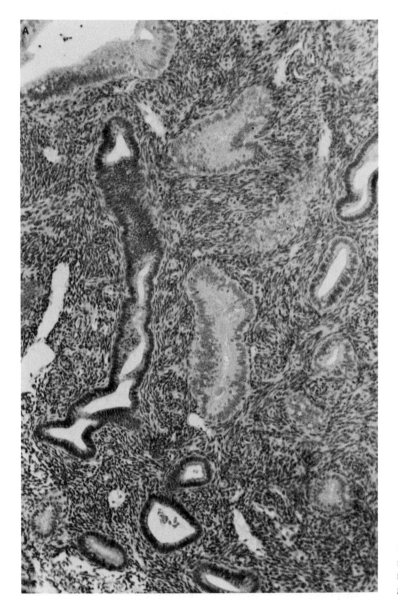

FIGURE 11-32. Adenocarcinoma in situ, Hertig type. Pale glands are surrounded by basophilic proliferative glands. (A) (X104) (B) (X260)

Membranous Dysmenorrhea

Some investigators consider this condition a variant of irregular shedding. As its name implies, it is associated with pain during menstruation. The patients discharge the whole endometrium in the form of a decidual cast or in fragments thereof. Again, like irregular shedding, the endometrium in membranous dysmenorrhea is secretory. These changes can be seen extending to and including the basalis. Pain may be related to the involvement of nerve endings by the abnormal menstrual period.

ORGANIC PATHOLOGY

Endometritis

The endometrium can be affected by a multitude of agents eliciting acute, chronic and/or granulomatous inflammation. The infections may follow ascending, descending, or hematogenous pathways or may be implanted during manipulations. Acute and chronic physiological endometritis occurs normally in each menstrual cycle and every pregnancy. Other common nonspecific chronic in-

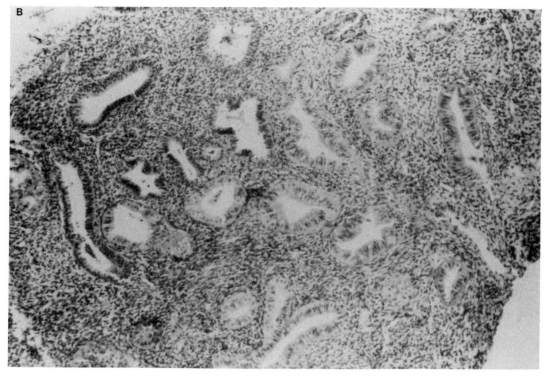

FIGURE 11-32. (*Continued*)

flammatory conditions associated with myomas or hemorrhages are recognized by the presence of mild plasma cell infiltrates. The clinical significance of these is at best controversial. For the pathologist, however, all specific and nonspecific endometritides are important, inasmuch as they alter the endocrine responses of the target organ, making the dating of the endometrium unreliable, if not impossible. It is our practice not to date endometria so affected. Curettage of the endometrium will often resolve the problem.

More important is the inflammation induced specifically by physical or physicochemical agents (irradiation, IUD, radiodiagnostic materials) and infections (viral, bacterial, fungal, or parasitic), and inflammation associated with neoplasms. The type and severity of the inflammatory response depend on the pathogenic agent, its virulence, and the susceptibility and defenses of the host. Acute endometritis can be produced by microorganisms from the vaginal flora gaining access to the endometrium during complications of puerperium, abortions and manipulations of pregnancy. Among numerous other pyogenic agents, gonococcus also can induce acute endometritis. However, acute gonococcal endometritis, relative to gonococcal salpingitis, is

usually mild. It seems as though the *Gonococcus* licks the endometrium and bites the fallopian tube.

In acute endometritis, whatever its cause, numerous polymorphonuclear leukocytes infiltrate glands and stroma associated with abscesses and necrosis. As the process becomes chronic, lymphocytes and plasma cells are attracted to the sites of inflammation. Thrombophlebitis of small venules may take place, produce septic emboli, and spread the infection to other pelvic organs (e.g., cause PID) and to distant sites.

The gynecologist must be alerted to the possibility of severe clostridium infections that may rarely complicate pregnancy with dramatic consequences if not promptly identified and treated. This necrotizing and hemolyzing infection may kill the patient in a matter of a few days. With the introduction of the IUD in gynecological practice, as well as immunosuppressive therapy, a series of unusual infections and infestations by opportunistic microorganisms are being reported.[128-131]

Chronic granulomatous inflammation may be seen as a response to foreign bodies in tuberculosis and sarcoidosis. Tuberculosis of the endometrium is rarely seen in the United States, since it more frequently follows a bovine tubercle bacillus infec-

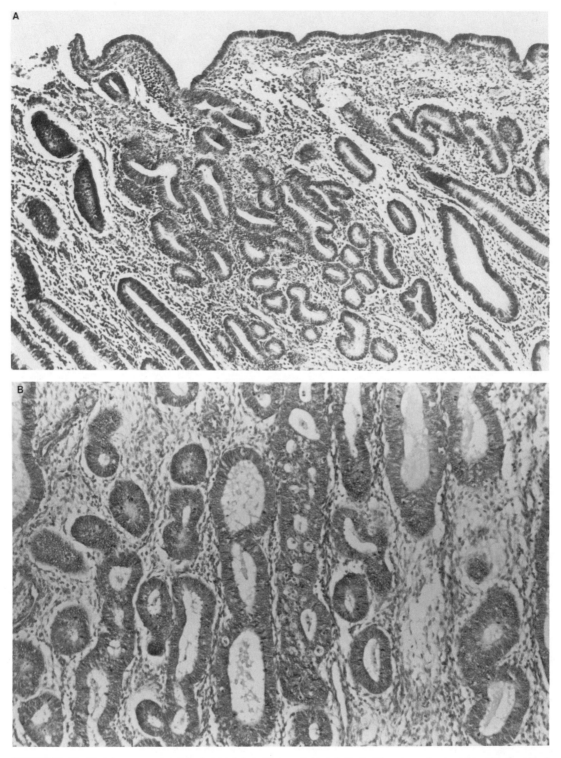

FIGURE 11-33. (A) Adenomatous hyperplasia (glandular). Cluster of glands is flanked by apparently normal proliferative glands. (X104) (B) Same case. Adenocarcinoma in situ, cribriform pattern. Photograph taken just below toward the basalis. (X104) (C) Same

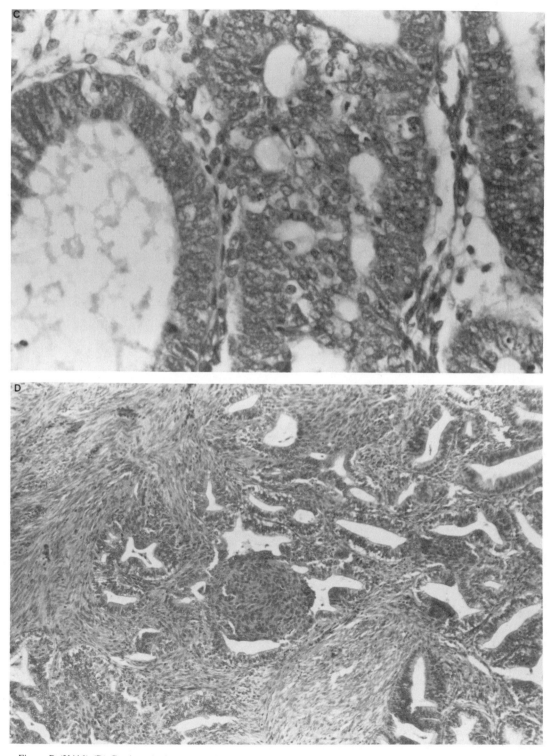

as Figure B (X416) (D) Cystic and adenomatous hyperplasia with a squamous morula at center. This case could be considered an adenocanthoma in situ (controversial). (X104)

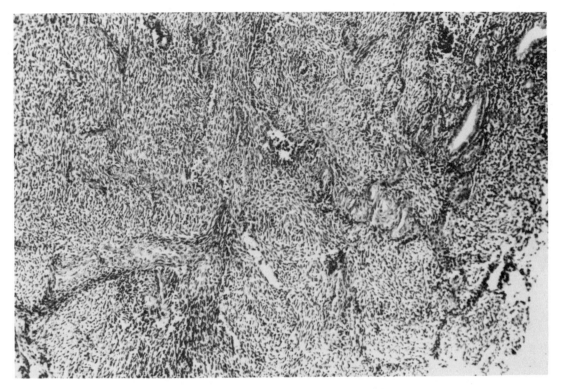

FIGURE 11-34. Stromal hyperplasia, pure. (X104)

tion. It is occasionally seen in immigrants from countries in which unpasteurized milk is consumed. Histologically, the disease is characterized by caseating granulomas or Köster follicles. Epithelioid cell reaction with or without giant cells associated with lymphocytic infiltration is seen (Fig. 11-36). Tubercle bacillus should be demonstrated by special stains, cultures, and innoculation into susceptible animals. Not all granulomas are tuberculous in nature.

The disease is usually descending from a peritoneal or salpingeal focus. Granulomas shed with the menstrual endometrium. Since it takes at least 7 days for a tubercle to develop, it is advisable to time the diagnostic curettage of suspected patients at least 7 days, preferably longer, after cessation of menses.

Endometrial Metaplasias

Epithelial metaplasias of the endometrium are relatively common. Squamous metaplasia is frequently seen in adenocarcinomas and also in noncycling endometrium of young women with various ovarian abnormalities. Tubal metaplasia is another common occurrence in the noncycling endometrium, as is mucus metaplasia.

Stromal metaplasias such as bony and cartilaginous are rare.[132] They also occur in association with malignancies, such as sarcomas with heterologous components. More infrequently they may be seen in nonmalignant forms, such as prolonged progestin administration and remote sequelae of abortions.

Adenomatous Polyps

During routine examination of uteri, one finds on occasions, in an otherwise normal endometrium, an intramural focus of cystic and/or adenomatous hyperplasia apparently emerging from the basalis. This type of lesion may represent either a developing or an incipient polyp. The cause of this lesion, as in endometrial polyps, is unknown, nor is their fate known. Its focal nature argues against a generalized endocrinopathy.

Fully developed polyps are common, may be pedunculated or sessile, single or multiple, and may

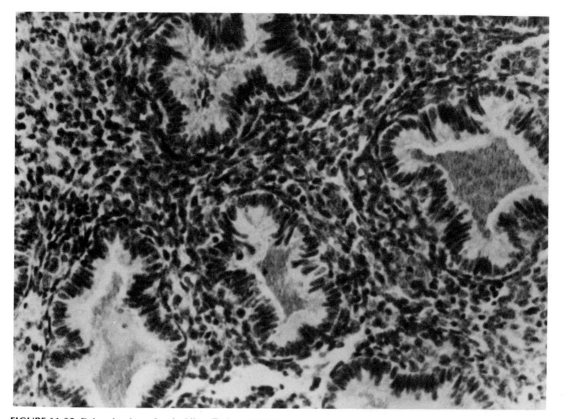

FIGURE 11-35. Delayed or irregular shedding. Endometrial biopsy taken on fifth day of cycle. Note irregular contour glands, tall columnar epithelium and inspissated luminal secretion. Hematoxylin and eosin. (X250) (From Abell.[50])

range from a few millimeters to 2 cm in maximum diameter. They are more common at the fundus, particularly at the cornual areas. Microscopically, polyps characteristically show a conjury of thick blood vessels extending from the pedicle or base toward the center of the lesion. The glandular and stromal elements may be nearly normal and functional, or they may be nonfunctional, revealing any of the pathological varieties, including cystic and/or adenomatous hyperplasia and even, on occasion, a carcinoma (Fig. 11-37). Endometrial polyps are better recognized in specimens obtained by sharp curettage. The vabra aspiration procedure is notoriously inadequate for sampling polyps.

Carcinoma

Carcinoma of the endometrium is the most common malignant neoplasia of the female genital tract. Its frequency in recent years has surpassed that of the uterine cervix. In the United States, the ex-

pected number of new cases per annum approximates 27,000, with 3000 expected deaths. Patients in the sixth decade are at higher risk. The etiology of endometrial carcinoma is unknown. However, since it is preceded by endometrial hyperplasia in a large number of cases, the role of prolonged noncyclical estrogenic states, as in hyperplasias, must also play an important role in carcinoma.[103,111,133–137] Additional risk factors are endocrinopathies (diabetes mellitus), obesity, hypertension, nulliparity, and genetic predisposition.

Grossly, carcinomas may be diffuse and superficial (cases related to high estrogen intake), polypoid and friable, or ulcerative and infiltrating. Their most common site is the fundus, but it may occur anywhere in the endometrium.

Several microscopic varieties are described, namely (1) adenocarcinoma, (2) adenoacanthoma, (3) adenosquamous, (4) pure squamous, (5) secretory carcinoma, (6) papillary, (7) serous papillary, (8) clear cell carcinoma, (9) mucinous, and

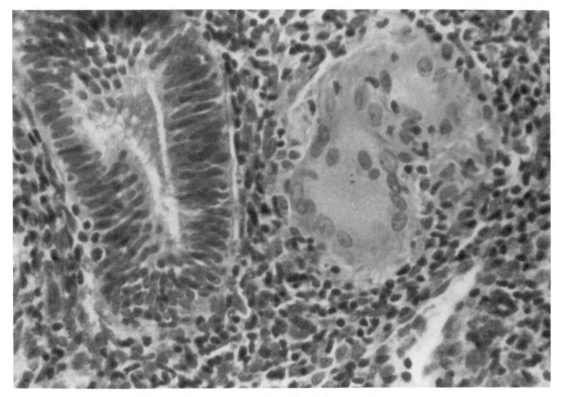

FIGURE 11-36. Granulomatous endometritis. Patient had tuberculosis. (X416)

(10) mixed carcinoma with a variety of sarcomatous components.

Adenocarcinoma

Adenocarcinoma is the most common malignant tumor of the endometrium. The tumor differentiates into well-formed or bizarre-shaped glands (Figs. 11-33a and 11-38). Foci of squamous metaplasia are extremely common. When the squamous components are well differentiated, the tumor is called adenoacanthoma (Fig. 11-42B) and when poorly differentiated, adenosquamous carcinoma.[138,139] Pure squamous carcinoma arising de novo in the endometrium is extremely rare. More often it is associated with cervical stenosis and pyometra. Figure 11-39 depicts a case of squamous cell CIS in the endometrium extending from the cervix and covering the entire surface of the endometrium.

It is our experience that the degree of anaplasia of the squamous epithelium parallels the grade of the glandular component and that the prognosis depends on the grade and stage of the tumor, irrespective of the presence or absence of the squamous elements.[135]

Well-differentiated adenocarcinomas may rarely show evidence of secretory activity. At times, this recapitulates the appearance of the day-17 endometrium so closely that it requires an alert and experienced pathologist to make the proper diagnosis. This variant is called secretory adenocarcinoma (Fig. 11-42D,E).

The occurence of a well-differentiated tumor secreting copious amounts of mucus constitutes a mucinous adenocarcinoma. This tumor often makes the differential diagnosis between endocervical and endometrial carcinoma in curettage material difficult, even if histochemical and immunochemical stains are used. The relative frequency of this variety is approximately 5%.

Papillary Carcinoma

This variety comprises approximately 10% of malignant epithelial neoplasias of the endometrium. As its name implies, the tumor organizes

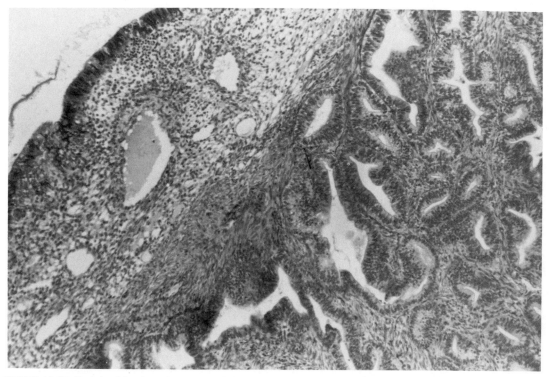

FIGURE 11-37. Endometrial polyp with adenocarcinoma. Note well-differentiated adenocarcinoma extending to nonmalignant endometrium. (X104)

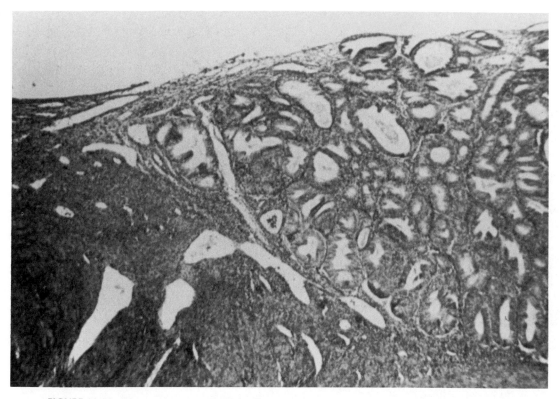

FIGURE 11-38. Adenocarcinoma, well differentiated. Neoplasia seen at right of a senile endometrium. (X260)

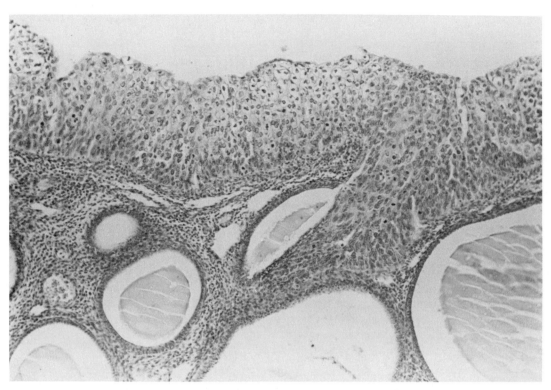

FIGURE 11-39. Squamous cell carcinoma in situ, endometrium. Malignant squamous epithelium (malignant icthyosis) lining the entire endometrial cavity. Tumor originated from a similar lesion in the cervix. (X104) (From St. Bernard's Hospital, Chicago, S-84-166. Courtesy of Dr. K. Karachorlu.)

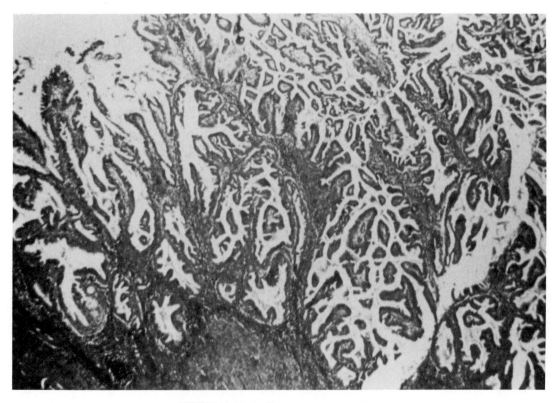

FIGURE 11-40. Papillary carcinoma. (X260)

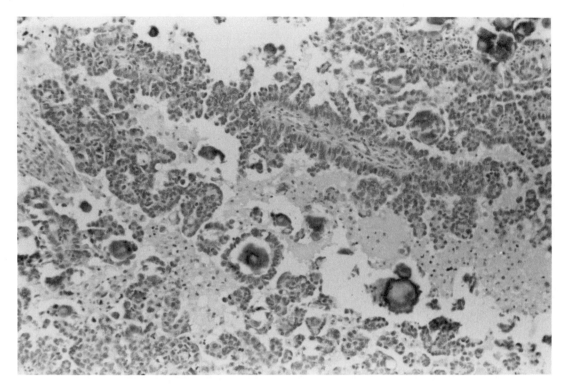

FIGURE 11-41. Papillary serous carcinoma with psammoma bodies. (X104)

in fronds supported by a thin vascular stroma (Fig. 11-40).

One subvariety of papillary carcinoma associated with psammoma bodies has been described. This tumor bears a striking microscopic similarity to the ovarian papillary serous carcinoma and carries a grave prognostic value equivalent to a grade III carcinoma[140,141] (Fig. 11-41).

The clear cell carcinoma, or mesonephroid, was formerly believed to derive from mesonephric rests. It is composed of uniform cuboidal cells with large, clear, glycogen-rich cytoplasm. Their nuclei sometimes protrude under the membrane in a hobnail appearance. This tumor carries a high-grade prognosis.

Adenocarcinomas may arise in or involve endometrial polyps (Fig. 11-37).

All the varieties of carcinomas described above can be seen in pure or mixed forms in variable proportions reflecting the totipotentiality of the mullerian tissue that originates them (Fig. 11-42).

Prognosis in general is directly related to the grade and stage of the tumor. Carcinomas are graded, depending on the degree of cellular atypia, rate of growth, patterns, and ratios of solid to non-solid growth as: moderately, poorly differentiated,

and undifferentiated (according to Broders) or as I, II, and III (according to FIGO). Determination of estrogen and progesterone receptors on these tumors may be a useful guide to therapy.[57]

Histochemical studies of endometrial carcinomas have not revealed any consistent pattern. In fact, there is no consistency even within different areas of the same tumor. On occasion, some tumors recapitulate the histochemical pattern of the secretory endometrium. Because of this, the progesterone role in pathogenesis of the tumors has been suggested.[51] These findings are at best inconstant and are therefore controversial.

Localization of carcinoembryonic antigen (CEA) may be useful in differentiating endometrial from endocervical carcinoma. The latter shows nearly 100% positivity, while CEA positivity in the former ranges from 0 to 30% in most studies, although some authors have found it to be as high as 60%.

Although TEM and SEM have been magnificent tools in broadening our knowledge of the normal and malignant endometrial tissues, they have not proved useful practical tools in the diagnosis of endometrial malignancies. They do show the bizarre shapes and types of growth that characterize these malignancies.

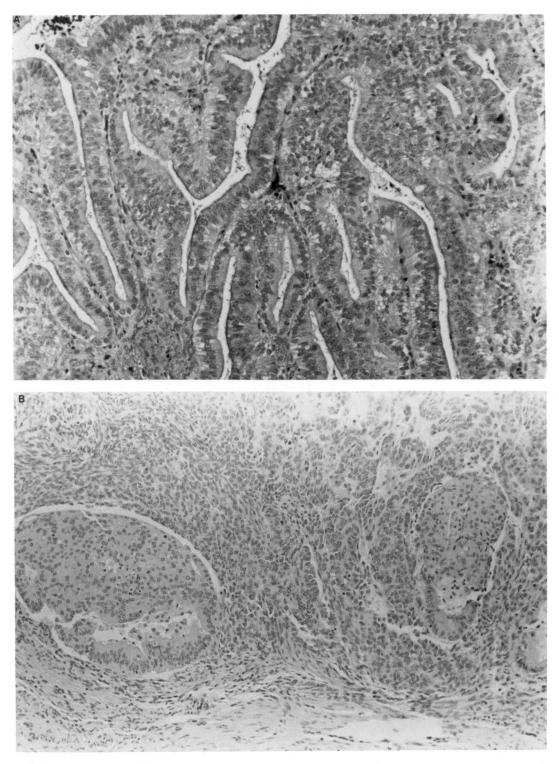

FIGURE 11-42. Tissue curetted from a 24-year-old obese woman with metrorrhagia taking Provera on a long-term basis, showing multiple patterns of malignancy: (A) Adenocarcinoma, well-differentiated, some secretory vacuoles. (X416) (B) Adenoacanthoma (X104) (C) Papillary pattern. (X104) (D) Secretory pattern. (X416) (E) Secretory pattern (observe mitosis in gland left lower corner)

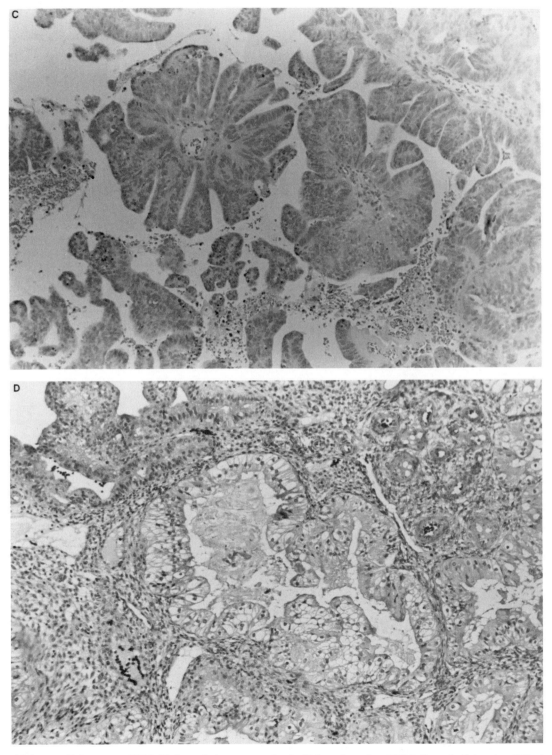

with foamy cells in stroma. (X416) (F) Stromal sarcoma, associated with bone formation. (X104) (From the University of Illinois, Chicago, S-83-8497.)

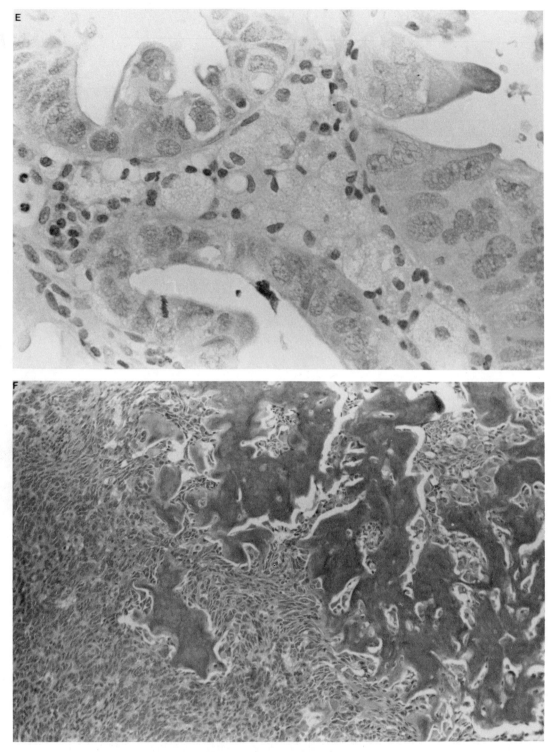

FIGURE 11-42. *(Continued)*

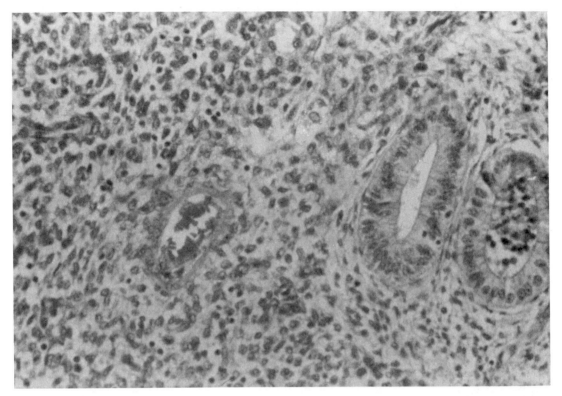

FIGURE 11-43. Endometrial stromal sarcoma. Sarcoma, left side, encroaching on nonmalignant glands and stroma, right. (X260)

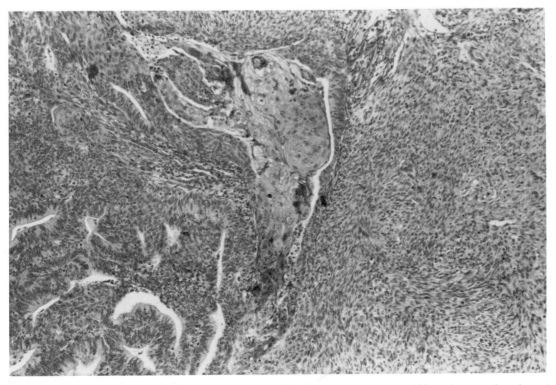

FIGURE 11-44. Carcinosarcoma endometrium. Adenocarcinoma, left side, squamous elements middle, and sarcoma (homologous) right. (X104) (From Free Hospital for Women, Brookline, Mass, S-52-4198.)

Endometrial Sarcoma

Endometrial sarcomas are less common malignant tumors of the endometrium whose relationship to endocrine influences is not clear. So are the low-grade sarcomas (endolymphatic stromal myosis), the highly malignant variants pure (Fig. 11-43) or mixed with either homologous or heterologous elements, and carcinosarcomas with homologous (Fig. 11-44) or heterologous components (mixed malignant mullerian tumors).

SUMMARY

This chapter presents a succinct description of the anatomy and physiology of the endometrium with a rather detailed description of the anatomic–physiologic bases for dating the endometrium during the normal menstrual cycle.

This has served as the foundation for the identification of endometrial responses as influenced by external factors (iatrogenic) or internal factors (pathological) bearing a relationship to contraception, infertility, dysfunctional disorders, and organic diseases. Some of the abnormal menstrual cycle syndromes have been discussed, with recommendations in each instance, to the proper timing for biopsy of the endometrium.

The different procedures for endometrial biopsy and the indications for using sharp versus aspiration curettage, office procedure versus hospital-confinement curettage have not been discussed in detail. The reader is referred to refs. 142–154.

Finally, organic diseases of the endometrium, which are important because of their frequency and severity, have either been discussed superficially or omitted, in line with the original purpose of emphasizing pathologic entities with endocrine relationships.

ACKNOWLEDGMENTS. The author gratefully acknowledges the assistance of Ms. Cynthia Davis and Ms. Rose Hozzian in the preparation of this manuscript.

QUESTIONS

1. In a patient with ectopic tubal pregnancy, the endometrial types that may be found by histopathological examination include

    a. menstrual.
    b. proliferative.
    c. hypersecretory.
    d. atypical secretory.
    e. any of the above.

2. A 25-year-old woman, married for 5 years (G0, P0, LMP 25 days prior to curettage), was found to have a biphasic temperature chart. A biopsy of the endometrium obtained at the onset of menstruation was reported by the pathologist as secretory endometrium equivalent to day 23 of the cycle with menstrual changes, with no predecidua seen. The diagnosis that applies is

    a. anovulatory cycle.
    b. luteal-phase defect.
    c. normal cycle.
    d. irregular shedding.
    e. hyperplasia.

3. Timing of the endometrial biopsy is paramount for diagnosis. In a suspected case of irregular shedding, the best time to perform this procedure is

    a. onset of menstruation.
    b. time of ovulation.
    c. 15–20 days into the cycle.
    d. 5–7 days into menstruation.
    e. any time.

4. A 45-year-old woman (G3, P3, LMP 27 days before) had a diagnostic endometrial curettage because of and during bleeding. The histopathological examination was reported as proliferative endometrium. The most likely interpretation of this finding is

    a. normal menstrual cycle.
    b. luteal-phase defect cycle.
    c. anovulatory cycle.
    d. irregular shedding.
    e. Asherman's syndrome.

REFERENCES

1. Ober WB: The endocrine pathology of the female reproductive system, in Velardo JT (ed): *Essentials of Human Reproduction—Clinical Aspects: Normal and Abnormal.* New York, Oxford University Press, 1950, pp 190–233.*
2. Hitschmann F, Adler L: Der Bau der Uterusschleimhaut des geschlechtsreifen Weibes mit besonderer Berucksichtigung der Menstruation. *Mscher Geburtsh Gynäkol* 27:1, 1908.
3. Allen E, Doisy EA: An ovarian hormone: Preliminary report on its localization, extraction and purification, and action in test animals. *JAMA* 81:819–821, 1923.

*Review article or chapter.

4. Corner GW, Allen WM: Physiology of the corpus luteum. II. Production of a special uterine reaction (progestational proliferation) by extracts of the corpus luteum. *Am J Physiol* 88:326–339, 1929.

5. Allen E: Menstrual cycle of monkey, Macacus rhesus: Observations on normal animals, effects of removal of ovaries and effects of injections of ovarian and placental extracts into spayed animals. *Contrib Embryol* 19:1–44, 1927.

6. Allen E, Hisaw FL, Gardner WU: Endocrine functions of ovaries, in Allen E, Danforth CH, Doisy EA (eds): *Sex and Internal Secretions,* 2nd ed. Baltimore, William & Wilkins, 1939, pp 452–629.

7. Allen WM: Physiology of corpus luteum. V. Preparation and some chemical properties of progestin, hormone of corpus luteum which produces progestational proliferation. *Am J Physiol* 92:174–188, 1930.

8. Bartelmez GW: Histologic studies on menstruating mucous membrane of the human uterus. *Contrib Embryol* 24:141–186, 1933.

9. Bartelmez GW, Corner GW, Hartman CG: Cyclic changes in the endometrium of the rhesus monkey (Macaca mulata). *Contrib Embryol* 34:99–144, 1951.

10. Bartelmez GW: Premenstrual and menstrual ischemia and the myth of endometrial arteriovenous anastomosis. *Am J Anat* 98:69–75, 1956.

11. Bartelmez GW: Form and function of uterine blood vessels in rhesus monkey. *Carnegie Inst Wash Publ No 611. Contrib Embryol* 37:153–182, 1957.

12. Daron GH: The arterial pattern of the tunica mucosa of the uterus in Macacus rhesus. *Am J Anat* 58:349–419, 1936.

13. Daron GH: The veins of the endometrium (Macacus rhesus) as a source of the menstrual blood. *Anat Rec* (suppl 3) 67:13, 1937.

14. Corner GW: Ovulation and menstruation in Macacus rhesus. *Contrib Embryol* 15:73–101, 1923.

15. Corner GW: Our knowledge of the menstrual cycle, 1910–1950. *Lancet* 1:919–923, 1951.

16. Hartmann CG: Studies in reproduction of monkey Macacus (pithecus) rhesus, with special reference to menstruation and pregnancy. *Contrib Embryol* 23:1–61, 1932.

17. Hertig AT: Diagnosing the endometrial biopsy, in Engle ET (ed): *Proceedings of the Conference on Diagnosis in Sterility.* Springfield, IL, Charles C Thomas, 1946, pp 93–128.

18. Hertig AT: The evolution of a research program. *Am J Obstet Gynecol* 76:252–270, 1958.*

19. Hisaw FL: Interaction of ovarian hormones in experimental menstruation. *Endocrinology* 30:301–308, 1942.

20. Phelps D: Physiology of menstruation and ovulation, in Council on Pharmacy and Chemistry of the AMA: *Glandular Physiology and Therapy,* 5th ed., Philadelphia, Lippincott, 1954, pp 162–199.*

21. Phelps D: Menstruation, in Velardo JT (ed): *Essentials of Human Reproduction. Clinical Aspects: Normal and Abnormal.* New York, Oxford University Press, 1958, pp 55–87.*

22. Ramsey EM: Vascular patterns in the endometrium and the placenta. *Angiology* 6:321–338, 1955.

23. Wislocki GB, Dempsey EW: Remarks on lymphatics of reproductive tract of female rhesus monkey (Macaca mulata). *Anat Rec* 75:341–363, 1939.

24. Velardo JT (ed): *Essentials of Human Reproduction. Clinical Aspects: Normal and Abnormal.* New York, Oxford University Press, 1958.*

25. Velardo JT, Rosa CG: Female genital system, in Graumann W, Neumann K (eds): *Handbuch der Histochemie.* Vol. VII/3: *Enzyme.* Stuttgart, Gustav Fischer, 1963, pp 54–88.

26. Velardo JT: An experimental model system for the detection of early uterine growth, in Campos A, da Paz T, Hasegawa T, Notake Y, Hayashi M (eds): *Human Reproduction.* Tokyo, Igaku Shoin, 1974, pp 54–67.*

27. Kasprow BA: Early uterine growth horizons, in Campos da Paz A, Hasegawa T, Notake Y, Hayashi M (eds): *Human Reproduction,* Tokyo, Igaka Shoin, 1974, pp 68–77.

28. Schröeder R: Anatomische Studien zur normale und pathologischen Physiologie des menstruationszyklus. *Arch Gynäkol* 104:55–82, 1915.

29. Rock J, Bartlett MK: Biopsy studies of human endometrium. Criteria of dating and information about amenorrhea, menorrhagia and time of ovulation. *JAMA* 108:2022–2028, 1937.

30. Noyes RW, Hertig AT, Rock J: Dating the endometrial biopsy. *Fertil Steril* 1:3–25, 1950.*

31. Hellweg G, Sandritter W: Ultraviolettmikrospektrophotometrische Untersuchungen an den körnchen der endometrialen körnchenzellen. *Klin Wochenschr* 34:1040, 1956.

32. Dallenbach FD, Dallenbach-Hellweg G: Immunohistologische Untersungen zur Lokalisation des Relaxins in menschlicher Plazenta und Dezidua. *Virchows Arch Pathol Anat* 337:301, 1964.

33. Daly DC, Maslar IA, Riddick DH: Prolactin production during in vitro decidualization of proliferative endometrium. *Am J Obstet Gynecol* 145:672–678, 1983.

34. Sekeba D: Zur morphologie und histologie des menstruationszyklus. *Arch Gynäkol* 121:36–60, 1923.

35. Craig JM, Danziger S: Reticulin and collagen in the human endometrium. *Am J Obstet Gynecol* 86:421–429, 1963.

36. McKay DG: Metachromasia in the endometrium. *Am J Obstet Gynecol* 59:875–882, 1950.

37. Hamperl H: Über endometriale Granulocyten (endometriale Körnchenzellen). *Klin Wochenschr* 29/30:665–668, 1954.

38. Hellweg G: Über endometriale körchenzellen (endometriale Granulocyten). *Arch Gynäkol* 185:150–166, 1954.

39. Okkels H, Engle ET: Studies on finer structure of uterine vessels of macacus monkey. *Acta Pathol Microbiol Scand* 15:150–168, 1938.

40. Markee JE: Relation of blood flow to endometrial growth and the injection of menstruation, in Engle ET (ed): *Menstruation and Its Disorders.* Springfield, IL, Charles C Thomas, 1950, pp. 165–185.

41. Robbard S, McMahon NJ, Denk M: Uterine structure and lymphatics. *Obstet Gynecol* 38:171–179, 1971.

42. Okkels H: Histophysiology of human endometrium, in Engle ET (ed): *Menstruation and its Disorders.* Springfield, IL, Charles C Thomas, 1950, pp 139–163.

43. Pribor HE: Innervation of the uterus. *Anat Rec* 109:339, 1951.

44. Krantz K: Innervation of the human uterus. *Ann NY Acad Sci* 75:770–784, 1959.

45. Markee JE: Menstruation in intraocular endometrial transplants in rhesus monkeys. *Contrib Embryol* 28:219–308, 1939.

46. McKay DG, Hertig AT, Bardawil WA, Velardo JT: Histochemical observations on the endometrium. I. Normal endometrium. *Obstet Gynecol* 8:22–39, 1956.

47. McLennan CE, Koets P: Chemical study of human endo-

metrium throughout menstrual cycle. *West J Surg Obstet Gynecol* 61:169–175, 1953.

48. Sturgis SH: In discussing Southam, AL. The natural history of menstrual disorders. *Ann NY Acad Sci* 75:840–854, 1959.

49. Noyes RW, Haman JO: Accuracy of the endometrial dating. Correlation of endometrial dating with basal body temperature and menses. *Fertil Steril* 4:504–517, 1953.

50. Abell MR: Endometrium, in Gold JJ, Josimovich JB (eds): *Gynecologic Endocrinology*, 3rd ed. Hagerstown, MD, Harper & Row, 1980, pp 232–270.

51. McKay DG, Hertig AT, Bardawil WA, Velardo JT: Histochemical observations on the endometrium. II. Abnormal endometrium. *Obstet Gynecol* 8:140–156, 1956.

52. Dallenbach-Hellweg G: *Histopathology of the Endometrium*, 3rd ed. Heidelberg and New York, Springer-Verlag, 1981.*

53. McLennan CE, Rydell AH: Extent of endometrial shedding during normal menstruation. *Obstet Gynecol* 26:605–621, 1965.

54. Noyes RW: Uniformity of secretory endometrium, multiple sections removed from 100 uteri. *Fertil Steril* 7:103–108, 1956.

55. Noyes RW: Normal phases of the endometrium, in Norris HJ, Hertig AT, Abell MR (eds): *The Uterus. International Academy of Pathology Monograph*. Baltimore, Williams & Wilkins, 1973, pp 110–135.*

56. Noyes RW: The underdeveloped secretory endometrium. *Am J Obstet Gynecol* 77:929–945, 1959.

57. Ehrlich CE, Young PCM, Cleary RE: Cytoplasmic progesterone and estradiol receptors in normal, hyperplastic and carcinomatous endometria: Therapeutic implications. *Am J Obstet Gynecol* 141:539–546, 1981.

58. Tsibris JCM, Cazanave CR, Cantor B, et al: Distribution of cytoplasmic estrogen and progesterone receptors in human endometrium. *Am J Obstet Gynecol* 132:449–454, 1978.

59. Tsibris JCM, Fort FL, Cazanave CR, et al: The uneven distribution of estrogen and progesterone receptors in human endometrium. *J Steroid Biochem* 14:997–1003, 1981.

60. Kreitmann-Gimbel B, Bayard F, Hodgen GD: Changing ratios of nuclear estrone to estradiol binding in endometrium at implantation: Regulation by chorionic gonadotropin and progesterone during rescue of the primate corpus luteum. *J Clin Endocrinol Metabol* 52:133–137, 1981.

61. Press MF, Greene GL: An immunochemical method for demonstrating estrogen receptor in human uterus using monoclonal antibodies to human estrophilin. *Lab Invest* 50:480–486, 1984.

62. Press MF, Nousek-Goebl N, King WJ, Greene GL: Immunohistochemical assessment of estrogen receptor distribution in the human endometrium throughout the menstrual cycle. *Lab Invest* 51:495–503, 1984.

63. Greene GL, Nolan C, Engler JP, Jensen EV: Monoclonal antibodies to human estrogen receptor. *Proc Natl Acad Sci USA* 77:5115–5119, 1980.

64. Dawood MY: Hormones, prostaglandins and dysmenorrhea, in Yusoff Dawood M (ed): *Dysmenorrhea*. Baltimore, Williams & Wilkins, 1981, pp 21–52.*

65. Press MF, De Sombre ER, Talerman A: Epithelial peroxidase and endometrial granulocytes in normal cyclic human endometrium. *J Clin Endocrinol Metab* 56:254–261, 1983.

66. Tsibris JCM, Trujillo YP, Fernandez BB, et al: Distribution of guaiacol peroxidase in human endometrium and endocervical epithelium during the menstrual cycle. *J Clin Endocrinol Metab* 54:991–997, 1982.

67. Nordqvist S: The synthesis of DNA and RNA in normal human endometrium in short term incubation in vitro and its responses to estradiol and progesterone. *J Endocrinol* 48:17–28, 1970.

68. MacDonald RG, Okulicz WC, Levitt WW: Progesterone-induced inactivation of nuclear estrogen receptor in the hamster uterus is mediated by acid phosphatase. *Biochem Biophys Res Commun* 104:570–576, 1982.

69. Sawaragi I, Wynn RM: Ultrastructural localization of metabolic enzymes during the human menstrual cycle. *Obstet Gynecol* 34:50–59, 1969.

70. Stuermer VM, Stein RJ: Cytodynamic properties of the human endometrium. V. Metabolism and enzymatic activity of the human endometrium during the menstrual cycle. *Am J Obstet Gynecol* 63:359–370, 1952.

71. Boutselis JG: Histochemistry of the normal endometrium, in Norris HJ, Hertig AT, Abell MR (eds): *The Uterus. International Academy of Pathology Monograph*. Baltimore, Williams & Wilkins, 1973, pp 175–184.*

72. Hagerman DD, Villee CA: Effects of the menstrual cycle on the metabolism of the human endometrium. *Endocrinology* 53:667–673, 1953.

73. Okagaki T, Richart RM: Oxygen consumption of human endometrium during the menstrual cycle. *Fertil Steril* 21:595–598, 1970.

74. Cavazos F, Lucas FV: Ultrastructure of the endometrium, in Norris HJ, Hertig AT, Abell MR (eds): *The Uterus. International Academy of Pathology Monograph*. Baltimore, Williams & Wilkins, 1973, pp 136–174.*

75. Ferenczy A, Richart RM: Female reproductive system: Dynamics of scan and transmission electron microscopy. New York, Wiley, 1974.*

76. Wynn RM, Wooley RS: Ultrastructural changes in the human endometrium. I. Normal post-ovulatory phase. *Fertil Steril* 18:721–738, 1973.

77. Clyman MJ: A new structure observed in the nucleolus of the human endometrial cells. *Am J Obstet Gynecol* 86:430–432, 1963.

78. Armstrong EM, More IAR, Seveney DM, Corty M: The giant-mitochondrion–endoplasmic reticulum unit of the human endometrial glandular cell. *J Anat* 116:375–383, 1973.

79. Armstrong EM, More IAR, Seveney DM, Corty M: The giant-mitochondrion–endoplasmic reticulum unit of the human endometrial glandular cell. *J Obstet Gynecol Br Commonw* 81:337–347, 1973.

80. Ober WB, Bernstein J: Observations on the endometrium and ovary in the newborn. *Pediatrics* 16:455–460, 1955.

81. Valdes-Dapena MA: The development of the uterus in late fetal life, infancy and childhood, in Norris HJ, Hertig AT, Abell MR (eds): *The Uterus. International Academy of Pathology Monograph*. Baltimore, Williams & Wilkins, 1973, pp 40–67.*

82. Hertig AT: Gestational hyperplasia of the endometrium: A morphologic correlation with ova, endometrium and corpora lutea during early pregnancy. *Lab Invest* 13:1153–1191, 1964.*

83. Somerville BW: Daily variations in plasma levels of progesterone and estradiol throughout the menstrual cycle. *Am J Obstet Gynecol* 111:419–426, 1971.

84. Arias-Stella J: Frecuencia y significado de las atipias endo-

metriales en el embarazo ectopico. *Rev Latinoam Anat Pathol* 1:81–91, 1957.

85. Arias-Stella J: Gestational endometrium, in Norris HJ, Hertig AT, Abell MR (eds): *The Uterus. International Academy of Pathology.* Baltimore, Williams & Wilkins, 1973, pp 185–212.*

86. Romney SL, Hertig AT, Reid DE: The endometria associated with ectopic pregnancy. *Surg Gynecol Obstet* 91:605–611, 1950.

87. Holmstrom EG, McLennon CE: Menorrhagia associated with irregular shedding of the endometrium: A clinical and experimental study. *Am J Obstet Gynecol* 53:727–748, 1947.

88. Driscoll SG: Placental–uterine relationships, in Norris HJ, Hertig AT, Abell MR (eds): *The Uterus. International Academy of Pathology.* Baltimore, Williams & Wilkins, 1973, pp 213–226.*

89. Jones GES: Some newer aspects of the management of infertility. *JAMA* 141:1123–1129, 1949.

90. Moszkowski E, Woodruff JD, Seegar Jones GE: The inadequate luteal phase. *Am J Obstet Gynecol* 83:363–372, 1962.

90a. Levy C, Robel P, Gautrey JP, et al: Estradiol and progesterone receptors in human endometrium: Normal and abnormal menstrual cycles. *Am J Obstet Gynecol* 136:646–651, 1980.

90b. Daly DC, Masler IA, Rosenberg SM, Tohan N, Riddick DH: Prolactin production by luteal phase defect endometrium. *Am J Obstet Gynecol* 140:587–591, 1981.

91. Dizerega GS, Ross GT: Luteal phase dysfunction. *Clin Obstet Gynecol* 8:733–751, 1981.*

92. Jones GES, Madrigal-Castro V: Hormonal findings in association with abnormal corpus luteum functions in the human. *Fertil Steril* 21:1–13, 1970.

93. Goutray JP, de Brux J, Tajchner G, et al: Clinical investigation of the menstrual cycle. III. Clinical, endometrial, and endocrine aspects of luteal defect. *Fertil Steril* 35:296–303, 1981.

94. Coutts JRT, Adam AH, Fleming R: The deficient luteal phase may represent an anovulatory cycle. *Clin Endocrinol* 17:389–394, 1982.

95. DeMoraes-Rueksen Jones GS, Barnett LS: The aluteal phase: A severe form of the luteal phase defect. *Am J Obstet Gynecol* 103:1059–1077, 1969.

96. Jones GES: Luteal phase defect. *Fertil Steril* 27:351–356, 1976.

97. Kistner RW: Further observations on the effect of clomiphene citrate in anovulatory females. *Am J Obstet Gynecol* 92:380–412, 1965.

98. Charles D, Barr W, Bell ET, et al: Clomiphene in the treatment of oligomenorrhea and amenorrhea. *Am J Obstet Gynecol* 86:913–922, 1963.

99. Charles D: MRL. 41 in the treatment of secondary amenorrhea and endometrial hyperplasia. *Lancet* 2:278–280, 1962.

100. Ober WB: Synthetic progestagen–estrogen preparations and endometrial morphology. *J Clin Pathol* 19:138–147, 1966.

101. Maqueo M, Becerra C, Mungia H, et al: Endometrial histology and vaginal cytology during oral contraception with sequential estrogen and progestin. *Am J Obstet Gynecol* 90:395–400, 1964.

102. Ludwig H: The morphologic response of the human endometrium to long term treatment with progestational agents. *Am J Obstet Gynecol* 142:796–808, 1982.

102a. Borushek S, Abell MR, Smith L, et al: The effects of Provest on the endometrium, *Int J Fertil* 8:605–618, 1963

103. Silverberg SG, Makoski EL: Endometrial carcinoma in young women taking oral contraceptives. *Obstet Gynecol* 46:503, 1975.

104. Gold JJ, Borushek S, Smith L, et al: Synthetic progestins: A review. *Int J Fertil* 10:99–113, 1965.

105. Umapathysivam K, Jones WR: Effects of contraceptive agents on the biochemical and protein composition of the endometrium. *Contraception* 22:425–441, 1980.

106. Whitehead MI, Townsend PT, Pryse-Davis J, et al: Actions of progestins on the morphology and biochemistry of the endometrium of postmenopausal women receiving low-dose estrogen therapy. *Am J Obstet Gynecol* 142:791–795, 1982.

107. Kokko E, Janne O, Kauppila A, et al: Effects of Tamoxifen, medroxyprogesterone acetate and their combination on endometrial estrogen and progestin receptor concentrations, 17 beta-hydroxysteroid dehydrogenase activity, and serum hormone concentrations. *Am J Obstet Gynecol* 143:382–388, 1982.

108. Sedlis A, Kim NG: Significance of the endometrial collagen band. *Obstet Gynecol* 38:264–268, 1971.

109. Alvizouri M: Effect of estradiol in experimental endometrial hyperplasia. *Am J Obstet Gynecol* 82:1224–1227, 1961.

110. Gerschenson LE, Fennell R Jr: A developmental view of endometrial hyperplasia and carcinoma based on experimental research. *Pathol Res Pract* 174:285–296, 1982.

111. Cramer DW, Knapp RC: Review of epidemiologic studies of endometrial cancer and exogenous estrogen. *Obstet Gynecol* 54:521, 1979.*

112. Fenoglio CM, Crum CP, Ferenczy A: Endometrial hyperplasia and carcinoma: Are ultrastructural, biochemical and immunocytochemical studies useful in distinguishing them? *Pathol Res Pract* 174:257–284, 1982.

113. Novak ER, Woodruff JD: *Gynecologic and Obstetric Pathology* 5th ed. Philadelphia, Saunders, 1962.*

114. Gore H, Hertig AT: Premalignant lesions of the endometrium. *Clin Obstet Gynecol* 5:1148–1165, 1962.

115. Gore H: Hyperplasia of the endometrium, in Norris HJ, Hertig AT, Abell MR (eds): *The Uterus, International Academy of Pathology Monograph.* Baltimore, Williams & Wilkins, 1973, pp 255–275.*

116. Hertig AT, Sommers SC, Bengloff H: Genesis of endometrial carcinoma. III. Carcinoma in situ. *Cancer* 2:964–971, 1949.

117. Gore H, Hertig AT: Carcinoma in situ of endometrium. *Am J Obstet Gynecol* 94:135–155, 1966.

118. Abell MR: Adenocarcinoma (Gland-cell carcinoma) in situ of endometrium. *Pathol Res Pract* 174:221–236, 1982.

119. Kurman RJ, Norris HJ: Evaluation of criteria for distinguishing atypical endometrial hyperplasia from well-differentiated carcinoma. *Cancer* 49:2547–2559, 1982.

120. Campbell PE, Barter RA: The significance of atypical endometrial hyperplasia. *J Obstet Gynaecol Br Commonw* 68:668–672, 1961.

121. Gusberg SB, Kaplan AL: Precursors of corpus cancer. IV. Adenomatous hyperplasia as stage 0 carcinoma of the endometrium. *Am J Obstet Gynecol* 87:662–678, 1963.

122. Gusberg SB: Current concepts in cancer: The changing nature of endometrial cancer. *N Engl J Med* 302:729–731, 1980.

123. Hertig AT, Sommers SC: Genesis of endometrial carcinoma. I. Study of prior biopsies. *Cancer* 2:946–956, 1949.

124. Beutler HK, Dockerty MB, Randall LM: Precancerous lesions of the endometrium. *Am J Obstet Gynecol* 86:433–443, 1963.*

125. Novak E, Yui EY: Relation of endometrial hyperplasia to adenocarcinoma of the uterus. *Am J Obstet Gynecol* 32:674–698, 1936.

126. Asherman S: Amenorrhoea traumatica (atretica). *J Obstet Gynaecol Br Commonw* 55:23–30, 1948.

127. McKelvey JL, Samuels LT: Irregular shedding of the endometrium. *Am J Obstet Gynecol* 53:627–636, 1947.

128. Czernobilsky B, Rothenstreich L, Mass N, et al: Effects of intrauterine device on histology endometrium. *Obstet Gynecol* 45:64–66, 1975.

129. Schiffer MA, Elquezabal A, Sultana M, et al: Actinomycosis infection associated with intrauterine contraceptive devices. *Obstet Gynecol* 45:67–72, 1975.

130. Dehner LP, Askin FB: Cytomegalovirus endometritis. Reports of a case associated with spontaneous abortion. *Obstet Gynecol* 45:211–214, 1975.

131. Saw EC, Smale LE, Einstein H, et al: Female genital coccidioidomycosis. *Obstet Gynecol* 45:199–202, 1975.

132. Ganem KJ, Parsons L, Friedell GH: Endometrial ossification. *Am J Obstet Gynecol* 83:1592–1594, 1962.

133. Jafari K, Jafaheri G, Ruiz G: Endometrial adenocarcinoma and the Stein-Leventhal syndrome. *Obstet Gynecol* 51:97–100, 1978.

134. Tsoutsoplides GC: Endometrial adenocarcinoma and the Stein-Leventhal syndrome. *Am J Obstet Gynecol* 147:844–845, 1983.

135. Robboy SJ, Miller AW III, Kurman RJ: The pathologic features and behaviour of endometrial carcinoma associated with exogenous estrogen administration. *Pathol Res Pract* 174:237–256, 1982.

136. Woll E, Hertig AT, Smith VSG, et al: The ovary in endometrial carcinoma. *Am J Obstet Gynecol* 56:617–633, 1948.

137. Fechner RE, Kaufman RH: Endometrial adenocarcinoma in Stein-Leventhal syndrome. *Cancer* 34:444–452, 1974.

138. Ng ABP, Reagan JW, Storaasli JP, et al: Mixed adenosquamous carcinoma of the endometrium. *Am J Clin Pathol* 59:765–781, 1973.

139. Silverberg SG, Bolin MG, DeGiorgi LS: Adenoacanthoma and mixed adenosquamous carcinoma of the endometrium. *Cancer* 30:1307–1314, 1972.

140. Hameed K, Morgan DA: Papillary adenocarcinoma of endometrium with psammoma bodies. *Cancer* 29:1326–1335, 1972.

141. Hendrickson MR, Ross JC, Kempson RL, et al: Uterine papillary serous carcinoma. *Lab Invest* 44:27A, 1981.

142. Delke I, Veridano NP, Diamond B: Vabra aspiration in office gynecology. *Gynecol Oncol* 10:329–336, 1980.

143. Einerth Y: Vacuum curettage by the Vabra method. A simple procedure for endometrial diagnosis. *Acta Obstet Gynecol Scand* 61:373–376, 1982.

144. Grimes DA: Diagnostic dilatation and curettage: A reappraisal. *Am J Obstet Gynecol* 142:1–6, 1982.

145. Haak-Sorensen PE, Starklint H, Aronsen A, et al: Diagnostic Vabra (aspiration) curettage. An evaluation of the diagnostic certainty, efficacy, acceptability, indication

146. Hale RW, Reich LA, Joiner JM, et al: Histopathologic evaluation of uteri curetted by flexible suction cannula. *Am J Obstet Gynecol* 125:805–808, 1976.

147. Jensen JA, Jensen JG: Abrasio mucosae uteri et aspiratione. *Ugeskr Laeg* 130:1224, 1968.

148. Jensen JG: Vacuum curettage. Out patient curettage without anesthesia. A report of 350 cases. *Dan Med Bull* 17:199, 1970.

149. Kelly HA: Curettage without anesthesia on the office table. *Am J Obstet Gynecol* 9:78–80, 1925.

150. Kriseman M: Description of a new disposable uterine sampler (the accurette) for endometrial cytology and histology. *S Afr Med J* 61:107–108, 1982.

151. MacKenzie IZ, Bibby JG: Critical assessment of dilatation and curettage in 1029 women. *Lancet* 2:566–568, 1978.

152. Nussler E, Thomsen PB, Weeth R: Vacuum curettage of the uterus: Vabra aspiration curettage in 1,370 cases in a gynaecological department. *Dan Med Bull* 22:165–168, 1975.

153. Page EW: In reply to Dr. Hale, R. W. et al. (editorial). *Am J Obstet Gynecol* 125:805–808, 1976.

154. Vassilakos P, Wyss R, Wenzer D, et al: Endometrial cytohistology by aspiration technic and by Gravlee jet washer: A comparative study. *Obstet Gynecol* 45:320–324, 1975.

155. Ober WB, Grady HG: Subinvolution of the placental site. *Bull NY Acad Med* 37:713–730, 1961.

156. Demopoulos RI: Endometrium, in Blaustein A (ed): *Pathology of the Female Genital Tract*. New York, Springer-Verlag, 1977, pp 211–242.*

157. Ehrmann RL, McKelvey HA, Hertig AT: Secretory behavior of endometrium in tissue culture. *Obstet Gynecol* 17:416–433, 1961.

158. More IAR, Armstrong EM, Corty M, et al: Cyclical changes in the ultarstructure of the normal human endometrial stromal cell. *J Obstet Gynecol Br Commonw* 81:337–347, 1974.

159. Rock J, Garcia CR, Menkin MF: Menstruation and menstrual disorders. A theory of menstruation. *Ann NY Acad Sci* 75:831–839, 1959.

160. Studd, JW, Thom MH, Paterson MEL: The prevention and treatment of endometrial pathology in postmenopausal women receiving exogenous estrogens, in Pasetto N, Paoletti R, Ambrus JL (eds): Lancaster, MTP Press, 1980, pp 127–139.

161. Thrasher TV, Richart RM: An ultrastructural comparison of endometrial adenocarcinoma and normal endometrium. *Cancer* 19:1713–1723, 1972.

162. Tsang BK, Ooi TC: Prostaglandin secretion by human endometrium. *Am J Obstet Gynecol* 142:626–632, 1982.

163. Tseng L, Gurpide E: Effects of progestins on estradiol receptor levels in human endometrium. *J Clin Encocrinol Metab* 41:402–404, 1975.

164. White AJ, Buchsbaum HJ: Scanning electron microscopy of the human endometrium. I. Normal. *Gynecol Oncol* 1:330–339, 1973.

165. White AJ, Buchsbaum HJ: II. Hyperplasia and adenocarcinoma. *Gynecol Oncol* 2:1–8, 1974.

166. Cane EM, Villee CA: The synthesis of prostaglandin F by human endometrium in organ culture. *Prostaglandins* 9:281–288, 1975.

and sociomedical importance. *Dan Med Bull* 26:1–6, 1979.*

ANSWERS

1. e

2. b

3. d

4. c

12

Diagnostic Imaging

BERTRAM LEVIN

INTRODUCTION

This chapter can do little more than present an overview of the wide variety of imaging procedures now available to the endocrinologist and gynecologist as well as some illustrative material showing the "readouts" of these techniques. Conventional radiography, fluoroscopy with spot films, ultrasonograms, ultrasound-guided biopsy, high-resolution computed tomography (CT), angiography, and nuclear imaging using a variety of scanning agents are all parts of the radiologist's armamentarium. With this wide selection available, it has become increasingly important that there be close cooperation among the endocrinologists, gynecologists, and radiologists to determine the proper techniques to be used and the most logical sequence of imaging studies.

SKELETAL AGE

Determination of skeletal age can be a useful tool for pediatricians and endocrinologists. Unfortunately, since it is often indiscriminately requested,

BERTRAM LEVIN • Department of Diagnostic Radiology, Michael Reese Hospital and Medical Center; and Department of Radiology, Pritzker School of Medicine, University of Chicago, Chicago, Illinois 60618

since most radiologists get little feedback as to the accuracy of their assessment of bone age, and since radiologists are often insufficiently disciplined and concerned about accurate determination of bone age, a time-consuming exercise, the examination too often leads to misleading interpretation.

It is beyond the scope of this chapter to analyze the many radiographic methods for assessment of bone age. The interested reader can find many scholarly essays on the subject. The radiologic methods used depend on the appearance of the bones of the wrist and hand, customarily the left side. The standard most commonly used is that of Greulich and Pyle's[1] modification of Todd's hand and wrist atlas.[2] Each roentgenogram in the atlas represents the modal film of all normal healthy children of the same chronologic age. When the patient's film matches an atlas picture, the chronologic age assigned to the picture becomes the skeletal age of the patient. It is essential to appreciate that there are relatively wide and differing ranges, depending on the atlas age. Likewise, it must be remembered that there are different standards for genetic males and for genetic females, and care must be exercised to use the proper set of standard films. Throughout childhood, girls have advanced bone ages compared with boys. It must also be understood that the Greulich and Pyle atlas is that of Caucasian American children and may not be appropriate for application to populations of other countries and other races. The use of an atlas to determine skeletal age is subject to systematic and variable errors; nevertheless, the reliability of the method has been shown to be consistently high when applied by those experienced with its use.[3-9]

Recently, Tanner et al.[10] revised an older Tanner and Whitehouse method of determination of bone age.[11] Both systems depend on carefully scoring the stage of bony development of each of 20 bones of the wrist and hand by comparison with a series of standards. These values are then totaled to give a skeletal score from which a skeletal age may be determined by use of a table. The system is a more time-consuming one than is the Greulich and Pyle atlas, requires meticulous radiographic technique and considerable experience by the radiologist with a significant interobserver error. Furthermore, it must be understood that the system is based on British children's standards.

In making a clinical application of the concept of the skeletal age, it must be remembered that two sets of factors control the growth process. As Johnston[5] observed, "One set of factors determines the ultimate size of the individual in any dimension; the other determines the speed at which the individual will attain that size." Johnston clearly demonstrated that because the growth time available is directly related to the degree of skeletal maturity exhibited, one can determine which individual will have more and which will have less growth time "in the bank." Since the speed and time of growth spurts vary appreciably among individuals, the concept of skeletal age is important in predicting ultimate stature.

The Roche–Wainer–Thissen (RWT) method for predicting adult stature, developed at the Fels Research Institute, was designed to "develop a prediction method that would be applicable when a child and his parents enter a physician's office for the first time."[12] The data required are recumbent length, nude weight, mid-parent stature, and hand–wrist skeletal age. With this method, the prediction errors are smaller than with the earlier used Bayley and Pinneau method.[13] It predicts stature at age 18 years. The skeletal age is assessed by bone-by-bone analysis of the radiograph of the left hand and wrist, using the Greulich and Pyle atlas. The method can be applied only to white children, since the atlas films are those of white children only. Furthermore, the RWT method is not applicable to children in whom more than one-half the bones of the hand and wrist are of adult maturity. Greulich and Pyle noted that the onset of menstruation usually occurs soon

after fusion of the epiphysis of the distal phalanges with their shafts. Thus, one is often able to predict the onset of menarche from a roentgenogram during the prepubertal period. Simmons and Greulich[14] noted that such a prediction based on skeletal age is about twice as accurate as that based on chronologic age. Graham[4] devised a bone-age sampling method that has yielded satisfactory results, a compromise between the single film hand–wrist study and the study of all hemiskeleton ossification centers. Appropriate radiographs are made of six body regions, different films made for genetic males and females, depending on age, up to 18 years. Film findings are then matched with the tables compiled by Garn et al.[15] The reader is referred to Graham's report for details of the areas to be radiographed at a given age.

The skeletal age of a child at a given examination shows if she is advanced or delayed in the particular time. Follow-up examinations are necessary to establish the rate at which she will attain full adulthood. Johnston[5] warns against the danger of inferring too much from a single wrist–hand x-ray examination. He has shown that the rates of growth in children vary greatly; one individual may be a year retarded at age 7, a year advanced at age 15, and still be completely normal, simply growing at a rate faster at 15 than that shown in the atlas standard. "The skeletal ages do not follow chronological ages at 1 : 1 ratio; fluctuations within the individual cause differences in his rate of development from the average. Successive x-rays therefore become of distinctive value here." Graham,[4] in his splendid review article on assessment of bone maturation, adds the caveat that many textbooks promote "normal ranges" that are only one-half or even one-fourth as wide as the actual ranges. Buckley[3] noted that it "is probable that 75% of paediatricians may receive very misleading information which they would probably be better without."

HYSTEROSALPINGOGRAPHY

Pelvic pneumography has given way to laparoscopy and ultrasonography, but hysterosalpingography (HSG) remains an important procedure in the study of primary or secondary infertility (see Figs. 12-1 through 12-13). In a series of 505 consecutive HSGs for the evaluation of infertility, a tubal abnormality was found in 37.2% and a uterine abnormality in 8.5% of cases. In 7.3%, both uterine and tubal abnormalities were found.[16] Pontifey et

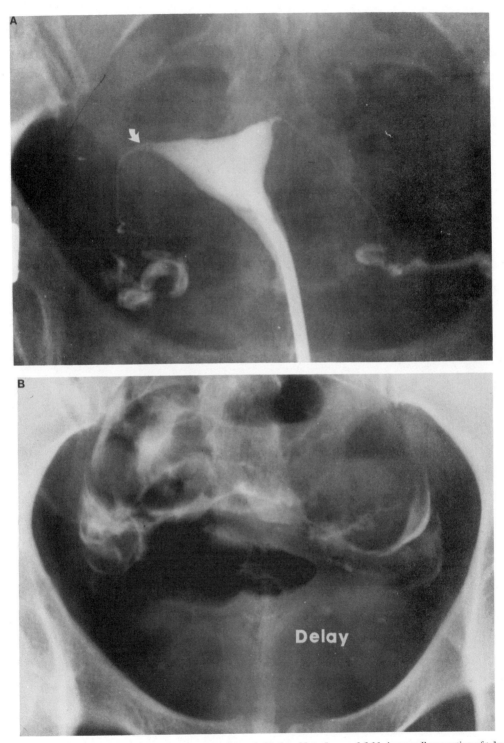

FIGURE 12-1. (A) Normal HSG. Arrow points to normal pretubal bulge. Note the rugal folds in ampullary portion of tubes. (B) Delayed upright film demonstrates contrast material within the peritoneal cavity coating surfaces of bowel.

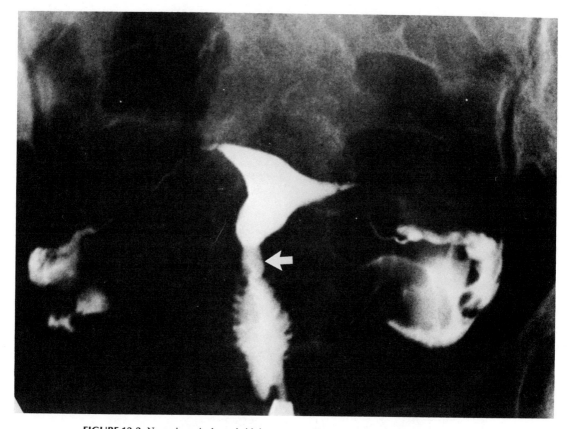

FIGURE 12-2. Normal cervical canal ridging pattern. The isthmus (arrow) is of normal diameter.

al.[17] reviewed 3697 HSGs for primary and secondary infertility and found 35.8% of the former and 22.6% of the latter to be normal. Contraindications to HSG are few: pregnancy, active uterine bleeding, and acute pelvic inflammatory disease (PID). Fortunately, complications are likewise few: between 0.3 and 1.7% of patients will develop serious pelvic infections following HSG, almost exclusively in women with dilated tubes.[18,19] Pittaway et al.[18] reported that oral doxycycline prophylaxis was effective in reducing post-HSG infection in women with dilated tubes. Nonallergic vasomotor reactions (flushing, dizziness, transient hypotension) are usually self-limiting and not serious. Oil embolism has been eliminated with the use of water-soluble contrast media, as have tubal and peritoneal granulomas.

Careful attention must be paid to performing the examination to achieve maximum information at the lowest radiation exposure. Thus, it is of utmost importance that the gynecologist and the radiologist know what to expect from the examination. Is there concern for a congenital defect? Is there suspicion of fallopian tube obstruction? Has there been prior surgery involving tubes or uterus? Is there concern about cervical os insufficiency? The examination should be tailor-made for each patient; there is no satisfactory routine amount of contrast material to be injected, nor should there be a limiting routine number of x-ray films taken. The examination should be carried out under fluoroscopic guidance with the patient having been advised and reassured as to the technique of the study and thereby one can generally expect greater relaxation and cooperation from her.

The amount of radiation to the ovaries will vary with the fluoroscopic unit used, the size of the patient, and the duration of fluoroscopy. With proper

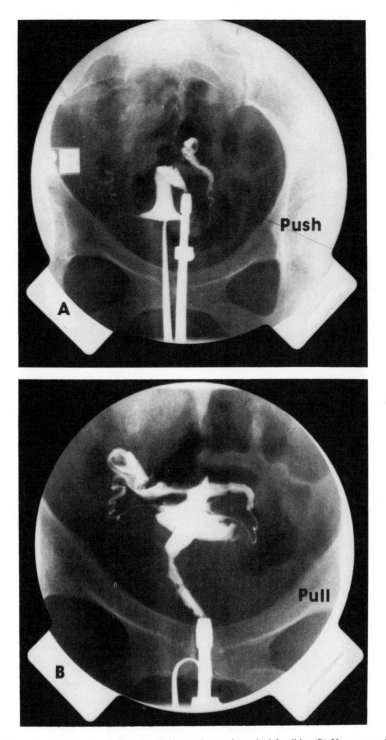

FIGURE 12-3. (A) Uterus displaced (anteverted) by tenaculum and cannula pushed forcibly. (B) Uterus repositioned by pull on instruments.

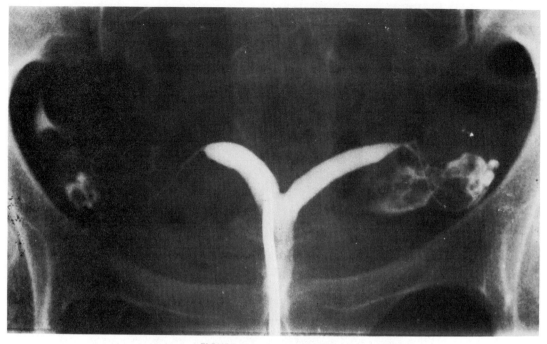

FIGURE 12-4. Bicornuate uterus.

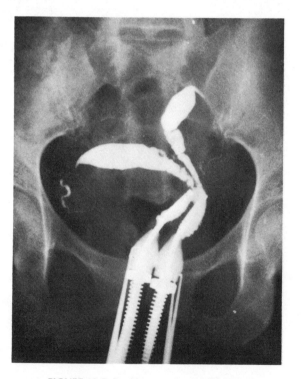

FIGURE 12-5. Double uterus (uterus didelphys).

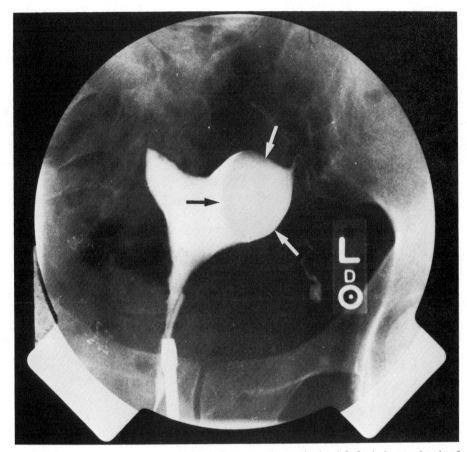

FIGURE 12-6. Uterus deformed by fibromyomas. Right tube is obstructed at proximal end. Left tube is patent in spite of a large mass in the cornu (arrows).

collimation, short bursts of fluoroscopy, and 100- or 105-mm camera spot films, the amount of radiation is small for the examination yield, up to 750 mrad.

A variety of instruments are in use for cannulating the cervical os and obstructing it for forward flow during injection, and for injecting the contrast material to outline the uterine canal and fallopian tubes. In recent years, Foley catheters (No. 8–10) are being used with increasing frequency, particularly if there is no concern about seeing anatomic detail of the lower uterine segment and cervical os. These require less of the painful manipulation for insertion, especially if a flexible stiffener is used to facilitate its introduction.[20]

Water-soluble contrast material is favored over oil-based media to avoid complications of intra-vasation (i.e., pulmonary emboli) and tubal or peritoneal granuloma formation. By contrast, oil-based agents appear to have a better record of post-HSG pregnancy. This beneficial effect of HSG might be produced by dislodging mucous plugs within the lumen of the tubes, breaking down of fine adhesions, stimulation of ciliary action, bacteriostatic properties of contrast agents, and psychic effects.[21] There is as yet no adequate clinical or laboratory investigation to support any of these possible causes. The incidence of pregnancy following HSG has been reported to range from 13 to 58%[21–28] To take advantage of the properties of water-soluble and of oil-soluble contrast media, DeCherney et al.[23] have recommended that HSG be performed with a water-soluble medium and once tubal patency has been established, 3 ml of an oil-soluble contrast agent be then

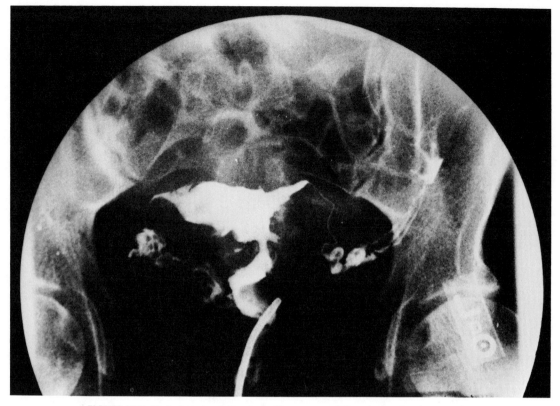

FIGURE 12-7. Marked uterine deformity by fibromyomas. Bilateral normal and patent tubes.

injected for its possible therapeutic effect to increase subsequent fertility.

For clinical applications of HSG, the reader is referred to the excellent reviews by Barnett,[21,29] Parekh and Arronet,[30] and Siegler.[19] A few details of the examination merit special note.

1. HSG should be performed only during the preovulatory period. During other phases of the menstrual cycle, the injection may cause endometrial tissue to be pushed into the tubes, causing occlusion and possibly tubal endometriosis. Also, the chances of intravasation of injected contrast media will be lessened.
2. It is important for the determination of tubal patency that the urinary bladder be empty. Bligh and Williams[31] reported on the effects of a distended bladder during HSG. They concluded that (1) the position of the tubes can be influenced by a full bladder and that a distended bladder may cause a picture mimicking hydrosalpinx; and (2) much valuable information regarding tubal motility may be obtained by noting the influence of a full bladder on tubal position. They advise that if a significant degree of bladder filling is noted the bladder should be emptied by catheterization before the examination is completed.
3. If a Foley catheter is used, care must be exercised that the tip of the catheter not be lodged in a cornu and thus obstruct a tube.
4. Tubal spasm may mimic organic obstruction. The patient should therefore be advised beforehand of the details of the examination to lessen apprehension. Glucagon, 1–2 mg, given intravenously is often useful in abating tubal spasm.
5. Fluoroscopy must be carefully performed to see what is happening at the moment to decide, in the light of the particular case, what should be done the next moment in terms of amount injected and position of the patient. The fluoroscope should not be used merely to aim the spot-filming device. Ordinarily, 1–2

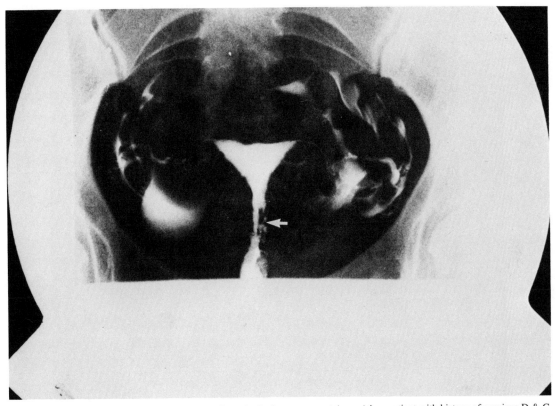

FIGURE 12-8. Intrauterine adhesions most prominent in the lower segment (arrow) in a patient with history of previous D & C.

min fluoroscopy time is required for the examination.

6. A scout film should be taken to avoid those errors that might result from misinterpreting shadows cast by bone structures, bowel content, or retained contrast material. The insurance against these errors is well worth the minimal additional radiation.

7. When there is a question of tubal patency, hydrosalpinx, or peritubal adhesions, a 20–30-min delayed film, preferably with the patient upright, should be taken.

GENITOGRAPHY

Properly applied, radiologic techniques can be of great importance in the clinical assessment of intersexual states, particularly in assessing the gross morphology of the internal genitalia (see Figs. 12-14 through 12-16). In 1963 Shopfner[32] reported on the use of genitography in intersexual states. The procedure is simple but must be meticulously ex-

ecuted to permit "the prompt assignment of a particular sex before gender role complicates matters and subsequent treatment is necessary, to give the patient sexual adequacy in the assigned sex." The examination should be performed in every "male" with hypospadias and with ambiguous genitalia to exclude a complicated intersexual state. Shopfner notes that the following two methods may be used for opaque contrast genitography: (1) the flushing technique, and (2) the multiple-catheter technique, both performed under fluoroscopic control.

The flushing technique is used according to the method of Tristan et al.[33] Opaque contrast material is injected through the perineal opening, flushing the material in and out in order to accomplish filling of all orifices. The nose of the syringe must be held firmly against the perineum to ensure a tight seal.

Cremin[34] and this author prefer the multiple catheter technique, care being taken to place the catheters into all possible passages. The contrast material is flushed through the catheters into the orifices simultaneously with careful fluoroscopic

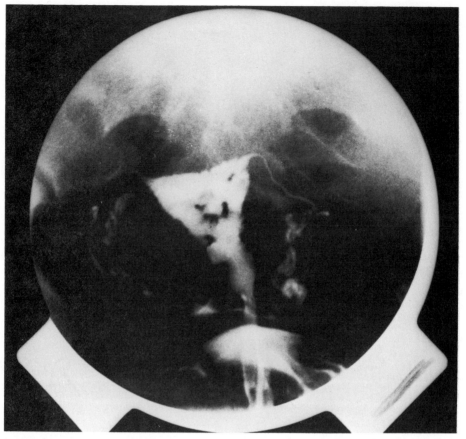

FIGURE 12-9. Extensive intrauterine adhesions throughout the uterine cavity in a patient with history of previous D & C.

observation and spot filming. The external genitalia must be carefully examined to seek out orifices. Those most often present are a hypospadic urethra and a single urogenital sinus opening, which may be at the base of the phallus or in the perineum. Rarely, there are two openings entering a small vestibule which exit to the perineum by a single opening. Peck and Poznanski[35] described a simple device made up of a nipple and an infant tube which can be used to create an effective seal at the perineal or other openings and thus prevent leakage around the injection site.

NEUROENDOCRINOLOGIC IMAGING (Figs. 12-17 to 12-20)

Pituitary Adenomas

Neoplasms of the pituitary gland have been classified as both functioning and nonfunctioning. They have been further classified by size into microadenomas (<1 cm) and macroadenomas. The neoplasms of the pituitary gland must be differentiated from empty sella as well as from parasellar and suprasellar lesions such as craniopharyngioma, meningioma, aneurysm, hypothalamic lesions, ectopic pinealoma, and arachnoidal cyst.[36,37]

Microadenomas are usually confined within a normal-sized sella, with or without subtle radiographic changes. Macroadenomas usually enlarge and deform the sella turcica so as to produce changes generally demonstrable on coned frontal and lateral views of the sella. Until recently subtle bone changes were evaluated by thin section pleuridirectional tomography. This permitted demonstration of secondary bone changes produced by primary lesions of the soft tissue arising from the pituitary gland as well as of other perisellar structures. High-resolution CT with contrast enhancement by intravenous injection now demonstrates

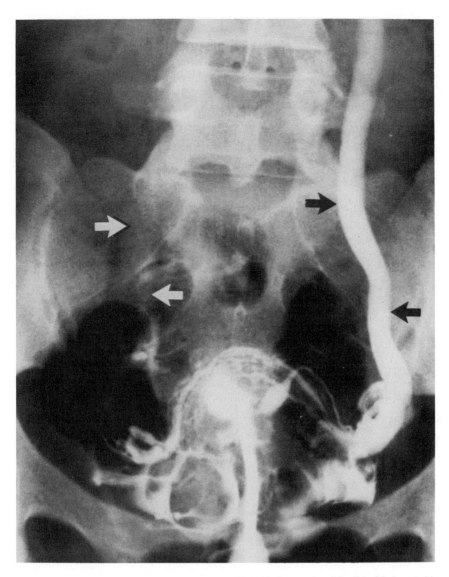

FIGURE 12-10. Intravasation. The left ovarian vein is densely opacified (black arrows) and the right faintly so (white arrows). The myometrium is irregularly opacified.

the pituitary gland, internal carotid arteries, cavernous sinus and its content, suprasellar cisterns, optic chiasms, and gray and white matter as well as the cerebrospinal fluid (CSF) spaces, in addition to bone detail. For these reasons, CT has proved more sensitive and more specific than pleuridirectional tomography in the diagnosis of pituitary adenomas and other sellar and perisellar lesions.[37,38]

Coned views of the sella turcica and high-resolution CT should be the primary imaging modalities

for sellar and perisellar lesions. CT may be performed with and without contrast enhancement in axial and coronal projections; computer reconstruction permits sagittal viewing as well.

A study of normal female volunteers of childbearing age proved that less variation in the size of the pituitary gland is present during the postovulation period of the menstrual cycle than during the preovulation period.[39] Thus, wherever possible, CT studies of the pituitary gland should be done

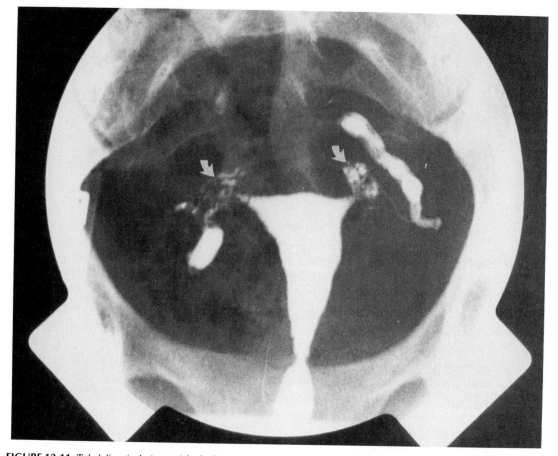

FIGURE 12-11. Tubal diverticula (arrows) in the intramural segments. There is also bilateral hydrosalpinx with tubal obstruction.

during the postovulation period to minimize the errors associated with the subtle enlargement of the gland often associated with microadenomas.

The radiologist must be aware that pituitary adenomas may be of equal, lower, or higher density than the pituitary gland itself.[37] Careful attention to the scanning technique must be given in order to accommodate this range of density. Low-density adenomas are often difficult to differentiate from empty sella syndrome, craniopharyngioma, and arachnoidal cysts. High-density adenomas, on the other hand, may be difficult to separate from aneurysms and meningiomas.[39,40]

Recent studies have shown that most prolactin-secreting microadenomas present a focal low density in a slightly enlarged contrast-enhanced pituitary gland.[41] These low-density microadenomas cannot be differentiated radiologically from pars intermedia cysts, metastases, epidermoid cysts, infarcts, or abscesses.[39,42]

Conventional cerebral angiography may be needed to differentiate pituitary adenomas from intra- and parasellar aneurysms. Angiography is also helpful in differentiating sellar and parasellar lesions from pituitary adenomas.[36,37,43]

Recently introduced digital subtraction angiography is an imaging technique of visualizing arteries by intravenous injection of contrast medium. The examination is usually performed by placing a catheter in either the superior vena cava, inferior vena cava, right atrium, or cephalic vein. The technique is safer than the conventional arteriogram and may be performed on an outpatient basis. However, the visualization of intracranial vessels is not selec-

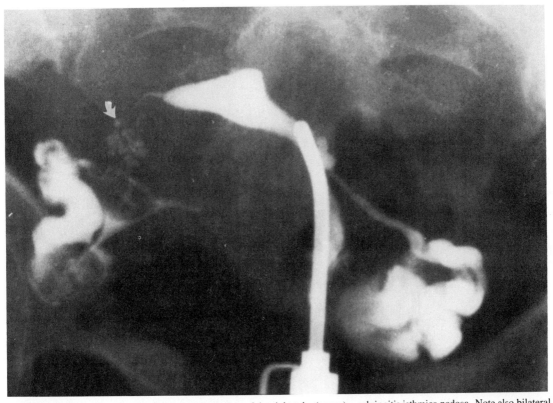

FIGURE 12-12. Tubal diverticula in the isthmic portion of the right tube (arrow)—salpingitis isthmica nodosa. Note also bilateral hydrosalpinx.

tive and subtle small vessel detail is poor. It has been shown to outline large parasellar vessels and their displacements. Large aneurysms can also be confirmed or excluded by this method.[43]

Empty Sella Syndrome

Normally, the pituitary gland located within the sella turcica takes up almost the entire intrasellar volume. It is attached to the base of the brain by the pituitary stalk, which passes through the sellar diaphragm made up of reflections of dura. The opening of the diaphragm is variable in size. The diaphragm with an opening of normal size (approximately 3 mm) is referred to as complete, and this is seen in 42% of the population. The others have openings through the diaphragm of varying size.[44]

The empty sella refers to that anatomic condition in which the sellar diaphragm is incomplete and permits the subarachnoid space to herniate in vary-ing degrees into the sella. This may lead to flattening of the pituitary gland, usually posteriorly and inferiorly, as well as enlargement of the sella.[44-46] Busch,[44] in 1951, was the first to refer to this state as the empty sella.

The primary or idiopathic empty sella syndrome is the result of the anatomic variation in the sellar diaphragm. Most reported cases have been obese, middle-aged women, with headaches as the most common symptom. The clinical appearances have varied, with normal endocrine function in approximately 75% of patients with empty sella syndrome. Impaired growth hormone secretion in response to hypoglycemia and decreased gonadotropic secretion are the most frequent abnormalities observed. Microadenomas in association with empty sellas have been found.[47-52]

The secondary empty sella syndrome results from surgery or from irradiation of an intrasellar tumor, with consequent loss of tissue volume. En-

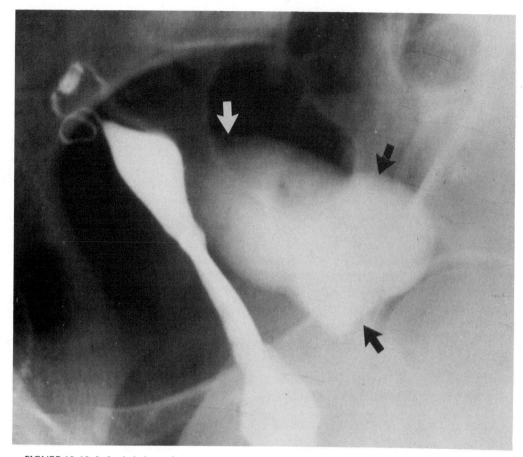

FIGURE 12-13. Left tubal obstruction at cornu. Note far-advanced left hydrosalpinx (at surgery, pyosalpinx).

docrine dysfunction is of the same degree in these cases as in patients treated for pituitary tumors in whom an empty sella does not develop. Rare cases of symptomatic visual-field defects have been found in association with empty sella syndrome.[53–55]

Enlargement of the sella is readily detected on plain films. However, this imaging technique does not differentiate the enlarged empty sella from enlargement due to an intrasellar mass. Such differentiation is now made with CT, where intrasellar herniation of the subarachnoid space can be identified, as can the pituitary stalk coursing through it.[56] The pituitary gland, which is flattened and displaced posteriorly and inferiorly, is often difficult to see. If the changes are subtle and doubtful, confirmation is obtained by performing high-resolution CT after intrathecal introduction of water-soluble contrast material (metrizamide cisternography).[37,55,56]

Post-treatment Evaluation of Pituitary Tumors

High-resolution CT is the imaging method of choice for evaluation of structural changes in patients who have been treated by either chemotherapy, surgery, or irradiation. In postsurgical and radiation therapy patients, a baseline examination is recommended should there later be a need for evaluation for recurrence. Reduction in size of the gland and complete resolution of pituitary adenomas have been shown in patients treated with bromocriptine or pergolide.[57,59]

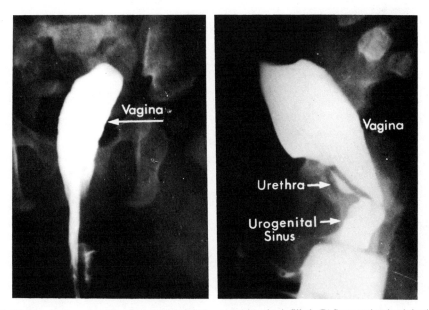

FIGURE 12-14. (A) Injection is made with a single catheter. Only a normal vagina is filled. (B) Same patient but injection is made by the flushing method. The tip of the syringe is in a urogenital sinus. A normal vagina and urethra enter the sinus near the end of the syringe, the anatomy of a female pseudohermaphrodite (From Shopfner.[32])

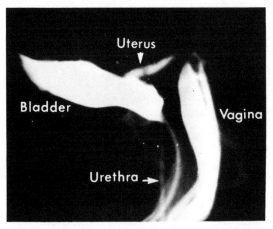

FIGURE 12-15. A 7-month-old child with ambiguous external genitalia. The injection was made with two catheters. The urethra, normal-size vagina, and uterus are filled. The urethra and vagina open together into a shallow vestibule, which was the only perineal opening. Above this opening was the phallus. Such anatomy can be seen with true hermaphroditism or male pseudohermaphroditism. This patient proved to have testicular tissue and a gonadal streak, indicating a male pseudohermaphrodite (From Shopfner.[32])

Magnetic Resonance Imaging

Magnetic resonance imaging (MRI) is in its infancy as a technique for imaging the pituitary and juxtapituitary region. Utilizing nuclear magnetic resonance (NMR) properties and without the use of ionizing radiation, MRI has the potential of displaying sagittal, coronal, and axial images of masses; it will more than replace CT for study of most patients with sellar tumors once the resolution of MRI is improved and the time for recording the image is significantly reduced.

ADRENALS

In the search for causes of gynecologic endocrine disorders, attention may center on the adrenal glands. Adrenal tumors may rarely be manifest on simple roentgenologic examinations, or they may require special techniques for demonstrations (see Figs. 12-21 through 12-27).

Some adrenal tumors, particularly pheochromocytomas and cortisol-secreting adenomas, may be

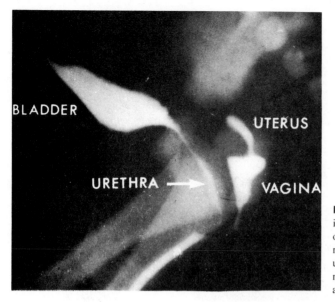

FIGURE 12-16. Newborn infant had ambiguous genitalia consisting of a phallus and a single perineal opening. Injection by catheter using a flushing technique was performed. The catheter is in a male-type urethra, with a verumontanum. At the site of the old müllerian tubercle is a hypoplastic vagina capped by a small uterus. (From Shopfner.[32])

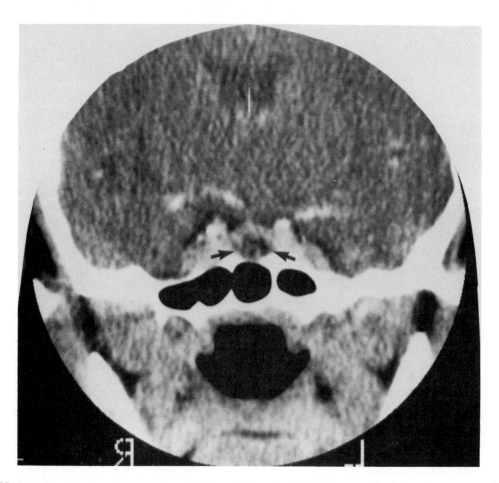

FIGURE 12-17. Coronal section of contrast-enhanced CT scan. Pituitary gland is slightly enlarged. Prolactinoma with a low-density center (arrows).

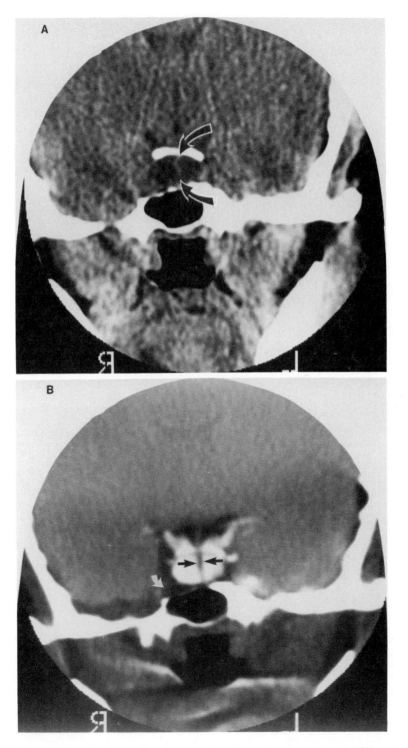

FIGURE 12-18. (A) Patient with hyperprolactinemia and suspected of having a microadenoma. Coronal CT scan shows a low density in an asymmetrically enlarged sella turcica. The pituitary stalk (arrows) is coursing through the low density. (B) Metrizamide CT cisternography confirms the partially empty sella with a pituitary microadenoma. Pituitary stalk (black arrows) courses through the contrast-enhanced cerebrospinal fluid. Defect due to pituitary microadenoma (white arrow) is present on the right with depression of the floor of the sella.

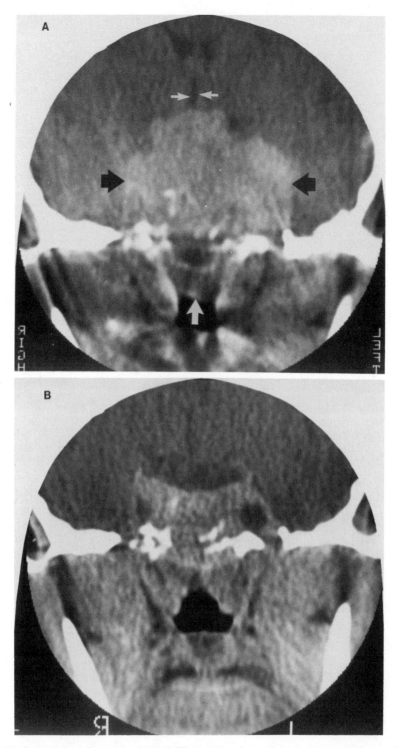

FIGURE 12-19. (A) Coronal view of contrast-enhanced CT scan. Note huge pituitary adenoma with extension upward in the suprasellar cistern with displacement of the third ventricle (white arrows), laterally (black arrows), and inferiorly into the nasopharynx (broad white arrow). (B) Coronal view of contrast enhanced CT scan at the same level approximately 5 months after bromocryptine therapy. Note the marked decrease in the size of the pituitary adenoma. There was a corresponding dramatic decrease in the prolactin level.

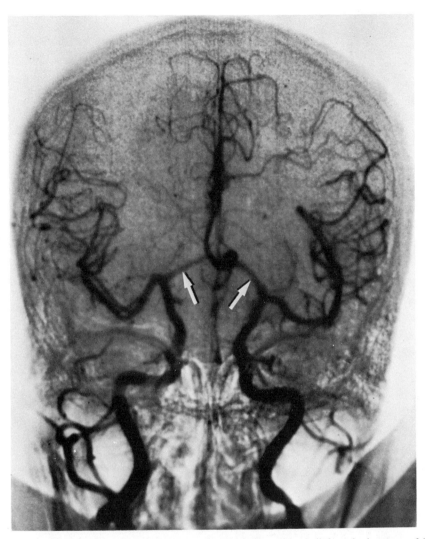

FIGURE 12-20. A 53-year-old female with chromophobe adenoma. Plain films of the skull showed enlargement of the sella turcica. Cerebral angiogram (subtraction film) shows appreciable elevation of the first portion of the anterior cerebral arteries (arrows) indicating extrasellar extension of tumor.

highly vascular and thus may be demonstrated by aortography and selective adrenal arteriography.[60,61] Since each adrenal is served by three arteries, delicate catheterization, injection, and filming techniques are required to identify tumor or adrenal hyperplasia.

In some instances, adrenal venography may be a useful technique for studying patients with suspected adrenal disease. The method has been particularly useful in studying patients with primary aldosteronism and in selected patients with Cushing's syndrome and with pure virilization.[62,63] Tumors smaller than 1 cm in diameter have been diagnosed by this technique. The method permits collection of adrenal venous blood for aldosterone assay during the course of the x-ray examination. Since this can be done selectively, it can facilitate the location of functioning tumors. Adrenal venography permits demonstration of adrenal tumors that are smaller or insufficiently vascularized to be detected by arteriography.

Radionuclide Adrenal Scan

The use of radionuclide imaging of the adrenal glands is an effective diagnostic procedure, es-

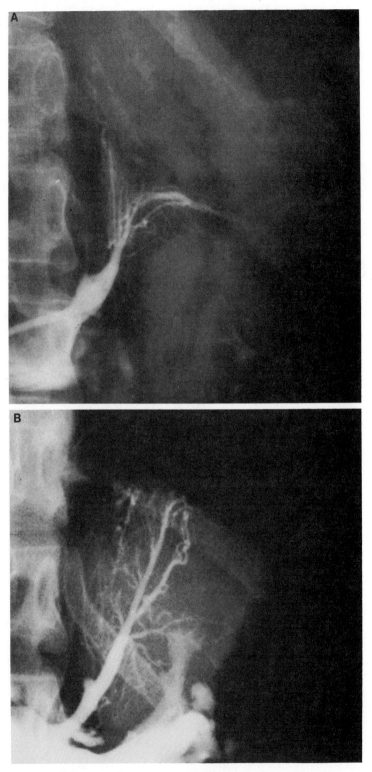

FIGURE 12-21. Adrenal venograms demonstrating normal venous patterns.

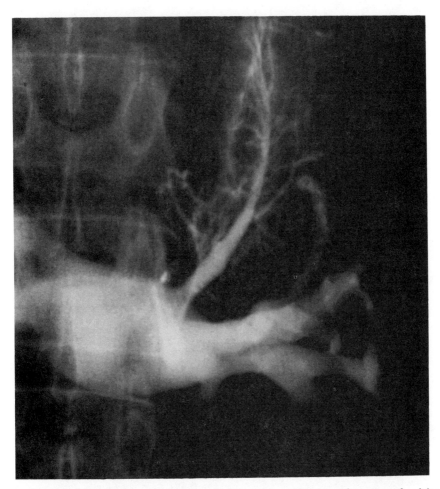

FIGURE 12-22. Left adrenal venogram demonstrating a stretched, irregular, and hypervascular pattern of nodular hyperplasia, proved at surgery. (Larger opacified vessels are renal veins.)

pecially with the new imaging agents,[131]I-6β-iodomethyl norcholesterol (^{131}I-6-iodocholesterol) for adrenal cortex and ^{131}I-metaiodobenzylguanidine (^{131}I-MIBG) for the adrenal medulla.[64,65] Radionuclide scan of the adrenals is unique among adrenal imaging procedures in that both adrenal structure and adrenal function are demonstrated.[64,66]

The indications for adrenal scanning have steadily increased. It is particularly useful in differentiating the various forms of adrenal cortical hyperplasia and hyperfunctioning adrenal adenomas.[66] The technique has the advantage of being noninvasive and free of complications. Limitations of the procedure are limited availability of the scanning agent, the relatively high radiation dose, and the necessity of waiting several days between the injection of the radionuclide and imaging.

Normal Adrenal Scan

A normal adrenal scan shows fairly symmetric uptake in both adrenals, although there are large variations in the uptake and in the gland locations. Usually the liver and part of the intestine are visualized because the ^{131}I-iodocholesterol is mainly metabolized by the liver and a large part of the radioiodine is excreted through the intestinal tract.

Cushing's Syndrome

A cortisol-producing adenoma shows unilateral increased uptake with suppression of the con-

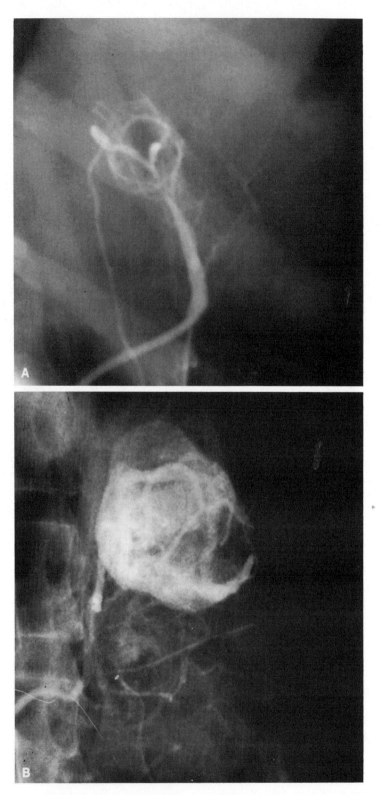

FIGURE 12-23. (A) Left adrenal venogram demonstrating veins circumscribing an avascular mass that proved to be an aldosteronoma. (B) Left adrenal venogram revealing a large, highly vascular mass with an avascular zone, which proved to be a large adenoma with a blood clot.

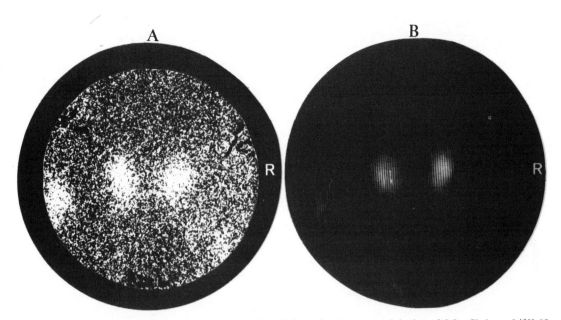

FIGURE 12-24. Normal radionuclide adrenal scan, obtained 5 days after intravenous injection of 0.8-mCi dose of ^{131}I-6β-iodomethylnorcholesterol. Both glands show symmetric, normal uptake. (A) Analogue image taken from gamma scintillation camera. Diffuse background activity in right side of field represents uptake by the liver. Focal activity in the edge of left field represents radionuclide activity in large intestine. (B) Digital image, the same image shown in (A) processed with contrast enhancement and smoothing, using a computer, PDP-11-34.

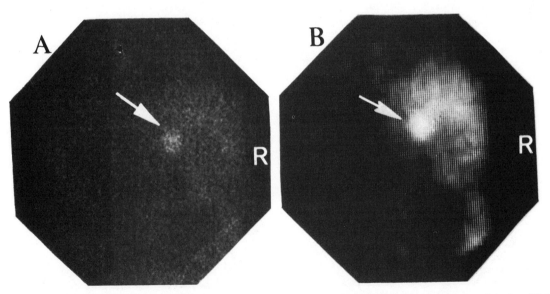

FIGURE 12-25. Radionuclide adrenal scan in a patient with adrenal adenoma, obtained 2 days after an intravenous injection of 0.6-mCi dose of ^{131}I-6β-iodomethylnorcholesterol in a patient with Cushing's syndrome. The scans, analogue image (A) and digital image (B), show abnormally increased uptake in right adrenal gland (arrow) and completely suppressed left gland. Uptake by the adrenals was 0.41% and 0.0% by right and left adrenal gland, respectively (normal range: 0.08–0.18%). A 3.5-cm cortical adenoma was removed from the right adrenal gland.

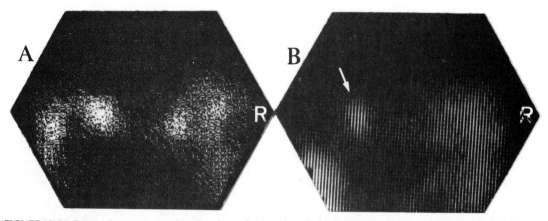

FIGURE 12-26. Dexamethasone suppression adrenal scan for detection of primary aldosteronoma. (A) Adrenal scan, digital image, obtained 4 days after intravenous injection of 1.0-mCi dose of [131]I-6β-iodomethylnorcholesterol in patient with hyperaldosteronism. Scan shows slightly increased uptake in left adrenal gland, while right gland appears to be smaller or suppressed. Note diffuse activity in liver (right) and intense activity in intestine (left). (B) Repeat scan obtained 5 days after intravenous injection of 0.9-mCi dose of [131]I-6β-iodomethylnorcholesterol. This time the patient was placed on oral dexamethasone medication, 2 mg every day beginning 3 days before the injection. The dexamethasone suppression scan shows the right adrenal gland to be completely suppressed while the left gland remains unsuppressible (arrow). A 1.1-cm small aldosterone-producing adenoma was removed from the left adrenal gland.

tralateral normal gland. The diagnosis may be made on the first scan obtained 2 days after the injection because the hyperfunctioning adenomas concentrate the ^{131}I-iodocholesterol faster than normally and thus are visualized earlier.[64,66] By contrast, bilateral adrenocortical hyperplasia shows diffusely increased bilateral uptake. In order to differentiate this condition from normal adrenals, the adrenal uptake measurement becomes useful.[66]

Adrenal Hyperandrogenism

Evaluation of women with hyperandrogenism is complicated because sources of elevated androgens can be ovaries, adrenals, or both. The radionuclide adrenal scan has been reported as useful in the evaluation of adrenal hyperandrogenism.[64]

Dexamethasone suppression scanning is also recommended for adrenal hyperandrogenism. Early

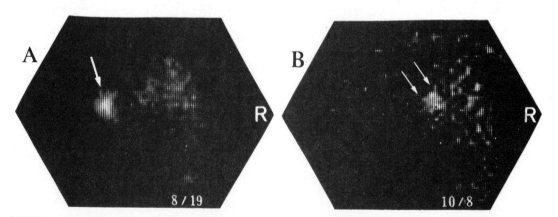

FIGURE 12-27. Radionuclide adrenal scan represents functional status of the gland. (A) Adrenal scan obtained 5 days after intravenous injection of 1.2-mCi dose of [131]I-6β-iodomethylnorcholesterol in a patient with Cushing's syndrome. The scan shows abnormally increased uptake in the left adrenal adenoma (arrow), and the right adrenal is completely suppressed. (B) Second adrenal scan obtained in the same patient 50 days after removal of the left adrenal gland. Note normal uptake in the right adrenal (thin arrows), which was completely suppressed on previous scan. The patient had normal corticosteroid levels at the time of the second imaging.

visualization of one adrenal on the suppression scan indicates adrenocortical adenoma, and early visualization of both glands indicates hyperplasia of the adrenals.[67]

The radionuclide adrenal scan is regarded as the most sensitive technique in the evaluation of functional abnormality of the adrenals. The uptake rate of ^{131}I-iodocholesterol by the adrenal gland reflects the functional status of the gland. Hyperfunctioning adrenals with slightly hyperplastic cortical structures such as in early stages of Cushing's disease or with a very small adenoma, can be better demonstrated by the radionuclide scan than by other noninvasive or invasive procedures.

Determination of whether an adrenal gland is functioning or is suppressed can best be made by either adrenal venous blood study for measurement of steroids or by radionuclide adrenal scanning.

GYNECOLOGIC ULTRASOUND

Since the initial reports of the value of ultrasound in the evaluation of pelvic pathology, this technique has undergone rapid advances that have permitted broad applications in the evaluation of gynecologic pathology.[68–70] Although ultrasound has widespread applications in the assessment of the presence, absence, and extent of disease, its ability to point to a specific histologic diagnosis is limited. Real-time ultrasonography is the imaging modality of choice for the evaluation of pelvic gynecologic pathology (see Figs. 12-28 through 12-36).

The widespread use of real-time ultrasonography has raised questions concerning the safety of this technique. However, research into the bioeffects of this modality have been conducted over the past 50 years, and to date there has been no demonstrated

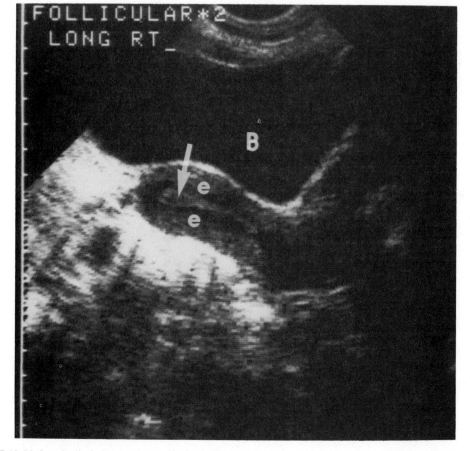

FIGURE 12-28. Longitudinal ultrasound scan. Uterine bull's eye (arrow) due to mucus in uterine canal surrounded by edematous endometrium (e). B, urinary bladder.

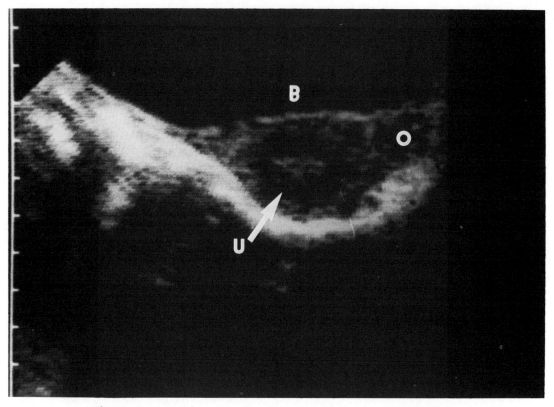

FIGURE 12-29. Transverse scan with uterine bull's-eye (arrow). B, bladder; O, ovary.

adverse effect related to diagnostic ultrasound.[71–74] Nevertheless, this procedure should be reserved for those patients in whom there is specific clinical indication.

In order to appreciate the clinical value of this modality, the sonographer must be aware of the normal anatomic and physiologic changes of both the uterus and ovaries, readily demonstrated with real-time ultrasonography.

Normal Anatomy and Physiology

Uterus

The sonographer must be aware of the patient's menstrual history prior to examination. It has been demonstrated that there are typical changes observed within the uterus during the course of the normal menstrual cycle.[75,76] A thin high-amplitude linear echo, representing the two opposed walls of the endometrial cavity, is normally seen. Absence

of this echo may indicate significant pathology. At mid-cycle, in response to endocrine changes, the central uterine echoes become dense and are surrounded by a hypoechoic halo of endometrium. The histologic correlates of the inner "bull's eye" are the vascular and glandular engorgement of the endometrium surrounding echogenic mucus within the central uterine cavity. Just before menses, the echogenic linear echo may decrease, reflecting sloughing of the endometrium.

The actual size of the uterus will vary with the patient's age and obstetric history; however, there are characteristic size relationships. In the prepubertal female, the cervix is typically thicker than that of the uterine corpus. This relationship rapidly changes following the menarche with the uterine corpus becoming thicker after puberty.[77] This relationship is thought to be due to the onset of estrogen stimulation. The knowledge of this physiologic alteration is useful in the evaluation of children with precocious puberty or adolescents with amenor-

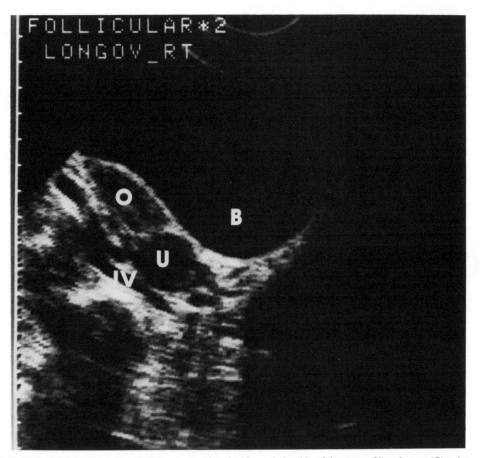

FIGURE 12-30. Longitudinal scan, day 8 of the menstrual cycle. Note relationship of the uterus (U) and ovary (O) to internal iliac vessels (IV).

rhea. Knowledge of the presence or absence of a uterus is useful for the evaluation of infants with ambiguous external genitalia.[77,79]

Ovaries

Ultrasound visualization of both ovaries has been reported in 73–100% of patients with at least one ovary being observed in 100% of patients examined.[69,77,80] The potential pitfalls in observation of the ovaries are primarily lack of adequate bladder distention, obesity, and the fact that the ovaries are freely mobile and frequently located posterior, anterior, or superior to the uterine corpus. Scanning from the contralateral side and angling the transducer properly will aid in satisfactorily delineating the ovaries in most patients.

The normal ovaries are echogenic and almond-shaped. They are only rarely visualized in patients under 2 years of age because of the lack of adequate bladder distention and poor patient cooperation.[77,79] In the prepubertal age group, ovarian volume ranges from 0.1 to 0.9 ml, with a median size of 0.5 ml. In the postpubertal female, the ovarian volume ranges from 1.5 to 5.7 ml, with a mean volume of 4.0 ml.[77,79]

Of particular interest is the ultrasonic assessment of the mature ovarian follicle and its role in the evaluation of the infertile patient. The presence and number of follicles are readily demonstrated with ultrasound.[81–85] The mature follicle ranges from 1.0 to 2.5 cm in diameter. The measurements in the nonoval follicle are the averages of the largest diameters visualized in two perpendicular scan plans. Several authors have examined correlation of follicular size and biochemical assessment of fol-

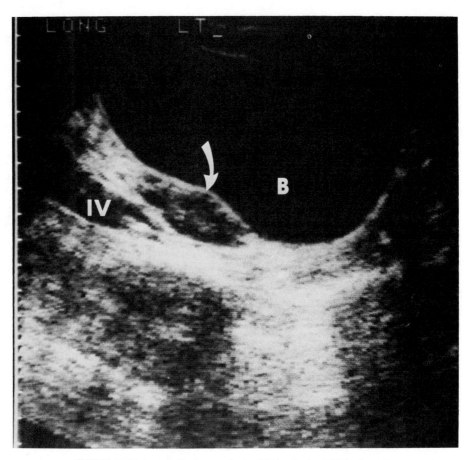

FIGURE 12-31. Longitudinal scan, day 9 with developing follicles (arrow).

licular maturity and have found the combination of techniques to be superior to biochemical analysis alone.[86-91] The minimum size of a follicle that will yield a mature ovum is 15 mm.[92] This information is important in the evaluation of the infertile patient because the presence and size of the ovarian follicle as determined by ultrasound may be used to predict the number of mature follicles and, therefore, predict the likelihood of obtaining a multiple gestation.[69,92] The presence of multiple follicles does not guarantee a multiple ovulation. Ultrasound is also useful in predicting the presence of ovarian stimulation when cystic ovarian enlargement is greater than 5 cm.[93,94] In addition, there is a characteristic of ultrasound that reflects actual ovulation. This consists of a sudden decrease in the follicular volume, the appearance of free fluid within the pouch of Douglas, and the sudden appearance of multiple low-level echoes within the mature folli-

cles.[76,81,95] Although absence of these findings does not exclude ovulation, their presence in any combination will certainly confirm ovulation. Ultrasound monitoring assumes importance with Pergonal therapy and in vitro fertilization techniques (see Chapter 32).

Pathology

Occasionally, sonographic features are specific for certain types of pelvic masses. Unfortunately, acoustical similarity or poor scanning technique not infrequently prevents diagnosis of a specific histologic entity. Ultrasonography is, however, extremely useful in answering the following major questions:

1. The presence or absence of a clinically suspected mass lesion

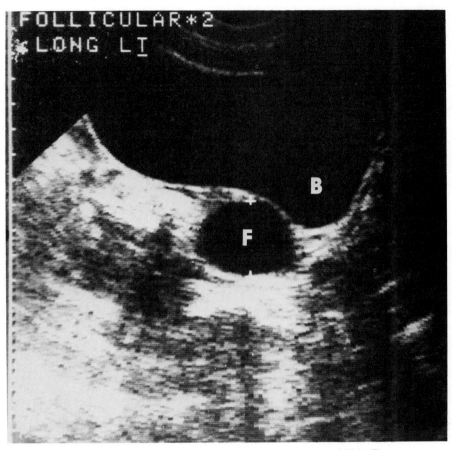

FIGURE 12-32. Longitudinal scan, day 14, with a dominant follicle (F).

2. The size, contour, and the internal consistency of the mass
3. The organ of origin
4. The involvement of surrounding structures, and
5. The presence or absence of fluid within the peritoneal cavity

These features combined with the clinical features of the case frequently considerably narrow the differential diagnostic possibilities.

In patients with either ovarian dysfunction or hyperfunction, knowledge of the presence of and the sonographic appearance of the normal ovary can be quite helpful in determining the presence of an abnormal one. There is a broad spectrum of ultrasound characteristics that may occasionally be present in varying types of ovarian lesions, thereby making the ultrasound findings nonspecific. It has been noted that in patients with polycystic ovarian disease some will show multiple small cysts measuring less than 1 cm with either normal or increased ovarian volume, while others may show a normal ovarian volume and normal acoustical architecture.[96,97] A benign or a malignant lesion may present the entire spectrum of an echogenic to an anechoic pattern.[69,98–103] However, a purely echo-free lesion is almost universally benign (cystic) whereas a solid or complex pattern may reflect either a benign or malignant lesion.

The value of ultrasound with respect to endocrinologically significant uterine abnormalities is restricted primarily to the presence or absence of the uterus in those patients with sex differentiation problems. For the evaluation of structural anomalies of the uterus, contrast radiography remains the imaging modality of choice. It has recently been noted that there are alterations in the normal acous-

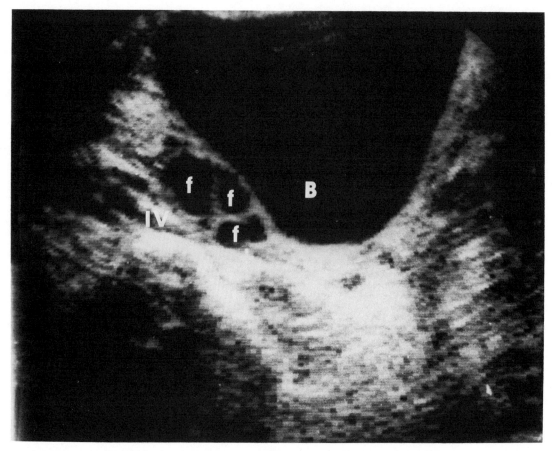

FIGURE 12-33. Longitudinal scan, day 14, in patient taking Pergonal. f, follicles.

tical appearance of the central uterine cavity in infertile patients.[104] The significance of the findings is yet to be determined.

GONADAL DYSGENESIS (Figs. 12-37 to 12-44)

The basic clinical elements of Turner's syndrome (gonadal dysgenesis) are sexual infantilism, primary amenorrhea, and short stature. In addition, a wide variety of congenital anomalies may occur separately or in combination.[105–114]

Among the anomalies reported are webbing of the neck, short phalanges of the hands or feet, cubitus valgus, wide arm span, medial femoral and tibial condyle defects, osteoporosis, some delay in bone maturation, cardiac defects, shield-shaped chest, renal anomalies, and low hairline. Additional anomalies include fused cervical vertebrae, scoliosis, spina bifida occulta, visual defects, deafness of various degrees, high-arched palate, low-placed ears, hypoplasia of the mandible, mongoloid features, syndactylism, Madelung's deformity, pes cavus, blue sclerae, hypertension of unknown cause, mental retardation, lymphangiectatic edema, telangiectasis, and pigmented nevi. Anomalies affecting almost every organ of the body have been described. Forbes and Engel[115] made note of the high incidence of diabetes mellitus in patients with gonadal dysgenesis and their relatives. Attention has been called to the high incidence of thyroiditis.[116] Pai et al.[117] summarized their findings as follows: (1) patients with Turner's syndrome are at a higher than average risk of developing thyroid disease even during childhood and adolescence; (2)

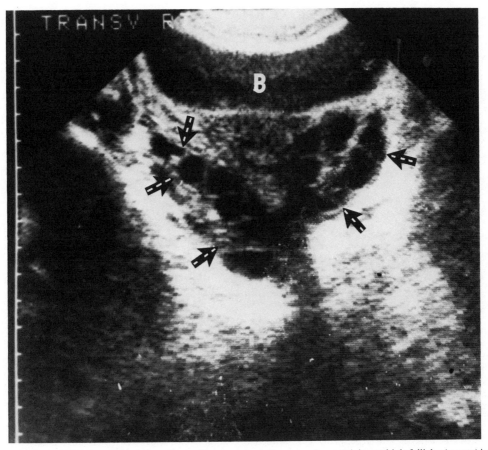

FIGURE 12-34. Ovarian hyperstimulation syndrome. Transverse scan. Large ovaries containing multiple follicles (arrows) in patient taking Pergonal.

the incidence is age related, as in the normal population; (3) elevated antibody titer alone does not indicate the thyroid function status of the patient but may indicate the need for careful periodic evaluation of the thyroid; and (4) since growth retardation is characteristic of Turner's syndrome, a further compromise due to hypothyroidism may not be noted. Polani et al.[118] have noted the high frequency of red-green color blindness in Turner's syndrome. There have also been cases of true gonadal dysgenesis without obvious associated congenital anomalies.

As would be expected in a condition having such widespread organ involvement, the radiologic findings are many. These can be best classified into skeletal and visceral abnormalities.

SKELETAL ABNORMALITIES

Bone Demineralization

A striking feature noted in most patients with gonadal dysgenesis is bone demineralization. Rarefaction of bone structures is most conspicuous in the bones of the hands, feet, and vertebrae, although it may also be present elsewhere. The trabeculae appear thin and widely spaced. In fact, Bercu et al.[119] believe that the most characteristic radiographic finding of Turner's syndrome is the coarse reticular pattern of the carpal bones due to this demineralization. There has been no complaint of pain, and no pathologic fractures have been encountered. Concentration of calcium and phos-

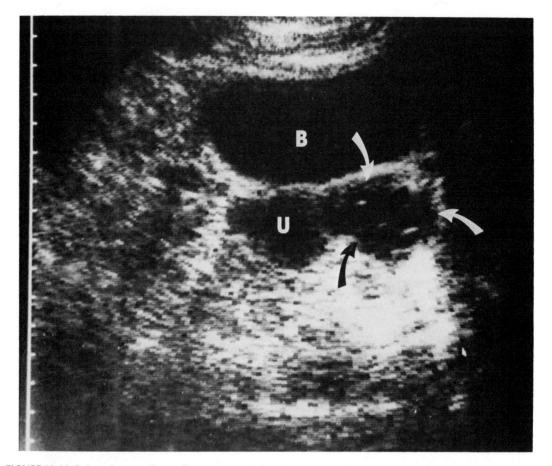

FIGURE 12-35. Polycystic ovary disease. Transverse scan in female with infertility and menstrual irregularity. Note multiple small cysts within the ovary (arrows).

phorus in the serum are normal in all patients studied. No apparent change has been reported after prolonged administration of estrogens. Whether this can be properly referred to as osteoporosis is debatable. Adequate biopsies that might explain the nature of the condition have not been performed. It has been suggested that these changes merely reflect the thinness of the bony matrix.

Osseous Maturation

There are differences in opinion in the literature as to whether delayed osseous maturation accompanies gonadal dysgenesis. Many reports do make direct reference to delayed epiphyseal closure in male and female patients. Lisser et al.[112] noted that "retardation of the epiphyseal closure is not the usual finding in this syndrome which is surprising

in view of the striking genital infantilism." Furthermore, Tanner et al.[120] concluded that "though in Turner's syndrome there is probably some slight retardation compared with girls' standards, together with abnormal asymmetry of development, in general XO leads to approximately the same bone age as XX." Keats and Burns,[110] Acheson and Zampa,[121] and Del Castillo et al.[122] indicate that the maturation of the skeletal system is normal up to 15 years of age. McDonough and Byrd[123] noted that the bone age of children with gonadal dysgenesis progresses satisfactorily until expected endocrine menarche, at which time it stops, usually at the chronologic age of 11–12 years. Bone age arrest dates the onset of gonadal failure. It is common to find late fusion of the apophyses of the iliac crest and of the ischia.[111] The development of these apophyses depends on ovarian steroid secretion and

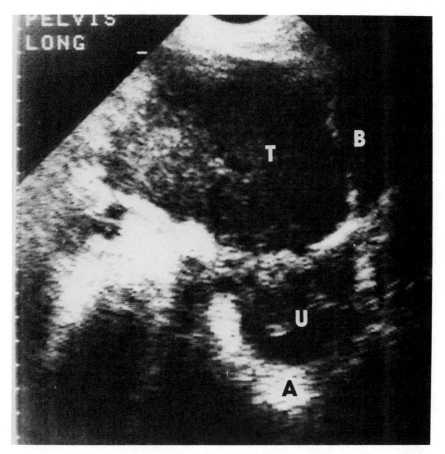

FIGURE 12-36. Longitudinal scan in patient with a Krukenberg tumor (T) and malignant ascites (A).

fusion with the body of bone further depends on continued release of these steroids. Where there is absence of ovarian function these apophyses do not undergo normal ossification. If ossification appears, this indicates that ovarian steroids have been or are being released. Limited ossification appears in those forms of gonadal dysgenesis with limited estrogenic ridge activity.[123]

Cubitus Valgus

Many investigators have stressed the frequency of cubitus valgus (increase in carrying angle of the arm) in patients with gonadal dysgenesis. Hoffenberg and Jackson,[124] however, found only one patient with cubitus valgus in their series of 27 patients, and the valgus deformity was minimal at that. These workers question whether this anomaly really exists in a gonadal dysgenesis syndrome.

Scoliosis

The most common vertebral abnormality encountered is scoliosis. This is generally slight, not apparent clinically, and only evident on roentgenographic examination. However, it may indeed be marked. There have been reports of irregularity and fragmentation of vertebral epiphyseal plates.[106,109,122]

Hands and Wrists

The hands have received much attention in the study of gonadal dysgenesis. Archibald et al.[125] studied the hands of 2594 patients, including 17 with gonadal dysgenesis, both clinically and roentgenographically. Their findings indicate that shortness of the fourth metacarpal relative to the fifth is of frequent occurrence in patients with gonadal dys-

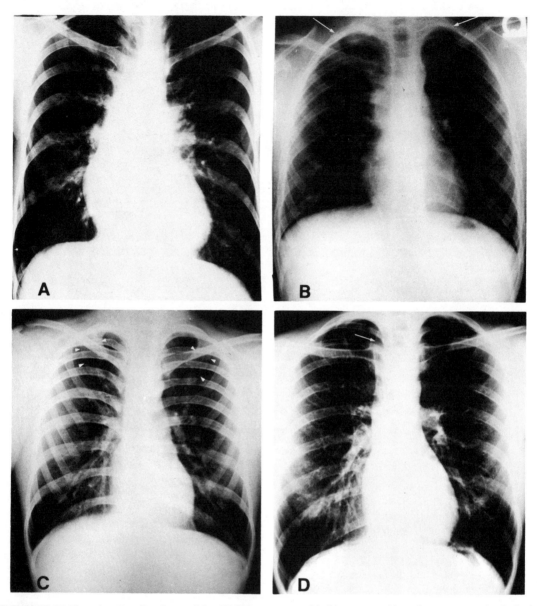

FIGURE 12-37. Thoracic and cardiac abnormalities. (A) Thirty-two-year-old white woman with cardiac murmurs and arrhythmias was acyanotic. After sudden death, postmortem examination revealed a large endocardial cushion defect (atrioventricularis cummunis). (B) Ten-year-old white girl with coarctation of the aorta. Bilateral supernumerary cervical ribs (arrows) are present. (C) Twenty-three-year-old black woman. The first rib bilaterally is markedly expanded (arrows). (D) Twenty-one-year-old white woman who was moderately hypertensive with no abnormality noted to account for it. Arrow points to an azygous fissure. (From Levin.[111]) (E) Twenty-one-year-old white woman with moderate thoracic spine scoliosis. (From Levin.[111]) (F) Seventeen-year-old black girl with minimal scoliosis. This patient also had supernumerary cervical ribs. The left twelfth rib is hypoplastic. (G) Forty-one-year-old white woman with moderate dorsal kyphoscoliosis. Note anterior wedging of the body of T-5 (arrow) and moderate bone demineralization.

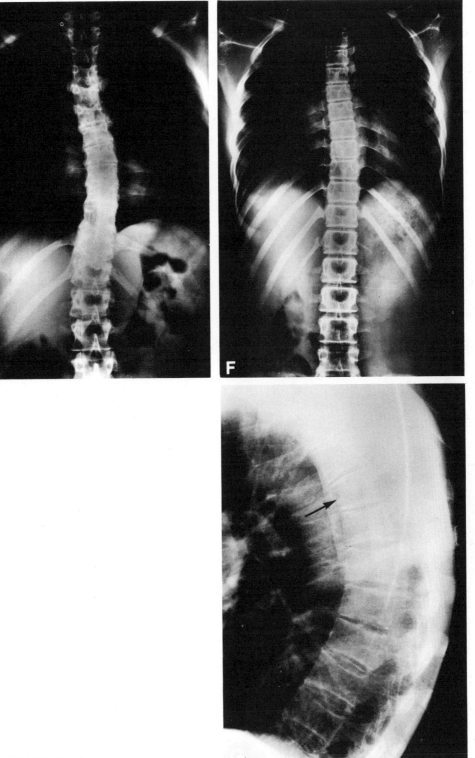

FIGURE 12-37. (*Continued*)

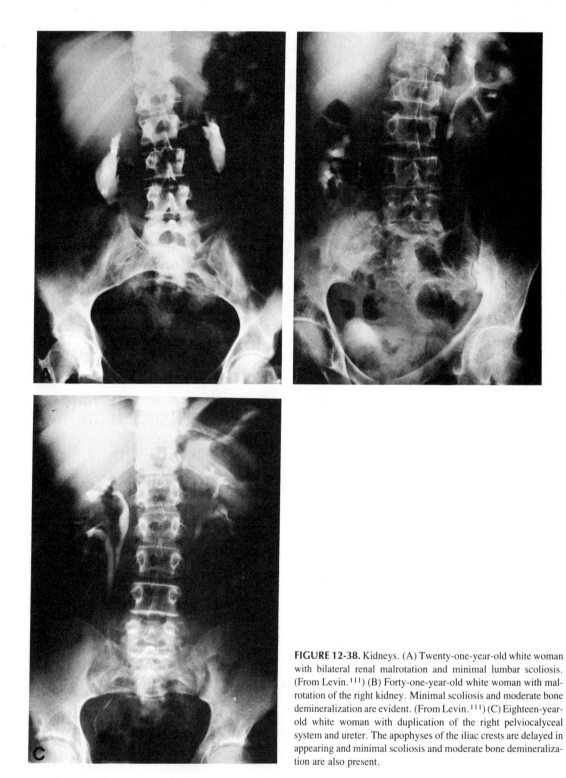

FIGURE 12-38. Kidneys. (A) Twenty-one-year-old white woman with bilateral renal malrotation and minimal lumbar scoliosis. (From Levin.[111]) (B) Forty-one-year-old white woman with malrotation of the right kidney. Minimal scoliosis and moderate bone demineralization are evident. (From Levin.[111]) (C) Eighteen-year-old white woman with duplication of the right pelviocalyceal system and ureter. The apophyses of the iliac crests are delayed in appearing and minimal scoliosis and moderate bone demineralization are also present.

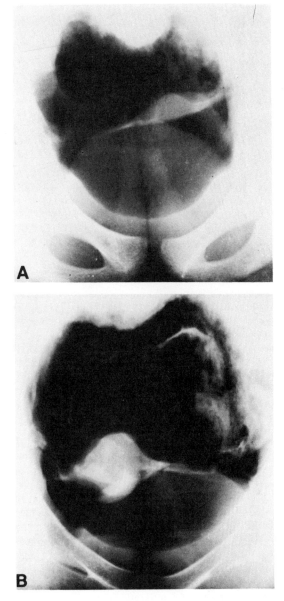

FIGURE 12-39. Pelvic pneumograms. (1) Seventeen-year-old black girl with an infantile uterus. No ovary is present. (B) Twenty-one-year-old white woman. No ovary is present. The uterus is near normal in size, perhaps as a result of 4 years of estrogen therapy.

genesis, having either female or male sex chromatin. Normally a line drawn tangentially to the distal ends of the heads of the fifth and fourth metacarpals extends distal to the third metacarpal. A positive metacarpal sign is present when the line passes through the head of the third metacarpal. When the line is tangential to the head of the third metacarpal, the sign is considered borderline. Of 17 female patients with gonadal dysgenesis, 11 had a positive metacarpal sign, and 3 had a borderline one. The positive sign is usually bilateral. The left side is the one of most frequent occurrence and degree of positiveness; this apparently is not related to hand dominance. It is of interest that two male patients with primary hypogonadism and four of six patients with hypophyseal hypogonadism had positive or borderline metacarpal signs in one or both hands.

Those investigators[125] also concluded that the metacarpal sign is without significance as far as

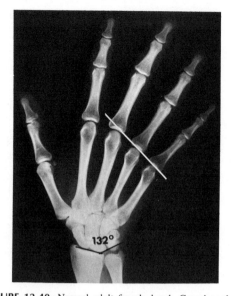

FIGURE 12-40. Normal adult female hand. Carpal angle is formed by intersection of a line touching the proximal border of the triquetrum and lunate bones. Normally this angle is 131.5°, with a standard deviation of ±7.2°. The angle is reduced in gonadal dysgenesis. The metacarpal line, drawn tangential to the distal ends of the fifth and fourth metacarpals, normally extends distal to the third metacarpal (negative metacarpal sign).

gonadal development is concerned when found in more than one generation of the same family. When found in only one generation, the sign is frequently associated with gonadal anomaly.

Kosowicz[126] not only confirmed the findings of Archibald et al. but pursued the study further and described a "carpal sign." He noted abnormally shaped bones in the proximal carpal row to be present frequently in gonadal dysgenesis. These bones did not form a slight arch, as is normal, but were often angular. This roentgenographic finding is noted on films of hands and wrists taken in the neutral position. When two tangents are drawn, the first one touching the proximal border of the navicular and lunate bones and the second one the proximal border of the triquetral and lunate bones, the angle formed by the intersection of these lines is called the "carpal angle." In normal subjects, this angle measures 131.5°, with a standard deviation of ±7.2°. In 23 patients with gonadal dysgenesis, the angle was found to be reduced, ranging from 102° to 117°, hence smaller by more than 2 SD from normal. In other patients with gonadal dysgenesis, the carpal angle was slightly decreased, ranging

from 118° to 131°, but never exceeding the mean value of this angle in normal subjects.

Kosowicz[127] made a number of other observations in his concern with the roentgen palmistry of gonadal dysgenesis. He noted that distal phalanges often had a drumstick appearance, phalangeal shafts were often slender, metaphyses sometimes appeared convex, epiphyses were flattened, and brachyphalangia and brachycarpia were often present. Madelung's deformity and protruding ulnae and nail anomalies were also encountered. Bercu et al.[119] believe that a coarse reticular pattern of carpal bones is the most characteristic radiologic sign of Turner's syndrome. This is a nonspecific finding, however, and is certainly subject to observer definition.

Necic and Grant[128] studied hand films from 17 patients with Turner's syndrome and 17 age-matched girls with constitutional short stature. They reported that while none of the radiological signs clearly distinguished between the two groups, ballooning of the tips of the terminal phalanges with a high ratio between the tip and mid-shaft diameters seemed to be the most useful sign of Turner's syndrome.

Roentgenograms of the feet often show similar changes to those in the hands.

Knees

Changes found in the roentgenograms of the knees were also noted by Kosowicz,[129] who reported the presence of a deformity of the medial tibial condyle in 12 of 18 cases of Turner's syndrome studied, in patients aged 8–42 years. Clinical examination did not reveal any lateral bowing of the tibia or other knee deformity.

These changes are bilateral and generally symmetric. The medial femoral condyle is larger than the lateral and extends downward below the level of the lateral condyle. The medial tibial condyle is enlarged and projects medially. In some instances a beaklike exostosis projects from the medial tibial condyle. The tibial epiphyseal plate is angled obliquely, medially and downward. The proximal tibial epiphysis is likewise deformed; its medial aspect spreads pointedly toward the enlarged and depressed metaphysis. In addition to the skeletal findings, there have been many reports of various skeletal abnormalities in patients with Turner's syndrome. These have little diagnostic significance, since they may occur as isolated findings in otherwise normal persons and are generally discovered

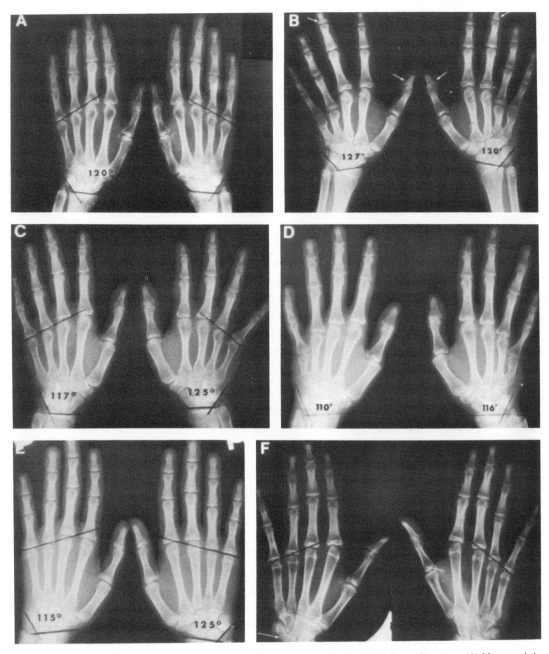

FIGURE 12-41. Hands of six patients with gonadal dysgenesis, each with a male (negative) chromatin pattern. (A) Metacarpal sign borderline on the left and positive on the right. The carpal angle is 120° bilaterally. Bone demineralization is evident. (B) The fourth and fifth metacarpals are short bilaterally. The terminal phalanges of the thumbs and middle fingers are also short (arrows). The epiphyses of the short phalanges are incompletely formed and fused with the shafts of the phalanges. The carpal angle is slightly decreased on the left, more on the right. (C) The metacarpal sign is negative on the right and positive on the left. The carpal angles are decreased, more so on the left. (D) The carpal angles are markedly decreased bilaterally. The fifth metacarpals are markedly shortened, the fourth moderately so. (E) The metacarpal sign is positive bilaterally and the carpal angles are decreased. (F) Borderline metacarpal sign on the left, positive on the right. The shafts of the terminal phalanges are slender and the tufts relatively broad (''drumsticks''). On the left, the triquetrum and lunate are congenitally fused (arrow).

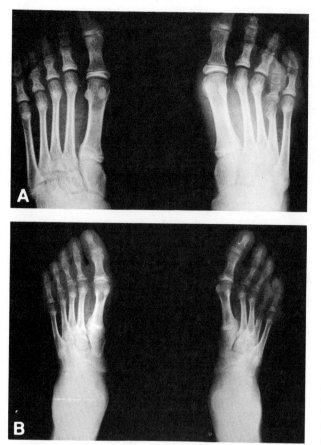

FIGURE 12-42. (A) Feet of two patients with gonadal dysgenesis, each with a male (negative) chromatin pattern. The right fourth metatarsal is shorter than normal. The proximal phalanx of the left fourth toe is short. There is slight hallux valgus deformity. (B) The right fourth metatarsal is short and there is moderate hallux valgus.

only when one looks for them in patients with more obvious roentgenographic signs of gonadal dysgenesis; they are roentgenologic ornamentations. Among these are lack of modeling of the clavicles, unevenness of rib caliber, narrowing of the pubic arch and sacrosciatic notch, hypoplasia of the body of the first cervical vertebra, anomalous development of the first and second cervical vertebrae, tilting of the articular surface of the trochlea, and bridging of the sella turcica.

VISCERAL ANOMALIES

Cardiovascular Malformations

Abnormalities of the cardiovascular system are often encountered in patients with Turner's syndrome. In a study of 55 patients with this disorder, Haddad and Wilkins[107] found eight patients with coarctation of the aorta, two of whom also had subaortic stenosis. Also noted were subaortic stenosis in one patient without coarctation, ventricular septal defect in another, and dextrocardia in a third patient. Thus 20% of this series had definite cardiovascular anomalies. Heart murmurs considered functional were present in eight patients. Rainier-Pope et al.[113] studied 36 patients with Turner's syndrome. Sixteen (44%) had cardiac anomalies, of whom seven had coarctation of the aorta, seven pulmonic stenosis, one an endocardial cushion defect, and one a ventricular septal defect with a patent ductus arteriosus. Two of those with coarctation had associated cardiovascular defects (one with patent ductus arteriosus and one with aortic stenosis). Of the seven patients with pulmonic stenosis, three had associated atrial septal defects and one a ventricular septal defect. Nora et al.[130] stud-

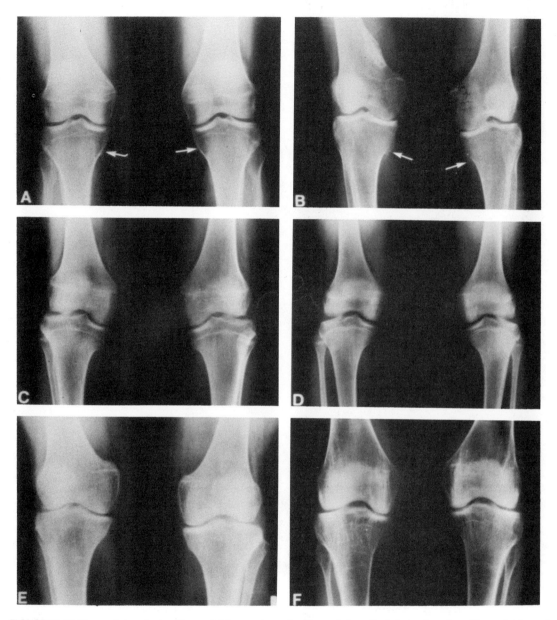

FIGURE 12-43. Knees of six patients with gonadal dysgenesis, each with a male (negative) chromatin pattern. The medial femoral condyle is prominent in each case, as is downward and medial angulation of the medial articulating surface. Tibial spurs are present in (A) and (B) (arrows). A benign cortical defect is present in the medial aspect of the right femur in (B). (From Levin.[111])

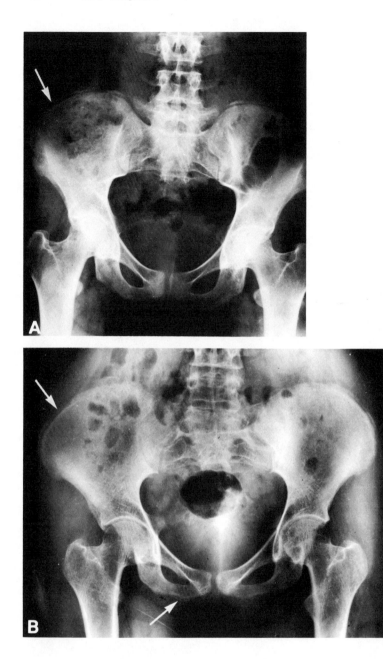

FIGURE 12-44. (A) Twenty-one-year-old woman with delayed fusion of the iliac crest apophyses (arrow). (From Levin.[111]) (B) Twenty-three-year-old woman with unfused iliac crest and ischial apophyses (arrows).

ied 40 patients with unequivocal Turner's stigmata and cardiovascular disease. Two distinct clusters of cardiovascular lesions were observed. Coarctation of the aorta was present in 11 of 16 patients with XO Turner's syndrome but in none of those with Turner's phenotype or Turner's mosaic constitution. Of 24 patients with Turner's phenotype or mosaic constitution, 21 had pulmonic stenosis. No pulmonic stenosis was found in any with XO Turner's syndrome. Another study of nine patients with 45, XO karyotype and nine with Turner's phenotype and normal karyotype shows that of the nine XO patients four had coarctation of the aorta, four had aortic stenosis, and the remaining patient had both.

Each of the nine others had pulmonic stenosis.[131] Many other reports of coarctation of the aorta associated with Turner's syndrome have appeared in the literature.[112,132–134]

Ravelo et al.[131] reported that children with Turner's syndrome who have coarctation of the aorta have significant risk of perioperative hemorrhage from aortic rupture. These workers recommended that consideration be given to angioplasty rather than to resection of the coarcted segment because of friability of the aortic wall.

Idiopathic Hypertension

Idiopathic hypertension is occasionally found in gonadal dysgenesis.[135] Some patients have been carefully studied for associated adrenal abnormality, renal disease, and renal vascular disease, but the cause has not been uncovered.[107] The hypertension does generally respond to antihypertensive drug therapy.

Renal Anomalies

In 1966 Hortling[108] noted a significant increase in the number of congenital kidney anomalies in patients with Turner's syndrome. These anomalies may be represented as aberrations of renal rotation, fused kidneys, or absence of a kidney. Since then, a number of other authorities have confirmed these findings.[111,136,137] Approximately 25% of persons with Turner's syndrome have significant renal abnormalities, the most frequent of which is horseshoe kidney.

Lymphedema

One of the prominent clinical manifestations of Turner's syndrome during infancy and early childhood is puffy edema, especially over the dorsum of the hands and feet. This lymphedema may be recognizable in utero by ultrasonic imaging as fetal hydrops.[138,139] This condition subsides spontaneously as the child gets older. No cause had been found until Benson et al.[140] reported on their investigation of six phenotypic females with lymphedema. Lymphangiography proved these patients to have hypoplasia or aplasia of the superficial lymphatics of the legs. In addition, two patients were found to have anomalous lymphatic vessels connecting the hypoplastic superficial lymphatic vessels to the deep systems. It was suggested that

these channels may contribute to the disappearance of the edema in patients with gonadal dysgenesis.

Intestinal Telangiectasis

There is a relatively high incidence of intestinal telangiectasis in patients with Turner's disease, in some instances leading to gastrointestinal bleeding. In a study of 55 patients with gonadal dysgenesis conducted by Haddad and Wilkins,[107] multiple intestinal telangiectasis was suspected in three. In two cases, the diagnosis was verified by exploratory laparotomy, and in the third the appearance of the intestinal mucosa on proctoscopic examination was very suspicious. Other isolated cases of multiple intestinal telangiectasis in patients with gonadal dysgenesis have been reported.[141] Barreto et al.[142] reported on the value of abdominal angiography in Turner's syndrome in instances of gastrointestinal bleeding, in order to establish a preoperative diagnosis of intestinal telangiectasis.

SUMMARY

The determination of skeletal age may be important in the study of a patient with growth retardation. Accurate assessment requires proper radiography and skillful interpretation by the radiologist. The determined bone age must then be coupled with other data about the patient and parents in order to arrive at a clinically useful prediction of adult stature. A number of caveats should be considered before embarking on a bone age study, as noted in the section on determination of skeletal age.

Hysterosalpingography is an important diagnostic technique for the study of infertility. Uterine, tubal, and peritubal abnormalities accounting for infertility may be demonstrated. Proof of absence of such abnormalities is also of importance.

Radiologic study contributes significantly to the assessment of intersexual states. Familiarity with the intersex anomalies and proper radiographic technique permits the radiologist to assess intersex states with accuracy.

Studies of the sella turcica and perisellar structures are important in the evaluation of women with possible pituitary adenomas, other tumors, or empty sellae. The radiologist has at his command a variety of techniques to choose from, including plain films, pluridirectional tomography, computed tomography (with and without contrast enhancement), arteriography, subtraction angiography, and magnetic resonance imaging. In consultation with the endocrinologist or gynecologist, the radiologist can select the most appropriate approach.

The most efficacious imaging technique for studying the adrenal glands is radionuclide scanning. This technique permits evaluation of both adrenal structure and adrenal function. The method is particularly useful in differentiating among various forms of adrenocortical hyperplasia and hyperfunctioning of adrenal adenoma. Adrenal arteriography and venography are other imaging techniques useful in selected patients with Cushing's syndrome and with pure virilization.

Ultrasonography is a useful diagnostic imaging technique; its value is enhanced in that it does not expose the patient to ionizing radiation. The ovaries are easily imaged, and their size can be readily determined, as can diagnosis of cysts or tumor of the organs. Assessment of follicle maturation is easily accomplished by ultrasonography. The uterus can likewise be readily imaged and masses identified. Changes relating to physiologic and anatomic differences occurring in various phases of the menstrual cycle are readily displayed.

ACKNOWLEDGMENTS. The author would like to thank Drs. U. Yun Ryo, Dushyant V. Patel, and Thomas D. Brandt for assisting in the preparation of this chapter.

QUESTIONS

1. A 48-year-old obese woman with headaches and decreased gonadotropin is suspected of having empty sella syndrome. Which imaging method is the one of choice as the first procedure?

2. A 26-year-old woman with pure virilization is suspected of having an abnormality of the adrenal gland. Which imaging method is the one of choice as the first procedure?

3. A 12-year-old girl with gonadal dysgenesis is found to have a palpable midline abdominal mass. What is the mass most likely to be?

4. To assess ovulation and follicle size and number, which imaging technique is the most reliable?

REFERENCES

1. Greulich WW, Pyle SI: *Radiographic Atlas of Skeletal Development of the Hand and Wrist*, 2nd ed. Stanford, CA, Stanford University Press, 1959
2. Todd TW: *Atlas of Skeletal Maturation (Hand)*. St. Louis, Mosby, 1937
3. Buckler JMH: How to make the most of bone ages. *Arch Dis Child* 58:761–763, 1983
4. Graham CB: Assessment of bone maturation—methods and pitfalls. *Radiol Clin North Am* 10:185–202, 1972*
5. Johnston FE: The concept of skeletal age. *Clin Pediatr* 1:133–144, 1962
6. Mainland D: Evaluation of the skeletal age method of estimating children's development. I. Systematic errors in the assessment of roentgenograms. *Pediatrics* 12:114–128, 1953
7. Mainland D: Evaluation of the skeletal age method of estimating children's development. II. Variable errors in the assessment of roentgenograms. *Pediatrics* 13:165–172, 1954
8. Mainland D: Evaluation of the skeletal age method of estimating children's development. III. Comparison of measurement and inspection in the assessment of roentgenograms. *Pediatrics* 20:979–992, 1957
9. Mellman WJ, Bongiovanni AM, Hope JW: The diagnostic usefulness of skeletal maturation in an endocrine clinic. *Pediatrics* 23:530–544, 1959
10. Tanner JM, Landt KW, Cameron N, et al: Prediction of adult height from height and bone age in childhood: A new system of equations (TW Mark II) based on a sample including very tall and very short children. *Arch Dis Child* 58:767–776, 1983
11. Tanner, JM, Whitehouse RH, Marshall WA, et al: *Assessment of Skeletal Maturity and Prediction of Adult Height. (TW 2 Method)*. London, Academic, 1975
12. Roche AF, Wainer H, Thissen D: The RWT method for the prediction of adult stature. *Pediatrics* 56:1027–1033, 1975
13. Bayley N, Pinneau SR: Tables for predicting adult height from skeletal age: Revised for use with Greulich-Pyle hand standards. *J Pediatr* 40:423–441, 1952
14. Simmons K, Greulich WW: Menarcheal age, and the height, weight, and skeletal age of girls age 7–17 years. *J Pediatr* 22:518–548, 1943
15. Garn SM, Rohmann CG, Silverman FN: Radiographic standards for postnatal ossification and tooth calcification. *Med Radiogr Photogr* 43:45–66, 1967
16. Sanfilippo JS, Yussman MA, Smith O: Hysterosalpingography in the evaluation of infertility: A six-year review. *Fertil Steril* 30:636–643, 1978
17. Pontifex G, Trichopoulous D, Karpathios S: Hysterosalpingography in the diagnosis of infertility. *Fertil Steril* 23:829–833, 1972
18. Pittaway DE, Winfield AC, Maxson W, et al: Prevention of acute pelvic inflammatory disease after hysterosalpingography: Efficacy of doxycycline prophylaxis. *Am J Obstet Gynecol* 147:623–626, 1983
19. Siegler AM: Hysterosalpingography. *Fertil Steril* 40:139–158, 1983

*Review article or chapter.

20. O'Connor KM, Hull MCR: Towards painless hysterosalpingography. *Br J Radiol* 56:690, 1983
21. Barnett E: The clinical value of hysterosalpingography. Part I. *J Fac Radiol* 7:115–129, 1955
22. Cooper RA, Jabamoni R, Pieters CH: Fertility rate after hysterosalpingography with Sinografin. *AJR* 141:105–106, 1983
23. DeCherney AH, Kort H, Barney JB, et al: Increased pregnancy rate with oil-soluble hysterosalpingography dye. *Fertil Steril* 33:407–410, 1980
24. Green-Armytage VB: The lessons and virtues of salpingography: An improved technique. *J Obstet Gynaecol Br Emp* 50:23–26, 1943
25. Horbach JGM, Maathuis JB, Van Hall EV: Factors influencing the pregnancy rate following hysterosalpingography and their prognostic significance. *Fertil Steril* 24:15–18, 1973
26. Mackey RA, Glass RH, Olson LE, et al: Pregnancy following hysterosalpingography with oil and water soluble dye. *Fertil Steril* 22:504–507, 1971
27. Robins SA, Shapira AA: The value of hysterosalpingography. *N Engl J Med* 205:380–395, 1931
28. Rubin IC: *Uterotubal Insufflation: A Clinical Diagnostic Method of Determining the Tubal Factor in Sterility Including Therapeutic Aspects and Comparative Notes on Hysterosalpingography.* St. Louis, Mosby, 1947
29. Barnett E: The clinical value of hysterosalpingography. II. Tubal conditions. *J Fac Radiol* 7:184–196, 1956
30. Parekh MC, Arronet GH: Diagnostic procedures and methods in the assessment of the female pelvic organs with specific reference to infertility. *Clin Obstet Gynecol* 15:1–104, 1972
31. Bligh AS, Williams EO: The effect of the full bladder in hysterosalpingography. *Br J Radiol* 29:99–102, 1956
32. Shopfner CE: Genitography in intersexual states. *Radiology* 82:664–674, 1964
33. Tristan TA, Everlein WR, Hope JW: Roentgenologic investigation of patients with heterosexual development. *AJR* 76:562–568, 1956
34. Cremin BJ: Intersex states in young children: The importance of radiology in making a correct diagnosis. *Clin Radiol* 25:63–73, 1974
35. Peck AG, Poznanski AK: A simple device for genitography. *Radiology* 103:212–213, 1972
36. Daniels DL, Williams AL, Thornton RS, et al: Differential diagnosis of intrasellar tumors by computed tomography. *Radiology* 141:697–701, 1981
37. Taylor S: High resolution computed tomography of the sella. *Radiol Clin North Am* 20:207–236, 1982
38. Syvertsen A, Haughton VM, Williams AL, et al: The computed tomography appearance of the normal pituitary gland and pituitary microadenomas. *Radiology* 133:385–391, 1979
39. Swartz JD, Russell KB, Basile BA, et al: High-resolution computed tomographic appearance of the intrasellar contents in women of childbearing age. *Radiology* 147:115–117, 1983
40. Khangure MS, ApSimon HT: Some pitfalls in the diagnosis of pituitary tumours: The importance of carotid angiography. *Surg Neurol* 16:300–308, 1981
41. Hemminghytt S, Kalkhoff RK, Daniels DL, et al: Computed tomographic study of hormone-secreting microadenomas. *Radiology* 146:65–69, 1983
42. Chambers EF, Turski PA, LaMasters D, et al: Regions of low density in the contrast-enhanced pituitary gland: Normal and pathologic processes. *Radiology* 144:109–113, 1982
43. Modic MT, Weinstein MA, Chilcote WA, et al: Digi431 subtraction angiography of the intracranial vascular system: Comparative study in 55 patients. *AJR* 138:299–306, 1982
44. Busch W: Die Morphologie der Sella Turcica und Ihre Beziehungen zur Hypophyse. *Arch Pathol Anat* 320:437–458, 1951
45. Jordan RM, Kendall JW, Kerber CW: The primary empty sella syndrome. *Am J Med* 62:569–580, 1977
46. Kaufman B: The "empty" sella turcia—a manifestation of the intrasellar subarachnoid space. *Radiology* 90:931–941, 1968
47. Barrow DL, Tindall GT, Kovacs K, et al: Clinical and pathological effects of bromocriptine on prolactin-secreting and other pituitary tumors. *J Neurosurg* 60:1–7, 1984
48. Ganguly A, Stanchfield JB, Roberts TS, et al: Cushing's syndrome in a patient with empty sella turcica and a microadenoma of the adenohypophysis. *Am J Med* 60:306–309, 1976
49. Gharib H. Frey HM, Laws ER Jr, et al: Coexistent primary empty sella syndrome and hyperprolactinemia. Report of 11 cases. *Arch Intern Med* 143:1383–1386, 1983
50. Hsu T-H, Shapiro JR, Tyson JE, et al: Hyperprolactinemia associated with empty sella syndrome. *JAMA* 235:2002–2004, 1976
51. Schaison G, Metzger J: The primary empty sella: An endocrine study on 12 cases. *Acta Endocrinol (Copenh)* 83:483–492, 1976
52. Swanson JA, Sherman BM, Van Gilder JC, et al: Coexistent empty sella and prolactin-secreting microadenoma. *Obstet Gynecol* 53:258–263, 1979
53. Buckman MT, Husain M, Carlow TJ, et al: Primary empty sella syndrome with visual field defects. *Am J Med* 61:124–128, 1976
54. Cupps TR, Woolf PD: Primary empty sella syndrome with panhypopituitarism, diabetes insipidus, and visual field defects. *Acta Endocrinol (Copenh)* 89:445–460, 1978
55. Sage MR, Chan ES, Reilly PL: The clinical and radiological features of the empty sella syndrome. *Clin Radiol* 31:513–519, 1980
56. Haughton VM, Rosenbaum AE, Williams AL, et al: Recognizing the empty sella by CT: The infundibulum sign. *AJR* 136:293–295, 1981
57. Horowitz BL, Hamilton DJ, Sommers CJ, et al: Effect of bromocriptine and pergolide on pituitary tumor size and serum prolactin. *Am J Neuroradiol* 4:415–417, 1983
58. Kleinberg DL, Boyd AE III, Wardlaw S, et al: Pergolide for the treatment of pituitary tumors secreting prolactin or growth hormone. *N Engl J Med* 309:704–709, 1983
59. Parkes D: Drug therapy: Bromocriptine. *N Engl J Med* 301:873–878, 1979
60. Kahn PC, Kelleher MD, Egdahl RH, et al: Adrenal arteriography and venography in primary aldosteronism. *Radiology* 101:71–78, 1971
61. Kahn PC, Nickrosz LV: Selective angiography of the adrenal glands. *AJR* 101:739–749, 1967
62. Blair AJ Jr, Reuter SR: Adrenal venography in virilized women. *JAMA* 213:1623–1629, 1970
63. Nicolis GL, Mitty HA, Modlinger RS, et al: Percutaneous adrenal venography. *Ann Intern Med* 76:899–910, 1972
64. Gross MD, Valk TW, Swanson DP, et al: The role of

pharmacologic manipulation in adrenal cortical scintigraphy. *Semin Nucl Med* 9:128–148, 1981
65. Thrall JH, Gross M, Freitas JE, et al: Clinical applications of adrenal scintigraphy. *Appl Radiol NM* 9:115–122, 1980
66. Ryo UY, Johnston AS, Kim I, et al: Adrenal scanning and uptake with 131-I-6β-iodomethyl-nor-cholesterol. *Radiology* 128:157–161, 1978
67. Gross MD, Freitas JE, Swanson DP, et al: Dexamethasone-suppression adrenal scintigraphy in hyperandrogenism: Concise communication. *J Nucl Med* 22:12–17, 1981
68. Donald I, MacVicar J, Brown TG: Investigation of abdominal masses by pulsed ultrasound. *Lancet* 2:1188–1195, 1958
69. Fleischer AC, James AE Jr, Millis JB, et al: Differential diagnosis of pelvic masses by gray-scale sonography. *AJR* 131:469–476, 1978
70. Walsh JW, Taylor KJW, Wasson JFM, et al: Gray-scale ultrasound in 204 proved gynecologic masses: Accuracy and specific diagnostic criteria. *Radiology* 130:391–397, 1979
71. Baker ML: Biological effects of diagnostic ultrasound: A review. *Radiology* 126:479–483, 1978
72. Hellman LM, Duffus GM, Donald I, et al: Safety of ultrasound in obstetrics. *Lancet* 1:1133–1134, 1970
73. Martin AO: Can ultrasound cause genetic damage? *J Clin Ultrasound* 12:11–19, 1984
74. Communication from the AIUM Bioeffects Committee. *J Clin Ultrasound* 5:2–4, 1977
75. Callen PW, De Martrie WJ, Filly RA: The central uterine cavity echo: A useful anatomic sign in the ultrasonographic evaluation of the female pelvis. *Radiology* 131:187–190, 1979
76. Hall DA, Hann LE, Ferrucci JT, et al: Sonographic morphology of the normal menstrual cycle. *Radiology* 133:185–188, 1979
77. Sample WF, Lippe BM, Gyepes MT: Gray scale ultrasonography of the normal female pelvis. *Radiology* 125:477–483, 1977
78. Haller JO, Schneider M, Kassner, EG, et al: Ultrasonography in pediatric gynecology and obstetrics. *AJR* 128:423–429, 1977
79. Lippe BM, Sample WF: Pelvic ultrasonography in pediatric and adolescent endocrine disorders. *J Pediatr* 92:897–902, 1978
80. Campbell S, Goessens L, Goswamy R, et al: Real time ultrasonography for determination of ovarian morphology and volume. *Lancet* 1:425–426, 1982
81. Nitscke-Dabelstein S, Hackeloer BJ, Sturm G: Ovulation and corpus luteum formation observed by ultrasonography. *Ultrasound Med Biol* 7:33–39, 1981
82. Fleischer AC, Daniell JF, Rocher J, et al: Sonographic monitoring of ovarian follicular development. *J Clin Ultrasound* 9:275–280, 1981
83. Hill LM, Breckle R, Coulam CB: Assessment of human follicular development by ultrasound. *Mayo Clin Proc* 57:176–180, 1982
84. O'Herlihy C, DeCrespigny LC, Lopata A, et al: Preovulatory follicular size: A comparison of ultrasound and laparoscopic measurements. *Fertil Steril* 34:24–26, 1980
85. Queenan JT, O'Brien GD, Bains LM, et al: Ultrasound scanning of ovaries to detect ovulation in women. *Fertil Steril* 34:99–105, 1980
86. Fink RS, Bowes LP, Mackintosh CE, et al: The value of

ultrasound for monitoring ovarian responses to gonadotrophin stimulant therapy. *Br J Obstet Gynecol* 89:856–861, 1982
87. Hackeloer BJ, Fleming R, Robinson HP, et al: Correlation of ultrasonic and endocrinologic assessment of human follicular development. *Am J Obstet Gynecol* 135:122–128, 1979
88. Reeves RD, Drake TS, O'Brien WF: Ultrasonographic versus clinical evaluation of a pelvic mass. *Obstet Gynecol* 55:551–554, 1980
89. Sallam HN, Marinho AO, Collins WP, et al: Monitoring gonadotrophin therapy by real-time ultrasonic scanning of ovarian follicles. *Br J Obstet Gynecol* 89:155–159, 1982
90. Smith DH, Picker RH, Sinosich M, et al: Assessment of ovulation by ultrasound and estradiol levels during spontaneous and induced cycles. *Fertil Steril* 33:387–390, 1980
91. Ylostalo P, Ronnberg L, Jouppila P: Measurement of the ovarian follicle by ultrasound in ovulation induction. *Fertil Steril* 31:651–655, 1979
92. McArdle CR, Sacks BA: Ovarian hyperstimulation syndrome. *AJR* 135:835–836, 1980
93. McCardle CR, Seibel M, Weinstein F, et al: Induction of ovulation monitored by ultrasound. *Radiology* 148:809–812, 1983
94. Rankin RN, Hutton LC: Ultrasound in the ovarian hyperstimulation syndrome. *J Clin Ultrasound* 9:473–476, 1981
95. Hann LE, Hall DA, Black EB, et al: Mittelschmerz. Sonographic demonstration. *JAMA* 241:2731–2732, 1979
96. Hann LE, Hall DA, McArdle CR, et al: Polycystic ovarian disease: Sonographic spectrum. *Radiology* 150:531–534, 1984
97. Parisi L, Tramonti M, Casciano S, et al: The role of ultrasound in the study of polycystic ovarian disease. *J Clin Ultrasound* 10:167–172, 1982
98. Cochrane WJ, Thomas MA: Ultrasound diagnosis of gynecologic pelvic masses. *Radiology* 110:649–654, 1974
99. Lawson TL, Albarelli JN: Diagnosis of gynecologic pelvic masses by gray scale ultrasonography: Analysis of specificity and accuracy. *AJR* 128:1003–1006, 1977
100. Levi S, Delval R: Value of ultrasonic diagnosis of gynecologic tumors in 370 surgical cases. *Acta Obstet Gynecol Scand* 55:261–266, 1976
101. Morley P, Barnett E: The use of ultrasound in the diagnosis of pelvic masses. *Br J Radiol* 43:602–616, 1970
102. Requard CK, Mettler FA Jr, Wicks JD: Preoperative sonography of malignant ovarian neoplasms. *AJR* 137:79–82, 1981
103. Sandler M, Silver TM, Karo JJ: Gray scale ultrasonic features of ovarian teratomas. *Radiology* 131:705–709, 1979
104. Brandt TD, Grant TH, Marut E, et al: Endometrial echo and its significance in female infertility. *Radiology* 157:225–229, 1985
105. Chokas WV: Gonadal dysgenesis, rheumatoid spondylitis, hypertension and multiple congenital anomalies. *Am J Med* 28:963–968, 1960
106. Finby N, Archibald RM: Skeletal abnormalities associated with gonadal dysgenesis. *AJR* 89:1222–1235, 1963
107. Haddad HM, Wilkins L: Congenital anomalies associated with gonadal aplasia: Review of 55 cases. *Pediatrics* 23:885–902, 1959
108. Hortling H: Congenital kidney anomalies in "Turner's syndrome." *Acta Endocrinol (Copenh)* 18:548–554, 1955

109. Jackson WPU, Sougin-Mibashan R: Turner's syndrome in female: Congenital agonadism combined with developmental abnormalities. *Br Med J* 2:368–371, 1953

110. Keats TE, Burns TW: The radiographic manifestations of gonadal dysgenesis. *Radiol Clin North Am* 2:297–313, 1964

111. Levin B: Gonadal dysgenesis: Clinical and roentgenologic manifestations. *AJR* 87:1116–1127, 1962

112. Lisser H, Curtis LE, Escamilla RF, et al: The syndrome of congenitally aplastic ovaries with sexual infantilism, high urinary gonadotropins, short stature and other congenital abnormalities: Tabular presentation of twenty-five previously unpublished cases. *J Clin Endocrinol Metab* 7:665–687, 1947

113. Rainer-Pope CR, Cunningham RD, Nadas AS, et al: Cardiovascular malformations in Turner's syndrome. *Pediatrics* 33:919–925, 1964

114. Turner HH: Syndrome of infantilism, congenital webbed neck, cubitus valgus. *Endocrinology* 23:566–574, 1938

115. Forbes AP, Engel E: The high incidence of diabetes mellitus in 41 patients with gonadal dysgenesis, and their close relatives. *Metabolism* 12:428–439, 1963

116. Williams ED, Engel E, Forbes AP: Thyroiditis and gonadal dysgenesis. *N Engl J Med* 270:805–810, 1964

117. Pai GS, Leach DC, Weiss L, et al: Thyroid abnormalities in 20 children with Turner's syndrome. *J Pediatr* 91:267–269, 1977

118. Polani PE, Lessof MH, Bishop PMF: Color blindness in "ovarian agenesis" (gonadal dysplasia). *Lancet* 271:118–120, 1956

119. Bercu BB, Kramer SS, Bode HH: A useful radiologic sign for the diagnosis of Turner's syndrome. *Pediatrics* 58:737–739, 1976

120. Tanner JM, Prader A, Habich H, et al: Genes on Y chromosome influencing rate of maturation in man. *Lancet* 2:141–144, 1959

121. Acheson RM, Zampa GA: Skeletal maturation in ovarian dysgenesis and Turner's syndrome. *Lancet* I:917–920, 1961

122. Del Castillo EB, De La Balze FA, Argonz J: Syndrome of rudimentary ovaries with estrogenic insufficiency and increase in gonadotropins. *J Clin Endocrinol Metab* 7:385–422, 1947

123. McDonough PG, Byrd JR: Gonadal dysgenesis. *Clin Obstet Gynecol* 20:565–579, 1977

124. Hoffenberg R, Jackson WPU: Gonadal dysgenesis in normal-looking females: Genetic theory to explain variability of syndrome. *Br Med J* 1:1281–1284, 1957

125. Archibald RM, Finby N, De Vito F: Endocrine significance of short metacarpals. *J Clin Endocrinol Metab* 19:1312–1322, 1959

126. Kosowicz J: The carpal sign in gonadal dysgenesis. *J Clin Endocrinol Metab* 22:949–952, 1962

127. Kosowicz J: The roentgen appearance of the hand and wrist in gonadal dysgenesis. *AJR* 93:354–361, 1965

128. Necic S, Grant DB: Diagnostic value of hand x-rays in Turner's syndrome. *Acta Paediatr Scand* 67:309–312, 1978

129. Kosowicz J: Changes in medial tibial condyle—common finding in Turner's syndrome. *Acta Endocrinol (Copenh)* 31:321–323, 1959

130. Nora JJ, Torres FG, Sinha AK, et al: Characteristic cardiovascular anomalies of XO Turner syndrome, XX and XY phenotype and XO/XX Turner mosaic. *Am J Cardiol* 25:639–641, 1970

131. Ravelo HR, Stephenson LW, Friedman S, et al: Coarctation resection in children with Turner's syndrome. *J Thorac Cardiovasc Surg* 80:427–430, 1980

132. Polani PE, Hunter WF: Chromosomal sex in Turner's syndrome with coarctation of the aorta. *Lancet* 2:120–121, 1954

133. Van Buchem FSP, Homan BPAA, Dingemanse E, et al: Endocrine disturbances in coarctation of aorta. *Acta Med Scand* 143:399–414, 1952

134. Van Der Hauwaert LG, Fryns JP, Dumoulin M, et al: Cardiovascular malformations in Turner's and Noonan's syndrome. *Br Heart J* 40:500–509, 1977

135. Strader WJ III, Wachtel HL, Lundberg GD Jr: Hypertension and aortic rupture in gonadal dysgenesis. *J Pediatr* 79:473–475, 1971

136. Litvak AS, Rousseau TG, Wrede LD, et al: The association of significant renal anomalies with Turner's syndrome. *J Urol* 120:671–672, 1978

137. Matthies F, Macdiarmid WD, Rallison ML, et al: Renal anomalies in Turner's syndrome. *Clin Pediatr* 10:561–565, 1971

138. Hunter AGW, DesLauriers GL, Gillieson MS, et al: Prenatal diagnosis of Turner's syndrome by ultrasonography. *Can Med Assoc J* 127:401, 1982

139. Robinow M, Spisso K, Buschi AJ et al: Turner syndrome: Sonography showing fetal hydrops simulating hydramnios. *AJR* 135:846–848, 1980

140. Benson PF, Gough MH, Polani PE: Lymphangiography and chromosome studies in females with lymphoedema and possible ovarian dysgenesis. *Arch Dis Child* 40:27–32, 1965

141. Rutter AG: Submucous telangiectasis of the colon. *Lancet* 271:1077–1079, 1956

142. Barreto A, Castaneda-Zuniga WR, Velasquez G, et al: The value of abnormal angiography in Turner's syndrome: A case report. *Cardiovasc Intervent Radiol* 4:97–98, 1981

ANSWERS

1. High-resolution CT scanning

2. Radionuclide adrenal scan

3. Horsehoe kidney or ectopic kidney

4. Ultrasonography

13

Endoscopic Procedures

ROBERT S. NEUWIRTH

HISTORY AND BACKGROUND

Gynecologic endoscopy had its origins in the early attempts to perform hysteroscopy by Pantaleone in 1867. Laparoscopy first appeared in the early twentieth century, and culdoscopy was developed by Decker around 1940. Historically, the utilization of hysteroscopy, laparoscopy, and culdoscopy relate to the comparative success of the equipment and techniques to overcome problems in the lighting, imaging, and distention of the cavities to be examined. Before the incandescent bulb, none of these procedures was very useful. With Edison's contribution, laparoscopy was feasible, although lack of a satisfactory pneumoperitoneum hampered this procedure until Palmer's work immediately after World War II. Culdoscopy, which used the knee–chest position, was an adequate substitute, as it could be performed with an incandescent bulb and did not require special pneumoperitoneum apparatus. Nevertheless, it was highly skill dependent and never gained widespread use.

The development of high-quality, cold light transmission systems, initially with the quartz rod, and later with fiberoptic bundles, was a major

ROBERT S. NEUWIRTH • Department of Obstetrics and Gynecology, Columbia University College of Physicians and Surgeons; and Department of Obstetrics and Gynecology, St. Luke's/Roosevelt Hospital, New York, New York 10025.

breakthrough for laparoscopy and hysteroscopy. Recognizing the need for an illumination system that would not burn the bowel, Palmer first used the quartz rod system. Fiberoptic lighting, which was less cumbersome, replaced the quartz system during the mid-1960s. The introduction of fiberoptic light was a major step in hysteroscopy, as the distal incandescent bulb not only occupied space in the uterine cavity limiting the ability to introduce the objective lens but risked burning the tissues.

Systems to distend the cavity to be examined were equally important to the development of optimal gynecologic endoscopy. The early pneumoperitoneum control systems for laparoscopy were fragile and inaccurate. More sophisticated systems now control the pressure and volume of gas and include double-lumen insufflation needles as well as excellent pressure–volume control devices. Laparoscopy is now a widely used procedure because of these technical developments, while culdoscopy, with its restricted views and high skill requirement, has almost disappeared because laparoscopic equipment and techniques make it clearly superior for most cases.

Hysteroscopy has also benefited from the refinement of techniques to distend the endometrial cavity. The use of carbon dioxide gas regulated to limit flow to 100 ml/min and pressure to 150 mm Hg has made the procedure in gas satisfactory and safe. The use of a contracervical cap with suction seal is necessary with gas, and sometimes with low-viscosity liquids such as 5% dextrose in water, in order to maintain distention. Thirty-two percent dextran, or Hyskon has also been a breakthrough for uterine distention. This liquid is a nonelectrolyte, is viscous, and provides a good view for diagnosis and many intrauterine surgical procedures.

Whereas culdoscopy has waned, laparoscopy and hysteroscopy are procedures currently adopted by many. These techniques have changed infertility and gynecologic practices very significantly by making diagnosis easier, more accurate, and precise. Both procedures have also developed a variety of therapeutic applications since 1970 that will be briefly explored later (see Laparoscopy: Technical Considerations and Hysteroscopy: Applications).

LAPAROSCOPY

Technical Considerations

The technique of diagnostic laparoscopy has been amply described elsewhere.[1,2] The key points include the insertion of the needle, which should be directed away from the areas of the great vessels. The pneumoperitoneum, which can employ CO_2, N_2O, or air[3] should develop with pressure of less than 20 mm Hg and usually requires 1.5 to 3 liters of gas. The insertion of the trochar should always avoid the course of the great vessels and should be inserted in a tangential path through the abdominal wall in order to avoid subsequent wound herniation. Once satisfactory entry is made, secondary instruments should be inserted under direct view with transillumination of the abdominal wall to avoid epigastric vessels. Single- and multiple-puncture approaches to laparoscopy should be selected on considerations of safety and the requirements to perform a specific procedure. It is important to remember that the laparoscope provides a two-dimensional view and that optical depth of field comes from the lens quality of the endoscope as noted in Figure 13-1. The skill of the laparoscopist must compensate for this limitation in both single- and double-puncture procedures.

Instrument care is very important for optimal endoscopy. Few institutions have organized the support staff into a team to assist with endoscopy or clean endoscopic instruments. Consequently, fiberoptic cables are fractured, leading to reduced light transmission, misplaced or broken pieces of equipment, damaged and electrical cords and in-

sulation, leading to errors or accidents. A group comprising a surgeon, nurse, and operating room aid should be specifically responsible for endoscopic procedures with authority over equipment management and the purchase of instruments. Not only will endoscopy go more smoothly, but the risk of injury will be reduced by proper instrument selection, maintenance, and utilization.

Applications

Few new diagnostic applications for laparoscopy have been found beyond those reported in the early 1970s. There is no doubt that the laparoscope had an historical rendezvous with the increasing demand for female sterilization as well as the rise in venereal diseases in the United States. More recently, the laparoscope has played a central role for in vitro fertilization programs serving as the vector for ovum retrieval. Not only is it useful to free adhesions around the ovaries, but it is used to control and stabilize the ovary, follicle puncture, and ovum collection. Another more recently proposed application has been the laparoscopic removal of early tubal gestation arising from the early diagnosis with the combination of radioimmunoassay (RIA) of chorionic gonadotropin and ultrasound diagnosis of extrauterine gestation. Aspiration of the tubal gestation from a salpingotomy done under laparoscopic control and bipolar tubal cautery for hemostasis has been reported by A. DeCherney (personal communication) to avoid laparotomy at a time unfavorable for tubal repair. Another new surgical application by Semm is the removal of subserous fibroids by a rongeur-like ancillary instrument. The laparoscope is also useful to the gynecologic oncologist at laparotomy or laparoscopy to examine the right subphrenic diaphragm with biopsy for microscopic ovarian cancer metastases. Tubal sterilization continues to be a mainstay of laparoscopic surgery. The nonelectrical techniques are slowly increasing their impact, as they avoid electrical injuries to the skin, viscera, and the surgeon. Bands and clips are not a panacea, however. They have also been inadvertently misapplied and have led to injuries as well as failure of the tubal sterilization. More recent applications include control of hysteroscopic surgery and of uterine perforation during curettage or early abortion. Retrieval of intrauterine devices (IUDs) displaced into the peritoneal cavity has also been reported more frequently, thereby avoiding laparotomy. Not all these new applications are nec-

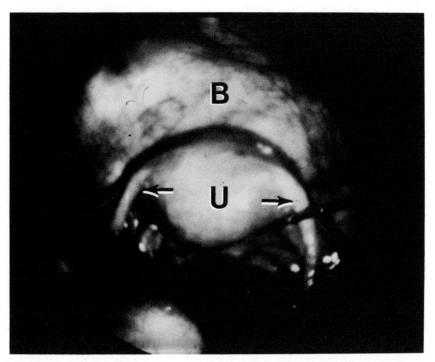

FIGURE 13-1. Laparoscopic view of the pelvis. Arrows indicate fallopian tubes. B, bladder; U, uterus.

essarily worth adopting or even prudent unless case selection is careful and the procedure well chosen and performed.

Complications

While laparoscopy has been an extraordinarily useful procedure, it has been associated with several groups of complications. Anesthetic accidents have been principally associated with failure to use endotracheal anesthesia, which is mandatory when general anesthesia is to be used. If local anesthesia is employed, excess sedation has also led to hypercarbia, hypoxia, dysrhythmia, and, at times, cardiac arrest. Sedation is usually satisfactory with 10 mg diazepam and 50 mg meperidine. Higher doses should be used with caution.

Visceral injury to bowel, bladder, and ureter have also been seen. These have usually been related to the use of cautery, although trochar and needle lacerations occur as well. Indeed, excessive or imprudent cauterization of the tubes or broad ligament for sterilization or control of hemorrhage carries the risk of burn to the ureteral wall with ureteroperitoneal fistula formation. Bipolar cautery has improved the safety of cautery, but operator error is ever-present, particularly if the problem is control of bleeding. Cautery injury to intestine noted during laparoscopy requires careful, experienced judgment. If the injury involves the muscularis of bowel or deeper, wide resection and repair of the injury is appropriate. For lesser degrees of injury, such as serosal effects only, close observation for up to 7 days in necessary to be sure that necrosis and peritonitis have been avoided.

Vascular injury is fortunately uncommon but can be very dramatic. The vena cava, aorta, common, external, and internal iliac vessels are at risk. Recognition and prompt laparotomy may be life saving. Primary repair and grafts have been employed to manage these injuries. Immediate control of the hemorrhage is the critical step.

HYSTEROSCOPY

Technical Considerations

Although the applications of laparoscopy are now well established and only a few new developments have occurred, the applications of hysteroscopy are still very much under development and evaluation. It appears that the use of liquid distention systems is proving more useful, as it can be employed easily for diagnosis and is more adaptable to various surgical procedures.

The techniques for diagnoses have been well described.[3] Two approaches to intrauterine surgery have thus far developed. Special endoscopic instrumentation has been developed to accept rigid scissors, clamps, and diathermic instruments to be passed through the hysteroscope itself. Aside from the resectoscope, all these instruments basically must have offset ocular optical systems, which are more expensive. The alternative has been the adaptation of microlaryngeal instruments to be passed through the cervix adjacent to the standard diagnostic hysteroscope. This latter system requires the use of liquids of high viscosity, such as Hyskon, in order to reduce fluid losses, as the cervical canal cannot be easily blocked with this approach, while uterine distention must be maintained.

Applications

Early applications of hysteroscopy included tubal sterilization,[4] the diagnosis and treatment of Asherman's syndrome, the location and removal of foreign bodies such as IUDs, the definition of local causes of abnormal bleeding such as polyps and submucous fibroids, and the staging of early endometrial carcinoma. The technique has been most useful for verification of abnormal hysterograms or diagnostic curettage. Sterilization has been evaluated by a variety of approaches including cautery, injection of caustic chemicals, and insertion of tubal plugs. None of these techniques has moved beyond clinical trials. Most recently, the insertion of custom-molded silicone plugs has achieved approximately 80% bilateral tubal obstruction and follow-up fertility control appears to be safe, reasonably effective, and therefore promising. This method requires skill, patience, and a trained assistant familiar with hysteroscopy as well as silicone rubber formation. Because of the appeal of a transcervical safe technique it appears to be developing acceptance in spite of its skill requirements and modest rate of success.

Asherman's syndrome is undoubtedly the condition for which hysteroscopy is most positively associated. The use of hysteroscopy has confirmed the finding originally noted by Zondek and Rozin[5] that hysterosalpingography can produce factitious filling defects leading to an erroneous diagnosis of intrauterine adhesions. If scar is confirmed at hysteroscopy the lesions can be transected or resected accurately and the normal contours of the endometrial cavity restored, as illustrated in Figure 13-2. The raw surfaces will often repair rather than scar if high doses of estrogen are used. One regimen is 1.25 mg Premarin for two 3-week courses. The use of an IUD or balloon to keep the endometrial walls separate is not as widely accepted. Where there are scars abutting the myometrium, it is prevalent to perform simultaneous laparoscopy to avoid visceral injury should inadvertent perforation of the uterus occur. It is important to bear in mind that the myometrium normally is 1 cm thick. Complications beyond perforation from this surgery have been rare. Recovery time has been brief—one or two postoperative hospital days and a few days of convalescence. Pregnancy rates are about 50% of the total group. It is clear, however, that the extent of the scar and its collagen content or thickness bear heavily on the outcome. Obviously, open continuity of the endometrial cavity with the tubes is an important feature of outcome. Should a successful result yield a pregnancy that aborts and formation of another scar, it is worthwhile to repeat the procedure, as the recurrent damage can also be repaired successfully. The ability of the endometrium to resurface denuded areas under estrogen stimulation has been a most impressive lesson from this experience.

Most recently the management of abnormal uterine bleeding in the absence of malignancy has been approached by hysteroscopic techniques. Where the uterus is not significantly enlarged, such as a 10-cm cavity or less, laser destruction and cautery excision of the endometrium have been attempted.[6] Initially, submucous myomata were excised if pedunculated. This was very effective in the control of bleeding or in the prevention of recurrent abortion. Then partial resection of the sessile type submucous fibroid was found to be feasible using a resectoscope technique. This appears to be worthwhile as well, as 80% of patients had no further difficulties and several desirous of pregnancy conceived and carried their pregnancy to term. Laser destruction of the endometrium combined with laparoscopic tubal banding also proved feasible and efficacious in women not desiring further pregnancy who were bleeding from dysfunctional or local causes and who had no other indication for hysterectomy. Hysteroscopic resection of the endometrium and superficial myometrium with laparo-

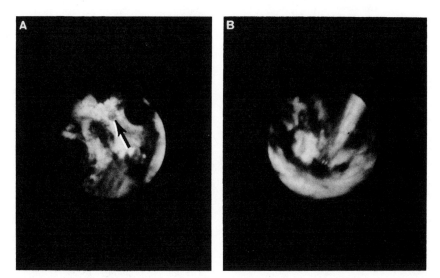

FIGURE 13-2. Hysteroscopic views of intrauterine synechiae (A) Arrow indicates scar mass before surgery. (B) Dissection of synechiae.

scopic tubal ligation too are feasible for the same indications, but the effectiveness awaits longer patient follow-up. Further positive experience with these approaches could signal a change in the customary management of women with this common problem.

Complications

Complications from hysteroscopy have been uncommon. For diagnosis, complications have been rare with the hysteroscope. Perforation of the uterus is seen during surgery for Asherman's syndrome and makes simultaneous laparoscopy a worthwhile safety feature. Hemorrhage and infection have been unusual even during significant surgery inside the uterus. Absorption of the distending media into the vascular system has been seen with gas, 5% dextrose in water, and Hyskon. The gas has produced cardiac dysrhythmia and, rarely, serious clinical embolism with death. Dextrose in water has produced edema if used in quantities of several liters. Hyskon has occasionally produced pulmonary edema when used in volumes over 500 ml during intrauterine surgery. Therefore, when significant intrauterine manipulation is associated with larger fluid volumes, one must monitor for cardiovascular disturbances to avoid difficulty.

CONTACT HYSTEROSCOPY

Contact hysteroscopy is a recently developed technique that provides magnified images of the tissues of the endocervix and endometrium. The procedure offers little of a panoramic view. The in vivo histology of the endometrium has considerable interest but still requires pathologic examination and confirmation before therapy can be offered. The contact hysteroscopes are clearly useful for examination of the endocervical canal for malignant and premalignant tissue. The instruments can also be used to observe the early gestational sacs. At the moment, other clinical applications, short of the endocervical evaluation, are not clear, although additional experience may give further utility to the procedure.

While panoramic hysteroscopic techniques are very new and require experience to do well, the potential advantages to the patient are significant. More accurate diagnosis is possible, surgical treatment may be less painful, and recovery is significantly shorter both in the hospital as well as during the convalescent period. It is certain that the management of retained IUDs, Asherman's syndrome, and selected anomalies are preferable with hysteroscopy. Less certain applications are sterilization, removal of submucous fibroids, and control of benign perimenopausal bleeding. The evidence suggests that the advantages outweigh the disadvantages and that wider introduction awaits dissemination of the skills and maturation of the techniques required to perform surgical hysteroscopy.

SUMMARY

During the past decade, gynecologic endoscopy has come to mean primarily laparoscopy and hysteroscopy. The impact of these procedures on gynecology and reproductive medicine has been enormous. New understanding of physiology, pathology, and pharmacology of the female genital tract has emerged through the use of improved techniques. The clinical application of these techniques has been extensive and continues to grow. The face of clinical practice has changed and promises to change even further as new refinements expand the applications. Ovum retrieval for in vitro fertilization has probably been the most dramatic example to date, although tubal sterilization and the management of benign gynecologic bleeding may produce a less dramatic but broader impact on clinical practice.

Although diagnostic imaging technology has rapidly advanced during the past decade as well, it does not seem likely that laparoscopy or hysteroscopy will be replaced by other forms of imaging. In particular, the surgical interventions permitted by the gynecologic endoscopic techniques will very likely earn laparoscopy and hysteroscopy a long-term place in the practice of gynecology and reproductive medicine.

QUESTIONS

1. Should diathermic cautery burns of the bowel seromuscularis be observed closely in the hospital?

2. Is laparoscopy necessary during hysteroscopic dissection of Ascherman's syndrome only when the scar blends into the wall?

3. Should diagnostic hysteroscopy be covered by antibiotics to avoid infection?

REFERENCES

1. Palmer R: Mon historie de la celioscopie in endoscopie ginecologie. Albano V, Cittadine E, Quartararo P (eds): *International Symposium on Gynecological Endoscopy*, Palermo, Italy, Oct. 1980
2. Steptoe P: *Laparoscopy in Gynecology*. Edinburgh, Livingstone, 1967
3. Neuwirth RS: *Hysteroscopy*. Philadelphia, Saunders, 1974
4. Reed TP: Hysteroscopic sterilization: Silicone elastic plugs. *Clin Obstet Gynecol* 26(2): 313 1983
5. Zondek B, Rozin S: Filling defects in the hysterogram simulating intrauterine synechiae which disappear after denervation. *Am J Obstet Gynecol* 88:123, 1964
6. Goldrath MH, Fuller TA, Segal S: Laser photovaporization of endometrium for the treatment of menorrhagia. *Am J Obstet Gynecol* 140:24, 1981

ANSWERS

1. No. If the muscularis is visibly burned, the area should be promptly excised and repaired.

2. Yes.

3. No. Infection is almost never seen after diagnostic hysteroscopy.

IV

Endocrine Disorders in the Female

14

Ovarian Dysgenesis and Related Genetic Disorders

JOE LEIGH SIMPSON

INTRODUCTION

Individuals with ovarian dysgenesis lack germ cells. Although showing a female phenotype, they lack secondary sexual characteristics and have streak gonads in lieu of normal gonads. These features usually result from either sex chromosomal abnormalities or mutant genes.

This chapter reviews the clinical features of individuals with monosomy X (45,X) and other chromosomal complements associated with gonadal dysgenesis. We shall also use the differences existing among individuals with various complements to deduce the number and location of determinants (genes) necessary for normal ovarian differentiation. Material reviewed in this chapter updates previous communications by the author.[1-3]

GENETIC CONTROL OF TESTICULAR AND OVARIAN DEVELOPMENT

An axiom of reproductive biology is that 46,XX zygotes differentiate into females, whereas 46,XY

zygotes differentiate into males. Both 46,XX and 46,XY zygotes (and early embryos) are morphologically indistinguishable. Sexual differentiation requires various genes. Determinant(s) on the Y chromosome are responsible for testicular differentiation and are located near the centromere on the short arm.[1] The Y short arm (Yp) and proximal long arm (Yq) are nonfluorescent, unlike the brilliantly fluorescent distal Yq. The latter is responsible for Y chromatin during interphase. These seemingly esoteric observations are clinically important because absence of Y chromatin would thus not necessarily signify a female fetus. It is well known that embryonic testes produce hormones that result in male reproductive morphology (Fig. 14-1).

The manner by which the testicular determinant(s) acts is not completely understood, but a cell-surface antigen, H-Y antigen, seems to be integrally involved in testicular differentiation.[4,5] Both circumstantial as well as direct evidence suggests that H-Y antigen can direct testicular differentiation. Surprisingly, both 45,X as well as 46,X,i(Xq) individuals show H-Y,[5,6] albeit at titers lower than in normal 46,XY. Since 45,X individuals obviously lack testes, it follows that H-Y antigen is not the gene product of the Y-linked testicular determinant. Instead, H-Y must be the gene product of an autosomal or X-linked structural locus. Pre-

JOE LEIGH SIMPSON • Department of Obstetrics and Gynecology, University of Tennessee, Memphis, Memphis, Tennessee 38163.

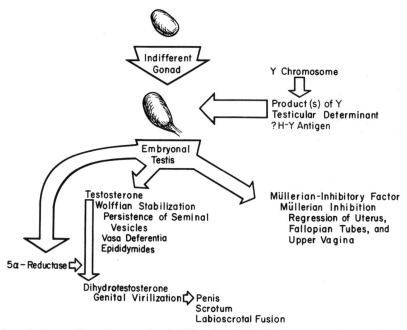

FIGURE 14-1. Schematic diagram illustrating normal male differentiation. The Y chromosome elaborates factors responsible for transformation of the indifferent gonad into a testis. Hormones synthesized by the fetal testes accomplish subsequent steps. (From Simpson.[99])

sumably the Y-testicular determinant is regulatory, assuming that H-Y is indeed primary to testicular differentiation. Also relevant is that ovaries have been detected in a phenotypic female with a normal Y and an X characterized by a duplication of Xp.[7] This is best explained by assuming that Xp contains

loci capable of suppressing H-Y. Absence of Xp (e.g., 45,X) permits expression of some H-Y, although not enough to permit testicular differentiation. Duplication of Xp must suppress H-Y despite a normal Y.

In the absence of the testicular determinant and

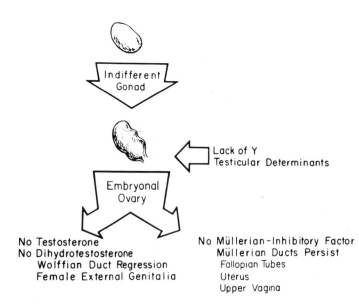

FIGURE 14-2. Schematic diagram illustrating the hypothesis that all reproductive systems in the embryo will differentiate in female fashion—ductal, genital, *and* gonadal—unless directed to do otherwise by a determinant on the Y chromosome. (From Simpson.[99])

the H-Y antigen (or its receptor) the indifferent gonad develops into an ovary (Fig. 14-2). This occurs not only in 46,XX, but also in 45,X germ cells.[8,9] However, if two intact X chromosomes are not present most ovarian follicles degenerate by the time of birth. Thus, X-ovarian determinants are responsible for oocyte maintenance, not initial oocyte differentiation. We devote considerable effort in this chapter toward localizing these determinants on the X. It may also be deduced that the constitutive path of gonadal differentiation is ovarian. Neonates with XY gonadal dysgenesis actually form transient ovaries, although adults show streak gonads (see the section on miscellaneous conditions). Thus, presence of an intact Y (a reasonable assumption, since XY gonadal dysgenesis is an X-linked recessive mutant) does not preclude ovarian differentiation. Further support for this hypothesis is provided from experiments in mice. A Y capable of directing normal male differentiation in some mouse strains may, when transferred to another genetic background (strain), result in Y-bearing progeny incapable of normal male development.[10] True hermaphroditism and complete sex reversal (XY females) result. Again, ovarian follicles form in the presence of the Y, supporting female constitutive development.

Finally, not only the X but various autosomal loci must be intact to permit normal ovarian development. The number and action of these loci are discussed in XX gonadal dysgenesis (see the section on gonadal dysgenesis in 46,XX individuals).

GENERAL CONSIDERATIONS

Historical Aspects

Gonadal dysgenesis and the somatic features characteristic of 45,X individuals have been recognized for centuries, but modern studies date from 1938. At that time, Turner[11] described seven girls with sexual infantilism, short stature, and certain skeletal anomalies. Turner apparently believed that the sexual infantilism in these patients was of pituitary origin. In 1942 Albright et al.[12] and Varney et al.[13] recognized that patients with Turner's syndrome had increased urinary excretion of gonadotropin, suggesting that gonadal failure was the cause of sexual infantilism. This observation was verified by Wilkins and Fleischmann,[14] who first visualized streak gonads in an affected patient. In 1959 Ford et al.[15] reported that the complement

45,X was associated with gonadal dysgenesis and the Turner stigmata. Additional complements later reported to be associated with gonadal dysgenesis included structural rearrangements of the X and Y chromosomes, autosomal abnormalities, and apparently normal male (46,XY) or female (46,XX) complements.

Turner's syndrome is probably the term most frequently applied to individuals with gonadal dysgenesis. However, this designation is confusing because it connotes different features to different investigators. For these and other reasons, the present author applies the term *gonadal dysgenesis* to any individual with streak gonads, reserving the term *Turner stigmata* for individuals with short stature and selected other somatic anomalies.[16] The term Turner stigmata, by itself, does not imply the presence of streak gonads.

Incidence of 45,X and Related Complements

About 50% of spontaneous abortions occurring during the first 3 months of gestation are associated with a chromosomal abnormality; 20% of chromosomally abnormal abortuses are 45,X. Of all pregnancies, 12–15% terminate in the first-trimester spontaneous abortion; thus 1–2% of all conceptions are 45,X. Sex chromosomal mosaicism or structural rearrangements are rarely detected among early abortuses. Since the incidence of 45,X newborns is only about 1 per 10,000 females, more than 99% of all 45,X embryos must have been aborted. Other complements associated with gonadal dysgenesis are rarely detected in prospective studies of liveborn neonates. It would not be possible to identify neonates with 46,XX or 46,XY gonadal dysgenesis, and mosaicism is difficult to detect in all surveys because few cells are counted. Since 45,X accounts for only about one-half of all patients with gonadal dysgenesis, underascertainment of other complements in neonatal surveys seems likely.

The proportion of 45,X individuals in a given sample will depend on ascertainment. Gynecologists will diagnose almost all cases with 46,XX or 46,XY complements, but pediatricians ordinarily will identify 45,X individuals. Relatively fewer 45,X individuals will be detected if primary amenorrhea is the presenting complaint, in contrast to short stature. Overall, approximately 50% of all patients with gonadal dysgenesis have a 45,X complement, 25% have sex chromosomal mosaicism without a structural abnormality (e.g.,

45,X/46,XX), and the remainder have either a structurally abnormal X or Y or no detectable chromosomal abnormality.[1]

Cytologic Origin of 45,X

Monosomy X (45,X) could originate during oogenesis, during spermatogenesis, or after fertilization. In humans the cytologic origin of 45,X aneuploidy can be deduced on the basis of familial distribution of alleles at X-linked loci, such as Xg or colorblindness.

About 70% of 45,X individuals arise as result of loss of a paternal sex chromosome.[17] In both 45,X liveborns and 45,X embryos maternal age is not increased, consistent with the abnormality arising during paternal meiosis. Similarly, 46,X,i(Xq) appears to arise in paternal meiosis.[17]

In the mouse the paternal X is nearly always the chromosome lost.[18] Murine monosomy (39,X) appears to arise at fertilization because irradiation between sperm entry and first cleavage increases the frequency of 39,X.[19] By contrast, irradiation of males before copulation does not increase the frequency of 39,X progeny.[20]

Detection of Mosaicism

The presence of two or more cell lines (mosaicism) implies nondisjunction or anaphase lag in the zygote or embryo. Although nondisjunction or anaphase lag may be the most common mechanisms, the high frequency of structurally abnormal X or Y chromosomes (isochromosomes, dicentrics, deletions) raises the possibility that in some cases the initial cytologic abnormality was not nondisjunction but production of a structurally abnormal sex chromosome that secondarily led to mosaicism. Irrespective, two or more cell lines ordinarily result. The final complement will depend on the time at which abnormal cell division occurs and on whether or not all daughter cells survive.

The ability to detect mosaicism is clinically important because management is altered by the presence or absence of certain cell lines, i.e., 46,XY. Moreover, the possibility of an undetected normal cell line always renders scientific (phenotypic–karyotypic) correlations hazardous. Detection of mosaicism depends on (1) the frequency of the minority cell line, (2) the number of cells analyzed per tissue, and (3) the number of tissues analyzed. Analysis of lymphocytes will ordinarily suffice for clinical purposes, provided predicted and observed phenotypes are not discordant. The

most common discrepancy warranting further cytogenetic studies is that of normal stature in an individual said to be 45,X; another cell line should be sought, particularly 46,XY.

PATHOLOGIC FEATURES OF MONOSOMY X (45,X)

Various pathologic features are associated with 45,X, and sometimes with other complements. These features are described by organ system.

Gonads and Genital Organs

Gonadal and genital features of individuals with gonadal dysgenesis can be considered irrespective of the associated chromosomal complement, for almost all streak gonads appear identical histologically. Individuals with a Y chromosome may develop gonadoblastomas or dysgerminomas (see the sections on Gonadal Dysgenesis in 46,XY Individuals and Miscellaneous Conditions).

However, before neoplastic transformation, their streak gonads are indistinguishable from those of 45,X individuals.

Gonads

In adults with gonadal dysgenesis, the normal gonad is replaced by a white fibrous streak, 2–3 cm long and about 0.5 cm wide, located in the position ordinarily occupied by the ovary (Fig. 14-3). A streak gonad is characterized histologically by interlacing waves of dense fibrous stroma, indistinguishable from normal ovarian stroma (Fig. 14-4). Oocytes are ordinarily absent. Ovarian rete tubules, which probably originate from either mesonephric tubules or medullary sex cords, are present in the median portion of most streak gonads. Hilar cells are usually detected in streak gonads removed from patients who are past the age of expected puberty. Both rete tubules and hilar cells are present in normal ovaries, indicating that gonadal development proceeded normally through the medullary cord stage. This is consistent with observations that germ cells are present in 45,X embryos.[8,9] Since the pathogenesis of germ cell failure in 45,X is increased rate of atresia, not failure of formation, it follows that those portions of the X which cause gonadal dysgenesis when deleted must be necessary for ovarian (oocyte) maintenance, as opposed to differentiation.

That 45,X oocytes fail to persist is actually less predictable than one might expect. X chromosomes

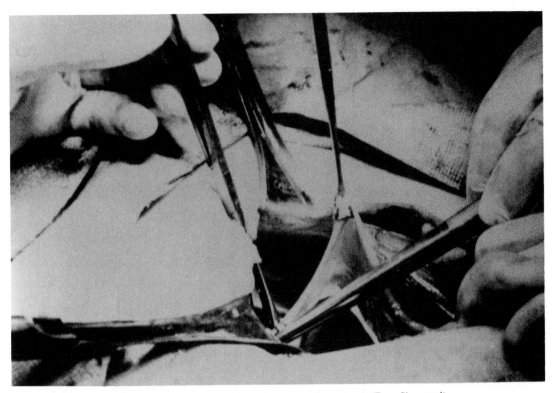

FIGURE 14-3. Streak gonad (arrow), as seen at laparotomy. (From Simpson.[1])

in excess of one are known to be genetically inactivated (Lyon hypothesis), and ovarian development is relatively normal in most monosomy X mammals (e.g., mice). There are several explanations for the phenotypic abnormalities in 45,X humans. First, in humans not all loci on the heterochromatic (inactive) human X are inactivated (e.g., steroid sulfatase), and loci influencing maintenance could similarly escape inactivation. In fact, distal Xp is known to escape inactivation.[21] Second, X inactivation also never occurs in human oocytes, unlike the situation in somatic tissues.[22] Other possibilities, plausable but unproved, include X inactivation occurring only after some crucial time during differentiation, beyond which only a single euchromatic (active) X is necessary for continued oogenesis, or reactivation of all or a portion of the heterochromatic X.

External Genitalia and Vagina

In gonadal dysgenesis, external genitalia usually differentiate as expected for females. However, genitalia remain infantile because ovarian sex steroid secretion is inadequate. If a patient with gonadal dysgenesis has an enlarged clitoris, one should suspect a cell line containing a Y chromosome. Occasionally 45,X or 45,X/46,XX individuals have an enlarged clitoris without demonstrable tumor or testicular tissue, possibly the result of elevated gonadotropin levels stimulating Leydig cells in the streak gonads to produce androgens.

Mullerian Derivatives

Mullerian derivatives (uterus, cervix, fallopian tubes, upper vagina) are usually structurally normal. Because uterine growth depends on steroids, however, the uterus is smaller than usual.

Endometrial carcinoma has occurred in 45,X patients treated with diethylstilbestrol (DES). However, the prevalance of carcinoma in estrogen-treated 45,X patients is extremely low, and estrogen replacement should not be withheld. It is preferable to administer both progestins as well as estrogens.

Secondary Sex Characteristics

Failure of sex steroid secretion results in the following picture: (1) pubic hair remains sparse and is fine rather than coarse in consistency (however,

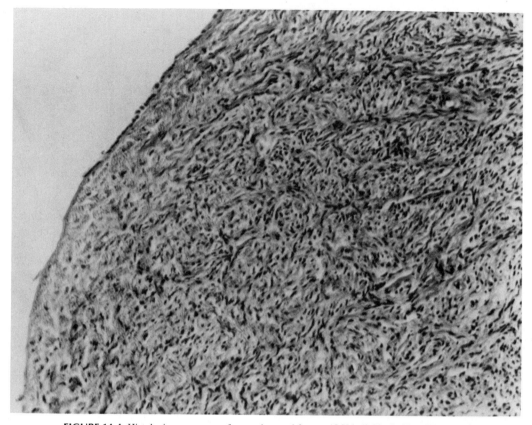

FIGURE 14-4. Histologic appearance of a streak gonad from a 45,X individual. (From Simpson.[1])

adrenal androgens also influence pubic growth); (2) axillary hair is sparse; (3) breasts contain little parenchymal tissue, and areolar tissue may be only slightly darker than the surrounding skin; and (4) external genitalia, vagina, and mullerian derivatives remain small.

Nongonadal Features (Turner Stigmata)

Certain somatic anomalies are associated with monosomy X (Table 14-1). These anomalies represent the Turner stigmata, the presence of which suggests the coexistence of gonadal dysgenesis. Individuals with the Turner stigmata form a clinical continuum with respect to the presence or absence of certain anomalies; however, not every anomaly will be present in every 45,X individual, nor is any particular anomaly pathognomonic.

Growth

45,X individuals have a low mean birth weight (adjusted mean 2851.1 ± 65.1 g).[23] Total body length at birth is sometimes less than normal, but often it is normal. Because more than 99% of 45,X embryos undergo spontaneous abortion, it is not surprising that growth may be abnormal in the rare surviving 45,X neonate.

Height velocity before puberty is in the tenth through twenty-fifth percentile,[24] and the mean height of 45,X adults (16 years or older) is 141 ± 0.62 cm.[16] Heights of 97% are below the third percentile; most of the remainder are only 152–155 cm tall.[16] Epiphyses remain open, and some additional growth usually occurs when sex steroids are administered. The final adult height depends on the parental heights but apparently not on the age at which hormone replacement is begun.[24] To increase height some physicians administer oxandrolone or growth hormone. However, the efficacy of treatment is actually not established because controlled studies have not yet been published.

The cellular basis for short stature is not known. That not all patients with gonadal dysgenesis are short shows that the explanation is not merely sex steroid deficiency. For example, normal stature is

TABLE 14-1. Somatic Anomalies Associated with 45,X Chromosomal Complement[a,b]

Growth
  Decreased birth weight
  Decreased adult height (mean 141 ± 0.62 cm)
Intellectual function
  Verbal IQ > performance IQ
  Cognitive deficits (space-form-blindness)
  Immature personality, probably secondary to short stature
Craniofacial
  Premature fusion spheno-occipital and other sutures,
    producing brachycephaly
  Abnormal pinnae
  Retruded mandible
  Epicanthal folds (25%)
  High-arched palate (36%)
  Abnormal dentition
  Visual anomalies, usually strabismus (22%)
  Auditory deficits: sensorineural or secondary to middle ear
    infections
  "Woolly" hair
Neck
  Pterygium coli (46%)
  Short broad neck (74%)
  Low buccal hair line (71%)
Chest
  Rectangular contour (shield chest) (53%)
  Apparent widely spaced nipples
  Tapered lateral ends of clavicle
Cardiovascular
  Coarctation of aorta or ventricular septal defect (10–16%)
Renal (38%)
  Horseshoe kidneys
  Unilateral renal aplasia
  Duplication ureters
Gastrointestinal
  Telangiectasias
Skin and lymphatics
  Pigmented nevi (63%)
  Lymphedema (38%) due to hypoplasia of superficial
    vessels
Nails
  Hypoplasia or malformation (66%)
Skeletal
  Cubitus valgus (54%)
  Radial tilt of articular surface of trochlear
  Clinodactyly
  Short metacarpals, usually IV (48%)
  Decreased carpal arch (mean angle 117°)
  Deformities of medial tibial condyle
Dermatoglyphics
  Increased total digital ridge count (mean 166.1 ± 8.62)
  Increased distance between palmar triradii a and b
  Distal axial triradius in position t'

[a]From Simpson.[1]
[b]Many other anomalies have been reported in 45,X individuals.

characteristic of 46,XX gonadal dysgenesis. Growth hormone levels are normal;[25] however, cellular resistance to growth hormone has been suggested. Indeed, growth hormone antibodies have been observed[26] and growth hormone reserve may be decreased.[27] Another potential explanation is that the epiphyses are structurally abnormal, compatible with observations that decreased growth occurs not only in long bones but in teeth[28] and the skull.[29] However, neither hormonal nor epiphyseal abnormalities are likely to explain high embryonic lethality. Thus, it is relevant that we have shown that the cell cycle is prolonged in 45,X, 46,X, del(X)(p11), and 46,X, del(X)(q22) fibroblasts,[30] all complements associated with short stature. (See section on Specific Sex Chromosomal Abnormalities.) A prolonged cell cycle is an attractive explanation not only for short stature, but also for the high embryonic lethality and intrauterine growth retardation (IUGR). Somatic anomalies are also explanable because anomalies usually originate during embryogenesis as result of a given organ having too few cells to sustain differentiation. Such a situation could be due to retardation of cell division. The mechanism(s) by which deletion of one or more determinants on the X chromosome causes prolonged cell generation time remains obscure, but confirmation of our data could provide an in vitro method for evaluating efficacy of therapeutic regimes to increase heights.

Intelligence

Most 45,X patients have normal intelligence, but any given 45,X patient has a slightly higher probability of being retarded than a 46,XX individual. The frequency of retardation is 11–17%.[16] However, biases of ascertainment dictate that this prevalence is likely to represent maximum risks. Performance IQ appears lower than verbal IQ.[31] 45,X individuals have an unusual cognitive defect characterized by an inability to appreciate the shapes and relationships of objects with respect to one another (space-form blindness).[32,33] 45,X patients usually appear socially immature, probably because they are short and sexually immature.

Craniofacial Structure

Premature closure of the spheno-occipital sutures, condylar cartilage, and sometimes other cranial sutures produced a short, wide skull (brachycephaly). The mandible appears recessed (retrognathia), although it is not necessarily small in proportion to the rest of the skull. The combination of a brachycephalic skull and a recessed mandible may impart to the facies a triangular appearance, the apex inferior. The ears are sometimes low set, usually in association with a short neck or pterygium coli (webbing of the neck). The pinnae may be malformed or small. Hearing may be decreased as result of either recurrent middle ear infections or congenital neurosensory deafness.

Of 45,X individuals, 22% have an ocular anomaly.[16] Strabismus is most common. Other common ocular abnormalities include epicanthal folds and ptosis.

The hard palate is said to be highly arched in about 36% of 45,X individuals. Dental anomalies include small teeth, persisting deciduous teeth, and an increased frequency of root absorption.[28]

Neck

A well-known feature of the Turner stigmata is webbing of the neck (pterygium coli), actually present in only 46% of 45,X individuals.[16] More common neck anomalies include a short broad neck (74%) and a low posterior hair line (71%). Cervical vertebrae may be hypoplastic, but rarely fused. Redundant skin folds may overlie the neck, especially in neonates. Because hygromatous neck masses are frequently present in 45,X abortuses, it is tempting to postulate that the pathogenesis of neck anomalies is related to excess fluid in utero.

Chest

45,X individuals often have a rectangular, rather than a sloping, chest. A shield chest is said to be present. Because of this contour, the nipples may appear widely separated.

Cardiovascular System

About 10–16% of reported 45,X individuals have a cardiac anomaly. Because of biases of ascertainment or reporting, this frequency (like that of mental retardation) probably represents the maximum risk. Coarctation of the aorta and ventricular septal defects are most frequent. Pulmonic stenosis, a defect frequently present in the Noonan syndrome, is rarely associated with monosomy X.

Vertebrae

Of 45,X individuals, 16% have a vertebral anomaly detectable upon physical examination.

Kyphosis and scoliosis are the most frequent abnormalities. Additional minor anomalies can often be detected by roentgenography. For example, the lumbar vertebral bodies tend to be relatively square.

Pelvis

The pelvic inlet may be android (heart-shaped) rather than gynecoid in contour. Small iliac wings, narrow sacrosciatic notches, and a narrow pubic arch are common.[34]

Urologic System

Renal anomalies are present in 40–60% of 45,X patients. The most frequent anomalies are horseshoe kidney, ureteral duplication, or absence of one kidney. It is often stated that the occurrence of renal anomalies in 45,X individuals is not unexpected because of the close embryologic relationship between the urinary and genital systems. However, in gonadal dysgenesis structural anomalies are limited to germ cells, which originate in the yolk sac some distance from anlage that will differentiate into the kidney and internal ducts (uterus). Mullerian derivatives, which *are* related embryologically to the kidney, are usually normal in individuals with gonadal dysgenesis. Thus, the occurrence of renal anomalies in 45,X is probably part of the generalized pattern of malformations (Turner stigmata), without a special relationship to dysgenetic gonads.

Gastrointestinal System

Telangiectasias of the small intestine occur more often than would be expected by chance.[35] Similarly, inflammatory bowel disease (Crohn's disease)[36] occurs with increased frequency.

Skin

Pigmented nevi occur in 63% of 45,X individuals. These nevi are very dark, about 0.5 mm in diameter, and are most likely to be located on the face, arms and chest. Capillary hemangiomas have also been described. Nails are often hypoplastic or malformed. Scalp hair may have a "wooly" consistency.

Lymphatic System

In 45,X individuals, 36% have lymphedema of the lower extremities or dorsum of the hands or feet. Lymphedema usually does not persist beyond 18 months except for dorum of the hands and feet.

Extremities

Cubitus valgus is present in 54% of 45,X individuals. Another useful diagnostic sign, detectable by roentgenograms, is a radial tilt to the articular surface of the trochlear.[37] Distal to the trochlear the forearm may deviate to the ulnar side, as if to compensate for cubitus valgus.

Hands

Of 45,X individuals, 48% have a short fourth metacarpal. A plane tangential to the circumference of the distal ends of the fourth and fifth metacarpals usually passes distal to the end of the third metacarpal. If the tangential line intersects the third metacarpal, a positive metacarpal sign is said to be present. The metacarpals may also curve radially. The distal phalangeal heads are relatively large and the shafts thin.[34] The carpal bones may be displaced. The third and fourth metacarpals may also be short, analogous to shortening of the metacarpals.

Metabolic Changes and Adult-Onset Diseases

Sex Steroids and Gonadotropin Levels. Endocrine studies reveal the findings to be expected of females who lack gonads. These data are predictable and need not be discussed in detail. As result of low estrogen levels, lack of normal feedback inhibition leads to increased levels of follicle-stimulating hormone (FSH) (>40 mIU/ml) and luteinizing hormone (LH).

Diabetes Mellitus. The frequency of diabetes is probably increased in 45,X patients. Engel and Forbes[38] detected diabetes in 8 of 45 adults with gonadal dysgenesis, and Polychronakos et al.[39] found an abnormal oral glucose tolerance test in 16 of 41 patients. AvRuskin et al.[40] showed decreased immunoreactive insulin in response to glucose and growth hormone. On the other hand, the frequency of overt diabetes is not increased in many other series of adults with gonadal dysgenesis.

Thyroiditis. Autoimmune thyroiditis occurs in patients with the Turner stigmata more often than expected by chance.[41] Grave's disease has also been observed in 45,X individuals.[42]

Hypertension. About one-third of adult 45,X patients have essential hypertension. Although more common in adults, hypertension may also occur in young 45,X patients. Therapy is not unique, although exogenous hormones may need to be reduced or carefully monitored.

SPECIFIC SEX CHROMOSOMAL ABNORMALITIES

45,X

45,X adults (Fig. 14-5) usually show the clinical features described above. However, not all 45,X individuals show complete absence of secondary sexual development. About 3–5% menstruate spontaneously, and slightly more show breast development.[16] Menstruation is usually not normal, but a few fertile patients have been reported.[43,44] An undetected 46,XX cell should always be the first suspicion when encountering a menstruating 45,X patient. It is not unreasonable, however, to expect that a few 45,X individuals could be fertile because germ cells are present in 45,X embryos and neonates. Recall that the pathogenesis of streak gonads is an increased rate of oocyte attrition, not failure of germ cell formation.

Previously we reviewed somatic anomalies characteristic of monosomy X. At least some of these anomalies, including short stature, are usually evident. Prepubertal patients thus deserve careful assessment for renal, cardiac, auditory, and vertebral anomalies. Hypertension should be sought in older patients. Mean adult height is 141 cm.[16]

45,X/46,XX Mosaicism

Not surprisingly, 45,X/46,XX individuals have fewer anomalies than do 45,X individuals. A survey by the author revealed that 12% of 45,X/46,XX individuals menstruated, compared with only 3% of 45,X individuals.[16] Pregnancies have been reported.[43,44] From another perspective, secondary amenorrhea is not uncommon in 45,X/46,XX. Evaluation of secondary amenorrhea should include FSH levels, which if elevated warrants chromosomal studies. In fact, at our institution most 45,X/46,XX cases presented with secondary amenorrhea.

The mean adult height is also greater in 45,X/46,XX (147 ± 1.7 cm) than in 45,X individuals (141 ± 0.6 cm), and more mosaic (25%) than nonmosaic (5%) individuals reach adult heights greater than 152 cm. Somatic anomalies seem less likely to exist in 45,X/46,XX than in 45,X, but those anomalies that do occur reflect the same spectrum as in 45,X.[16]

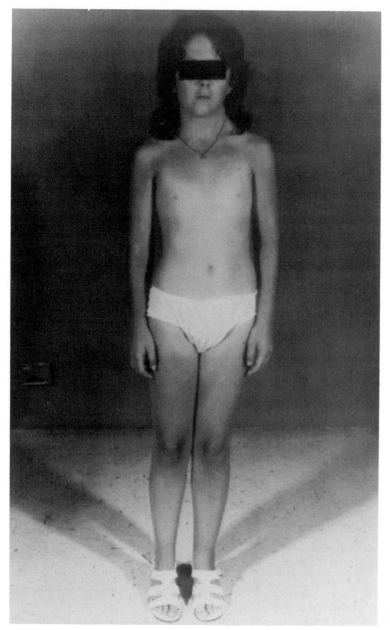

FIGURE 14-5. 45,X individual. Patient of the author. (From Sutton.[100])

Deletion of the X Short Arm [del(Xp)]

A deletion of the X short arm (Fig. 14-6) may or may not cause gonadal dysgenesis, short stature and other features of the Turner stigmata, depending on the amount of Xp that is deficient. Almost 50 nonmosaic cases have been reported, as tabulated elsewhere by the author.[1,3] Interstitial deletions, insertions, and X/autosomal translocation also occur, but discussion of these entities is beyond the scope of this chapter.

Two general types of short-arm deletions occur, those with breakpoints at Xp11 and those with break points at Xp21.[3,30,45-47] If the breakpoint

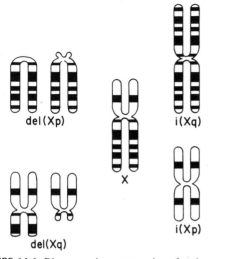

del(Xp)

i(Xq)

X

i(Xp)

del(Xq)

FIGURE 14-6. Diagrammatic representation of various structurally abnormal X chromosomes. (Modified from Simpson.[1])

occurs at Xp11 (Figs. 14-6 and 14-7), only the proximal portion of the Xp remains. The chromosome appears acrocentric or occasionally telocentric. Primary amenorrhea often occurs, but at least limited spontaneous menstruation occurs in almost 40% (13/36) of 46,X, del (X)(p11) individuals. More distal breaks occur at Xp21 or Xp22; 90% of cases with a more distal breakpoint (Xp21 or Xp22) show normal menstruation and fertility (11/12) cases) (Fig. 14-8). Amenorrhea thus occurs only if both the proximal (centromeric) and distal (telomeric) portions of Xp are deleted, not if only the distal portion (i.e., Xp21 → ter) is deleted. However, Maraschio and Fraccaro[47] caution that apparent differences in phenotype between del(Xp) and del(Xq) may reflect biases of ascertainment because many del (Xp) cases are ascertained through X-autosomal translocations.

All 45,X,del(Xp) individuals are short. A tabulation by the author reveals a mean adult height of 148 cm in 46,X,del(X)(p11) ($N=11$) and 55 cm on 46,X,del(Xp21) ($N=12$). Since 46,X,del(X)(p21) individuals are short but do not usually manifest gonadal abnormalities, ovarian determinants and statural determinants are obviously distal to ovarian determinants (Fig. 14-9).

Isochromosome for the X Long Arm [i(Xq)]

Division of the centromere in the transverse rather than in the longitudinal plane results in an isochromosome, a metacentric chromosome consisting of isologous arms (Fig. 14-6). Both arms are structurally identical and contain the same genes. An isochromosome for the X long arm [i(Xq)] consists of duplication for all of Xq and deficiency for all of Xp. Nonmosaic 46,X,i(Xq) is considerably less common than 45,X/46,X,i(Xq) mosaicism.

An isochromosome for the X long arm is the most common X-structural abnormality, much more frequent than 46,X,i(Xp). Almost all 46,X,i(Xq) patients seem to have streak gonads, short stature and some features of the Turner stigmata. Occasionally, 46,X,i(Xq) individuals menstruate, but surveys seem to confirm that of Simpson[16] in showing rarity of menstruation. The more complete lack of gonadal development in 46,X,i(Xq) contrasts with 46,X,del(X)(p11). In the former not only the terminal portion but all of Xp is deleted. This difference could reflect gonadal determinants being located at several different locations on Xp. A locus on Xp might be deficient in i(Xq), yet retained if a break at Xp11 produced 46,X,del(X)(p11). Irrespective, duplication of Xq (i.e., 46,X,i(Xq) does not compensate for deficiency of Xp; thus, gonadal determinants on Xq and Xp must have different functions.

An i(Xq) chromosome is usually paternal in origin.[17] Coupled with the high frequency of associated mosaicism, this suggests that the paternal X undergoes rearrangement early in embryogenesis.

Deletion of the X Long Arm [del(Xq)]

About 40 nonmosaic cases of this deletion provide data for analysis. Breakpoints have been observed at bands Xq13, 22, 24, and 26[3,30,45–47] (Figs. 14-6 and 14-7). In the next section will be raised the possibility that further cases could exist, namely those claimed to be 46,X,i(Xp) but actually 46,X,del(Xq).

Most patients with a deletion of the X long arm have primary amenorrhea and presumably streak gonads (Fig. 14-8). Moreover, X/autosomal translocations involving the region extending from Xq13 to Xq26 usually are associated with sterility.[48,49] In aggregate, the above indicate that important ovarian determinants exist in this region of Xq. However, menstruation and breast development may occur. Figure 14-8 shows that 3 of 21 46,X,del(X)(q13) individuals menstruated as did 6 of 19 46,X,del,X(q)(22 or 21). At least six Xq/autosomal translocations occurring in the (Xq13 → 26) region are compatible with fertility, usually involving Xq22.[48,49] In aggregate, these observa-

A

DEL (X) (p 11)

B

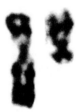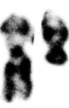

DEL (X) (q13)

C

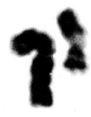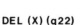

DEL (X) (q22)

FIGURE 14-7. Pairs of X chromosomes from three individuals with deletions of the X chromosome. (From Simpson and LeBeau.[30])

tions indicate that absence of a portion of the X is less deleterious than complete monosomy X. Very distal [46,X,del(X)(q26)] deletions are usually,[50,51] but not always,[52] compatible with menstruation. Otherwise, the presence or absence of gonadal function cannot to date be correlated readily with the amount of Xq that is absent. For example, menstruation or breast development has occurred in individuals deficient for most of Xq [46,X,del(X)(q13)] whereas individuals with less extensive deletions [(46,X,del(X)(q24)] have manifested primary amenorrhea. Irrespective, the precise location of Xq ovarian determinant(s) remains uncertain.

Relevant to this issue, the X/autosome translocations involving Xq13 → 26, usually disrupt ovarian maintenance,[53] despite the exceptions earlier. By contrast, X-autosome translocations in-

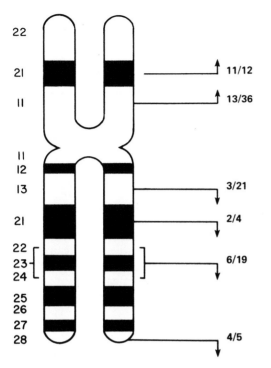

FIGURE 14-8. Relationship between break points for X deletions and frequencies of spontaneous menstruation and breast development. The tabulation assumes that purported 46,X,i(Xp) cases are actually 46,X,del(X)(q22 or 24). (From Simpson.[3])

volving Xp have produced del(Xp) offspring, especially del(Xp21 or 22).[47] This suggests either existence of ovarian determinants in Xq13 → 26 or necessity for the region to remain undisturbed (position effect).

Initially, deletion of Xq did not seem to result in short stature. It is now clear that 46,X,del(Xq) shows decreased mean heights,[30] indicating presence of a statural determinant on Xq. Mean adult heights are 151.3 cm for 46,X,del(X)(q13) (N=20), 149.3 for 46,X,del(X)(q21) (N=7), 150.8 for 46,X,del(X) (q22 or q24) (N=16), and 158.5 for 46,X,del(X)(q26) (N=4). Analogous to uncertainty about ovarian determinants on Xq, the precise location of the Xq statural determinant(s) is uncertain. Statural heterogeneity ostensibly cannot be explained on the basis of the length of Xq that is deficient. However, this author suspects that contradictory data could be explained by some purported 46,X,del(X)(q13) patients actually being 46,XY (Y mounted upside down in karyotype).

Isochromosome for the X Short Arm [i(Xp)]

It is difficult in practice to distinguish i(Xp) from del(X)(q22 or 24) chromosomes. Fryns[54] published i(Xp) chromosomes that could represent del(Xq), but other individuals originally reported to be 46,X,i(Xp) were later shown to be 46,X,del(Xq).[55] The consensus is that 46,X,i(Xp) is lethal, for which reason Figure 14-8 is prepared under the assumption that these cases are 46,X,del(q22). Indi-

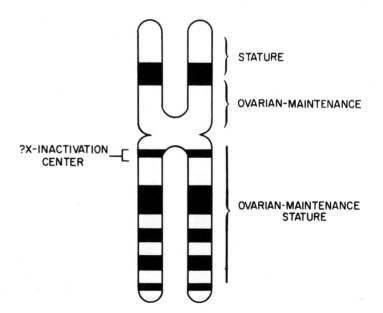

FIGURE 14-9. Relative location of ovarian maintenance and statural loci on the X chromosome. (From Simpson and LeBeau.[30])

viduals claimed to be 46,X,i(Xp) show primary amenorrhea and normal stature. Reinvestigation with current cytogenetic techniques would be helpful.

Other X Abnormalities

Centric fragments and ring [r(X)] chromosomes are often mitotically unstable; thus, phenotypic–karyotypic correlations are hazardous because monosomic cells are frequently associated. One potentially informative case, however, showed menstruation, normal breast development and a 46,X/46,X,r(X),r(X) complement.[56] The r(X) was so large that only its most telomeric regions could have been deleted. My colleagues and I have studied a similar case. This is consistent with other data.[45–50] One can conclude that gonadal determinants on Xp and Xq are not telomeric.

Autosomal Abnormalities

Autosomal abnormalities are occasionally associated with gonadal dysgenesis, but a causal relationship has not been proved. It is relevant, however, that autosomal recessive genes cause XX gonadal dysgenesis (see the section on Gonadal Dysgenesis in 46,XY Individuals). If autosomal abnormalities occur in individuals heterozygous for XX gonadal dysgenesis, the abnormality might cause deletion of a normal allele at the XX gonadal dysgenesis locus. This would result in hemizygosity and, hence, XX gonadal dysgenesis; however, involvement of different autosomes renders such a possibility unlikely.

Isochromosome for the Y Short Arm [i(Yq)]

46,X,i(Yq) individuals are female in appearance and have bilateral streak gonads.[16] Thus, testicular determinants can be deduced to be located on the Y short arm. Combined with other data, the testicular determinant(s) can be deduced to be located near the centromere on Yp.[1]

45,X/46,XY Mosaicism

Individuals with both a 45,X cell line and at least one line containing a Y chromosome may manifest a variety of phenotypes, ranging from almost normal males with cryptorchidism or penile hypospadias to females indistinguishable from those with the 45,X Turner syndrome. The different phenotypes presumably reflect different tissue distribu-

tions of the various cell lines; however, this assumption is unproved.

45,X/46,XY individuals may show (1) unambiguous female external genitalia; (2) ambiguous external genitalia, i.e., the sex of rearing is in doubt; or (3) almost normal male external genitalia. It is the first group that concerns us most in the present context.

Some 45,X/46,XY individuals with female external genitalia may have the Turner stigmata and thus be clinically indistinguishable from 45,X individuals. However, others are normal in stature and have no somatic anomalies. As in other types of gonadal dysgenesis, the external genitalia, vagina, and mullerian derivatives remain unstimulated because of deficient sex steroids. Breasts fail to develop, and little pubic or axillary hair develop. In fact, if breast development occurs in a 45,X/46,XY individual, one should suspect an estrogen-secreting tumor.

The streak gonads of 45,X/46,XY individuals are usually histologically indistinguishable from the streak gonads of individuals with 45,X gonadal dysgenesis. However, gonadoblastomas or dysgerminomas develop in about 15–20% of 45,X/46,XY individuals.[57] These neoplasias may arise during the first two decades of life. Gonadoblastomas occur almost exclusively in 46,XY or 45,X/46,XY individuals and are usually benign. However, they may be associated with dysgerminomas or other germ cell tumors which may be malignant. Thus, gonads should be extirpated in 45,X/46,XY individuals, regardless of their age. Because of the risk of neoplasia, one should distinguish patients with 45,X/46,XY gonadal dysgenesis from those who have complements lacking a Y chromosome. Analysis of buccal epithelial cells for the presence or absence of X-chromatin constitutes inadequate evaluation for patients with gonadal dysgenesis because X-chromatin is present in neither 45,X nor 45,X/46,XY individuals.

The terms asymmetric gonadal dysgenesis or mixed gonadal dysgenesis are often applied to individuals who have one streak gonad and one dysgenetic testis. Individuals with mixed gonadal dysgenesis usually have ambiguous external genitalia and a 45,X/46,XY complement, although occasionally only 45,X or only 46,XY cells can be demonstrated. Many investigators believe that the phenotype is almost always associated with 45,X/46,XY mosaicism, ostensible nonmosaic cases merely reflecting an inability to analyze appropriate tissues. Most 45,X/46,XY individuals with ambiguous external genitalia have Mullerian derivatives (e.g., a uterus). Presence of a uterus is helpful diagnostically because a uterus is absent in most genetic forms of male pseudohermaphroditism. If an individual has ambiguous external genitalia, bilateral testes, and a uterus, it is therefore reasonable to infer that such a person has 45,X/46,XY mosaicism (regardless of whether both lines can be demonstrated cytogenetically). Occasionally the uterus is rudimentary, or a fallopian tube may fail to develop ipsilateral to a testis. Less commonly, 45,X/46,XY mosaicism has been detected in individuals with almost normal male external genitalia.

45,X/47,XXY and 45,X/46,XY/47,XYY complements exist but are rarer than 45,X/46,XY. They are associated with the same phenotypic spectrum. Of particular interest is one family in which two and possibly three sibs had 45,X/46,XY/47,XYY mosaicism.[58] The parents were second cousins.

GONADAL DYSGENESIS IN 46,XX INDIVIDUALS

DeCourt et al.[59] were the first to report an individual with gonadal dysgenesis who had an apparently normal female (46,XX) complement. By 1971, Simpson et al.[60] accumulated 61 individuals with XX gonadal dysgenesis and concluded that the disorder was inherited in autosomal recessive fashion. External genitalia and the streak gonads in XX gonadal dysgenesis are indistinguishable from those of individuals who have gonadal dysgenesis and an abnormal chromosomal complement. Likewise, endocrine findings do not differ from those of other individuals with streak gonads. However, individuals with XX gonadal dysgenesis are usually normal in stature (mean height 165 cm). In at least 20 families, more than one sib has had XX gonadal dysgenesis, often with coexisting parental consanguinity (Fig. 14-10). Concordantly affected monozygotic twins have been reported.[61] Of

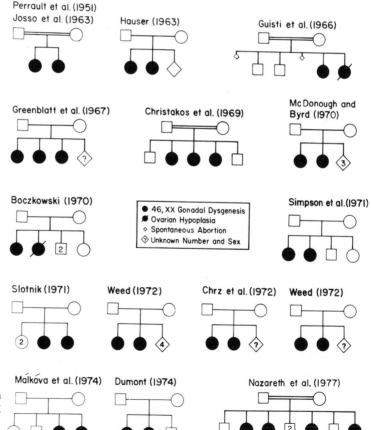

FIGURE 14-10. Pedigrees of kindreds in which multiple family members had XX gonadal dysgenesis, as tabulated in 1979. (From Simpson.[2])

course, not every 46,XX individual with streak gonads or ovaries devoid of oocytes is abnormal as result of a mutant gene. Teratogenic factors exist, as reviewed by Verp.[62] However, segregation analysis by our group suggests that gondal dysgenesis in 46,XX individuals usually results from an autosomal recessive gene(s).

Varied Expressivity

Varied expressivity exists with respect to gonadal development. For example, in one family one 46,XX sib had streak gonads, whereas another had primary amenorrhea and extreme ovarian hypoplasia (a few ova were detected).[63] In a second family, one sib had streak gonads, whereas another menstruated spontaneously despite increased urinary excretion of gonadotropin.[64] The present author has also studied slightly discordant 46,XX sibs. One showed streak gonads, whereas the other showed small rounded rudimentary ovaries with no functioning ova. Thus, individuals carrying the abnormal allele need not necessarily show complete absence of oocytes. If this reasoning is correct, the presenting complaint in XX gonadal dysgenesis might sometimes be secondary rather than primary amenorrhea. It follows that the XX gonadal dysgenesis mutant could be responsible for familial (sibship) aggregates of premature ovarian failure.

XX Gonadal Dysgenesis and Deafness

Both XX gonadal dysgenesis and neurosensory deafness have occurred in multiple sibs in several families.[65] This coexistence of features could be explained in several ways: (1) varied expressivity for the single (pleiotropic) gene that produces XX gonadal dysgenesis without deafness or (2) existence of two separate mutant genes (genetic heterogeneity), one associated with XX gonadal dysgenesis alone, and another associated with XX gonadal dysgenesis and deafness. The latter seems more likely. Males inheriting the mutation are deaf but have normal testes.[65]

Malformation Syndromes Associated with 46,XX Gonadal Dysgenesis

In other families, a mutant gene distinct from those already discussed has caused gonadal dysgenesis in 46,XX individuals. Maximilian et al.[66] reported sibs with gonadal dysgenesis, short stature, microcephaly, mental retardation, and arachnodactyly. Hamet et al.[67] described three sibs with

renal failure and adrenal hyperplasia; the one male showed abnormalities of spermatogenesis, whereas both his sisters had bilateral streak gonads. Skre[68] observed sibs with cerebral ataxia and hypergonadotropic hypogonadism. Lundgren[69] reported three sibs with mental retardation, streak gonads, myopathy and various neurological abnormalities. These syndromes further indicate that autosomal loci are integral to ovarian development.

GONADAL DYSGENESIS IN 46,XY INDIVIDUALS

Gonadal dysgenesis can occur in 46,XY individuals. Affected individuals are phenotypic females who show sexual infantilism and bilateral streak gonads that may undergo neoplasia transformation. The tumors occurring are gonadoblastomas and dysgerminomas, considered above in the context of 45,X/46,XY mosaicism. Neoplasia occurs in 20–30% of individuals with XY gonadal dysgenesis,[57] high enough to justify gonadal extirpation. Many familial aggregates have been recognized, and it is well accepted that at least one form of XY gonadal dysgenesis results from an X-linked recessive or male-limited autosomal dominant gene.[70-74] (Fig. 14-11).

The pathogenesis of XY gonadal dysgenesis involves failure of testicular differentiation, which as expected would result in nonvirilized female external genitalia and persistent mullerian derivatives. An analogous disorder in Swedish wood lemmings (*Myopus schistocolor*) is the result of an X-linked mutant that apparently suppresses H-Y antigen. In humans about two-thirds of affected individuals are H-Y positive and one-third H-Y negative. The only family with X-linked recessive inheritance that has been studied[72] showed H-Y positive individuals with neoplasia.

Genetic Heterogeneity on the Basis of Different Modes of Inheritance

In at least one type of XY gonadal dysgenesis, inheritance is definitely X-linked recessive or male-limited autosomal dominant (Fig. 14-11). Distinction between these two modes is not yet possible because the locus has not been shown to be linked to other loci.

Inheritance in X-linked fashion does not exclude the simultaneous existence of a clinically indistinguishable disorder resulting from an autosomal recessive gene (male-limited) (i.e., genetic hetero-

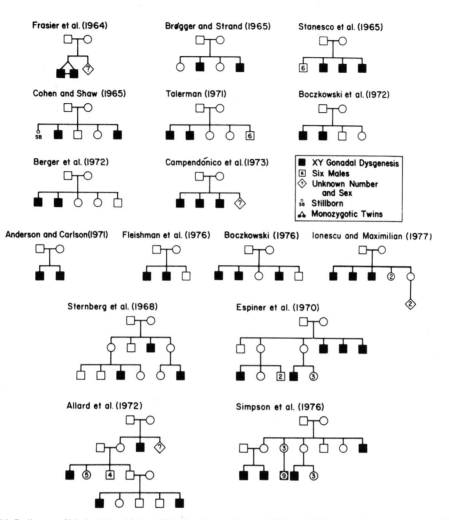

FIGURE 14-11. Pedigrees of kindreds in which multiple family members had XY gonadal dysgenesis, as tabulated in 1981. (From Simpson.[2])

geneity). Indeed, autosomal recessive inheritance could not only explain some unusual kindreds[76] but is also consistent with observations that some affected individuals are the products of consanguineous unions. If a male-limited autosomal recessive form of XY gonadal dysgenesis exists, 25% of male sibs of the proband should be affected, compared with 50%, if X-linked recessive inheritance were operative. Indeed, segregation analysis (incomplete ascertainment, single selection) by Simpson et al.[73] showed that the proportion of affected sibs was not statistically different from that expected (25%) on the basis of autosomal recessive inheritance. If genetic heterogeneity exists, a search for clinical differences between X-linked recessive and autosomal recessive XY gonadal dysgenesis is in order. The X-linked recessive form would seem to be characterized by H-Y positivity and a tendency toward neoplasia,[72] but an autosomal recessive form might show opposite characteristics.

XY Gonadal Dysgenesis and Campomelic Dwarfism

In campomelic dwarfism, short-limbed dwarfism and bowing of the long bones occurs. XY gonadal dysgenesis and campomelic dwarfism have coexisted in several individuals.[77,78] In some cases, gonads are indistinguishable from a streak gonad, whereas in others they resemble an ovary (sex reversal). H-Y antigen is not detected.[77,78]

Other Malformations Associated with XY Gonadal Dysgenesis

In addition to campomelic dwarfism, other somatic anomalies may be associated with XY gonadal dysgenesis. Some anomalies probably represent only coincidental associations. However, for other anomalies a more solid relationship exists.[79] For example, renal parenchymal abnormalities frequently occur.

In addition, Brosnan et al.[80] reported a distinctive syndrome in which two 46,XY sibs with streak gonads displayed unusual facies, cardiac anomalies, renal anomalies, ectodermal abnormalities such as scalp defects, and mental retardation. Similar cases have been reported by others.[7,81] The above suggest the existence of a distinct form of XY dysgenesis; the malformations are relatively nonspecific, however, for which reason additional data seems necessary.

MISCELLANEOUS CONDITIONS

This section calls attention to a few selected conditions not otherwise emphasized.

Rudimentary Ovary Syndrome and Unilateral Streak Gonad Syndrome

The rudimentary ovary syndrome is a poorly defined entity of unknown etiology said to be characterized by decreased numbers of follicles. This "syndrome" is certainly heterogeneous and is thus not a valid single entity. Many cases have been associated with sex chromosomal abnormalities, particularly 45,X/46,XX mosaicism. Similar statements apply also to individuals with the so-called unilateral streak ovary syndrome. For example, our group observed unilateral streak gonad and contralateral polycystic ovary in a 46,XX/46,X,i(Xq) individual who became pregnant.

Premature Ovarian Failure

Diagnosis of premature ovarian failure (POF) requires elevated FSH ($>$40 mIU/ml) in a patient before age 35 or 40 years. Ovaries are not usually streaklike

but are rather small and rounded like postmenopausal ovaries. The etiology is heterogeneous.[82] Indeed, one should recall the relationship of POF to XX gonadal dysgenesis, 45,X/46,XX mosaicism, 46,X,del(Xp) and 46,X,del(Xq). In addition, separate mutant genes could still be responsible for other cases. For example, Smith et al.[83] reported sibs affected with POF, and Mattison et al.[84] observed five families in which women in more than one generation were affected. The prevalence of such mutant genes is unknown.

Galactosemia and Gonadal Failure

Gonadal dysgenesis (streak gonads) may occur in galactosemia (galactose 1-phosphate uridyltransferase deficiency), an autosomal recessive trait. Kaufman et al.[85] observed hypergonadotropic hypogonadism in 9 of 12 galactosemics, and further cases continue to be recognized.[86] Optimal dietary treatment may or may not prevent this complication.

Adrenal 17α-Hydroxylase Deficiency and Gonadal Dysgenesis

Females affected with adrenal 17α-hydroxylase deficiency fail to undergo secondary sexual development because the enzymatic block precludes estrogen production. Ovarian differentiation should be normal; indeed, unstimulated but morphologically normal ovaries are usually observed. However, Tvedgaard et al.[87] observed streak gonads in two patients.

Agonadia

Agonadia warrants consideration in the differential diagnosis of XY gonadal dysgenesis. In this condition, 46,XY individuals show absent or abnormal external genitalia and rudimentary mullerian or wolffian derivatives. External genitalia usually consist of (1) a phallus about the size of a clitoris, (2) nearly complete fusion of the labioscrotal folds, and (3) often a persistent urogenital sinus. By definition, gonads cannot be detected (agonadia). Likewise, neither normal mullerian derivatives nor normal wolffian derivatives are present, although structures resembling a rudimentary fallopian tube, an epioophoron, or an epididymis may be present along the lateral pelvic wall. Somatic anomalies are common—craniofacial anomalies, vertebral anomalies, dermatoglyphic anomalies, and mental retardation.[1,88,89]

Any explanation for agonadia must explain not only the absence of gonads, but abnormal external genitalia and lack of normal internal ducts as well. One possible explanation is that fetal testes functioned sufficiently long to inhibit mullerian development, yet not sufficiently long to complete male differentiation. Alternatively, the entire gonadal, ductal, and genital systems developed abnormally, as result of defective anlage, defective connective tissue, or a teratogen. The frequent coexistence of somatic anomalies favors either a teratogen or defective connective tissue. In one and possibly other kindreds affected sibs have been reported; thus, a genetic etiology should be considered.[1] Schulte[90] detected H-Y antigen, suggesting that pathogenesis does not involve an abnormality of this system. Although agonadia is usually associated with 46,XY individuals, 46,XX individuals may show the same phenotype.[91]

Leydig Cell Agenesis

A few 46,XY patients have been reported to have complete absence of Leydig cells, precluding embryonic virilization.[92] As predicted, they show normal female external genitalia or minimal posterior labial fusion, no uterus and bilateral testes devoid of Leydig cells. Absence of a uterus excludes XY gonadal dysgenesis; absence of breast development excludes complete androgen insensitivity (testicular feminization). Presence of testes excludes agonadia.

Polycystic Ovary Syndrome

Stein–Leventhal syndrome is a common gynecologic disorder characterized by polycystic ovaries, obesity, hirsutism, and infertility due to anovulation. Detailed clinical considerations are provided elsewhere in this volume. Affected individuals usually have hirsutism and either secondary amenorrhea or oligomenorrhia, but it remains uncertain as to whether this defect is primary or merely an effect secondary to hyperandrogenism.

This varied expressivity, so well accepted by gynecologists, is genetically significant. Varied expressivity is characteristic of dominant but not recessive inheritance. Indeed, dominant tendencies have been suggested. In studying male and female relatives of 12 probands with Stein-Leventhal syndrome, Cooper et al.[93] concluded that the disorder results from an incompletely penetrant autosomal dominant gene. Based on a study of 48 sibships, Cohen et al.[94] likewise concluded that the trait was also dominant, albeit X-linked. Of female offspring of affected females, 47% were considered affected. Of female offspring of males with elevated LH/FSH ratios, 87% showed oligomenorrhea or hirsutism. These findings suggested X-linked dominant inheritance. On the other hand, most gynecologists observe symptomatic polycystic ovarian disease less often in relatives. Clinically symptomatic polycystic changes seem to occur in far fewer than 50% of relatives. Mandel et al.[95] found only 4 of 23 females to have an affected sib.

The genetics of polycystic ovarian disease are thus uncertain. Genetic tendencies clearly exist. Moreover, support for a dominant gene would exist if elevated LH/FSH ratio is indeed of primary etiology. By contrast, the much lower frequency of symptomatic relatives suggests that clinical expectations in surveillance of a proband's family should be based on far fewer than 50% cases. Recurrence risks for symptomatic cases is nearer polygenic/multifactorial expectations. Genetic heterogeneity also exists, for which reason studies in different geographic locations are desirable. Evidence for genetic heterogeneity includes patients showing abnormalities of the X chromosome and those having adult-onset 21-hydroxylase deficiency.

Ovarian Unresponsiveness to Gonadotropin

Although belying the title of this chapter, this rare disorder deserves mention. End-organ resistance to various pituitary trophic hormones is well documented. It was thus not completely unexpected when Jones and Moraes-Ruebsen[96] reported three females with primary amenorrhea, elevated gonadotropin levels, and histologically normal ovaries. All three had normal breasts, normal pubic hair, and normal overall appearance. Other patients with ovarian unresponsiveness have subsequently been reported. The ovaries of these patients may be longer and thinner than normal ("fat streaks"). About 20 cases have been claimed,[97] although some individuals claimed as "affected" strangely presented with secondary amenorrhea.

The mechanism of ovarian resistance remains unknown. Possibilities include functionally abnormal FSH or LH or an autoimmune phenomenon. However, FSH and LH are normal by both immunoassay and bioassay, and there is no evidence for autoimmunity. Although no familial aggregates have been reported, receptor defects involving other organ systems invariably prove genetic (usually a single mutant gene, as in androgen insensitivity). If affected individuals cannot reproduce, dominant inheritance will be difficult to recognize. However, recessive factors would clearly be shown if affected sibs are observed.

MANAGEMENT

Gynecologists usually detect patients with gonadal dysgenesis because of their ovarian failure. Primary treatment is not possible, but secondary complications may be addressed.

Psychologic Considerations

These patients are often socially immature, especially if short; however, they should obviously be treated as adults. This author prefers to explain pathogenesis by relating that "ovaries failed to persist." Realization that pathogenesis involves increased rate of attrition, as opposed to failure of germ cell formation, seems well-received by patients (and parents). Those with elevated gonadotropin are counseled to anticipate sterility, except perhaps by embryo-transfer techniques.

Chromosomal Studies

Cytogenetic studies are obligatory to exclude a 46,XY line. A study of 50 lymphocytes should suffice, unless phenotype and karyotype are discordant. If they are discordant, additional tissues should be studied. If a "45,X" patient is tall, we prefer buccal smear for X or Y chromatin, skin cultures and finally streak gonad cultures. Detection of a Y necessitates gonadal extirpation, but in its absence laparatomy is not necessary.

Somatic Anomalies

In addition to a general physical examination, every patient with gonadal dysgenesis should have excretory urography to exclude renal anomalies. Vertebral roentgenograms are also recommended, and audiograms are useful in children. Blood pressure monitoring deserves special attention.

Hormonal Replacement

Hormonal replacement therapy requires cyclic estrogen supplement by a progestogen. The present author prefers to initiate therapy with 0.625 mg conjugated estrogens on the first 20 or 25 days of each calendar month. This dosage is later increased to 1.25 mg/day, and if tolerated occasionally to a maximum of 2.50 mg/day. After an initial 6–12-month period with estrogen alone, 10–20 mg medroxyprogesterone acetate can be added on days 16–25. Other regimens and other hormones are entirely satisfactory, although progestins should be used with estrogens in cyclic fashion.

Adequacy of hormone therapy is monitored by assessment of withdrawal flow, intermittent endometrial biopsy, and FSH levels. Breast development should occur, although varying in degree between individuals. The rectangular (shield) chest contour perceptually augments breast development. Use of high collars or surgery is cosmetically helpful for patients with webbed necks, and nevi require surveillance. Periodic evaluation should emphasize emotional support, pelvic examination, cervical cytology, blood pressure assessment, urine cultures if renal anomalies exist, and perhaps endometrial biopsy to verify progestational effect.

Occasionally, gynecologists encounter 45,X patients. Although sterility is the likely outcome, I prefer to initiate hormonal therapy only after verifying gonadal failure with elevated FSH (>40 mIU/ml). Increasing uterine size (ultrasonography) and normal bone age between ages 10 and 14 years predict spontaneous puberty. Such approaches are especially desirable for 46,X,del(Xp) or 46,X,del(Xq) individuals, who may menstruate spontaneously. One might also recall the instructive report of Starup et al.,[98] who achieved pregnancies in two hypergonadotropic females treated first with estrogens and then ovulation-inducing agents. Similarly, the occurrence of short stature and Turner stigmata should not lead to the conclusion that gonadal failure is inevitable, given expected phenotype in 46,X,del(X)(q21).

Finally, many physicians administer anabolic steroids (e.g., oxandrolone) or growth hormone to short patients, but the efficacy of this approach has not been established.

Surgical Considerations

Gonadal extirpation may be necessary if a 46,XY or 45,X/46,XY complement is detected. In such circumstances, this author believes that only the streaks should be removed. Sequential clamping and suture ligation will extirpate the tissue. Identification of the entire specimen requires inspection of the infundibular pelvic ligament, into which extension may occur. Presence of gonadoblastoma or dysgerminoma usually requires unilateral salpingectomy and the usual precautions to exclude metastases (peritoneal cytology, palpation of aortic nodes and upper abdomen). However, in my opinion the technically easier hysterectomy should be avoided. Not only is there a psychological advantage to withdrawal of uterine bleeding, but embryo-transfer techniques (donor ova) may now make possible pregnancies in women having an intact uterus but lacking ovaries.

SUMMARY AND CONCLUSIONS

Monosomy X(45,X) is usually associated with streak gonads, short stature, and certain other anomalies that make up the Turner stigmata. Phenotypic expression varies more often than generally appreciated, as evidenced by observations that 45,X individuals occasionally menstruate or become pregnant. This is actually not surprising because pathogenesis of germ cell failure involves increased rate of oocyte atresia, not failure of germ cell formation. The short stature may reflect the prolonged 45,X cell cycle, a phenomenon that could also explain high embryonic lethality and IUGR.

Deletions of most [del(Xp)] or all [i(Xq)] of the X short arm are usually associated with short stature and certain features of the Turner stigmata. Menstruation or breast development occurs in approximately 40% of 46,X,del(X)(p11) individuals, but less often in 46,X,i(Xq). Deletions limited to only the distal (telomeric) end of Xp [del(X)(p21 or 22)] seem compatible with normal ovarian function, although short stature still occurs.

Deletions of most [del(q13)(q22) or (q24)] of the X long arm are often associated with gonadal dysgenesis, menstruation occurring in only 20% of adult 46,X,del(Xq) cases. Distal deletions [46,X,del(X)(q26)] are much more likely to be associated with normal menstruation. 46,X,del(Xq) leads to a decreased mean height.

The above findings permit one to conclude that determinants essential for ovarian (oocyte) maintenance exist on both the X short arm (Xp) and the X long arm (Xq). Duplication of one arm (i.e., an isochromosome) fails to compensate for loss of the other arm; thus, determinants on Xp and Xq have different functions, each essential to normal ovarian development. Each arm may contain more than a single determinant.

Both the X short arm and the X long arm contain determinants that, if deleted, result in short stature and possibly other features of the Turner stigmata. The statural determinant on Xp is distal (telomeric) to the ovarian determinant on that arm. The precise location of the Xq statural determinant is unknown.

Gonadal dysgenesis in 46,XX individuals (XX gonadal dysgenesis) usually results from an autosomal recessive gene. Genetic heterogeneity exists, with one relatively common form associated with deafness.

Gonadal dysgenesis in 46,XY individuals (XY gonadal dysgenesis) most often results from an X-linked recessive or male-limited autosomal dominant allele. The prevalence of gonadoblastomas or dysgerminomas is 20–30%. Most subjects with tumors show H-Y antigen.

Clinical management of patients with ovarian failure should emphasize (1) open discussion and emotional support, (2) exclusion of somatic anomalies (renal, cardiac, vertebral, auditory), (3) hormonal replacement therapy, and (4) extirpation of streak gonads (but not the uterus) in 46,XY and 45,X,/46,XY individuals.

QUESTIONS

1. Short stature in patients with gonadal dysgenesis is *not* characteristic of

    a. 45,X.
    b. 46,XX.
    c. 46,X,i(Xq).
    d. 46,X,del(X)(p21).
    e. 46,X,del(X)(q22).

2. The streak gonads of individuals with gonadal dysgenesis show increased propensity for neoplastic transformation. The chromosomal complement often associated with gonadoblastomas or dysgerminomas, if detected in individuals with gonadal dysgenesis, is

    a. 45,X.
    b. 46,X,del(X)(p21).
    c. 46,XY.
    d. 46,X,del(X)(q22).
    e. 46,XX.

3. The human Y chromosome

    a. is fluorescent throughout the entire long arm.
    b. contains a testicular determinant near the centromere.
    c. contains the structural locus for H-Y antigen.
    d. none of the above.

4. A 45,X chromosomal complement

    a. accounts for 10–15% of all first-trimester spontaneous abortuses.

    b. usually causes ovarian dysgenesis, but not other anomalies.

    c. is usually associated with normal stature.

    d. is the only chromosomal complement commonly associated with ovarian dysgenesis.

5. The structural locus for H-Y antigen is located on

    a. the short arm of the Y chromosome near the centromere.

    b. the X chromosome.

    c. an autosome.

    d. cannot exclude a, b, or c.

    e. can exclude a but not b or c.

6. The pathogenesis of germ cell failure in 45,X most accurately can be said to involve

    a. failure of germ cell formation.

    b. failure of germ cell migration from yolk sac to genital ridge.

    c. increased oocyte attrition.

    d. increased secretion of H-Y antigen.

REFERENCES

1. Simpson JL: *Disorders of Sexual Differentiation: Etiology and Clinical Delineation.* New York: Academic, 1976
2. Simpson JL: Gonadal dysgenesis and sex chromosomal abnormalities. Phenotypic–karyotypic correlations, in Porter I, Vallet HL (eds): *Genetic Mechanism of Sexual Development.* New York: Academic, 1979, p 365
3. Simpson JL: Disorders of sex chromosomes and sexual differentiation, in Kirstner R, Grant P (eds): *Progress in Infertility,* 3rd ed. Boston, Little, Brown, 1985
4. Wachtel SS, Chervenak FA, Brunner M, et al: Notes on the biology of the H-Y antigen. *J Pediatr Endocrinol* (in press)
5. Wachtel SS: H-Y Antigen and the Biology of Sex Determination. New York: Grune and Stratton, 1983
6. Wolf U, Fraccaro M, Mayerova A, et al: Turner syndrome patients are H-Y positive. *Hum Genet* 54:315, 1980
7. Bernstein R, Jenkins T, Dawson B, et al: Female phenotype and multiple abnormalities in sibs with a Y chromosome and partial X chromosome duplication: H-Y antigen and Xg blood group findings. *J Med Genet* 17:291, 1980
8. Singh RP, Carr DH: The anatomy and histology of XO human embryos and fetuses. *Anat Rec* 155:369, 1966
9. Jirasek J: Principles of reproductive embryology, in Simpson JL (ed): *Disorders of Sexual Differentiation: Etiology and Clinical Delineation.* New York, Academic, 1976, p 51
10. Washburn LL, Eicher EM: Sex reversal in XY mice caused by dominant mutation on chromosome 17. *Nature (Lond)* 303:338, 1983
11. Turner HH: A syndrome of infantilism, congenital webbed neck and cubitus valgus. *Endocrinology* 23:566, 1938
12. Albright F, Smith PH, Fraser R: A syndrome characterized by primary ovarian insufficiency and decreased stature. Report of 11 cases with a depression on hormonal control of axillary and pubic hair. *Am J Med Sci* 204:625, 1942
13. Varney FF, Kenyon AT, Koch FC: An association of short stature, retarded sexual development and high urinary gonadotropin titers in women; ovarian dwarfism. *J Clin Endocrinol* 2:137, 1942
14. Wilkins L, Fleischmann W: Ovarian agenesis. Pathology, associated clinical symptoms and the bearing on the theories of sex differentiation, *J Clin Endocrinol* 4:357, 1944
15. Ford CE, Jones KW, Polani PE, et al: A sex-chromosome anomaly in a case of gonadal dysgenesis (Turner's syndrome). *Lancet* 1:711, 1959
16. Simpson JL: Gonadal dysgenesis and abnormalities of the human sex chromosomes: Current status of phenotypic–karyotypic correlations. *Birth Defects* 11(4):23, 1975
17. Sanger R, Tippett P, Gavin J, et al: Xg groups and sex chromosome abnormalities in people of northern European ancestry: An addendum. *J Med Genet* 14:210, 1977
18. Russell LB: Chromosome aberrations in experimental mammals. *Prog Med Genet* 2:230, 1962
19. Russell LB, Saylors CL: Factors causing a high frequency of mice having the XO sex-chromosome constitution. *Science* 131:1321, 1960
20. Russell LB, Montgomery CS: The incidence of sex-chromosome anomalies following irradiation of mouse spermatogonia with single or fractionated doses of X-rays. *Mutat Res* 25:367, 1974
21. Mohandes T, Shapiro LJ, Sparkes RC: Regional assignment of the steroid sufatase-X-linked ichthyosis locus: Implications for a noninactivated region on the short arm of human S-chromosome. *Proc Natl Acad Sci USA* 76:5779, 1979
22. Gartler SM, Liskay, RM, Campbell BK, et al: Evidence of two functional X chromosomes in human oocytes. *Cell Diff* 1:125, 1972
23. Chen ATL, Chan Y-KM, Falek A: The effects of chromosome abnormalities on birth weight in man. I. Sex chromosome disorders. *Hum Hered* 21:543, 1971
24. Brook CGD, Murset G, Zachman M, et al: Growth in children with 45,XO Turner's syndrome. *Arch Dis Child* 49:789, 1974
25. Donaldson CL, Wegienko LC, Miller D, et al: Growth hormone studies in Turner's syndrome. *J Clin Endocrinol Metab* 28:383, 1968
26. Bottazzo GF, McIntosh C, Stanford W, et al: Growth hormone cell antibodies and partial hormone deficiency in a girl with Turner's syndrome. *Clin Endocrinol* 12:1, 1980
27. Laczi F, Julesz J, Janaky T, et al: Growth hormone reserve capacity in Turner's syndrome. *Horm Metab Res* 11:664, 1979
28. Filipsson R, Lindsten J, Almqvist S: Time of eruption of the permanent teeth, cephalometric and tooth measurement and sulphation factor activity in 45 patients with Turner's syndrome with different types of X chromosome aberration. *Acta Endocrinol (Copenh)* 48:91, 1965
29. Lindsten J, Fraccaro M: Turner's syndrome, in Rashad MN, Morton WRM (eds): *Genital Anomalies.* Springfield, IL, Thomas, 1969, p 396
30. Simpson JL, LeBeau MM: Gonadal and statural determinants on the X chromosome and their relationship to in vitro studies showing prolonged cell cycles in 45,X; 46,X.del(X)(p11); 46,X,del(X)(q13); and 46,X,del(X)(q22) fibroblasts. *Am J Obstet Gynecol* 141:930, 1981

31. Garron DC, Vander Stoep LR: Personality and intelligence in Turner's syndrome. *Arch Gen Psychiatry* 21:339, 1969

32. Money J: Two cytogenetic syndromes: Psychologic comparisons. I. Intelligence and specific-factor quotients. *J Psychiatr Res* 2:223, 1964

33. Shaffer JW: A specific cognitive defect observed in gonadal aplasia (Turner's syndrome). *J Clin Psychol* 18:403, 1962

34. Keats TE, Burns TWL: The radiographic manifestations of gonadal dysgenesis. *Radiol Clin North Am* 2:297, 1964

35. Passarge E: Gastrointestinalblutung beim Turner-syndrom in infolge telangiektasien in der Darmwand. *Dtsch Med Wochenschr* 93:204, 1968

36. Arulanantham K, Kramer MS, Gryboski JD: The association of inflammatory bowel disease and X chromosomal abnormalities. *Pediatrics* 66:53, 1980

37. Astley R: Chromosomal abnormalities in childhood with particular reference to Turner's syndrome and Mongolism. *Br J Radiol* 36:2, 1963

38. Engel E, Forbes AP: Cytogenetic and clinical findings in 48 patients with congenitally defective or absent ovaries. *Medicine (Baltimore)* 44:135, 1965

39. Polychronakos C, Letarte J, Collu R, et al: Carbohydrate intolerance in children and adolescents with Turner syndrome. *J Pediatr* 96:1009, 1980

40. AvRuskin TW, Crigler JF Jr, Soeldner JS: Turner's syndrome and carbohydrate metabolism. I. Impaired insulin secretion after tolbutamide and glucagon stimulation tests: Evidence of insulin deficiency. *Am J Med Sci* 277:153, 1979

41. Doniach D, Roitt IM, Polani PE: Thyroid antibodies and sex-chromosome anomalies. *Proc R Soc Med* 6:278, 1968

42. Brooks WH, Meek JC, Schimke RN: Gonadal dysgenesis with Grave's disease. *J Med Genet* 14:468, 1977

43. Dewhurst J: Gonadal dysgenesis and X chromosome deletion. *Br J Obstet Gynecol* 88:944, 1981

44. Simpson JL: Pregnancies in women with chromosomal abnormalities, in Schulman JD, Simpson JL (eds): *Genetic Diseases in Pregnancy.* New York, Academic, 1981, p 440

45. Fraccaro M, Maraschio P, Pasquali F, et al: Women heterozygous for deficiency of the (p21 → pter) region of the X chromosome are fertile. *Hum Genet* 39:283, 1977

46. Goldman B, Polani PE, Daker MG, et al: Clinical and cytogenetic aspects of X-chromosome deletions. *Clin Genet* 21:36, 1982

47. Maraschio P, Fraccaro M: X Chromosome abnormalities and female fertility, in Crosignani PG, Rubin BL, Fraccaro M (eds): *Genetic Control of Gamete Production and Function.* London, Academic, 1982, p 275

48. Madan K: Balanced structural changes involving the human X: Effect on sexual phenotype. *Hum Genet* 63:216, 1983

49. Mattei M, Mattei JF, Vidal I, et al: Structural anomalies of the X chromosome and the inactivation center. *Hum Genet* 56:401, 1981

50. Fitch N, Richer CL, de St Victor J, et al: Premature menopause due to a small terminal deletion of the long arm of the X chromosome. *Am J Hum Genet* 33:103A, 1981

51. Fryns JP, Petit P, Van Den Berghe H: The various phenotypes in Xp deletion. Observations in eleven patients. *Clin Genet* 22:76, 1982

52. Palmer CG, Reichmann A: Chromosomal and clinical findings in 110 females with Turner's syndrome. *Hum Genet* 35:35, 1976

53. Therman E, Sarto GE, Palmer CG, et al: Position of the human X inactivation center on Xq. *Hum Genet* 50:59, 1979

54. Fryns JP: Sex chromosomes: New data, in Armendares S, Lister R, Ebling FJG, Henderson IW (eds): *Human Genetics.* Amsterdam, Excerpta Medica, 1977, p 114

55. De La Chapelle, Schroeder J: Reappraisal of a 46,X,i(Xp) karyotypes 46,X,del(Xq). *Hereditas* 80:137, 1975

56. Lindsten J, Tillinger KG: Self-perpetuating ring chromosome in a patient with gonadal dysgenesis. *Lancet* 1:593, 1962

57. Simpson JL, Photopulos G: The relationship of neoplasia to disorders of abnormal sexual differentiation. *Birth Defects* 12(1):15, 1976

58. Hsu LY, Hirschhorn K, Goldstein A, et al: Familial chromosomal mosaicism, genetic aspects. *Ann Hum Genet* 33:343, 1970

59. De Court J, Michaud JP, Delzant G: Syndrome de Turner avec caryotype feminin normal. *Rev Fr Endocrinol Clin Nutr Metab* 1:321, 1960

60. Simpson JL, Christakos AC, Horwith M, et al: Gonadal dysgenesis in individuals with apparently normal chromosomal complements: Tabulation of cases and compilation of genetic data. *Birth Defects* 7(6):215, 1971

61. Youlton R, Michelsen H, Be C, et al: Pure XX gonadal dysgenesis in identical twins. *Clin Genet* 21:262, 1982

62. Verp MS: Environment causes of ovarian failure. *Semin Reprod Endocrinol* 1:101, 1983

63. Guisti G, Borghi A, Salti M, et al: Disgenesia gonadica pura, con cariotippo 44A + XX in sorelle figlie di cugini. *Acta Genet Med Gemellol* 15:51,1966

64. Boczkowski K: Pure gonadal dysgenesis and ovarian dysplasia in sisters. *Amer J Obstet Gynecol* 106:626, 1970

65. Pallister PD, Opitz JM: The Perrault syndrome: Autosomal recessvie-ovarian dysgensis with facultative, non-sex limited sensorineural deafness. *Amer J Med Genet* 4:239, 1979

66. Maximilian C, Ionescu B, Bucur A: Deux soers avec dysgenesie majeure, hypotrophic staturale, microcephalie, arachnodactylie et caryotype 46,XX. *J Genet Hum* 18:365, 1970

67. Hamet P, Kuchel O, Nowacinski W, et al: Hypertension with adrenal, genital, renal defects and deafness. *Arch Intern Med* 131:563, 1973

68. Skre H, Bassoe HH, Berg K, et al: Cerebellar ataxia and hypergonadotropic hypogonadism in two kindreds. Chance concurrence, pleiotropism or linkage. *Clin Genet* 9:234, 1976

69. Lundgren PO: Hereditary myopathy, oligophrenia, cataract, skeletal abnormalities and hypergonadotropic hypogonadism; a new syndrome. *Eur Neurol* 10:261, 1973

70. Espiner EA, Veale AMO, Sands VE, et al: Familial syndrome of streak gonads and normal male karyotype in five phenotypic females. *N Engl J Med* 283:6, 1970

71. German J, Simpson JL, Chaganti RSK, et al: Gentically determined sex-reversal in 46,XY humans. *Science* 202:53, 1978

72. Mann JR, Corkery JJ, Fisher HJW, et al: The X linked recessive form of XY gonadal dysgenesis with high incidence of gonadal germ cell tumors: Clinical and genetic studies. *J Med Genet* 20:264, 1983

73. Simpson JL, Blagowidow N, Martin AO: XY gonadal dysgenesis: Genetic heterogeneity based upon clinical observations, H-Y antigen status and segregation analysis. *Hum Genet* 58:91, 1980

74. Sternberg WH, Barclay DL, Kloepfer HW: Familial XY gonadal dysgenesis. *N Engl J Med* 278:695, 1976

75. Wachtel SS, Koo GC, Breg WR: H-Y antigen in X,i(Xq) gonadal dysgenesis: Evidence of X-linked genes in testicular differentiation. *Hum Genet* 56:183, 1980

76. Allard S, Codotte M, Boivin Y: Disgénésie gonadique pure familiale et gonadoblastome. *Un Med Can* 101:448, 1972

77. Bricarelli FD, Fraccaro M, Lindsten J, et al: Sex-reversed XY females with campomelic dysplasia are H-Y negative. *Hum Genet* 57:15, 1981

78. Puck SM, Haseltine FP, Francke U: Absence of H-Y antigen in an XY female with campomelic dysplasia. *Hum Genet* 57:23, 1981

79. Simpson JL, Chaganti RSK, Mouradian J, et al: Chronic renal disease, myotonic dystrophy, and gonadoblastoma in an individual with XY gonadal dysgenesis. *J Med Genet* 19:73, 1982

80. Bronson PG, Lewandowski RC, Toguri AG, et al: A new familial syndrome of 46,XY gonadal dysgenesis with anomalies of ectodermal and mesodermal structures. *J Pediatr* 97:586, 1980

81. Silengo M, Kaufman RL, Kissane J: A 46,XY infant with uterus, dysgenetic gonads and multiple anomalies. *Humangenetik* 25:65, 1974

82. Rebar RW: Premature menopause. *Semin Reprod Endocrinol* 1:161, 1983

83. Smith A, Fraser IS, Noel M: Three siblings with premature gonadal failure. *Fertil Steril* 32:528, 1979

84. Mattison DR, Evans MI, Schwimmer WB, et al: Familial premature ovarian failure. Abstracts, *Am J Hum Genet* 36:1341, 1984

85. Kaufman F, Kogut MD, Donnell GN, et al: Ovarian failure in galactosemia. *Lancet* 2:737, 1979

86. Robinson ACR, Dockeray CJ, Cullen MJ, et al: Hypergonadotrophic hypogonadism in classical galactosemia. Evidence for defective oogenesis. Case report. *Br J Obstet Gynaecol* 91:199, 1984

87. Tvedgaard E, Fredericksen V, Olgaard K, et al: Two cases of 17β-hydroxylase deficiency—One combined with complete gonadal agenesis. *Acta Endocrinol (Copenh)* 98:267, 1981

88. Coulam CB: Testicular regression syndrome. *Obstet Gynecol* 53:45, 1979

89. Sarto GE, Opitz JM: The XY gonadal agenesis syndrome. *J Med Genet* 10:288, 1973

90. Schulte MJ: Positive H-Y antigen testing in a case of XY gonadal absence syndrome. *Clin Genet* 16:438, 1979

91. Duck SC, Sekhon GS, Wilbois R, et al: Pseudohermaphroditism with testes and a 46,XX karyotype. *J Pediatr* 87:58, 1975

92. Brown DM, Markland C, Dehner LP: Leydig cell hypoplasia. A cause of male pseudohermaphroditism. *J Clin Endocrinol Metab* 46:1, 1978

93. Cooper HE, Spellacy WN, Prem KA, et al: Hereditary factors in the Stein-Leventhal syndrome. *Am J Obstet Gynecol* 100:317, 1968

94. Cohen BN, Givens JR, Wiser WL, et al: Polycystic ovarian disease, maturation arrest of spermatogenesis and Klinefelter's syndrome in siblings of a family with familial hirsutism. *Fertil Steril* 26:1228, 1975

95. Mandel FP, Chang RJ, DuPont B, et al: HLA genotyping in family members and patients with familial polycystic ovarian disease. *J Clin Endocrinol Metab* 56:862, 1983

96. Jones GES, de Moraes-Ruebsen M: A new syndrome of amenorrhea in association with hypergonadotropism and apparently normal ovarian follicular apparatus. *Am J Obstet Gynecol* 104:597, 1969

97. Maxson W, Wentz AC: The gonadotropin resistant ovarian syndrome. *Semin Reprod Endocrinol* 1:47, 1983

98. Starup J, Philip J, Sele V: Oestrogen treatment and subsequent pregnancy in two patients with severe hypergonadotropic ovarian failure. *Acta Endocrinol (Copenh)* 89:149, 1978

99. Simpson JL: Genetics of human reproduction, Hafez ESE (eds): in *Human Reproduction,* 2nd ed, Hagerstown, MD, Harper & Row, 1980, p 395

100. Sutton E: *An Introduction to Human Genetics,* 2nd ed. New York, Holt, Rinehart, and Winston, 1975

ANSWERS

1. b

2. c

3. b

4. a

5. e

6. c

15

Female Pseudohermaphroditism in 21-Hydroxylase Deficiency

MARIA I. NEW

INTRODUCTION

Congenital adrenal hyperplasia (CAH) is a family of inherited disorders of adrenal steroidogenesis. Each of these disorders has a characteristic pattern of hormonal abnormalities caused by an inherited deficiency of one of the several enzymes necessary for normal steroid synthesis. The most common form of CAH is caused by a deficiency of the 21-hydroxylase enzyme. Virilization is the foremost clinical symptom of 21-hydroxylase deficiency, as was first documented by the Neapolitan anatomist DeCrecchio in 1865.[1] Since his report, numerous investigators have unravelled the mechanism of adrenal steroid synthesis and the associated enzyme defects responsible for CAH. A brief review of the mechanism and regulation of adrenal steroidogenesis is given below to aid in the understanding of the pathophysiology of CAH.

STEROIDOGENESIS AND ENZYMATIC CONVERSIONS OF ADRENAL STEROID HORMONES

Steroidogenesis

Figure 15-1 shows a simplified scheme of adrenal steroidogenesis; each hydroxylation step is indicated, and the newly added hydroxyl group is circled. The three main classes of hormones synthesized by the adrenal cortex are mineralocorticoids (17-deoxy pathway), glucocorticoids (17-hydroxy pathway), and sex steroids.

A detailed discussion of steroidogenesis is omitted here, since it has been extensively reviewed in other texts[2,3] and in Chapter 4. For the purpose of understanding the clinical manifestations of CAH, reference to the scheme in Figure 15-1 will suffice.

Mineralocorticoids (17-Deoxy Pathway)

Pregnenolone, a Δ^5-steroid, is converted to a biologically active Δ^4-steroid, progesterone, by the enzymes 3β-hydroxysteroid dehydrogenase (3β-HSD) and an isomerase. Progesterone is then hydroxylated at the C-21 position to form deoxycorticosterone (DOC), an active salt-retaining hor-

MARIA I. NEW • Department of Pediatrics, Division of Pediatric Endocrinology, Pediatric Clinical Research Center, The New York Hospital–Cornell Medical Center, New York, New York 10021.

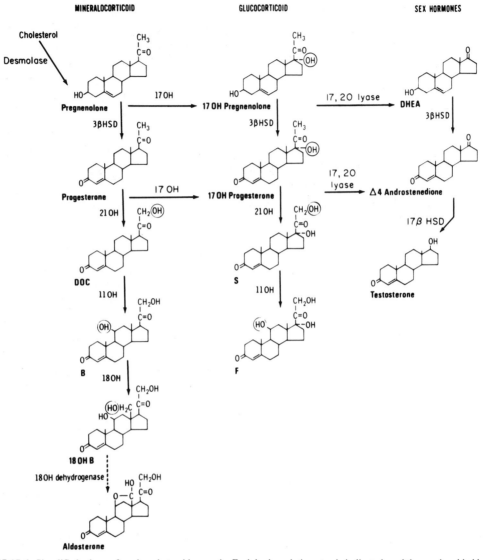

FIGURE 15-1. Simplified scheme for adrenal steroidogenesis. Each hydroxylation step is indicated, and the newly added hydroxyl group is circled. (From New and Levine.[42])

mone. When DOC is hydroxylated at the C-11 position, corticosterone (B) is formed, which is a weak mineralocorticoid, but is the precursor of aldosterone, the most potent salt-retaining hormone. Synthesis of aldosterone, a unique hormone because of the aldehyde group at C-18, occurs in the zona glomerulosa of the adrenal cortex. Regulation of the zona glomerulosa differs from that of the other zones, as discussed below. The mechanism of the synthesis of aldosterone from corticosterone has not been entirely elucidated.

Glucocorticoids (17-Hydroxy Pathway)

Glucocorticoid synthesis requires 17α-hydroxylation at the C-17 position. Negligible 17α-hydroxylase activity has been found in the zona glomerulosa, in contrast to the active 17α-hydroxylation occurring in the zona fasciculata. It is generally accepted that glucocorticoids and sex steroids, both of which require 17α-hydroxylation for their synthesis, originate predominantly in the zona fasciculata and zona reticularis. Pregnenolone and progesterone yield 17-hydroxypregnenolone and 17-hydroxyprogesterone (17-OHP), respectively, when acted upon by the 17α-hydroxylase enzyme. The Δ^5-steroid 17-hydroxypregnenolone is converted to 17-OHP, a Δ^4-steroid, by enzymatic steps similar to those that convert pregnenolone to progesterone. When 17-OHP undergoes 21-hydroxylation, 11-deoxycortisol (S) is formed, and this is further hydroxylated to form cortisol (F), the most potent glucocorticoid in humans. Thus, it can be seen from Figure 15-1 that parallel hydroxylation steps in progesterone and 17-OHP result in corticosterone (B) and cortisol (F), respectively. Although these steps are parallel, it has not been proved that the enzymes are identical for both the 17-hydroxy and the 17-deoxy substrates.

Sex Steroids

Dehydroepiandrosterone (DHEA) is the main unconjugated C-19 steroid secreted by the adrenal cortex. It results from the side-chain cleavage of the steroid, 17-hydroxypregnenolone, by the action of a desmolase enzyme. DHEA, a Δ^5-steroid with little androgenic activity, is converted to Δ^4-androstenedione, a moderately active androgen, by 3β-HSD and an isomerase enzyme. When Δ^4-androstenedione is reduced, testosterone, the most potent secreted androgen, is formed.

Mechanism of Adrenal Steroid Regulation

The circulating level of plasma cortisol mediates the hypothalamic–pituitary–adrenal feedback system. The central nervous system (CNS) controls the secretion of ACTH, its diurnal variation, and its increase in stress via corticotropin-releasing factor

(CRF).[4] Any condition that decreases cortisol secretion will result in increased ACTH secretion. In those forms of CAH in which an enzyme deficiency causes impaired cortisol synthesis, there is excessive ACTH secretion and hyperplasia of the adrenal cortex (Fig. 15-2).

Aldosterone secretion is primarily regulated via the renin-angiotensin system, which is responsive to the state of electrolyte balance and plasma volume (Fig. 15-3). Aldosterone secretion is also stimulated directly by high serum K^+ concentration. The enzyme renin, which arises from the renal juxtaglomerular apparatus, reacts with an α_2-globulin produced in the liver to release angiotensin I. Angiotensin I is then enzymatically converted to angiotensin II, a potent stimulator of aldosterone secretion. This mechanism is generally accepted, but many aspects of aldosterone regulation remain unexplained.

It has been proposed by New and Seaman[5] that the zona glomerulosa and the zona fasciculata behave as two separate glands with respect to regulation and secretion. According to this concept, steroidogenesis in the fasciculata is regulated by ACTH, while that in the glomerulosa is regulated by the renin-angiotensin system such that (1) ACTH stimulates secretion of cortisol, corticosterone, and androgens by the zona fasciculata and zona reticularis, and (2) angiotensin stimulates aldosterone secretion by the zona glomerulosa, with ACTH presumably exerting only a secondary influence on the glomerular secretion of aldosterone (Fig. 15-4). Whereas the zona fasciculata lacks the enzyme necessary for the terminal step of aldosterone synthesis, the zona glomerulosa lacks the 17α-hydroxylase activity required for the production of 17-hydroxycorticoids and androgens.

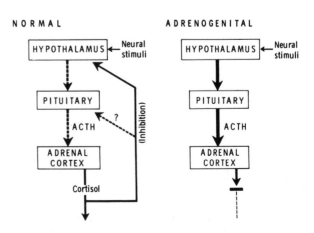

FIGURE 15-2. Regulation of cortisol secretion in normal subjects and in patients with congenital adrenal hyperplasia. (From New and Levine.[42])

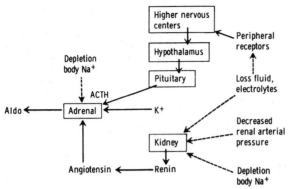

FIGURE 15-3. Regulation of aldosterone secretion. (From New and Peterson.[48])

FETAL SEXUAL DEVELOPMENT

In order to understand the pathophysiology of CAH, it is necessary to discuss normal sexual differentiation briefly. According to the hypothesis developed by Jost,[6] normal differentiation of male

genitalia is dependent on two functions of the fetal testes:

1. Secretion of the androgen testosterone, which stimulates the wolffian ducts to develop into the male internal genitalia (the epi-

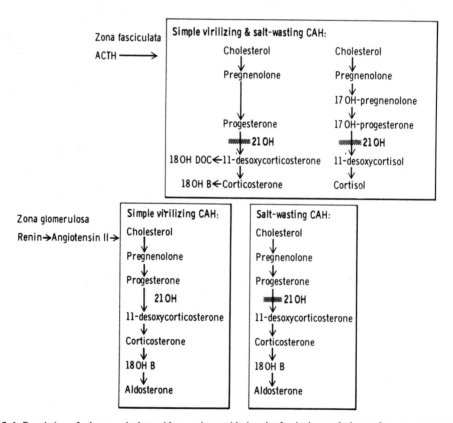

FIGURE 15-4. Regulation of adrenocortical steroidogenesis considering the fasciculata and glomerulosa as two separate glands. Dotted arrows indicate negative feedback. P, progesterone; DOC, deoxycorticosterone; B, corticosterone; 17-OHP, 17-hydroxyprogesterone; S, 11-deoxycortisol; F, cortisol; Δ4, Δ⁴-androstenedione; DHEA, dehydroepiandrosterone; T, testosterone; 18OHDOC, 18-hydroxydeoxycorticosterone; 18OHB, 18-hydroxycorticosterone; ALDO, aldosterone. (From New et al.[49])

didymis, vas deferens, seminal vesicles, and ejaculatory ducts): The secreted testosterone is also reduced in the target tissue to dihydrotestosterone, which acts on the undifferentiated tissues to cause differentiation to the male external genitalia, including midline fusion of the labioscrotal folds and swellings to form the shaft of the penis and the scrotal sacs, and elongation of the genital tubercle to form the glans penis. If male differentiation is complete, the urethra opens at the tip of the penis; if it is not, hypospadias results. In the male, the normal source of androgen is the fetal testis, but androgen from the adrenal or exogenous sources can cause masculinization of the external genitalia.

2. Secretion of a nonsteroidal substance[7] that inhibits mullerian duct development such that normal males are born without a uterus. Since the fetal ovary secretes neither testosterone nor the inhibiting factor necessary to inhibit mullerian structures, the normal female is born without male differentiation of external genitalia (i.e., with female external genitalia) and without mullerian repression (i.e., with a uterus and fallopian tubes). This process is shown schematically in Figure 15-5.

Thus, in the above scheme, the ovary does not play a determining role in sex differentiation. Female fetuses exposed to high levels of androgen consequent to CAH, an androgen-producing tumor in the mother, or administration of androgens to the mother manifest virilization of the external genitalia but normal internal female genitalia.[8]

21-HYDROXYLASE DEFICIENCY

Impairment of 21-hydroxylation is the most common enzymatic deficiency observed in CAH. Figure 15-1 shows that an enzymatic deficiency of 21-hydroxylase results in decreased cortisol synthesis. The decreased cortisol synthesis induces increased ACTH secretion, which has been demonstrated in the blood.[9] Increased ACTH secretion leads to overproduction of cortisol precursors and sex steroids (e.g., testosterone), which do not require 21-hydroxylase for their biosynthesis.

Early studies showed that in patients with 21-hydroxylase deficiency, there is excessive urinary excretion of pregnanetriol, the metabolite of 17-OHP. Urinary 17-ketosteroids, which result from the metabolism of DHEA, Δ^4-androstenedione and testosterone, are also present in increased amounts.

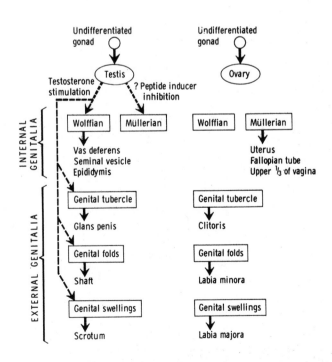

FIGURE 15-5. Fetal sex differentiation. (From New and Levine.[42])

More recently, newly developed simple and reliable radioimmunoassays for circulating serum levels of adrenal steroids have provided a more accurate laboratory method for the diagnosis of CAH than can be provided by urinary steroid measurement alone.

Simple Virilizing Congenital Adrenal Hyperplasia

The most prominent feature of this form of 21-hydroxylase deficiency is virilization. Since adre-

nocortical function begins in the third month of gestation, the fetus is exposed at the critical time of sexual differentiation to the overproduced fetal adrenal androgens resulting from 21-hydroxylase deficiency.

From the previous discussion of normal and abnormal sexual differentiation, it is apparent that excessive androgens will cause virilization of external genitalia. Thus, in the female fetus, the external genitalia are masculinized by excessive fetal adrenal androgens resulting in female pseudohermaphroditism (Fig. 15-6). In rare cases, the mas-

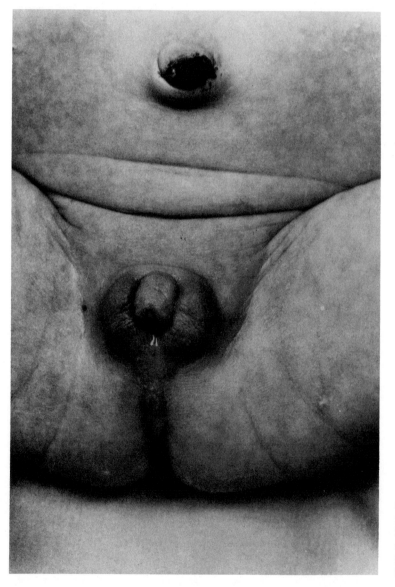

FIGURE 15-6. Ambiguous genitalia in a newborn female with CAH due to 21-hydroxylase deficiency. Note the enlarged clitoris, single orifice on the perineum, and scrotalization of the labia majora. (From New et al.[49])

culinization may be so profound that the urethra is penile.[10] Since the female fetus does not possess a testis, mullerian inhibiting factor is not produced, and the female with CAH is born with a uterus and fallopian tubes. The absence of the wolffian system, despite increased androgen levels, suggests that the level of androgen necessary for wolffian development is higher than that produced in CAH.

Because CAH due to 21-hydroxylase deficiency is the most common cause of ambiguous genitalia in the newborn, and because the female pseudohermaphrodite with this disorder has the capacity for an entirely normal female sex role, including fertility, it is very important to consider this disorder in any intersex problem presenting at birth.

Males with this disorder do not manifest genital abnormalities at birth. Without treatment, both males and females manifest progressive virilization, resulting in early fusion of the epiphyses and eventual short stature.

Salt-Wasting Congenital Adrenal Hyperplasia

A salt-wasting form of CAH is also associated with 21-hydroxylase deficiency. The feature of virilism is the same as in simple virilizing CAH, but in addition there is profound aldosterone deficiency, which may present with low serum sodium, high serum potassium, vomiting, diarrhea, and vascular collapse. The salt-wasting form of 21-hydroxylase CAH may present with life-threatening crisis within the first few weeks of life, and therefore must be recognized soon after birth in order for treatment to be administered prior to adrenal crisis.

Genetics of 21-Hydroxylase Deficiency

Population Studies

Several surveys have established that the 21-hydroxylase deficiency is transmitted as an autosomal recessive trait, with males and females equally at risk. With few exceptions,[11] either the simple virilizing or salt-wasting form is found consistently within one family.

In Europe and the United States, recent estimates of the incidence of CAH have been between $1:5000$ and $1:15,000$. In Alaska, the incidence in Yupik-speaking Eskimos is unusually high, while the low incidence reported in Maryland may have been due to inadequate case ascertainment. The gene frequency is estimated as approximately $1:100$.[12] The salt-wasting variety occurs in about 50–80% of patients with 21-hydroxylase deficiency.[13] In Alaska, the Yupik Eskimos exhibit a very high incidence of the salt-wasting variety.[14]

Screening for CAH and Future Population Studies

In 1977, neonatal screening for CAH became possible by the development of a microfilter paper method for measuring 17-OHP.[15] This method uses a heel stick blood specimen that is spotted onto filter paper and then analyzed for 17-OHP by radioimmunoassay (RIA). The hormone is stable on filter paper, and the filter paper specimens can be sent to an appropriate laboratory by surface mail. A screening program for hypothyroidism and phenylketonuria has been successful and is mandated in most states. On the basis of population surveys indicating that the incidence of 21-hydroxylase deficiency is approximately $1:15,000$ before screening (an incidence equal to that of phenylketonuria after screening), we and others have proposed that the newborn population be screened for 21-hydroxylase deficiency. Both classical and cryptic 21-hydroxylase deficiency have gone unrecognized in families in the general population.[16]

The reliability and feasibility of the 17-OHP microfilter paper screening method were recently proved by a pilot study screening of all infants born in Alaska in a 30-month period.[17] A total of 19,677 consecutive newborns were screened on their third day of life. Four of 1131 newborn Yupik Eskimos screened were found to be affected with CAH, and 1 of 13,733 newborn Caucasians screened were found to be affected. All five affected patients had the salt-wasting form of CAH. According to these data, a 95% confidence limit establishes a range for the incidence of salt-wasting CAH of between $1:110$ and $1:1038$ live births in Yupiks, and between $1:2465$ and $1:524,000$ live births in Caucasians. The incidence of salt-wasting CAH in Yupiks agrees with the incidence previously predicted by case survey (between $1:292$ and $1:896$) in this population.[14] In Caucasians, the highest incidence of salt-wasting CAH allowed at the 95% confidence level based on screening data ($1:2465$) is far greater than the highest possible incidence predicted by case surveys ($1:18,454$ for salt-wasting CAH and $1:14,798$ for salt-wasting and simple virilizing CAH combined). A larger screening sample size is needed, however, to permit more definite conclusions about the frequency of this disorder in Caucasians. The false-positive and recall rates for the

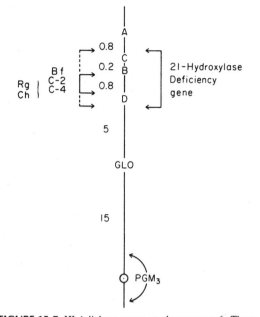

FIGURE 15-7. HLA linkage group on chromosome 6. The recombinant fractions for the known linkages between A : C, C : B, B : D, B : GLO, and GLO : PGM₃ are shown. The position of the genes for factor B (Bf), complement C-2, complement C-4, and Rodgers (Rg) and Chido (Ch) blood groups is also indicated. The 21-hydroxylase deficiency gene can be mapped between HLA-A and glyoxalase I (GLO). The most likely position of the 21-hydroxylase deficiency gene is very close to HLA-B. (From Levine et al.[20])

pilot screening program were 0.05% and 0.1%, respectively,[17] figures that compare favorably with the rates in currently enacted screening programs for other disorders.[18]

HLA Linkage

The genes for HLA (human leukocyte antigens), cell-surface antigens important in transplantation, are located on chromosome 6. The HLA complex consists of at least four genetic loci that code for the antigens HLA-A, HLA-B, HLA-C, and HLA-D/DR. Multiple alleles have been demonstrated for each locus. In addition to the HLA loci, several other loci have been mapped on chromosome 6 in close linkage with HLA (Fig. 15-7). Each individual inherits one chromosome 6 from his father and one from his mother. The HLA genes are codominantly expressed as follows:

$$\frac{A3;Bw47(w4);Cw6;DR7}{A28;Bw35(w6);Cw4;DR5}$$

in which one haplotype, the set of A3;Bw47(w4); Cw6;DR7, is inherited from one parent, while the other haplotype, A28;Bw35(w6);Cw4;DR5, is inherited from the other parent.

Close genetic linkage between HLA and CAH due to 21-hydroxylase deficiency was first described in 1977.[19] In this initial study, HLA genotyping of parents and children in six families with one or more child affected with CAH due to 21-hydroxylase deficiency was performed. In five of these families, all the affected offspring were HLA identical, and all were HLA different from their unaffected sibs. In the sixth family, the two affected sibs were HLA-B identical. Subsequently, studies of 34 unrelated families with a total of 48 patients were reported from New York and Zurich.[20] The findings of this study are illustrated in the two typical pedigrees shown in Figure 15-8. As can be observed in family 7, the three affected sibs are HLA identical. In family 16, the unaffected sibs are all HLA different from their affected sister. Each parent is an obligate heterozygote carrier and has transmitted one HLA haplotype carrying the gene for 21-hydroxylase deficiency to the patient. The brother and sister having only one haplotype linked to the gene for CAH are presumed heterozygotes. The sib sharing neither haplotype with the patient is presumed not to carry the gene for 21-hydroxylase deficiency. Thus, the HLA genotype is a marker for the CAH genotype.

Recent international studies reported at the Eighth International Histocompatibility Workshop have provided more detailed genetic mapping of the specific location of the 21-hydroxylase deficiency gene relative to the different loci that constitute the HLA complex. These studies have established that the 21-hydroxylase deficiency gene is located between the HLA-A locus and the centromere but is farther away from the centromere than the glyoxalase I (GLO) locus (21). The gene is thus mapped to within 3–4 centimorgans.

Statistical methods of genetic analysis have more formally demonstrated close genetic linkage between the 21-hydroxylase deficiency gene and HLA. The studies reported at the Eighth International Histocompatibility Workshop found a peak LOD score of 15.65 at a recombination frequency of $\theta = 0.00$ for linkage between HLA and 21-hydroxylase deficiency CAH.[21] The LOD score is a statistical index of the certainty with which one can arrive at a conclusion of genetic linkage. A score of 15.65 means that the odds are $10^{15.65}$ to 1 that linkage exists. In humans, genetic linkage is considered established if the LOD score exceeds 3.00.

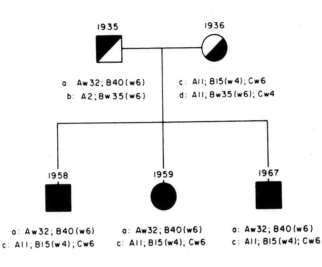

A.   FAMILY Zurich 7 (21-Hydroxylase Deficiency)

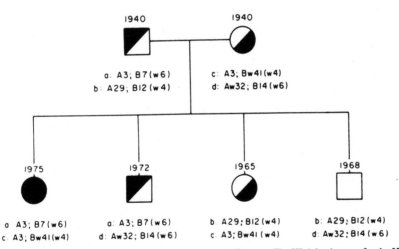

B.   FAMILY N.Y. 16 (21-Hydroxylase Deficiency)

FIGURE 15-8. Pedigrees for two families with classical 21-hydroxylase deficiency. The HLA haplotypes for the HLA-A, HLA-B, and HLA-C alleles are given in each family. The paternal haplotypes are labeled a and b and the maternal haplotypes c and d. The parents are obligate heterozygous carriers for the 21-hydroxylase deficiency gene (denoted by the half-black symbols). The affected children are denoted by black symbols. (A) Three affected siblings are HLA genotypically identical. (B) One affected child is HLA genotypically different from the three unaffected siblings. One sibling who carries the parental a and d haplotypes is presumed to be a heterozygous carrier for 21-hydroxylase deficiency because he shares the a haplotype with the patient. Another sibling has the parental b and c haplotypes and shares the c haplotype with the patient, and should be a carrier of the classical 21-hydroxylase deficiency gene. The child with the b and d haplotypes should be normal for the gene. (From Levine et al.[20])

Genetic Linkage Disequilibrium

In genetic studies, it is important to distinguish between genetic linkage, which we have described for the HLA loci and the 21-hydroxylase deficiency locus, and genetic linkage disequilibrium, which is the nonrandom association of particular alleles of different genetic loci. In patients with classical and nonclassical 21-hydroxylase deficiencies, certain HLA antigens appear with either a significantly increased or decreased frequency relative to their frequency in the general population. Thus, not only are 21-hydroxylase deficiency and HLA genetically linked, but there is genetic linkage disequilibrium between the 21-hydroxylase deficiency and specific HLA genes.

The most significant association for classical 21-hydroxylase deficiency has been found for HLA-Bw47, for which the combined relative risk is 15.4.[21] Slight increases have also been reported for Bw51, Bw53, Bw60, and DR7. A review of the Bw47 positive haplotypes in patients with 21-hydroxylase deficiency reveals that this antigen frequently occurs on one particular haplotype: A3; Cw6; Bw47; DR7. Although the gene frequency for Bw47 in different Caucasian populations is always very low (<0.005), international studies have found that Bw47 appears with remarkable frequency among 21-hydroxylase CAH patients; in one particular region of England, the Bw47 frequency among CAH patients is nearly 50%. Several studies have also demonstrated that the haplotype A1;B8; DR3 is consistently decreased among 21-hydroxylase-deficient patients.[20,25,38,39]

Genetic linkage disequilibrium has also been reported for the nonclassical forms of 21-hydroxylase deficiency.[29,32,33] Our latest studies document the significantly increased frequency of HLA-B14; DR1, and complement factor BfS in both late onset and cryptic 21-hydroxylase deficiency.[29,35] These alleles tend to appear together on the same haplotype in patients with late-onset or cryptic 21-hydroxylase deficiency, suggesting that the haplotype segment HLA-B14;DR1;BfS—rather than the individual alleles—is highly associated with both these nonclassical forms of 21-hydroxylase deficiency.

The finding that both the late-onset and cryptic 21-hydroxylase-deficiency genes are associated with the same haplotype segment (B14; DR1; BfS) suggests that these two variant genes are highly related. It is possible that individuals with highly similar or identical nonclassical 21-hydroxylase deficiency alleles may have different clinical manifestations of their 21-hydroxylase defect, expressing either the late-onset or the cryptic disorder. Similarly, the clinical difference between the late-onset and cryptic disorders no longer appears as distinct as initially appreciated.

We have found marked variability in the symptoms of the late-onset patients we have recently examined, ranging from precocious pubic hair growth without subsequent symptoms of virilization, to more severe degrees of hirsutism, acne, menstrual disturbances, and stunted growth. In one patient (Fig. 15-9), the symptoms of late-onset 21-hydroxylase deficiency, including pubic hair and advanced growth, were evident at 6 months of age. The symptoms subsequently disappeared, but the biochemical abnormality persisted. Thus the clinical classification for this patient changed from late-onset to cryptic 21-hydroxylase deficiency within a span of 10 years.

Heterozygote Detection

Attempts to detect heterozygosity for the 21-hydroxylase gene by hormonal tests before the discovery of HLA linkage were only partially successful. In studying the obligate heterozygote parents of children with CAH, a mild deficiency of 21-hydroxylase was demonstrated in several studies.[22,23] However, similar studies in the sibs of patients with CAH were difficult to interpret because of the inability to ascertain which sibs were carriers of the gene and which were unaffected. With the demonstration of linkage between the genes for HLA and 21-hydroxylase deficiency, HLA genotyping makes it possible to predict which sibs are carriers and which sibs are genetically unaffected. The method for utilizing HLA genotyping in this prediction is shown in Figure 15-8, family 16. The validity of the prediction of heterozygosity by HLA genotyping is supported by hormonal studies.

Thus in family studies, the response of 17-OHP to ACTH stimulation was higher in family members predicted by HLA genotyping to be heterozygotes than in family members predicted to be unaffected.[24] No other hormonal measurement was as useful in discriminating heterozygotes from normals.[16,24] Other investigators observed similar correlations between HLA genotyping and hormonal measurements.[25] Grosse-Wilde et al.[25] and Lejeune-Lenain[26] recently reported obtaining improved distinction of CAH heterozygotes from unaffected subjects in the adult population by admin-

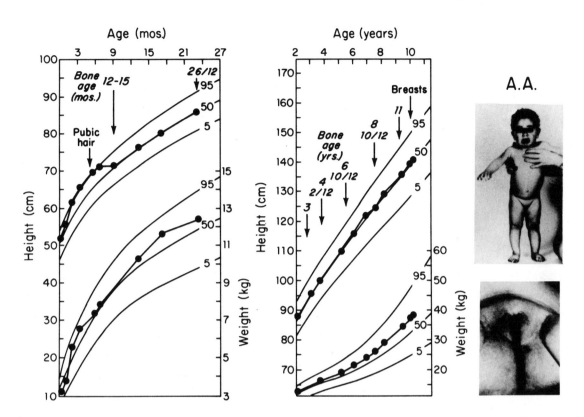

FIGURE 15-9. The changing clinical profile from late-onset to cryptic 21-hydroxylase deficiency. In this female, postnatal onset of virilization and growth acceleration was followed by a remission of symptoms during childhood despite persistence of hormonal abnormalities. (From New et al.[49])

istration of dexamethasone before ACTH stimulation.

Hormonal Standards for Genotyping 21-Hydroxylase Deficiency

We have developed nomograms relating the baseline and ACTH-stimulated levels of 17-OHP, Δ^4-androstenedione (Δ^4), DHEA, the ratio DHEA/Δ^4, and testosterone (T).[40] The 17-OHP and Δ^4 nomograms provide hormonal standards for assignment of the 21-hydroxylase deficiency genotype; i.e., patients whose hormonal values fall on the regression line within a defined group are assigned to that group. Figures 15-10 and 15-11 present the hormonal reference data for the 60-min ACTH test. Figures 15-12 and 15-13 present data for the 360-min test. There is a strong correlation for the prediction of CAH genotype between the 60-min and 360-min ACTH stimulation tests, so that the shorter and less cumbersome 60-min test may be

used with the same confidence as the longer test. Clinical symptoms and signs must distinguish between the symptomatic and asymptomatic non-classical forms of 21-hydroxylase deficiency, which are indistinguishable biochemically. The nomograms document that both of these patient groups show the biochemical defect to the same degree, providing further evidence that both the symptomatic and asymptomatic nonclassical forms of 21-hydroxylase deficiency result from the same genetic mutation. Heterozygotes for classical and nonclassical 21-hydroxylase deficiencies all demonstrate a similar hormonal response and are thus phenotypically indistinguishable from one another.

The distribution of responses along a regression line suggests that there is a spectrum of enzymatic deficiency in these groups. Patients with classical CAH have the most severe deficiency, patients with nonclassical forms have a less severe deficiency, while heterozygotes for both forms have an even milder deficiency that is unmasked only upon

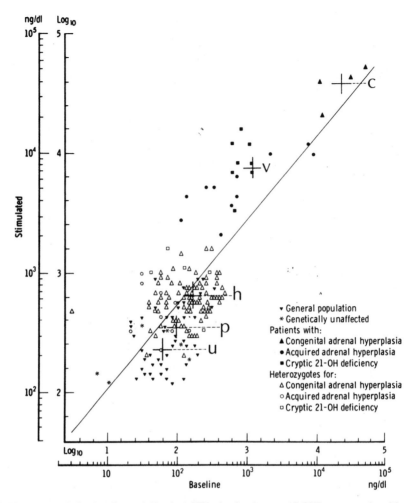

FIGURE 15-10. Nomogram relating baseline and 60-min ACTH stimulated serum 17-OHP concentration. Mean values for each group are indicated as follows: c, congenital adrenal hyperplasia; v, patients with nonclassical symptomatic or asymptomatic (cryptic, acquired or late onset) 21-hydroxylase deficiency; h, heterozygotes for classical congenital adrenal hyperplasia, nonclassical symptomatic congenital adrenal hyperplasia, (acquired or late-onset adrenal hyperplasia), nonclassical asymptomatic congenital adrenal hyperplasia (cryptic 21-hydroxylase deficiency); u, family members predicted by HLA genotyping to be unaffected; and p, general population (not HLA genotyped).

ACTH stimulation. Hormonal values in family members predicted by HLA genotyping to be unaffected for 21-hydroxylase deficiency fall at the lowest point of the regression line and serve as the best control population for normal 21-hydroxylase activity. Those members of the general population whose responses are in the heterozygote range may actually be carriers of a gene for 21-hydroxylase deficiency. The incidence of classical 21-hydroxylase deficiency in a homogeneous Caucasian population has been estimated by screening to be between 1 : 5000 and 1 : 10,000. The corresponding carrier frequency is calculated to be 1 : 35. However, this estimate of heterozygote frequency is only for classical 21-hydroxylase deficiency. The gene frequency for nonclassical 21-hydroxylase deficiency remains to be determined, but our experience suggests that the nonclassical defect may be more frequent than the classical defect.

Nonclassical Variants of 21-Hydroxylase Deficiency

Nonclassical symptomatic (late-onset) CAH is a syndrome characterized by virilization, menstrual disturbances, and endocrinologic features con-

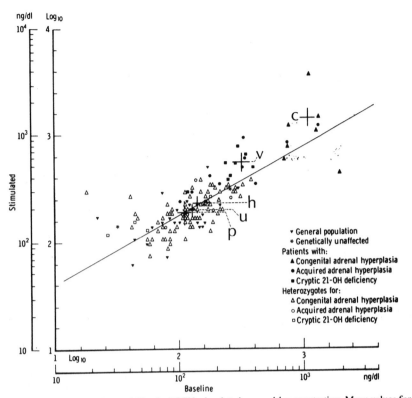

FIGURE 15-11. Nomogram relating baseline and 60-min ACTH stimulated serum Δ⁴ concentration. Mean values for each group are indicated as for Figure 15-10.

sistent with 21-hydroxylase deficiency that presents in later childhood or adolescence.[27-29] Unlike females with classical 21-hydroxylase deficiency, females with late-onset 21-hydroxylase deficiency demonstrate no evidence of in utero virilization, and are born with normal vaginal and urethral orifices and no labial fusion. Both types of patients respond similarly to glucocorticoid treatment. The late presentation of a biochemical defect has raised the question as to whether this is the same inherited disorder as CAH with delayed presentation or is an acquired disorder distinct from CAH. Although initial studies suggested that the late-onset disorder was not HLA linked,[30,31] more recent reports have provided evidence that this disorder is in fact also genetically linked to HLA,[32-35] and it has been proposed that classical and late-onset 21-hydroxylase deficiencies are allelic variants.[29,34-36] This disorder is discussed more fully in Chapter 19 of this volume.

Our HLA studies of families with classical 21-hydroxylase deficiency have also led us to uncover a new, cryptic form of 21-hydroxylase deficiency. During the course of HLA genotyping and hormon-

al testing, we encountered family members whose biochemical profiles were characteristic of a mild 21-hydroxylase deficiency, although the clinical hallmarks commonly accompanying the disorder (e.g., virilization, abnormal puberty and growth, infertility) were absent. The presence of hormonal abnormalities without clinical stigmata led us to designate this disorder as cryptic 21-hydroxylase deficiency. The hormonal abnormalities that these nonclassical, asymptomatic patients demonstrated were similar to those observed in those with the nonclassical, symptomatic form of 21-hydroxylase deficiency.[37] LOD score analysis established close genetic linkage between HLA and the gene for the mild 21-hydroxylase deficiency.[37]

An interesting biologic paradox is the absence of clinical signs in patients with cryptic 21-hydroxylase deficiency, in contrast to the severe virilization noted in patients with late-onset 21-hydroxylase deficiency, despite the fact that both patient groups demonstrate similar biochemical abnormalities. In the group with late-onset 21-hydroxylase deficiency, the excessive androgen levels produce virilization, while in the other group no such

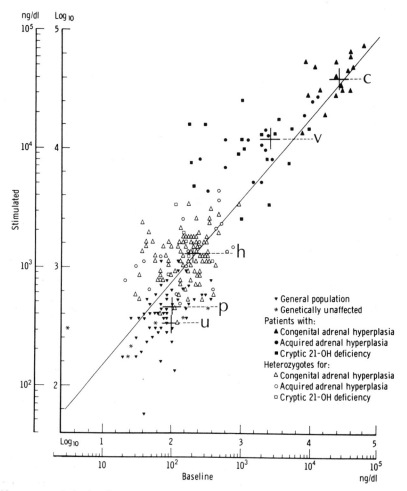

FIGURE 15-12. Nomograms relating baseline and 360-min ACTH-stimulated serum 17-OHP concentration. Mean values for each group are indicated as for Figure 15-10.

hormonal effect is observed—hence the term "cryptic" 21-hydroxylase deficiency. Patients with the late-onset disorder are detected because of their clinical symptoms, whereas cryptic 21-hydroxylase deficiency has been detected only as a result of genetic and hormonal studies of classical CAH families.

Clinical Spectrum of 21-Hydroxylase Deficiency: Phenotypic Variability

It appears that 21-hydroxylase deficiency has a spectrum of clinical manifestations, as well as a spectrum of enzymatic deficiency, as reflected in the hormonal findings presented in Figures 15-10 through 15-13. If 21-hydroxylase deficiency is sim-

ilar to other autosomal recessive enzyme defects, we would predict that further studies will reveal patients whose clinical and biochemical abnormalities will be intermediate to those currently described. It may also be possible that the assignments made by clinical criteria may change in the course of a lifetime.

Prenatal Diagnosis of Congenital Adrenal Hyperplasia: 21-Hydroxylase Deficiency

Since the report by Jeffcoate et al.[41] of the prenatal diagnosis of CAH by elevated concentrations of 17-ketosteroids and pregnanetriol in the amniotic fluid of the affected fetus, several investigators have attempted the prenatal diagnosis by measure-

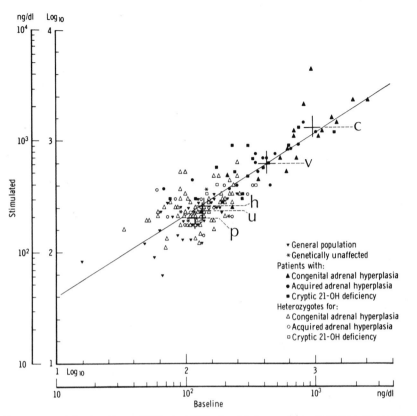

FIGURE 15-13. Nomograms relating baseline and 360-min ACTH-stimulated serum Δ^4 concentration. Mean values for each group are indicated as for Figure 15-10.

ment of various hormones.[42] Most recently, elevated levels of 17-OHP and Δ^4 in the amniotic fluid of fetuses affected with CAH due to 21-hydroxylase deficiency have been reported.[43] HLA genotyping of amniotic cells has provided an additional method for prenatal diagnosis of 21-hydroxylase deficiency in an at-risk pregnancy and has made possible the prediction of a heterozygous fetus.[39] When HLA genotyping of amniotic cells demonstrates that the fetus is HLA identical to the affected sib, the fetus is predicted to be affected. The HLA prediction of CAH genotype should always be corroborated by hormonal measurement of 17-OHP and Δ^4 in amniotic fluid. Caution must be exercised in interpreting results if multiple births are expected or if there is antigen sharing in the parents.

Treatment of Congenital Adrenal Hyperplasia

The virilization caused by CAH can be remedied by surgical correction of the ambiguous genitalia, but the decision to do so must take into account an assessment of the patient's potential for future sexual function and fertility. In cases of female pseudohermaphroditism due to 21-hydroxylase deficiency, the aim of surgical repair should be to remove the redundant erectile tissue, preserve the sexually sensitive glans clitoris, and provide a normal vaginal orifice that will function adequately for menstruation and intromission.[44] When there is early therapeutic intervention in these patients, because of the normal internal genitalia, normal puberty, fertility, and childbearing are possible. Full correction of vaginal defects must in many cases be deferred until after puberty.

The aim of endocrine therapy in CAH is to provide replacement of the deficient hormones. Glucocorticoid therapy has been the keystone of treatment for this disorder. Glucocorticoid administration both replaces the deficient cortisol and suppresses ACTH overproduction.

Plasma renin activity (PRA) has long been recog-

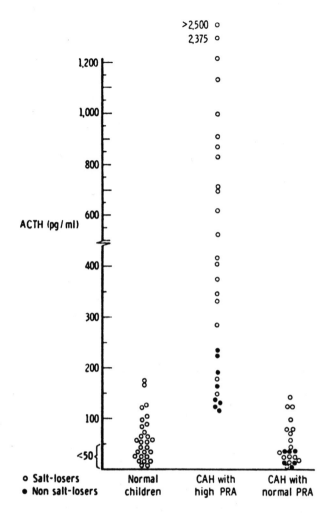

FIGURE 15-14. Correlation between ACTH and plasma renin activity (PRA) levels in patients with CAH treated with constant replacement doses of glucocorticoids equivalent to 25 mg/m^2 per day of hydrocortisone. Patients were studied during different states of sodium balance. (From Rosler et al.[46])

nized to be elevated in the simple virilizing form as well as in the salt-wasting form,[36,45] although aldosterone levels have not been reported as being deficient in the simple virilizing form of 21-hydroxylase deficiency.[36] Despite the observation of elevated PRA, it has not been customary to supplement conventional glucocorticoid replacement therapy with the administration of salt-retaining steroids in cases of simple virilizing 21-hydroxylase deficiency. In a recent clinical study, however, Rosler et al.[46] demonstrated that the addition of salt-retaining hormone to glucocorticoid therapy in simple virilizing patients with elevated PRA does in fact improve the hormonal control of the disease.

Rosler showed that in patients with CAH due to 21-hydroxylase deficiency, the PRA was closely correlated to the ACTH level (Fig. 15-14). Thus,

when PRA was normalized by the added administration of 9α-fluorocortisone acetate, a steroid with salt-retaining activity, the ACTH level fell, and excessive androgen stimulation by ACTH decreased (Fig. 15-14). The addition of salt-retaining steroids to the therapeutic regimen often made possible a decrease in the glucocorticoid dose. Normalization of PRA also resulted in improved statural growth[36] (Fig. 15-15).

In the past, urinary 17-ketosteroids and pregnanetriol excretion were the biochemical monitors of hormonal control. Since the advent of radioimmunoassay, it has been possible to establish normal serum androgen concentrations for children of various ages.[47] Recent studies have indicated that serum 17-OHP and Δ^4-androstenedione (Δ^4) levels provide a sensitive index of biochemical control.

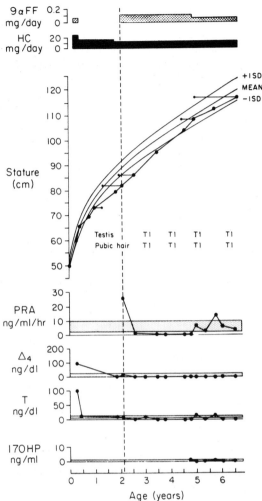

♂ J.W 8/3/73

FIGURE 15-15. Growth curve of a patient with salt-wasting CAH before and after therapeutic control of plasma renin activity. Note that with renin suppression, hydrocortisone dose could be lowered; also, growth improved and androgen suppression was maintained despite the decrease in hydrocortisone dose. (From New et al.[36])

The serum testosterone is useful in females and prepubertal males, but not in newborn and pubertal males.

The combined laboratory determinations of PRA, 17-OHP, and serum androgens, and the clinical assessment of growth and pubertal status must all be considered in adjusting the dose of glucocorticoid and salt-retaining steroid. In our clinic, we employ hydrocortisone and 9α-fluorocortisone acetate as treatment modalities.

SEX ASSIGNMENT IN CONGENITAL ADRENAL HYPERPLASIA

Ambiguous sex in the newborn infant constitutes a medical emergency. The decision as to sex assignment at birth has obvious long-term implications. A rational approach permits a careful assessment of the problem and choice of sex assignment.

Early sexual identification can be divided into several aspects, which appear in chronologic order, as shown in Figure 15-16. Note that the nursery room sex, which is the key to the child's later gender role, depends on the external genitalia, generally evaluated by an obstetrician's examination in the delivery room. When all aspects of sexual identification are the same (isosexual), the nursery room sex assignment is correct. However, in situations in which all aspects of sexual identification are not alike, the external body sex may be misleading.

A male sex assignment to a female pseudohermaphrodite with CAH due to 21-hydroxylase deficiency is particularly tragic, since with proper treatment, the infant could become a reproductive female, capable of normal sexual function and childbearing. The error can be avoided by a systematic approach to the problems of ambiguous genitalia in the newborn. With the ascertainment of female genetic sex by means of buccal smear or

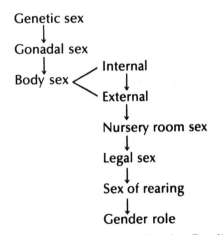

FIGURE 15-16. Development of sexual identity. (From New and Levine.[42])

karyotype, the diagnosis of female pseudohermaphroditism is established and the previously discussed laboratory tests define the etiology and treatment.

In rare cases, female infants have been so virilized as to have a penile urethra. In these infants, surgical correction of the external genitalia to conform to the female sex presents a much greater challenge to the skill and experience of the surgeon. Before undertaking corrective surgery, several questions must be raised and answered. First, what is the radiographic and endoscopic appearance of the proximal urethra and its spatial relationship to the vaginal "diverticulum"? In order to have a functioning and competent postoperative female urethra, the distance between internal bladder neck and point of juncture of urethra and vaginal diverticulum (the future vaginal introitus) must be at least 2.0 cm in the newborn. Second, how well developed is the vaginal "diverticulum"? A shallow vaginal pocket will demand extensive augmentation vaginoplasty in the future, thereby presenting a potential hazard to continence should the urethra and bladder base have to be undermined extensively during such a surgical procedure. Should there be serious doubt as to the eventual outcome of corrective surgery as far as urinary continence is concerned, on the basis of the above considerations and the ready availability of surgical expertise, due consideration should be given to a male sex assignment in such a newborn with a prominent phallus and a completely formed male-type urethra. Of course, fertility would be sacrificed in the female given the male sex assignment, as a complete hysterectomy and oophorectomy would have to be done to complete such a sex reversal.

Treatment with hydrocortisone is necessary in both sex assignments for growth and prevention of early epiphyseal fusion, whereas treatment with testosterone is necessary after puberty to induce male secondary sex characteristics in the castrated genetic female raised as a male. In the case of female sex assignment, the surgery for phallic correction must be carried out in early infancy, whereas in the case of male sex assignment, hysterectomy and oophorectomy, relatively simple procedures, can be delayed until prepuberty. The hysterectomy and oopherectomy are necessary in genetic females raised as males in order to avoid menstrual flow at puberty. This often presents as cyclic hematuria. The function of the urethra is not compromised in the male assignment, while it may be in the female. The certain loss of fertility in the case of male sex

assignment and the ease of surgical correction must be balanced against possible urologic complications in the potentially difficult surgical correction when the female sex is assigned to the baby. A rational and judicious choice of sex assignment is a critical aspect of treatment, since the sex assignment has life-long implications.

SUMMARY

Congenital adrenal hyperplasia (CAH) due to 21-hydroxylase deficiency is a disorder of adrenal steroidogenesis. Oversecretion of ACTH secondary to impairment of cortisol synthesis leads to two abnormalities: (1) excessive synthesis of the steroid precursors proximal to the enzyme defect, and (2) accumulation of the products of those adrenal hormones, the synthesis of which is unimpaired by the enzyme deficiency.

Female pseudohermaphroditism presenting at birth is the most prominent clinical feature of CAH due to 21-hydroxylase deficiency, as a result of excessive prenatal secretion of adrenal androgens. Salt wasting may be associated with 21-hydroxylase deficiency and may present as a life-threatening adrenal crisis in the neonatal period.

The adrenal zona fasciculata and zona glomerulosa appear to function as two separate glands; the fasciculata is primarily regulated by ACTH and the glomerulosa by the renin-angiotensin system. A new hypothesis to explain the presence or absence of salt-wasting signs in 21-hydroxylase deficiency is as follows: (1) in both simple virilizers and salt-wasters there is a fasciculata defect of 21-hydroxylation in both the 17-hydroxy and 17-deoxy pathways, and (2) in salt-waters there is also a 21-hydroxylase defect in the glomerulosa, while in simple virilizers the glomerulosa is spared this defect. The ability of simple virilizers, but not salt-wasters, to respond to renin-angiotensin stimulation with an increase in aldosterone secretion supports this hypothesis.

The 21-hydroxylase deficiency is inherited as an autosomal recessive trait. Close genetic linkage between the HLA complex and the 21-hydroxylase deficiency gene has been demonstrated, and the 21-hydroxylase deficiency gene has been mapped in close proximity to the HLA-B genetic locus on chromosome 6.

Two nonclassical, HLA-linked forms of 21-hydroxylase deficiency are described: a symptomatic late-onset form and an asymptomatic cryptic form.

The degree of enzymatic deficiency ranges from severe in the classical form to milder in the late-onset and cryptic disorders, to a still milder deficiency, detectable only with ACTH stimulation, in heterozygotes for all three forms. It is proposed that there are allelic variants at the 21-hydroxylase genetic locus that produce different degrees of 21-hydroxylase deficiency, resulting in the phenotypic diversity of classical, late-onset, and cryptic 21-hydroxylase deficiencies.

HLA genotyping, in addition to hormonal testing, is useful for the detection of heterozygote carriers for 21-hydroxylase deficiency and for prenatal diagnosis in families with an affected index case.

A microfilter paper method for measuring 17-hydroxyprogesterone (17-OHP) for the neonatal diagnosis of 21-hydroxylase deficiency is described. The results of a pilot newborn screening program for CAH using the 17-OHP microfilter paper method has demonstrated that screening for this disorder is feasible. Furthermore, 21-hydroxylase deficiency occurs with sufficient frequency to warrant screening. Measurement of 17-OHP and Δ^4-androstenedione levels in amniotic fluid makes the prenatal diagnosis of 21-hydroxylase deficiency possible.

The fundamental aim of therapy in CAH is to provide replacement of the deficient hormones. Glucocorticoid administration both replaces the deficient cortisol and suppresses ACTH overproduction, resulting in a decrease in excess adrenal androgens, which leads to virilization and ultimately short stature. Mineralocorticoid supplements are required in the salt-wasting disorders. Mineralocorticoid administration is also recommended for patients with elevated plasma renin activity but no evident symptoms of salt-wasting, in order to improve the control of androgen oversecretion. Recognition of this disorder is important in the sex assignment of newborns with ambiguous genitalia. Surgical correction of the genitalia may be necessary to remove redundant tissue and permit normal female sexual function. Early therapeutic intervention in these patients makes normal puberty, fertility and childbearing possible.

The early detection of 21-hydroxylase deficiency of the adrenal gland, whether congenital or acquired, overt or cryptic, is essential to permit proper sex assignment in newborns, life sustenance, and avoidance of further virilization. Newer techniques of detection in utero by individual and familial genetic analysis of steroid hormone metabolites, renin levels and transplantation antigens have added to

our understanding of the variety of defects present, as well as the forms of medical and surgical treatment best suited to the patient.

ACKNOWLEDGMENTS. Much of the work described in this review was done with the support of NIH grants HD-00072 and HD-15084, and of a grant (RR 47) from the General Clinical Research Centers Program of the Division of Research Resources, National Institutes of Health. I wish to express my sincere gratitude to Ms. Robin Grimm for her editorial assistance in the preparation of this chapter.

QUESTIONS

1. Which of the following are correct?

    I. ACTH stimulates glucocorticoid synthesis.
    II. Renin stimulates mineralocorticoid synthesis.
    III. Angiotensin stimulates sex steroid and mineralocorticoid synthesis.

    a. I
    b. II
    c. I and II
    d. I and III

2. The nature of female pseudohermaphroditism in 21-hydroxylase deficiency is such that

    a. internal genitalia are normal.
    b. external genitalia are masculinized.
    c. there are no wolffian duct derivatives present.
    d. all of the above

3. The most accurate diagnostic test for 21-hydroxylase deficiency CAH is

    a. urinary 17-hydroxycorticoid levels.
    b. serum 17-OHP levels.
    c. urinary 17-ketosteroid levels.
    d. serum aldosterone levels.

4. If untreated, patients with 21-hydroxylase deficiency may manifest

    a. menstrual irregularities.
    b. acne and hirsutism.
    c. early fusion of the epiphyses.
    d. all of the above.

5. Genetic studies of families of patients with 21-hydroxylase deficiency have shown

    a. no genetic linkage between the 21-hydroxylase deficiency gene and HLA complex.

    b. genetic linkage between the 21-hydroxylase deficiency gene and HLA complex.

    c. genetic linkage disequilibrium but no genetic linkage between the 21-hydroxylase deficiency gene and the HLA complex.

    d. both genetic linkage and genetic linkage disequilibrium between the 21-hydroxylase deficiency gene and the HLA complex.

6. Which of the following is useful for identification of heterozygotes for 21-hydroxylase deficiency in a family at risk:

    I. Measurement of 24-hr urinary hormone levels
    II. ACTH stimulation tests
    III. HLA genotyping
    IV. Examination of internal and external genitalia

      a. I
      b. II and III
      c. I and III
      d. I and IV

7. A young women first presents with hirsutism, acne, and menstrual irregularities in the pubertal period. She may be affected with

    a. symptomatic, late-onset, nonclassical 21-hydroxylase deficiency.
    b. asymptomatic, cryptic, nonclassical 21-hydroxylase deficiency.
    c. cryptic, classical 21-hydroxylase deficiency.
    d. classical 21-hydroxylase deficiency.

8. A screening program for 21-hydroxylase deficiency

    a. can be performed using a heel-stick specimen blotted onto a microfilter paper disk.
    b. has shown a higher incidence than predicted by case survey.
    c. can identify affected infants before salt-wasting adrenal crisis.
    d. all of the above.

9. Prenatal diagnosis of 21-hydroxylase deficiency may be carried out by:

    I. HLA genotyping of the fetus and family members
    II. Hormonal measurements of the fetus
    III. Plasma renin activity measurements of the mother

      a. I
      b. II
      c. I and II
      d. I and III

10. The treatment for female pseudohermaphroditism due to 21-hydroxylase deficiency usually includes

    a. glucocorticoid therapy.
    b. mineralocorticoid therapy.
    c. surgical correction of the genitalia.
    d. all of the above.

REFERENCES

1. Decrecchio L: Sopra un caso di apparenze virile in una donna. *Morgagni* 7:1951, 1865
2. Bongiovanni, AM, Eberlein WR, Goldman AS, et al: Disorders of adrenal steroid biogenesis. *Recent Prog Horm Res* 23:375–439, 1967
3. Finkelstein, M, Shaefer JM: Inborn errors of steroid biosynthesis. *Physiol Rev* 59:353–406, 1979
4. Ganong WF: Neurotransmitters and pituitary function: Regulation of ACTH secretion. *Fed Proc* 39:2923–2930, 1980
5. New MI, Seaman MP: Secretion rates of cortisol and aldosterone precursors in various forms of congenital adrenal hyperplasia. *J Clin Endocrinol Metab* 30:361–371, 1970
6. Jost A: Embryonic sexual differentiation, in Jones HW, Scott WW (eds): *Hermaphroditism, Genital Anomalies and Related Endocrine Disorders*, 2nd ed. Baltimore, Williams & Wilkins, 1971, pp 16–64
7. Josso N, Picard JY, Tran D: The antiMullerian hormone. *Recent Prog Horm Res* 33:117–168, 1977
8. Federman DD: *Abnormal Sexual Development*. Philadelphia, Saunders, 1968, pp 121–133
9. Binoux M, Pham-Huu-Trung MT, Gourmelen M, et al: Plasma ACTH in adrenogenital syndrome. *Acta Paediatr (Stockh)* 61:269–270, 1972
10. Wilkins L: Adrenal disorders. II. Congenital virilizing adrenal hyperplasia. *Arch Dis Child* 37:231–241, 1962
11. Rosenbloom AL, Smith DW: Varying expression for salt losing in related patients with congenital adrenal hyperplasia. *Pediatrics* 38:215–219, 1966
12. Muller W, Prader A, Kofler J, et al: Frequency of congenital adrenal hyperplasia. *Padiatr Padol* 14:151–155, 1979
13. Cohen JM: Salt-losing congenital adrenal hyperplasia. *Pediatrics* 44:621–622, 1969
14. Hirschfeld AJ, Fleshman JK: An unusually high incidence of salt-losing congenital adrenal hyperplasia in the Alaskan Eskimo. *J Pediatr* 75:492–494, 1969
15. Pang S, Hotchkiss J, Drash AL, et al: Microfilter paper method for 17α-progesterone radioimmunoassay: Its application for rapid screening for congenital adrenal hyperplasia. *J Clin Endocrinol Metab* 45:1003–1008, 1977
16. Lorenzen F, Pang S, New MI, et al: Hormonal phenotype and HLA-genotype in families of patients with congenital adrenal hyperplasia (21-hydroxylase deficiency). *Pediatr Res* 13:1356–1370, 1979
17. Pang S, Murphey W, Levine LS, et al: A pilot newborn screening for congenital adrenal hyperplasia in Alaska. *J Clin Endocrinol Metab* 55:413–420, 1982
18. LaFranchi SH, Murphey WH, Foley TP Jr, et al: Neonatal hypothyroidism detected by the northwest regional screening program. *Pediatrics* 63:180–191, 1979
19. Dupont, B, Oberfield, SE, Smithwick EM, et al: Close genetic linkage between HLA and congenital adrenal hyperplasia (21-hydroxylase deficiency). *Lancet* 2:1309–1311, 1977

20. Levine LS, Zachmann M, New MI, et al: Genetic mapping of the 21-hydroxylase deficiency gene within the HLA linkage group. *N Engl J Med* 299:911–915, 1978

21. Dupont B, Pollack MS, Levine LS, et al: Congenital adrenal hyperplasia, in Teraski PI (ed): *Histocompatibility Testing.* Los Angeles, UCLA Tissue Typing Laboratory, 1980, pp 693–706

22. Gutai JP, Kowarski AA, Migeon CJ: The detection of the heterozygous carrier for congenital adrenal hyperplasia. *J Pediatr* 90:924–929, 1970

23. Knorr D, Bidlingmaier F, Butenandt O, et al: Test for heterozygosity of congenital adrenal hyperplasia, in Lee PA, Plotnick LP, Kowarski AA, Migeon CJ (eds): *Congenital Adrenal Hyperplasia.* Baltimore, University Park Press, 1977, pp 495–500

24. Lorenzen F, Pang S, New MI, et al: Studies of the C-21 and C-19 steroids and HLA genotyping in siblings and parents of patients with congenital adrenal hyperplasia due to 21-hydroxylase deficiency. *J Clin Endocrinol Metab* 50:572–579, 1980

25. Grosse-Wilde HJ, Weil J, Albert E, et al: Genetic linkage studies between congenital adrenal hyperplasia and the HLA blood group system. *Immunogenetics* 8:41–49, 1979

26. Lejeune-Lenain C, Cantraine F, Dufrasnes, M, et al: An improved method for the detection of heterozygosity of congenital virilizing adrenal hyperplasia. *Clin Endocrinol (Oxf)* 12:525–535, 1980

27. Newmark S, Dluhy RG, Williams GH, et al: Partial 11- and 21-hydroxylase deficiencies in hirsute women. *Am J Obstet Gynecol* 127:594–598, 1977

28. Rosenwaks Z, Lee PA, Jones GS, et al: An attenuated form of congenital virilizing adrenal hyperplasia. *J Clin Endocrinol Metab* 49:335–339, 1979

29. Kohn B, Levine LS, Pollack MS, et al: Late-onset steroid 21-hydroxylase deficiency: A variant of classical congenital adrenal hyperplasia. *J Clin Endocrinol Metab* 55:817–827, 1982

30. New MI, Lorenzen F, Pang S, et al: "Acquired" adrenal hyperplasia with 21-hydroxylase deficiency is not the same genetic disorder as congenital adrenal hyperplasia, *J Clin Endocrinol Metab* 48:356–359, 1979

31. Morillo E, Gardner, LI: Genetics of acquired and congenital adrenal hyperplasia. *Lancet* 2:202–203, 1979

32. Laron Z, Pollack MS, Zamir R, et al: Late onset 21-hydroxylase deficiency and HLA in the Ashkenzai population: A new allele at the 21-hydroxylase locus. *Human Immunol* 1:55–66, 1980

33. Blankstein J, Faiman C, Reyes FI, et al: Adult-onset familiar adrenal 21-hydroxylase deficiency. *Am J Med* 68:441–448, 1980

34. Migeon CJ, Rosenwaks, Z, Lee PA, et al: The attenuated form of congenital adrenal hyperplasia as an allelic form of 21-hydroxylase deficiency. *J Clin Endocrinol Metab* 51:647–649, 1980

35. Pollack MS, Levine, LS, O'Neill GJ, et al: HLA linkage and B14, DR1, Bfs haplotype association with the genes for late onset and cryptic 21-hydroxylase deficiency, *Am J Hum Genet* 33:540–550, 1981

36. New MI, Dupont B, Pang S, et al: An update of congenital adrenal hyperplasia. *Recent Prog Horm Res* 37:105–181, 1981

37. Levine LS, Dupont B, Lorenzen F, et al: Cryptic 21-hydroxylase deficiency in families of patients with classical congenital adrenal hyperplasia. *J Clin Endocrinol Metab* 51:1316–1324, 1980

38. Klouda PT, Harris R, Price DA: HLA and congenital adrenal hyperplasia. *Lancet* 2:1046, 1978

39. Pollack MS, Levine LS, Pang S, et al: Diagnosis of congenital adrenal hyperplasia (21-hydroxylase deficiency) by HLA typing. *Lancet* 1:1107–1108, 1979

40. Levine, LS, Dupont, B, Lorenzen F, et al: Genetic and hormonal characterization of cryptic 21-hydroxylase deficiency. *J Clin Endocrinol Metab* 53:1193–1198, 1981

41. Jeffcoate TNA, Fliegner JRH, Russell SH, et al: Diagnosis of the adrenogenital syndrome before birth. *Lancet* 2:553–555, 1965

42. New MI, Levine LS: Congenital adrenal hyperplasia, in Harris H, Hirschhorn K (eds): *Advances in Human Genetics.* New York, Plenum, 1973, pp 251–326

43. Pang S, Levine LS, Cederqvist LL, et al: Amniotic fluid concentrations of Δ^5 and Δ^4 steroids in fetuses with congenital adrenal hyperplasia due to 21-hydroxylase deficiency and in anencephalic fetuses. *J Clin Endocrinol Metab* 51:223–229, 1980

44. Mininberg DT, Levine LS, New MI: Current concepts in congenital adrenal hyperplasia. *Invest Urol* 17:169–175, 1979

45. Bartter FC, Albright F, Forbes AP, et al: The effects of adrenocorticotropic hormone and cortisone in the adrenogenital syndrome associated with congenital adrenal hyperplasia: An attempt to explain and correct its disordered hormonal pattern. *J Clin Invest* 30:237–251, 1951

46. Rosler A, Levine LS, Schneider B, et al: The interrelationship of sodium balance, plasma renin activity and ACTH in congenital adrenal hyperplasia. *J Clin Endocrinol Metab* 45:500–512, 1977

47. Korth-Schutz S, Levine LS, New MI: Serum androgens in normal prepubertal and pubertal children and in children with precocious adrenarche. *J Clin Endocrinol Metab* 42:117–124, 1976

48. New MI, Peterson RE: Disorders of aldosterone secretion in childhood. *Pediatr Clin North Am* 13:43–58, 1966

49. New MI, Dupont B, Grumbach K, et al: Congenital adrenal hyperplasia and related conditions, in Stanbury JB, Wyngaarden JB, Frederickson DS, Goldstein JL, Brown MS (eds): *The Metabolic Basis of Inherited Disease,* 5th ed. New York, McGraw-Hill, 1982, pp 973–1000

ANSWERS

1. c

2. d

3. b

4. d

5. d

6. b

7. a

8. d

9. c

10. d

16

Hypothalamic–Pituitary Disease

FRANCISCO I. REYES

INTRODUCTION

The pituitary gland arises from the conjunction of an evagination of the oral cavity (Rathke's pouch) and a process of neural ectoderm growing down from the ventral portion (hypothalamic region) of the diencephalon. The former becomes the adenohypophysis (anterior pituitary) and the latter the neurohypophysis (posterior pituitary); by 10–12 weeks of fetal life, both appear to be functionally linked to the hypothalamus.[1]

The main body of the pituitary gland (intrasellar portion), which includes the anterior lobe (pars distalis) with the vestigial intermediate zone (pars intermedia), and the posterior lobe (pars nervosa or infundibular process), is linked to the tuber cinereum of the hypothalamus by the pituitary stalk or infundibular stem (suprasellar portion) (Fig. 16-1). The link structure or median eminence (of the tuber cinereum) consists of a neurovascular complex for transfer of hypophysiotropic secretions, and the supraoptic and paraventricular–hypophyseal tracts for oxytocin, vasopressin, and neurophysins I and II transport; (Figs. 16-1 and 16-2). Hypophysiotropic and inhibitory hormones, produced in dis-

crete areas of the medial basal hypothalamus (parvicellular nuclear system), are released from neural endings (tuberoinfundibular or tuberohypophyseal) into the capillary loop system (external and internal plexuses) of the median eminence. From this capillary network, these neurohormones reach their specific pituitary target cells through the long portal vessels running on the surface of the median eminence and pituitary stalk.[2]

The pars distalis secretes several hormones and factors: follicle-stimulating hormone (FSH); luteinizing hormone (LH); prolactin (PRL); thyrotropin or thyroid-stimulating hormone (TSH); somototropin or growth hormone (GH); and derivatives of the precursor pro-opiomelanocortin (POMC). From the derivatives of POMC, the melanocyte-stimulating hormones (α-, β-, and γ-MSH) and the corticotropin-like intermediate lobe peptide (CLIP) appear to be normally secreted in humans only during fetal life. In the adult pituitary gland, the final products of POMC processing are corticotropin (ACTH) and β-lipoprotein (β-LPH), as well as the cleavage products of the latter: γ-LPH and β-endorphin. Each of the anterior pituitary hormones is synthesized by a single specific cell type, except that gonadotropic cells (gonadotrophs) produce both FSH and LH, as well as chorionic gonadotropinlike substance, and the corticotrophs process all the POMC derivatives.[3,4] Hormone secretion by these cells depends directly on stimula-

FRANCISCO I. REYES • Division of Reproductive Endocrinology, Department of Obstetrics and Gynecology, State University of New York, Downstate Medical Center, Brooklyn, New York 11203.

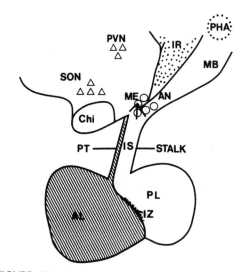

FIGURE 16-1. Diagram of the hypothalamic–pituitary unit. SON, supraoptic nucleus; PVN, paraventricular nucleus; PHA, posterior hypothalamic area; Chi, optic chiasm; ME, median eminence of the tuber cinereum; IR, infundibular recess of the third ventricle; AN, arcuate nucleus; MB, mammilary body; PT, pars tuberalis; IS, infundibular stem; AL, anterior lobe (pars distalis); IZ, intermediate zone (vestigium of intermediate lobe); PL, posterior lobe (infundibular process).

tion by the hypothalamic neurohormones, except for the lactotrophs, which are mainly regulated by dopamine (PRL inhibitory factor) inhibition. Synthesis and release of anterior pituitary hormones are further regulated by the products of their own target glands (long feedback mechanism). In addition, because of the interlacing vascular connections between the adenohypophysis and neurohypophysis,[2] both oxytocin and vasopressin also influence gonadotropin and ACTH secretion. On the other hand, anterior pituitary hormones may be secreted directly into the brain through several routes *via* the neurohypophyseal capillary bed, and influence hypophysiotropic neuron secretion (short feedback mechanism).[5]

The concept of the hypothalamic–pituitary unit has been established because of the intimate anatomic and functional relationships between the pituitary gland and hypothalamus. It is also valid in pathologic terms, since lesions in one of these two organs generally affect the function of the other, and most developmental, as well as many acquired abnormalities involve both organs simultaneously. Furthermore, in many instances our diagnostic tools do not permit the distinction between a primary pituitary or hypothalamic origin of pituitary dysfunction. The corollary is that hypothalamic or pituitary disease implies dysfunction of the hypothalamic–pituitary unit.

To be in a better position in assessing clinical problems, this chapter presents a review of the hypothalamic–pituitary disorders affecting reproductive function, followed by an outline of the investigative approach and management of the patient with neuroendocrine disease.

HYPOTHALAMIC–PITUITARY DISORDERS

There is no completely satisfactory classification of hypothalamic–pituitary disorders.[6-8] For descriptive and clinical purposes, it remains appropriate to retain the classic division into two broad categories: hypopituitarism and hyperpituitarism. It must be emphasized, however, that coexistence of hormonal excess and deficiency states is common and is well exemplified in patients with pituitary adenomas. Excessive or deficient pituitary hormone production may be related to a distinct pituitary or hypothalamic abnormality; accordingly, the hyperpituitarism or hypopituitarism can be further defined as primary or secondary (or hypothalamic).

Hypopituitarism

This may be caused by a variety of hereditary, congenital, or acquired factors. Many are rare pathologic entities, and a number of clinical syndromes bear little or no relevance to reproductive processes.

Hereditary and Congenital Disorders

Absence or maldevelopment of the pituitary gland and hypothalamus usually occurs in combination with other severe cephalic malformations (anencephaly and holoprosencephaly–hypopituitarism syndrome) and results almost invariably in neonatal death[9,10] (see Table 16-1). Mild cases of mid-line anomalies (e.g., cleft palate and harelip) are rarely associated with pituitary hormone deficiency.[11] Few cases of isolated pituitary maldevelopment have been documented but, if recognized shortly after birth, they can be treated successfully.[12]

Genetic deficiency of two or more pituitary hormones not associated with somatic malformations is rare and most cases fall within the category of familial panhypopituitary dwarfism. Growth hor-

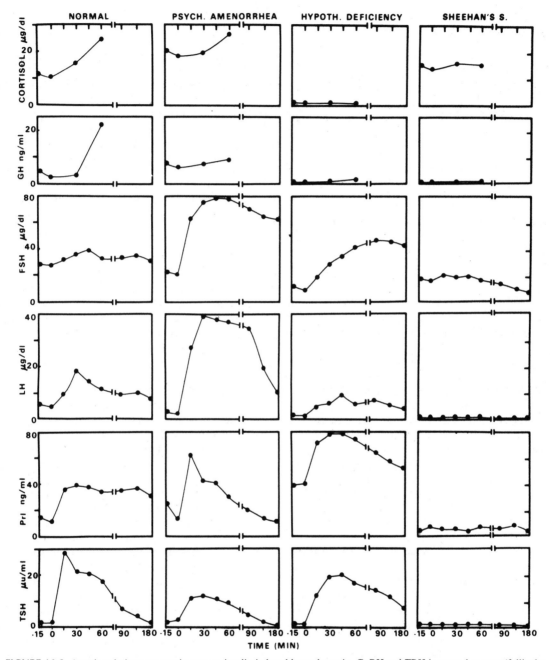

FIGURE 16-2. Anterior pituitary responsiveness to insulin-induced hypoglycemia, GnRH and TRH in normal women (follicular phase) and in patients with psychogenic amenorrhea, hypothalamic infarction (cardiac arrest), and postpartum pituitary necrosis (Sheehan's syndrome; on cortisol replacement). To convert from micrograms (μg) LER-907/d to mIU 2nd IRP-hMG/ml, multiply FSH values by 0.5 and LH values by 0.8.

TABLE 16-1. Hypopituitarism: Hereditary Disorders and Congenital Abnormalities of the Hypothalamic–Pituitary Unit

Pituitary and/or hypothalamic agenesis, aplasia, and
   hypoplasia
   Isolated forms
   Associated with midline craniofacial defects and
      anencephaly
Hereditary polytropic hypopituitarism
   Familial panhypopituitary dwarfism
Hereditary monotropic hypopituitarism
   Isolated FSH-LH, PRL, GH, and TSH deficiencies
Hypopituitarism associated with complex genetic syndromes
   Hypogonadotropic hypogonadism with anosmia
   Laurence-Moon-Bardet-Biedl and related syndromes
   Prader-Willi syndrome
   Ataxia-telangiectasia
   Bloom's syndrome
   Fanconi's syndrome
   Hemochromatosis

mone (GH) deficiency may be combined with deficiency of any other tropic hormone(s), gonadotropin being the most common.

Acquired forms of monotropic hypopituitarism are being recognized more frequently, but largely it has a genetic origin.[9,13] Children with isolated GH deficiency undergo puberty spontaneously, although it tends to be delayed. GH replacement causes rapid development of pubertal changes in these children. Thus, failure of this sexual development initially suggests hypopituitary disproportionate short stature combined with gonadotropin deficiency.[14] Reproductive capacity in GH-deficient men and women is normal. Untreated women have to be delivered by cesarean section, however, since their offspring are of normal average size. GH deficiency does not interfere with lactation. Isolated gonadotropin deficiency is the most commonly reported form of monotropic hypopituitarism, but a large number of cases have not been thoroughly documented. The defect is frequently inherited as an autosomal trait or occurs sporadically, and it involves either follicle-stimulating hormone (FSH), luteinizing hormone (LH), or, more frequently, both. Hypothalamic failure to secrete gonadotropin-releasing hormone (GnRH) explains the hypogonadotropism in most cases, but a primary defect in pituitary gonadotropin synthesis could

be the cause in some patients.[15] The characteristic clinical features are partial or complete failure of pubertal development, primary amenorrhea, and frequently eunuchoidism. A particular syndrome of isolated LH deficiency has been recognized in males with clinical and biochemical evidence of hypoandrogenism, who although infertile, have active spermatogenesis as shown by testicular biopsy ("fertile eunuch" syndrome).[16]

Hereditary forms of isolated prolactin (PRL) and thyroid-stimulating hormone (TSH) deficiency have been found to be associated with pseudohypoparathyroidism, but not as a single entity.[17] There are no reports of familial cases of isolated ACTH deficiency.

Sexual immaturity is the common characteristic of a group of rare complex genetic syndromes whose endocrine features remain largely undefined. The clinical significance concerning reproductive function in most cases is limited by the nature and severity of their neurologic or somatic abnormalities (e.g., Laurence-Moon-Bardet-Biedl and Prader-Willi syndromes). Aside from rare mild cases,[18] an exception to this observation is the syndrome of hypogonadotropic hypogonadism with anosmia or hyposmia, also known as olfactogenital dysplasia, or Kallman's syndrome.[19] This disorder affects males more frequently than females, and it appears to be most often inherited as an X-linked recessive or autosomal dominant trait, but nonfamilial sporadic cases also have been reported. Deficiency of FSH and LH in this syndrome appears to be mainly due to a hypothalamic defect, since patients respond to exogenous GnRH but not to clomiphene citrate or estrogen. This is supported by the finding of hypothalamic dysplasia in some, but not all, of the few postmortem cases examined. The anosmia is due to agenesis or maldevelopment of the olfactory bulbs and tracts. Other abnormalities such as color blindness and renal agenesis have been described in some cases. The gonads in both sexes show arrest at the primary follicle or spermatocyte stage, but otherwise they appear normal.

Iron deposition in endocrine glands, including the pituitary, is common in hereditary hemochromatosis. Clinical manifestations of pituitary or gonadal iron overload do not generally occur until the fifth decade of life or later. Therefore, female reproductive function is not affected.[20] By contrast, acquired transfusional iron overload in young adults with anemia (e.g., thalassemic patients) may produce gonadotropin deficiency.[21]

TABLE 16-2. Hypopituitarism: Acquired Disorders of the Hypothalamic–Pituitary Unit

Functional hypopituitarism
  Psychogenic
    Hypothalamic amenorrhea
    Anorexia nervosa
    Pseudocyesis
  Malnutrition and starvation
  Exogenous hormones
  Drugs affecting neurotransmitters
Vascular and/or coagulation disorders
  Postpartum pituitary necrosis
  Nonpuerperal pituitary necrosis
Inflammatory disorders
  Acute and chronic infections
  Autoimmune hypophysitis
  Sarcoidosis
  Histiocytosis-X
Non-neoplastic tumors
  Pituitary cysts
  Aneurysms
  "Empty sella" syndrome
Neoplasms
  Pituitary adenomas
  Craniopharyngioma
  Meningioma
  Germinomas
  Gliomas
  Others
Surgical, irradiation, and traumatic injury
  Hypophysectomy
  Adenomectomy
  Stalk section
  Radiation necrosis
  Cranial trauma

Acquired Disorders

Acquired deficiencies of pituitary function are far more commonly the result of nonorganic abnormalities (hypothalamic–pituitary dysfunction)[6–8] (see Table 16-2). Hypopituitarism due to acquired structural abnormalities is most often due to pituitary adenomas and postpartum pituitary necrosis, but it can be caused by a large number of different etiologic factors. Monotropic hypopituitarism has been documented with increasing frequency over the past 10 years, however, polytropic hypopituitarism, either partial or complete, is more common. Concurrent deficiency and hypersecretion of pituitary hormones occur frequently in cases of pituitary adenoma and may also be found in other conditions, such as stalk section and anorexia nervosa.

Emotional disorders primarily affect gonadotropic function, which results in anovulation and loss of menses (psychogenic or hypothalamic amenorrhea) or may delay puberty. Psychic trauma-related amenorrhea may develop as a consequence of acute minor or major stresses, such as change in environment or rape; it is usually temporary. Chronic stressful life events associated with certain behavioral and social patterns may also lead to psychogenic amenorrhea.[22,23] Psychogenic disorders not only affect gonadotropin secretion,[24] but also the production of other anterior pituitary hormones. For example, children with emotional deprivation syndrome show GH and ACTH deficiency, which is reversible. In pseudocyesis, or imaginary pregnancy, a well-defined psychogenic syndrome, hypogonadotropism, may be associated with elevated PRL secretion.[25]

Another well-defined psychogenic syndrome characterized by deficient gonadotropin secretion is anorexia nervosa.[26,27] The incidence of anorexia nervosa remains uncertain, as there is no widely accepted definition of this condition, but it is not rare. It mainly affects young women and is uncommon in males. Abnormal eating and self-perception behavior leading to progressive weight loss and amenorrhea are the dominant clinical features of anorexia nervosa. Starvation or malnutrition and even simple weight loss by itself, may also lead to hypopituitarism[28,29]. Anovulation and amenorrhea also occur in other nutrition-related syndromes with psychosocial components: bulimia and physical hyperactivity (e.g., ballet dancing; long-distance running).[27] (See Chapter 21.)

Chronic suppression of hypothalamic–pituitary function, e.g., exogenous glucocorticoids and steroid contraceptives, may persist for a variable time after discontinuation of therapy. Postpill amenorrhea over a 6-month duration rarely, if at all, represents a distinct pathologic entity; in most patients careful investigation reveals a different underlying disorder.

Postpartum pituitary necrosis[30,31] has been ranked after pituitary adenoma as the most common cause of hypopituitarism. It is difficult, however, to ascertain its present true incidence. Nevertheless, it is quite apparent that an improvement of obstetric care has made it less frequent. Nonpuerperal pituitary necrosis[32] remains less often recognized; it has been found as a complication of diabetes mellitus, nonobstetric shock, increased intracranial pressure, cerebrovascular accidents (CVAs), and other entities. Whether associated with pregnancy or not, ischemia frequently involves not only the adenohypophysis but also the hypothalamus, and occasionally the neurohypophysis. Necrosis may cause complete hypopituitarism (panhypopituitarism) with diabetes insipidus, but small lesions result in selective hormone deficiency or reduced pituitary functional reserve.[33,34] The precise mechanism of the ischemia remains unsettled. Sheehan[35] championed the hypothesis of selective spasm of the hypophyseal vessels resulting from circulatory collapse. Bergland and Page[2] speculated about the possible effects of vasoconstriction and dilatation at different levels of the hypothalamic–pituitary circulatory systems, but experimental evidence is lacking. By contrast, Beernink and McKay,[36] explain the ischemia as a manifestation of disseminated intravascular coagulation. Thrombosis has been found to account for the hypothalamic pituitary necrosis seen in patients with sickle cell anemia.

Earlier reports indicate that hypopituitarism secondary to pyogenic infections of the central nervous system (CNS) is an uncommon complication and as a rule is seen following subacute and chronic types of sepsis (tuberculous, fungus, or syphylitic meningitis). In recent years isolated reports describe cases of pituitary deficiencies following encephalitis (e.g., measles, epidemic hemorrhagic fever, and postvaccinial). Autoimmune disease may destroy any gland, but so far few cases of hypophysitis have been described that fit into this category.[37,38] Circulating immunoglobulins may prevent hormone receptor binding,[39] or the autoimmune process may destroy glandular tissue and affect the secretion of one or more pituitary hormones. Hypophysitis is usually associated with other endocrinopathies (insulin-dependent diabetes mellitus and chronic thyroiditis); i.e., it belongs to the polyglandular failure syndrome. This autoimmune syndrome has been linked to the HLA B-8 loci, suggesting that this condition is genetically determined. Hypopituitarism may also result from the induction of antibodies to hypothalamic or pituitary hormones by hormone therapy.[40] Intracranial sarcoidosis preferentially involves the hypothalamic–pituitary region and produces diabetes insipidus and anterior pituitary deficiency. These manifestations seldom occur in the absence of other systemic features.[41] Histiocytosis-X[42,43] is the generic term for a group of uncommon disorders (eosinophilic

granuloma, Hand-Schüller-Christian disease, and Letterer-Siwe disease) found predominantly in children but often seen first in adults. The distinctive lesion is inflammatory histiocytosis (granulomatosis), which may be found in bones, viscera, and skin. Involvement of the hypothalamic–pituitary region results most often in diabetes insipidus and short stature, but amenorrhea and other features of pituitary hormone deficiencies may also occur.

Pituitary deficiency due to Rathke cleft cysts or intrasellar or parasellar aneurysms is quite rare and, like the empty sella syndrome, their finding is often incidental. The latter entity corresponds to an arachnoid herniation, containing cerebrospinal fluid (CSF), into the pituitary fossa, which enlarges the sella turcica and flattens the pituitary gland against the posteroinferior wall. It occurs as a congenital defect or secondary to pituitary infarction or to surgical or radiation therapy. This abnormality seldom causes endocrine dysfunction, by itself, but it may coexist with other conditions such as adenoma, which may produce hypopituitarism or hyperpituitarism.[44]

Neoplasms[45-47] of the hypothalamus and the pituitary gland are the most frequent organic cause of pituitary dysfunction. Although these include a wide variety of unusual tumors, the bulk are pituitary adenomas. (Since these are frequently characterized by hormone hypersecretion, they are discussed in the section of hyperpituitary syndromes.) Most of the other neoplasms develop in the suprasellar region and therefore tend to produce early neurologic effects and diabetes insipidus by tissue destruction and compression or displacement of neighbouring structures. Craniopharyngioma[48,49] is the most common neoplasm in this region. It usually arises from the stalk, but it may also have an intrasellar origin. Most are cystic and almost always calcified in children, but in adults one out of three shows no calcification. It is diagnosed most often in children or young adults, but it can first be detected in any age group. In children it is the most common neoplasm associated with pituitary failure. Gliomas of the optic chiasm or hypothalamus are usually associated with neurofibromatosis. Less common neoplasms in this region that cause hypopituitarism include germinomas (ectopic pinealoma) and teratomas, which usually become symptomatic during the first two decades of life.[50] (It is important to remember, however, that tumors involving the hypothalamic region in children are most frequently associated with precocious puberty.) By contrast, meningiomas and metastatic neoplasms tend to appear late in life and thus have less clinical significance in relationship to reproductive processes.

Hypophysectomy and stalk section have been performed extensively during recent years. Most patients are at or beyond reproductive age, since the common indications are carcinoma of the breast or prostate and advanced diabetic retinopathy. By contrast, excision or irradiation of pituitary adenomas and hypothalamic neoplasms is frequently carried out in children and young adults and may result in a new or further impairment of pituitary function that affects reproductive function.[49,51] The irradiation effect on hypothalamic or pituitary hormone secretion tends to be slow progressing and manifests itself within years. Cranial trauma, with or without an associated fracture of the base of the skull, may occasionally result in hypopituitarism due to hypothalamic or pituitary damage secondary to vascular lesions or stalk section. A number of cases labeled idiopathic hypopituitarism may in fact be secondary to obstetric trauma at birth.[52]

Hyperpituitarism (Hyperpituitary Syndromes)

Excluding peripheral target organ failure, pituitary hormone hypersecretion can be the result of hypothalamic lesions or, more often, pituitary adenomas[45–47] (Table 16-3).

True precocious puberty is caused by an excessive pituitary gonadotropin production for age. It may be induced by neoplasms, hypothyroidism, infections, degenerative lesions, and other rare disorders involving the hypothalamus, but more commonly it develops, particularly in young girls, in the absence of an obvious hypothalamic lesion (idiopathic true precocious puberty). It has been proposed that the presence of a mass may passively trigger the release of hypothalamic secretion. However, in the case of hamartomas, it has been shown

that the aberrant tissue secretes GnRH autonomously,[53] suggesting an active mechanism for premature development. Women with polycystic ovary syndrome and other hyperandrogenic conditions may show mildly increased LH levels associated with normal or low FSH concentrations, arguing in favor of a causal primary hypothalamic abnormality. Hypothalamic neoplasms that disrupt the tuberoinfundibular pathway (e.g., pituitary stalk compression) are associated with hypopituitarism, as well as with hyperprolactinemia. Oversecretion of other pituitary hormones due to organic hypothalamic abnormalities is most unusual. On the other hand, it has been suggested that sustained functional disturbances of the hypothalamus could be primarily responsible for the development of pituitary cell hyperplasia and/or neoplasia leading to Cushing's disease.[54] Intracranial germinomas may secrete human chorionic gonadotropin (hCG), resulting in incomplete sexual precocity in boys rather than true precocious puberty; females are not affected, since follicular development depends on the activity of both FSH and LH.[55]

Pituitary adenomas[47,56–58] make up 3–10% of all intracranial tumors and are found in adults of all ages in both sexes, but seldom in children. Classically, they have been classified according to their tinctorial affinity as eosinophilic, basophilic, or chromophobic. This classification is misleading and of limited clinical value. Pituitary adenomas should be classified according to functional categories related to the particular hormone(s) produced. Histopathologic confirmation can be obtained by electron microscopy and immunologic methods.[3] GH-, ACTH-, and PRL-secreting adenomas produce distinct syndromes.

FSH–LH and TSH-secreting adenomas not only appear to be less common than other varieties of pituitary adenomas but are also more difficult to recognize. Most gonadotropin-producing tumors hypersecrete only FSH. They are found mostly in males and may be associated with hypogonadism.[59,60] Pituitary adenomas producing excessive amounts of TSH cause secondary hyperthyroidism.[61] Hypersecretion of the nonspecific α-subunits of the glycoprotein hormones has been found in association with FSH-, LH-, and TSH-secreting tumors. However, isolated α-subunit overproduction has also been recognized in patients with nonfunctioning pituitary adenomas.[62]

A large number of previously labeled "functionless pituitary adenomas," which failed to stain by conventional histologic methods, have been

TABLE 16-3. Hyperpituitarism

Hormone(s) excess	Disorder
FSH–LH	True precocious puberty
PRL	Delayed puberty, amenorrhea–galactorrhea, male hypogonadism
GH	Acromegaly-gigantism
ACTH	Cushing's disease
	Nelson's syndrome
TSH	Hyperthyroidism

found to secrete prolactin (PRL-cell adenomas); they are frequently associated with the amenorrhea–galactorrhea syndrome. Although these adenomas are the most common cause of hyperpituitarism, hyperprolactinemia results more often from idiopathic hypothalamic dysfunction not associated with structural abnormalities, or as a result of other endocrine and nonendocrine disorders and a number of PRL secretion-inducing drugs (see Chapter 24).

High basal GH levels occur in almost any condition associated with malnutrition, such as anorexia nervosa and hepatic cirrhosis. GH hypersecretion is otherwise most likely due to GH-producing adenomas and associated with hypersomatotropism (acromegaly-gigantism syndrome). Although normal gonadal function may persist for several years in the face of readily recognizable acral changes, some patients may show early signs of impairment. These may be explained by hyperprolactinemia since at least 30% of GH-secreting adenomas also produce PRL, or by mild hyperandrogenism of adrenal or ovarian origin. By contrast, late disturbances of reproductive function are more likely to be the result of impaired gonadotropin secretion secondary to pituitary compression by tumor proliferation.

Excessive pituitary ACTH secretion (Cushing's disease) is the most frequent cause of endogenous hypercortisolism.[54] Patients with Cushing's syndrome may become pregnant, but menstrual dysfunction, usually in the form of amenorrhea, is present at the time of diagnosis in a large majority. Ovarian hypofunction might result from increased adrenal androgen or glucocorticoid secretion. The mechanism for the deleterious effects of androgen excess remains unclear; cortisol excess has been shown to result in diminished gonadotropin release after exogenous GnRH stimulation. Pituitary ACTH-secreting adenomas are most often subclinical (microadenomas), but tend to enlarge after adrenalectomy (Nelson's syndrome) and may cause deficiency of other pituitary hormones.

DIAGNOSIS OF HYPOTHALAMIC–PITUITARY DISEASE

The possibility of hypothalamic–pituitary disease is usually suspected by the presence of clinical evidence of peripheral gland failure or hyperfunction. Sometimes this possibility arises instead from the occurrence of neurologic abnormalities or,

more infrequently, nonendocrine manifestations of hypothalamic dysfunction. In some cases, recognition of a causal disorder (i.e., obstetric shock) raises the possibility of hypothalamic–pituitary disease. From the reproductive endocrinologic viewpoint, manifestations of gonadotropin deficiency and PRL oversecretion are the main clues of possible hypothalamic–pituitary abnormality.

A patient suspected of hypothalamic–pituitary disease should be approached considering the endocrine and the nonendocrine manifestations of hypothalamic–pituitary abnormalities at a time. Although both aspects are interrelated, this division has practical advantages. A detailed clinical examination will not only often bring out features of abnormal endocrine and/or neurologic function but also may help define the primary cause. Together these may provide strong evidence of a hypothalamic–pituitary disorder. However, a definite diagnosis of hypothalamic–pituitary disease depends on specific endocrine and other special investigations.

Endocrine Manifestations of Pituitary Disease

Hypopituitarism

Mild pituitary hyposecretion may become evident only under stressful conditions or may be recognized only by pituitary function challenge tests (limited pituitary reserve) (see Fig. 16-3). Characteristically, however, hypopituitarism results in hypotrophy and a diminished hormonal secretion of the various target glands. In general, clinical manifestations of primary and secondary peripheral gland failure are similar. The possibility of primary versus secondary peripheral gland failure is greater when there is no evidence of impairment of other glandular function. Primary peripheral gland failure is characteristically associated with high circulating concentrations of the corresponding pituitary hormone in contrast to normal, low, or undetectable levels in pituitary or hypothalamic disorders. Diagnosis of isolated pituitary hormone deficiency can be made with certainty only if intact responses to appropriate stimulation are demonstrated for all but one of the pituitary hormones. Sometimes an apparent monotropic hypopituitarism of either hypothalamic or pituitary origin may be found coexisting with limited pituitary reserve of other tropic hormones. Furthermore, in some patients with isolated pituitary deficiency polytropic hypopituitarism may eventually develop.

Failure of lactation and rapid mammary gland

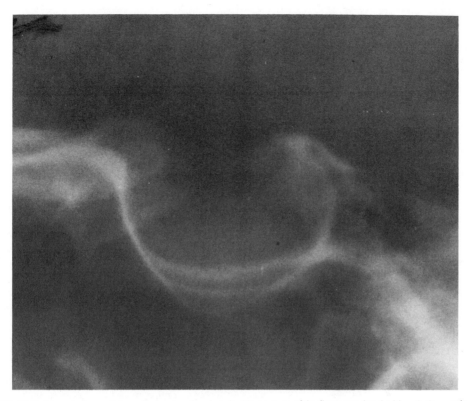

FIGURE 16-3. Lateral view of the sella turcica showing double contour of the floor associated with a pituitary microadenoma.

involution (PRL deficit) are usually the initial features following a large postpartum pituitary infarct. Menses do not resume thereafter (FSH–LH deficit), and if pubic hair had been shaved it fails to regrow. Weakness, lethargy, apathy, and anorexia may be recognized early (ACTH deficiency) and become more obvious within weeks, whereupon cold intolerance may also be noted (TSH deficit). Rarely polyuria may develop shortly after delivery (vasopressin deficit), but this feature may be masked by an accompanying ACTH-cortisol deficit. The sequence of these hormonal events, as well as the onset of manifestations is variable not only in postpartum necrosis but also in polytropic hypopituitarism resulting from other causes. Moreover, specific effects of any particular hormone deficiency may predominate over those of others, and many can be influenced by age and sex.

During childhood, FSH and LH deficiency shows no clinical manifestations, but later it is associated with pubertal failure and eunuchoidism.[63,64] This may be complete or partial; that is, females may show a variable degree of breast development,

sexual hair, and, although primary amenorrhea is the rule, occasionally menses may occur. Low basal FSH and LH values differentiate these children from those with hypergonadotropic hypogonadism (e.g., gonadal dysgenesis and agonadism), although not uncommonly single gonadotropin determinations may fall within the normal pubertal range. In the absence of extraendocrine characteristic features, such as the lack of the sense of smell (hypogonadotropic hypogonadism with anosmia) or radiologic evidence of an abnormality, hypogonadotropic hypogonadism is difficult to differentiate from constitutional delay of puberty unless prolonged observation is carried out. Low gonadotropin levels and a blunted or prepubertal type of response to GnRH are seen in both. Increasing FSH and LH levels and GnRH responsiveness within months or a few years point to a constitutional type of delay. A computed tomography (CT) scan of the brain is, however, a most valuable tool for early identification of an organic lesion.

In females amenorrhea, or oligomenorrhea and anovulation in milder forms, in males loss of libido and potency, and infertility in both sexes are the most prominent features of hypogonadotropism in adults. A diminished rate of sexual hair growth is more apparent in males, but it may also occur in females, especially with coexisting ACTH deficiency. Longstanding hypogonadotropism also results in genital hypotrophy in both sexes. All these clinical manifestations are also found in primary hypogonadism; even hot flushes, which are characteristic of primary ovarian failure may also occur uncommonly in hypogonadotropic females.[65] Clinical evidence of hypogonadism, together with inappropriately low circulating FSH and LH levels, indicates a hypothalamic or pituitary disorder. The failure to find an increment in FSH and LH levels following both acute and chronic GnRH stimulation indicates an abnormality at the pituitary level. However, some patients with definite pituitary lesions may show normal GnRH responses. Subnormal and normal or even exaggerated responses to standard tests may be seen in patients with hypothalamic disorders; thus differentiation of hypothalamic (tertiary hypogonadism) versus pituitary (secondary hypogonadism) deficiency may be difficult.[66,67] Chronic intermittent GnRH stimulation appears to be more helpful to localize the origin of the problem.[15,68] The finding of a normal response to GnRH, however, does not exclude a small pituitary or a hypothalamic lesion; it indicates only that sufficient gonadotropic cells are present. Patients who respond to GnRH but fail to release gonadotropins following estrogen or clomiphene citrate presumably have a primary hypothalamic impairment.

Diagnosis of psychogenic (hypothalamic) amenorrhea can be reached only after exclusion of organic lesions. In these patients serum FSH and LH levels are low normal or low and the gonadotropin response to GnRH may be exaggerated.[23,24] Undetectable circulating hCG levels confirm the clinical impression of pseudocyesis. Induction of withdrawal uterine bleeding with exogenous hormones may convince some patients that they were not pregnant. Anorexia nervosa may be distinguished from other types of psychogenic amenorrhea by the clinical features of exaggerated concern regarding diet and figure, history of weight loss, constipation, bradycardia, and the presence of lanugo hair. Patients with anorexia nervosa or undernourished show similar endocrine features.[26–28] Aside from low gonadotropin and sex steroid levels, in both conditions there is a reversion to the pubertal LH secretion pattern; that is, a decrease in magnitude of episodic release and nocturnal en-

hancement, and delayed FSH and LH responsiveness to GnRH stimulation (Fig. 16-2). The TSH response to thyrotropin-releasing hormone (TRH) is also delayed, and the serum levels of 3,5,3'-triiodothyronine (T3) are reduced. By contrast, serum GH levels are high. In addition, evidence of mild diabetes insipidus may be present in both conditions.

Prolactin deficiency can be recognized clinically only during the puerperium by lactational failure. It is one of the cardinal features of Sheehan's syndrome, but it may be absent, since some patients do lactate.[33] Prolactin deficiency is confirmed by low endogenous levels that fail to increase following TRH or chlorpromazine stimulation.[17]

Clinical effects of GH hyposecretion are evident only in infants and children. Deficiency states in adults, though relatively common, can be documented only by reduced or absent GH release responses to provocative agents such as insulin hypoglycemia or arginine hydrochloride.[67] Hypothyroid, hypogonadal, and obese subjects also show subnormal GH responses, but these normalize after hormone replacement, weight normalization, or the use of combined provocative stimuli. Basal GH concentrations are not useful in the diagnosis of deficiency, since values in normal subjects are often undetectable.

Patients with TSH deficiency present the typical clinical features of hypothyroidism: fatigue, cold intolerance, constipation, hoarse voice, and menstrual disturbances. An inappropriately low serum TSH level differentiates with certainty pituitary (secondary) or hypothalamic (tertiary) from primary hypothyroidism which characteristically shows high TSH levels in association with low concentrations of thyroxine (T4) and T3. The TRH stimulation test may be helpful in differentiating hypothalamic versus pituitary TSH deficiency; that is, a normal or a delayed response suggests a hypothalamic defect, whereas an absent response tends to be associated with pituitary lesions.[67]

Weakness, hypotension, anorexia, and weight loss should be considered results of adrenal insufficiency until proved otherwise. These features are common to primary, secondary, or tertiary hypocortisolism.[67]

Amenorrhea develops independent of origin, especially with long-standing cortisol deficiency. Menstrual function and fertility may be maintained in less severe cases. Hyperpigmentation is a useful clue for the diagnosis of primary adrenal disease. The possibility of ACTH deficiency should be ruled out in hypopituitary patients even when no clinical evidence of hypoadrenalism exists, since stressful situations may prove life threatening. Serum ACTH levels are low or undetectable in secondary and tertiary, and high in primary (Addison's disease) hypocortisolism.[69] Until recently, differentiation of cortisol deficiency origin depended on adrenal responsiveness to exogenous ACTH and indirect assessment of pituitary ACTH reserve (e.g., insulin hypoglycemia, metyrapone).[67] If serum or urinary cortisol levels show an appropriate rise after administration of ACTH but fail to increase after metyrapone or insulin, adrenal hyposecretion is due to pituitary or hypothalamic impairment. The adrenal responses to ACTH in long-standing cases of secondary hypoadrenocorticism may be subnormal and delayed. Therefore, a 3-day stimulation test with long-acting corticotropin should be used.

These tests, particularly insulin hypoglycemia, may be hazardous and should be done only under strict supervision and avoided absolutely in the presence of cardiac disease. Corticotropin releasing factor (CRF) has been recently characterized, but its clinical application remains to be determined.

Diabetes insipidus in a patient with anterior pituitary deficiency suggests that the primary lesion involves the hypothalamus or the upper stalk. Loss of large amounts of urine or low osmolality suggests the diagnosis, but polyuria may be absent initially if hypovolemia is present (e.g., postpartum necrosis, or ACTH-cortisol deficiency); polyuria may not appear until the circulation volume has been expanded and renal function improved or cortisol replacement initiated. Diagnosis must be confirmed by demonstrating under close and experienced supervision the inability to conserve water on a dehydration test and by the responsiveness to exogenous vassopressin.[66]

Diagnosis of Hyperpituitarism[6–8,47,56]

The sequence of pubertal changes in children with true precocious puberty[63] is usually similar to the normal pattern. Urine or serum FSH and LH, and serum estradiol levels in these young females are most of the time above the normal range for age. The gonadotropin response to GnRH is increased in keeping with the attained stage of sexual maturation, as well as the ovarian responsiveness to gonadotropins. Differential diagnosis should exclude organic causes and the possibility of pseudoprecocious puberty (see Chapter 14).

Increased gonadotropin secretion in adults is almost always the result of primary gonadal failure. Isolated high FSH levels may be found in infertile men with oligospermia and denotes severe spermatogenetic damage. Similarly, a transient elevation of FSH levels in females, which may reach castrate levels and later is associated with high LH levels, indicates waning ovarian function. These changes occur even in women with apparent normal menstrual cycles, and they signal the approach of either premature or a normal menopause.[70] High circulating FSH and LH levels are also found in patients with the gonadotropin-resistant ovary syndrome, most probably as a result of inhibition of ovarian follicle FSH receptors by antibodies.[39]

Pituitary FSH-LH, like α-subunit-secreting adenomas are not associated with any clinical evidence of hyperpituitarism. Isolated elevation of LH levels raises the possibility of a hCG-producing tumor, since hCG shows cross reactivity in most LH assays.

The somatic features of acromegaly are readily recognizable when reproductive endocrine disturbances arise, but characteristic high basal serum GH levels not suppressible by a glucose load[67] are present before acral changes become obvious.

Centripetal obesity, plethoric round face, purple striae, hypertension, hirsutism, and oligomenorrhea, associated with impaired glucose tolerance and mild erythrocytosis, eosinopenia, and lymphopenia, are associated with excessive cortisol secretion, but in early or mild cases these features are mild or may not be present.

More often than not, cushingoid changes are found in primary obesity, and Cushing's syndrome can readily be excluded in most cases by measuring serum cortisol levels eight hours after oral administration of 1 mg dexamethasone at midnight (normal < 5 μg/dl).

Inappropriate pituitary ACTH secretion (Cushing's disease) must be differentiated from other varities of Cushing's syndrome (adrenal neoplasms and ectopic ACTH syndrome).[71] Patients with Cushing's disease show normal or borderline high ACTH levels, and distinct cortisol suppression with large (2 mg dexamethasone every 6 hr for 8 doses), but not with moderate (0.5 mg dexamethasone every 6 hr for 8 doses) amounts of exogenous corticoids.

Nonpuerperal galactorrhea associated with oligomenorrhea or amenorrhea raises the possibility of a PRL-secreting adenoma. Galactorrhea is commonly not recognized by the patient and may be found only upon proper breast examination. Since many patients fail to develop galactorrhea, routine serum PRL determinations in all amenorrheic or oligomenorrheic women are needed to recognize these tumors and other disorders causing hyperprolactinemia.[72] Although high serum PRL levels (>100 ng/ml) strongly suggests the possibility of a PRL cell adenoma, tumors are found associated with lesser degrees of hyperprolactinemia, and definitive diagnosis depends on nonendocrine tests (see Chapter 24).

Nonendocrine Features of Pituitary Disease

Neurologic manifestations of hypothalamic–pituitary disease[6,45,47,73] are by no means solely the result of damage, either local or to neighboring structures by destruction, compression, or vascular compromise. For example, mental alertness in hypopituitary patients may be restored by thyroid and cortisol replacement, and sex steroid administration may increase sexual desire. Similarly, alterations in sleep–wakefulness, behavior (apathy and lack of motor activity), autonomic function, appetite, and libido may arise from high CNS center lesions, although the hypothalamus plays a primary controlling role of these functions.

Somnolence is rather common with hypothalamic lesions; it may be also present with pituitary disease. Reversal of day–night rhythm tends to occur in patients with posterior hypothalamic damage. Apathy and depression are seen more frequently than aggressive behavior with hypothalamic lesions. Decreased libido is characteristically present in hyperprolactinemic males, but it is also a feature of secondary hypogonadism in both sexes. Rarely, hypothalamic lesions have been associated with hypersexuality. Hypothermia appears to be more common than hyperthermia in hypothalamic disorders. Increased perspiration is a frequent complaint in acromegalics, and some hypopituitary patients develop hot flushes. Both compulsive eating and dieting are associated with diverse hypothalamic syndromes. Thirst and fluid intake disturbances are more often than not linked to diabetes insipidus.

All large reported series of pituitary adenomas indicate that most were first recognized because of visual symptoms.[74] Nonetheless endocrinologic disturbances precede neurologic manifestations in most instances. By contrast, neurologic changes tend to develop earlier in patients with hypothalamic lesions. The most common presenting neurologic symptom caused by pituitary tumors and craniopharyngioma is headache of variable character. Headaches from rapidly growing hypothalamic tumors (e.g., glioma) or raised intracranial pressure may also be variable but tend to be more severe.

Pressure on the sellar diaphragm by an enlarging pituitary adenoma may give rise to blurring of vision and slight visual-field defects.[75] The latter become more obvious when the tumor gains access to the suprasellar region. Thus, even early recognition of a visual-field defect has to be considered as an advanced stage of pituitary tumor growth. Dimness of vision and bitemportal hemianopsia occur early in craniopharyngiomas due to their close proximity to the optic chiasm. But hypothalamic neoplasms frequently expand inferiorly or laterally, and it is not uncommon to find gross visual defects due to compromise of the optic chiasm (bitemporal hemianoptic deficits) or the optic tracts (homonymous hemianoptic defects). Assessment of visual fields by confrontation should not be omitted, but it is not a substitute for a complete ophthalmologic examination. Formal perimetry is not only helpful in demonstrating peripheral or central visual defects but also in ruling out other possible neuroopthalmological abnormalities. Minimal chiasmal abnormalities may first be recognized by testing the visual fields with a red object. It is worth emphasizing that visual-field defects are in large measure unreliable in assessing the size or precise localization of the primary lesion and that the classic bitemporal hemianopsia observed is more often than not asymmetric in patients with pituitary tumors.

Other neuro-ophthalmologic manifestations such as optic atrophy, papilledema, and extraocular paralysis are more frequently seen as a consequence of craniopharyngioma or intrinsic hypothalamic lesions.[45,76] Lateral extension of intrasellar neoplasma, however, predisposes to extraocular motor nerve palsy, since the cavernous sinuses which flank the pituitary fossa enclose cranial nerves III, IV, V-1, and VI, as well as the carotid arteries within their dural folds. Except for massive suprasellar extension of pituitary tumors, optic atrophy, anosmia, facial paralysis, pyramidal signs, ataxia, and other neurologic signs are usually the result of expanding hypothalamic lesions.

Radiologic Features

High-resolution CT (thin-slice CT scanning) has established itself as the most reliable radiologic technique for the detection of hypothalamic and pituitary neoplasms and other lesions.[77,78] It has drastically limited the use of other diagnostic procedures, particularly invasive techniques such as pneumoencephalography and angiography.

Plain skull X-ray films (coned-down lateral and anteroposterior projections) may be still helpful for initial assessment of patients with suspected hypothalamic–pituitary disease. Roentgenograms may assist for definition of optimal angulation or the need of less slices for CT scan studies. Also gross sellar and parasellar abnormalities may be readily recognized, as well as lesions in other areas of the skull (e.g., old fractures, metastatic lytic lesions). Since small lesions are not detected and this technique yields a large number of both false-positive and false-negative results, confirmation of the presence or absence of hypothalamic–pituitary disease must be pursued with other procedures.[79,80] Hypocycloidal polytomography provides a more detailed visualization of the sella turcica and contiguous regions than conventional radiography; therefore, it can help detect or clarify questionable findings observed in plain films. Although a high diagnostic accuracy rate for pituitary small adenomas (microadenomas) can be obtained by this technique,[77] interpretation is difficult and has produced high numbers of false-positive and -negative results.[82] Pituitary microadenomas are first recognized in tomograms by localized demineralization, "blistering," erosion, or a tilt of the floor of the sella turcica (Fig. 16-4). Continued tumor growth

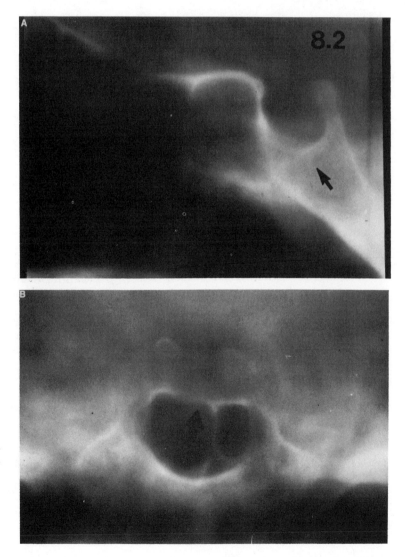

FIGURE 16-4. Hypocycloidal tomographic study of the sella turcica. (A) Lateral tomogram showing a normal-size sella turcica with inferior bulging of the right hemicellar floor (8.2-cm cut). (B) Anteroposterior tomogram showing blistering on the right side of the floor. A 6-mm pituitary microadenoma was selectively excised through the transsphenoidal route.

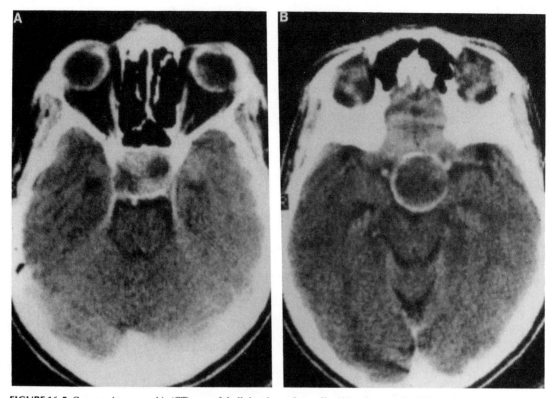

FIGURE 16-5. Computed tomographic (CT) scan of skull showing an intrasellar (A) and suprasellar (B) round mass corresponding to a craniopharyngioma. The mass shows solid and cystic components, as well as a peripheral ring of calcification.

produces further demineralization and erosion of the bone, and if expansion is asymmetric it will result in a double contour (double floor) demonstrable on plain X-ray films. When the tumor further enlarges the classical features are uniform expansion (ballooning) or distinct enlargement, with distortion in shape often associated with thinning or destruction of the sella. Abnormalities of the sella turcica can also be caused by suprasellar neoplasms or raised intracranial pressure. For example, craniopharyngiomas tend to widen the outlet of the sella and destroy the clinoid processes (Fig. 16-5). Moreover, other lesions, such as eosinophilic granuloma, may also cause bone destruction. X-ray films and tomograms of the skull are also helpful in delineating intrasellar and suprasellar soft tissue calcification. Its demonstration during childhood almost invariably indicates a craniopharyngioma. In adults, too, it is the most likely diagnosis, although it is less frequently calcified than in children. Gross calcification may also occur in teratomas, aneurysms, meningiomas, tuberculosis, and, rarely, in pituitary adenomas.

Pituitary microadenomas appear on CT scans[77,78,83] with IV contrast enhancement as areas of low density as compared with the surrounding normal tissue. Sometimes, however, they may show up as contrast-enhanced areas. One should be aware that focal areas of low density may occasionally represent abnormalities of no clinical significance, such as nonfunctioning microadenomas or cysts, or even artifacts. Additional diagnostic clues for microadenoma are an increase in height of the pituitary gland (>8 mm), and convexity of its superior margin (normally it appears flat or concave). High-resolution CT scanning not only provides a precise determination of the size of macroadenomas but also delineates suprasellar or lateral neoplastic extension and rules out the presence of an empty sella turcica or an aneurysm.[84] Thus, it permits accurate diagnosis before surgery or radiotherapy is attempted, and offers an objective measurement for follow-up management.

High-resolution CT scanning is also the most sensitive procedure to define structural anomalies in the suprasellar area. Aside from delineation of location and extension of hypothalamic masses, CT scanning often helps define their nature and the affect of neighboring structures. However, the use of magnetic resonance imaging (MRI) tomography appears more promising. It does not only offer the option for optimal demonstration of brain lesions and its anatomic relationships, but avoids radiation.[85]

Biopsy

Definitive diagnosis of suprasellar and sometimes intrasellar lesions ultimately depends on histopathological diagnosis. Biopsy of hypothalamic neoplasms remains helpful in determining the appropriate modality of treatment.

Treatment

Hypopituitarism

True replacement of anterior pituitary hormone deficiency is practical and effective only for growth retardation in children or delayed puberty in young adults, and for the induction of ovulation in women. The conventional alternative is direct replacement of the peripheral gland hormones. It should be emphasized that treatment of the causal disorder should always be considered in all cases of hypopituitarism.

In teenagers with hypothalamic hypogonadotropism, induction of puberty may be accomplished by pulsatile administration of GnRH.[86] Otherwise, pubertal failure as adult hypogonadism with severe hypotrophic genital changes may be treated initially with estrogen alone (ethinyl estradiol 20–50 μg/day). In order to maintain secondary sexual characteristics and libido as well as reduce carcinogenic potential, a combined estrogen–progestin preparation (oral contraceptive) is most adequate for these patients, as well as for younger ones once induced puberty is complete. Inherent risks of this therapy, such as coagulation complications, should be considered as when given for contraceptives purposes. Ovulation and pregnancy in these women may be accomplished by stimulation with human menopausal or pituitary gonadotropins (hMG; hPG) and hCG or GnRH therapy.[65]

ACTH-deficient patients are well maintained chronically on 25 mg (15–37.5 mg) cortisone acetate orally per day or on an equivalent dose of other corticoid given in 2–3 equally divided doses. It is mandatory to instruct corticoid-dependent patients to carry identification (bracelet, necklace, wallet card) with them to alert others in case of an accident. They must also be aware of the need to increase their corticoid dose twofold to threefold during conditions of stress and to call the physician's office or hospital to get parenteral replacement if they are unable to take medication orally. Larger parenteral doses of a soluble hydrocortisone ester are needed for more stressful situations (e.g., trauma, surgery, and serious medical disorders). Salt-retaining hormone therapy is seldom required by these patients. Harmful effects (e.g., iatrogenic Cushing's syndrome) are seldom seen with these maintenance dosages of glucocorticoid.

Thyroid replacement should be avoided until adrenal insufficiency has been excluded or glucocorticoid therapy has begun. It is usually initiated with 25–50 μg/day L-thyroxine and gradually increased to maintenance dosage (150–200 μg/day in a single dose).

Hyperpituitarism and Pituitary Adenomas

The treatment of hyperpituitarism is aimed to abort hormone oversecretion and, in the case of neooplasia, its removal or reduction in size and/or growth to abolish or refrain further advancement of their clinical manifestations.[8,47,56–58] These aims should be attained without further impairment of hypothalamic–pituitary or neurologic function.

The management of hyperpituitary patients involves pharmacologic treatment, surgery, and radiotherapy, or a combination of these modalities. Choice of treatment depends on the nature of the hyperpituitary problem (e.g., absence or presence of tumor, type of neoplasm, the presence of local or general complications) and the availability of therapeutic resources (e.g., neurosurgical skills, radiation equipment).

Several hormones have been tried in patients with idiopathic true precocious puberty. Therapy with progestins (e.g., medroxyprogesterone acetate) and antiandrogens or with cyproterone acetate is effective in arresting menses and breast growth but not in regard to bone maturation and growth rate. Preliminary results indicate that administration of long-acting analogues of GnRH not only abolishes menses and breast growth but retards bone maturation increasing the rate of growth as well.[87]

Other hypergonadotropic conditions, such as GnRH hypersecretion by hamartoma or FSH–LH secreting adenomas, have been mainly managed by surgical means.[53,60] By contrast, irradiation appears to be the treatment of choice for patients with a CNS hCG-secreting germinoma.[50]

Medical treatment is particularly effective for hyperprolactinemia syndrome, including cases of PRL-cell adenoma. Ergot alkaloids with long-acting dopamine agonist activity, such as bromocriptine, lisuride, and pergolide, diminish rapidly PRL hypersecretion and restore pituitary–gonadal function.[88] These alkaloids administered to patients with large pituitary adenomas by reducing tumor size can help accomplish a more complete surgical excision. Ergot derivatives are also helpful in normalizing PRL hypersecretion in cases of incomplete tumor removal by surgery as well as in accelerating clinical recovery postirradiation. About 95% of patients with PRL cell microadenomas respond effectively to these agents, that is they go into clinical remission as a result of normalization of PRL secretion. Moreover, they frequently show shrinkage of their tumors. Unfortunately, immediately after discontinuation of treatment, the clinical and mass responses are reversed (i.e., medical treatment achieves no cure); therefore, it must be given chronically.[89] Furthermore, tumor enlargement may occur during ergot derivative treatment.[90] The best immediate results following prolactinoma transsphenoidal microsurgical excision are seen in patients with microadenomas.[91] Postadenomectomy results deteriorate with increasing tumor size. Long-term follow-up after adenomectomy indicates a high recurrence rate of hyperprolactinemia, however, but without radiologic evidence of tumor reappearance.[92] Local mass effects of tumoral extension remains as a standard indication for surgical management. Primary radiation therapy is a reasonable approach for patients with PRL cell adenomas with no major suprasellar extension in whom other treatment modalities are either unacceptable or at high risk (for further details, see Chapter 24).[93]

The main modalities of treatment for acromegaly and Cushing's disease are surgery and radiotherapy. Bromocriptine reduces GH hypersecretion but seldom normalizes it; therefore, medical treatment has only a secondary role. Cyproheptadine, a serotonin antagonist, produces remission in about 50% of patients with Cushing's disease.[54]

QUESTIONS FOR THE FUTURE

It is clear that our knowledge about hypothalamic–pituitary function has changed profoundly during the last decade. However, innumerable questions remain for elucidation. For example, a good number of cases of hypopituitarism still fall under the idiopathic category. Similarly, we do not know which factor(s) trigger the development of pituitary adenomas. Moreover, it is still unsettled if these neoplasms are the result or not of a hypothalamic disturbance. The radiologic diagnosis of sellar and parasellar lesions has advanced rapidly. Will the application of MRI scanning provide better definition of hypothalamic–pituitary disease? Most probably the answer will be affirmative; therefore, we will have a tool free of irradiation hazards for diagnosis and follow-up evaluation. The availability of effective drugs to control hypothalamic–pituitary secretion has certainly produced a basic change in the management of hyperpituitarism. Thus, will the rapid progress in physiologic and pharmacologic knowledge of hypothalamic–pituitary function provide more specific and less expensive drugs capable of not only suppressing but curing hyperpituitarism? The application of microsurgery has produced not only better results in the excision of hypothalamic and pituitary neoplasm but has markedly reduced the surgical morbidity as well. It is possible that the use of new therapeutic techniques (e.g., laser) will result in further improvement.

CONCLUSION

It is evident that pituitary disorders cannot be approached in the isolation of one's own field of interest. The diagnosis and management of these conditions optimally should be carried out using a multidisciplinary approach. Nevertheless, best results will depend very much on the awareness of the gynecologist to identify these patients and enlist the help of other team physicians early on, since the most common presenting features of hypothalamic–pituitary disease in women are menstrual dysfunction and infertility.

QUESTIONS

1. Primary hypopituitarism is characterized by

    a. decreased hormone production by specific pituitary hormone target tissue.

    b. decreased circulating concentrations of corresponding pituitary hormone(s).

    c. failure to respond to both acute and chronic

stimulation with hypothalamic releasing hormone(s).

    d. all the above.

2. Bone erosion or destruction of the sella turcica may be associated with

    a. Empty sella syndrome.
    b. PRL-producing microadenoma.
    c. craniopharyngioma.
    d. all the above.

3. GnRH or its analogues are therapeutically effective for

    a. ovulation induction in primary hypogonadotropism.
    b. induction of puberty in gonadal dysgenesis.
    c. arresting menses and breast growth in idiopathic true precocious puberty.
    d. all the above.

4. The condition commonly associated with delayed puberty is

    a. isolated GH deficiency.
    b. hereditary hemochromatosis.
    c. intracranial sarcoidosis.
    d. all the above.

5. The tumors capable of secreting protein hormones are

    a. craniopharyngioma.
    b. hamartoma.
    c. germinoma.
    d. all the above.

6. It is characteristic of pituitary gonadotropin producing adenomas to

    a. secrete FSH more frequently than LH or both.
    b. be found mainly in males.
    c. be associated with hypogonadism.
    d. all the above.

REFERENCES

1. Reyes FI, Faiman C, Winter JSD: Development of the regulatory mechanisms of the hypothalamic–pituitary–gonadal system in the human fetus, in Resko J, Novy M (eds): *Fetal Endocrinology* New York, Academic, 1981, pp 285–302
2. Bergland RM, Page RB: Pituitary–brain vascular relations: A new paradigm. *Science* 204:18–24, 1979
3. Pelletier G, Robert R, Hardy J: Identification of human anterior pituitary cells by immunoelectron-microscopy. *J Clin Endocrinol Metab* 46:534–542, 1978
4. Liotta AS, Falaschi P, Krieger DT: Characterization of pro-opiomelanocortin (POMC)-related peptides in fresh human (H) anterior pituitary (AP), in *Proceedings of the Sixty-fourth Annual Meeting of the Endocrine Society* p 135
5. Bergland RM, Page RB: Can the pituitary secrete directly to the brain? (Affirmative anatomical evidence). *Endocrinology* 102:1325–1338, 1978
6. Martin JB, Reichlin S: *Clinical Neuroendocrinology,* 2nd ed. Philadelphia, Davis, 1984
7. Besser GM (ed): The hypothalamus and pituitary. *Clin Endocrinol Metab* 6:1–275, 1977
8. Tolis G, Labrie, F, Martin JB, et al (eds): *Clinical Neuroendocrinology: A Pathophysiological Approach.* New York, Raven Press, 1979
9. Rimoin DL, Schimke RN: *Genetic Disorders of the Endocrine Glands.* St Louis, Mosby, 1971, pp 11–78
10. Fisher DA, Hughes ER: Disorders of the hypothalamus, in Kelley VC (ed): *Endocrine and Genetic Disorders in Children.* Hagerstown, MD, Harper & Row, 1974, pp 143–166
11. Gendrel D, Chaussain JL, Job JC: Les hypopituitarismes congenitaux par anomalie de la ligne mediane. *Arch Fr Pediatr* 38:227–232, 1981
12. Sadeghi-Nejad A, Senior B: A familial syndrome of isolated "aplasia" of the anterior pituitary. *J Pediatr* 84:79–84, 1974
13. Odell WD: Isolated deficiency of anterior pituitary hormones. *JAMA* 197:176–186, 1966
14. Sauder SE, Corley KP, Hopwood, NJ, et al: Subnormal gonadotropin responses to gonadotropin-releasing hormone persist into puberty in children with isolated growth hormone deficiency. *J Clin Endocrinol Metab* 53:1186–1192, 1981
15. Yoshimoto Y, Moridera K, Imura H: Restoration of normal pituitary gonadotropin reserve by administration of luteinizing-hormone-releasing hormone in patients with hypogonadotropic hypogonadism. *N Engl J Med* 292:242–245, 1975
16. Faiman C, Hoffman DL, Ryan RJ, et al: The "fertile eunuch" syndrome: Demonstration of isolated hormone deficiency by radioimmunoassay technique. *Mayo Clin Proc* 43:661–667, 1968
17. Carlson HE, Brickman AS, Bottazzo GF: Prolactin deficiency in pseudohypoparathyroidism. *N Engl J Med* 296:140–144, 1977
18. Chang RJ, Davidson BJ, Carlson HE, et al: Hypogonadotropic hvpogonadism associated with retinitis pigmentosa in a female sibship: Evidence for gonadotropin deficiency. *J Clin Endocrinol Metab* 53:1179–1185, 1981
19. Lieblich JM, Rogol AD, White BJ, et al: Syndrome of anosmia with hypogonadotropic hypogonadism (Kallman syndrome). *Am J Med* 73:506–519, 1982
20. Feller RE, Pont A, Wands JR, et al: Familial hemochromatosis: Physiologic studies in the precirrhotic stage of the disease. *N Engl J Med* 296:1422–1426, 1977
21. Kletzky OA, Costin G, Marrs RP, et al: Gonadotropin insufficiency in patients with thalassemia major. *J Clin Endocrinol Metab* 48:901–905, 1979
22. Fries H, Nillius SJ, Pettersson F: Epidemiology of secondary amenorrhea. II. A retrospective evaluation of etiology with special regard to psychogenic factors and weight loss. *Am J Obstet Gynecol* 118:473–479, 1974
23. Lachelin GCL, Yen SSC: Hypothalamic chronic anovulation. *Am J Obstet Gynecol* 130:825–831, 1978
24. Rebar RW, Harman SM, Vaitukaitis JL: Differential responsiveness to LRF after estrogen therapy in women with

hypothalamic amenorrhea. *J Clin Endocrinol Metab* 46:48–54, 1978

25. Yen SSC, Rebar RW, Quesenberry W: Pituitary function in pseudocyesis. *J Clin Endocrinol Metab* 43:132–136, 1976

26. Vigersky R (ed): *Anorexia Nervosa.* New York, Raven, 1977

27. Warren MP: Effects of undernutrition on reproductive function in the human. *Endocrine Rev* 4:363–377, 1983

28. Pimstone B: Endocrine function in protein-calorie malnutrition. *Clin Endocrinol* 5:79–95, 1976

29. Vigersky RA, Andersen AE, Thompson RH, et al: Hypothalamic dysfunction in secondary amenorrhea associated with weight loss. *N Engl J Med* 297:1141–1145, 1977

30. Kovacs K: Necrosis of anterior pituitary in humans. *Neuroendocrinology* 4:170–241, 1969

31. Daughaday WH: Sheehan's syndrome, in Givens JR (ed): *Endocrine Causes of Menstrual Disorders.* Chicago, Year Book Medical Publishers, 1978, pp 143–164

32. Veldhuis JD, Hammond JM: Endocrine function after spontaneous infarction of the human pituitary: Report, review and reappraisal. *Endocr Rev* 1:100–107, 1980

33. Purnell DC, Randall RV, Rynearson EH: Postpartum pituitary insufficiency. *Mayo Clin Proc* 39:321–331, 1964

34. Martin JE, McDonald PC, Kaplan NM: Successful pregnancy in a patient with Sheehan's syndrome. *N Engl J Med* 282:425, 1970

35. Sheehan HL, Stanfield JP: The pathogenesis of postpartum necrosis of the anterior lobe of the pituitary gland. *Acta Endocrinol (Copenh)* 37:479–510, 1961

36. Beernik FG, McKay DG: Pituitary insufficiency associated with pregnancy, panhypopituitarism, and diabetes insipidus. *Am J Obstet Gynecol* 84:318–338, 1962

37. Asa SL, Bilbao JM, Kovacs K, et al: Lymphocytic hypophysitis of pregnancy resulting in hypopituitarism: A distinct clinicopathological entity. *Ann Intern Med* 95:166–171, 1981

38. Kojima I, Nejima I, Ogata E: Isolated adrenocorticotropin deficiency associated with polyglandular failure. *J Clin Endocrinol Metab* 54:182–186, 1982

39. Chiauzzi V, Cigorraga S, Escobar ME, et al: Inhibition of follicle-stimulating hormone receptor binding by circulating immunoglobulins. *J Clin Endocrinol Metab* 54:1221–1228, 1982

40. Lindner J, McNeil LW, Marney S, et al: Characterization of human antiluteinizing hormone-releasing hormone (LRH) antibodies in the serum of a patient with isolated gonadotropin deficiency treated with synthetic LRH. *J Clin Endocrinol Metab* 52:267–270, 1981

41. Vesely DL, Maldonado A, Levey GS: Partial hypopituitarism and possible hypothalamic involvement in sarcoidosis. *Am J Med* 62:425–431, 1977

42. Zinkham WH: Multifocal eosinophilic granuloma: Natural history, etiology and management. *Am J Med* 60:457–463, 1976

43. Braunstein DG, Kohler PO: Pituitary function in Hand-Schuler-Christian disease. *N Engl J Med* 286:1225–1229, 1972

44. Jordan RM, Kendall JW, Kerber CW: The primary empty sella syndrome: Analysis of the clinical characteristics, radiographic features, pituitary function and cerebrospinal fluid adenohypophysial hormone concentrations. *Am J Med* 62:569–580, 1977

45. Locke W, Schally AV (eds): *The Hypothalamus and Pituitary in Health and Disease.* Springfield, IL, Charles C Thomas, 1972

46. Carmel PW: Surgical syndromes of the hypothalamus. *Clin Neurosurg* 27:133–159, 1980

47. Post K, Jackson I, Reichlin S (eds): *Pituitary Adenoma.* New York, Plenum, 1980

48. Jenkins JS, Gilbert CJ, Ang V: Hypothalamic–pituitary function in patients with craniopharyngiomas. *J Clin Endocrinol Metab* 43:394–399, 1976

49. Thomsett MJ, Conte FA, Kaplan SL, et al: Endocrine and neurologic outcome in childhood craniopharyngioma: Review of effect of treatment in 42 patients. *J Pediatr* 97:728–735, 1980

50. Sklar CA, Grumbach MM, Kaplan SL, et al: Hormonal and metabolic abnormalities associated with central nervous system germinoma in children and adolescents and the effect of therapy: Report of 10 patients. *J Clin Endocrinol Metab* 52:9–16, 1981

51. Huang K-E: Assessment of hypothalamic–pituitary function in women after external head irradiation. *J Clin Endocrinol Metab* 49:623–627, 1979

52. Craft WH, Underwood LE, Van Wyk JJ: High incidence of perinatal insult in children with idiopathic hypopituitarism. *J Pediatr* 96:397–402, 1980

53. Judge DM, Kulin HE, Page R, et al: Hypothalamic hamartoma: A source of luteinizing-hormone-releasing factor in precocious puberty. *N Engl J Med* 296:7–10, 1977

54. Krieger DT: Physiopathology of Cushing's disease. *Endocrine Rev* 4:22–43, 1983

55. Sklar CA, Conte FA, Kaplan SL, et al: Human chorionic gonadotropin-secreting pineal tumor: Relation to pathogenesis and sex limitation of sexual precocity. *J Clin Endocrinol Metab* 53:656–660, 1981

56. Tindall GT, Collins WF: *Clinical Management of Pituitary Disorders.* New York, Raven, 1979

57. Laws ER Jr, Randall RV, Kern EB, et al (eds): *Management of Pituitary Adenomas and Related Lesions with Emphasis on Transphenoidal Microsurgery.* New York, Appleton-Century-Crofts, 1982

58. Cook DM: Pituitary tumors: Diagnosis and therapy. *CA-A* 33:215–236, 1983

59. Wide L, Lundberg PO: Hypersecretion of an abnormal form of follicle-stimulating hormone associated with suppressed luteinizing hormone secretion in a woman with a pituitary adenoma. *J Clin Endocrinol Metab* 53:923–930, 1981

60. Harris RI, Schatz NJ, Gennarelli T, et al: Follicle-stimulating hormone-secreting pituitary adenomas: Correlation of reduction of adenoma size with reduction of hormonal hypersecretion after transphenoidal surgery. *J Clin Endocrinol Metab* 56:1288–1293, 1983

61. Tolis G, Bird C, Bertrand G, et al: Pituitary hyperthyroidism. *Am J Med* 64:177–181, 1978

62. Ridgway EC, Klibanski A, Ladenson PW, et al: Pure alpha-secreting pituitary adenomas. *N Engl J Med* 304:1254–1259, 1981

63. Brasel JA, Wright JC, Wilkins L, et al: An evaluation of seventy-five patients with hypopituitarism beginning in childhood. *Am J Med* 38:484–498, 1965

64. Winter JSC, Faiman C, Reyes FI: Normal and abnormal pubertal development. *Clin Obstet Gynecol* 21:67–86, 1978

65. Meldrum DR, Erlik Y, Lu JKH, et al: Objectively recorded hot flushes in patients with pituitary insufficiency. *J Clin Endocrinol Metab* 52:684–687, 1981

66. Mortimer CH: Clinical applications of gonadotropin releasing hormone. *Clin Endocrinol Metab* 6:167–179, 1977

67. Cryer PE: *Diagnostic Endocrinology,* 2nd ed. London, Oxford University Press, 1979

68. Leyendecker G, Wildt L: Induction of ovulation with chronic intermittent (pulsatile) administration of GnRH in women with hypothalamic amenorrhea. *J Reprod Fertil* 69:397–409, 1983

69. Krieger DT, Liotta AS, Suda T, et al: Human plasma immunoreactive lipotropin and adrenocorticotropin in normal subjects and in patients with pituitary–adrenal disease. *J Clin Endocrinol Metab* 48:566–571, 1979

70. Reyes FI, Winter JSD, Faiman C: Pituitary ovarian relationships preceding the menopause. *Am J Obstet Gynecol* 129:557–565, 1977

71. Crapo L: Cushing's syndrome: A review of diagnostic tests. *Metabolism* 28:955–977, 1979

72. Gomez F, Reyes FI, Faiman C: Nonpuerperal galactorrhea and hyperprolactinemia. *Am J Med* 62:648–660, 1977

73. Bauer HG: Endocrine and other clinical manifestations of hypothalamic disease: A survey of 60 cases, with autopsies. *J Clin Endocrinol Metab* 14:13–31, 1954

74. Hollenhorst RW, Younge BR: Ocular manifestations produced by adenomas of the pituitary gland: Analysis of 1000 cases. *Excerpta Medica Int Cong Ser* 303:53–64, 1973

75. Wilson P, Falconer M: Patterns of visual failure with pituitary tumors. *Br J Ophthalmol* 52:94–110, 1978

76. Neetens A, Selosse P: Oculomotor abnormalities in sellar and parasellar pathology. *Ophthalmologica* 175:80–104, 1977

77. Cohen WA, Pinto RS, Kricheff II: The value of dynamic scanning. *Radiol Clin North Am* 20:23–35, 1982

78. Taylor S: High resolution computed tomography of the sella. *Radiol Clin North Am* 20:207–236, 1982

79. Muhr C, Bergstrom K, Grimelius L, et al: A parallel study of the roentgen anatomy of the sella turcica and the histopathology of the pituitary gland in 205 autopsy specimens. *Neuroradiology* 21:55–65, 1981

80. Burrow GN, Wortzman G, Rewcastle NB, et al: Microadenomas of the pituitary and abnormal sellar tomograms in an unselected autopsy series. *N Engl J Med* 304:156–158, 1981

81. Vezina JL: Prolactin-secreting pituitary adenomas: Radiologic diagnosis, in Robyn C, Harter M (eds): *Progress in Prolactin Physiology and Pathology*. Amsterdam, Elsevier/North-Holland Biomedical Press, 1978, pp 351–360

82. Raji MR, Kishore PRS, Becker DP: Pituitary microadenoma: A radiological-surgical correlative study. *Radiology* 139:95–99, 1981

83. Bonneville J-F, Cattin F, Moussa-Bacha K, et al: Dynamic computed tomography of the pituitary gland: The "tuft sign." *Radiology* 149:145–148, 1983

84. Macpherson P, Anderson DE: Radiological differentiation of intrasellar aneurysms from pituitary tumors. *Neuroradiology* 21:177–183, 1981

85. Hawkes RC, Holland GN, Moore WS, et al: Nuclear magnetic resonance (NMR) tomography of the brain: A preliminary clinical assessment with demonstration of pathology. *J Comput Assist Tomogr* 4:577–586, 1980

86. Wildt L, Marshall G, Knobil E: Experimental induction of puberty in the infantile female rhesus monkey. *Science* 207:1373–1375, 1980

87. Mansfield MJ, Beardsworth DE, Loughlin JS, et al: Long-term treatment of central precocious puberty with a long-acting analogue of luteinizing hormone-releasing hormone. *N Engl J Med* 309:1286–1290, 1983

88. Wass JAH, Besser GM: The medical management of hormone-secreting tumors of the pituitary. *Annu Rev Med* 34:283–294, 1983

89. Thorner MO, Perryman RL, Rogol AD, et al: Rapid changes of prolactinoma volume after withdrawal and re-institution of bromocriptine. *J Clin Endocrinol Metab* 53:480–483, 1981

90. Crosignani PG, Mattei A, Ferrari C, et al: Enlargement of a prolactin-secreting pituitary microadenoma during bromocriptine treatment. *Br J Obstet Gynaecol* 89:169–70, 1982

91. Hardy J, Beauregard H, Robert F: Prolactin-secreting pituitary adenomas: Transphenoidal microsurgical treatment, in Robyn C, Harter M (eds): *Progress in Prolactin Physiology and Pathology*. Amsterdam, Elsevier/North-Holland, 1978, pp 361–370

92. Serri O, Rasio E, Beauregard H, et al: Recurrence of hyperprolactinemia after selective transphenoidal adenomectomy in women with prolactinoma. *N Engl J Med* 309:280–283, 1983

93. Mehta AE, Reyes FI, Faiman C: Primary radiotherapy of prolactinoma: Long follow-up, in *Proceedings of the Sixty-fifth Annual Meeting of the Endocrine Society, San Antonio*, 1983, p 82

ANSWERS

1. a, b
2. b, c
3. c
4. a
5. b, c
6. d

17

Secondary Amenorrhea and the Menopause

ANTONIO SCOMMEGNA and SANDRA ANN CARSON

SECONDARY AMENORRHEA

Are regular cyclic menses the unnatural state for a healthy, normal female? During her reproductive years, nature may have intended her to have only a few menstrual periods interspersed with pregnancies followed by lactation. The reproductive system may not have been designed for long-term monthly menstruation. In the absence of pregnancy or lactation, it is surprising that secondary amenorrhea develops in so few women. Nonetheless, the absence of previously regular menses for 6 months or three menstrual cycles is defined as secondary amenorrhea and warrants investigation.

As described in earlier chapters, the menstrual cycle results from the coordinated integration of a functioning hypothalamus, pituitary, ovary, and uterus and is affected by the input of higher cortical centers. Disorders at any of these levels may result in secondary amenorrhea, and treatment focuses on eliminating the cause.

ANTONIO SCOMMEGNA and SANDRA ANN CAR-SON • Department of Obstetrics and Gynecology, Michael Reese Hospital and Medical Center, University of Chicago, Chicago, Illinois 60616.

Pregnancy

The most common cause of secondary amenorrhea in the reproductive age group is pregnancy. Before any further diagnostic procedures or therapeutic measures are undertaken, pregnancy must be ruled out. Menses resume by 3 months after delivery in more than 90% of nonlactating women[1] and by 6 months in more than 90% of women who breast feed[2].

Uterine Factors

Intrauterine synechiae (Asherman's syndrome) are fibrous bands formed in the uterus that replace normal endometrial tissue. The synechiae are often the result of a previous uterine curettage, either postpartum, abortal, or therapeutic for dysfunctional uterine bleeding. The diagnosis is confirmed by hysteroscopic visualization of the bands or filling defects on hysterosalpingogram (honeycomb pattern) (Fig. 17-1).

Intrauterine synechiae may be lysed under direct hysteroscopic vision,[3] and an IUD is placed in an attempt to prevent reformation of the adhesions. Of 69 patients undergoing hysteroscopic synechiolysis,[3] 28 had no postoperative IUD placed; in

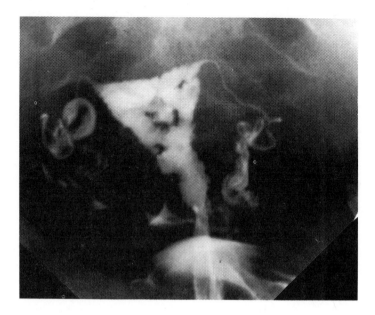

FIGURE 17-1. Hysterosalpingogram illustrating intrauterine filling defects (Asherman's syndrome) in a patient with secondary amenorrhea.

5 of these patients, adhesions recurred. By contrast, only 3 of 41 patients who had postoperative IUD placement had recurrent adhesions; two of these three had a history of pelvic tuberculosis. In addition, these patients should be given high-dose estrogen therapy in an effort to stimulate endometrial proliferation. A minimum of 5 mg/day conjugated estrogens should be administered orally for 2 months, followed by 7–10 days on progestogen therapy.

The endometrial lining may also be replaced by granulomas resulting from tuberculosis. The diagnosis is made by histologic examination of an endometrial biopsy, repeated cultures of menstrual blood, and a tuberculin test (PPD). Tuberculous endometritis is secondary to an infection elsewhere. Treatment is with appropriate antibiotics.

Obstruction of the endocervical canal after scarring from a cone biopsy or, more rarely, a tumor, may be ruled out by history and pelvic examination. These patients often experience severe monthly cramping presumably resulting from uterine contractions and retrograde menstruation.

Ovarian Factors

Anovulation and amenorrhea may result from Polycystic ovarian disease, a disorder that includes a spectrum of abnormalities ranging from hyperthecosis to large sclerocystic ovaries with multiple cysts. The ovarian cysts are multiple follicles in

various stages of development. Usually no corpora lutea are found. This, together with stromal and capsular hyperplasia and luteinization suggests acyclic gonadotropin stimulation. The stimulation may be afforded by the elevated luteinizing hormone/follicle-stimulating hormone (LH/FSH) ratio characterizing this disorder. The normal hormonal fluctuations are replaced by constant, steady-state levels. Ovarian androgens are usually elevated.[4]

Amenorrhea was present in about one-half of patients with polycystic ovaries in a literature review by Goldzieher and Green.[5] Infertility, hirsutism, obesity, and irregular bleeding were other common symptoms.

Polycystic ovarian disease resulting in anovulation is at times associated with endometrial carcinoma,[6] perhaps resulting from unopposed estrogen. Therefore, patients not desiring a pregnancy should be treated with a progestogen to induce cyclic bleeding. The interval between courses of progesterone is debatable. Therapy every 4 weeks may be physiologic, but therapy every 8 weeks will permit detection of spontaneous ovulation. On the other hand, 8 weeks of unopposed estrogen stimulation will result in heavy withdrawal bleeding. Our compromise is to give progestogen 6 weeks after spontaneous or progestogen-induced withdrawal bleeding.

Patients desiring contraception may be treated with a combination oral contraceptive containing 50 μg estrogen. These preparations will decrease the LH, increase the sex hormone binding globulin (SHBG), thus reducing free androgens, and also ensure cyclic endometrial bleeding.

Patients desiring pregnancy may be treated with clomiphene citrate to induce ovulation. Efficacy ranges from 47%[7] to 85%.[8] About one-half of the ovulating patients become pregnant. Women who fail to ovulate with clomiphene citrate may be treated with human menopausal gonadotropins. Ovarian wedge resection for treatment of polycystic ovaries has been replaced by medical induction of ovulation.

Gonadal dysgenesis usually causes primary amenorrhea, However, some patients with gonadal dysgenesis may experience menstrual periods for a few years before complete ovarian failure. In fact, these patients do have a reduced number of primordial follicles that may be stimulated to develop and permit pregnancy.[8] Of the reported cases of gonadal dysgenesis who became pregnant, 7 have had 45,X karyotype and 24 were mosaics carrying a 45,X cell line.[9]

Patients with gonadal dysgenesis who have a history of menstruation may have follicles that can be stimulated to ovulate. These patients should have weekly blood sampling drawn and saved over a period of 4 weeks. The collected samples should be assayed individually in one assay for LH, FSH, and E_2.[10] If the gonadotropins remain elevated and the estrogen remains low, the patient is considered to have ovarian failure and she should be given cyclic estrogen/progesterone replacement therapy. On the other hand, if the gonadotropins decrease in association with an estrogen rise, this is taken as evidence of ovarian follicular activity with intact negative feedback of estradiol on pituitary gonadotropin secretion. These patients may be treated with hMG to induce further follicle growth and ovulation.

Idiopathic Premature Menopause

This is the cessation of ovarian function before age 40 without apparent cause. These patients have elevated gonadotropins, low estrogens, and apparent lack of ovarian follicles. This disorder has been suggested to be reversible,[11] as some patients with premature ovarian failure have become pregnant.[12-15] One patient treated with human menopausal gonadotropins[15] later conceived in a nontreated cycle. The others became pregnant during or after estrogen replacement therapy.

Idiopathic premature menopause in 46,XX individuals may actually occur as an end point of

46,XX gonadal dysgenesis. Patients with 45,X or mosaic gonadal dysgenesis may display evidence of ovarian folliculogenesis before gonadal failure.[16] It is therefore conceivable that ovaries of patients with 46,XX gonadal dysgenesis may display similar activity. Because these patients have no cytogenetic abnormality, they would be thought to simply be undergoing menopause at an early age. Similarly, those cases with elevated gonadotropins and a normal karyotype may be at the end point of the gonadotropin-resistant ovary syndrome (GROS), in which the follicles have become atretic. Perhaps all these disorders, which we now clinically separate, are merely the same disorder seen at different stages.

Patients with idiopathic premature menopause may be fertile, prompting Rebar et al.[10] to suggest that weekly serum gonadotropin and estrogen be drawn. A concomitant decrease in gonadotropins and increase in estrogens lends evidence to ovarian follicular activity. If such is the case, patients may be given a course of estrogen–progesterone replacement therapy in an attempt to increase follicular FSH receptors and spur follicular growth and ovulation. Similarly, those who do not desire a pregnancy and are given estrogen–progesterone replacement therapy further development of amenorrhea requires ruling out a pregnancy.

Gonadotropin-Resistant Ovaries

Patients with Savage syndrome have ovarian follicles that do not respond to FSH and LH. These patients have secondary sexual characteristics, primary or secondary amenorrhea, elevated gonadotropins, and a 46,XX karyotype. The follicles are within the ovarian medulla, and the diagnosis is made by measuring elevated gonadotropin levels in the presence of primordial follicles on ovarian wedge biopsy. A laparoscopic biopsy is insufficient to make the diagnosis, as the follicles are deep within the ovarian stroma.[17-19] In a recent review by Maxson and Wentz,[20] 14 cases were cited as having findings sufficient for the diagnosis of gonadotropin-resistant ovaries. Fifty-seven percent of these patients had secondary amenorrhea, and 43% had primary amenorrhea. All cases were particularly resistant to stimulation with clomiphene citrate or human menopausal gonadotropins. One patient in the reviewed series conceived while being given cyclic estrogen–progesterone replacement therapy.[19]

The etiology of this syndrome remains obscure.

Jones[21] suggested that these patients have an FSH receptor defect. If this is the case, however, none of these patients would be able to develop follicles or conceive. Another hypothesis is suggested by Irvine et al.,[22] who have reported a patient with Addison's disease in whom autoimmune ovarian failure developed. Similar antibodies directed against the ovarian FSH receptor or the gonadotropin itself may result in the gonadotropin-resistant ovarian syndrome, but no evidence for such exists. Finally, this syndrome may simply be a point in the spectrum of idiopathic premature ovarian failure, as described above.

Patients with this syndrome have low estrogen and are at risk for the consequences of estrogen deprivation. These patients should therefore be treated with cyclic estrogen–progesterone replacement. Since this is the only treatment that has resulted in pregnancy,[19] patients who desire a pregnancy may be treated with estrogen–progesterone combinations for three cycles. After that time, the patient is given estrogen alone and asked to record her basal body temperature. Progesterone is added after 20 days if she does not ovulate. Similarly, in those patients who are on cyclic replacement therapy and who do not have a withdrawal bleed, a pregnancy should be suspected.

Pituitary Factors

Hyperprolactinemia

Hyperprolactinemia is present in 13–30% of patients who present with secondary amenorrhea. Although the precise mechanism is unknown, high levels of this hormone are thought to inhibit ovarian steroidogenesis directly, inhibit pituitary gonadotropin release, and interfere with ovarian steroid modulation of pituitary function. Prolactin secretion from the pituitary is normally inhibited by hypothalmic inhibitory factors, one of which is dopamine.[23] Histamine also inhibits prolactin secretion,[24] whereas serotonin and thyrotropin-releasing hormone (TRH) stimulate its release.[23] Therefore, hyperprolactinemia may result from lesions obstructing the inhibitory influence from the hypothalamus (e.g., craniopharyngioma, sarcoidosis, surgical ablation), increased stimulation (elevated TRH in primary hypothyroidism), or prolactin-secreting pituitary adenomas. Exogenous sex steroids, phenothiazines, certain antidepressants, and antihypertensives may also cause hypoprolactinemia.[24,25]

Patients with hyperprolactinemia should have a thyroid function screen and computed tomograph (CT) scan of the sella turcica with 1.5-mm cuts. Pituitary tumors greater than 1 cm in diameter (macroadenomas) are best treated with combination medical/surgical therapy, although recent evidence indicates that medical therapy alone will shrink these tumors.[26] On the other hand, microadenomas (<1 cm) may be treated either surgically or medically. The current trend is medical therapy.

Hyperprolactinemia may be treated with bromocriptine, an ergot alkaloid that directly inhibits pituitary prolactin secretion. The drug is initially given in a dose of 2.5 mg q HS and increased weekly as necessary to 7.5 mg bid. This gradual increase causes less nausea than does initiation of therapy with the full dose. Prolactin levels should be monitored weekly. Bromocriptine will decrease prolactin levels by 75% within 6 hr.

Patients with ameonorrhea secondary to hyperprolactinemia usually respond within 8 weeks of initiation of therapy. About 80% of these patients resume ovulatory menstruation.[25]

Pituitary Necrosis

Pituitary necrosis secondary to previous postpartum hemorrhage or cerebral radiation will result in ablation of pituitary function. These patients will have no tropic hormones for the gonads, adrenal, and thyroid. They should therefore be treated with thyroid and adrenal replacement.

Ovulation induction in these patients requires hMG. If no pregnancy is desired, these patients may need estrogen–progesterone replacement therapy for, in the absence of gonadotropins, follicular development will be arrested.

Hypothalamic Factors

Hypothalamic amenorrhea is the second most frequent cause of secondary amenorrhea. It is associated with stress, severe weight loss, or vigorous athletic participation. Although the association is well known, its etiology remains diffuse.

Dopamine, serotonin, and opioids are involved in the neuroendocrine regulation of GNRH.[27] Dopamine decreases GNRH pulses and inhibits LH release from the pituitary. Opioids inhibit LH release while augmenting PRL secretion. It is therefore not surprising that psychotropic and antihypertensive agents that alter the secretion, synthesis, or action of the neurotransmitters will cause hypothalamic amenorrhea. Similarly, psychological stress exemplified in the extreme by anorexia nervosa may alter the neuroamines and opioids and result in amenorrhea.

Anorexia Nervosa

This condition occurs primarily in middle- to upper-class women younger than 25. These patients exhibit a prepubertal LH and FSH response to GNRH (FSH response greater than LH response) and lose gonadotropin pulsatility.[28] The postpubertal response can be attained by pulsatile GNRH stimulation, suggesting that the primary disorder lies in the hypothalamus or higher centers. As the patient gains weight, the gonadotropin response gradually assumes the adult pattern in a way that mimics pubertal changes. However, only 70% of patients resume menstruating.[29]

Weight Loss

Loss of weight to less than 30% of ideal body weight results in secondary amenorrhea. It seems that women need a fat content equal to about 22% of body weight to maintain menstrual function. Although the mechanism is unknown, amenorrhea may result in part from increased catechol estrogen production. Estradiol, normally metabolized to 16-OH-estradiol is converted to 2-OH-estrone in patients who have decreased body stores of fat. This catechol estrogen has no intrinsic estrogenic activity despite its binding to the cytoplasmic estrogen receptor.[30] In addition, low fat stores reduce the contribution of peripheral androgen aromatization to total circulating estrogen. In those patients recovering from severe weight loss, menses return when body fat reaches about 90% of ideal body weight. This may not be true, however, in patients recovering from anorexia nervosa, as this disease seems to involve more factors than merely weight loss.[31]

Traumatic or Exudative Processes

Traumatic or exudative processes disrupting the hypothalamic–pituitary axis will result in secondary amenorrhea. Craniopharyngioma, gummas, teratomas, and gliomas are examples. Tuberculosis, sarcoidosis, and other infiltrative diseases may also interrupt the hypothalamic–pituitary connection. These diseases rarely present with amenorrhea alone.

Hypothalamic disorders are initially treated by an attempt to remove the primary process such as stress or weight loss. Ovulation induction and pregnancy in patients with hypothalamic amenorrhea has been achieved by chronic intermittent administration of exogenous GNRH. An automatic infusion pump (Zyklomat: Ferring GmbH, Kiel, FRG), or an autosyringe can be used to deliver intravenous GNRH every 90 min in doses of 10–20 μg.[32] Patients not desiring pregnancy should be cycled with estrogen–progestin replacement therapy.

Thyroid Disease

Hypothyroidism results in secondary amenorrhea. Low thyroxine levels fail to inhibit TSH and TRF, which become elevated. TRF stimulates prolactin secretion, which itself causes normal metabolism and balance of the sex steroid. The higher free androgens and lower estradiol may alter pituitary gonadotropin release and result in anovulation.[33] Treatment is with thyroid replacement therapy.

Postpill Amenorrhea

The return of normal menstrual cycles is delayed in some women discontinuing oral contraceptives (OCP). Menses usually return in 6 months. One study has demonstrated that the incidence of secondary amenorrhea following OCP use is not significantly different from the incidence in women not previously using OCPs.[34]

In a 10-year retrospective study comparing women with secondary and postpill amenorrhea, March and Mishell[35] concluded that although OCP does not cause secondary amenorrhea, therapy may mask the development of this symptom in women who have oligomenorrhea. This study further points out that although the OCP does not increase the incidence pituitary adenomas, the incidence of hyperprolactinemia and of galactorrhea was significantly higher in the group with postpill amenorrhea.

Patients who do not begin menstruating within 6 months after discontinuing OCPs should be considered to have secondary amenorrhea and undergo the diagnostic workup outlined below.

Clinical Evaluation

A careful history and physical examination is the first step in clinical evaluation of a patient with secondary amenorrhea. Pregnancy, chronic disease, and stressful influences may be elicited.

TABLE 17-1. Hormone Choices for Endometrial Challenge

Progestin challenge	Estrogen challenge[a]
Progesterone in oil, 100 mg IM	Estrace, 2 mg qd
Medroxyprogesterone acetate, 10 mg PO qd × 7 days	Conjugated equine estrogen, 0.625 mg qd
Norethindrone acetate, 5 mg PO qd × 7 days	Diethylstilbestrol, 0.25 mg qd
	Ethinyl estradiol, 10 μg qd

[a] ×21 days.

A serum prolactin level and TSH will screen for hyperprolactinemia and hypothyroidism. The treatment of both conditions is discussed in previous chapters.

After these basic tests, the patient is given a progesterone challenge. The doses of the various progestins that may be used are listed in Table 17-1. A patient with sufficient estrogen to permit endometrial stimulation and growth will bleed within 7–10 days after completion of her progesterone challenge. Indeed, such a bleed suggests that the patient was lacking progesterone, confirming a diagnosis of anovulation.

Failure of withdrawal bleeding suggests either uterine unresponsiveness or estrogen levels too low to provoke endometrial proliferation. To distinguish these possibilities, the patient is given a course of estrogen (Table 16-1) followed again by the progestin. Failure to withdraw suggests endometrial unresponsiveness most likely due to intrauterine synechia (Asherman's syndrome). This diagnosis is confirmed by hysteroscopy or hysterosalpingography.

The patient who does withdraw from combined therapy is estrogen deficient. To distinguish between an ovarian disorder and a pituitary disorder, gonadotropin levels are drawn. If elevated (FSH > 40 mIU/ml, LH >30 mIU/ml), the patient's pituitary is functioning normally and she has ovarian failure with lack of estrogen feeding back to inhibit gonadotropin secretion. Patients who are younger than 35 years of age with ovarian failure should be karyotyped to rule out the presence of a Y chromosome. Patients with a Y chromosome are at risk for gonadal tumors and require a gonadectomy. When the gonadotropins are low (LH<5, FSH<5), the patient has a pituitary or hypothalamic disorder. Pituitary insufficiency cannot be distinguished from hypothalamic dysfunction in most cases. Even those patients with normal serum prolactin levels should have a computed tomograph (CT) scan to rule out a pituitary lesion (see Fig. 17-2).

Treatment of secondary amenorrhea is influenced by the patient's desire for fertility as well as the diagnosis. In summary, patients who have low endogenous estrogen and desire no pregnancy should be treated with estrogen/progestogen replacement therapy. Replacement therapy for patients younger than 40 requires more estrogen than postmenopausal replacement therapy: The equivalent of 1.25 mg conjugated equine estrogen is administered daily for the first 25 days of the month, and 10 mg medroxyprogesterone acetate is added daily from day 16 to 25. If endogenous estrogen is normal and the patient desires no pregnancy, she should be treated with either periodic progestogen withdrawal or oral contraceptives. Finally, if the patient desires pregnancy, ovulation induction should be initiated, unless the diagnosis makes such a course impossible (see Chapter 31).

THE CLIMACTERIC AND MENOPAUSE

Definitions

Menopause is the last menstrual period. It is a single point in the climacteric, which is that part of the natural aging process between the woman's reproductive and nonreproductive years. Perimenopause refers to the period before and just after the menopause, during which the decline and cessation of ovarian function occurs.

Epidemiology

Unlike the age at menarche, which is falling, the age at menopause does not reflect a secular trend and has been remarkably stable over the years. There is a general consensus that natural menopause occurs at a median age of about 50 years,[36] and it has not changed for hundreds of years.[37]

The 1982 U.S. Census showed that 47.9 million women living in the United States are 55 years of

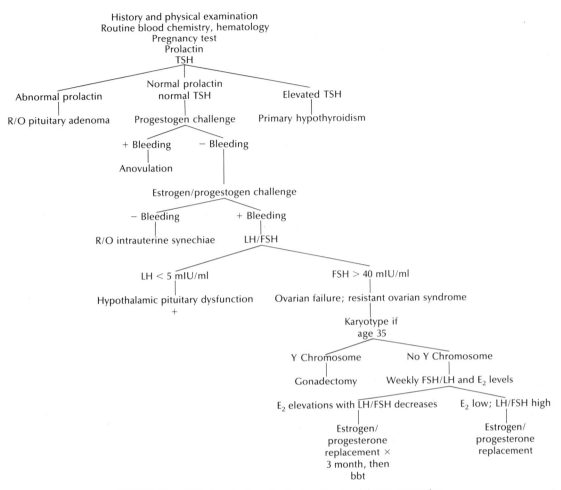

FIGURE 17-2. Clinical evaluation of patients with second-degree amenorrhea.

age and over. They represent one-seventh of the total U.S. population.[38] This number is bound to increase at a rate higher than the increase in the general population with the graying of the baby boom generation and the continuing practice of family limitation by U.S. couples. Thus, with changing population trends and increasing life expectancy, the physician will be confronted with an increasing number of women who will spend more than one-third of their lives in their postmenopausal years.

Endocrinology of the Climacteric

The climacteric and menopause are both expressions of the gradual senescence of the ovary and decreased estrogen production. This endocrine picture is somewhat unique for *Homo sapiens*. In most

animals, fecundity is impaired and then lost because uterine factors increase fetal losses.[39]

In women the reproductive years are followed by an infertile phase of life associated with low estrogen production. Fertility begins to decline approximately 10 years before the menopause and by age 50 almost all germ cells and follicles are lost.[40]

Atresia, the progressive loss of germ cells and follicles from the ovaries, is a continuous process initiated during intrauterine life and continuing throughout the life of the woman until menopause. The rate of atresia is determined by the intrinsic genetic program of the ovary; it is not influenced by the endogenous or exogenous hormonal milieu. The gradual loss of primordial follicles and oocytes continues as the menopause approaches, and the few remaining follicles become increasingly resistant to the gonadotropins.[41] A few immature fol-

TABLE 17-2. Serum Estrogen Values[a]

	Estradiol (pg/ml ± SE)	Estrone (pg/ml ± SE)
Premenopausal women		
Early follicular	63 ± 8	52 ± 5
Late follicular	235	170 ± 13
Oophorectomy	17.9 ± 3.9	26.7 ± 7.2
Postmenopausal women		
Intact ovaries	14.6 ± 2.9	30.3 ± 3.4
Oophorectomized	14.1 ± 1.7	37.6 ± 7.1

[a]Data based on refs. 119, 120, and 121.

licles will undergo maturation and atresia up to a few years after the menopause.[42]

The ovary becomes smaller and fibrotic with atrophy of the ovarian cortex that contained the oocytes and the follicles. The ovarian medulla becomes more abundant with active stromal cells, which are probably the source of androgens. During the late postmenopausal years, even those stromal cells become atrophic so that the ovary is completely replaced by a small mass of fibrotic tissue.

Gonadotropin Secretion

As women approach menopause, the first detectable endocrine manifestation is a gradual increase in plasma FSH.[43] This striking increase of FSH can be noted about a decade before menopause despite apparently normal ovulation. Some time after the rise in FSH, estradiol production decreases slightly and serum LH levels rise. Increased resistance to the gonadotropins of the remaining follicles[41] may explain the decreased estrogen production. Also, the progressive decline in the number of ovarian follicles may be responsible for decreased production of ovarian inhibin and explain this early elevation of FSH.[43] Eventually as estradiol secretion falls to very low levels, both FSH and LH concentrations rise to postmenopausal levels and remain elevated for many years.[44]

Sex Steroids

The single most important factor in the evolution of the physiological changes at menopause is the decrease in estrogen production. With menopause, the amount of estrogen produced is decreased, the cyclicity is lost, and estrone (not estradiol) is the major circulating estrogen.

In premenopausal women, the ovary is the major source of estrogen, and estradiol is the major circulating estrogen derived almost entirely from the secretion of the maturing follicle (see Table 17-2).

During the perimenopausal years, even before the cyclicity of estradiol secretion is lost, there is a slight decrease in estradiol production,[43,45] probably reflecting the waning steroidogenic capability of the aging follicles.

After menopause, both the levels of estradiol and estrone drop, but estrone to a lesser extent than estradiol (Table 17-2) reflecting the absence of maturing ovarian follicles. With the decrease of direct ovarian secretion, alternate sources of estrogen production become important. Androstenedione converted to estrone in the fat and in the liver becomes the primary source of estrogen precursor. Thus, estrone is the most abundant circulating unconjugated estrogen.

At menopause, androstenedione is secreted mainly by the adrenal and thus under ACTH control. The ovarian contribution to this steroid decreases from 30% during the early menopausal years to less than 5% late in the menopause (Fig. 17-3). The rate of conversion of androstenedione to estrone increases with age.[46] Liver disease, hyperthyroidism, and obesity[47] also increase androstenedione to estrone conversion. Estradiol is produced after the menopause by extraglandular conversion of estrone and testosterone.

In summary, as the ovary fails, a major decline of estrogen production takes place. Androgen production continues for a fairly long interval after menopause, and some of these androgens are converted to estrogens in peripheral tissues. However, the

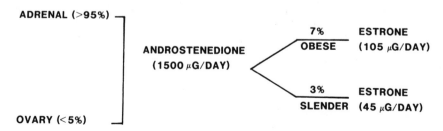

FIGURE 17-3. Production of estrone in postmenopausal women.

concentration of biologically active estrogen is significantly decreased.

Symptomatology

Menstrual Irregularities

Before the establishment of permanent secondary amenorrhea, which is the hallmark of menopause, climacteric women experience menstrual irregularities lasting for several months. Unusually short cycles are particularly frequent and may be one of the earliest signs of perimenopause. They result most often from a shortening in the length of the follicular phase,[48] probably related to increased FSH secretion. Alternatively, short cycles, although still ovulatory, may be related to inadequate luteal phase[49] caused by decreased estrogen production by the aging follicles and thus defective development of LH receptors in the corpus luteum.

Eventually ovulation will fail and uterine bleeding will occur after an estradiol peak[43] without progesterone production. Without progesterone, unopposed estrogens lead to unusually long cycles with episodes of profuse blood loss (dysfunctional uterine bleeding). With fewer follicles capable of development, intervals between menstrual bleeding become increasingly prolonged. Not unusually, after several months of amenorrhea and hot flashes women may experience one or two menstrual periods along with temporary disappearance of the hot flashes before menopause sets in permanently.

Changes in the Reproductive Tract

With the decline of hormonal support, the uterus becomes smaller and the endometrium atrophic. However, prolonged estrogen stimulation (endogenous or exogenous) unopposed by progesterone will increase the risk of endometrial hyperplasia, atypia and endometrial carcinoma. In the vagina the lack of estrogens renders the epithelium thinner and superficial cells disappear from the vaginal smear replaced by intermediate and parabasal cells. Atrophic vaginitis, vaginal dryness, and dyspareunia are the results of estrogen lack. The bladder and urethra are lined by transitional epithelium, which like the vaginal mucosa is sensitive to ovarian steroids. Atrophic distal urethritis in the climacteric may lead to urgency, incontinence, and ascending infections.

Skin Changes

It is difficult to differentiate between the effect of aging and the decrease levels of estrogen on the skin. Estrogen receptors are present in the skin, and estrogen administration will cause edema of the dermis and increased proliferation of the epidermis.[50] With menopause, the skin becomes dry, the epidermis becomes thinner, and the rate of production of melanin increases.

Cardiovascular Changes

Hypertension and atherosclerosis increase in women after menopause. During their premenopausal years, women are relatively free from these diseases as compared with men of similar age. After menopause, the incidence of such conditions becomes similar in both sexes. Early castration increases the risk of coronary atherosclerosis in women.[51] However, the relationship of these conditions to ovarian hormones is not clearly understood. It was thought that young women are protected from coronary heart disease by ovarian hormones and that they lose this protection after menopause or at a younger age after removal of the ovaries. However, Heller and Jacobs[52] suggested that it is men that are at higher risk than are women before age 50. Around the age of 50, men begin to lose a factor that had previously put them at increased risk for coronary heart disease as compared with the incidence in women, hence the apparent increased risk in postmenopausal women. We now know these factors to be low-density lipoprotein (LDL) and high-density lipoprotein (HDL). Yet when women of the same age are compared for risks of major cardiovascular events, premenopausal women have only one-third the risk of postmenopausal women.[53]

Vasomotor Instability

One of the earlier symptoms of estrogen deprivation is vasomotor instability manifested as hot flashes. More than any other symptom climacteric hot flashes will motivate women to seek medical help. Hot flashes are described as a sudden feeling of heat about the face, neck and chest accompanied by flushing of the skin and perspiration. As many as 85% of women in the climacteric suffer from hot flashes,[54] which may start a few years before menopause and continue for many years afterward. They may occur any time, day or night, the latter termed "night sweats."

Hot flashes are associated with an increase in skin temperature, peripheral vasodilation, increase in heart rate and decreased skin resistance.[55] Recent evidence has linked the flushing episode temporally

TABLE 17-3. Symptoms Asociated with the Climacteric

Improved by estrogen therapy	Not improved by estrogen therapy
Insomnia	Joint pain
Irritability	Decreased physical activity
Headache	Backache
Anxiety	Skin changes
Worry about oneself	Decreased coital frequency

with pulsatile release of LH but not FSH.[56,57] However, the LH or GnRH pulses are not directly related to the flush, since untreated women with gonadal dysgenesis do not experience hot flashes, although LH and GnRH secretions closely resemble those of menopausal women. Hot flashes have been objectively documented in women with pituitary insufficiency.[58]

Prior exposure to estrogens appears necessary for the development of hot flashes, since women with gonadal dysgenesis will experience hot flashes after being exposed to estrogen therapy. Hypothalamic neurons, which produce GnRH and the anterior hypothalamic nuclei regulating body temperature, are in close anatomical proximity.[59] Thus neurotransmitter signals associated with GnRH release may affect thermoregulating neurons and trigger the vasomotor flush.

Other Climacteric Symptoms

While hot flashes and menstrual irregularities are the most prominent complaints in a climacteric woman, other symptoms and complaints affect the woman at this age (Table 17-3). Some of these symptoms are related to the natural aging process modified by the individual lifestyle. Others are related to estrogen deprivation and respond to estrogen therapy.

It has been postulated that hot flashes may be responsible for most of the psychological symptoms that occur at the time of menopause. The so-called domino theory proposes that if a woman has severe hot flashes that wake her up several times during the night, night in and night out, it would be likely that she would suffer from insomnia, be irritable, and develop anxiety and worry about herself. Estrogen administration, by abolishing the hot flashes, would indirectly correct the rest of the symptoms.

However, Campbell and Whitehead[60] have shown that such psychological symptoms are corrected by estrogen administration even in those women who are not afflicted by hot flashes. Thus we have to postulate a direct effect of estrogen on the central nervous system (CNS) modulating behavior and other psychological symptoms.

How estrogens affect the CNS is open to speculation. Biogenic amines have long been implicated in the pathogenesis of affective disorders.[61] Modifications in the brain metabolism of serotonin by ovarian steroids have been implicated in estrous behavior.[62] The metabolism of tryptophan, a serotonin precursor, seems to be affected by estrogens. Moreover, catechol estrogens (estrogens with an hydroxyl function in position 2 of the steroid nucleus) share a structural similarity to the catecholamines (Fig. 17-4), and they are found in the brain in concentrations 10 times higher than the parent steroids.[63] Thus they serve as a substrate for the enzyme catechol-O-methyl transferase, the same enzyme that inactivates catecholamines. Thus catechol estrogens can serve as competitive inhibitors of the normal degradation of circulating catecholamines.[64]

Prostaglandins may also play a role in the integration of neuroendocrine function,[65] and estrogens may affect the synthesis and release of prostaglandins in the brain.[66]

In summary, although the evidence is mostly circumstantial, estrogen deficiency may play a role in psychological changes associated with the climacteric by modulating biogenic amines and prostaglandins at the level of the CNS.

Osteoporosis

After the menopause, cortical thickness and tensile strength of bones are reduced, resulting in osteoporosis. With the decrease in bone mass, the bones become more susceptible to fracture. Bone is not a static tissue but it undergoes continuous remodeling throughout life. Osteoclasts reabsorb bone in microscopic cavities; osteoblasts then reform the bone filling the cavities. Normally this remodeling process is closely regulated by mechanical, hormonal, and local factors.

Peak bone mass is achieved by age 30 in females and 40 in males; it is influenced by sex, race, exercise, health, and nutrition. Men have 30% more bone mass than women and blacks 10% more than whites and orientals. In women, bone mass declines rapidly for 3–7 years after the menopause. Bone loss with age is a universal phenomenon. After

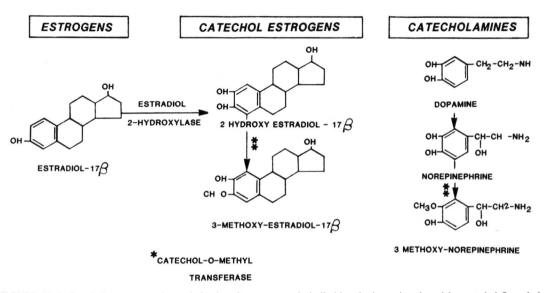

FIGURE 17-4. Catecholestrogens and catecholamines have structural similarities; both are inactivated by catechol-O-methyl transferase.

menopause, bone mass is lost at a rate of 1–1.5% per year. Low bone mineral mass carries an increased risk of fracture.

Characteristically fractures occur in the thoracic and lumbar vertebral bodies, the neck and intertrochanteric regions of the femur and the distal radius. However, osteoporotic individuals may fracture any bone easily. Spine and radial fractures are frequent about the age of 60 and may develop during routine activities such as bending or lifting. Local back pain often is immediate and severe. By contrast, some vertebral fractures do not cause pain and become apparent only because of loss of body heights and the development of kyphosis. As many as 50% of women will develop vertebral fractures by age 75.[67]

Hip fractures are more frequent somewhat later about the age of 70. Among the women who live to be 90, as many as one-third will develop hip fractures. Most patients fail to recover completely, and as many as one-fifth are dead within 1 year.[68]

Physiopathology of Osteoporosis

The cause of osteoporosis is multifactorial. Complex cellular, physiological and metabolic factors underly its pathogenesis. Since many factors regulate normal bone metabolism, multiple etiologies may be possible. In addition to race, other factors possibly implicated include a poor diet low in vitamin D, high in caffeine and alcoholic intake, and high in animal protein. Cigarette smoking and a sedentary lifestyle also have been implicated. Some of these factors may act indirectly through their effects on calcium, estrogen metabolism, or body weight. Current data, however, point to two principal causes: estrogen deficiency and calcium deficiency.

Menopause is often followed by rapid bone loss, but estrogen replacement prevents it.[69,70] Premature osteoporosis follows bilateral oophorectomy but is prevented by estrogen therapy.[71] In experimental animals, calcium deficiency causes osteoporosis. The elderly in the USA often consume a diet deficient in calcium but calcium supplementation reduces the bone loss.

The relationships between calcium balance, vitamin D metabolism, estrogen and aging have been more clearly defined in the past several years.[72] A negative mineral bone loss, serum calcium, phosphorus, parathyroid hormone and 1,25-dihydroxy vitamin D all decrease. The intestinal absorption of calcium also decreases with age. While estrogen administration improves calcium balance, it does so without a direct effect on the bone.

A simplified view of calcium bone homeostosis is shown in Figure 17-5. Estrogen sets the level of bone sensitivity to parathyroid hormone (PTH). In the presence of estrogens larger amounts of PTH are needed to mobilize a given amount of calcium from the bone stores. Increased circulating PTH will promote 25-hydroxylation and 1-hydroxylation of vi-

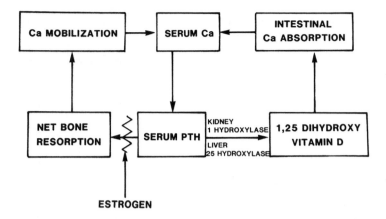

FIGURE 17-5. Simplified view of calcium homeostasis. Levels of parathyroid hormone (PTH) affect serum calcium homeostasis by mobilizing calcium from the bone and by increasing hydroxylation of vitamin D in the kidney. 1,25-Dihydroxy vitamin D increases absorption of dietary calcium from the gut. Estrogen sets the level of bone sensitivity to PTH. In the absence of estrogen, a small amount of PTH mobilizes a greater amount of calcium from bone.

tamin D in the liver and kidney respectively, thereby increasing the circulating levels of 1,25-dihydroxy vitamin D_3, the most active vitamin D metabolite. This will favor increased intestinal absorption of calcium, thereby maintaining ionized serum calcium homeostasis.

Estrogen removal increases bone sensitivity to PTH without changing the sensitivity of its other target organs, the kidneys and, indirectly through vitamin D metabolites, the gut. Thus, the bone becomes a more dominant and easily available source of calcium, while the kidney and intestine become less efficient in conserving calcium.

Diagnosis

In the presence of atraumatic fractures, the diagnosis of osteoporosis is easily made. Identification of women who have milder forms of bone loss is more taxing. As with any other condition an accurate history and physical examination are essential. Attention should be paid to physical activity, diet, and body weight–height ratio. The physician should look for and exclude other causes of secondary osteoporosis, such as hyperparathyroidism, hyperthyroidism, multiple myeloma, metastatic disease, osteomalacia, and hypercortisolism.

No laboratory test will establish the diagnosis of primary osteoporosis, but it may help exclude secondary causes. Thus laboratory studies should include a CBC, urinalysis, total serum calcium, inorganic phosphate, alkaline phosphatase, serum protein, and parathyroid hormone.

Several noninvasive methods are available to evaluate bone density. Standard radiographs of the vertebral spine are available but they are not sensitive to bone loss of less than 30%. More precise but less available techniques include radiogramme-

try for measurements of bone cortical thickness,[73] x-ray photodensitometry,[74] photon absorptiometry,[75] neutron activation analysis,[76] and computed tomography.[77] Although available at some centers, further studies are needed to determine whether these techniques are capable of early identification of women at risk.

Management

Estrogen therapy is highly effective in preventing osteoporosis in women. Estrogen reduces bone resorption and retards or halts bone loss associated with natural or surgical menopause.[78] However, estrogen therapy does not abolish all age-related bone loss and is more effective when administered early in the menopause.[79] Once discontinued, bone loss resumes at an accelerated pace.[71]

Loss of bone density by itself would be of little clinical significance; however, its importance lies in its increased predisposition to fractures. During the past few years, accumulating data have shown a substantial reduction in hip and wrist fractures in women on estrogen replacement therapy. In a case-controlled study, Weiss et al.[80] showed in 1980 that the risk of hip and lower forearm fractures in postmenopausal women taking estrogen for 6 years or more was 50–60% lower than that of women who did not take estrogens.

The rate of vertebral fractures are also reduced by estrogen therapy. Even when started late in the climacteric estrogen prevents further bone loss, but it does not restore bone mass to premenopausal levels.[81] Only small doses of oral estrogens are needed,[80] such as 0.625 mg conjugated equine estrogens, 20 μg ethinyl estradiol, or 2 mg micronized estradiol daily. In women with a contraindication to estrogen treatment, progestins may be useful, although they are not as effective as estrogens[82] in preventing calcium loss.[83]

Other Therapeutic Agents

The elemental calcium intake in the usual American diet averages between 450 and 550 mg, well below the dietary allowance of 800 mg recommended by the National Research Council.[84] Metabolic balance studies indicate that healthy premenopausal women may require about 1 g calcium daily to maintain a positive calcium balance, while postmenopausal women not treated with estrogens may require about 1.5 g calcium per day.[85,86] Thus, the recommended dietary allowance for calcium is evidently too low, particularly for postmenopausal women.

Some studies have shown that postmenopausal bone loss can be delayed by high intake of dietary calcium.[87] However, daily calcium intake higher than 1000–1500 mg may cause hypercalcemia, hypercalciuria, and kidney stones in susceptible people. Other possible therapeutic agents such as vitamin D analogues, calcitonin, diphosphonates, 1–34 fragment of synthetic PTH, thiazides, and sodium fluoride are currently under investigation; however, their efficiency and safety are unproven.

Risks of Estrogen Therapy

Numerous potential benefits may be gained with estrogen therapy of the climacteric. However, the benefits should be balanced against the potential risks of such therapy.

The estrogen content of the oral contraceptives is responsible for many of the risks associated with this form of contraception. Postmenopausal estrogen therapy is different from oral contraceptives because of the significantly lower dosage and different estrogens used. Postmenopausal estrogen therapy is physiological estrogen replacement as opposed to pharmacologic suppression of ovulation by an estrogen–progestogen combination of oral contraceptive. Thus many of the complications seen with oral contraceptives are not present with noncontraceptive estrogen replacement.

The risk of hypertension, stroke, or thromboembolism is not increased in women on replacement estrogen therapy.[88,89] The risk of myocardial infarction may possibly be decreased.[90,91] This is not surprising, since oral contraceptives and noncontraceptive estrogens differ in their effect on blood lipids. Noncontraceptive hormones have been associated with lowered low-density lipoprotein (LDL) and very-low-density lipoprotein (VLDL) cholesterol and triglyceride levels and with an increase in high-density lipoprotein (HDL) cholesterol.[92] A strong and inverse correlation exists between HDL cholesterol and coronary heart disease.[93,94] Given the high prevalence of death from coronary heart disease in the U.S. population, the use of replacement estrogen in the menopause would be of great public health benefit.

Endometrial Cancer

In 1975 Smith and co-workers[95] first pointed out the association of exogenous estrogens and endometrial carcinoma. Since then, this relationship has been confirmed by several studies.[96,97] Although all reports consist of retrospective case-control studies and are thus open to some criticism because of possible bias in the diagnosis, selection of controls and presence of other confounding variables,[98] the available evidence is convincing: Estrogen replacement therapy is associated with an increased risk of endometrial cancer ranging between 2 and 10 times that of untreated controls.

The risk is related to the duration of exposure, the dose and the schedule of administration (i.e., continuous versus cyclic).[97] The increase in endometrial cancer seems limited to early, highly localized, well-differentiated easily treated cancers.[99] Thus, despite the increased incidence of endometrial cancer in the United States, the mortality from the disease has decreased. More recent studies have placed the problem of sex steroid replacement therapy and endometrial cancer in clinical perspective.[100,101] The risk can be reduced or eliminated by the addition of a progestin.[102–104] This is not surprising, for although estrogens stimulate endometrial growth, progestins inhibit such growth. This antiestrogenic effect is mediated by a decrease in the synthesis of estrogen receptors and an increase in estradiol dehydrogenase, an enzyme which converts estradiol to estrone.

Small doses of progestin are sufficient provided they are administered for at least 10 days.[105] Moreover, the addition of the progestin to the estrogen regime did not reduce the metabolic benefit of estrogen treatment.[106]

Breast Cancer

The association between estrogen and breast cancer in experimental animals is well known. Since breast cancer is a frequent and lethal disease in women, the possibility that estrogen use increases the risk of breast cancer requires close scrutiny.

The hormonal dependency of breast tissue and the increased incidence of breast cancer in conditions associated with unopposed estrogen have suggested a permissive or supportive role for this hormone in the pathogenesis of cancer of the breast.[107]

However, careful review of several well-conducted case-control studies has failed to demonstrate any association between exogenous estrogen use and increased incidence of breast cancer. More recent studies have also confirmed that noncontraceptive estrogens do not increase the risk of breast cancer,[108,109] and one study suggests a decrease risk for this malignancy in women taking both estrogen and progestin.[110] Thus, it may be prudent to use a program of estrogen–progestin therapy even in women who have undergone a hysterectomy.

Current Recommendations

After considering all available evidence, the balance of risks and benefits of hormonal replacement therapy does favor therapeutic intervention. Estrogen administration does prevent osteoporosis, controls vasomotor symptoms, alleviates atrophic changes of the urogenital system, and may provide some protection against coronary artery disease. It may also maintain the integrity of the skin and breasts.

Estrogens should be administered in a cyclical fashion and concomitantly with a progestin. This approach is probably more important than the type of estrogen administered, although some evidence would favor the use of "natural estrogens." Ethinyl estradiol and diethylstilbestrol (DES) seem to produce a more marked effect on liver proteins as compared with their effect on gonadotropin sup-

TABLE 17-4. Estrogen Bioequivalence[a,b]

End point	E_2V (mg)	EE (μg)	Conj. E (mg)	E_2 (mg)
Endometrium	2	20	1.25	2
Coagulation system	2	50	2.50	2
Liver	1	10	1.25	1
Lipids	2	20	2.50	2
Bone	1	20	0.625	1

[a]From Upton.[46]
[b]E_2V, estradiol valerate; EE, ethinyl estradiol; Conj. E, premarin; E_2, 17β-estradiol.

TABLE 17-5. Current Recommendations for Hormonal Replacement Therapy of the Menopause

History, physical examination, and pap smear
CBC, urinalysis, total serum calcium, inorganic phosphate, alkaline phosphatase, parathyroid hormone, and lipid profile
Screening mammography
Progesterone challenge test—if positive: endometrial sampling
Conjugated estrogen, 0.625 mg, or micronized estradiol, 1 mg from first through twenty-fifth day of month
Medroxyprogesterone acetate, 5 mg from sixteenth through twenty-fifth day of month
Calcium carbonate, 600 mg, 2 tablets at bedtime daily
Diet and moderate exercise

pression.[111] Table 17-4 shows the approximate bioequivalence of some commonly used estrogens, although the exact potency of each preparation is difficult to ascertain.[112]

Equivalent amounts of estrogen necessary to prevent osteoporosis with the least endometrial stimulation are 0.625 mg conjugated estrogen or 1 mg micronized estradiol.[112] Whatever estrogen is chosen, it should be given in cyclical fashion, usually from the 1st through the 25th day of the month (Table 17-5). To decrease the risk of endometrial hyperplasia, a progestin must be administered for at least the last 10 days of estrogen administration. Medroxyprogesterone acetate in doses of 5 mg is sufficient to suppress the endometrial receptor.[113] In vivo studies are needed to confirm the adequacy of this dose. The 19-nortestosterone progestins may be less desirable, since they reverse the beneficial increase in HDL-cholesterol induced by estrogens.[114] If chosen, norethindrone 2.5 mg or norgesterel 150 μg, will probably suffice.[115] Higher doses are often associated with depression, edema and weight gain. There is a difference of opinion whether to perform an endometrial sampling before the initiation of sequential estrogen–progesterone therapy. Some authors[116] suggest aspiration endometrial biopsy to identify those cases in whom endometrial hyperplasia is present. Others[117] find it unnecessary unless other indications exist such as postmenopausal bleeding. Since it has been estimated that more than 3000 biopsies would be needed to uncover an invasive lesion in an asymptomatic woman, we suggest that prior to therapy a progestin challenge test be performed.[117] Women with chronic estrogen exposure will respond with a withdrawal bleeding. Endometrial sampling can thus be limited to those women at higher risk for endometrial pathology. Many women on sequential estrogen–progestin therapy will experience withdrawal vaginal bleeding during the last days of the month upon discontinuation of the medication. Women should be alerted to this possibility and counseled to consider scheduled bleeding as a normal event. Breakthrough bleeding at any other time warrants endometrial sampling. Some authors also suggest that endometrial biopsy be performed every 2 or 3 years even in the absence of unscheduled bleeding.[117] We believe that, in absence of abnormal bleeding and if a progestin is administered for at least 10 days of each month, routine endometrial sampling may be unnecessary.

Calcium supplementation is also useful in preventing bone loss. This is best accomplished by the administration of 500 mg elementary calcium given as a single dose at bedtime.[118] Calcium loss is maximal during the night. An adequate diet containing approximately 600 U vitamin D and a program of moderate exercise should also be encouraged.

When estrogens are contraindicated, progestin alone may be used to relieve vasomotor symptoms and inhibit bone loss although less effective than estrogens.[82] Oral Provera (30 mg/day) and Depoprovera (150 mg IM every 2 months) are equally useful. If estrogens are not used, calcium supplementation should be increased to 1 g/day, and atrophic dyspareunia may be partially relieved by the use of vaginal lubricants.

SUMMARY

Loss of cyclic menses occurs physiologically during pregnancy, lactation, and the climacteric. The most common cause of nonphysiological secondary amenorrhea is hypothalamic amenorrhea, but disorders of the pituitary, ovaries, uterus, and thyroid can also result in secondary amenorrhea. Treatment of these disorders is influenced by the patient's desire for fertility as well as the level of her endogenous estrogen.

Women in the climacteric years develop physiological secondary amenorrhea. The lack of ovarian estrogen biosynthesis results in signs and symptoms which include hot flashes, urogenital atrophy, mood changes, and osteoporosis. The significant health risk posed by osteoporosis mandates estrogen/progestin replacement therapy. The risks of replacement therapy must be weighed against its significant benefits. When contraindications to es-

trogen therapy exist, other therapeutic modalities are chosen.

This chapter discusses the differential diagnosis, evaluation and treatment of secondary amenorrhea as well as the climacteric syndrome. The indications for, dosage of, and risks of estrogen/progestogen replacement therapy are described.

QUESTIONS

1. A 52-year-old woman with previously regular cyclic menses presents with 8 weeks of secondary amenorrhea, mood changes, and feeling warm. What must be done before initiating treatment?

2. A 28-year-old woman had no menses since her elective abortion 3 years ago. She is not pregnant and has normal prolactin and TSH levels. Her basal body temperature chart reveals a thermal shift and her progesterone level is in the ovulatory range. What is her diagnosis and how should it be confirmed?

3. A patient with ovarian failure is found to have a mosaic karyotype with only 20% of her cells being 46,XY and 80% 46,XX. Does she need a gonadectomy?

4. Can oral contraceptives be used for estrogen/progesterone replacement therapy after the menopause?

5. What is the most sensitive noninvasive technique of determining bone density?

REFERENCES

1. Sharman A: Menstruation after childbirth. *J. Obstet Gynaecol Br Emp* 58:440, 1951
2. Perez A, Vela P, Masnic GS, et al: First ovulation after childbirth: The effect of breastfeeding. *Am J Obstet Gynecol* 114:1041, 1972
3. Hamou J, Salat-Baroux J, Siegler AM: Diagnosis and treatment of intrauterine adhesions by microhysteroscopy. *Fertil Steril* 39:321, 1983
4. Raj SG, Thompson IE, Berger MJ, et al: Clinical aspects of the polycystic ovary syndrome. *Obstet Gynecol* 49:552, 1977
5. Goldzieher JW, Green JA: The polycystic ovary: Clinical and histologic features. *J Clin Endocrinol Metab* 22:325, 1962
6. Chamlian DL, Taylor HB: Endometrial hyperplasia in young women. *Obstet Gynecol* 36:659, 1970
7. Garcia J, Jones GS, Wentz AC: The use of clomiphene citrate. *Fertil Steril* 28:707–717, 1977

8. Reyes FI, Koh KS, Farman C: Fertility in women with gonadal dysgenesis. *Am J Obstet Gynecol* 126:668, 1976

9. Kable WT, Yussman, MA: Pregnancy in mosaic Turner patients: Case report and a guide to reproductive counseling. *Fertil Steril* 35:477–478, 1981

10. Rebar RW, Erickson GF, Yen SSC: Idiopathic premature ovarian failure: Clinical and endocrine characteristics. *Fertil Steril* 37:35, 1982

11. Szlachter BN, Nachitgall LE, Epstein J, et al: Premature menopause: A reversible entity? *Obstet Gynecol* 54:396–398, 1979

12. Starup J, Philip J, Sele V: Oestrogen treatment and subsequent pregnancy in two patients with severe hypergonadotropic ovarian failure. *Acta Endocrinol (Copenh)* 89:149–157, 1978

13. Shapiro AG, Rubin A: Spontaneous pregnancy in association with hypergonadotropic ovarian failure. *Fertil Steril* 28:500–501, 1977

14. Schreiber JR, Davajan V, Kletzky OA: A case of intermittent ovarian failure. *Am J Obstet Gynecol* 132:698–699, 1978

15. Johnson TR Jr, Peterson EP: Gonadotropin-induced pregnancy following "premature ovarian failure." *Fertil Steril* 31:351–352, 1979

16. Gordon DL, Paulsen CA: Premature menopause in XO/XX/XXX/XXXX mosaicism. *Am J Obstet Gynecol* 97:85–90, 1967

17. Polansky S, dePapp EW: Pregnancy associated with hypergonadotropic hypogonadism. *Obstet Gynecol* 47:475–515, 1976

18. O'Herlihy C, Pepperell RJ, Evans JH: The significance of FSH elevation in young women with disorders of ovulation. *Br Med J* 281:1447–1450, 1981

19. Shangold MM, Turksoy RN, Bashford RA, et al: Pregnancy following the insensitive ovary syndrome. *Fertil Steril* 28:1179–1181, 1977

20. Maxson WS, Wentz AC: The gonadotropin resistant ovary syndrome. *Semin Reprod Endocrinol* 1(2):147–160, 1983

21. Jones GS: Editorial comment. *Obstet Gynecol Surv* 30:700, 1975

22. Irvine WJ, Chan MMW, Scarth L, et al: Immunological aspects of premature ovarian failure associated with idiopathic Addison's disease. *Lancet* 2:883–884, 1968

23. Zacur HA, Foster GV, Tyson JE: Multifactorial regulation of prolactin secretion. *Lancet* 1:140, 1976

24. Carlson HF, Ippoliti AF: Cimetidine, an H2 antihistamine stimulates prolactin secretion in man. *J Clin Endocrinol Metab* 45:367, 1977

25. Chang RJ: Hyperprolactinemia and menstrual dysfunction. *Clin Obstet Gynecol* 26:736–748, 1983

26. Chiodine P, Luizzi A, Cozzi R, et al: Size reduction of macroprolactinomas by bromocryptine or lisuride treatment. *J Clin Endocrinol Metab* 53:737, 1981

27. Yen SSC, Lasley BL, Wang CF, et al: The operating characteristics of the hypothalamic–pituitary system during the menstrual cycle and observations of biological actions of somatostatin. *Recent Prog Horm Res* 31:321, 1975

28. Marshall JC, Kelch RD: Low dose pulsatile gonadotropin-releasing hormone in anorexia nervosa: A model of human pubertal development. *J Clin Endocrinol Metab* 49:712, 1979

29. Starkey TA, Lee RA: Menstruation and fertility in anorexia nervosa. *Am J Obstet Gynecol* 105:374, 1969

30. Gordon S, Cantrall EW, Leklenick WP, et al: Steroid and lipid metabolism: The hypocholesterolaemic effects of estrogen metabolites. *Steroids* 4:267, 1964

31. Eisenberg E: Toward an understanding of reproductive function in anorexia nervosa. *Fertil Steril* 36:543, 1981

32. Leyendecker G, Wildt L: Induction of ovulation with chronic intermittent (pulsatile) administration of Gn-RH in women with hypothalamic amenorrhea. *J Reprod Fertil* 69:397, 1983

33. Fishman J, Hellman I, Zumoff B: Influence of thyroid hormone in estrogen metabolism in man. *J Clin Endocrinol Metab* 22:389, 1962

34. MacLeod SC: Endocrine effects of oral contraception. *Int J Gynaecol Obstet* 16:518, 1979

35. March CM, Mishell DR Jr: A 10-year comparison of post oral contraceptive amenorrhea with amenorrhea unrelated to use of drugs, in *Endocrinology of Human Infertility: New Aspects, Serono Symposium, Oxford,* 1980, p 207.

36. McKinlay S, Jefferys M, Thompson B: An investigation of the age at menopause. *J Biosoc Sci* 4:161, 1972

37. Amundsen DW, Diers CJ: The age of menopause in medieval Europe. *Human Biol* 45:605, 1973

38. US Bureau of the Census: Current Population Reports, Series P-25, No. 952, Projections of the Population of the United States, by Age, Sex, and Race: 1983 to 2080. Washington, DC, US Government Printing Office, 1984

39. Talbert GB: Effect of maternal age on reproductive capacity. *Am J Obstet Gynecol* 102:451, 1968

40. Costoff A: An ultrastructural study of ovarian changes in the menopause, in Greenblatt RB, Mahesh UB, McDonough PG (eds): *The Menopausal Syndrome.* New York, Medcom, 1974, p 12

41. Van de Wiele R, Bogumil J, Dyrenfurth I, et al: Mechanisms regulating the menstrual cycle in women. *Recent Prog Horm Res* 26:63, 1970

42. Ross GT, Van de Wiele RL, Frantz AG: The ovaries and breasts, in Williams RH (ed): *Textbook of Endocrinology,* Ed. 5, Philadelphia, Saunders, 1974, p 360

43. Sherman BM, West JH, Korenman SG: The menopausal transition: Analysis of LH, FSH, estradiol and progesterone concentrations during menstrual cycles of older women. *J Clin Endocrinol Metab* 42:247, 1976

44. Chakravarti S, Collins WP, Forecast JD, et al: Hormonal profiles after the menopause. *Br Med J* 2:784, 1976

45. Reyes FI, Winter SD, Faiman C: Pituitary–ovarian relationships preceding the menopause. *Am J Obstet Gynecol* 129:557, 1977

46. Upton GV: Therapeutic considerations of the management of the climacteric. *J Reprod Med* 29:71, 1984

47. McDonald PC, Edman CD, Hemsell DL, et al: Effect of obesity on conversion of plasma androstenedione to estrone in postmenopausal women with and without endometrial cancer. *Am J Obstet Gynecol* 130:448, 1978

48. Treloar AE, Boynton RE, Behn BG, et al: Variability of the human menstrual cycle through reproductive life. *Int J Fertil* 12:77, 1967

49. Sherman BM, Korenman SG: Hormonal characteristics of the human menstrual cycle throughout reproductive life. *J Clin Invest* 55:699, 1975

50. Stumpf WE, Madhabananda S, Joshi SG: Oestrogen target cells in the skin. *Experientia* 30:196, 1974

51. Parrish HM, Carr CA, Hall DG, et al: Time interval from castration in premenopausal women to development of excessive coronary atherosclerosis. *Am J Obstet Gynecol* 99:155, 1967

52. Heller RJ, Jacobs HS: Coronary heart disease in relation to age, sex, and the menopause. *Br Med J* 1:472, 1978

53. Shurtleff D: Some characteristics related to the incidence

of cardiovascular disease and death: Framingham study, 18 year follow up, in Kannel WB, Gordon T (eds): *The Framingham Study*, Section 30. Washington, DC, Department of Health, Education and Welfare publication 74-599, 1974

54. Thompson B, Hart SA, Durno D: Menopausal age and symptomatology in general practice. *J Biosoc Sci* 5:71, 1973

55. Molnar GW: Body temperatures during menopausal hot flashes. *J Appl Physiol* 38:499, 1975

56. Tataryn IV, Meldrum DR, Frumar AM, et al: LH, FSH, and skin temperature during the menopausal hot flash. *J Clin Endocrinol Metab* 49:152, 1979

57. Casper RF, Yen SSC, Wilkes MM: Menopausal flashes: A neuroendocrine link with pulsatile luteinizing hormone secretion. *Science* 205:823, 1979

58. Meldrum DR, Erlik Y, Lu JKH, et al: Objectively recorded hot flushes in patients with pituitary insufficiency. *J Clin Endocrinol Metab* 52:684, 1981

59. Reaves TA, Hayward JM: Hypothalamic and extrahypothalamic thermoregulatory centers, in Lomax P, Schonbaum E (eds): *Body Temperature: Regulation, Drug Effects and Therapeutic Implications*. New York, Dekker, 1979, p 45

60. Campbell S, Whitehead M: Estrogen therapy and the menopausal syndrome. *Clin Obstet Gynecol* 4:31, 1977

61. Schildkraut JJ: The catecholamine hypothesis of affective disorders: A review of supporting evidence. *Am J Psychiatry* 122:509, 1965

62. Munaro NI: The effect of ovarian steroids on hypothalamic 5-hydroxytryptamine neuronal activity. *Neuroendocrinology* 26:270, 1978

63. Paul SM, Axelrod J: Catecholestrogens: Presence in brain and endocrine tissues. *Science* 197:657, 1977

64. Ball P, Knuppen R, Haupt M, et al: Interactions between estrogens and catecholamines: III. Studies on the methylation of catechol estrogens, catecholamines and other catechols by the catechol-O-methyl-transferase of human liver. *J Clin Endocrinol Metab* 34:736, 1972

65. Brody MJ, Kadowitz PJ: Prostaglandins as modulators of the autonomic nervous system. *Fed Proc* 33:48, 1974

66. Roberts JS, McCracken JA: Prostaglandin $F_{2\alpha}$ production by the brain during estrogen-induced secretion of luteinizing hormone. *Science* 190:894, 1975

67. Iskrant AP: The etiology of hip fractures in females. *Am J Public Health* 58:485, 1968

68. National Institutes of Health: *Consensus Development Conference on Osteoporosis, Washington, DC, April 2, 1984*

69. Lindsay R, Hart DM, Aitken JM, et al: Long-term prevention of postmenopausal osteoporosis by oestrogen: Evidence for an increased bone mass after delayed onset of oestrogen treatment. *Lancet* 1:1038, 1976

70. Lindsay R, Hart DM, MacLean A, et al: Bone response to termination of oestrogen treatment. *Lancet* 1:1325, 1978

71. Lindsay R et al: Prevention of spinal osteoporosis in oophorectomized women. *Lancet* 2:1151, 1980

72. Gallagher JC, Riggs BL, Eisman J, et al: Intestinal calcium absorption and serum vitamin D metabolites in normal subjects and osteoporotic patients: Effect of age and dietary calcium. *J Clin Invest* 64:729, 1979

73. Gallagher JC, Nordin BEC: Oestrogens and calcium metabolism. *Front Horm Res* 2:98, 1973

74. Anderson JB, Shimmins J, Smith DA: A new technique for the measurement of metacarpal density. *Br J Radiol* 39:443, 1966

75. Boyd RM, Cameron EC, McIntosh HW, et al: Measurement of bone mineral content in vivo using photon absorptiometry. *Can Med Assoc J* 111:1201, 1974

76. Cohn SH, Ellis KJ, Wallach S, et al: Absolute and relative deficit in total-skeletal calcium and radial bone mineral in osteoporosis. *J Nucl Med* 15:428, 1974

77. Cann CE, Genart HK: Precise measurement of vertebral mineral content by computed tomography. *J Comput Assist Tomogr* 4:493, 1980

78. Meema S, Bunker ML, Meema HE: Preventive effect of estrogen on postmenopausal bone loss. *Arch Intern Med* 135:1436, 1975

79. Nachtigall LE, Nachtigall RH, Nachtigall RD, et al: Estrogen replacement therapy. I: A 10-year prospective study in the relationship to osteoporosis. *Obstet Gynecol* 53:277, 1979

80. Weiss NS, Ure CL, Ballard JH, et al: Decreased risk of fractures of the hip and lower forearm with postmenopausal use of estrogen. *N Engl J Med* 303(21):1195, 1980

81. Recker RR, Saville PD, Heaney RP: Effect of estrogens and calcium carbonate on bone loss in postmenopausal women. *Ann Intern Med* 87:649, 1977

82. Lindsay R, Hart DM, Purdie D, et al: Comparative effects of oestrogen and a progestogen on bone loss in postmenopausal women. *Clin Sci Mol Med* 54:193, 1978

83. Davidson BJ, Deftos LJ, Meldrum DR, et al: Effect of medroxyprogesterone acetate (MPA) on bone metabolism of postmenopausal women. The Society for Gynecologic Investigation, abst 279, 1980

84. National Research Council: *Recommended Dietary Allowances*, 9th ed. Washington, DC: National Academy of Sciences, 1980, p 129

85. Heaney RP, Recker RR, Saville PD: Calcium balance and calcium requirements in middle-aged women. *Am J Clin Nutr* 30:1603, 1977

86. Heaney RP, Recker RR, Saville PD: Menopausal changes in calcium balance performance. *J Lab Clin Med* 92:953, 1978

87. Horsman A, Gallagher JC, Simpson M, et al: Prospective trial of oestrogen and calcium in postmenopausal women. *Br Med J* 2:789, 1977

88. Pfeffer RI, Kurosaki TT, Charlton SK: Estrogen use and blood pressure in later life. *Am J Epidemiol* 110:469, 1979

89. Pfeffer RI, Van Den Noort: Estrogen use and stroke risk in postmenopausal women. *Am J Epidemiol* 103:445, 1976

90. Rosenberg L, Armstrong B, Jick H: Myocardial infarction and estrogen therapy in postmenopausal women. *N Engl J Med* 294:1256: 1976

91. Ross RK, Mack TM, Paganini-Hill A, Arthur M, et al: Menopausal oestrogen therapy and protection from death from ischaemic heart disease. *Lancet* 1:858, 1981

92. Wallace RB, Hoover J, Barrett-Conner E, et al: Altered plasma lipid and lipo-protein associated with oral contraceptive and oestrogen use. *Lancet* 2:112, 1979

93. Gordon T, Castelli WP, Hjortland MC, et al: High density lipoprotein as a protective factor against coronary heart disease. *Am J Med* 62:707, 1977

94. Miller NE, Thelle DS, Forde OH, et al: The Tromso heart study. High-density lipoprotein and coronary heart disease: A prospective case-control study. *Lancet* 1:965, 1977

95. Smith DC, Prentice R, Thompson DJ, et al: Association of exogenous estrogens and endometrial carcinoma. *N Engl J Med* 293:1164, 1975

96. Ziel AK, Finkle WD: Increased risk of endometrial car-

cinoma among users of conjugated estrogens. *N Engl J Med* 293:1167, 1975

97. Mack TM, Pike MC, Henderson BE, et al: Estrogens and endometrial cancer in a retirement community. *N Engl J Med* 294:1262, 1976

98. Horwitz RI, Feinstein AR: Alternative analytic methods for case control studies of estrogens and endometrial cancer. *N Engl J Med* 299:1089, 1978

99. Hulka BS: Effect of exogenous estrogen on postmenopausal women: The epidemiological evidence. *Obstet Gynecol Surv* 35:389, 1980

100. Cramer DW, Knapp RC: Review of epidemiologic studies of endometrial cancer and exogenous estrogen. *Obstet Gynecol* 54:521, 1979

101. Sturde DW, Wade-Evans T, Paterson MEL, et al: Relations between bleeding pattern, endometrial histology, and oestrogen treatment in menopausal women. *Br Med J* 1:1575, 1978

102. Hammond CB, Jelovsek FR, Lee KL, et al: Effects of long-term estrogen replacement therapy. II. Neoplasia. *Am J Obstet Gynecol* 133:537, 1979

103. Gambrell RD Jr, Massey FM, Castaneda TA, et al: Reduced incidence of endometrial cancer among postmenopausal women treated with progestogens. *J Am Geriatr Soc* 27:389, 1979

104. Paterson MEL, Wade-Evans T, Sturdee DW, et al: Endometrial disease after treatment with oestrogens and progestogens in the climacteric. *Br Med J* 1:822, 1980

105. Whitehead MI, Townsend PT, Pryse-Davies J, et al: Effects of estrogen and progestins on the biochemistry and morphology of the postmenopausal endometrium. *N Engl J Med* 305:1599, 1981

106. Hammond CB, Jelovsek FR, Lee KL, et al: Effects of long-term estrogen replacement therapy. I. Metabolic effects. *Am J Obstet Gynecol* 133:525, 1979

107. Korenman SG: Oestrogen window hypothesis of the aetiology of breast cancer. *Lancet* 1:700, 1980

108. Kaufman DW, Miller DR, Rosenberg L, et al: Noncontraceptive estrogen use and the risk of breast cancer. *JAMA* 252:63, 1984

109. Hulka BS, Chambless LE, Deubner DC, et al: Breast cancer and estrogen replacement therapy. *Am J Obstet Gynecol* 143:638, 1982

110. Gambrell RD, Maier RC, Sanders BI: Decreased incidence of breast cancer in postmenopausal estrogen–progestogen users. *Obstet Gynecol* 62:435, 1983

111. Mashchak CA, Lobo RA, Dozono-Takano R, et al: Comparison of pharmacodynamic properties of various estrogen formulations. *Am J Obstet Gynecol* 144:511, 1982

112. Upton GV: Therapeutic considerations in the management of the climacteric: A critical analysis of prevalent treatments. *J Reprod Med* 29:71, 1984

113. Gibbons WE, Lobo RA, Roy S, et al: Evaluation of estrogen receptor status in the endometria of postmenopausal women on sequential estrogen–progestin therapy. The Endocrine Society Program, abst 1079, 1982

114. Hirvonen E, Malkonen M, Manninen V: Effects of different progestogens on lipoproteins during postmenopausal replacement therapy. *N Engl J Med* 304:560, 1981

115. Whitehead MI, Townsend PT, Pryse-Davies, J, et al: Effects of estrogens and progestins on the biochemistry and morphology of the postmenopausal endometrium. *N Engl J Med* 305:1599, 1981

116. Judd HL, Cleary RE, Creasman WT, et al: Estrogen replacement therapy. *Obstet Gynecol* 58:267, 1981

117. Gambrell RD Jr, Massey FM, Castenda TA, et al: Use of the progestogen challenge test to reduce the risk of endometrial cancer. *Obstet Gynecol* 55:732, 1980

118. Belchetz PE, Lloyd MW, Johns RGS, et al: Effect of late night calcium supplements on overnight urinary calcium excretion in premenopausal and postmenopausal women. *Br Med J* 2:510, 1973

119. Judd HL: Hormonal dynamics associated with the menopause. *Clin Obstet Gynecol* 19:775, 1976

120. Judd HL, Judd GE, Lucas WE, et al: Endocrine function of the postmenopausal ovary: Concentration of androgens and estrogens in ovarian and peripheral vein blood. *J Clin Endocrinol Metab* 39:1020, 1974

121. Baird DT, Guevara A: Concentration of unconjugated estrone and estradiol in peripheral plasma in nonpregnant women throughout the menstrual cycle, castrate and postmenopausal women and in men. *J Clin Endocrinol Metab* 29:149, 1969

ANSWERS

1. Pregnancy must be ruled out.

2. Intrauterine synechiae/HSG or hysteroscopy.

3. Yes. Any percentage of cells with a Y chromosome poses a risk of the development of gonadal tumors.

4. No. The estrogen dose is too high and the progestin may adversely affect the lipid profile. In addition, the progestin need not be given every day of therapy.

5. CT scan of lumbar vertebrae, however it exposes the patient to about 250 mrem radiation.

18

Endometriosis

M. YUSOFF DAWOOD

HISTORICAL BACKGROUND

The original histological description of endometriosis dates back to 1860 by von Rokitansky.[1] In 1899 Russell described the disease. However, it was not until six decades ago that the term "endometriosis" was coined by Sampson.[2] Although significant advances have been made in many aspects of endometriosis, its etiology and pathogenesis remain poorly understood.

During the 1950s, Karnaky[3] employed progressively increasing doses of estrogen to suppress ovulation for the treatment of endometriosis and thereby established the concept of ovarian suppression for the treatment of endometriosis. This was quickly followed by the pseudopregnancy regimen introduced by Kistner in 1958.[4] During the 1970s, danazol therapy quickly gained widespread acceptance because of its effectiveness in relieving symptoms of endometriosis and promoting fertility.[5] During the present decade promising preliminary data have ushered in the potential use of reversible "medical oophorectomy" with the gonadotropin-releasing hormone (GnRH) analogue for the medical management of endometriosis.

M. YUSOFF DAWOOD • Department of Obstetrics and Gynecology, Division of Reproductive Endocrinology, University of Illinois College of Medicine, Chicago, Illinois 60612.

DEFINITION

Endometriosis is the condition wherein endometrial tissue is found to be established in sites outside the endometrial cavity. Ectopic endometrium found in the uterine wall is referred to as endometriosis interna or adenomyosis. Ectopic endometrium located at sites other than the uterus is referred to as endometriosis externa or generally referred to as endometriosis. Since adenomyosis appears to behave quite differently and for all purposes is a different disorder, this chapter deals exclusively with endometriosis externa.

INCIDENCE

The incidence of endometriosis appears to be increasing; such an increase is both real and apparent. While the real increase is due to the current trend of postponing conception well into the fourth decade of life, the apparent increase is due to both the frequent and justifiable use of diagnostic laparoscopy as well as the heightened awareness of this disease complex by the gynecologist.

In 1949, Meigs[6] found that 5–15% of patients undergoing pelvic operations had endometriosis. This incidence increased to 18% of all gynecological laparotomies in 1978.[7] It is currently estimated that at least one-third to one-half of all patients undergoing major gynecological procedures have findings of endometriosis.[8] With increasing numbers of women working and pursuing careers and the accompanying deferment of pregnancies into the fourth decade of life, the incidence of endometriosis is likely to increase further.

Contrary to traditionally held views, endometriosis is more common than hitherto believed. Teenagers accounted for 8.5% of the patients with endometriosis in one group.[9] In more recent series, endometriosis accounted for 65%[9,10] and 47%[11] of 43 and 140 symptomatic teenagers, respectively, who underwent laparoscopy.

Endometriosis was found in 21% of 54 women who had elective sterilization[12] and in another study in 74% if the tubes were sterilized within 4 cm and 20% in women whose tubes were sterilized more than 4 cm from the proximal end.[13] Although endometriosis regresses with the menopause when ovarian cyclical activity ceases, the frequency of postmenopausal endometriosis was 1.3% in a series of 903 patients operated on for endometriosis.[14]

There is a familial incidence of endometriosis. While there is a 7% relative risk of developing endometriosis if a first degree female relative has it,[15] the incidence of severe endometriosis in the familial group was 61.1% as opposed to 23.8% in the non-familial group.[16] A recent study on HLA in patients with endometriosis showed no particular distribution of HLA type in women with endometriosis.[17] Contrary to the former belief that endometriosis affects whites more often than blacks, it is now clear that black women are as frequently affected by endometriosis as their white counterparts.[9]

PATHOGENESIS

The pathogenesis of endometriosis remains uncertain and abounds with theories. At least 12 theories have been advanced with the principal ones being:

Retrograde Menstruation

The most widely accepted explanation of the initiation of endometriosis is the retrograde flow of menstrual fluid with subsequent implantation of viable fragments of endometrium within the pelvic cavity,[17] known as Sampson's theory. Retrograde menstruation has been observed in a majority of otherwise normal women undergoing peritoneal dialysis during menstruation.[18] Similar observations have been made in women undergoing laparoscopy during menstruation and also in rhesus monkeys.[19] The blood may appear during the few days before menstruation and usually persists during the first day of menstrual flow. Retrograde menstruation can account for the frequent sites of endometriosis in the posterior aspects of the pelvis. Women with endometriosis often have a long history of dysmenorrhea. The excessive uterine contractions characteristic of primary dysmenorrhea[20,21] may further contribute to a bidirectional menstrual flow from the uterus. However, Sampson's theory of retrograde menstruation does not explain the extrapelvic sites of endometriosis such as endometriosis of the limbs, thoracic cavity and elsewhere. Retrograde menstruation *per se* is unlikely to produce endometriosis by itself. It is most probable that a genetic factor or susceptibility as well as a favorable hormonal mileau are necessary for successful implantation and growth of the transported fragments of endometrium.

Celomic Metaplasia

All tissues in which endometriosis arises can be traced to be embryologically derived from celomic epithelium. It has been suggested that chronic irritation of the peritoneum by menstrual blood may cause celomic metaplasia, which may subsequently result in endometriosis. Alternatively, mullerian tissue remnants trapped within the peritoneum could undergo metaplasia and be transformed into endometriosis.[22] This theory can account for all the sites of endometriosis so far described.

Direct Implantation

According to this theory, endometrial tissues are displaced into an implant in the new sites. In women, endometriosis seen in scars as a result of direct seeding of the new sites at surgery lends support to this theory. In rabbits, endometriosis is produced in the pelvic peritoneum by direct subperitoneal implantation of surgically excised endometrial tissue segments. This model has been employed for a number of studies on endometriosis. In order for successful implantation to occur, ovarian estrogens or exogenous estrogens are necessary. In rhesus monkeys, bilateral oophorectomy without estrogen replacement produced significantly less direct implantation of endometrium for production of endometriosis while replacement with exogenous estrogens produced a significantly higher rate of induction of endometriosis.[23] While direct implantation may explain many of the endometriosis sites, it does not explain the occurrence of endometriosis in the limbs and the thoracic cavity.

Genetic and Immunological Factors

There is a 5.8% familial incidence among immediate female siblings, an 8.1% risk if the mother has endometriosis, and a 7% risk of endometriosis if the female sibling or mother has endometriosis. This would suggest a polygenic and multifactorial inheritance for endometriosis.[15,16] The genetic basis of endometriosis probably accounts for the small segment of patients with endometriosis who have a family history but not the majority of those without.

Recent findings in monkeys with spontaneous endometriosis suggest that a defect of cellular immunity may be the basis for the ectopic tissue being allowed to grow in abnormal locations only in certain persons.[24] It may explain why cervical endometriosis is rare in spite of regular exposure of the cervix to menstrual fluid.

Luteinized Unruptured Follicle Syndrome

Luteinized unruptured follicle (LUF) syndrome is reportedly more common in women with endometriosis.[25-27] The high concentrations of steroid hormones in peritoneal fluid after ovulation are postulated to inhibit and inactivate the endometrial tissues reaching the peritoneum in normal women. In women with LUF syndrome, the peritoneal fluid steroid hormone content is suboptimal and therefore implantation of retrograde endometrial tissue may occur by the absence of the inhibitory and inactivating effects of steroid hormones. In monkeys[28] and rabbits[29] with experimental endometriosis, LUF has been found to be a common correlate of infertility, suggesting that the presence of pelvic endometriosis may cause an attenuation of follicular rupture.

Elevated Prostaglandin Levels

The ectopic endometrial implants have been found to have higher prostaglandin $F_{2\alpha}$ ($PGF_{2\alpha}$) concentrations in women with endometriosis.[30] Indeed if the increased prostaglandins are present and could therefore alter tubal motility depending on the relative composition of the different prostaglandins, further retrograde showering of menstrual endometrial tissue into the peritoneal cavity may oc-

cur as a result of tubal dyskinesia. However, early observations that peritoneal fluid prostaglandins and prostanoids are elevated in women with endometriosis[31] have been recently refuted by several larger and well controlled studies.[32-35] Nevertheless, the increased production of $PGF_{2\alpha}$ by the ectopic endometrium itself could lead to exposure of the tube to increased local blood levels of prostaglandins.

Other Theories

Other theories for the pathogenesis of endometriosis include lymphatic and hematogenous spread of normal endometrium to distant sites where implantation then occurs.[36] Although this theory explains the presence of endometriosis in distant sites such as the limbs and thoracic cavity, it is not well supported by both direct clinical observation and experimental data.

CLINICAL FEATURES

The symptoms and clinical findings on examination of the woman with endometriosis are summarized in Table 18-1. It is not uncommon for patients with endometriosis to be without symptoms and to have endometriosis suspected only on pelvic examination or incidentally at laparoscopy or laparotomy.

Infertility

While infertility is commonly associated with endometriosis, interpretation of the frequency of in-

TABLE 18-1. Signs and Symptoms of Endometriosis

Common	Less common
Symptoms	
Infertility	Premenstrual spotting
Dysmenorrhea	Menstrual dysfunction
Pelvic pain	Urinary symptoms
Dyspareunia	(dysuria, urgency, hematuria)
Signs	
None	Intestinal obstruction
Tender, enlarged ovary	Hemoperitoneum
Pelvic nodularities	Torsion of ovarian cyst
Pelvic thickenings	Catamenial pneumothorax
Fixed retroverted uterus	

fertility in women with endometriosis on the basis of series with no matched controls must be taken with caution. The incidence of infertility of greater than 1 and 2 years duration was as high as 100% and 79%, respectively.[37] The duration of infertility was unrelated to the severity of the endometriosis, and primary infertility was twice as frequent as secondary infertility. Recent findings indicate that mild endometriosis does not interfere with female infertility[38] and that pregnancy rates were similar without treatment and with treatment by medication or surgery.[39,40]

Mechanism for Infertility

The physiological bases for infertility in women with endometriosis are probably multifactorial. In some women, the mechanism(s) responsible for infertility are self-evident and readily explicable. However, the physiological basis for infertility is less readily explained when the mechanism cannot be easily traced to a macroscopically visible abnormality. The various etiological factors include adhesions, tubal occlusion, prostaglandins and tubal dyskinesia, anovulation, luteinized unruptured follicle, luteal-phase defects, autoimmunity, decreased sperm transport, and finally spontaneous abortions.

When there are obvious adhesions involving the fallopian tubes, ovaries, and uterus, the tubes may be occluded or stenosed, tubal motility and transtubal ovum or embryo transport may be altered, and ovarian function may be compromised.

Recent findings suggest that there is increased $PGF_{2\alpha}$ content and production in endometriotic tissues[30] and that 6-ketoprostaglandin $F_{1\alpha}$ (6-keto-$PGF_{1\alpha}$) and thromboxane B_2 (TxB_2), the stable metabolites of prostacyclin and thromboxane A_2, are increased in the peritoneal fluid of women with endometriosis but without obvious and readily explicable infertility.[31] Such alterations in composition or content of either prostaglandins or prostanoids or both may explain the associated infertility observed in mild or moderate cases of endometriosis that do not involve the fallopian tubes or ovaries. Thus it was hypothesized that altered tubal function could result in inappropriate tubal transit of either ovum or blastocyst and, therefore, account for the pregnancy failure. $PGF_{2\alpha}$ induces tubal contractions, whereas PGE_2 induces relaxation. Thromboxane A_2 (TxA_2) is expected to stimulate tubal muscle contractions, since it has been shown to stimulate contractions in all types of

smooth muscles studied thus far. By contrast, prostacyclin will relax human fallopian tubes, whereas 6-keto-$PGF_{1\alpha}$ induces mild contractions of the tubal musculature.

The initial findings on prostaglandins and prostanoids in endometriosis indirectly supported the above mechanism of infertility.[31] However, the balance of evidence from recent data on peritoneal fluid prostaglandins and prostanoids indicates no change in these compounds in the peritoneal fluid of women with endometriosis.[32-35] In rabbits, surgically induced endometriosis produced a significant increase in $PGF_{2\alpha}$ concentration in peritoneal fluid.[29] In women, the endometriotic tissue itself was found to have high concentrations of $PGF_{2\alpha}$ and a significantly enhanced capacity to produce $PGF_{2\alpha}$ in vitro.[30]

A preliminary study showed an apparent increase in the metabolite of $PGF_{2\alpha}$, and more recently the peritoneal fluid contents of TxB_2 and 6-keto-$PGF_{1\alpha}$ were found to be elevated in women with endometriosis.[31] In contrast to these two observations, recent studies on larger numbers of patients and better controlled phases of the menstrual cycle, could not find any significant elevation in peritoneal fluid concentration of either the prostaglandins or prostanoids.[32-35] During the proliferative phase, peritoneal fluid concentrations of PGE_2, $PGF_{2\alpha}$, 15-keto-13,14-dihydro-$PGF_{2\alpha}$, and TxB_2 from women with endometriosis were similar to those from normal women.[32] Other studies at different phases of the menstrual cycle showed no increase in peritoneal fluid PGE_2, $PGF_{2\alpha}$, and TxB_2 in women with endometriosis.[33-35] Data from our laboratory showed that in women with endometriosis, the total content of PGE_2, $PGF_{2\alpha}$, TxB_2, and 6-keto-$PGF_{1\alpha}$ in peritoneal fluid was not significantly different from that of normal women.[35] Thus, peritoneal fluid prostaglandins and prostanoids are not elevated and probably do not have an important role in the mechanism of infertility in endometriosis. Nevertheless, the excess prostaglandins produced by ectopic endometrium in sites near the tube, such as the ovaries, may expose the fallopian tubes to high or inappropriate levels of prostaglandins, resulting in tubal dyskinesia. Data on prostaglandin content and production of such endometriotic tissues must be interpreted with caution, as these tissues often contain cryptic menstrual fluid and thus much blood and platelets, which are rich sources of thromboxanes and prostaglandins.

Ovulatory dysfunction can be present in up to 27% of women with endometriosis.[41,42] The types of ovulatory dysfunction include anovulation and severe oligoovulation. Correct treatment of the ovulatory dysfunction can produce good pregnancy rates. The mechanisms responsible for the anovulation are unknown but may include (1) severe periovarian adhesions with disruption of ovarian blood flow, function and steroidogenesis; (2) alteration in ovarian prostaglandin production and ovulation or on the effects of prostaglandins on ovarian blood flow and function; and (3) effects *via* alteration of the hypothalamic endocrine function, such as hyperprolactinemia, and therefore ovarian function.

In one study, LUF was observed in 79% of patients with endometriosis by virtue of absence of the ovulation stigma.[25] In LUF syndrome, there is regular menstruation, presumptive evidence of ovulation without release of the ovum, and therefore absence of the ovulation stigma. Nevertheless, the existence of LUF is still debatable, and it is unclear whether LUF occurs sporadically or repetitively. Recently, LUF was found to be frequently correlated with infertility in monkeys[28] and rabbits[29] with experimentally induced endometriosis. This finding would suggest that the presence of endometrium in pelvis may attenuate follicular rupture. Because follicular fluid contains an inhibitor of luteinization, failure to ovulate may cause a delay of progesterone secretion.

Both the duration and magnitude of progesterone secretion are decreased in women with endometriosis compared with normal cycles[25,43] and are similar to changes in progesterone secretion seen with LUF syndrome.[26] A secondary increase in luteinizing hormone (LH) is seen 2–3 days after the main mid-cycle LH surge, with a delay in the rise in serum progesterone.[43] The true incidence of LUF associated with endometriosis is probably much lower than reported earlier[25–27,44] and is refuted by some investigators.[45]

Several studies have reported a higher incidence of luteal-phase defects, as high as 25–45%, in patients with endometriosis.[4,46–48] However, a recent observation suggests that the luteal-phase defect may not be more frequent in patients with endometriosis than in those without it.[49]

Autoimmunity is certainly a possible mechanism for infertility in women with endometriosis but without significant pelvic abnormality to readily account for their infertility. Several pathophysiological mechanisms may be responsible for an autoimmune cause of infertility in these women.[50,51] Circulating antibodies of the IgA and IgG types to endometrial and whole ovarian tissues, granulosa, and theca cells are increased.[51] There is deposition of complement in the endometrium, hence reduced serum complement levels in women with endometriosis.[51] Proteins from the endometriotic tissues are thought to be phagocytosed and absorbed by the host, giving rise to an autoimmune response. Recent studies have shown that peritoneal fluid macrophages are increased in women with endometriosis as compared with other infertile women without endometriosis.[52] The increased numbers of peritoneal fluid macrophages in these women have an enhanced capacity to phagocytose and degrade spermatozoa in vitro.[53] In addition, the activation of the macrophages is accompanied by increased release of acid phosphatase and neutral protease activity.[54] The activated peritoneal macrophages may act as antifertility effector leukocytes and render toxicity to the microenvironment in which fertilization occurs. Thus if these macrophages gain entry into the fallopian tubes *via* the fimbrial end, fertilization could be prevented. The peritoneal fluid of women with endometriosis was also found to inhibit in vivo human sperm penetration of zona-free hamster ova.[55]

There is an increased incidence of spontaneous abortion (22–49%) in women with endometriosis, but both surgical and medical therapies of the underlying endometriosis can reduce the incidence of spontaneous abortion.[56–59] However, the observations are generally not well controlled. The mechanisms responsible for the spontaneous abortion are not known although decreased progesterone secretion (see above) may partially account for it. Decreased sperm transport secondary to changes in cervical mucus has been suggested as contributory to the infertility in endometriosis but this is at best speculative.

Pelvic Pain and Dysmenorrhea

In Sampson's original report, 50% of patients had dysmenorrhea.[60] The overall occurrence of dysmenorrhea in a recent report was 63% in women with endometriosis.[37] The frequency of severe dysmenorrhea in endometriosis has, however, been shown to be 27% in mild cases, 26% in moderate cases and 35% in severe disease.[37] Initially, pain characteristically occurs for several days before menstruation, followed by dysmenorrhea. As endometriosis progresses, the pain extends over the entire luteal phase, leaving only a few days of pain-free interval postmenstrually. Dysmenorrhea due to endometriosis usually occurs some time after menarche; this historical feature is an important diagnostic clue. With more frequent use of laparoscopy, however, it is clear that endometriosis can begin with the first menstrual flow and the accompanying dysmenorrhea may be strikingly similar to that seen in primary dysmenorrhea. Classically, the extent of pelvic pain and dysmenorrhea does not correlate with the amount of disease; severe incapacitating dysmenorrhea and pelvic pain are often observed with minimal endometriosis, while extensive disease is, at times, symptom free and found on routine examination. This tendency to an inverse relationship has led to the suggestion that the extensive disease may eventually destroy nerve endings in the tissues.

Mechanisms for Pelvic Pain

The mechanisms for pelvic pain in endometriosis are again poorly understood and probably multifactorial. They include adhesions, scarring, stretching of the peritoneum, alteration in pelvic blood flow, impingement of pelvic nerve pathways, and possibly pelvic prostaglandins. The extent, vascularity, fibrosis, and distortion of pelvic structures caused by the adhesions secondary to the endometriosis are important factors in pelvic pain. With cryptic menstruation of ectopic endometrium in confined spaces between or beneath peritoneal layers, pelvic pain can result from peritoneal stretching and irritation. With healing and dense scarring of the endometriotic implants, pain may arise. This may be secondary to scar tissue contraction and distortion of the surrounding structures or impingement on nerve pathways. Alteration of pelvic blood flow secondary to the adhesions, scarring, elevated or altered pelvic prostaglandins, or inflammatory response to the ectopic endometrium can give rise to pelvic congestion and pelvic discomfort. Impingement of pelvic nerve pathways, such as those around the uterosacral ligaments, the ovarian nerve supply, and the hypogastric nerve plexus, from scarring, bleeding, or fibrosis can certainly give rise to pelvic pain. Uterosacral and presacral neurectomies have been employed with moderate success in overcoming the pelvic pain. PGE_2 and $PGF_{2\alpha}$ levels have been found to be increased in uterine endometrial tissues as well as endometriotic tissues.[30] While prostaglandins may contribute to some degree to the pelvic pain or dysmenorrhea in endometriosis, they are less likely to be a significant physiological basis of the pain in most instances. Indeed, a clinical trial with several non-

steroidal anti-inflammatory agents showed no significant relief of the pelvic pain in women with endometriosis.[62] Pelvic peritoneal defects, one of the features of the Allen-Masters syndrome, including dysmenorrhea, may be causally related to endometriosis. As many as 68% of peritoneal defects in women with pelvic pain were found to be associated with endometriosis.[63] However, we have found these peritoneal defects in women with no pelvic pain, dysmenorrhea, or endometriosis at routine laparoscopy for other indications.

Dyspareunia

Dyspareunia due to pelvic endometriosis is usually deep dyspareunia, and the pain often intensifies with vigorous intercourse during rapid to-and-fro intravaginal movement of the penis. The dyspareunia probably arises from the tenderness elicited by the stretching of the structures in the cul-de-sac by the penis or by direct-contact tenderness. Thus, the dyspareunia may sometimes be relieved or even eliminated by a change in coital position. In one series, 27% of patients with endometriosis reported dyspareunia that appeared to have no relationship with the severity of the endometriosis.[37]

Menstrual Irregularities

Menstrual irregularities were noted in 12–14% of patients with endometriosis irrespective of the severity of their disease.[37] Recently, premenstrual spotting was found to be significantly more common in women with endometriosis compared with women with luteal-phase defects without endometriosis.[63] Therefore, regular premenstrual spotting in an infertile woman should be a helpful clue to the likelihood of endometriosis. With ovarian endometriotic cyst (chocolate cyst), menstrual disorders and lower abdominal pain were the two most common symptoms in 72% of cases.[64]

Clinical Findings

The clinical findings on examination of the woman with endometriosis are summarized in Table 18-2. It is not uncommon for pelvic examination to be completely within normal limits. Specific abnormalities to look for include the presence of tender enlarged ovaries, an adnexal mass as is the case with ovarian chocolate cyst, nodularities with or without tenderness in the cul-de-sac, the uterosacral ligaments nearer to the uterine end and rectovaginal

TABLE 18-2. Classification of Endometriosis^a

		Peritoneum	
Endometriosis	<1 cm	1–3 cm	>3 cm
	1	2	3
Adhesions	Filmy	Dense with partial cul-de-sac obliteration	Dense with complete cul-de-sac obliteration
	1	2	3
		Ovary	
Endometriosis	<1 cm	1–3 cm	>3 cm or ruptured endometriosis
Right	2	4	6
Left	2	4	6
Adhesions	Filmy	Dense with partial ovarian enclosure	Dense with complete ovarian enclosure
Right	2	4	6
Left	2	4	6
		Tube	
Endometriosis	<1 cm	>1 cm	Tubal occlusion
Right	2	4	6
Left	2	4	6
Adhesions	Filmy	Dense with tubal distortion	Dense with tubal enclosure
Right	2	4	6
Left	2	4	6

Stage I	Mild	1–5
Stage II	Moderate	6–15
Stage III	Severe	16–30
Stage IV	Extensive	31–54

Total _____

septum, and finally a fixed retroverted uterus. Less frequent findings may include torsion of an ovarian cyst, catamenial pneumothorax, hemoperitoneum from rupture of a chocolate cyst, and signs of intestinal obstruction if the bowel is significantly infiltrated by endometriosis.

DIAGNOSIS

It is apparent that endometriosis is more common than generally realized. Unless thought of, endometriosis can be missed and the diagnosis delayed or never made. Endometriosis should be differentiated from primary dysmenorrhea and other causes of secondary dysmenorrhea (see Chapter 19), pelvic inflammatory disease (PID), and other causes of adnexal mass(es).

In primary dysmenorrhea, the pain usually begins immediately before the onset of menstruation, is usually gone within 48 hr and is accompanied by nausea, vomiting, diarrhea, and tiredness. With endometriosis, the pain often may start several days before and persist throughout menstruation and even for a few days thereafter. The pain of primary dysmenorrhea is crampy or laborlike, while the pain associated with endometriosis is usually dull, dragging, and referred to the rectum. Historically primary dysmenorrhea begins with or a few months after the menarche when ovulatory cycles are established but the dysmenorrhea of endometriosis often sets in a few years after the menarche. Nevertheless, in the absence of positive physical findings, the dysmenorrhea of endometriosis can mimic primary dysmenorrhea so strikingly that only failure to respond to oral contraceptives and to the nonsteroidal anti-inflammatory agents[20,21,65,66] should prompt laparoscopy.

Endometriosis may present so subtly that it is not uncommonly confused with PID, and the patient is given repeated courses of antibiotic therapy. This diagnostic trap is often true in patients who have pelvic pain and who may have minimal pelvic tenderness and adnexal thickenings, but without fever or other signs. With florid acute PID or an acute exacerbation, the diagnosis may more readily be apparent by a previous history of pelvic infection and the presence of chills, fever, purulent vaginal discharge, adnexal masses (usually bilateral), and pelvic tenderness. Failure to respond to appropriate antibiotic therapy should arouse suspicion of endometriosis, especially if a pelvic abscess has been ruled out. With pelvic infection, the adnexal masses, if present, are usually bilateral. Although unilateral inflammatory adnexal mass, has been shown to be present in women using the intrauterine device (IUD),[67] endometriosis should be considered. In one series of 263 patients with ovarian endometriotic cysts, the diagnosis was made on admission and prior to surgery in only 7% of cases.[64] Thus, in the presence of a unilateral adnexal mass in a premenopausal women, endometriosis should always be considered.

Endometriosis involving the bowel and or urinary tract with bowel or urinary symptoms needs to be differentiated from other gastrointestinal (GI) and urinary tract symptoms.

Diagnosis by visual inspection is necessary before commencing therapy. This is carried out with the laparoscope unless a laparotomy is indicated or if the endometriosis involves structures such as the skin, vagina, or cervix which are readily visible on routine gynecologic examination. The gross appearance of endometriosis is so characteristic that histological confirmation is generally unnecessary. We have biopsied the lesion for histological documentation only if the site of the lesion is not hazardous. The extent of diagnostic workup depends on the stage of the disease and structures involved. Intravenous pyelography (IVP) and/or cystoscopy becomes necessary if ureteral or bladder involvement is suspected. Barium enema, sigmoidoscopy, and upper GI series are indicated if the bowels are suspected to be involved with endometriosis. Endocrine evaluation is usually not helpful unless the patient is suffering from menstrual dysfunction, ovulatory dysfunction, or luteal-phase defects. In such cases, either endometrial biopsy or mid-luteal-phase serum progesterone, or both, will be useful. Hysterosalpingogram may be necessary in patients suspected of having tubal involvement but can be obviated if laparoscopy is contemplated soon.

At laparoscopy, the pathognomonic appearance of endometriosis is due to blood deposition into the tissues thus giving a rust-colored appearance with time (Fig. 18-1). Older endometriotic deposits will appear yellowish-brown or even gray as the blood is resorbed (Fig. 18-2). Healed areas may show puckering with fibrosis and even adhesions. With larger endometriotic deposits in the ovary, the characteristic "chocolate cyst" may be seen. With severe disease, extensive adhesions may develop with the cul-de-sac completely obliterated and the sigmoid colon and other loops of bowel stuck to the uterus.

All cases of diagnosed endometriosis should be classified and staged as an aid to predicting prognosis, choosing therapy, and managing the disease. Several classifications have been introduced, with the Acosta classification[41] popularly used until recently. The official classification of the American Fertility Society[68] (Table 18-2) is preferred and currently the Revised Classification by the American Fertility Society (Table 18-3) is in use.

MANAGEMENT

Endometriosis can be treated surgically or medically or by a combination of both modalities. There is continuing controversy as to which type of therapy produces better results. It is clear, however, that both medical and surgical therapies have their place in the management of the woman with endometriosis, depending on her age, reproductive status, presenting complaints, need for fertility, and extent and location of disease. The only method of treatment which offers permanent cure is castration. All other methods offer temporary remission at best.

Surgical Management

Surgery is clearly indicated in the management of endometriosis in the following situations: (1) for diagnosis; (2) tubal occlusion, peritubal, pelvic, and ovarian adhesions (when fertility is desired); (3) chocolate cysts of the ovary; (4) intractable pelvic pain unrelieved by medical management; and (5) failed medical management. However, when the patient is asymptomatic or the disease is mild or moderate, it is less clear whether surgical ablative therapy gives better results than medical therapy. Recent data have clearly shown that with mild disease (Acosta classification) and in the absence of tubal occlusion, pregnancy rates were similar with surgical, medical, or no treatment.[38-40]

Definitive surgery for management of endometriosis can be subdivided as either conservative surgery or complete surgery.

Conservative Surgery

The conservative approach is indicated in women who want to become pregnant or who wish to pre-

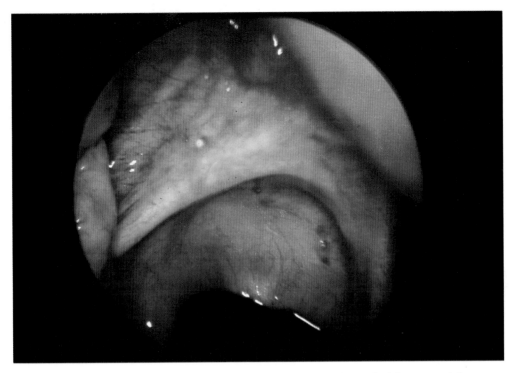

FIGURE 18-1. Small rust-colored deposits of endometriosis in the cul-de-sac and over the left uterosacral ligaments seen at laparoscopy.

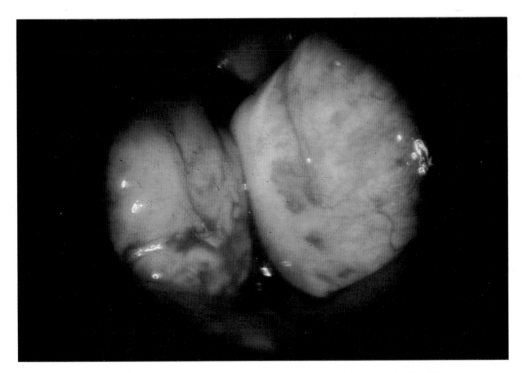

FIGURE 18-2. Characteristic appearance of endometriosis deposits on the surface of the ovary visualized through the laparoscope.

TABLE 18-3. The American Fertility Society Revised Classification of Endometriosis

Stage I   (Minimal) - 1–5
Stage II (Mild)   - 6–15
Stage III (Moderate) - 16–40
Stage IV (Severe)   - >40

Total _____

	Peritoneum		
Endometriosis	<1cm	1-3cm	>3cm
Superficial	1	2	4
Deep	2	4	6
	Ovary		
R Superficial	1	2	4
Deep	4	16	20
L Superficial	1	2	4
Deep	4	16	20
Posterior culdesac	Partial		Complete
obliteration	4		40
	Ovary		
Adhesions	<1/3 Enclosure	1/3-2/3 Enclosure	>2/3 Enclosure
R Filmy	1	2	4
Dense	4	8	16
L Filmy	1	2	4
Dense	4	8	16
	Tube		
R Filmy	1	2	4
Dense	4[a]	8[a]	16
L Filmy	1	2	4
Dense	4[a]	8[a]	16

[a]If the fimbriated end of the fallopian tube is completely enclosed, change the point assignment to 16.

serve their reproductive function. Ovarian cystectomy is done for chocolate cysts, lysis of adhesions and salpingoplasty for tubal complications, and cauterization of pelvic peritoneal lesions if they are not at critical sites. Microsurgical techniques should be employed. With adhesive disease, plication of the round ligament, approximation of the uterosacral ligaments posteriorly, or even ventrosuspension of the uterus may be necessary to prevent the uterus from becoming adherent in the cul-de-sac or posteriorly.

Some of these procedures may be carried out with the laparoscope; the Argon laser has recently been employed to photocoagulate the endometriosis deposits through the laparoscope.[69,70] With the appropriate adapters and instruments, the CO_2 laser is also being used for vaporizing endometriosis through the laparoscope. The advantages of laser photocoagulation of endometriosis through the laparoscope include reduced morbidity; less likelihood of adhesions, since the abdomen is not opened; reduced tissue injury necrosis; and vaporization of the endometriosis including its proteins, which are thought to be antigenic and to cause autoimmunity. Such treatment appears to extirpate the lesion completely and reduces the risks of autoimmunity. Specifically, lysis of adhesions and cauterization of pelvic peritoneal endometriotic deposits can be performed through the laparoscope. However, it is prudent not to cauterize lesions that are close to or on critical structures, since undesirable postoperative thermal necrosis and its complications may arise. The CO_2 laser has been used together with the laparoscope for lysis of adhesions, cauterization of peritoneal endometriosis, and neosalpingostomies in patients with endometriosis.

While this technique has definite advantages, long-term success rates in terms of fertility remain to be evaluated.

Complete Surgery

In patients who have completed their family or if medical therapy has failed, extensive surgery may be indicated. In this setting, the surgery should include total hysterectomy and bilateral salpingo-oophorectomy. Oophorectomy is necessary to remove the source of endogenous ovarian estrogens which are the cause of continued stimulation and growth of the endometriosis. Dissection may be difficult in patients with extensive adhesions and bowel involvement. In patients with pelvic pain or dysmenorrhea unresponsive to medical therapy, bilateral uterosacral neurectomy and presacral neurectomy may be performed. Although some centers may do these procedures as an integral part of surgery for endometriosis, there appears to be little or no indication for these procedures in the absence of pelvic pain or intractable dysmenorrhea.

Estrogen replacement therapy can be started for menopausal symptoms within a few days after surgery if all endometriosis has been removed. The dose of estrogen employed, usually conjugated equine estrogens (Premarin) 0.625–1.25 mg/day or ethinyl estradiol 5–10 μg is sufficiently low enough not to be a major concern for its effects on endometriosis. Nevertheless, postmenopausal endometriosis has been reported in as many as 2% of patients with endometriosis, usually in association with either endogenous estrogen sources or exogenously administered estrogens. Therefore, if there is any likelihood of endometriosis still left behind or of restimulation of the endometriosis with estrogens, the menopausal symptoms as well as the endometriosis can be readily controlled with medroxyprogesterone acetate.[71] After 3–6 months, estrogen replacement therapy may then be initiated, and long-term prevention of osteoporosis can still be accomplished.

On the basis of retrospective analysis and only those patients who had repeat surgery for symptoms, the annual recurrence rates after surgery ranged from 0.9% in the first postoperative year to 13.6% in the eighth postoperative year.[71,72] However, the cumulative 3- and 5-year recurrence rates were 13.5% and 40.3%, respectively,[71] similar to the recurrence rates seen after medical treatment. With recurrent abortions associated with endometriosis, published data suggest that surgical therapy gives better results in terms of reducing the abortion rate than medical therapy.[58,59]

Combined Surgery and Medical Therapy

Surgery and danazol have been used in combination. The best means of combining the two remains uncertain. Danazol has been employed preoperatively for 6 weeks or more followed by surgery. It appears that for technically difficult cases danazol therapy induces regression of the endometriosis and renders surgical dissection easier. In addition, conservative surgery following hormonal treatment permits lysis of any adhesions that might have formed during healing of the disease. Danazol therapy has also been employed postoperatively, especially when all the endometriosis could not be removed by surgery.

Medical Management

Medical management can offer significant relief of endometriosis. Several new novel approaches to medical management of endometriosis based on advances in endocrinology are evolving.

Current Therapies

Hormonal therapy is clearly indicated in patients whose disease may not be extensive, when there is a need to conserve reproductive function, where the disease may be located at critical sites and surgery could be mutilating or technically difficult, where there is a need to ''reduce'' the endometriosis and render the subsequent surgery easier for relief of pelvic pain, and for suppression or eradication of the endometriosis until ready for childbearing.

There are two basic approaches to the medical management of endometriosis, both of which are hormonal therapies: (1) pseudopregnancy therapy, and (2) pseudomenopause therapy. The ideal therapy is to induce pregnancy. The progesterone produced by the placenta and suppression of the ovarian function will induce regression of the endometriosis, but pregnancy is not always readily achievable in women with endometriosis. Hormonal therapy is aimed at (1) suppressing ovarian function and thus reducing the growth promoting effects of ovarian estrogen, (2) directly inhibiting endometrial growth, and (3) converting the endometrium to a secretory or pseudodecidual type of tissue, with resultant glandular atrophy.

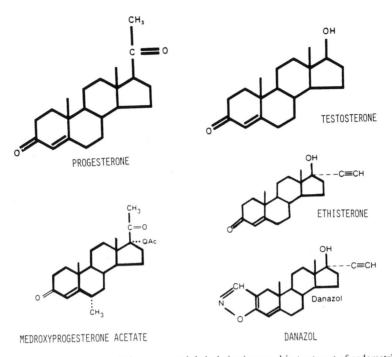

FIGURE 18-3. Chemical formula for some steroid hormones and their derivatives used in treatment of endometriosis. Note that danazol is the isoxazole derivative of 17α-ethinyl testosterone (Ethisterone).

Pseudopregnancy Therapy. In this type of therapy, the woman is rendered pseudopregnant through the use of one of several gestagens currently available, including norethindrone, oral medroxyprogesterone acetate,[73] Depo-Provera,[74] and the 6-retroprogesterone. Medroxyprogesterone acetate (Provera) and norethindrone are given orally. For norethindrone, the initial dose is 5 mg twice a day and increased at 1–2 weekly intervals until symptoms are relieved or the patient is intolerant of the dose. The dose is then reduced by 5 mg/day. The usual daily maintenance dose is 20–30 mg/day. For Provera, the usual dose is 30–40 mg/day. For Depo-Provera, the dose is 100 mg IM every 2 weeks for four doses and then 200 mg every month. Treatment should be continuous for 6–9 months. Besides inhibiting pituitary gonadotropin secretion, progestogens induce excessive secretory and pseudodecidual changes of the endometrium, including the endometriosis, resulting in glandular atrophy, increased macrophage activity, and fibrosis. Side effects of progestogen therapy include water retention and weight gain, oily skin, acne, and infrequently mild hirsutism. Breakthrough bleeding may occur if the dose is inadequate, With both oral medroxyprogesterone acetate and Depo-Provera, spotting and breakthrough bleeding are common side effects in spite of adequate dosage.[73] The 6-retroprogesterone has been used in Europe as a progestin for the treatment of endometriosis. The advantage apparently rests with no inhibition of ovulation.

Oral contraceptives may be used to suppress ovarian function and endometrial growth. Any oral contraceptive can be used, but one with a higher progestogen content is preferable. The oral contraceptive agent is given continuously so as to render the patient amenorrheic and therefore pseudopregnant. The effect of continuous exposure to a combined estrogen–progesterone preparation is suppression of endometrial growth (including the endometriosis) leading to an inactive and atrophic endometrium. This is then resolved by macrophage activity and engulfed in fibrosis. The oral contraceptive pill will also suppress pituitary gonadotropins and thereby inhibit ovulation and ovarian function. Treatment is usually continued for 9 months. If pain or dysmenorrhea is unrelieved or if breakthrough bleeding occurs, the dose of the pill may be increased to 2 tablets or more per day. Side effects are those usually associated with oral contraceptive therapy.

The results of pseudopregnancy treatment, if continued to completion, have been found satisfactory by many investigators. With progestin-induced pseudopregnancy, improvement in symptoms may be as high as 94%.[75] Although the corrected pregnancy rate achieved with medroxyprogesterone acetate was as high as 90% in those with fertile husbands,[73] the pregnancy rates are generally lower than those after conservative surgery.[76] The usual pregnancy rate after pseudopregnancy therapy is 43–55%.[77–79]

Recurrence rates after pseudopregnancy therapy are similar regardless of the medication employed for pseudopregnancy. The recurrence rate is 5–10% annually with rates of 17–18% being reported 1 year after treatment.[80,81]

Pseudomenopause Therapy

Danazol. This is probably the most effective hormonal therapy for endometriosis currently available. However, danazol is expensive compared with the other hormones used. It is a modified androgen, an isoxazole derivative of 17α-ethinyl testosterone (Table 18-4), and is therefore mildly androgenic and anabolic. It is an antigonadotropin and was originally thought to suppress pituitary gonadotropins completely. It is now clear, however, that gonadotropin concentrations remain nor-

mal, while the pulsatile release of, and therefore the peaks, of gonadotropin and ovulation are suppressed by danazol.[82,83] The usual dose is 800 mg/day given orally, although preliminary data suggest that 600 mg/day may be effective as well. Danazol binds to progesterone receptors[86] and inhibits ovarian steroidogenesis at a point distal to the gonadotropin-receptor action in the ovary[85] by interfering with gonadotropin action. Danazol is also antiestrogenic and inhibits the enzymes of steroidogenesis in the ovary and endometrium.[86,87] It induces an atrophic endometrium similar to that of postmenopausal women. Thus, danazol therapy has been inappropriately referred to as "pseudomenopause therapy," although the endocrine changes induced by danazol are not similar to those of the menopause. With danazol therapy, total serum estrone, estradiol, and free estradiol concentrations were reduced to the low follicular phase range for premenopausal women, but free testosterone levels increased twofold secondary to marked suppression of sex hormone binding globulin.[88]

To avoid irregular bleeding and inadvertent exposure of an early conceptus to danazol, therapy should begin with the first day of the menstrual cycle. Therapy should last at least 3 months, but usually 6–9 months, depending on the extent of endometriosis. The daily dose is 800 mg and is best given as four divided doses because of the short plasma half-life (4.5 hr).[89] Although lower daily doses of danazol (100–600 mg) have been used for treating endometriosis, the results are variable, with a lower pregnancy rate and a higher rate of recurrence of symptoms within 1 year of discontinuation.[90–93] Effective treatment is heralded by prompt relief of symptoms, amenorrhea, and gradual decrease in size of palpable lesions. In patients with palpable lesions, the length of time for treatment may be guided by the time to complete disappearance of the lesion. Danazol is especially effective for relief of pelvic pain and dysmenorrhea. The beneficial effects of danazol in the treatment of endometriosis have been well documented.[94–100] With danazol treatment, symptomatic improvement was noted in 70–93% of patients, while pelvic findings improved in 80%. Objective improvement was found in 85–95% of patients at repeat laparoscopy on completing danazol therapy.[95] The uncorrected fertility rate was 40–50%,[100] while the corrected fertility rate was 76% after treatment with danazol.[95] Thus the pregnancy rate compares favorably with that achieved with conservative surgery. Most of the conceptions occurred within the

TABLE 18-4. Adverse Reactions to Danazol (800 mg/day)

Type reaction	%
Androgenic effects	
Acne	17
Edema	6
Weight gain	5
Hirsutism	6
Voice changes	3
Skin oiliness	3
Antiestrogenic effects	
Flushes and sweats	15
Uterine spotting	10
Decreased breast size	5
Change in libido	5
Atrophic vaginitis	3
Idiopathic drug reactions	
Gastrointestinal disturbances	8
Weakness, dizziness	8
Muscle aches or cramps	4
Skin rashes	3
Headaches	2
Sleep disturbances	Occasional

first year after stopping medication and early post-treatment conception appears to confer further protection from recurrence of the endometriosis.

Danazol is usually well tolerated with few side effects. Side effects include nausea, vomiting, weight gain, breakthrough bleeding with lower doses (below 600 mg/day), acne, oily skin, reversible hyperlipidemias,[101] and infrequently hirsutism and deepening of the voice (Table 18-3). Other reported side effects include decrease in libido (6% of patient), decrease in breast size, and hot flashes (8%). Recurrence of symptoms occurs in 5–15% of patients 1 year after completing treatment.

Testosterone and methyltestosterone have been widely used in the past and are highly effective in relieving the pain of endometriosis. The usual dose of methyltestosterone is 5–10 mg/day sublingually. Testosterone probably inhibits the endometriotic lesion directly, since ovulation may not be inhibited by these doses. With low doses, side effects are infrequent but may include facial hair growth, acne, and infrequently jaundice. Conception rates were higher with 10 mg/day testosterone but with 5 mg/day, pregnancy rates declined to 30%.[102] Remissions tend to be transient. Because of the undesirable side effects of testosterone and the availability of danazol, however, testosterone is seldom required for treatment of endometriosis.

Future Therapies

Possible future medical therapies for endometriosis include the use of GnRH or its analogues, antiestrogen therapy using estrogen blockers, prostaglandin synthetase inhibitors, and manipulation of the autoimmune mechanism.

GnRH or GnRH Analogues. This is by far the most promising therapy of the future. Preliminary observations suggest that GnRH agonists can induce "medical oophorectomy," which is reversible and may offer a less permanent and non-invasive form of ovarian ablation for endometriosis. The potent long-acting GnRH-agonist, D-Tr$_p$^{6}-Pro-Net-LRHR (GnRH-a), was able to suppress ovarian function, follicle-stimulating hormone (FSH) secretion, ovulation, and menstruation in monkeys[103] and in women with endometriosis.[104] In women, circulating estrogen levels were markedly suppressed by the GnRH-a to concentrations normally found in oophorectomized women.[88] While GnRH agonists can clearly induce effective and reversible "medical oophorectomy," long-term studies are needed to evaluate such therapy for both relief of pain and regression of the endometriosis before this type of therapy can be established. Another GnRH agonist analogue, buserelin, has also been tested in a limited number of patients with endometriosis and can be given intranasally[105,106] or by subcutaneous injections. In a recent study,[106] 6 months of therapy with 200 μg buserelin administered intranasally three times a day showed improvement or complete resolution of their endometriosis laparoscopically in five of six patients. One patient became pregnant. The efficacy of GnRH agonists on pregnancy rates remains unestablished. Because of the potential of hot flashes occurring with GnRH agonist treatment, the addition of a progestin such as medroxyprogesterone acetate is being examined.

Antiestrogen Therapy. Newer approaches to anti-estrogen therapy include receptor blockers at the estrogen receptors in the endometrium or the use of specific antiestrogen compounds. Recent studies have shown that the ectopic endometrium has reduced cytosol estrogen and progesterone receptors compared with normal endometrium, suggesting dissimilar control mechanisms of estrogen and progesterone receptors between normal and ectopic endometrium.[108–110] This autonomy in the estrogen receptors of endometriotic tissue may account for poorer therapeutic results with methods employing suppression of the pituitary–gonadal axis. Therefore, direct action on the estrogen or progesterone receptors with antiestrogen or antiprogesterone may offer a new approach to therapy. A synthetic antiestrogen, antiprogesterone, gestrinone (R-2323) has been tested in 20 women with endometriosis with good pain relief, encouraging results, and good subsequent pregnancy rates.[111] Another antiestrogen that could be employed for further evaluation is tamoxifen.

Prostaglandin Inhibition. The future of prostaglandin inhibition in the management of endometriosis is much less clear than that of GnRH analogues and antiestrogens. Suppression of prostaglandin biosynthesis with an effective nonsteroidal anti-inflammatory drug (NSAID) may offer additional pain relief if excess prostaglandins contribute to the pelvic pain; however, studies with such compounds have yielded disappointing results.[61] If increased and/or altered prostaglandin production by the ectopic endometrium contributes to abnormal tubal motility and accounts for the so-called "unexplained infertility" of endometriosis, perhaps an NSAID could normalize the tubal motility and permit pregnancy; this hypothesis is yet to be tested in vivo; the drawback is the non-selective inhibition of prostaglandin biosynthesis by most of the available NSAIDs. During the next few years, understanding of the leukotriene pathway and its role in reproduction and specifically in endometriosis may open up new approaches to therapy.

Suppression of the Autoimmune Mechanism. While several studies have shown evidence of autoimmunity[50,51] and specific increased peritoneal fluid macrophage number and activity, which are cytotoxic to spermatozoa,[52–55] an understanding of these changes has not been exploited for therapeutic gains. Perhaps pharmacological manipulation of the macrophage activity could be employed to restore the fertility of these patients.

Other Possible Approaches. It is conceivable that the mechanism(s) contributing to the infertility and other symptoms of endometriosis could be worked out for each patient by performing some of the tests to determine the mechanisms referred to. The management could then be specifically tailored to the patient's individual pathophysiology. Finally, combination therapy using different "lines of attack" could be employed in some patients and permit potentiation of the individual therapeutic modalities resulting in lower doses of each medication used.

SUMMARY

The incidence of endometriosis is increasing. It is not uncommon among teenagers and black females. Theories of pathogenesis of endometriosis include retrograde menstruation with implantation, celomic metaplasia, direct implantation, immunological or genetic defects, luteinized unruptured follicle with reduced peritoneal fluid steroid hormones and failure to inhibit endometrial implants, elevated prostaglandins with tubal dyskinesia and retrograde menstruation, and lymphatic and hematogenous spread. A recent study indicates that there is no HLA relationship in patients with endometriosis.[112]

Common symptoms of endometriosis include infertility, dysmenorrhea (63%), pelvic pain, and dyspareunia (27%), while premenstrual spotting, menstrual dysfunction, and urinary symptoms are less common complaints. Often there may be no abnormal physical signs, or the ovary may be enlarged or tender; pelvic nodularities or thickenings and a fixed retroverted uterus may be present as well. Less frequent physical signs include intestinal obstruction, hemoperitoneum, torsion of ovarian cyst, and catamenial pneumothorax. The mechanisms for infertility in women with endometriosis are multifactorial, including pelvic adhesions, tubal occlusion, abnormal prostaglandins levels and release, tubal dyskinesia, anovulation, luteinized unruptured follicle, luteal-phase defects, autoimmunity with increased peritoneal macrophage activity and phagocytosis of sperms, decreased sperm transport, and spontaneous abortions. The mechanisms for dysmenorrhea and pelvic pain include excessive prostaglandin production and release, fibrosis, adhesions with distortion and disruption of vascular flow, and cryptic menstruation with peritoneal irritation.

Diagnosis of endometriosis requires visualization of the characteristic endometriotic deposits—a rust-colored appearance, yellowish-brown or gray deposits with puckering, fibrosis, and even adhesions. This is usually done by laparoscopy.

Management of endometriosis must take into account the patient's main complaints, her need for further childbearing, and the extent and sites of her endometriosis. Complete surgery, that is, hysterectomy and bilateral salpingo-oophorectomy, is reserved for those who have completed their family, failed medical therapy, and present with intractable pain. Endometriotic ovarian cysts require surgical removal. Conservative surgery is reserved for those with (1) a desire for childbearing, (2) extensive pelvic adhesions or tubal occlusions due to the endometriosis, or (3) recurrent spontaneous abortion.

Medical management is accomplished with pseudopregnancy therapy using a combined oral contraceptive pill or a progestin. It is somewhat less effective than pseudomenopause therapy, especially for pelvic pain. For pseudomenopause therapy, danazol, a modified androgen with antigonadotropic and antiestrogen properties, is generally used for 6–9 months. Symptomatic and objective (laparoscopic) improvements occur in up to 95% of patients. The corrected fertility rate was 76% with danazol therapy, which is similar to that with conservative surgery. Recurrence rates after medical therapy is similar to that after conservative surgery.

Future therapies of endometriosis that show promise include the use of GnRH analogues to induce reversible "medical oophorectomy" and the antiestrogens, such as gestrinone. Other possible future approaches include manipulation of the pelvic tissue prostaglandin levels or the autoimmune mechanisms.

ACKNOWLEDGMENT. The author wishes to thank Winthrop–Breon Laboratories, New York, New York, for their generous contribution toward the color reproduction of Figures 18-1 and 18-2.

QUESTIONS*

1. The following statements about endometriosis are true except:

   a. Endometriosis is more common in white women and therefore occurs infrequently in black women.
   b. Endometriosis may present as early as at the time of the menarche.
   c. There is an 8% risk of developing endometriosis in a woman if she has one female sib or a mother who suffers from endometriosis.
   d. Current evidence suggests that the inheritance of endometriosis is polygenic.
   e. Infertility is a frequent accompaniment of endometriosis.

2. In patients with endometriosis the following are true except:

   a. Dysmenorrhea is present in 63% of patients with endometriosis.
   b. Severe dysmenorrhea occurs equally frequently in mild, moderate, or severe endometriosis.
   c. Pelvic pain and dysmenorrhea due to endometriosis can be adequately and significantly improved with a prostaglandin synthetase inhibitor.
   d. The recurrence rates of endometriosis after conservative surgery or after pseudomenopause therapy are not significantly different.
   e. Dyspareunia is deep seated rather than superficial.

3. The following are characteristics of Danazol.

   a. Danazol is an isoxazole derivative of 17a-ethinyl testosterone (ethisterone).
   b. Danazol is used as pseudomenopausal thera-

py, effectively relieves pelvic pain and dysmenorrhea due to endometriosis in more than 90% of patients.
   c. Danazol induces transient reversible hyperlipidemias while the patient is on it.
   d. Danazol suppresses only pulsatile but not basal secretion of pituitary gonadotropins.
   e. All of the above.

4. Which of these statements is true?

   a. Endometriosis in the postmenopausal woman does not require estrogens.
   b. The growth, proliferation, and maintenance of endometriotic tissues require stimulation with estrogen.
   c. The ectopic endometrium in endometriotic tissues have been shown to have increased cytosol estrogen and progesterone receptors.
   d. All patients with endometriosis always have ovulatory cycles.
   e. Premenstrual spotting does not occur in women with endometriosis.

5. These statements are concerned with the treatment of endometriosis. Select only one answer.

   a. Gonadotropin hormone releasing hormone agonist analogue can induce "medical oophorectomy" and resolution of endometriosis.
   b. When reproductive function is no longer desired, endometriosis which fails to respond to medical treatment requires definitive surgery with total abdominal hysterectomy and bilateral salpingo-oophorectomy.
   c. Laser can be employed to vaporize pelvic endometriosis through the laparoscope.
   d. All of the above.
   e. None of the above.

REFERENCES

1. von Rokitansky C: 1860, quoted by Ridley JH: The histogenesis of endometriosis: A review of facts and fancies. *Obstet Gynecol Surv* 23:1, 1968
2. Sampson JA: Perforating hemorrhagic (chocolate) cysts of the ovary, their importance and especially their relation to pelvic adenomas of the endometrial type. *Arch Surg* 3:245, 1921
3. Karnaky KH: The use of stilbestrol for endometriosis. *South Med J* 41:1109, 1948
4. Kistner RW: The use of progestins in the treatment of endometriosis. *Am J Obstet Gynecol* 75:264, 1958
5. Greenblatt RB, Dmowski WT, Mahesh VB, et al: Clinical

*Choose only one answer for each question.

*Review article or chapter.

studies with an antigonadotropin—Danazol. *Fertil Steril* 22:102, 1971

6. Meigs JV: Medical treatment of endometriosis and significance of endometriosis. *Surg Gynecol Obstet* 19:317, 1949

7. Kistner RW: *Gynecology: Principles and Practice,* 3rd ed. Chicago, Yearbook, 1978*

8. Williams TJ, Pratt JH: Endometriosis in 1000 consecutive celiotomies: Incidence and management. *Am J Obstet Gynecol* 129:245, 1977

9. Chatman DL: Endometriosis and the black women. *Am J Obstet Gynecol* 125:987, 1976

10. Chatman DL, Ward AB: Endometriosis in adolescents. *J Reprod Med* 27:156, 1982

11. Goldstein DP, De Cholnoky C, Emans JS: Adolescent endometriosis. *J Adolescent Health Care* 1:37, 1980

12. Stock RJ: Postsalpingectomy endometriosis: A reassessment. *Obstet Gynecol* 60:560, 1982

13. Rock JA, Parmley TH, King TM, et al: Endometriosis and the development of tuboperitoneal fistulas after tubal ligation. *Fertil Steril* 35:16, 1981

14. Punnonen R, Klemi PJ, Nikkanen V: Postmenopausal endometriosis. *Eur J Obstet Gynecol Reprod Biol* 11:195, 1980

15. Simpson JL, Elias S, Malinak LR, et al: Heritable aspects of endometriosis. I. Genetic studies. *Am J Obstet Gynecol* 137:327, 1980

16. Malinak LR, Buttram VC, Elias S, et al: Heritable aspects of endometriosis. II. Clinical characteristics of familial endometriosis. *Am J Obstet Gynecol* 137:332, 1980

17. Simpson JL, Malinak LR, Elias S, et al: HLA associations in endometriosis. *Am J Obstet Gynecol* 148:395, 1984

18. Sampson JA: Development of the implantation theory for the origin of peritoneal endometriosis. *Am J Obstet Gynecol* 40:549, 1940

19. Blumenkrantz MJ, Gallagher N, Bashore RA, et al: Retrograde menstruation in women undergoing chronic pelvic dialysis. *Obstet Gynecol* 57:667, 1981

20. Scott RD, Telinde RW: Clinical external endometriosis. *Obstet Gynecol* 4:502, 1954

21. Dawood MY: Dysmenorrhea. *Clin Obstet Gynecol* 26:719, 1983

22. Dawood MY: Choosing the correct therapy for dysmenorrhea. *Contemp Obstet Gynecol* 19:235, 1982

23. DiZerega GS, Barber DL, Hodgen GD: Endometriosis: role of ovarian steroids in initiation, maintenance, and suppression. *Fertil Steril* 33:649, 1980

24. Scott BR: External endometriosis: mechanism of origin, theoretical and experimental. *Clin Obstet Gynecol* 3:429, 1960

25. Dmowski WP, Steele WR, Baker FG: Deficient cellular immunity in endometriosis. *Am J Obstet Gynecol* 141:377, 1981

26. Brosens IA, Koninckx PR, Corvelyen PA: A study of plasma progesterone, oestradiol-17β, prolactin and LH levels and of the luteal phase appearance of the ovaries in patients with endometriosis and infertility. *Br J Obstet Gynecol* 85:246, 1978

27. Koninckx PR, DeMoore P, Brosens IA: Diagnosis of the luteinized unruptured follicle syndrome by steroid hormones assays on peritoneal fluid. *Br J Obstet Gynaecol* 87:929, 1980

28. Donnez J, Thomas K: Incidence of the luteinized unruptured follicle syndrome in fertile women and in women with endometriosis. *Eur J Obstet Gynecol Reprod Biol* 14:187, 1982

29. Schenken RS, Asch RH, Williams RF, et al: Etiology of infertility in monkeys with endometriosis. *Fertil Steril* 39:393, 1983

30. Schenken RS, Asch RH: Surgical induction of endometriosis in rabbit: effects on fertility and concentration of peritoneal fluid prostaglandins. *Fertil Steril* 34:581, 1980

31. Moon YS, Leung PCS, Yuen BH, et al: Prostaglandin F in human endometriotic tissue. *Am J Obstet Gynecol* 141:344, 1981

32. Drake TS, O'Brien WF, Ramwell PS, et al: Peritoneal fluid thromboxane B_2 and 6-ketoprostaglandin $F_{1\alpha}$ in endometriosis. *Am J Obstet Gynecol* 140:40, 1981

33. Rock JA, Dubin NH, Ghodgaonkar RB, et al: Cul-de-sac fluid in women with endometriosis: fluid volume and prostanoid concentration during the proliferative phase of the cycle—day 8 to 12. *Fertil Steril* 37:747, 1982

34. Badawy SZA, Marshall L, Gabal AA, et al: The concentration of prostaglandin $F_{2\alpha}$ and prostaglandin E_2 in peritoneal fluid in infertile patients with and without endometriosis. *Fertil Steril* 38:166, 1982

35. Sgarlata CS, Hertelendy F, Mikhail G: The prostanoid content in peritoneal fluid and plasma of women with endometriosis. *Am J Obstet Gynecol* 147:563, 1983

36. Dawood MY, Khan-Dawood FS, Wilson L: Peritoneal fluid prostaglandin and prostanoids in women with endometriosis, chronic pelvic inflammatory disease and pelvic pain. *Am J Obstet Gynecol* 148:391, 1984

37. Halban J: Hysteroadenosis metastatica: Die lympogene gense der sog. Adenofibromatosis heterotopia. *Arch Gynaekol* 124:457, 1925

38. Buttram VC:.Conservative surgery for endometriosis in the infertile female: A study of 206 patients with implications for both medical and surgical therapy. *Fertil Steril* 31:117, 1979

39. Portuondo JA, Echanojauregui AD, Herran C, et al: Early conception in patients with untreated mild endometriosis. *Fertil Steril* 39:22, 1983

40. Seibel MM, Berger MJ, Weinstein FG, et al: The effectiveness of danazol on subsequent fertility in minimal endometriosis. *Fertil Steril* 38:534, 1982

41. Schenken RS, Malinak LR: Conservative surgery versus expectant for the infertile patient with mild endometriosis. *Fertil Steril* 37:183, 1982

42. Acosta AA, Buttram VC, Besch PK, et al: A proposed classification of pelvic endometriosis. *Obstet Gynecol* 42:19, 1973

43. Soules MR, Malinak LR, Bury R, et al: Endometriosis and anovulation: A coexisting problem in the infertile female. *Am J Obstet Gynecol* 125:412, 1976

44. Cheeseman KL, Ben-Nun I, Chatterton RT, et al: Relationship of luteinizing hormone, pregnanediol-3-glucuronide, and estriol-16-glucuronide in urine in infertile women with endometriosis. *Fertil Steril* 38:542, 1982

45. Koninckx PR, Heyns WJ, Corvelyn PA, et al: Delayed onset of luteinization as a cause of infertility. *Fertil Steril* 29:266, 1978

46. Dmowski WP, Rao R, Scommegna A: The luteinized unruptured follicle syndrome and endometriosis. *Fertil Steril* 33:30, 1980

47. Grant A: Additional sterility factors in endometriosis. *Fertil Steril* 17:514, 1966

48. Hargrove JT, Abraham GK: Abnormal luteal function in endometriosis. *Fertil Steril* 34:302, 1980

49. Levine B, Eisenberg E, Wallach EE: Luteal phase defect: An association with endometriosis. *Fertil Steril* 39:394, 1983

50. Pittaway DE, Maxson W, Daniel J, et al: Luteal phase

defects in infertility patients with endometriosis. *Fertil Steril* 39:712, 1983

51. Mathur RS, Peress MR, Williamson HO, et al: Autoimmunity to endometrium and ovary in endometriosis. *Clin Exp Immunol* 50:259, 1982

52. Weed JC, Arquembourg PC: Endometriosis: Can it produce an autoimmune response resulting in infertility? *Clin Obstet Gynecol* 23:885, 1980

53. Haney AF, Muscato JJ, Weinberg JB: Peritoneal fluid cell populations in infertility patients. *Fertil Steril* 35:696, 1981

54. Muscato JJ, Haney AF, Weinberg JB: Sperm phagocytosis by human peritoneal macrophages: A possible cause of infertility in endometriosis. *Am J Obstet Gynecol* 144:503, 1982

55. Halme J, Becker S, Hammond MG, et al: Increased activation of pelvic macrophages in infertile women with mild endometriosis. *Am J Obstet Gynecol* 145:333, 1983

56. Halme J, Hall JL: Effect of peritoneal fluid from endometriosis patients on human sperm penetration of zona-free hamster ova. *Fertil Steril* 37:573, 1982

57. Petersohn L: Fertility in patients with ovarian endometriosis before and after treatment. *Acta Obstet Gynecol Scand* 49:331, 1970

58. Rock JA, Guzik DS, Sengos C, et al: The conservative surgical treatment of endometriosis: evaluation of pregnancy success with respect to the extent of disease as categorized using contemporary classification systems. *Fertil Steril* 35:131, 1981

59. Naples JD, Batt RE, Sadigh H: Spontaneous abortion rate in patients with endometriosis. *Obstet Gynecol* 57:509, 1981

60. Wheeler JM, Johnston BM, Malinak RL: The relationship of endometriosis to spontaneous abortion. *Fertil Steril* 39:656, 1983

61. Sampson JL: Peritoneal endometriosis due to menstrual dissemination of endometrial tissue into the peritoneal cavity. *Am J Obstet Gynecol* 14:442, 1927

62. Kauppila A, Puolakka J, Ylikorkala O: Prostaglandin biosynthesis inhibitors and endometriosis. *Prostaglandins* 18:665, 1979

63. Chatman DL: Pelvic peritoneal defects and endometriosis: Allan-Masters syndrome revisited. *Fertil Steril* 36:751, 1981

64. Wentz AC: Premenstrual spotting: Its association with endometriosis but not luteal phase inadequacy. *Fertil Steril* 33:605, 1980

65. Egger H, Weigmann P: Clinical and surgical aspects of ovarian endometriotic cysts. *Arch Gynecol* 233:37, 1982

66. Dawood MY: Overall approach to the management of dysmenorrhea. In Dawood MY (ed): *Dysmenorrhea.* Baltimore, Williams & Wilkins, 1981, p 261

67. Dawood MY: Dysmenorrhea and prostaglandins: Pharmacological and therapeutic considerations. *Drugs* 122:42, 1981*

68. Dawood MY, Birnbaum SJ: Unilateral tubo-ovarian abscess and intrauterine contraceptive device. *Obstet Gynecol* 46:429, 1975

69. American Fertility Society: Classification of endometriosis. *Fertil Steril* 32:633, 1979

70. Keye WR, Dixon J: Photocoagulation of endometriosis by the Argon laser through the laparoscope. *Obstet Gynecol* 62:383, 1983

71. Keye WR, Matson GA, Dixon J: The use of the Argon laser in the treatment of experimental endometriosis. *Fertil Steril* 39:26, 1983

72. Wheeler JM, Malinak LR: Recurrent endometriosis: Incidence, management and prognosis. *Am J Obstet Gynecol* 146:247, 1983

73. Punnonen R, Klemi, Nikkanen V: Recurrent endometriosis. *Gynecol Obstet Invest* 11:307, 1980

74. Moghissi KS, Boyce CR: Management of endometriosis with oral medroxyprogesterone acetate. *Obstet Gynecol* 47:265, 1976

75. Gunning, TE, Moyer D: The effect of medroxyprogesterone acetate on endometriosis in the human. *Fertil Steril* 18:759, 1967

76. Andrews MC, Andrew WC, Strauss F: Effects of progestin-induced pseudopregnancy on endometriosis: Clinical and microscopic studies. *Am J Obstet Gynecol* 78:776, 1959

77. Hammond CB, Haney AF: Conservative treatment of endometriosis: 1978. *Fertil Steril* 30:497, 1978

78. Kistner RW: Infertility with endometriosis. A plan of therapy. *Fertil Steril* 13:237, 1962

79. Kistner RW: The effects of new synthetic progestogens on endometriosis in the human female. *Fertil Steril* 16:61, 1965

80. Kourides IA, Kistner RW: Three new synthetic progestins in the treatment of endometriosis. *Obstet Gynecol* 31:821, 1968

81. Andrews WC, Larsen GD: Endometriosis: Treatment with hormonal pseudopregnancy and/or operation. *Am J Obstet Gynecol* 118:643, 1974

82. Riva HL, Wilson JH, Kawaski DM: Effect of norethynodrel on endometriosis. *Am J Obstet Gynecol* 82:109, 1961

83. Luciano AA, Hauser KS, Chapter FK, Sherman BM: Danazol: Endocrine consequences in healthy women. *Am J Obstet Gynecol* 141:723, 1981

84. Hirschowitz, JS, Soler NG, Wortsman J: Sex steroid levels during treatment of endometriosis. *Obstet Gynecol* 54:449, 1979

85. Chamness GC, Asch RH, Pauerstein CJ: Danazol binding and translocation of steroid receptors. *Am J Obstet Gynecol* 136:426, 1980

86. Menon M, Azhar S, Menon KMJ: Evidence that danazol inhibits gonadotropin-induced ovarian steroidogenesis at a point distal to gonadotropin-receptor interaction and adenosine $3'5'$ cyclic monophosphate formation. *Am J Obstet Gynecol* 136:524, 1980

87. Barbieri RL, Canick JA, Makris A, et al: Danazol inhibits steroidogenesis. *Fertil Steril* 28:809, 1977

88. Musich R, Behrman SJ, Menon KMJ: Estrogenic and antiestrogenic effects of danazol administration in studies of estradiol receptor binding. *Am J Obstet Gynecol* 140:62, 1981

89. Meldrum DR, Pardridge WM, Karow WG, et al: Hormonal effects of danazol and medical oophorectomy in endometriosis. *Obstet Gynecol* 62:480, 1983

90. Davison C, Banks W, Fritz A: The absorption, distribution and metabolic fate of danazol in rats, monkeys and human volunteers. *Arch Int Pharm Ther* 221:294, 1976

91. Moore EE, Harger JH, Rock JA, et al: Management of pelvic endometriosis with low-dose danazol. *Fertil Steril* 36:15, 1981

92. Dmowski WP, Kapetamakis E, Scommegna A: Variable effects of danazol on endometriosis at 4 low-dose levels. *Obstet Gynecol* 59:408, 1982

93. Chalmers JA: Treatment of endometriosis with reduced dosage schedules of danazol. *Scott Med J* 27:143, 1982

94. Moore EE, Harger JH, Rock JA, et al: Management of

pelvic endometriosis with low-dose danazol. *Fertil Steril* 36:15, 1981

95. Greenblatt RB, Dmowski WP, Mahesh VB, et al: Clinical studies with an antigonadotropin-danazol. *Fertil Steril* 22:102, 1971

96. Dmowski WP, Cohen MR: Treatment of endometriosis with an antigonadotropin, danazol. A laparoscopic and histologic evaluation. *Obstet Gynecol* 46:147, 1975

97. Laursen NH, Wilson KH, Birnbaum SJ: Danazol: An antigonadotropic agent in the treatment of pelvic endometriosis. *Am J Obstet Gynecol* 123:742, 1975

98. Dmowski WP, Cohen MR: Antigonadotropin (danazol) in the treatment of endometriosis. Evaluation of post-treatment fertility and three-year follow-up data. *Am J Obstet Gynecol* 130:41, 1978

99. Greenblatt RB, Tzingounis V: Danazol treatment of endometriosis: long-term follow-up. *Fertil Steril* 32:518, 1979

100. Buttram VC, Belue JB, Reiter R: Interim report of a study of danazol for the treatment of endometriosis. *Fertil Steril* 37:478, 1982

101. Barbieri RL, Evans S, Kistner RW: Danazol in the treatment of endometriosis: Analysis of 100 cases with a 4-year follow-up. *Fertil Steril* 37:737, 1982

102. Allen JK, Fraser IS: Cholesterol, high density lipoprotein and danazol. *J Clin Endocrinol Metab* 53:149, 1981

103. Katayama PK, Manuel M, Jones HW, et al: Methyltestosterone treatment of infertility associated with pelvic endometriosis. *Fertil Steril* 27:83, 1976

104. Werlin LB, Hodgen GD: Gonadotropin-releasing hormone agonist suppresses ovulation, menses and endometriosis in monkeys: An individualized intermittent regimen. *J Clin Endocrinol Metab* 56:844, 1983

105. Meldrum DR, Chang RJ, Lu J, et al: "Medical oophorectomy" using a long-acting GnRH agonist—a possible new approach to the treatment of endometriosis. *J Clin Endocrinol Metab* 54:1081, 1982

106. Lemay A, Quesnel G: Potential new treatment of endo-
metriosis: Reversible inhibition of pituitary-ovarian function by chronic intranasal administration of a luteinizing hormone-releasing hormone (LH-RH) agonist. *Fertil Steril* 38:376, 1982

107. Shaw RW, Fraser HM, Boyle H: Intranasal treatment with luteinizing hormone releasing hormone agonist in women with endometriosis. *Br Med J* 287:1667, 1983

108. Tamaya T, Motoyama T, Ohono Y, et al: Steroid receptor levels and histology of endometriosis and adenomyosis. *Fertil Steril* 31:396, 1979

109. Bergqvist A, Rannevik G, Thorell J: Estrogen and progesterone cytosol receptor concentration in endometriotic tissue and intrauterine endometrium. *Acta Obstet Gynecol Scand [Suppl]* 101:53, 1981

110. Janne O, Kauppila A, Kokko E, et al: Estrogen and progestin receptors in endometriosis lesions: Comparison with endometrial tissue. *Am J Obstet Gynecol* 141:562, 1981

111. Gould SF, Shannon JM, Cunha GR: Nuclear estrogen binding sites in human endometriosis. *Fertil Steril* 39:520, 1983

112. Coutinho EM: Treatment of endometriosis with gestrinone (R-2323), a synthetic antiestrogen, antiprogesterone. *Am J Obstet Gynecol* 144:895, 1982

ANSWERS

1. a

2. c

3. e

4. b

5. d

19

Dysmenorrhea and Prostaglandins

M. YUSOFF DAWOOD

HISTORICAL ASPECTS

In the folklore of many cultures, the menstrual fluid is believed to be endowed with magical properties. The concept of toxins in the menstrual fluid is evident in many historical writings. Schick[1] remarked that his maidservant caused withering of cut flowers when she touched them during her menstrual period. Similar observations were noted by Macht and colleagues.[2,3] Acetone extracts of menstrual fluid were found toxic to primulas and could potentiate the epinephrine-induced contractions of the rat vas deferens in vitro.[4] Pickles[5] ushered in the era of prostaglandins in menstrual fluid when he showed that menstrual fluid extracts induced smooth muscle contractions in vitro; the term ''menstrual stimulant'' was coined, and this was later shown to be prostaglandins F and E.[6] Later, women with primary dysmenorrhea were collectively shown to have a higher amount of menstrual fluid prostaglandins than normal women.[7] During the 1970s, a few groups, including our laboratory, showed that endometrial and menstrual fluid prostaglandins were increased in dysmenorrheic women and could be reduced to below normal levels with nonsteroidal

anti-inflammatory drugs while concomitant relief of the dysmenorrhea occurred.[8-11]

DEFINITION AND CLASSIFICATION

The term dysmenorrhea, derived from Greek, means difficult monthly flow but is commonly used to refer to painful menstruation. Dysmenorrhea is best classified as primary and secondary dysmenorrhea, In primary dysmenorrhea, there is no macroscopically identifiable pelvic pathology. By contrast, macroscopically identifiable pelvic pathology is present in secondary dysmenorrhea. Such a classification permits an approach to management based on the etiologic mechanism.

INCIDENCE

Dysmenorrhea is one of the most frequently encountered gynecologic disorders; it has been recognized as an extensive personal and public health problem for women. However, with the advent of oral contraceptive and nonsteroidal anti-inflammatory drug therapy, dysmenorrhea can be significantly and readily relieved. It is estimated that more than 50% of menstruating women are affected by dysmenorrhea, about 10% of whom have severe dysmenorrhea with incapacitation for 1–3 days

M. YUSOFF DAWOOD • Department of Obstetrics and Gynecology, Division of Reproductive Endocrinology, University of Illinois College of Medicine, Chicago, Illinois 60612.

each month.[12] In the United States, women constitute 42% of the adult workforce.[13] Thus, about 600 million working hours will be lost annually because of incapacitating dysmenorrhea if adequate relief is not provided. In addition, this problem causes considerable personal and family disruption. Dysmenorrhea occurs most commonly between the ages of 20 and 24, with women in this age group more severely disabled.[14] For those over 25 years of age, the incidence of disabling dysmenorrhea is reduced. Primary dysmenorrhea occurs more frequently in unmarried than in married women (61% versus 51%).[15] The incidence of primary dysmenorrhea decreases with age more rapidly in married than in unmarried women, possibly related to child bearing. However, pregnancy and vaginal delivery do not necessarily cure primary dysmenorrhea.[16,17] The frequency of disabling dysmenorrhea does not appear to be related to the type of occupation or physical condition of the woman. Bergsjo[18] found that 50% of menstruating women in Norway experience dysmenorrhea, with 30% being disabled at least one day each month. His group also found that whereas many women are absent from work during days of severe dysmenorrhea, their reduced working capacity results in lower work output during the discomfort days when they do work.

The incidence of dysmenorrhea in adolescents is estimated to be 5–50%.[19,20] In a study of 5485 adolescent girls aged 10–20 years, 46% had completely painless menstruation, and 13% invariably had dysmenorrhea.[20] During the first year after menarche, 7.2% of adolescent girls had dysmenorrhea, but the incidence tripled to 26% by 5 years after menarche. Seventy-five percent of these adolescents reported the onset of painful menstruation before the end of the first year after menarche. There was good correlation between mothers and daughters for dysmenorrhea, with 7.9% of the mothers of dysmenorrheic girls also having had dysmenorrhea. If female adolescents are analyzed according to chronologic age at 13–20, the frequency of dysmenorrhea increased from 36% at age 13 to 56% at age 20, with an average of 47%,[20] which is similar to the overall frequency of dysmenorrhea in all menstruating women.[12] Overall absenteeism in dysmenorrheic adolescents was about 24%, with only 3% absent frequently and 12% absent sometimes.[20] Women experiencing dysmenorrhea were found to have lower marks and more school adjustment problems than among nondysmenorrheic students.[21] Exercise does not appear to have any significant effect on the incidence of dysmenorrhea because the frequencies of dysmenorrhea among gymnastic and nongymnastic students were found to be similar. Students who had dysmenorrhea did not notice any attenuation of their symptoms during the time when they attended regular gymnastic classes.

CLINICAL FEATURES

Primary Dysmenorrhea

Primary dysmenorrhea occurs almost invariably in ovulatory cycles and usually appears shortly or within 6–12 months after menarche when ovulatory cycles have been established. About 88% of adolescents with dysmenorrhea experienced their first painful menstruation within the first 2 years after menarche.[20] Dysmenorrhea usually begins a few hours before or just after the onset of menstruation. Discomfort is most severe and may be incapacitating on the first or second day of menstruation. The pains are characteristically spasmodic in nature and are strongest over the lower abdomen, although they may also radiate to the back and along the inner aspects of the thighs. Usually uterine cramp is accompanied by one or more systemic symptoms that include nausea and vomiting (89%), fatigue (85%), diarrhea (60%), lower backache (60%), and headache (45%). Nervousness, dizziness, and in some severe cases even syncope and collapse can be associated with dysmenorrhea. The symptoms may last from a few hours to 1 day but seldom persist for more than 2–3 days. In some patients, primary dysmenorrhea may disappear after the first childbirth but the relief may be temporary. Symptoms often decrease with age.

Primary dysmenorrhea is often diagnosed through exclusion of other causes of dysmenorrhea and serves as a repository for many forms of dysmenorrhea or even pelvic pain. However, primary dysmenorrhea should be diagnosed by its positive clinical features, the hallmarks of which are as follows:

1. *Initial onset of primary dysmenorrhea:* The condition dates back to the menarche or shortly therafter. A previous history of dysmenorrhea starting 2 years or more after menarche should arouse suspicion of secondary dysmenorrhea. Endometriosis can be extremely difficult to exclude, since the dysmenorrhea of endometriosis can remarkably resemble

that of primary dysmenorrhea. In a study of adolescent girls with endometriosis, dysmenorrhea typically began at 2.9 years after menarche.[22]

2. *Duration of the dysmenorrhea:* It usually lasts 48–72 hr, with the pain starting a few hours before or more often just after the onset of menstrual flow. Thus, dysmenorrhea that starts more than just a few hours and extending into several days before the onset of menstrual flow is less likely to be primary dysmenorrhea. The duration of pain in primary dysmenorrhea correlates very closely with the period of maximum prostaglandin release in the menstrual fluid.[23]

3. *Character of the pain:* It is described as cramping or laborlike.

4. *Pelvic examination:* No abnormal findings should be found during the pelvic–rectovaginal examination.

Differential diagnosis of primary dysmenorrhea includes all the causes of secondary dysmenorrhea. The causes of secondary dysmenorrhea are listed in Table 19-1. Endometriosis should always be considered, since it can closely mimic primary dysmenorrhea and can clearly begin with the onset of menarche or shortly thereafter. Contrary to conventional thinking, endometriosis occurs frequently enough in teenagers and in black women, as shown with the increasingly frequent use of laparoscopy.[24] Therefore, in those patients with a strong index of suspicion for endometriosis such as those with a family history of endometriosis in an immediate female sibling or the mother,[25] laparoscopy should be undertaken fairly early during the course of management of the patient, once medical therapy has failed.

TABLE 19-1. Causes of Secondary Dysmenorrhea

Endometriosis
Intrauterine device (IUD)
Pelvic inflammatory disease and infections (PID)
Adenomyosis
Uterine myomas, uterine polyps, uterine adhesions
Congenital malformations of the mullerian system (bicornuate and septate uterus; transverse vaginal septum)
Cervical structures or stenosis
Ovarian cysts
Pelvic congestion syndrome
Allen-Masters syndrome

Secondary Dysmenorrhea

The appearance of dysmenorrhea years after the menarche may be a sign of secondary dysmenorrhea, which is most frequently caused by endometriosis. Dysmenorrhea in women with anovulatory cycles is also more likely to be of the secondary type.

Although the age of onset of dysmenorrhea often distinguishes primary from secondary dysmenorrhea, endometriosis can also occur with or soon after the onset of menarche. A history of recurrent pelvic inflammatory disease (PID), irregular menstrual cycles especially associated with anovulation, menorrhagia, use of an intrauterine device (IUD), and infertility problems suggest secondary dysmenorrhea. The differential diagnosis of secondary dysmenorrhea includes primary dysmenorrhea and chronic pelvic pain. There is no time relationship between chronic pelvic pain and the menstrual cycle, but in dysmenorrhea the pain is confined to the menstrual phase or shortly before menstruation.

Physical examination, especially a pelvic examination including a rectovaginal examination, is likely to reveal causes of secondary dysmenorrhea, such as uterine malformations, uterine myomas, presence of an IUD, PID, and some cases of endometriosis. In women over 40 years of age, adenomyosis should be considered a cause of the dysmenorrhea. This diagnosis can be made only on the basis of a uterine specimen evaluation, but clinically the dysmenorrhea will be associated with a dull, pelvic dragging discomfort and a uniformly enlarged, boggy uterus, about the size of an 8–10-week gestation. In these cases, hysterectomy should be considered only after all other causes of dysmenorrhea have been eliminated.

Investigations that may be useful in determining the cause of the secondary dysmenorrhea include a complete blood count, erythrocyte sedimentation rate, pelvic ultrasonography, hysterosalpingography, and genital cultures for pathogens. The final diagnosis can usually be confirmed with diagnostic laparoscopy, hysteroscopy, or dilatation and curettage.

ETIOLOGY OF DYSMENORRHEA

Primary Dysmenorrhea

The etiology of primary dysmenorrhea has been attributed to many factors, including behavioral and psychological factors, uterine ischemia, cervical factors, increased vasopressin release, and increased uterine prostaglandin production and release. Although psychological factors have not been convincingly demonstrated to be the *ab initio* mechanism in primary dysmenorrhea, their contribution should be considered in those patients who have not responded to medical therapy. Whereas many psychoanalytic phenomena have been advanced to explain the basis of the dysmenorrhea, none of the reports dealing with this has studied the patients prior to the development of their primary dysmenorrhea, so that the observations made are either an accompaniment to or the result of the dysmenorrhea.[12] Undoubtedly psychological factors that modulate the pain of primary dysmenorrhea and therefore influence the pain perceived by the woman should be taken into consideration. However, such factors are no more unique to the pain of primary dysmenorrhea than to the pain arising from any other pathology.

A demonstrable cervical factor giving rise to primary dysmenorrhea does not appear to exist. There are no objective data to support the suggestion that women with primary dysmenorrhea have a relative stenosis or narrowing of their cervical canal. Hence there is no basis for these two mechanisms as major etiologic factors contributing to the pain of primary dysmenorrhea.

Some preliminary studies suggest that there may be an increase in circulating vasopressin levels in women with primary dysmenorrhea during their menstruation.[26] However, these studies have not demonstrated serial levels before and during menstruation in these women. An increase in circulating vasopressin levels without a concomitant and proportional increase in oxytocin levels may give rise to dysrhythmic uterine contractions, which are more likely to cause uterine hypoxia and ischemia. Primary dysmenorrhea occurs only in ovulatory cycles; therefore, exposure to progesterone after adequate estrogen effect appears to be mandatory for whatever the causal factor responsible for primary dysmenorrhea.

Primary dysmenorrhea occurs almost exclusively in ovulatory cycles. Women on oral contraceptive to suppress ovulation are relieved of their primary dysmenorrhea. Whereas dysmenorrhea may occur in women with anovulatory cycles, it is almost certain that this is secondary dysmenorrhea. Earlier studies indicating that primary dysmenorrhea was found in some women with anovulatory cycles did not have any objective documentation

and it is, in all probability, due to failure to exclude rigorously other causes of secondary dysmenorrhea.

There is enough evidence to indicate that increased production and release of endometrial prostaglandins in many if not all women with primary dysmenorrhea gives rise to abnormal uterine activity and results in uterine hypoxia and ischemia. It is therefore appropriate at this point to discuss uterine activity and prostaglandins in primary dysmenorrhea.

Uterine Activity and Primary Dysmenorrhea

Changes in ovarian steroid hormone production as well as changes in endometrial prostaglandin levels bring about cyclic variation in the uterine activity during the normal menstrual cycle, as shown with a variety of intrauterine pressure monitoring techniques. Figure 19-1 shows the basal or resting tone, active pressure, and number of contractions per 10 min throughout the different phases of the menstrual cycle in normal women. In nondysmenorrheic women, during menstruation the uterine resting tone is lowest (10 mm Hg), the active pressure is maximal (120 mm Hg), and the number of contractions (3–4 every 10 min) is least compared with the rest of the menstrual cycle.

In dysmenorrheic women, no single consistent abnormality has been observed, but one or more of the following four abnormalities have been found in most cases: (1) increased uterine resting tone, (2) increased active pressure, (3) increased number of contractions, and (4) incoordinate or dysrhythmic uterine activity. When more than one of these abnormalities are present, they tend to potentiate each other; pain is experienced at a much smaller change than when only one abnormality is present. When uterine activity is abnormal and increased, uterine blood flow has been shown to be reduced.[27] When the abnormal uterine activity is suppressed, uterine blood flow is enhanced and returns to normal. Clearly, one contributory mechanism to the pain of primary dysmenorrhea is uterine ischemia or uterine hypoxia. The increased uterine activity is secondary to increased endometrial prostaglandin production and release during menstruation.

Prostaglandins and Primary Dysmenorrhea

The evidence for prostaglandin involvement in the pathogenesis of primary dysmenorrhea has been discussed in many recent reviews[12,23] and can be summarized as follows:

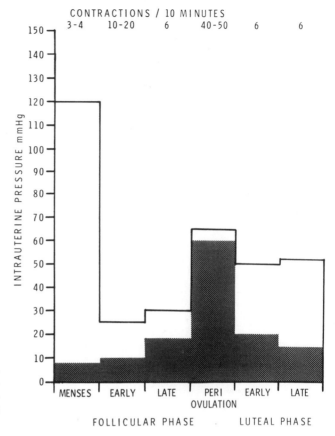

FIGURE 19-1. Uterine activity including active pressure and resting tone at various stages of the menstrual cycle. The hatched area represents uterine resting tone, while the clear areas represent uterine active pressure. (From Ylikorkala and Dawood.[12])

1. A striking similarity exists between clinical manifestations of primary dysmenorrhea and the symptoms induced when exogenous prostaglandin E_2 (PGE_2) or prostaglandin $F_{2\alpha}$ ($PGF_{2\alpha}$) is administered. The pain and contractions are described as laborlike under both circumstances. The associated symptoms of diarrhea, vomiting, and nausea are well recognized side effects commonly observed when either PGE_2 or $PGF_{2\alpha}$ is administered to induce labor or abortion.

2. The secretory endometrium has higher concentrations of prostaglandins than does the proliferative endometrium.[23] This is consistent with primary dysmenorrhea, occurring only during ovulatory cycles. In anovulatory cycles and in the absence of increased progesterone, there is no increase in endometrial prostaglandin concentrations[28]; therefore, the ensuing menstrual period is painless.

3. Many recent studies have documented painful primary dysmenorrhea in women who have a significantly higher than normal concentration of prostaglandins in their endometrium,[8,29] endometrial jet washings,[30] and menstrual fluids.[8–11,31,32]

4. Many prostaglandin synthetase inhibitors have been shown to be effective in the treatment of primary dysmenorrhea,[10,11,16,32–36] and many more are being evaluated for efficacy in relieving the symptoms of primary dysmenorrhea.

At this point, it is essential to examine briefly the biosynthesis of prostaglandins and the points of action of the nonsteroidal antiinflammatory drugs on this pathway. Figure 19-2 shows the structure of prostanoic acid, PGE_2 and $PGF_{2\alpha}$. Prostaglandins are C_{20} hydrocarbons with a cyclopentane ring; they are present in human tissues, where they are produced locally under the control of the microsomal enyzmes collectively called prostaglandin synthetase. The pathway for the biosynthesis of prostaglandins and other related compounds such as

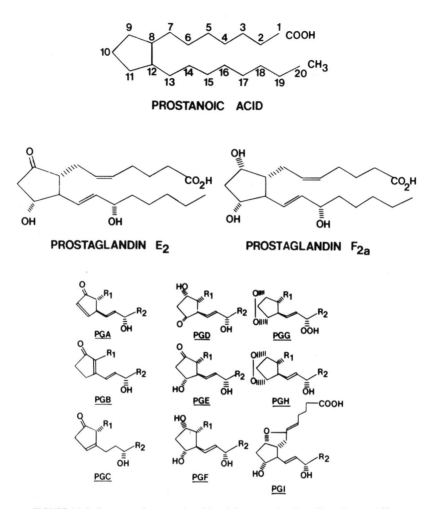

FIGURE 19-2. Structure of prostanoic acid and the prostaglandins. (From Dawood.[23])

prostacyclin (PGE$_2$) and thromboxanes is schematically shown in Figure 19-3. Prostaglandins are synthesized from free unesterified fatty acids, derived from conversion of phospholipids, triglycerides, and cholesterol esters by the acyl hydrolase enzymes. Free unsaturated fatty acids can serve as precursors for prostaglandin synthesis. Two such unesterified fatty acids involved in the production of prostaglandins are arachidonic and eicosatrienoic acids. PGF$_{2\alpha}$ and PGE$_2$ are usually produced from arachidonic acid. The factors controlling the conversion of arachidonic acid to PGE$_2$ and PGF$_{2\alpha}$ have not been fully elucidated, but two important factors include trauma and the availability of arach-

idonic acid. The availability of arachidonic acid appears to be the rate limiting step and trauma is a powerful stimulus favoring the production of PGE$_2$ and PGF$_{2\alpha}$. It has been suggested that the nonsteroidal anti-inflammatory drugs be divided into two types: (1) type I inhibitor, which inhibits cyclooxygenase and therefore prevents conversion of arachidonic acid to cyclic endoperoxides, and (2) type II inhibitor, which suppresses the arachidonic acid cascade after the formation of cyclic endoperoxides (Fig. 18.3). In tissues derived from the uterus, arachidonic acid is usually produced from phospholipids through hydrolysis by phospholipase A$_2$, a lysosomal enzyme. Since phospholipase A$_2$

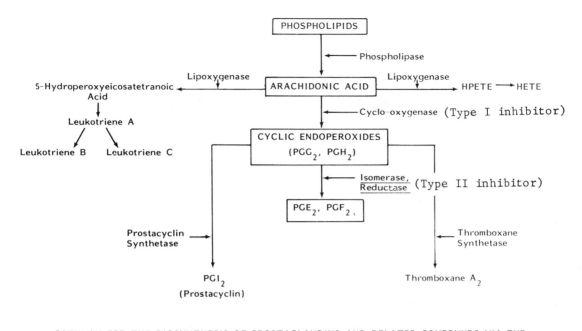

PATHWAY FOR THE BIOSYNTHESIS OF PROSTAGLANDINS AND RELATED COMPOUNDS VIA THE ARACHIDONIC ACID CASCADE.

FIGURE 19-3. Schematic representation of biosynthesis of prostaglandins from phospholipids and the sites of action of prostaglandin synthetase inhibitors (nonsteroidal anti-inflammatory agents). The type of prostaglandin inhibitor is shown in brackets next to the enzyme(s) it inhibits. (From Dawood.[23])

governs the hydrolysis of phospholipids, hence the availability of arachidonic acid, it is probable that the availability of phospholipase A_2 is an important rate-limiting step in the biosynthesis of PGE_2 and $PGF_{2\alpha}$.

The stability of lysosomes is controlled by a number of factors, one of which is the level of progesterone. A high level of progesterone tends to stabilize lysosomes, while a falling level of progesterone labilizes them. At the end of the luteal phase of the menstrual cycle, if pregnancy does not occur, the corpus luteum undergoes regression, progesterone levels decline, and lysosomal instability sets in. With labilization of the lysosomes, menstruation begins and phospholipase A_2 is released, resulting in hydrolysis of phospholipids from the cell membrane and generation of arachidonic acid. With the intracellular destruction and trauma accompanying the onset of menstruation, the stimulus for biosynthesis of prostaglandin favors the production of these compounds. In women with primary dysmenorrhea it has been shown that their endometrial tissue is capable of increased production and release of prostaglandins during menstruation.[9–11,32]

Pickles and colleagues were the first to identify and quantitate prostaglandins in menstrual fluids.[4–7,31] They found that dysmenorrheic women produced 8–13 times more PGF than do nondysmenorrheic women.[28] Subsequently, the endometrial content of PGE_2 and $PGF_{2\alpha}$ was found to be significantly elevated throughout the menstrual cycle of dysmenorrheic women.[29] In another study, uterine jet washings of a dysmenorrheic woman had significantly high concentrations of PGF.[30] With radioimmunoassay (RIA), the endometrial $PGF_{2\alpha}$ concentrations were reported to be significantly higher on or before the first day of menstruation in dysmenorrheic women than in nondysmenorrheic women.[37] In another study, circulating blood concentrations of 15-keto-13,14,-dihydro-$PGF_{2\alpha}$ and 13,14-dihydro-$PGF_{2\alpha}$ but not $PGF_{2\alpha}$ were found to be significantly higher on the first day of menstruation in dysmenorrheic women than in those with normal periods.[37] This is not surprising, since $PGF_{2\alpha}$ is rapidly metabolized to the 15-keto,13,14,-dihydrometabolite in a single passage through the lung.

Our studies on the continuous release of prostaglandins throughout menstruation have shown

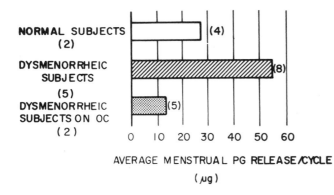

FIGURE 19-4. Menstrual fluid prostaglandins in normal subjects, dysmenorrheic women, and dysmenorrheic women treated with oral contraceptives. OC, oral contraceptive; PG, prostaglandin. (From Chan and Dawood.[11])

that significantly high quantities of prostaglandins are released per menstruation in women with primary dysmenorrhea[9–11,32] (Fig. 19-4). During menstruation, most of the production and release of prostaglandins occurs during the first 48 hr of menstrual flow, thereby explaining the intense pain experienced during the first or second day of menstruation in primary dysmenorrhea. There is also good correlation between the amount of prostaglandins released in the menstrual fluid per hour and the clinical symptoms of the dysmenorrhea during the first 48 hr of menstruation (Fig. 19-5). Clearly, the high concentrations of prostaglandins found in women with primary dysmenorrhea result from increased prostaglandin production rather than from altered metabolism or from other forms of abnormal prostaglandin release. In vitro studies of the production of $PGF_{2\alpha}$ production by human endometrium have shown that the endometrium of dysmenorrheic women biosynthesizes prostaglandin

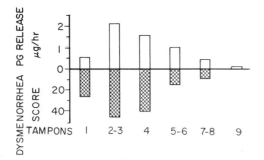

FIGURE 19-5. Relationship between the clinical symptoms of primary dysmenorrhea (dysmenorrhea score) and the amount of prostaglandin release per hour into the tampons used during menstruation in a dysmenorrheic woman. When the rate of prostaglandin release increased, the clinical symptoms (dysmenorrhea) increased as well. There is a direct relationship between the clinical symptoms and the amount of prostaglandin released over the same period of time (From Dawood.[23])

seven times faster than that of normal women.[38] It is unlikely that increased sensitivity to PGE_2 and $PGF_{2\alpha}$ by the myometrium is a significant contributing factor in dysmenorrhea, because the myometrial responses to intrauterine administration of either PGE_2 or $PGF_{2\alpha}$[39] are similar in both dysmenorrheic and nondysmenorrheic women.[31]

Thus, the presence of increased production and release of endometrial prostaglandins at menstruation is associated with increased abnormal uterine activity, accordingly giving rise to uterine hypoxia and therefore pain. The postulated mechanism for the generation of pain from the pelvic structures in primary dysmenorrhea has been discussed in detail by Dawood[23] and is summarized in Figure 19-6.

The roles of prostanoids, such as thromboxane A_2 (TxA_2) and prostacyclin (PGI_2) in primary dysmenorrhea have not been fully elucidated. Preliminary evidence suggests that PGI_2 is involved in the pathophysiology of primary dysmenorrhea.[23] PGI_2 is a potent vasodilator that relaxes uterine muscle in vitro; thus, a reduction in PGI_2 concentration could enhance uterine activity and vasoconstriction, in turn causing hypoxia, ischemia, and pain. Although endoperoxides and thromboxanes are potent uterotonic compounds, they have very short half-lives, rendering them difficult to quantitate. There is no published information on their concentrations in women with primary dysmenorrhea. Therefore, it is unclear whether any change occurs in the relative composition of the prostaglandins or prostanoids in the endometrium of women who suffer from primary dysmenorrhea. An imbalance in the concentration of different prostaglandins could be responsible for some forms of dysmenorrhea.

MANAGEMENT

For proper therapy with gratifying results, it is essential to identify whether the patient is suffering

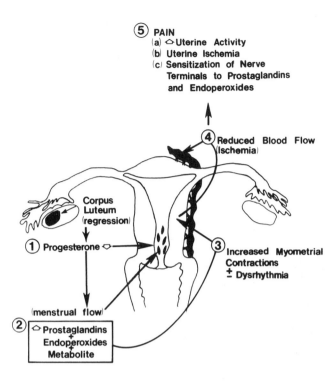

FIGURE 19-6. Postulated mechanism of pain generation from the pelvic structures in primary dysmenorrhea. Extrapelvic factors such as central modulation and perception of pain are not depicted (From Dawood.[23])

from primary or secondary dysmenorrhea. The differential diagnosis and distinguishing features of these two types of dysmenorrhea have already been discussed. The overall approach to management of both primary and secondary dysmenorrhea should include manipulation of the psychological and behavioral factors as well as the specific management be it pharmacologic or surgical.[16]

The pain associated with both primary and secondary dysmenorrhea is the sum total of the actual organic factors causing the pain as well as psychological components (the inherent factors that influence the response to pain and the recurring pain itself), which in turn influence the response to subsequent cycles of dysmenorrhea. A careful assessment of the proportion contributed by these various factors to the final pain experienced in each woman is essential to appropriate therapy or combination of therapies. While it is difficult to quantify pain or to identify the precise degree to which the various factors contribute to the total pain, in clinical practice an overall assessment can be made if the physician spends enough time taking a careful history. Obviously the efficacy of any modality of treatment for any type of dysmenorrhea can be greatly enhanced if some form of simple psychotherapy in the

form of doctor–patient dialogue, explanation, and reassurrance is informally given by the physician.

Specific Therapy

The specific therapy for dysmenorrhea depends on whether it is primary or secondary.

Primary Dysmenorrhea

Various modalities of treatment used in primary dysmenorrhea are summarized in Table 19-2. The two most effective medications are the oral contraceptives and the prostaglandin synthetase inhibitors. The choice of medication will depend on whether the woman prefers an oral contraceptive for birth control and whether there is any contraindication to the use of the combined oral contraceptive or the prostaglandin synthetase inhibitor.

Oral Contraceptives. If the patient desires birth control with the combined oral contraceptive pill, this would be the method of choice for the treatment of her primary dysmenorrhea. Combination-type

TABLE 19-2. Modalities Available for the Treatment of Primary Dysmenorrhea[a]

Approach	Specific methods
General measures	Psychotherapy, reassurance
Surgery	Dilatation and curettage, presacral neurectomy
Endocrine therapy	Oral contraceptive pills, inhibition of ovulation
Tocolysis	Alcohol, β-receptor stimulators
Analgesics	Non-narcotics, narcotics
Prostaglandin synthetase inhibitors	Type I inhibitors (aspirin, indomethacin, meclofenamic acid, ibuprofen); Type II inhibitors (phenylbutazone, p-chloromercuribenzoate)

[a]From Dawood.[16]

oral contraceptives are effective in the treatment of primary dysmenorrhea and have been the main method of treatment since their introduction. Menstrual fluid prostaglandin levels are reduced to below normal levels in women who use oral contraceptives.[11,32] These reduced levels are brought about through (1) a reduction in the menstrual fluid volume, which accompanies the use of birth control pills, since the suppression of endometrial tissue growth results in reduced menstrual fluid loss[11,32]; and (2) inhibition of ovulation, which results in an anovulatory cycle, an endocrine milieu that is essentially similar to the early proliferative phase of the menstrual cycle, when levels of prostaglandins are low. Furthermore, the absence of luteal-phase progesterone levels, which are necessary for increased prostaglandin biosynthesis, will contribute to the anovulatory mechanism of reduced menstrual fluid prostaglandins.

With birth control pills, more than 90% of dysmenorrheic women can be relieved of their primary dysmenorrhea. A trial of the oral contraceptive for a period of 3–4 months is worthwhile. Patients who respond to oral contraceptive therapy can be maintained on this regimen. If the dysmenorrhea is not adequately relieved, an appropriate prostaglandin synthetase inhibitor can then be added. It may be necessary to increase the dose of the prostaglandin synthetase inhibitor or to change the type of prostaglandin synthetase inhibitor if the patient does not obtain complete relief during the first couple of cycles of treatment.

Prostaglandin Synthetase Inhibitor. If an oral contraceptive is not desired for birth control, the drug of choice for the treatment of primary dysmenorrhea is a prostaglandin synthetase inhibitor. Unlike the oral contraceptives, the prostaglandin synthetase inhibitors are taken for the first 2–3 days

of the menstrual flow, there is no significant suppression of the pituitary ovarian axis, and there are none of the metabolic effects seen with oral contraceptives, which have to be taken for a minimum of 3 out of every 4 weeks. Selection of the most suitable or optimal prostaglandin synthetase inhibitor is based both on clinical evidence of its efficacy as well as some of the theoretical considerations listed in Table 19-3. A 6-month trial of prostaglandin synthetase inhibitors, with the necessary change in dosage and from one inhibitor to another should the one chosen not work satisfactorily, will be sufficient to determine whether relief can be obtained through this form of therapy.

If the patient does not respond to a prostaglandin synthetase inhibitor, it is necessary to reconsider whether a pelvic pathology and therefore secondary dysmenorrhea might have been missed. At this point, the patient merits having a laparoscopy to rule out or confirm pelvic disease. In the event that pelvic disease is discovered, the appropriate therapies directed toward the underlying pathology are instituted, thereby alleviating the dysmenorrhea.

TABLE 19-3. Suggested Criteria for Choosing an Ideal Prostaglandin Synthetase Inhibitor in the Treatment of Dysmenorrhea[a]

Effective in inhibiting endometrial prostaglandin synthesis
Type I prostaglandin synthetase inhibitor (i.e., a cyclooxygenase blocker)
Rapidly absorbed to achieve therapeutic blood levels quickly
Possess prostaglandin antagonist properties
Low ulcerogenicity
Minimal, tolerable, and inconsequential side effects
Long-term safety

[a]From Dawood.[16]

In the event that no pelvic pathology is found, the approach to management of the dysmenorrhea becomes one of trial and error, as it is unclear whether any specific pharmacotherapy could be of help. Several agents such as the β-mimetic agent[27] or a calcium antagonist as nifedipine[32] could be tried on an experimental basis, since preliminary studies suggest that they may provide some relief. These agents should probably not be used on a routine basis, however, and such attempts are best left to centers carrying out specific trials or studies on these agents. At this point, psychiatric help in the management of these patients might be appropriate. It should not be construed that the dysmenorrhea is wholly psychosomatic but, in the absence of an understanding of the basic pathophysiologic mechanisms of their dysmenorrhea, symptomatic treatment with analgesics and psychotherapy to modulate the psychologic factors that could be playing a significant or contributing role to the pain could ameliorate the dysmenorrhea to some extent. Very few patients with primary dysmenorrhea fall into this category if the correct diagnosis has been made and steps in the management of the patient have been undertaken.

The prostaglandin synthetase inhibitors appear to relieve primary dysmenorrhea through suppression of menstrual fluid prostaglandins. This has been adequately demonstrated in several studies.[10,11,32] An example of the suppression of menstrual fluid prostaglandins during therapy with the prostaglandin synthetase inhibitor, ibuprofen, during a controlled, double-blind, crossover study is shown in Figure 19-7. In addition, these compounds also have direct analgesic properties; it is unclear whether the relief of dysmenorrhea is also mediated through their direct analgesic effect. The reduction in menstrual fluid prostaglandin appears to be a direct suppression of the biosynthesis of prostaglandins in the endometrial tissue and release of prostaglandins, which normally occurs during the first 48 hr of menstruation.

It is important to remember that because primary dysmenorrhea is a cyclic phenomenon, treatment is necessary for each menstrual cycle. With the oral contraceptive agent, the elevated pretreatment levels of menstrual fluid prostaglandins and the dysmenorrhea return as soon as treatment is discontinued.[11]

Types of prostaglandin inhibitors. There are five major groups of prostaglandin synthetase inhibitors (Table 19-4). Based on their site of action, pros-

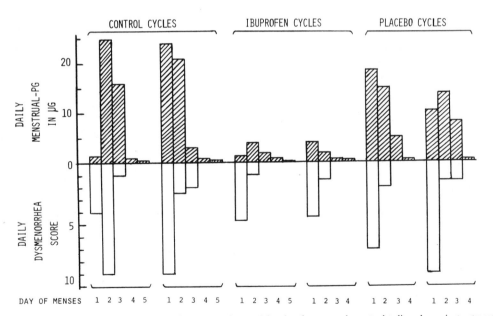

FIGURE 19-7. Relationship between severity of dysmenorrhea and levels of menstrual prostaglandin release in treatment and nontreatment cycles of a dysmenorrheic woman. The subject was studied for six successive menstrual cycles (two control, two ibuprofen-treated, and two placebo), using double-blind crossover procedures on the treatment cycles. Open bars show the daily global assessment of dysmenorrheic symptoms as recorded by the patient using a 10-point scale visual analogue method. Hatched bars represent the levels of menstrual prostaglandin release during the corresponding period. (From Chan et al.[10])

TABLE 19-4. Prostaglandin Synthetase Inhibitors Classified According to Structural Derivative and Clinical Efficacy in Dysmenorrhea[a]

Prostaglandin synthetase inhibitor group	Example	Dose	Clinical relief (%)
Benzoic acid deratives	Aspirin	500–600 mg, 4 times/day	No difference from placebo (except in one study)
Buterophenones	Phenylbutazone, oxyphenbutazone	No information available	
Indoleacetic acid derivatives	Indomethacin	25 mg, 3–6 times/day	73–90
Fenamates	Flufenamic acid	100–200 mg, 3 times/day	77–82
	Mefenamic acid	250–500 mg, 4 times/day	93
	Tolfenamic acid	133 mg, 3 times/day	88
Aryl propionic acid	Ibuprofen	400 mg, 4 times/day	66–100
	Naproxen sodium	275 mg, 4 times/day	78–90
	Ketoprofen	50 mg, 3 times/day	90

[a]From Dawood.[16]

taglandin synthetase inhibitors may work at two different sites in the arachidonic acid cascade: (1a) inhibition of cyclic endoperoxide synthesis at the cyclooxygenase level, or (2b) through the cyclic endoperoxide cleavage enzymes after the formation of cyclic endoperoxides. Most of the prostaglandin synthetase inhibitors work through inhibition of the enzyme cyclooxygenase (type I inhibitor), except the buterophenones, which act on the enzyme system after the formation of cyclic endoperoxide (type II inhibitor). Therefore, the buterophenones are less desirable than the other prostaglandin synthetase inhibitors, since they do not effectively inhibit cyclooxygenase and production of cyclic endoperoxides, which are potent uterotonic substances.

The benzoic acid derivative (e.g., aspirin), administered in doses of 500–650 mg four times per day, has generally proved no more effective than a placebo, with the exception of a single study.

The indoleacetic acid derivative (e.g., indomethacin), the fenamates (e.g., flufenamic acid, mefenamic acid, and tolfenamic acid), and the aryl propionic acid derivatives (e.g., ibuprofen and sodium naproxen) have all been shown to be highly effective in relieving primary dysmenorrhea. The efficacy rate for these three classes of prostaglandin synthetase inhibitors is in the range of 60–90% (Table 19-4). Suppression of endometrial tissue prostaglandins, resulting in significant inhibition of uterine activity with accompanying relief of primary dysmenorrhea, has been demonstrated with ibuprofen and sodium naproxen.

The physician should become familiarized with,

and use, a couple of the prostaglandin synthetase inhibitors that have been proved effective, that have been approved by the regulatory agency for such an indication, and that carry little or no side effects. More details about the pharmacology of the prostaglandin synthetase inhibitors are readily available in a recent review.[34,39] Although indomethacin is effective, the high incidence of gastrointestinal side effects cause many patients to discontinue its use during the clinical trials. Thus the inhibitor of choice in the treatment of primary dysmenorrhea would appear to be either a fenamate or an aryl propionic acid derivative.

It is now quite apparent that with these rapidly absorbed inhibitors, treatment before the onset of dysmenorrhea is not necessary.[32] This finding is important in clinical practice, since many women suffering from primary dysmenorrhea are young and sexually active. Because the time of onset of menstrual flow is variable, it is more practical to initiate medication at the beginning of menstruation and to continue therapy for 3 days if necessary.[34–36] It is the rapidity of drug absorption that determines how quickly relief of dysmenorrhea is obtained. The choice of the most suitable or satisfactory inhibitor is based on clinical evidence of its efficacy. The rationale behind giving a nonsteroidal anti-inflammatory agent for 48 hr or during the first 3 days of menstruation is based on the observation that prostaglandin release is maximal during the first 48 hr of the menstrual flow, as shown in studies from our laboratory.[9–11,23–32] If the response to treatment during the first cycle indicates that some degree of uterine cramps persists during the first

TABLE 19-5. Side Effects of Prostaglandin
Synthetase Inhibitors*a*

Gastrointestinal symptoms
    Indigestion
    Heartburn
    Nausea
    Abdominal pain
    Constipation
    Vomiting
    Anorexia
    Diarrhea
    Melena
CNS symptoms
    Headache
    Dizziness
    Vertigo
    Visual disturbances
    Hearing disturbances
    Irritability
    Depression
    Drowsiness
    Sleepiness
Other symptoms
    Allergic reactions
    Skin rash
    Edema
    Bronchospasm
    Hematologic abnormalities
    Effects on the eyes
    Fluid retention
    Effects on liver and kidney

*a*From Dawood.[16]

few hours or so after beginning oral medication, it is recommended that the starting dose be increased by 50% or doubled at the next cycle, but the maintenance dose can be kept essentially the same as before. If the patient reports no improvement, a trial of a new inhibitor may be necessary. Dosages for some of the inhibitors that have proved effective in treatment of dysmenorrhea are shown in Table 19.4.

Side effects of prostaglandin inhibitors. Although some of the newer nonsteroidal anti-inflammatory agents may have a much lower ulcerogenic index, it is probably prudent not to prescribe these medications to a patient with a definite history of gastric or duodenal ulcer. Another contraindication is a previous history of bronchospastic type of reaction after the ingestion of aspirin or aspirinlike drugs. Side effects of prostaglandin inhibitors and antagonists are relatively mild during therapy of primary dysmenorrhea and are usually reported to

be well tolerated. Some of the more frequent as well as uncommon side effects are listed in Table 19.5. There have been recent suggestions that the long-acting nonsteroidal anti-inflammatory agents might have an advantage over the currently available short-acting nonsteroidal anti-inflammatory agents, which require multiple doses. Nevertheless, the toxic side effects associated with some of the long-acting nonsteroidal anti-inflammatory agents suggest that significant problems need to be overcome before the marginal advantage of a single daily dose can be considered sufficiently acceptable.

Other Forms of Treatment. If the patient does not respond to either an effective prostaglandin synthetase inhibitor or an oral contraceptive, laparoscopy will become necessary to rule out a pelvic pathology and a possible cause of secondary dysmenorrhea. β-mimetic agents have generally been disappointing in efficacy and have many side effects, but they may be worth trying in these difficult cases.[16] Newer agents such as calcium antagonists have been tested and hold promise.[41]

During laparoscopy, dilatation of the cervix should be undertaken. However, cervical dilatation as a primary method of therapy before a trial of suitable medication is currently not warranted. Narrowing of the cervical canal has never been demonstrated in primary dysmenorrhea. Certainly dilatation of the cervix is indicated in secondary dysmenorrhea due to cervical stenosis. Dilatation of the cervix does relieve primary dysmenorrhea temporarily, but with a progressive return of the symptoms. The reason for the relief is unclear, but possible mechanisms include disruption of the paracervical nerve fibers and plexus with consequent neuropraxia or partial denervation of the cervix. Dilatation of the cervix will also probably increase the diameter of the cervical canal, culminating in enhanced menstrual fluid flow with a shorter contact time between the uterine wall and the menstrual fluid containing the prostaglandins.

Most β-mimetic agents, such as isoxsuprine[42] and hydroxyorciprenaline[43] have been shown to be no more effective than a placebo. Terbutaline is found to be more effective than a placebo,[27] but the use of β-receptor stimulators in dysmenorrhea is handicapped by the high incidence of side effects, some of which are troublesome. Consequently, their use in dysmenorrhea is limited and perhaps reserved to only those cases in which more effective and established methods of therapy have failed or are contraindicated.

Alcohol, a tocolytic agent, certainly diminishes the severity of dysmenorrhea, but the quantity that must be taken to obtain complete relief produces a state of inebriation that may be as incapacitating as the dysmenorrhea. The side effect mitigates against recommending alcohol as a method of therapy for primary dysmenorrhea.

The progesterone-medicated IUD (Progestasert) was found to reduce menstrual fluid prostaglandin and relieve primary dysmenorrhea in one study.[44] Nevertheless, the advisability of recommending the use of the IUD, which itself gives rise to dysmenorrhea, is seriously questioned in women with primary dysmenorrhea, as there are alternative methods of contraception and therapy of dysmenorrhea.

Presacral neurectomy is hardly ever required today in most forms of primary dysmenorrhea. The place of presacral neurectomy should be extremely limited, and this procedure should be reserved for (1) patients with chronic pelvic pain, where other methods of pain relief have failed, (2) patients with pelvic malignancy, and (3) patients with pelvic pathology, such as endometriosis, that is impinging on or involving the area of the presacral plexus.

More recently, transcutaneous nerve stimulation has been found experimentally to relieve primary dysmenorrhea (V Lundstrom, personal communication, 1983). The relief is temporary, however, and the transcutaneous nerve stimulation probably has to be applied for a longer period of time, making it unsuitable as a practical method of management.

Secondary Dysmenorrhea

Specific therapy for secondary dysmenorrhea is directed entirely toward the underlying cause of the condition. In contrast to primary dysmenorrhea, surgery is more definitive and has a relatively greater role in the treatment of most forms of secondary dysmenorrhea. In patients with an IUD, nonsurgical management is preferable. Women wearing the IUD should be treated for their dysmenorrhea with an effective prostaglandin synthetase inhibitor.

Studies both in animals and in women have demonstrated that the presence of an IUD provokes leukocytic infiltration in the vicinity of the IUD, resulting in an increase in prostaglandin production by the endometrial tissue.[45–47] In women endometrial prostaglandin levels were found to increase significantly 1–5 months after the insertion of an IUD as compared with levels before the use of the device. Most of the increase is in $PGF_{2\alpha}$. Several clinical trials have shown that nonsteroidal anti-inflammatory agents will not only effectively relieve the dysmenorrhea associated with the use of the IUD, but will also correct the menorrhagia associated with the IUD.[48–50] In this respect, flufenamic acid, ibuprofen, and naproxen have been found to relieve the dysmenorrhea and menorrhagia associated with the use of the IUD.[48–50] Therefore, in current clinical practice whenever an IUD is inserted, it is recommended that a prostaglandin synthetase inhibitor, rather than a nonspecific analgesic, be prescribed to combat the dysmenorrhea and menorrhagia that may occur.

Women with uterine myomas have been found to have increased endometrial prostaglandin levels.[29] However, prostaglandin synthetase inhibitors cannot be advocated as a definitive therapy for the relief of dysmenorrhea due to uterine myomas and should only be used as an interim measure for the relief of secondary dysmenorrhea while awaiting definitive myomectomy or hysterectomy.

There is much recent interest in the role of prostaglandins in endometriosis. Ectopic endometrial tissue may have a greater capacity to produce prostaglandins than does normal endometrium,[51] but the findings on peritoneal fluid prostaglandin levels are far more controversial.[52–56] The balance of evidence suggests that no significant increase occurs in the levels of $PGF_{2\alpha}$, PGE, 6-keto-$PGF_{1\alpha}$ (the stable metabolite of prostacyclin), and thromboxane B_2 (the stable metabolite of thromboxane A). Therefore, the role of peritoneal or peritoneal fluid prostaglandin in the pathogenesis of pelvic pain or dysmenorrhea associated with endometriosis is at best unclear and probably an insignificant one.

Finally, the pathogenesis of pain associated with endometriosis is likely to be multifactorial. Clinical trials with prostaglandin synthetase inhibitors such as aspirin, indomethacin, and tolfenamic acid have not provided significant relief of the premenstrual as well as the intramenstrual pain associated with endometriosis. Therefore, the nonsteroidal anti-inflammatory agents cannot be recommended as a suitable alternative to currently well-established methods of managing the pelvic pain and dysmenorrhea of endometriosis through hormonal manipulation.

SUMMARY

This chapter has discussed the incidence, etiology, clinical features, differential diagnosis, and management of primary and secondary dysmenorrhea. In primary dysmenorrhea, the patient has painful menstrual cramps but without any visible pelvic pathology. In secondary dysmenorrhea, there is visible pelvic pathology. Primary dysmenorrhea is a common complaint in 50% of postmenarcheal women, with 10% severely incapacitated, affecting their work, performance, and life-style.

In true primary dysmenorrhea, most patients have an increased abnormal uterine activity secondary to increased production and release of endometrial prostaglandins at the time of menstruation. The abnormality gives rise to uterine hypoxia. Characteristic features of primary dysmenorrhea include a history that dates back to shortly after the menarche, painful menstrual cramps occurring with or just shortly before the onset of menstrual flow and lasting only for 48 hr, associated symptoms of nausea, vomiting, diarrhea, headache, and tiredness, and a normal pelvic examination. Primary dysmenorrhea must be distinguished from endometriosis and other forms of secondary dysmenorrhea. The treatment of primary dysmenorrhea includes physician–patient dialogue and reassurance as well as specific pharmacotherapy. The drug of choice for treatment of primary dysmenorrhea is an effective prostaglandin synthetase inhibitor (PGSI) such as ibuprofen, sodium naproxen, naproxen, or indomethacin. If the patient desires birth control pills for contraception, this will be appropriate therapy for her primary dysmenorrhea as well. PGSIs should not be given to patients with gastrointestinal ulcers or with a history of bronchospastic reaction to aspirin and aspirinlike drugs. If a patient does not respond to either birth control pills or PGSIs, laparoscopy is indicated to rule out pelvic lesions as a cause of the dysmenorrhea.

Secondary dysmenorrhea may be attributed to the use of an IUD, to endometriosis, congenital malformations of the mullerian ducts, an occlusion of the genital outflow tract (e.g., imperforate hymen and transverse vaginal septum), ovarian cyst, pelvic adhesions, uterine polyps or submucus myoma, cervical stenosis, or Allen-Masters syndrome. With the exception of the IUD wearer, the treatment of secondary dysmenorrhea is directed toward the underlying pelvic pathology. For the IUD wearer, secondary dysmenorrhea and menorrhagia due to increased endometrial prostaglandin production and release are frequent accompaniments. PGSIs such as mefenamic acid, ibuprofen, and sodium naproxen are effective in relieving the dysmenorrhea and correcting menorrhagia caused by the IUD.

Our understanding of the pathophysiology of primary dysmenorrhea and of secondary dysmenorrhea due to the IUD has led to a rational and physiologic approach to the management of these patients by pharmacologic suppression of excessive uterine prostaglandin production. This has in turn brought about significant relief of pain, suffering, and economic loss to many women.

QUESTIONS

1. In women suffering from primary dysmenorrhea, it has been shown that

    a. menstrual fluid prostaglandins are significantly increased as compared with normal women.
    b. the uterine activity during menstruation is abnormal.
    c. endometrial tissue prostaglandin concentrations are significantly elevated.
    d. the oral contraceptive will suppress menstrual fluid prostaglandins and relieve the dysmenorrhea.
    e. all of the above.

2. In a woman who does not wish to take the oral contraceptive pill as a method of birth control, the treatment of choice for her primary dysmenorrhea is

    a. dilatation and curettage.
    b. the Progestasert intrauterine device.
    c. a suitable prostaglandin synthetase inhibitor.
    d. observation and follow-up.
    e. hysterectomy.

3. Prostaglandin synthetase inhibitors

    a. inhibit the activity of the prostaglandin synthetase enzyme system.
    b. are contraindicated in patients with gastric ulcers.
    c. are indicated for treatment of primary dysmenorrhea in women who do not want the oral contraceptive.
    d. all of the above.
    e. none of the above.

4. In women using the intrauterine contraceptive device

    a. there is an increase in endometrial prostaglandin levels which accounts for the dysmenorrhea.
    b. there is an increased incidence of menorrhagia.

c. the dysmenorrhea can be relieved by administration of a suitable prostaglandin synthetase inhibitor.

d. the dysmenorrhea can be relieved by using a progesterone-medicated intrauterine device.

e. all of the above.

5. All the following prostaglandin synthetase inhibitors have been shown to be significantly better than a placebo in most of the controlled double-blind studies in primary dysmenorrhea except

a. mefenamic acid.
b. ibuprofen.
c. naproxen.
d. aspirin.
e. flufenamic acid.

REFERENCES

1. Schick B: Das menstruationsgift. *Wien Klin Wochenschr* 33:395–397, 1920
2. Macht DI, Davis ME: Experimental studies, old and new, on menstrual toxin. *J Comp Physiol Psychol* 18:113–134, 1934
3. Macht DI, Lubin DS: A plyto-pharmacological study of menstrual toxin. *J Pharmacol Exp Ther* 22:413–466, 1923
4. Pickles VR: A plain-muscle stimulant in the menstruum. *Nature (Lond)* 180:1198–1199, 1957
5. Pickles VR: Myometrial responses to the menstrual plain muscle stimulant. *J Endocrinol* 19:150–157, 1959
6. Clitheroe HJ, Pickles VR: The separation of the smooth muscle stimulants in the menstrual fluid. *J Physiol (Lond)* 156:225–237, 1961
7. Pickles VR, Hall WJ, Best FA, et al: Prostaglandins in endometrium and menstrual fluid from normal and dysmenorrheic subjects. *J Obstet Gynecol Br Commonw* 72:185–192, 1965
8. Lundstrom, V Green K, Wiqvist N: Prostaglandins, indomethacin and dysmenorrhea. *Prostaglandins* 11:893–904, 1976
9. Chan WY, Hill JC: Determination of menstrual prostaglandin levels in non-dysmenorrheic and dysmenorrheic subjects. *Prostaglandins* 15:365–375, 1978
10. Chan WY, Dawood MY, Fuchs F: Relief of dysmenorrhea with the prostaglandin synthetase inhibitor ibuprofen: Effect on prostaglandin levels in menstrual fluid. *Am J Obstet Gynecol* 135:102–108, 1979
11. Chan WY, Dawood MY: Prostaglandin levels in menstrual fluid of non-dysmenorrheic and dysmenorrheic subjects with and without oral contraceptive or ibuprofen therapy. *Adv Prostaglandin Thromboxane Leukotriene Res* 8:1443–1447, 1980
12. Ylikorkala O, Dawood MY: New concepts in dysmenorrhea. *Am J Obstet Gynecol* 130:833–847, 1978*
13. Waite LJ: US women at work. *Pop Bull* 36(2):3–43, 1981
14. Svennerud S: Dysmenorrhea and absenteeism. *Acta Obstet Gynecol Scand* 38(Suppl 2):1–116, 1959

15. Widholm O: Dysmenorrhea during adolescence. *Acta Obstet Gynecol Scand (Suppl)* 87:61–66, 1979
16. Dawood MY: Overall approach to the management of dysmenorrhea, in Dawood MY (ed): *Dysmenorrhea*, Baltimore, Williams & Wilkins, 1981, p 261–279*
17. Robert DWT: Dysmenorrhea. *Br J Hosp Med* 20:716–718, 1978*
18. Bergsjo P: Socioeconomic implications of dysmenorrhea. *Acta Obstet Gynecol Scand (Suppl)* 87:67–68, 1979
19. Heald FP, Masland RP, Sturgis SH, et al: Dysmenorrhea in adolescence. *Pediatrics* 20:121–127, 1957
20. Widholm O: Epidemiology of Premenstrual tension syndrome and primary dysmenorrhea, in Dawood MY, McGuire JL, Demers LM (eds): *Premenstrual Syndrome and Dysmenorrhea*. Baltimore, Urban and Schwarzenberger, 1985, pp 3–12*
21. Frisk M, Widholm O, Hortling H: Dysmenorrhea—Psyche and soma in teenagers. *Acta Obstet Gynecol Scand* 44:339, 1965
22. Goldstein DP, Cholkony C, Emans JS: Adolescent Endometriosis. *J Adolescent Health Care* 1:37–41, 1980
23. Dawood MY: Hormones, prostaglandins and dysmenorrhea, in Dawood MY (ed): *Dysmenorrhea*. Baltimore, Williams & Wilkins, 1981, p 21–52*
24. Chatman DL: Endometriosis and the black woman. *Am J Obstet Gynecol* 125:987–989, 1976
25. Simpson JL, Elias S, Malinak LR, et al: Heritable aspects of endometriosis. I. Genetic Studies. *Am J Obstet Gynecol* 137:327–331, 1980
26. Akerlund M, Stromberg P, Forsling MD: Primary dysmenorrhea and vasopressin. *Br J Obstet Gynaecol* 86:484–487, 1979
27. Akerlund M, Andersson KE, Ingemarsson J: Effects of terbutaline on myometrial activity, uterine blood flow and lower abdominal pain in women with primary dysmenorrhea. *Br J Obstet Gynaecol* 83:673–678, 1976
28. Pickles VR: Prostaglandins in the human endometrium. *Int J Fertil* 12:335–338, 1967
29. Willman EA, Collins WP, Clayton SG: Studies in the involvement of prostaglandins in uterine symptomatology and pathology. *Br J Obstet Gynecol* 83:337–341, 1976
30. Halbert DR, Demers LM, Fontana J, et al: Prostaglandin levels in endometrial jet wash specimens in patients with dysmenorrhea before and after indomethacin therapy. *Prostaglandins* 10:1047, 1975
31. Pickles VR, Clitheroe HJ: Further studies of the menstrual stimulant. *Lancet* 2:959–960, 1960
32. Chan WY, Dawood MY, Fuchs F: Prostaglandin in primary dysmenorrhea: comparison of prophylactic and nonprophylactic treatment with ibuprofen and use of oral contraceptive. *Am J Med* 70:535–541, 1981
33. Chan WY: Prostaglandin inhibitors and antagonists in dysmenorrhea therapy, in Dawood MY (ed): *Dysmenorrhea*. Baltimore, Williams & Wilkins, 1981, p 209–246*
34. Dawood MY: Dysmenorrhea and prostaglandins: Pharmacological and therapeutic considerations. *Drugs* 22:42–56, 1981*
35. Dawood MY: Choosing the correct therapy for dysmenorrhea. *Contemp Obstet Gynecol* 19:235–249, 1982*
36. Dawood MY: Dysmenorrhea. *Comp Ther* 8:9–15, 1982*
37. Lundstrom V, Green K: Endogenous levels of prostaglandin $F_{2\alpha}$ and its main metabolites in plasma and endometrium of normal and dysmenorrheic women. *Am J Obstet Gynecol* 130:640–646, 1978
38. Walker SM: In vitro synthesis of prostaglandin $F_{2\alpha}$ by

*Review article/chapter.

human endometrium. Abstracts of the Twenty-First British Congress of Obstetrics and Gynaecology, Sheffield, 1977, p 37

39. Lundstrom V: The myometrial response to intra-uterine administration of $PGF_{2\alpha}$ and PGE_2 in dysmenorrheic women. *Acta Obstet Gynecol Scand* 56:167–172, 1977

40. Dawood MY: *Prostaglandin Inhibition in Obstetrics and Gynecology.* Kalamazoo, MI, Scope Publication, 1983*

41. Sandahl, B, Ulmsten U, Andersson KE: Trial of calcium antagonist nifedipine in the treatment of primary dysmenorrhea. *Arch Gynecol* 227:147–151, 1979

42. Nesheim BI, Walloe L: The use of isoxsuprine in essential dysmenorrhea. A controlled clinical study. *Acta Obstet Gynecol Scand* 55:315–316, 1976

43. Hansen MK, Secher NJ: Beta-receptor stimulation in essential dysmenorrhea. *Am J Obstet Gynecol* 121:566–567, 1975

44. Trobough G, Guderian AM, Erickson RR, et al: The effect of exogenous intrauterine progesterone on the amount and prostaglandin $F_{2\alpha}$ content of menstrual blood in dysmenorrheic women. *J Reprod Med* 21:153–158, 1978

45. Saksena SK, Lau IF, Castracane VD: Prostaglandin-mediated action of IUDs. II. F-prostaglandin (PGF) in the uterine horn of pregnant rats and hamsters with intrauterine devices. *Prostaglandins* 5:97–106, 1974

46. Spilman CH, Duby RT: Prostaglandin mediated luteolytic effect of an intrauterine device in the sheep. *Prostaglandins* 2:159–168, 1972

47. Hillier K, Kasonde JM: Prostaglandin E and F concentrations in human endometrium after insertion of intrauterine contraceptive device. *Lancet* 1:15–16, 1976

48. Anderson ABM, Gillebaud J, Haynes PJ, et al: Reduction of menstrual blood-loss by prostaglandin synthetase inhibitors. *Lancet* 1:774–776, 1976

49. Davies AJ, Anderson ABM, Turnbull AC: Reduction by naproxen of excessive menstrual bleeding in women using intrauterine devices. *Obstet Gynecol* 57:74–78, 1981

50. Roy S, Shaw ST Jr: Role of prostaglandins in IUD-associated uterine bleeding—Effect of a prostaglandin synthetase inhibitor (ibuprofen). *Obstet Gynecol* 58:101–106, 1981

51. Moon YS, Leung PCS, Yuen BH, et al: Prostaglandin F in human endometriotic tissue. *Am J Obstet Gynecol* 141:344–345, 1981

52. Drake TS, O'Brien WF, Ramwell PW, et al: Peritoneal fluid thromboxane B_2 and the 6-keto-prostaglandin $F_{1\alpha}$ in endometriosis. *Am J Obstet Gynecol* 140:401–411, 1981

53. Rock JA, Dubin NH, Ghodgaonkar RB, et al: Cul-de-sac fluid in women with endometriosis: Fluid volume and prostanoid concentration during the proliferative phase of the cycle—days 8 to 12. *Fertil Steril* 37:747–750, 1982

54. Badawy SZA, Marshall L, Gabal AA, et al: The concentration of 13,14-dihydro-15-keto prostaglandin $F_{2\alpha}$ and prostaglandin E_2 in peritoneal fluid of infertile patients with and without endometriosis. *Fertil Steril* 38:166–170, 1982

55. Sgarlata CS, Hertelendy F, Mikhail G: The prostanoid content in peritoneal fluid and plasma of women with endometriosis. *Am J Obstet Gynecol* 147:563–565, 1983

56. Dawood MY, Khan-Dawood FS, Wilson L Jr: Peritoneal fluid prostaglandins and prostanoids in women with endometriosis, chronic pelvic inflammatory disease and pelvic pain. *Am J Obstet Gynecol* 148:391–395, 1984

57. Kauppila A, Puolakka J, Ylikorkala O: Prostaglandin biosynthesis inhibitors and endometriosis. *Prostaglandins* 18:655–661, 1979

ANSWERS

1. e

2. c

3. d

4. e

5. d

Fertility following Steroidal Oral Contraception and Diethylstilbestrol Exposure

DAVID F. ARCHER

INTRODUCTION

Oral steroidal contraceptives were first introduced in the United States in 1960. They were met with great enthusiasm as a method of preventing pregnancy and enabling people to exercise control over reproduction. One of the early concerns was that the use of the exogenous steroids might result in decreased fertility, in response to the description in the mid-1960s of the so-called postpill amenorrhea syndrome.[1-5]

POSTPILL AMENORRHEA SYNDROME

At that time, it was believed that the use of the exogenous steroids would suppress the hypothalamus and/or pituitary and inhibit them such that on discontinuation of the oral contraceptive a transient or prolonged delay in resumption of ovulation

DAVID F. ARCHER • Department of Obstetrics and Gynecology, University of Pittsburgh School of Medicine; and Department of Obstetrics and Gynecology, Magee-Womens Hospital, Pittsburgh, Pennsylvania 15213.

would result. However, the postpill amenorrhea syndrome does not appear to be either epidemiologically or hormonally different from spontaneously occurring secondary amenorrhea.[1,2,4,6-8] The reported occurrence of secondary amenorrhea (anovulation) varies and reflects the population under investigation. In the general population, the incidence of spontaneous amenorrhea is reported to be 0.7–1.0% when lack of menstruation for more than 6 months is used as the criterion.[1,9] A survey using a questionnaire mailed to 1 of 15 women in Upsala, Sweden, found that 0.7% of subjects had experienced amenorrhea of more than 6 months duration.[9] Multivariant analysis of these data showed a statistical correlation only with the age of the individual, although there was a weak but insignificant correlation with smoking. Other studies reporting the occurrence of amenorrhea after discontinuation of oral contraceptives indicate a range of 0.2–3.1% (Table 20-1).[3,4,7,8,10]

Several definite causes or relationships have been found in women with amenorrhea in both the postpill and nonpill-use groups (Table 20-2).[4-6,11,12] Ovarian failure is present in approximately 5% of all cases. Elevated prolactin levels

TABLE 20-1. Incidence of Amenorrhea following Discontinuation of Oral Contraceptives

Investigator	Incidence %	Duration of amenorrhea	No. of women
Rice-Wray et al. (1967)[16]	2.8	>3 months	168
Larson-Cohn (1969)[19]	0.8	ND[a]	500
Shearman and Smith (1972)[10]	<1.0	>12 months	230
Golditch (1972)[3]	0.22	>6 months	20,000
Royal College of General Practitioners (1974)[8]	0.2–2.64[b]	ND	11,338

[a]ND, not described.
[b]Range of incidence is age related, with increased occurrence in older ages.

have been reported, ranging in incidence from 2–22% in these women.[13,14]

Polycystic ovarian disorders, perhaps best characterized as chronic anovulation with either obesity or androgen excess, has been found to occur in anywhere from 5 to 10% of cases under investigation. Anorexia nervosa and weight loss have been present in 10–25% of cases. A significant number of cases have been found showing no evidence of any definite endocrine disorder other than normal follicle-stimulating hormone (FSH) and luteinizing hormone (LH) levels associated with low 17β-estradiol levels. This group has been considered as

having functional or hypothalamic amenorrhea and has been best characterized in recent reports by Tolis and Hull and co-workers.[7,12] Again the discrepancy in the incidence of this condition found by these two groups probably represents the bias introduced by referral patterns as well as the small number of subjects studied (Table 20-2).

The report by Tolis et al.[12] identified 65 women of 106 total who were thought to have functional amenorrhea, 29 of whom were related to prior oral contraceptive use. In the report by Hull et al.[7] of 102 women with postpill amenorrhea, 29 women (30%) were found to have functional amenorrhea. However, Hull pointed out that significantly more women have no obvious cause for the amenorrhea upon discontinuation of the oral contraceptives as compared with women who were never users of oral contraceptives. The bias in these studies is that women with prior amenorrhea or menstrual irregularities may have been placed on oral contraceptives as a means of regulating or initiating menstrual bleeding. In fact, a significant percentage of women with postpill amenorrhea were found to have had menstrual irregularities before being placed on oral contraceptives.[2,15]

Clinical Assessment of the Return of Ovulation

Several studies have investigated the return of ovulation following the use of oral contraceptives based on hormonal or endometrial sampling. Rice-

TABLE 20-2. Occurrence (%) of Various Diagnostic Categories in Women with Secondary Amenorrhea

Diagnosis	Shearman and Fraser (1977)[5]	Jacobs et al. (1977)[4] NOC[a]	Jacobs et al. (1977)[4] OC[a]	Tolis et al. (1977)[11] NOC[a]	Tolis et al. (1977)[11] OC[a]	Hull et al. (1981)[7] NOC[a]	Hull et al. (1981)[7] OC[a]
Ovarian failure	4.9	12.7	5.8	3.8		11.0	8.0
Hyperprolactinemia	39.0	35.4	25.0	8.5	7.5	22.0	23.0
Anorexia	—	15.2	17.3	8.5		—	—
Weight loss	7.8	8.9	9.6	—	—	32.0	22.0
Psychiatric	30.0	19.0	17.3	—	—	10.0	10.0
Polycystic ovary syndrome	18.4	8.9[d]	25.0[d]	4.7[e]	—	8.0	4.0
Other	23.3[b]	—	—	27.4[b]	33.9[c]	—	—

[a]NOC, non-oral contraceptive user; OC, oral contraceptive use.
[b]This group was characterized as functional amenorrhea by the author.
[c]This group was called post-oral contraceptive amenorrhea by the author.
[d]This group was called clomiphene-responsive amenorrhea.
[e]These categories were not delineated as to prior oral contraceptive use.

Wray et al.[16] found that more than 80% of the women who discontinued oral contraceptives had a spontaneous menstruation within 42 days. In most of these women, ovulation occurred within 2–3 weeks of the last contraceptive tablet based on assessment of urinary pregnanediol concentrations and the finding of secretory endometrium when the biopsy was obtained within the 14 days before the onset of the spontaneous menstruation. These data are in agreement with the urinary excretion of gonadotropins and steroids reported by other investigators.[1,17,18]

Using plasma progesterone levels as an index of ovulation, Lähteenmäki et al.[18] found that 83% of women discontinuing oral contraceptives appeared ovulatory within 6 weeks. After following six women daily for 2 months after stopping oral contraceptives, Klein et al.[17] found the LH peak to occur 21–28 days after the ingestion of the last tablet. Serum progesterone levels and the duration of the luteal phase were entirely normal in these women, but the follicular phase was lengthened and unpredictable.[16,18,19]

Epidemiologic Studies Involving Oral Contraceptives

Several epidemiologic studies have investigated the return of fertility after the utilization of oral steroidal contraceptive agents. The largest of these is the ongoing study carried out by the Oxford Family Planning Association and reported between 1974 and 1977.[20–22] These reports indicate a lag in the return of fertility of approximately 3 months in women who have used oral contraceptives, compared with those individuals who have used either the intrauterine device (IUD) or barrier forms of contraception. This finding is based on the occurrence of pregnancy in women discontinuing oral contraceptives compared with either the IUD or barrier contraception. The differences between the oral contraceptive users versus other contraception in terms of percentage of women remaining undelivered was greatest at 12 months, 60% for oral contraceptive users versus 48% for IUD, and 39% for other methods.[22] These differences were less apparent at 18 months and insignificant at 24 months. Approximately 5% of both nulliparous and parous women who were prior contraceptive users had not established a pregnancy by 42 months after discontinuation of the contraceptive method (Fig. 20-1).[21] Comparable information regarding return of fertility is available from retrospective studies of women from Thailand, Mexico, and the United States.[16,23–25]

Many of these studies indicated an increased occurrence of conception at 3 months after discontinuation of oral contraceptives.[16,23] Janerich et

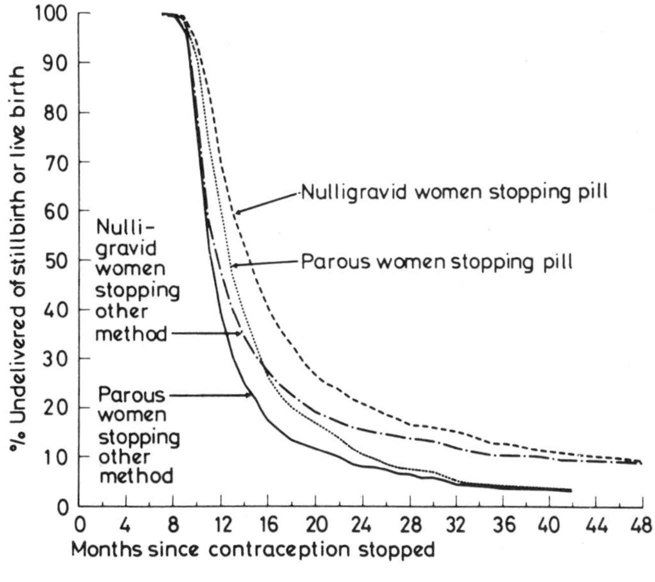

FIGURE 20-1. Return of fertility in nulligravid and parous women after discontinuing oral contraceptives. (From Vessey et al.[21])

al.[23] reevaluated their own data as well as those presented from the Oxford Family Planning Council to show that there appears to be a cyclic or rhythmic pattern of conceptions unique to those individuals who have discontinued oral contraceptives.[23] Peaks of the occurrence of conceptions occurred at 3, 7, and 11 months after discontinuation of the oral contraceptive agent. The etiology of this rhythmic occurrence of increased fecundity is unknown.

Linn et al.[26] documented the occurrence of pregnancy after discontinuation of oral contraceptives in women who ultimately became pregnant and delivered. Again, an initial 3-month interval of fewer than anticipated conceptions was found after discontinuation of oral contraceptives. In this study, all the women became pregnant, but Linn and colleagues admit that the bias of the study is attributable to their having interviewed only women who had delivered; that is, they were measuring the return of fertility in a group of fertile women following use of oral contraceptives. This study provides no information as to the incidence of infertility or to other problems in establishing pregnancy. It should be noted that in this study the delay in conceiving is such that by 1 year after discontinuation of the oral contraceptives, only 50% of the women were pregnant. This could be a cause of concern and particularly so if one uses the standard definition of infertility, which is 12 months of unprotected intercourse without conception. It does appear to require an additional 3–6 months to establish a pregnancy for women who have stopped using oral contraceptives. It should also be stressed that in these epidemiologic studies no cause of the failure to achieve a pregnancy is documented; nevertheless, they all support the fact that it requires 12 months or more for 90% of the "normal" population at risk to establish a pregnancy.[27]

Outcome of Pregnancy in Prior Users of Oral Steroidal Contraception

Despite the finding of a slight (<3-month) delay in the return of fertility in prior users of oral steroidal contraceptives, there is no evidence of any residual effect on the pregnancy.[22] Specifically addressed issues have involved the occurrence of chromosomal disorders (abnormalities in the baby) in the offspring of women who had used oral contraceptives.[8,29,30] No significant increased risk was present in any of these studies. There was no evidence for an increased occurrence of Down's syndrome and previous use of oral contraceptives.[28] There is no evidence for any significant deleterious effect of previous oral contraceptive use on miscarriages, ectopic pregnancies, stillbirth, or multiple births.[8,27,28,31,32]

Persistent Anovulation following Oral Steroidal Contraception

Resumption of menses and/or ovulation may be prolonged in some women after use of the oral contraceptive formulation. However, 95% of women with postpill amenorrhea were found to recover (resume menstruation) within 6 years.[32] Resumption of menses by 6 years occurred in 56% of women with anorexia nervosa, 72% of both psychogenic amenorrhea and weight loss amenorrhea, and 61% of functional amenorrhea.[32] In this investigation, where fertility was a concern, ovulation induction was carried out with either clomiphene citrate and/or menopausal gonadotropin therapy, with a 59% conception rate.[32] Other investigators have indicated that in these women with ovulatory dysfunction, a pregnancy rate comparable to the normal population (never users of oral contraceptives) can be expected by either expectant management or ovulation induction (Fig. 20-2).[7,22,25−27,32]

REPRODUCTIVE PERFORMANCE IN DIETHYLSTILBESTROL-EXPOSED WOMEN

Diethylstilbestrol (DES), a stilbene derivative, is a nonsteroidal estrogen synthesized during the 1930s by Dr. Charles Dodd. The structural formula is shown in Figure 20-3. DES is a potent estrogen when administered either orally or topically, the latter usually as a vaginal suppository or cream. Beginning in the 1940s, DES was used extensively in obstetrics and gynecology to inhibit lactation, manage menopausal symptoms, and treat for senile vaginitis. At that time, DES came into vogue as a treatment for threatened abortion (any vaginal bleeding in the first trimester), as well as prophylatically, to prevent abortion in women with poor obstetric history. Stilbestrol was administered to prevent premature labor and/or stillbirths. Although several studies had demonstrated what appeared to be an improvement in late pregnancy complications with the administration of DES, a prospective double-blind study performed by Dieckmann et al.[35] in 1952 from the Chicago

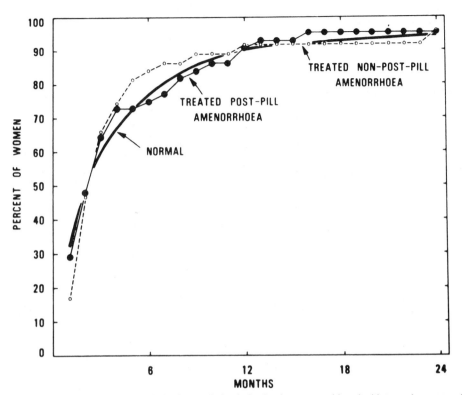

FIGURE 20-2. Cumulative conception rates following ovulation induction in women with and without oral contraceptive related amenorrhea. (From Hull et al.[56])

Lying-In Hospital failed to document any efficacy of DES in preventing pregnancy complications. In fact, a recalculation of Dieckmann's data in 1978 found a significantly increased occurrence of abortions, neonatal deaths, and premature births in the DES-exposed women.[34]

Despite the adverse nature of the report from the Chicago Lying-In Hospital study, the utilization of DES did not diminish in the United States. In fact, the discussion following the presentation of the Dieckmann paper attributed the failure to demonstrate an effect of DES on reproduction to the lack of a well-defined group such as primigravidas for evaluation.[35] However, the utilization of DES as a preventive therapeutic regimen in pregnancy waned over the succeeding 10–15 years.[34]

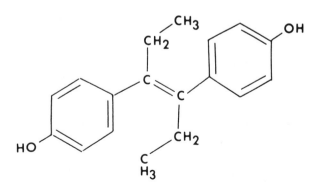

FIGURE 20-3. Structural formula of diethylstilbestrol, a nonsteroidal orally active estrogen.

Herbst et al.[36] in 1971 initially reported the association of maternal DES therapy with clear cell adenocarcinoma of the vagina in the daughters of these women. This report led to an extensive investigation of the children of women who had used DES during pregnancy in the United States. Current evidence indicates that the risk of clear cell adenocarcinoma of the vagina in the daughters of DES-exposed women is 1.4 in 1000.[37,38]

Other alterations in the reproductive tract, specifically physical changes in the vagina and uterus along with what appeared to be significant menstrual irregularities focused attention on the reproductive performance of these women. Changes in the cervix (cockscomb and cervical hood) and vaginal adenosis are part of the gross abnormalities that were initially documented.[37–39] These anatomic changes have been reported to occur from between 22 and 58% of DES-exposed women.[38,39] Upper genital tract alterations, specifically an abnormal configuration of the uterine cavity and/or fallopian tubes, have also been reported.[40,41] Hysterosalpingogram-documented changes in the uterus have been found to be present in approximately 69% of 267 DES-exposed women.[40,41]

Overall reproductive performance per se has been difficult to evaluate, and infertility is still being debated.[42] Bibbo et al.[43] reported decreased fertility in the DES-exposed individual as compared with controls (Table 20-3). This 1977 report fol-

lowed up the children of the women who had participated in the Chicago Lying-In study, 1950–1952. Sixteen hundred women had participated in this study during that period, and the 1977 report involved 163 DES-exposed males compared with 168 controls, and 229 DES females compared with 136 controls. The DES-exposed males were found to have an increased occurrence of epididymal cysts, hypertropic testes, and capsular induration as compared with controls. Semen analyses carried out on a much smaller subset of the exposed male population ($N = 39$) demonstrated a reduced ejaculate volume of less than 1.5 ml in 26% of DES-exposed males compared with none of the control males ($N = 25$). Also reported was a significantly decreased semen quality in the exposed males as compared with that of the unexposed controls. The clinical significance of these changes is still unclear, since other investigators have not found a significant change in age of puberty or postpubertal hormonal levels in DES-exposed males compared with controls.[44] The DES-exposed males in this study "tended to have smaller testes" than those of controls, but there were no data on semen parameters.

The report from the Chicago Lying-In Hospital further documented an increased occurrence of menstrual irregularities in the DES-exposed women compared with controls (18% vs. 10%, respectively). Also, a lower occurrence of pregnancy in

TABLE 20-3. Fertility in Diethylstibestrol-Exposed Women

Study	DES exposed	Controls	Patient population[e] DES	Patient population[e] Non-DES
Controlled (Chicago Lying-In Hospital)				
Bibbo et al. (1977)[43]	18% pregnant	33% pregnant	229	136
Herbst et al. (1980)[45]	19/226 = 8.4%[a]	4/203 = 1.8%[a]	226	203
Herbst et al. (1981)[38]	53/338 (15.7%)[a]	19/298 (6.4%)[a]	338	298
	31/338 (9.2%)[b]	5/298 (1.7%)[b]		
DESAD				
Barnes et al. (1980)[37]	46.8%[c]	50.2%[c]	618	618 (matched controls)
Cousins et al. (1980)[46]	4/71[d]	2/69[d]	71	69 (matched)
Uncontrolled				
Berger and Goldstein (1980)[47]	46/69 pregnant (66.7%)		69	
Schmidt et al. (1980)[48]	31/106 unsuccessful in established pregnancy	70.5% pregnant	276 total	

[a]Complaints of infertility.
[b]Never pregnant.
[c]Percentage pregnant.
[d]Difficulty conceiving; no difference in "ever pregnant"; 46% of each group.
[e]DES, DES-exposed; non-DES; non-DES-exposed.

the DES-exposed group was found as compared with the controls 18% vs. 33% (Table 20-3). It should be noted that other later reports of menstrual function in women exposed to DES do not appear to document a significant increase in the occurrence of menstrual irregularity over the unexposed population.[37,39]

This initial report was subsequently expanded using the same Chicago Lying-In Hospital study group but increasing the number of controls. In this 1980 study, Herbst et al.[45] specifically addressed the reproductive performance, 226 DES-exposed daughters were compared with 203 non-DES-exposed daughters. Primary infertility was reported in 19 of the exposed and four of the unexposed women (Table 20-3). This study included only those women who had complete prenatal medication records (the total number potentially available were 389 DES-exposed and 395 unexposed daughters). The interviews were performed during gynecologic visits or by telephone or mail. The same report indicated that the number of women who had been pregnant at least once was higher in the unexposed group compared with the exposed group, 58% vs. 39%. This discrepancy between the unexposed and DES exposed in terms of pregnancy achieved becomes even larger when only sexually active noncontraceptive women are evaluated. It should be noted, however, that a specific cause of the infertility in these women had not been documented. In fact, the cause(s) of the infertility in all the reports are not apparent. A more recent update of this group of women in 1981 by Herbst et al.[38] indicated that "infertility" occurred in 53 of the exposed compared with 19 of the unexposed. This report defined infertility as no pregnancy after 1 year of unprotected intercourse. However, only 31 of the exposed and 5 of the unexposed have never been pregnant (Table 20-3), indicating that the use of the definition of infertility, although accurate, may require modification for this type of study.[27]

What makes the Chicago experience unique is that the control group consists of the daughters of the placebo-administered women. Also, the dosage of DES was standardized, as was the administration of the drug.

One other major study, the National Cooperative Diethylstilbestrol Adenosis (DESAD) project, documented the occurrence of pregnancy in daughters of women who received DES and compared them with either their un-exposed sisters or un-exposed age-matched controls (Table 20-3).[37] This study did not find any difference in the percentage of women who became pregnant, age at first pregnancy, number of pregnancies, or pregnancy rates. No information specifically addressed the issue of infertility in this study, since it was published in response to the first Chicago Lying-In Hospital study in 1977, which reported a reduced pregnancy occurrence, and Barnes et al. only speculated about infertility. One other controlled study of fertility in DES-exposed women is available using matched controls.[46] This investigation shows no evidence of infertility between the two groups. These data, reported by Cousins in Table 20-3, report "difficulty in conceiving." In this study, the incidence of pregnancy in the control and DES-exposed group is 46% and is comparable to the 46.8% in the DESAD report. The designation "difficulty in conceiving" has no clinical relevance and should be compared with the 1981 Chicago Lying-In Hospital report.

Two other reports of the incidence of pregnancy in DES-exposed women, although not controlled, indicated that 67–70% of DES-exposed women had established a pregnancy (Table 20-3).[47,48] These figures are higher than the pregnancy incidence reported by Barnes and Cousins but comparable to that found in the Herbst 1981 report, wherein 75% of DES-exposed women who were sexually active and noncontraceptive had had a pregnancy.

No specific cause of the infertility has been related to DES exposure. An anecdotal report found that preovulatory cervical mucus is poor in DES-exposed women with infertility, but this is a preliminary observation.[39] A retrospective study investigating the incidence of endometriosis in DES-exposed infertile women as compared with a larger group of non-DES exposed infertile women was unable to show a significant incidence in the exposed group, although a relatively greater percentage of the DES-exposed women were found to have endometriosis.[49]

Although most reports have assessed menstrual function in terms of age of menarche, menstrual regularity, and amount of bleeding, there is no consistent evidence of any significant alteration in this indirect assessment of ovarian function. Preliminary evidence has shown mice exposed in utero to DES to have impaired ovarian function.[50] This poor ovarian function was found to be principally a decrease in folliculogenesis with age. Also reported have been increased biosynthesis of progesterone, testosterone, and estrogen in ovarian tissue of DES-exposed mice incubated in vitro.[51] The increased steroidogenic capacity of the mouse ovary in vitro was related to an increased size of the interstitial

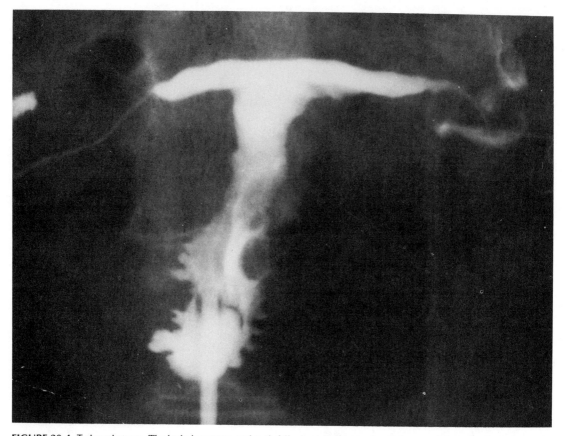

FIGURE 20-4. T-shaped uterus. The body is narrow, and each fallopian tube appears to originate at right angles from the uterine cavity.

compartment of the ovary. What relevance their findings have to human reproduction is unknown.

Despite the lack of clear-cut evidence for infertility due to a specific alteration in the female reproductive tract related to DES exposure, there is still concern over the reproductive performance of these women. Part of this stems from the anatomic changes in the uterus present on hysterosalpingography.[40,41,52] These changes are principally characterized by the T-shaped uterus. This anatomic alteration is a narrow uterine cavity, that is not triangular in shape, and the fallopian tubes appear to extend perpendicular to the uterine cavity. (see example in Fig. 20-4). Other uterine abnormalites are constrictions of the uterine cavity, a small uterine cavity, filling defects, synechia, diverticula, and uterine unicollis or bicornuas. A single case report has documented an atrophic-appearing "withered" fallopian tube.[39] DES exposure in experimental mice has been reported to result in

alteration of the uterine horns with anatomic changes, the relationship of the oviduct to the ovary being the principal alteration (short ovarian ligament and failure of the ovary to rotate into the normal adult position).[53] Also present was a marked inflammatory reaction in the endosalpinx with diverticula composed of nests of cells protruding through the muscularis of the oviduct. DES-exposed mice were also found to exhibit poor reproductive performance, most notably in the total number of offspring from "forced" breeding.[50] In this experiment, mothers were administered various doses of DES; their female offspring were then bred repetitively over an 8-month period. The total number of litters and the size of the litters were markedly reduced in the DES-exposed female mice.[50]

Reports in human reproductive performance have attempted to link the occurrence of the physical findings such as the T-shaped uterus, cervical hood or cuff, and adenosis to reproductive performance. No significant association between physical stigmata of DES exposure and reproductive wastage has been found.[37,45,52]

Premature Delivery

The Chicago Lying-In Hospital studies have shown a reduction in the number of term deliveries in DES-exposed daughters compared with non-DES-exposed controls (Table 20-4).[38,45] This is associated with an increased occurrence of premature deliveries in this population of approximately 50%. No significant differences in prematurity rates were found in the DESAD study group (Table 20-4).[37] The DESAD figure of 7.7% should be compared with the overall incidence of prematurity, reported to be 8.8% in the United States.[54] The U.S. data on the incidence of prematurity is the same as that found in the DES-exposed women and their controls in the DESAD study and the non-DES-exposed daughters from the Chicago Lying-In Hospital series (Table 20-4). However, in agreement with the Chicago Lying-In data, a statistically significant increase in premature deliveries (40%) was reported by Cousins.[46]

In the noncontrolled studies, the term pregnancy percentages range from 25 to 43% of the study population, while the premature rates were 9.5–36% (Table 20-4).[47,48,52]

These findings reflect the possibility of an increased risk of prematurity in the DES-exposed population. However, in the uncontrolled studies, selection bias could account for the markedly increased rate of premature deliveries. It should be reiterated that poor reproductive performance was found in the female offspring of the DES-exposed mice, especially a reduction in litter size arguing for an increased in utero pregnancy loss before parturition.[50] However, there is no correlation between the anatomic and reproductive performance of the rodent and the human subject.

Ectopic Pregnancy

The DESAD study and that reported by Cousins show a significant increase in ectopic pregnancy in DES-exposed women as compared with that in controls (Table 20-4).[37,47] This difference in ectopic pregnancy rates was also found in the Chicago Lying-In reports and the uncontrolled studies of reproductive performance in DES-exposed women (Table 20-4). The percentages are derived from the group of women who had been exposed to DES. These data for the most part are uncontrolled, and the range of 4–7% incidence in ectopic pregnancies

TABLE 20-4. Occurrence of Spontaneous Abortion, Extrauterine Pregnancy, and Premature Labor in Diethylstilbestrol-Exposed Women

Study	Spontaneous abortion (%)		Extrauterine pregnancy (%)		Premature (%)		Term (%)	
	DES	Non-DES	DES	Non-DES	DES	Non-DES	DES	Non-DES
Controlled (Chicago Lying-In Hospital)								
Bibbo et al. (1977)[43]	5.0	11.0	—	—	—	—	13.0	23.0
Herbst et al. (1980)[45a]	18.0	7.0	6.0	0	22.0	7.0	47.0	85.0
Herbst et al. (1981)[38a]	21.0	11.0	7.0	0	70.0	6.0	52.0	83.0
DESAD								
Barnes et al. (1980)[37]	26.0	16.0[b]	3.6[c]	1.3[c]	7.7[c]	4.5[c]	—	—
Cousins et al. (1980)[46]	12.0[c]	14.0[c]	4.6[c]	0	40.0[b]	0	—	—
Uncontrolled								
Berger and Goldstein (1980)[47d]	30.6	—	4.8	—	12.8	—	33.9	—
Schmidt et al. (1980)[48e]	17.3	—	4.0	—	9.5	—	25.3	—
Kaufman et al. (1980)[52e]	32.0	—	6.0	—	36.0	—	43.0	—

[a]Outcome of first pregnancy.
[b]Difference statistically significant.
[c]Not statistically significant.
[d]62 pregnancies in 32 DES-exposed women.
[e]For comparison purposes, only the outcome of the first pregnancy was used.

of the total group does not differ significantly from the 0.83 in 1000 incidence of ectopic pregnancy reported in women aged 15–44 in 1977 in the United States.[55] The incidence of ectopic pregnancy in the United States and the world has been increasing during the past 10 years. There is difficulty in calculating the true incidence of ectopic pregnancy in DES-exposed women, but it may be no higher than that in the unexposed population.

Spontaneous Abortion

In comparison with the control group, both the Chicago Lying-In study and the DESAD study show what appears to be a significant increase in the occurrence of spontaneous abortion.[37,38,45] Cousins did not find a significant increase in spontaneous abortions compared with the controls in his study.[46] By comparison, in the studies of DES-exposed women without controls, the occurrence of spontaneous abortion ranged from 17.3 to 32% (Table 20-4).[47,48,52] The true incidence of spontaneous abortion in the United States is unknown but is believed to be 10–20% of all pregnancies.

Of interest was the consistent finding throughout these studies of induced abortions ranging from 19 to 39% of the DES-exposed group. The figure for induced abortions in the control group from the DESAD study was 20.1% (Table 20-5).[37] Although these figures seem high, they may reflect the age of the study population.

SUMMARY

The available information does not indicate any significant impairment of either ovulation and/or fertility following discontinuation of oral steroidal contraceptives.[1,32] Pregnancy outcomes in terms of fetal anomalies, chromosomal defects, and complication of pregnancy, such as spontaneous abortion, stillbirth, or multiple births, are not increased in women who have previously used oral contraceptives as compared with never users of oral contraceptives.

Epidemiologic studies of users and never users of oral contraceptives indicate that fertility may be delayed in terms of number of months or years of unprotected intercourse but that this appears to be related more to maternal age than to prior use of steroidal contraceptives. There is a steady increase in involuntary infertility in women as they age. The use of appropriate pharmacologic agents for ovula-

TABLE 20-5. Incidence of Induced Abortion in Diethylstilbestrol-Exposed Women

Study	Abortion (%)	Abortion/total No.
Herbst et al. (1980)[45]	20.2	18/89[a]
Herbst et al. (1981)[38]	21.3	32/150[a]
Cousins et al. (1980)[46]	37.2	16/43
Berger and Goldstein (1980)[47]	30.4	14/46
Schmidt et al. (1980)[48]	38.7	29/75[a]
Kaufman et al. (1980)[52]	19.0	18/93[a]
Barnes et al. (1980)[37]	25.9	57/220

[a]Result of first pregnancy.
[b]Induced abortion in control 16.1% (36/224) not significantly different.

tion induction results in conception rates similar to those present in the "normal" population.

There is evidence for increased reproductive loss in DES-exposed women, principally premature labor, but there is no conclusive evidence that this is related to the uterine abnormalities. There does not seem to be a significant increase in infertility in DES-exposed women. Specifically, no etiology of the infertility could be linked directly to the DES exposure of these women.

QUESTIONS

1. Upon discontinuing steroidal oral contraceptives, there has been shown to be

    a. an increased incidence of chromosomal defects in subsequent conceptions.
    b. an increased incidence of spontaneous abortions in subsequent conceptions.
    c. a slight delay in return to fertility compared with patients using barrier contraceptive techniques.

2. Administration of DES to pregnant women appears to cause

    a. lessened ability of the female offspring to conceive
    b. an increased incidence of premature labor suffered by the female offspring.
    c. both a and b.

REFERENCES

1. Archer DF, Thomas RL: The fallacy of the post-pill amenorrhea syndrome. *Clin Obstet Gynecol* 24:943–950, 1981

2. Buttram VC Jr, Vanderheyden JD, Besch PK, et al: Post "pill" amenorrhea. *Int J Fertil* 19:37–44, 1974
3. Golditch IM: Postcontraceptive amenorrhea. *Obstet Gynecol* 39:903–908, 1972
4. Jacobs HS, Knuth UA, Hull MGR, et al: Post "pill" amenorrhea—cause or coincidence? *Br Med J* 2:940–942, 1977
5. Shearman RP, Fraser IS: Impact of new diagnostic methods on the differential diagnosis and treatment of secondary amenorrhea. *Lancet* 1:1195–1197, 1977
6. Harlap S: Are there two types of postpill anovulation. *Fertil Steril* 31:486–491, 1979
7. Hull MGR, Bromham DR, Savage PE, et al: Post-pill amenorrhea: A causal study. *Fertil Steril* 36:472–476, 1981
8. The Royal College of General Practitioners: Oral contraceptives and Health: An interim report. Tunbridge Wells, England, Pitman, 1974, p 71
9. Pettersson F, Fries H, Nillius SJ: Epidemiology of secondary amenorrhea. 1. Incidence and prevalence rates. *Am J Obstet Gynecol* 117:80–86, 1977
10. Shearman RP, Smith ID: Statistical analysis of relationship between oral contraception, secondary amenorrhea and galactorrhea. *J Obstet Gynaecol Br Commonw* 76:654–656, 1972
11. Tolis G, Ruggere D, Hendelman M, et al: Prolonged amenorrhea and oral contraceptives. *Fertil Steril* 32:265–268, 1979
12. Marshall JC, Reed PI, Gordon H: Luteinizing hormone secretion in patients presenting with post-oral contraceptive amenorrhea: Evidence for a hypothalamic feedback abnormality. *Clin Endocrinol (Oxf)* 5:131–143, 1976
13. Steele SJ, Mason B, Brett H: Amenorrhea after discontinuation combined oestrogen-progestogen oral contraceptives. *Br Med J* 4:343–345, 1973
14. Van Campenhout J, Blanchet P, Beauregard H, et al: Amenorrhea following the use of oral contraceptives. *Fertil Steril* 28:728–732, 1977
15. Starup J: Amenorrhea following oral contraception. *Acta Obstet Gynecol Scand* 51:341–345, 1972
16. Rice-Wray E, Corren S, Gorodoosky J, et al: Return of ovulation after discontinuation of oral contraceptives. *Fertil Steril* 18:212–218, 1967
17. Klein TA, Mishell DR Jr: Gonadotropin, prolactin, and steroid hormone levels after discontinuation of oral contraceptive. *Am J Obstet Gynecol* 127:585–589, 1972
18. Lähteenmäki P, Ylöstalo P, Sipinen S, et al: Return of ovulation after abortion and after discontinuation of oral contraceptives. *Fertil Steril* 34:246–249, 1980
19. Larsson-Cohn U: The length of the first three menstrual cycles after combined oral contraceptive treatment. *Acta Obstet Gynecol Scand* 48:196–204, 1969
20. Vessey M, Doll R, Peto R, et al: A long-term follow-up study of women using different methods of contraception—An interim report. *J Biosoc Sci* 8:373–427, 1976
21. Vessey MP, Wright NH, McPherson K, et al: Fertility after stopping different methods of contraception. *Br Med J* 1:265–267, 1978
22. Vessey MP, Lawless M, McPherson K, et al: Fertility after stopping use of intrauterine contraceptive device. *Br Med J* 286:106, 1983
23. Janerich DT, Lawrence CE, Jacobson HI: Fertility patterns after discontinuation of use of oral contraceptives. *Lancet* 1:1051–1053, 1976
24. Pardthaisong T, Gray RH: The return of fertility following discontinuation of oral contraceptives in Thailand. *Fertil Steril* 35:532–534, 1981
25. Westoff CF, Bumpass L, Ryder NB: Oral contraception, coital frequency and the time required to conceive. *Soc Biol* 29:157–167, 1982
26. Linn S, Schoenbaum SC, Monson RR, et al: Delay in conception for former "pill" users. *JAMA* 247:629–632, 1982
27. Cooke ID: The natural history and major causes of infertility, in Diczfalusy E, Diczfalusy A (eds): *Regulation of Human Fertility*, WHO symposium. Copenhagen, Scriptor, 1977, pp 88–110
28. Huggins GR: Contraceptive use and subsequent fertility. *Fertil Steril* 28:603–612, 1977
29. Rice-Wray E, Cervantes A, Gutierrez J, et al: Pregnancy and progeny after hormonal contraceptives—Genetic studies. *J Reprod Med* 6:101–104, 1971
30. Vessey M, Meisler L, Flavel R, et al: Outcome of pregnancy in women using different methods of contraception. *Br J Obstet Gynaecol* 86:548–556, 1979
31. Harlap S: Multiple births in former oral contraceptive users. *Br J Obstet Gynaecol* 86:557–562, 1979
32. Hirvonen E: Etiology, clinical features and prognosis in secondary amenorrhea. *Int J Fertil* 22:69–76, 1977
33. Fraser IS, Weisberg E: Fertility following discontinuation of different methods of fertility control. *Contraception* 26:389–415, 1982
34. Brackbill Y, Berendes HW: Dangers of diethylstilbestrol: Review of a 1953 paper. *Lancet* 2:520, 1978
35. Dieckman WJ, Davis ME, Rynklewicz LM, et al: Does the administration of diethylstilbestrol during pregnancy have therapeutic value. *Am J Obstet Gynecol* 66:1062–1081, 1953
36. Herbst AL, Ulfelder H, Poskanzer D: Adenocarcinoma of the vagina. *N Engl J Med* 284:878–881, 1971
37. Barnes AB, Colton T, Gundersen J, et al: Fertility and the outcome of pregnancy in women exposed in utero to diethylstilbestrol. *N Engl J Med* 302:609–613, 1980
38. Herbst AL, Hubby MM, Azizi F, et al: Reproductive and gynecologic surgical experience in diethylstilbestrol-exposed daughters. *Am J Obstet Gynecol* 141:1019–1028, 1981
39. Stillman RJ: In utero exposure to diethylstilbestrol: Adverse effects on the reproductive tract and reproductive performance in male and female offspring. *Am J Obstet Gynecol* 142:905–921, 1982
40. Haney AF, Hammond CB, Soules MR, et al: Diethylstilbestrol-induced upper genital tract abnormalities. *Fertil Steril* 31:142–146, 1979
41. Kaufman RH, Binder GL, Gray PM Jr, et al: Upper genital tract changes associated with exposure in utero to diethylstilbestrol. *Am J Obstet Gynecol* 128:51–59, 1977
42. Seigler AM, Wang CF, Friberg J: Fertility of the diethylstilbestrol-exposed offspring. *Fertil Steril* 31:601–607, 1979
43. Bibbo M, Gill WB, Azizi F, Blough R, et al: Follow-up study of male and female offspring of DES-exposed mothers. *Obstet Gynecol* 49:1–8, 1977
44. Ross RK, Garbeff P, Paganini-Hill A, Henderson BE: Effect of in utero exposure to diethylstilbestrol on age of onset of puberty and on postpubertal hormone levels in boys. *Can Med Assoc J* 128:1197–1198,1983
45. Herbst AL, Hubby MM, Brough RR, et al: A comparison of pregnancy experience in DES-exposed and DES-unexposed daughters. *J Reprod Med* 24:62–69, 1980
46. Cousins L, Karp W, Lacey C, et al: Reproductive outcome of women exposed to diethylstilbestrol in utero. *Obstet Gynecol* 56:70–76, 1980
47. Berger MJ, Goldstein DP: Impaired reproductive perfor-

mance in DES-exposed women. *Obstet Gynecol* 55:25–27, 1980

48. Schmidt G, Fowler WC Jr, Talbert LM, et al: Reproductive history of women exposed to diethylstilbestrol in utero. *Fertil Steril* 33:21–24, 1980

49. Stillman RJ, Miller LC: Diethylstilbestrol exposure in utero and endometriosis in infertile females. *Fertil Steril* 41:369–372, 1984

50. McLachlan JA, Newbold RR, Shah HC, et al: Reduced fertility in female mice exposed transplacentally to diethylstilbestrol (DES). *Fertil Steril* 38:364–371, 1982

51. Haney AF, Newbold RR, McLachlan JA: Changes in ovarian morphology and steroidogenesis *in vitro* in mice exposed to diethylstilbestrol (DES) in utero. *Biol Reprod* [Suppl 1] 24:130A, 1981

52. Kaufman RH, Adam E, Binder GL, et al: Upper genital tract changes and pregnancy outcome in offspring exposed in utero to diethylstilbestrol. *Am J Obstet Gynecol* 137:299–308, 1980

53. Newbold RR, Bullock BC, McLachlan JA: Exposure to diethylstilbestrol during pregnancy permanently alters the ovary and oviduct. *Biol Reprod* 28:735–744, 1983

54. Allegheny County Health Department, Division of Biostatistics, Health Indicator Series, *Selected Vital Statistics 1968–1983,* Pittsburgh, Pennsylvania, 1984

55. Sivin I: Copper T IUD use and ectopic pregnancy rates in the United States. *Contraception* 19:151–173, 1979

56. Hull MGR, Bromham DR, Savage PE, et al: Normal fertility in women with post pill amenorrhea. *Lancet* 1:1329–1332, 1981

ANSWERS

1. c

2. b

21

Anorexia Nervosa and Other Weight-Loss-Associated Amenorrheas

JOHN R. MUSICH

INTRODUCTION

The human female reproductive system is regulated by complex neuroendocrinological control mechanisms that are exquisitely sensitive to changes in both the endogenous central and peripheral endocrine milieus as well as to modifying factors in the environment. A loss of body weight is one such factor that may be induced by internal or external motivation and that may result in hypothalamic–pituitary–ovarian dysfunctions manifested by menstrual disturbances. The extent to which menstrual aberrations occur after weight loss is quite variable, ranging from the amenorrheas associated with anorexia nervosa to the lesser, concerning oligomenorrheas usually seen with bulimia, simple weight loss, or as part of exercise programs. To attribute menstrual changes in these situations solely to alterations in body weight, however,

JOHN R. MUSICH • Department of Obstetrics and Gynecology, William Beaumont Hospital, Royal Oak, Michigan 48072; and Department of Obstetrics and Gynecology, Wayne State University School of Medicine, Detroit, Michigan 48201.

would be unrealistically simplistic. Reproductive dysfunctions attributable to undernutrition are complicated in their etiology and, although poorly understood, are thought to involve not only peripheral endocrine changes due to a loss of weight, but also central modifications of neuroendocrine reproductive cycle control brought about by psychodynamic stress and metabolic and neural inputs to the hypothalamic–pituitary axis.[1] This chapter briefly considers the general pathophysiology of weight loss-associated amenorrheas and then describes the physiological and management aspects of four clinical entities of concern today that are characterized by weight loss and menstrual dysfunction: (1) anorexia nervosa (AN), (2) bulimia, (3) simple weight loss, and (4) exercise-induced amenorrhea.

PATHOPHYSIOLOGY

Frisch's theory[2] that a critical metabolic size or weight is required for a woman to initiate pubertal events and menarche is the background concept that has stimulated much of the interest, in recent years, in weight changes and menstrual disturbances. In

1970, Frisch and Revelle[2] collated information from three large longitudinal growth studies and proposed that the pubertal events of initiation of the weight spurt and initiation of the height spurt both began at a weight of 68 lb (30 kg). According to their findings, the only difference between the "early" and "late" maturer is the height at which this critical weight is attained, with the late maturer being taller when she reached the critical weight necessary for triggering the growth spurts. As their longitudinal studies were continued, it was seen that menarche was also related to an unchanging mean weight. Menarche began after the maximum rate of growth and height was attained, occurring at weight averages of 106 lb (46 kg), age 12.9 years, and height 63 inches (158 cm). Quantitatively as before, the late maturer at menarche, although taller, would exhibit the same critical weight as the shorter, earlier maturer.

In 1974 Frisch and McArthur[3] recognized that the critical weight at menarche more importantly represented a critical body composition of fat as a percentage of total body weight. According to this landmark theory, the body composition necessary for the initiation of menses may occur at varying heights and weights in a population, but the percentage of body fat is a constant figure. As such, the shortest, lightest girls and the tallest, heaviest girls at menarche have the same body fat percentage, although they may vary in height by as many as 8

inches (20 cm) and in weight by as much as 24 lb (11 kg). The study determined that the critical body fat percentage needed to initiate menses was 17% and that at age 18, when most women have ended their height growth and are likely to be stable from a weight standpoint, a 22% fat content would be necessary to maintain normal menstrual function. Also noted in the study was that the weight changes associated with the cessation and restoration of menstrual function were in the range of 10–15% of body weight, with a weight loss or gain of this magnitude being mainly a loss or gain of fat.

The foregoing thoughts of Frisch and colleagues can conveniently be conceptualized by the diagram in Figure 21-1. In order to initiate menstruation, a woman must have a minimum 17% body fat content. As she matures, she will require a 22% fat content to maintain normal menstruation and will likely reach the 25–27% fat content of the average adult woman. If she then undergoes a loss of weight for any reason, there will be a concomitant decrease in her fat content. As she passes back through the 22% mark, she may note the onset of lesser menstrual dysfunctions that may develop into more concerning amenorrhea as she passes below the critical 17% fat content level. To restore normal menstrual function, she will need to regain weight to a point representing at least a 22% fat content. Although Frisch's hypotheses have been criticized,[4–6] it is interesting to note the repetitiveness with which

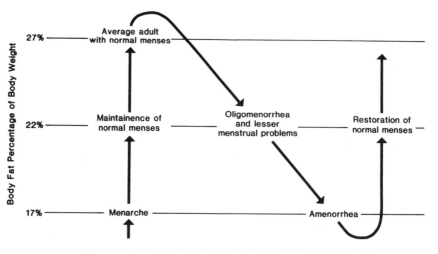

Progression of Menstrual Events Influenced By Body Fat

FIGURE 21-1. Relationship between body fat percentages and menstrual function. On the basis of Frisch's concepts,[2,3] the flow diagram depicts the proposed cycle of initiation, maintenance, loss, and restoration of menses that may be associated with the gain and loss of body weight and fat.

their fat percentage figures have been verified, especially in studies on exercise-induced amenorrhea.

In considering the physiological basis for the induction of pubertal events by the attainment of a critical metabolic size or weight and the pathophysiological mechanism accounting for the menstrual dysfunction consequent to weight loss, Frisch[2] could only speculate that hypothalamic sensitivity to ovarian estrogen would somehow be altered. A definitive link to estrogen involvement in these problems was provided by Fishman's important finding that estrogen metabolism was significantly influenced by changes in body weight.[7] Estradiol (E_2) is reversibly metabolized to estrone (E_1) in the liver, brain, and, more importantly, adipose tissue. E_1, in turn, can be metabolized *via* either one of two routes: (1) by 16-hydroxylation to estriol (E_3), or epiestriol; or (2) by 2-hydroxylation to the catecholestrogen 2-hydroxyestrone. In comparing urinary metabolites of E_2 in patients with AN or obesity, Fishman demonstrated that obese women preferentially metabolize E_2 to E_3, while patients with extensive weight loss due to AN preferentially metabolize estrogen to 2-hydroxyestrone.[7] As proposed by Fishman, 2-hydroxyestrone likely combines its very weak estrogenic biologic activity with its affinity for estrogen receptors to make it an endogenous antiestrogen.

Having apparently established then that a loss of body weight and adipose tissue shifts the metabolism of estrogen along the pathway to 2-hydroxyestrone, it is now necessary to consider the effect of this change on hypothalamic–pituitary function. Adashi and Yen[8] infused 2-hydroxyestrone into estrogen-primed hypogonadal women and found that luteinizing hormone (LH) was suppressed by approximately 40% of its base value over a 24-hr period. Follicle-stimulating hormone (FSH) was suppressed but to a lesser 20% degree. Their study, along with others,[9,10] suggest that the catecholestrogens centrally inhibit gonadotropin secretion and eventually may result in ovulatory disturbances. An alternative would be the possibility that such patients have a generalized lower estrogenic milieu which may make the pituitary gland less sensitive to stimulating amounts of gonadotropin-releasing hormone (GnRH). In either case, as catecholestrogen levels increase with increasing loss of body fat, the menstrual disturbances may become more severe or long lasting.

The shifting of the estrogenic metabolic pathway due to weight and fat loss eventually resulting in

possible catecholestrogenic suppression of gonadotropins and menstrual aberrations is a scenario that would certainly satisfy Frisch's speculation that estrogen is involved in weight-affected menstrual dysfunction. Other mechanisms must be considered, however and, as reviewed by Warren,[1] include (1) the differing effects of obesity and weight loss on the metabolism of androstenedione to E_1; (2) the effect of changes in blood flow and in tissue uptake of hormones in exercise-related weight loss problems; (3) alterations in the neuroendocrine mechanisms involving gonadotropins, GnRH, and endorphins that may be modulated by weight loss or exercise; and (4) possible thermogenic and adrenergic influences on hypothalamic–pituitary function induced by exercise or weight loss. With these pathophysiologic mechanisms in mind and possibly involved to some extent in all weight loss-associated amenorrheas, the specific clinical entities can be discussed.

ANOREXIA NERVOSA

Of the several weight-loss disorders associated with menstrual dysfunction, none is more life threatening and less understood than AN.[11-16] AN is a disorder thought to have biological and psychological causes that may result in severe self-imposed weight loss, a distorted attitude toward eating behavior and other weight-regulation functions, and abnormalities or distortions of mood, self-esteem, and body image. Bruch, who has been credited with ushering in the modern era of the study of AN,[17] has defined both primary and secondary forms of anorexia nervosa.[18] In primary AN, the striving toward a thin body habitus is a result of one's distorted sense of body image and self-control, while the secondary forms of AN are characterized by weight loss due to schizophrenia, depression, or other distinct psychiatric disorders. The etiology of AN has not been determined despite decades of research and clinical attention to this disorder; controversy persists regarding whether the various disturbances of hypothalamic–pituitary function seen in AN are etiologic to the disease process or secondary to the development of starvation and weight loss.

Feighner's diagnostic criteria (Table 21-1) are those usually used in defining AN clinically.[19] Although the clinical presentation of this disease may be quite variable (Table 21-2), the hallmark clinical features include amenorrhea, constipation, hypo-

TABLE 21-1. Feighner's Diagnostic Criteria for Anorexia Nervosa[a]

Age of onset prior to 25
Anorexia with accompanying weight loss of at least 25% of original body weight
A distorted implacable attitude toward eating, food, or weight
  Denial of illness
  Enjoyment in weight loss
  Desired body image of thinness
  Unusual hoarding or handling of food
No other medical illness that could account for the weight loss
No other known psychiatric illness
At least two of the following:
  Amenorrhea
  Lanugo
  Bradycardia
  Periods of overactivity
  Episodes of bulimia
  Emesis (may be self-induced)

[a]From Feighner JP, Robins E, Guze SB, et al.[19]

TABLE 21-2. Clinical Features of Anorexia Nervosa[a]

Demographic and historical features
  Female predominance
  Late childhood and adolescent onset
  Caucasian predominance
  Middle- to upper-class families
  History of overweight period in past
  Preoccupation with food and nutrition
  Preoccupation with exercise
Symptoms
  Amenorrhea, primary or secondary, in nearly all patients
  Constipation with complaints of abdominal pain
  Cold intolerance
  Agitation or lethargy
  Emesis
Physical findings
  Cachexia
  Increased lanugolike hair
  Skin abnormalities
  Hypotension
  Hypercarotenemic skin
  Peripheral edema
  Hypothermia
Laboratory findings
  Decreased thyroid function test values
  Abnormal cortisol and growth hormone secretion
  Decreased FSH and LH
  Hypercarotenemia
  Other evidence of hypothalamic dysfunction
  Elevated blood urea nitrogen

[a]Schwabe AD, Lippe BM, Chang RJ, et al.[12]

tension, hypothermia, bradycardia, leukopenia, azotemia, hypercarotenemia, and various endocrinological changes.[11] The diagnosis of AN is made many times more frequently in women than in men, and certainly the virtual 100% incidence of amenorrhea in anorexic women highlights the generally accepted notion that AN is a female-predominant problem.

Because of the nearly universal finding of amenorrhea in anorexic women, the function of the hypothalamic–pituitary–ovarian axis in AN has been the subject of much investigation. A review by Fries[20] has reported that 25% of the patients with AN developed amenorrhea after the establishment of weight loss, a finding consistent with the pathophysiology of Frisch's critical body weight hypothesis discussed earlier. In Fries's study, 55% of patients manifested simultaneous losses of body weight and normal menstrual function, while 16% of women developed amenorrhea before the onset of weight loss. Others have also shown that a large portion of anorectic women develop amenorrhea before a substantial loss of body weight,[21,22] a finding that suggests that the etiological factor resulting in amenorrhea or lesser menstrual disturbances may be psychogenic rather than metabolic in origin. The fact that amenorrhea can result from severe psychogenic stress is well accepted and frequently observed[23] and the finding that not all anorectic patients recover normal menstrual function after normalization of body weight gives support to the possibility that persistent psychologic stress may be the principal etiologic factor for the amenorrhea.[24] This supports the concept that psychogenic factors may be more important than metabolic factors. It is not uncommon to find that anorectic patients reestablish normal menstrual patterns after resolving their psychiatric problems in the absence of weight gain.[11]

Both urine and serum levels of FSH, LH, and E_2 are depressed in anorexic women,[11,25] and the cyclical characteristics of gonadotropin release regress to prepubertal patterns.[24,26,27] Instead of exhibiting the expected adult secretion pattern of slight LH pulsation throughout the entire sleep–wake cycle, LH secretion and levels are reduced to prepubertal nonpulsatile levels. After weight gain associated with recovery, the amenorrheic anorectic woman may exhibit gonadotropin secretion characteristics of normal pubertal development, i.e., an increase in LH secretion pulsatility and amplitude during sleeping hours, followed by similar secretion characteristics during the waking hours

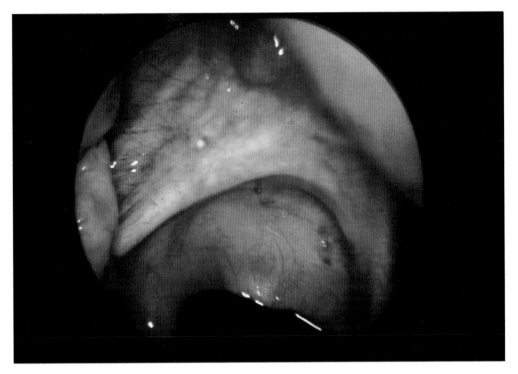

FIGURE 18-1. Small rust-colored deposits of endometriosis in the cul-de-sac and over the left uterosacral ligaments seen at laparoscopy.

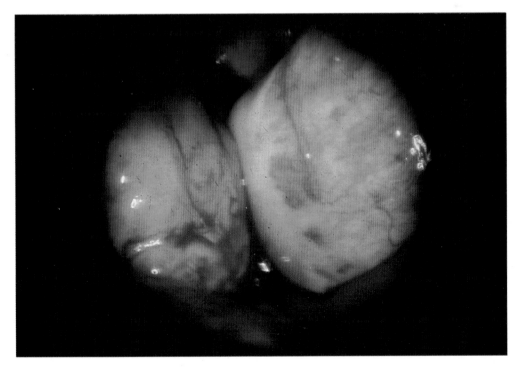

FIGURE 18-2. Characteristic appearance of endometriosis deposits on the surface of the ovary visualized through the laparoscope.

and eventual reestablishment of postpubertal or adult patterns associated with normal ovulatory and menstrual function. Patients who retain their behavioral and psychiatric disturbances, however, do not reestablish normal gonadotropin functions despite weight gain and will have continuing amenorrhea due to the persistent prepubertal state of gonadotropin release.[24] Similarly, menstrual recovery due to redevelopment of the adult pattern of gonadotropin release can also be seen in anorexics who regain minimal weight but who resolve their psychiatric problems.[24] Gonadotropin release following GnRH administration is usually suppressed in AN with evidence to suggest good correlation between the severity of the weight loss and the degree of suppression of gonadotropin release.[28] Impressively, however, Marshall and Kelch[29] demonstrated that low-dose GnRH administration in a repetitive, pulsatile manner to anorectic women can induce an FSH–LH release pattern that mimics the pubertal hypothalamic–pituitary–ovarian functions necessary to establish ovulatory cycles.

The cause of suppression of gonadotropin activity in AN is unknown, but it may involve one or all of several possible mechanisms. The suppressive effect on hypothalamic–pituitary function of increased catecholestrogen levels induced by severe weight loss has already been discussed. There is evidence that other neurotransmitters may be involved as well. An increase in central dopaminergic activity has been proposed as the cause of the psychiatric disturbances in AN,[30] and dopamine (DA) infusions have been shown to inhibit LH secretion.[31] Similarly, the DA agonists, bromocriptine and levodopa, depress LH activity.[32] The suppressive activity of DA may also be enhanced by the increased levels of catecholestrogens present in anorexic patients. Catecholestrogens inhibit the metabolic inactivation of DA and other catecholamines by inhibiting catechol-o-methyltransferase activity and may thereby enhance DA activity.[8] In addition, opiate peptide levels have been found to be increased in the cerebrospinal fluid (CSF) of anorexics and may be etiologically related to AN gonadotropin dysfunction.[33]

Changes in other endocrine systems in AN have been reviewed by Beumont and are less consistent.[25] Growth hormone (GH) levels may be normal or elevated and although inconclusive, there may be some dysfunction in the hypothalamic catecholaminergic control of GH secretion. Plasma cortisol levels are usually elevated due to both an increase in adrenal secretion and to a decrease in starvation-induced metabolic changes.[34] Prolactin levels are normal in AN, and there appears to be no relationship between body weight and prolactin levels.[35] Thyroid status is more complex. Bradycardia, increased serum cholesterol levels, and a low basal metabolic rate are common. Thyroxine (T4), the levels of which are normal or low-normal, is preferentially degraded to reverse triiodothyronine (RT3) rather than to the more bioactive T3, a process that conserves energy in the face of a catabolic state such as AN.

The diagnosis of AN is made by careful history-taking and physical examination and should not require an exhaustive endocrine evaluation. Laboratory confirmation, if needed, can usually be limited to the demonstration of decreased FSH and LH with an FSH : LH ratio of less than 1 and of elevated levels of carotene and GH. If the patient's history is compatible with AN, the finding of other biochemical or endocrinological abnormalities should only serve to support the diagnosis and not be reason to subject the patient to an extensive and unnecessary metabolic evaluation.

Because AN is such a poorly understood disease, many treatment programs have been advocated and tried.[36] After establishing the diagnosis, however, treatment should generally focus simultaneously on three considerations: (1) psychiatric counseling, (2) nutritional support, and (3) indicated endocrine replacement or stimulation therapy. Emergency nutritional support by nasogastric tube feeding or central vein hyperalimentation is mandatory for patients who have lost more than 40% of their ideal body weight, since metabolic derangements and cardiac arrhythmias may be life threatening in this situation. In cases of lesser weight loss, behavior modification should be attempted in an effort to encourage weight gain. At the same time, individual and family counseling should be pursued in an effort to delineate and hopefully gain acknowledgement of the patient's conceptual distortions and defects so that specific psychotherapeutic and behavioral modification programs can be initiated.

Hormonal therapy will depend on the severity of the menstrual problems and the specific desires of the patient but should likely be a tertiary therapeutic consideration after nutritional and psychiatric concerns. The reestablishment of ovulatory cycles and the achievement of pregnancy, if desired, are definitely possible after the normalization of body weight. During the recovery process, however, the patient's estrogen status can be determined by attempting to induce progestational withdrawal bleeding. In a patient with amenorrhea, such bleeding offers reassurance that the hypothalamic–pituitary–ovarian axis is recovering. If no bleeding occurs after progestin stimulation, estrogen replacement should be offered (see Chapter 16). In patients desiring pregnancy, the need for nutritional adequacy and weight gain must be encouraged, after which clomiphene citrate, human menopausal gonadotropins, or GnRH may be considered to induce ovulation if needed (see Chapter 30).

For a detailed look at treatment outcome in AN, the reader is referred to Hsu's exhaustive review.[37] Although acute nutritional therapy has been effective in reducing AN mortality to less than 5% overall, problems still present at long-term follow-up confirm that our understanding and management of AN still leave much to be desired. In summarizing Hsu's data, the following generalizations of treatment can be offered: (1) 75% of patients will show an improvement in body weight, defined as a weight gain equal to or greater than 75% of ideal body weight, while 15–25% of patients will continue to have body weight below 75% of their expected weight; (2) continuing menstrual abnormalities are common, with up to 50% of patients exhibiting amenorrhea even after appropriate weight gain; and (3) 50–75% of patients, with or without resolution of their nutritional and menstrual problems, will still exhibit unhealthy attitudes toward body image, obsessive-compulsive tendencies, drug dependence, or other types of sociopathological behavior.

BULIMIA

Bulimia, a term derived from the Greek meaning "ox hunger," refers both to a symptom and to an eating-disorder syndrome.[38] Bulimia as a symptom refers to the rapid gorging of large amounts of food over a short period of time, while the bulimic syndrome is an eating disorder with psychiatric overtones that is very difficult to diagnose and that may frequently (50%) be part of AN. Diagnostic criteria have been established for the bulimic syndrome (Table 21-3),[39] which is also known as the binge-eating syndrome, binge–purging, and the gorging–purging syndrome of young women.[38] In brief, the bulimic patient gorges herself and then self-induces vomiting or takes purgatives to prevent weight gain or to increase weight loss. Because up to 50% of anorectics exhibit bulimia as their means of losing weight, bulimia is considered by some to be a vari-

TABLE 21-3. Criteria for Bulimia (DSM III)

Recurrent episodes of binge eating
At least three of the following:
  Consumption of high-calorie, easily ingested food during a
    binge
  Inconspicuous eating during a binge
  Termination of binge episodes by abdominal pain, sleep,
    social interruption, or self-induced vomiting
  Repeated attempts to lose weight by severely restrictive
    diets, self-induced vomiting, cathartics, or diuretics
  Frequent weight fluctuation greater than 10 lb due to
    alternating binges and fasts
Awareness that eating pattern is abnormal and fear of not
    being able to stop eating voluntarily
Depression and self-deprecating thoughts after binges
Bulimic episodes not due to anorexia nervosa or other
    physical disorders

[a]From *Diagnostic and Statistical Manual of the American Psychiatric Association.*[39]

ant of AN[40] and may be referred to as bulimia nervosa or bulimarexia.

Bulimia usually occurs in late adolescence or early adulthood (average age 18 years) and, like AN, is distinctly a female-predominant problem (96% of bulimics).[1] Depression, considered to be an essential aspect of bulimia, is manifested by low self-esteem, low mood, and self-deprecating thoughts.[41] Like anorectics, bulimics have a distorted body image. While as many as 10% of bulimics may be overweight, the remainder are either of normal weight (50%) or below their ideal body weight (30%).[38] Medical complications associated with bulimia would generally be dependent on the severity of the individual's weight loss, and can include abdominal pain, lethargy, dehydration, and electrolyte imbalances as metabolic alkalosis, hypochloremia, hypokalemia, and hyponatremia.

Menstrual irregularities may occur in 50% of bulimics, although the problem is more likely to be oligomenorrhea rather than amenorrhea. Because many bulimics are of normal body weight, it is essential to inquire about eating behavior in all patients with menstrual irregularities in order to uncover those that may yet be found to have dietary deficiencies that might contribute to reproductive disorders even though they may have no history of weight loss.

The diagnosis of bulimia is entirely dependent on eliciting a history of the gorge–purge eating pattern. There are no specific endocrine laboratory alterations except those that may characterize the anorectic subgroup of bulimia. Treatment, as with AN, should focus on psychotherapy, behavior modification, dietary counseling, and oligoamenorrhea pharmacological manipulation as warranted.

SIMPLE WEIGHT LOSS

The quest for thinness among women, particularly in the adolescent age groups, is not without consequences in menstrual function. Severe weight loss that occurs for any reason, whether due to chronic illness, AN, bulimia, or dieting, can result in oligomenorrhea, primary or secondary amenorrhea, and delayed puberty.[42] Likewise, the simple weight loss (SWL) associated with dietary behavior and exercise activities intended to achieve a thin body habitus may lead to endocrine dysfunctions resulting in amenorrhea.[43] Such weight loss must also be covered in infertility evaluations, as anovulatory cycles or luteal phase inadequacies causing infertility may be due to caloric restriction in some patients.[44]

Although SWL patients do not by definition fulfill Feighner's criteria for AN, the amount of weight loss by them may be comparable to AN patients.[45] Wentz's study of SWL patients with amenorrhea found them, as a group, to be approximately 80% of their ideal body weight, with a minimum loss of 41% of their body fat.[45] This degree of body fat loss represents a loss of weight very comparable to the 10–15% weight loss thought by Frisch (discussed earlier) to represent a fat loss sufficient to induce amenorrhea.[3,46] Similar percentages of ideal body weight, approximately 80% and 90%, respectively, were found by Vigersky et al.[43] and Bates et al.[44] to be associated with their patients exhibiting menstrual dysfunction.

Vigersky's endocrine studies on SWL patients found hypothalamic and pituitary functions intermediate between those of normal and AN patients, and in some cases, very similar to AN patients.[43] In SWL patients with amenorrhea, FSH levels were found to be lower than in normal patients but higher than in AN, while LH levels, although higher than in AN, were indistinguishable from normal patients. Gonadotropin-secreting response to GnRH was also suppressed in SWL patients although not to the extent seen in AN.[43] Bates's study of gonadotropins in SWL patients found FSH levels to be decreased with a decreasing FSH : LH ratio as the ideal body weight percentage increased,[44]

which is in keeping with gonadotropin dynamics seen in recovering AN patients.[24]

It is important in the counseling of SWL patients with reproductive difficulties to note that pharmacological ovulation induction may be feasible, but any effort toward reestablishment of ideal body weight may, by itself, be salutary or even curative in achieving ovulatory cycles.[44] Except for its potential detrimental effects on menstruation and reproduction, SWL is of minimal medical concern unless the severity approaches that of AN, at which time the management of SWL should likewise approach that of AN.

EXERCISE-INDUCED AMENORRHEA

With participation by more women in strenuous exercise programs such as running, skiing, aerobic dancing, and ballet, there has been a clinical awareness of increased problems with amenorrhea, oligomenorrhea, and other menstrual disturbances in these women.[47] Since Erdelyi's report[48] of a 12% incidence of menstrual dysfunction in a large group of female athletes, there have been several reports, as reviewed by Baker,[47] suggesting that menstrual problems may occur in up to 50% of athletic women. As societal influences encourage the improvement of cardiovascular health and general well-being through exercise, the practicing gynecologist is thereby presented with further challenges in the realm of weight-loss reproductive disturbances.

Although young age, nulliparity, stress, and prior menstrual dysfunction may predispose female athletes to amenorrhea,[47] loss of body weight and changes in body fat percentages are strikingly associated with and likely causally related to the development of amenorrhea. Speroff[49,50] found that competitive female runners with weight loss between 10 and 20 lb had a 15% chance of developing amenorrhea while those with weight losses greater than 20 lb had a 20% incidence of secondary amenorrhea. Women at greatest risk for development of menstrual problems were those under 25 years of age who weighed 115 lb or less when they began running and subsequently lost more than 10 pounds. He also found, as would be expected, that the competitive runners had lesser body fat. Schwartz and associates[51] found that amenorrheic runners weighed less, lost more weight after the onset of running, and had a significantly lower percentage of body fat than did runners with regular menses. In a study of female distance runners, Dale et al.[52] found runners with the greatest incidence of oligo/amenorrhea to have an average body fat content of 17%, while runners with lesser degrees of menstrual problems had a 21% body fat percentage; the eumenorrheic control patients had a 24% body fat content. This study strikingly supports the body fat percentages of 17% and 22% that Frisch had claimed would be necessary to initiate and maintain normal menstrual function, and which, depicted in Figure 21-1, would be expected to be predictive of body fat percentages associated with the development of lesser (22%) and then more severe (17%) forms of menstrual dysfunction. Although others have found no difference in weight between eumenorrheic and amenorrheic runners,[53,54] the bulk of evidence does suggest a pattern of progressively worsening menstrual problems directly proportional to the degree of loss of body weight and fat.

Gonadotropin and sex steroid values in amenorrheic runners, although decreased in some women and therefore supportive of the earlier discussed physiology of weight loss amenorrhea, have been found to be normal or increased in other studies. Dale et al.[52,55] and Demers et al.[56] found suppressed FSH and LH levels in their oligomenorrheic runners with consequently suppressed E_2 and progesterone (P) levels.[52,55] While others have found no substantial change in gonadotropin values in either acute or chronic exercise,[57-59] Schwartz et al.[51] found increased LH levels and slightly decreased FSH levels in their amenorrheic runners. Schwartz's findings of an increased $E_1 : E_2$ ratio in these women, combined with the elevated LH : FSH ratio, suggest a possible polycystic ovarian-like hormonal profile in amenorrheic runners. Estrogen and P levels are increased during acute exercise,[57,59] but with the chronic exercise that better characterizes those with menstrual dysfunctions luteal phase P levels are decreased.[55,58] This suggests that if exercise does not lead to amenorrhea, it certainly can result in ovulatory disturbances characterized by an inadequate luteal phase.[58] The levels of androgens and prolactin in exercising women, reviewed by Baker,[47] have a tendency to be elevated during the acute phase of exercise, but basal levels are likely to be normal and of unknown consequence in the pathophysiology of exercise-induced amenorrhea.

Although the preceding findings generally support the concept that metabolic changes associated with the loss of weight and fat through exercise can result in amenorrhea, the etiology of reproductive dysfunction in female athletes is likely to be more complex. McArthur et al.[60] studied three amenorrheic runners with normal weight and fat composition and found that, although baseline GnRH stimulation studies resulted in variable gonadotropin responses in the three patients, all three runners responded with exaggerated LH release when repeat GnRH stimulation was carried out during a period of naloxone administration. The β-endorphin opiates, which can suppress gonadotropin function,[61] are elevated by running and exercise[62-64] and, in addition to being a possible etiology of disrupted thypothalamic–pituitary function in exercise-induced amenorrhea, endorphins may also be responsible for the euphoric "high" associated with running.[65] McArthur's study of the effect of the infusion of naloxone, which is an endorphin antagonist, is suggestive evidence that opiates may play a role in exercise-induced amenorrhea. The finding that amenorrheic runners associate stress with their physical activities[51] offers further support to the notion that endogenous opiates, which are elevated in a stress situation, may be causally related to the amenorrhea found in these women. Dietary changes,[51,66] alterations in thyroid function,[67] and augmented secretion of catecholamines[68] have also been etiologically implicated in exercise-induced menstrual problems. Finally, Warren[69] postulated that an energy drain associated with exercise may result in amenorrhea or menarcheal delay as evidenced by her study of ballet dancers who achieve cyclic menses in the absence of any weight gain when they were forced to stop exercising for extended intervals due to injuries.

Menstrual disorders precipitated by physical activity are easily diagnosed by virtue of their usual manifestation after the onset of exercise-induced weight loss. Because many of these women are hypoestrogenic, the threat of endometrial hyperplasia is virtually nonexistent. Therefore, the cyclic use of progestins to induce periodic bleeding is not necessary, although the progestin challenge test may be used periodically to ascertain an individual's relative state of estrogenicity. The hypoestrogenic state, however, may make the amenorrheic athlete more susceptible to osteoporotic bone loss and therefore estrogen replacement therapy should be considered.[70] Ovulation induction, if desired, is usually possible with clomiphene citrate, although some patients may be forced to lessen their activities if clomiphene is not readily effective. The most important aspect of the management of such patients is to make them aware of the consequences of exercise on their reproductive function, with the realization that cessation of their activities will likely restore cyclic menses.

SUMMARY

The amenorrhea and lesser menstrual disorders associated with anorexia nervosa, bulimia, simple weight loss, and exercise can certainly be due, in part, to alterations in estrogen metabolism induced by the loss of body weight and fat. Although such an etiology is in keeping with Frisch's critical metabolic size theory as it pertains to menarche and the maintenance of normal menstrual function, it is clear that the etiology of weight-loss amenorrhea is much more complex. As the complicated network of hormonal and neural influences on gonadotropin-controlling neurotransmitters is unraveled, the causation of these and other ''hypothalamic'' amenorrheas will be better understood and it is hoped, treated.

The seriousness of the anorectic's amenorrhea speaks for itself. Practicing clinicians, however, will be more commonly faced with lesser menstrual disturbances induced by milder forms of weight loss that must be carefully searched for historically to avoid being overlooked. Although hormonal and pharmacological manipulation will frequently restore normal menstrual function in these patients, they must clearly understand that dietary and activity modification may be necessary to achieve reproductive satisfaction.

QUESTIONS

1. Frisch's critical metabolic size theory of the initiation of puberty states that the acquisition of a critical body weight and fat content is responsible for

    a. adrenarche.
    b. thelarche.
    c. menarche.
    d. peak height.

2. According to Fishman's study of the influence of adipose tissue on estrogen metabolism, patients with anorexia nervosa preferentially metabolize estrogen to

    a. estriol.
    b. androstenedione.
    c. estrone.
    d. catecholestrogen.

3. Runner's amenorrhea is *not* attributable to

    a. loss of body weight and fat.
    b. alteration in dietary habits during training.
    c. stress-elevated endogenous opioids.
    d. chronic dopaminergic suppression of GnRH.

REFERENCES

1. Warren MP: Effects of undernutrition on reproductive function in the human. *Endocrine Rev* 4:363, 1983*
2. Frisch RE, Revelle R: Height and weight at menarche and a hypothesis of critical body weights and adolescent events. *Science* 169:397, 1970
3. Frisch RE, McArthur JW: Menstrual cycles: Fatness as a determinant of minimum weight for height necessary for their maintenance or onset. *Science* 185:949, 1974
4. Crawford JD, Osler DC: Body composition at menarche: The Frisch–Revelle hypothesis revisited. *Pediatrics* 58:449, 1975
5. Falk JK, Halmi KA: Amenorrhea in anorexia nervosa: Examination of the critical body weight hypothesis. *Biol Psychol* 17:799, 1982
6. Trussel J: Menarche and fatness: Re-examination of the critical body composition. *Science* 200:1506, 1978
7. Fishman J, Boyar RM, Hellman L: Influence of body weight on estradiol metabolism in young women. *J Clin Endocrinol Metab* 41:989, 1975
8. Adashi EY, Rakoff J, Divers W, et al: The effect of acutely administered 2-hydroxyestrone on the release of gonadotropins and prolactin before and after estrogen priming in hypogonadal women. *Life Sci* 25:2051, 1979
9. Schinfield JS, Tulchinsky D, Schiff I, et al: Suppression of prolactin and gonadotropin secretion in post-menopausal women by 2-hydroxyestrone. *J Clin Endocrinol Metab* 50:408, 1980
10. Fishman J, Tulchinsky D: Suppression of prolactin secretion in normal young women by 2-hydroxyestrone. *Science* 210:73, 1980
11. Eisenberg E: Toward an understanding of reproductive function in anorexia nervosa. *Fertil Steril* 36:543, 1981*
12. Schwabe AD, Lippe BM, Chang RJ, et al: Anorexia nervosa. *Ann Intern Med* 94:371, 1981*
13. Lester EP: Symposium: Anorexia nervosa and obesity—Recent developments. *Can J Psychol* 4:211, 1981*
14. Bruch H: Developmental considerations of anorexia nervosa and obesity. *Can J Psychol* 4:212, 1981*
15. Bruch H: Psychological antecedents of anorexia nervosa, in Vigersky RA (ed): *Anorexia Nervosa*. New York, Raven Press, 1977, pp 1–10*
16. Bruch H: *The Golden Cage*. Cambridge, MA, Harvard University Press, 1978*
17. Lucas AR: Toward the understanding of anorexia nervosa as a disease entity. *Mayo Clin Proc* 56:254, 1981
18. Bruch H: Anorexia nervosa: Therapy and theory. *Am J Psychiatry* 139:1531, 1982
19. Feighner JP, Robins E, Guze SB, et al: Diagnostic criteria for use in psychiatric research. *Arch Gen Psychiatry* 26:57, 1972
20. Fries H: Studies on secondary amenorrhea, anorectic behav-

*Review articles and chapters.

ior, and body-image perception: Importance for the early recognition of anorexia nervosa, in Vigersky RA (ed): *Anorexia Nervosa.* New York, Raven Press, 1977, p. 163–176

21. Silverman JA: Anorexia nervosa: Clinical observations in a successful treatment plan. *J Pediatr* 84:68, 1974

22. Halmi KA: Anorexia nervosa: Demographic and clinical features in 94 cases. *Psychosom Med* 36:18, 1974

23. Lachelin GC, Yen SSC: Hypothalamic chronic anovulation. *Am J Obstet Gynecol* 130:825, 1978

24. Katz JL, Boyar R, Roffwarg H, et al: Weight and circadian luteinizing hormone secretory pattern in anorexia nervosa. *Psychosom Med* 40:549, 1978

25. Beumont PJV: The endocrinology of anorexia nervosa. *Med J Aust* 1:611, 1979

26. Boyar RM, Katz J, Finkelstein JW, et al: Anorexia nervosa: Immaturity of the 24-hour luteinizing hormone secretory pattern. *N Engl J Med* 291:861, 1974

27. Boyar RM, Katz J: Twenty-four hour gonadotropin secretory patterns in anorexia nervosa, in Vigersky RA (ed): *Anorexia Nervosa.* New York, Raven Press, 1977, p 177

28. Warren MP, Jewelewicz R, Dyrenfurth I, et al: The significance of weight loss in the evaluation of pituitary response to LH-RH in women with secondary amenorrhea. *J Clin Endocrinol Metab* 40:601, 1975

29. Marshall JC, Kelch RP: Low dose pulsatile gonadotropin-releasing hormone in anorexia nervosa: A model of human pubertal development. *J Clin Endocrinol Metab* 49:712, 1979

30. Barry VC, Klawans HL: On the role of dopamine in the pathophysiology of anorexia nervosa. *J Neurol Trans* 38:107, 1976

31. Leblanc H, Lachelin GCL, Abu-Fadil S, et al: Effects of dopamine infusion on pituitary hormone secretion in humans. *J Clin Endocrinol Metab* 43:668, 1976

32. Lachelin GCL, Leblanc H, Yen SSC: The inhibitory effect of dopamine agonists on LH release in women. *J Clin Endocrinol Metab* 44:728, 1977

33. Kaye WH, Pickar D, Naber D, et al: Cerebrospinal fluid opioid activity in anorexia nervosa. *Am J Psychiatry* 139:643, 1982

34. Doerr P, Fichter M, Pirke KM, et al: Relationship between weight gain and hypothalamic pituitary adrenal function in patients with anorexia nervosa. *J Steroid Biochem* 13:529, 1980

35. Wakeling A, de Souza VFA, Gore MBR, et al: Amenorrhea, body weight and serum hormone concentrations, with particular reference to prolactin and thyroid hormones in anorexia nervosa. *Psychol Med* 9:265, 1979

36. Rockwell WJK, Ellinwood EH Jr, Dougherty GG, et al: Anorexia nervosa: Review of current treatment practices. *South Med J* 75:1101, 1982*

37. Hsu LKG: Outcome of anorexia nervosa. *Arch Gen Psychiatry* 37:1041, 1980*

38. Pyle RL, Mitchell JE: The bulimia syndrome. *Female Patient* 8:48, 1983*

39. *Diagnostic and Statistical Manual of the American Psychiatric Association,* 3rd ed. Washington, DC, American Psychiatric Association, 1980

40. Russell G: Bulimia nervosa: An ominous variant of anorexia nervosa. *Psychol Med* 9:429, 1979

41. Humphries LL, Wrobel S: Bulimia: The binge eating syndrome. *South Med J* 76:181, 1983

42. Warren MP: The effects of altered nutritional states, stress and systemic illness on reproduction in women, in Vaitukaitis J (ed): *Clinical Reproductive Neuroendocrinology.* New York, Elsevier Biomedical, 1982, pp 177–188

43. Vigersky RA, Andersen AE, Thompson RH, et al: Hypothalamic dysfunction in secondary amenorrhea associated with simple weight loss. *N Engl J Med* 297:1141, 1977

44. Bates GW, Bates SR, Whitworth NS: Reproductive failure in women who practice weight control. *Fertil Steril* 37:373, 1982

45. Wentz AC: Body weight and amenorrhea. *Obstet Gynecol* 56:482, 1980

46. Frisch RE, Revelle R, Cook S: Components of the critical weight at menarche and at initiation of the adolescent spurt: estimated total water, lean body mass, and fat. *Hum Biol* 45:469, 1973

47. Baker ER: Menstrual dysfunction and hormonal status in athletic women: A review. *Fertil Steril* 36:691, 1981*

48. Erdelyi GJ: Gynecological survey of female athletes. *J Sports Med Phys Fitness* 2:174, 1962

49. Speroff L, Redwine DB: Exercise and menstrual function. *Physician Sports Med* 8:42, 1980

50. Speroff L: Can exercise cause problems in pregnancy and menstruation? *Contemp Obstet Gynecol* 16:57, 1980

51. Schwartz B, Cumming DC, Riordan E, et al: Exercise-associated amenorrhea: A distinct entity? *Am J Obstet Gynecol* 141:662, 1981

52. Dale E, Gerlach DH, Wilhite AL: Menstrual dysfunction in distance runners. *Obstet Gynecol* 54:47, 1979

53. Baker ER, Mathur RS, Kirk RF, et al: Female runners and secondary amenorrhea: correlation with age, parity, mileage, and plasma hormonal and sex-hormone-binding globulin concentrations. *Fertil Steril* 36:183, 1981

54. Dale E, Gerlach DH, Martin DE, et al: Physical fitness profiles and reproductive physiology of the female distance runner. *Physician Sports Med* 7:83, 1979

56. Demers LM, Harrison TS, Halbert DR, et al: Cited by Grunby P: Increasing numbers of physical changes found in nation's runners (Medical News). *JAMA* 245:547, 1981

57. Jurkowski JE, Jones NL, Walker WC, et al: Ovarian hormonal responses to exercise. *J Appl Physiol* 44:109, 1978

58. Shangold M, Freeman R, Thysen B, et al: The relationship between long distance running, plasma progesterone and luteal phase length. *Fertil Steril* 31:130, 1979

59. Shangold M, Gatz ML, Thysen B: Acute effects of exercise on plasma concentrations of prolactin and testosterone in recreational women runners. *Fertil Steril* 35:699, 1981

60. McArthur JW, Bullen BA, Beitins IZ, et al: Hypothalamic amenorrhea in runners of normal body composition. *Endocr Res Commun* 7:13, 1980

61. Quigley ME, Sheehan KL, Casper RF, et al: Evidence for an increased dopaminergic and opioid activity in patients with hypothalamic hypogonadotropic amenorrhea. *J Clin Endocrinol Metab* 50:949, 1980

62. Carr DB, Bullen BA, Skrinar GS, et al: Physical conditioning facilitates the exercise-induced secretion of beta-endorphin and beta-lipotropin in women. *N Engl J Med* 305:560, 1981

63. Colt EWD, Wardlaw SL, Frantz AG: The effect of running on B-endorphin. *Life Sci* 28:1637, 1981

64. Bortz WM II, Angwin P, Mefford IN, et al: Catecholamines, dopamine, and endorphin levels during extreme exercise. *N Engl J Med* 305:466, 1981

65. Speroff L: Getting high on running. *Fertil Steril* 36:149, 1981

66. Frisch RE, Gotz-Welbergen AV, McArthur JW, et al: Delayed menarche and amenorrhea of college athletes in relation to age of onset of training. *JAMA* 246:1559, 1981
67. Irvine CHG: Effect of exercise on thyroxine degradation in athletes and nonathletes. *J Clin Endocrinol Metab* 28:942, 1968
68. Carr D, Arnold M, Bullen B: Abstract No. 466. Sixty-Third Annual Meeting, Endocrine Society, June 17–19, 1981, Cincinnati, 1981, p 199
69. Warren MP: The effects of exercise on pubertal progression and reproductive function in girls. *J Clin Endocrinol Metab* 51:1150, 1980
70. Cann CE, Martin MC, Genant HK, et al: Decreased spinal mineral content in amenorrheic women. *JAMA* 251:616, 1984

ANSWERS

1. c

2. d

3. d

Premenstrual Tension and Idiopathic Edema

EDWARD L. MARUT

PREMENSTRUAL TENSION: THE PROBLEM

Premenstrual tension or, more commonly premenstrual syndrome (PMS), is a long-recognized heterogeneous symptom complex that has defied adequate characterization, elucidation of pathophysiology, and treatment for many years. First described by Frank[1] in 1931, premenstrual syndrome has taken on a spectrum of presentations ranging from purely physiologic symptoms during the luteal phase (molimina) to a pattern of aberrant violent behavior that has apparently involved assault, child abuse, spouse battering, and murder.[2] The myriad of reported symptoms attributed to the premenstrual interval is pointless to list, but those most likely to be associated with endocrine changes in the premenstruum are noted in Table 22-1. In general, they most often involve breast symptoms, fluid retention, and emotional changes. The pattern of waxing and waning symptoms, which typically encompass approximately the last 7 days of a luteal phase, is

EDWARD L. MARUT • In Vitro Fertilization–Embryo Transfer Program, Division of Reproductive Endocrinology, Michael Reese Hospital and Medical Center; and Department of Obstetrics and Gynecology, Pritzker School of Medicine–University of Chicago, Chicago, Illinois 60616.

actually highly variable. It presents with a spectrum of symptoms starting from the periovulatory interval to only 1 or 2 days premenstrually, and with resolution occurring from initiation of menses to the end of the menstrual flow.[3] Thus, defining what ''PMS'' really means is not always clear cut. Documentation of cyclic symptomatology in relationship to the menses may require charting of symptoms on a menstrual calendar to determine whether such an association really exists. However, the problem of self-evaluation has been demonstrated by a study in which women reported ''premenstrual'' symptoms when they were falsely told their cycles would be shortened by medication, but menses did not actually occur until the expected time.[4] Generally, follicular phase symptoms or intermittent acyclic symptoms are unlikely to be due to endocrine changes related to the menstrual cycle. This is further compounded by the presence of apparent premenstrual symptoms in some women without evidence of ovulation as well as some receiving anovulatory steroids. The opposite effect may be obtained, on the other hand, where unexplained cyclic symptomatology is found to relate to the menstrual cycle when previously unexplained.

Thus, whether a symptom complex qualifies as being part of PMS or not may not be immediately

TABLE 22-1. Symptoms of PMS

Breast swelling and tenderness
Abdominal bloating
Edema
Headache
Fatigue
Depression
Irritability
Anxiety
Thirst
Hunger
Constipation
Allergic reactions

obvious. If the symptoms are to be related to some cyclic endocrine change, the temporal relationship must at least be set. The pathophysiology of premenstrual symptomatology has been the subject of many studies with conflicting results; the choice of therapeutic regimens has been marred by poorly controlled trials. The first question is, of course: What is normal, and what is abnormal? If premenstrual symptoms that accompany regular cycles are indicative of ovulation, they should be construed as being not only normal but desirable. However, just as mild menstrual cramping is suggestive of prior ovulation under the above criteria, exaggeration of these presumptive postovulatory stigmata may became pathologic, depending on the effect on the individual women. Herein lies the crux of the matter: Is there a unitary pathophysiologic event that covers all the variants of PMS, or are there as many etiologies as specific symptoms? Contrariwise, is the absence of cyclic somatic symptomatology actually abnormal? Attempts to identify the etiology of premenstrual syndrome begin with its description, which preceded the label by more than 20 years.[5] The magnitude of the health problem is uncertain, but rates of significant diminution of normal daily functioning occur during the premenstruum in up to 40% of women.[6]

The number of women who seek medical aid or volunteer information has been significantly smaller, however. Dissemination of information and awareness groups should change this pattern and encourage more women who have been suffering in silence to seek relief. While the sensationalistic aspects of PMS are newsworthy, absolving murder with a ''PMS defense'' is highly questionable. Concentrating on recognition of a constellation of symptoms related to endocrinologic events in contrast to the concept of ''rejection of femininity''

will provide women with a better understanding of their physiology. Better understanding should provide therapeutic relief from symptoms often chronically crippling to her 25% of the time.

PATHOPHYSIOLOGY

The first hypothesis on the etiology of PMS originated with Frank,[1] was championed by Dalton,[7] and is the most widely discussed. That is, an imbalance exists in the luteal phase of women with PMS between estrogen and progesterone. The exaggerated effects of estrogen and deficient actions of progesterone were thought to explain fluid retention, mastodynia, and impaired glucose tolerance, as well as central nervous system symptoms.[8] Although this theory is plausible (i.e., estrogen enhances the renin-angiotensin-aldosterone axis, whereas progesterone is natriuretic, and reports of women with PMS and decreased luteal progesterone have appeared in the literature),[9-12] the overall clinical experience completely speaks against progesterone deficiency as the cause for PMS. Women with florid PMS have been shown to have predominantly adequate luteal phases by basal body temperature graphs, serum progesterone, and endometrial histology and to lack an excess incidence of infertility.[13-18] The more likely role of progesterone and estrogen in PMS lies in drops from the midluteal peaks of these hormones, rather than their absolute levels.[5,19] One may, in fact, argue that higher peak luteal progesterone would give rise to greater premenstrual symptoms due to withdrawal phenomena. O'Brien reported a higher, earlier peak progesterone in PMS patients which gives rise to natriuresis followed by rebound hyperaldosteronism.[20] As discussed later, this may indirectly or directly be the case.

Treatment of PMS with progesterone based on the deficiency theory has been, at best, without benefit in the light of controlled studies. Despite the enthusiastic dispensing of progesterone as a treatment for PMS,[7] the only two controlled studies have demonstrated no difference in relief of symptoms when progesterone is compared with placebo.[21,22] Thus, clinical trials must be considered unreliable and the use of progesterone discouraged. Similarly, use of synthetic progestins has had variable effects.[23-26] Since synthetic compounds may actually lower endogenous progesterone, a pharmacologic effect cannot be ruled out. Certainly, it does not add to the prevailing progesterone level nor does it prevent the withdrawal from progestinlike effects.

Suppression of cyclic sex steroid changes by the use of oral contraceptives has been reported to have beneficial effects on premenstrual symptoms.[19,27-30] This makes sense if a fall from a mid-luteal progesterone–estrogen peak level is an operative factor. The suppression of gonadotropins and the resultant anovulatory cycle result in a more even state of steroid effects and potentially reduced slope of declining hormones during the week off the drug. However, many women without previous significant premenstrual symptoms develop them while on the pill due to the estrogen–progestin pharmacologic side effects.[27] Alternatively their prior PMS may be modified in the number of days they are symptomatic or in differential improvement/aggravation of specific symptoms. While relief of dysmenorrhea is more predictable when a woman takes oral contraceptives, pelvic pain is not uniformly considered to be part of the premenstrual syndrome, since primary dysmenorrhea has been shown to be due to increased effects of menstrual endogenous prostaglandin, and secondary dysmenorrhea is linked to underlying pelvic pathology. The latter is not significantly improved by oral contraceptives. Some believe that relief of menstrual pain is confused with relief of premenstrual symptoms, and this invalidates the PMS effect[31]; others have reported no difference in emotional lability when oral contraceptives were compared to placebos.[31,32] Anecdotally, many previous sequential oral contraceptive users gained improvement in premenstrual symptoms when switched to combination pills, but total dosage may have been as responsible as the absence of cyclicity. Although rejected as therapy by some, more recent studies demonstrate a clearly beneficial effect in selected women with PMS placed on oral contraceptives.[30]

Further suggestion that changes in luteal phase progesterone are important in the perception of premenstrual symptoms is exemplified by anovulatory women, in whom PMS does not tend to develop. This also speaks against the excess estrogen and deficient progesterone hypothesis, although individual cases of euestrogenic anovulation may find their premenstrual symptoms relieved by progestin administration. Others will develop temporary premenstrual symptoms while taking the medication.

These observations, and knowledge of endocrine profiles in women with and without PMS, do not necessarily confound the issue. While a single explanation of symptoms based on ovarian steroid se-cretion is not possible, the individual effects may be quite real and suggest a complex picture involving steroid metabolism, effect on other systems, and receptor number and sensitivity. For example, the divergent effects of estrogen and progesterone on the renin-angiotensin-aldosterone system, may only be relevant when the effects of the latter are considered. While estrogens increase renin substrate and thus angiotensin generation with its pressor and aldosteronogenic properties,[33-37] progesterone is natriuretic by virtue of its aldosterone antagonism[38]; however, a compensatory increase in aldosterone occurs after a few days.[20] In addition, estrogen may have an effect independent of aldosterone,[39] as demonstrated in patients with primary adrenal failure.[40]

In the normal luteal phase, the estrogen effect on renin substrate is not seen,[33] yet plasma-renin activity[41,42] (as measured by generation of angiotensin II) and aldosterone are increased.[41,43,44] This finding suggests that rebound from progesterone antagonism of aldosterone is most important. In anovulatory cycles, the increased plasma renin substrate is not accompanied by elevation of plasma-renin activity or aldosterone.[41] This is likely due to the acyclicity of estrogen levels in these women. Some investigators have noted elevated luteal-phase aldosterone levels or excretion in women with PMS,[45,46] whereas others have not found this difference.[12] In addition, 21-hydroxylation of progesterone to deoxycorticosterone, a potent mineralocorticoid, is increased in the luteal phase, confusing the balance between natriuresis and sodium retention further.[47] The symptom of fluid retention or bloating obviously relates to the above described parameters; treatment directed toward that symptom has largely been salt restriction and the use of diuretics.[48-50] Controlled studies comparing diuretics with placebo have had mixed results,[51,52] although others have noted clear improvement in fluid retention symptoms when these are isolated from other complaints.[53,54] However, generalized fluid retention can theoretically affect other aspects of the PMS, if one considers shifts in electrolytes. One study utilizing spironolactone, an antagonist of aldosterone, found improved specific fluid retention symptoms as well as emotional ones.[55] This finding suggests a beneficial effect of spironolactone on the basis of its fluid and electrolyte effects, but the androgen antagonism attributable to the drug may also play a role.[56]

Other hormones implicated in premenstrual fluid retention are vasopressin and prolactin. Vasopressin, or antidiuretic hormone (ADH), originates in the hypothalamic supraoptic and paraventricular nuclei and is ultimately released in response to several stimuli.[57] The primary role of vasopressin is in the regulation of intravascular osmolarity, so changes in secretion patterns may be expected to result in variable degrees of fluid retention. In addition, vasopressin can be transported to other parts of the brain including the anterior pituitary, so its role in higher-level function and trophic hormone release may be important.[58] Indeed, vasopressin affects memory function in humans (as does oxytocin), and serves as one corticotropin (ACTH) releasing factor.[59] Because the estrogen-sensitive neurophysin is associated with vasopressin,[60] one may hypothesize an estrogen-induced vasopressin increase that could cause fluid retention. However, no evidence exists that vasopressin levels change through the menstrual cycle, nor have levels in women with PMS been measured. The fact that vasopressin acts as a CRF may link vasopressin to release of proopiomelanocortin, the precursor molecule not only for ACTH, but for β-endorphin as well.

The role of prolactin in PMS is a potential two-edged sword. The levels of prolactin in the luteal phase have been reported to exceed those in the follicular phase;[44,61,62] this makes sense in light of studies in monkeys demonstrating synergism between estrogen and progesterone in elevating serum prolactin.[63] However, numerous reports documenting elevated prolactin levels in women with PMS[18,64,65] have been matched by others refuting this claim.[66–68] As expected, treatment directed at reducing prolactin levels in women with PMS has variable success in regard to fluid retention.[18,66–70] Because prolactin has not been conclusively shown to modulate osmoregulation in humans as it does in lower mammals, correlation of prolactin with symptoms of fluid retention should not realistically be expected.

Specific breast symptoms may be associated, however, with either hyperprolactinemia or an exaggerated response of the mammary tissue to prolactin in the premenstrual interval. Although galactorrhea is not a recognized component of PMS, it may accompany mastodynia, and suggest the use of bromocriptine. Studies performed to assess the utility of bromocriptine in PMS have isolated breast symptoms alone as being significantly responsive.[71,72] The greatest argument against prolactin being an important factor in PMS is the absence of typical PMS symptoms in women with hyperprolactinemia[71] who, as a group, will suffer from ovulatory dysfunction to some degree. It seems possible, however, that the addition of galactorrhea (or more specifically galactopoiesis) to steroid-primed luteal-phase breasts will increase the discomfort by increasing the intra-alveolar and intraductal volume.

A link between prolactin and PMS may be more indirect, as reflective of a generalized dopamine aberration. Dopamine, a neurotransmitter which functions as prolactin inhibitory factor, also is involved in the tonic suppression of aldosterone. Dopamine has been shown to be natriuretic with or without increases in renal plasma flow.[73,74] Thus, it seemed to fill a place in the etiology of fluid retention in PMS. Recent double-blind controlled studies have shown that bromocriptine may indeed be useful for more than breast symptoms; it has been studied more thoroughly in idiopathic edema but seems to correct symptoms in PMS unexplained by a placebo effect. When compared with placebo, bromocriptine has been shown to improve breast symptoms, bloating, and depression, with other symptomatic improvement more likely to be placebo effect.[75,76] In another study, in which bromocriptine was compared with norethisterone, bromocriptine improved breast symptoms, irritability, and weight gain in PMS patients, while progestin improved breast symptoms only in relationship to decreased luteal function.[26] No correlation of mood changes and luteal prolactin levels has yet been made. Recognition that vitamin B_6 acts as a coenzyme (pyridoxal phosphate) in the biosynthesis of dopamine as well as serotonin led to renewed enthusiasm in vitamin B_6 therapy, with its roots in the theory that estrogen metabolism is dependent on vitamin B_6.[77] This couples the role of dopamine to fluid metabolism, prolactin control, and an association with affective disorders, making this treatment logical to some practitioners. However, controlled studies involving B_6 therapy have not been in agreement. The early studies suggesting a suppressive effect of B_6 on prolactin and lactation were ultimately disproved, so the impetus for use of vitamin B_6 slowed.[78–82] Nonetheless, Abraham and Hargrove[83] expounded the use of high doses of vitamins and minerals, principally B_6 and magnesium, to counteract the deleterious effects of a poor diet on response to stress in PMS. However, a cyclic vitamin deficiency does not seem plausible to explain the symptoms of PMS.

Along dietary lines, hypoglycemia has been touted as a cause as well as an effect of PMS. An abnormal glucose tolerance has been used to explain premenstrual symptoms involving sugar craving, gastrointestinal complaints, emotional lability, and diaphoresis.[84] Several uncontrolled studies suggested an increased incidence of premenstrual hypoglycemia during glucose tolerance tests, but these women did not experience typical PMS symptoms. The relationship between reactive hypoglycemia and behavioral abnormalities has been noted nonetheless. One explanation resides in a relative decrease in glucose tolerance in the luteal phase due to progesterone, and thus a rebound sensitivity premenstrually when progesterone wanes.[85] The lack of correlation between detection of hypoglycemia and PMS symptoms, or correction of hypoglycemia and relief of PMS symptoms speak against this etiology.

Often mentioned in PMS reviews is progesterone autoimmunity.[6] Largely a dermatologic problem, a wide variation in allergic phenomena in the luteal phase has been noted, with multiple types of suggested therapy, ranging from ovulation suppression to immunosuppression to desensitization. Uncontrolled studies have noted increased cutaneous reactivity to skin testing with progesterone in PMS patients,[86] but the classic spontaneous cases do not convincingly make PMS a part of the allergic reaction.

Besides dopamine, abnormalities of catecholamine metabolism have been implicated in PMS. While adrenergic effects on renal function may cause salt loss or retention either directly or *via* the renin-angiotensin-aldosterone system, studies using blockade have not been performed in women with PMS as they have in those with idiopathic edema.[87] The opposite theory, one of catecholamine deficiency due to increased monoamine oxidase (MAO) in the brain, has been put forth to explain premenstrual depression under the control of progesterone.[88]

Recent reviews on PMS by Reid and Yen[3,6] have proposed a hypothesis of PMS based on the action of endogenous opioids (endorphins). These peptides are distributed throughout the brain as well as in extracranial sites. The modulation of gonadotropin secretion by opioids has been shown to be most prominent in the luteal phase by demonstrating increased pulsatility of LH in naloxone-treated women.[89,90] The pulse generator of GnRH in the hypothalamus is thought to be slowed by endogenous opioids due to high levels of both estrogen and progesterone.[91] In addition, endorphins stimulate prolactin and growth hormone from the anterior pitui-

tary,[92] vasopressin from the posterior pituitary,[93,94] and insulin and glucagon from the pancreas.[95] Exogenous endorphin will suppress LH in both males and females irrespective of steroid milieu.[92] These effects of the endorphins, as well as recognized involvement in pain perception, mood and behavior, make them as suitable a candidate for causing PMS as any other. Fluid retention and glucose abnormalities as well as breast symptoms and emotional swings all can be explained by endorphin action or withdrawal. β-endorphin in primate portal blood has been found highest in the luteal phase and lowest at menstruation, confirming others' findings that progesterone is necessary to achieve these elevations in an ovarian cycle.[96] While increases in endorphin may result in bloating, mastodynia, and hypoglycemia, withdrawal may cause affective changes. In addition, opioids may increase catecholamines and thus aggressive, irritable behavior, while reduction causes depression. Administration of naloxone has been shown to result in PMS-type symptoms in normal volunteers.[97]

Prostaglandins (PGs) may also play a role in PMS, alone or linked to endogenous opioids.[98] While clearly implicated in dysmenorrhea[99] (which is generally thought not to be part of PMS), many PG-associated symptoms such as gastrointestinal changes, salt and water handling, and central nervous system symptoms point to a possible association. Indeed, treatment of dysmenorrhea with PG synthetase inhibitors has been shown to alleviate other PMS conditions.[100] A well-controlled study using mefenamic acid, a prostaglandin blocker, showed relief of multiple PMS symptoms, excluding breast and bloating symptoms.[101]

EVALUATION OF THE PATIENT WITH PMS

The list of psychological and somatic complaints is highly variable, with severity and number differing with the individual. Assessing the existence of a premenstrual syndrome may require careful recording of symptoms on a menstrual calendar or even a basal body temperature chart. If there is no consistent symptom-free interval between menses and at least ovulation, it is not a premenstrual syndrome. Confusion of dysmenorrhea with PMS, especially when pain begins before menstrual flow, may actually be due to pelvic pathology, such as endometriosis. Documentation of physical changes may be necessary, such as weight changes or fluctuation of the fit of clothing. A predominant symptom may cause the patient to seek medical care; management should be focused rather than a ''shotgun'' approach.

It should be evident that there are only theoretical unifying etiologies explaining PMS. The diversity of symptoms and the diversity of probable causes have been emphasized, so selective therapy for the individual is appropriate for the individual patient and her individual problem or problems. The psychiatric and psychological approach to PMS will not be discussed here; to the endocrinologist, recognition of PMS as a pathophysiologic problem, with education, support, reassurance, and understanding, is the most important form of psychological therapy. High degrees of placebo success may be due merely to the sympathetic attention afforded a woman with PMS. The most difficult symptoms, the emotional and behavioral ones, may require psychiatric referral if not linked to treatable physical events or if reaction to somatic complaints is deemed disproportionate. The danger here is the dismissal of all symptoms as psychosomatic: While a psychosomatic element is present in any pathologic state, with a vicious circle of physical and mental ills perpetuating each other, it does not detract from the severity of the underlying endocrinologic disorder. The patient nonetheless should always be given the benefit of the doubt as to the physical source of the symptoms. However, PMS is not an excuse for violence, suicidal or homicidal ideation and behavior, or psychosis. Undoubtedly, hormonal changes may accentuate these psychiatric ones, but the more important problem here is protection of the patient (and others) from herself, and psychiatric referral is mandatory.

An approach to the patient with single or multiple PMS symptoms that are deemed treatable after careful discussion and counseling should begin with isolation of the prominent symptom or complex. Abraham and Lubran[102] divided PMS into four symptom groups which he feels can all be treated by balanced nutrition with vitamin and mineral supplementation. Their four groups are as follows: PMT A, including nervousness and moodiness; PMT B, with fluid retention and breast symptoms; PMT C, characterized by hypoglycemic changes; and PMT D, involving depressive symptoms. Unfortunately, the overlap between groups is great, and this division does not help the individualized therapy plan.

The prominent individual complaints are breast symptoms, hypoglycemic symptoms, fluid reten-

tion, behavioral and emotional changes, and pain, although inclusion of the latter as a PMS element is controversial. In the patient's complete history and physical examination, which may need to be done both premenstrually and postmenstrually, it is necessary to appreciate the changes first hand. Abnormalities found in the patient's history or physical examination should be dealt with appropriately, such as disease states that may be misinterpreted as PMS due to cyclic changes (including the aforementioned psychiatric aspect as well as cardiac, renal, hepatic, and immunologic disease).

Specific findings directly related to PMS, such as an abnormal pelvic examination, may require laparoscopic diagnosis or the finding or report of galactorrhea may require prolactin determination and evaluation of the pituitary. Treatment is very specific and direct toward an obvious cause, if detected.

THERAPY

The needs and desires of the patient are important in deciding on therapy. The woman requiring contraception with no medical contraindication to oral contraceptives could be tried on ovulation suppression; a positive effect should be noted with the first cycle, irrespective of symptom complex. Obviously, relief of dysmenorrhea is most likely to occur, but other cyclic symptoms related to progesterone fluctuation will be improved. O'Brien,[103] in fact, also suggests this as primary therapy. This may be especially true for other nonspecific symptoms, such as gastrointestinal, headache, pain, and sometimes moodiness. Patients who do not respond to ovulation suppression may have aggravation or initiation of certain symptoms, such as breast and fluid retention, if sensitive to the estrogenic component. This can be minimized by using 35 μg or less of estrogen in the compound. The use of progestational compounds alone, especially during the luteal phase, may be useful if progesterone levels are suppressed. Irregular bleeding and progestin side effects are possible.

For the patient with specific symptoms of breast tenderness, occasionally with normoprolactinemic galactorrhea, bromocryptine 2.5 mg once or twice a day is often successful. The orthostatic and gastrointestinal effects of the drug for a few patients may be intolerable, however. Other patients may be relieved of other symptoms, such as generalized fluid retention and emotional lability based on previously mentioned effects of dopamine on these parameters. In order to increase the likelihood of bromocriptine acceptability, a trial of once-daily dosage may be sufficient, taken at bedtime, or dividing the tablet. Obviously, the lowest dosage that will correct the unwanted symptoms is desirable.

Control of fluid retention symptoms may be achieved by the use of spironolactone, an aldosterone antagonist that conserves potassium. Given as 100 mg/day in divided doses to start, the drug may also alleviate breast symptoms as well as emotional effects. The androgen synthesis and receptor blocking effect may also play a role. Patients on spironolactone must be advised against conception while taking the medication, since safety in pregnancy has not been determined. It is a potential teratogen, as it interferes with steroid metabolism. The drug may be useful as well if only taken in the premenstruum.

Hypoglycemic symptoms manifesting as nausea, palpitations, sweet cravings, and sympathetic autonomic excitation are best controlled by maintaining a balanced diet, which prevents wide swings in blood sugar. Decreasing glucose tolerance may be a theoretical side effect of oral contraceptives.

Although the use of prostaglandin synthetase inhibitors, such as ibuprofen, naproxen, and mefenamic acid, is well founded in treating dysmenorrhea, the prostaglandin-related symptoms involving pain (including pelvic discomfort and headache) may be improved premenstrually, as well as menstrual diarrhea, by initiating treatment early. Separation of analgesic from specific antiprostaglandin effects is difficult. Selective decrease in certain prostaglandins is unlikely to be reliable.

More drastic pharmacotherapy includes the use of danazol, 200–800 mg/day, to reduce ovarian steroidogenesis as well as gonadotropin secretion when treating breast symptoms.[104] Unfortunately, danazol has its own side effects at the higher dosages, which include fluid retention, weight gain, acne, and hirsutism due to its androgenic properties and which may be worse than the beneficial effect.[105] Menstrual irregularities may or may not occur, and a pregnancy would be at risk of genital anomalies. Cyclic use of danazol would not be likely to be effective.

Other drugs that can be used to suppress ovarian function include the GnRH agonists[106]; also, antagonists, not available currently for clinical use, may provide an option of therapy in the future.

The remaining substances touted for use in PMS all have limited logical application. However,

rather than dismissing symptoms that may not obviously be due to specific endocrine events, the use of vitamins in conjunction with the aforementioned education and understanding may have some benefit. If pyridoxine (B_6) is indeed deficient in women with PMS, a vitamin with an excess of the recommended daily requirement of B_6 may be helpful. The placebo effect may be operative, but controlled amounts of vitamins are relatively harmless.

On the other hand, the use of progesterone has no rational place in PMS therapy, except as a last, desperate treatment. Although the placebo effect may be just as powerful, some women may respond. However, the cost and side effects of progesterone are often extraordinary, making it highly undesirable. Pharmacologic levels of progesterone may have unexplained central nervous system effects, since dosage up to thousands of milligrams daily have been used. The least treatable aspects of PMS again are the purely emotional ones, and failure of other regimens to improve these symptoms signals the indication for a psychiatric referral, when the use of psychoactive drugs may be prescribed. Waiting for an unproven mode of therapy to act is unfair to patient and physician.

The theory of endogenous opiates being involved in PMS brings up possible therapeutic possibilities. In the swing from endorphin effect to endorphin withdrawal, therapy with an opioid antagonist such as naloxone may prevent the hypothesized central and peripheral effects at mid-luteal phase as well as the "withdrawal" symptoms that occur immediately premenstrually. Clinical trials with the opioid antagonists are ongoing.

IDIOPATHIC EDEMA

Idiopathic or cyclic edema is mentioned here because of its confusion with, as well as similarity to, the fluid retention symptoms of PMS. Idiopathic edema is cyclic in a diurnal sense, not according to a menstrual cycle. The edema is postural, increased by orthostasis, heat, some drugs, and exaggerated by menstrual cyclicity. It is virtually unknown in males in whom cardiac, renal, hepatic, and immunologic etiologies have been ruled out. The subject has been thoroughly reviewed by Streeten,[107] who notes that vascular permeability may be the critical factor. Patients are marked by a decreased response of dopamine and sodium excretion to orthostasis or diuretics,[74,108] and they fail to adjust sodium retention on a high-sodium diet.[109] There is a decreased dopaminergic effect on the renin-angiotensin-aldosterone axis, resulting in higher aldosterone effects. Patients exaggerate the aldosterone effect of orthostasis without increasing renin.[110] The dissociation of plasma-renin activity from aldosterone and plasma 18-hydroxycorticosterone (18-OHB) from aldosterone is exaggerated in patients with idiopathic edema during orthostasis, but bromocriptine normalizes the effect. 18-OHB and corticosterone were suppressed and stimulated, respectively, in both patients and controls by bromocriptine, suggesting that dopamine modulates glomerulosa 18-hydroxylase activity.[111] This points to a decreased tonic suppression of this enzyme in idiopathic edema. The effects of this decreased tonic suppression—orthostatic weight gain and elevated prolactin and aldosterone—are corrected by bromocriptine as well.

This dopamine dysfunction may be linked to the hypothesized generalized dopamine dysfunction in PMS and may give a clue to the use of dopamine agonists in therapy. In addition, vasopressin metabolism has been shown to be abnormal in women with idiopathic edema; they have an impaired water excretion, especially orthostatic, and a failure of a water load to decrease urinary arginine vasopressin in the upright state.[112] Interestingly, 20% of cases of idiopathic edema are nonorthostatic, which may be similar to the fluid retention of PMS.[107]

Besides bromocriptine, found useful in these and other studies,[113] other therapies have included sympathetic amines and spironolactone, but a rebound aldosterone effect may occur after the latter. At least one authority believes that the use of diuretics leads to a rebound edema state that requires perpetuation of therapy. Only after discontinuing all natriuretic drugs do parameters of electrolyte and water metabolism return to normal.[114]

SUMMARY

Premenstrual syndrome has no proven unitary hypothesis. The multiplicity of symptoms is matched by the multiplicity of potential etiologies and further by attempted therapeutic regimens. The high placebo success rate and lack of sufficient controlled trials has confused the issue of treatment of PMS and given rise to highly illogical empiric treatment of varying benefit and risk. The mainstay of therapy is patient education, reassurance and sympathy, and identification of individual or clustered symptoms. Therapy directed toward the cyclicity of

sex steroid hormones or toward the individual symptoms may be highly successful in some patients but frustrating in others. It must be remembered that transference of a patient's underlying psychological need from psychosomatic symptoms to rigidity of treatment does her only apparent good, and a concerted effort to understand the separate fragments of PMS and how they can be approached is necessary to render the patient physically and emotionally healthy. The approach to idiopathic edema suggests ways to investigate further the edema of PMS; the overall syndrome demands research into the pathophysiology in order to develop a sound basis for future therapy.

QUESTIONS

1. Women with the premenstrual syndrome

    a. have low progesterone levels after ovulation.
    b. have decreased LH pulsatility in the luteal phase.
    c. usually have galactorrhea without hyperprolactinemia.
    d. may have emotional swings that respond to anovulatory steroids.
    e. tend to be poorly nourished.

2. Premenstrual syndrome

    a. results from identifiable alterations of specific neurotransmitters.
    b. requires pharmacotherapy or psychotherapy in every case.
    c. may extend past the actual menses.
    d. may be due to insufficient uterine vasculature.
    e. may be manifest as atypical cyclic somatic symptomatology.

3. Medical treatment of premenstrual syndrome

    a. often improves multiple symptoms, although it is aimed at specific ones.
    b. is most successful when edema is not present.
    c. tends to be free of side effects.
    d. should be directed toward improving ovulatory function.
    e. precludes psychiatric referral.

4. Progesterone therapy for premenstrual syndrome

    a. has proved successful in controlled studies.
    b. is supported by consistent findings of luteal dysfunction.

c. is safe and inexpensive, hence a reasonable first line of therapy.

d. may increase psychotic episodes.

e. has a likely placebo effect.

5. Idiopathic edema

a. reflects primary myocardial dysfunction.

b. always follows menstrual cyclicity.

c. seems to be related to decreased dopaminergic tone on aldosterone suppression.

d. is associated with high-renin hypertension.

e. has never been reported in men.

REFERENCES

1. Frank RT: The hormonal causes of premenstrual tension. *Arch Neurol Psychiatry* 26:1053, 1931
2. Dalton K: Cyclical criminal acts in premenstrual syndrome. *Lancet* 2:1070, 1980
3. Reid RL, Yen SSC: The premenstrual syndrome. *Clin Obstet Gynecol* 26:710, 1983*
4. Ruble DN: Premenstrual symptoms; a reinterpretation. *Science* 197:291, 1977
5. Greene R, Dalton K: The premenstrual syndrome. *Br Med J* 1:1007, 1953
6. Reid RL, Yen SSC: Premenstrual syndrome. *Am J Obstet Gynecol* 139:85, 1981*
7. Dalton K: *The Premenstrual Syndrome and Progesterone Therapy.* London, Heinemann, 1977*
8. Morton JH: Premenstrual tension. *Am J Obstet Gynecol* 60:343, 1950
9. Backstrom T, Carstensen H: Estrogen and progesterone in plasma in relation to premenstrual tension. *J Steroid Biochem* 5:257, 1974
10. Backstrom T, Mattsson B: Correlation of symptoms in premenstrual tension to oestrogen and progesterone concentrations in blood plasma. *Neuropsychobiology* 1:80, 1975
11. Munday M: Hormone levels in severe premenstrual tension. *Curr Med Res Opin* 4:16, 1977
12. Munday MR, Brush MG, Taylor RW: Correlations between progesterone, oestradiol and aldosterone levels in the premenstrual syndrome. *Clin Endocr (Oxf)* 14:1, 1981
13. Herzberg B, Coppen A: Changes in psychological symptoms in women taking oral contraceptives. *Br J Psychiatry* 116:161, 1970
14. Greenblatt RB: Syndrome of major menstrual molimina with hypermenorrhea alleviated by testosterone propionate. *JAMA* 115:120, 1940
15. Gray LA: The use of progesterone in nervous tension states. *South Med J* 34:1004, 1941
16. Bickers N, Wood M: Premenstrual tension—Rational treatment. *Tex Rep Biol Med* 9:406, 1951
17. Loraine JA, Bell ET: Ovarian steroids, in *Hormone Assays and their Clinical Application.* Baltimore, Williams & Wilkins, 1971, pp 408–409
18. Andersch B, Hahn L, Wendestam C, et al: Treatment of

*Review article/chapter.

premenstrual tension syndrome with bromocryptine. *Acta Endocrinol* 216(Suppl 88):165, 1978
19. Kutner SJ, Brown WL: Types of oral contraceptives, depression and premenstrual symptoms. *J Nerv Ment Dis* 155:153, 1972
20. O'Brien PMS, Selby C, Symonds EM; Progesterone, fluid and electrolytes in premenstrual syndrome. *Br Med J* 280:1161, 1980
21. Smith SL: Mood and the menstrual cycle, in Sachar B (ed): *Topics in Psychoendocrinology.* New York, Grune & Stratton, 1975, pp 19–58*
22. Sampson GA: Premenstrual syndrome; a double-blind controlled trial of progesterone and placebo. *Br J Psychiatry* 130:265, 1979
23. Parker AS: The premenstrual tension syndrome. *Med Clin North Am* 44:339, 1960*
24. Somerville BW: The role of progesterone in menstrual migraine. *Neurology (NY)* 21:853, 1971
25. Simmons RJ: Premenstrual tension. *Obstet Gynecol* 8:99, 1956
26. Ylostalo P, Kauppila A, Puolakka J, et al: Bromocriptine and norethisterone in the treatment of premenstrual syndrome. *Obstet Gynecol* 59:292, 1982
27. Moos RH: Psychological aspects of oral contraceptives. *Arch Gen Psychiatry* 19:87, 1968
28. Herzberg BN, Johnson AL, Brown S: Depressive symptoms and oral contraceptives. *Br Med J* 4:142, 1970
29. Nilson L, Solvell L: Clinical studies on oral contraceptives—A randomized double blind crossover study of four different preparations. *Acta Obstet Gynecol Scand* 46(Suppl 8):1, 1962
30. Andersch B, Hahn L: Premenstrual complaints. II. Influence of oral contraceptives. *Acta Obstet Gynecol Scand* 60:579, 1981
31. Cullberg J: Mood changes and menstrual symptoms with different estrogen combinations. *Acta Psychiatr Scand (Suppl)* 236:1, 1972
32. Goldzieher JW, Moses LE, Averkin E, et al: Nervousness and depression attributed to oral contraceptives: A double-blind, placebo-controlled study. *Am J Obstet Gynecol* 111:1013, 1971
33. Skinner SL, Lumbers ER, Symonds EM: Alteration by oral contraceptives of normal menstrual changes in plasma renin activity, concentration and substrate. *J Clin Sci* 36:67, 1969
34. Vander AJ, Geelhoed GW: Inhibition of renin secretion by angiotensin II. *Proc Soc Exp Biol Med* 120:399, 1965
35. Katz FH, Kappas A: The effects of estradiol and estriol on plasma levels of cortisol and thyroid hormone-binding globulins and on aldosterone and cortisol secretion rates in man. *J Clin Invest* 46:1768, 1967
36. Layne DS, Meyer CJ, Vaishwaner PS, et al: The secretion and metabolism of cortisol and aldosterone in normal and in steroid-treated women. *J Clin Endocrinol Metab* 22:107, 1962
37. Hodge RL, Lowe RC, Vane JR: The effects of alteration of blood volume on the concentration of circulating angiotensin in anaethetized dogs. *J Physiol (Lond)* 186:613, 1966
38. Landau RL, Lugibihl K: Inhibition of the sodium-retaining influence of aldosterone by progesterone. *J Clin Endocrinol Metab* 18:1237, 1958
39. Johnson JA, Davis JO, Baumber JS, et al: Effects of estrogens and progesterone on electrolyte balances in normal dogs. *Am J Physiol* 219:1691, 1970
40. Thorn GW, Engel IL: The effect of sex hormones on the

renal excretion of electrolytes. *J Exp Med* 68:299, 1938

41. Sundsfjord JA, Aakvaag A: Plasma renin activity, plasma renin substrate and urinary aldosterone excretion in the menstrual cycle in relation to the concentration of progesterone and oestrogens in the plasma. *Acta Endocrinol (Copenh)* 71:519, 1972

42. Brown JJ, Davies DL, Lever AF, et al: Variations in plasma renin during the menstrual cycle. *Br Med J* 2:1114, 1964

43. Oelkers W, Schoneshofer M, Blumel A: Effects of progesterone and four synthetic progestogens on sodium balance and the renin-aldosterone system in man. *J Clin Endocrinol Metab* 39:882, 1974

44. Kaulhausen H, Leyendecker G, Beuker A, et al: The relationship of the renin-angiotensin II and aldosterone excretion during the menstrual cycle. *Acta Endocrinol (Copenh)* 64:152, 1970

45. Perrini A, Piliego N: The increases of aldosterone in the premenstrual syndrome. *Minerva Med* 50:2897, 1959

46. Chiorboli E, Miller dePaiva L: Excretion of aldosterone in premenstrual tension. *Arq Bras Endocrinol Metab* 15:107, 1966

47. Parker CR, Winkel CA, Rush AJ, et al: Plasma concentrations of 11-deoxycorticosterone in women during the menstrual cycle. *Obstet Gynecol* 58:26, 1981

48. Ernest EM: Preliminary clinical report on trichlormethiazide in premenstrual tension. *Curr Ther Res* 3:221, 1961

49. Jungck EC, Barield WE, Greenblatt RB: Chlorothiazide and premenstrual tension. *JAMA* 169:96, 1952

50. Baden WF, Lizcano HR: Evaluation of a new diuretic drug (Quinethazone) in the premenstrual tension syndrome. *J New Drugs* 3:167, 1964

51. Mattson B, van Schoultz B: A comparison between lithium, placebo and a diuretic in premenstrual tension. *Acta Psychiatr Scand (Suppl)* 255:74, 1974

52. Reeves BD, Garvin JE, McElin TW: Premenstrual tension: Symptoms and weight changes related to potassium therapy. *Am J Obstet Gynecol* 109:1036, 1971

53. Coppen AJ, Milne HB, Outram DH, et al: Dytide, norethisterone and placebo in the premenstrual syndrome. *Clin Trial J* 6:33, 1969

54. Werch A, Kane RE: Treatment of premenstrual tension with metolazone: A double-blind evaluation of a new diuretic. *Curr Ther Res* 19:565, 1976

55. O'Brien PMS, Craven D, Selby C, et al: Treatment of premenstrual syndrome by spironolactone. *Br J Obstet Gynaecol* 86:142, 1979

56. Steelman SL, Brooks JB, Morgan EP, et al: Anti-androgenic activity of spironolactone. *Steroids* 14:449, 1969

57. Hays RM: Antidiuretic hormone. *N Engl J Med* 295:659, 1976*

58. Bergland RM, Page RB: Pituitary-brain vascular relations: A new paradigm. *Science* 204:18, 1979

59. Costovsky R, Wajchenberg BI, Nogneira O: Hyperresponsiveness to lysine-vasopressin in Cushing's disease. *Acta Endocrinol (Copenh)* 75:125, 1974

60. Zimmerman EA, Carmel PW, Husain MK, et al: Vasopressin and neurophysin: High concentrations in monkey hypophyseal portal blood. *Science* 182:925, 1973

61. Franchimont P, Dourey C, Legros JJ, et al: Prolactin levels during the menstrual cycle. *Clin Endocrinol (Oxf)* 5:643, 1976

62. Vekeman M, Delvoye P, L'Hermite M, et al: Serum prolactin levels during the menstrual cycle. *J Clin Endocrinol Metab* 44:989, 1977

63. Williams RF, Barber DL, Cowan BD, et al: Hyperprolactinemia in monkeys: Induction by an estrogen–progesterone synergy. *Steroids* 38:321, 1981

64. Halbreich U, Ben-David M, Assael M, et al: Serum-prolactin in women with premenstrual syndrome. *Lancet* 2:654, 1976

65. Cole EN, Everend D, Horrobin DF, et al: Is prolactin a fluid and electrolyte regulating hormone in man? *J Physiol (Lond)* 25:54p, 1975

66. Benedek-Jaszmann LJ, Hearn-Sturtevant MD: Premenstrual tension and functional infertility. *Lancet* 1:1095, 1976

67. Andersch B, Abrahamsson L, Wendestam C, et al: Hormone profile in premenstrual tension: Effects of bromocriptine and diuretics. *Clin Endocrinol (Oxf)* 11:657, 1979

68. Andersen AN, Larsen JF, Steenstrup OR, et al: Effect of bromocriptine on the premenstrual syndrome: A double blind clinical trial. *Br J Obstet Gynaecol* 84:370, 1977

59. Graham JJ, Harding PE, Wise PH, et al: Prolactin suppression in the treatment of premenstrual syndrome, *Med J Aust (Suppl)* 2:18, 1978

70. Ghose K, Coppen A: Bromocryptine and premenstrual syndrome: Controlled study. *Br Med J* 1:147, 1977

71. Andersen AN, Larsen JF: Bromocriptine in the treatment of premenstrual syndrome. *Drugs* 17:383, 1979

72. Mansel RE, Preece PE, Hughes LE: A double blind trial of the prolactin inhibitor bromocriptine in painful benign breast disease. *Br J Surg* 65:724, 1978

73. Fitzsimmons JT, Setler PE: The relative importance of central nervous catecholaminergic and cholinergic mechanisms in drinking in response to angiotensin and other thirst stimuli. *J Physiol (Lond)* 250:613, 1975

74. Kuchel O, Buu NT, Unger T: Dopamine-sodium relationship. Is dopamine a part of the endogenous natriuretic system? *Contrib Nephrol* 13:27, 1978

75. Kullander S, Svanberg L: Bromocriptine treatment of the premenstrual syndrome. *Acta Obstet Gynecol Scand* 58:375, 1979

76. Elsner CW, Buster JE, Schindler RA, et al: Bromocriptine in the treatment of premenstrual tension syndrome. *Obstet Gynecol* 56:723, 1980

77. Rose DP: The interactions between vitamin B_6 and hormones. *Vitam Horm* 36:53, 1978

78. Delitala G, Masala A, Alagna S, et al: Effect of pyridoxine on human hypophyseal trophic hormone release: A possible stimulation of hypothalamic dopaminergic pathway. *J Clin Endocrinol Metab* 42:603, 1976

79. McIntosh EN: Treatment of women with galactorrhea–amenorrhea syndrome with pyridoxine (vitamin B_6). *J Clin Endocrinol Metab* 42:1192, 1976

80. DeWaal JM, Steyn AF, Harms JHK, et al: Failure of pyridoxine to suppress raised serum prolactin levels. *S Afr Med J* 53:293, 1978

81. Husami N, Idriss W, Jewelewicz R, et al: Lack of acute effects of pyridoxine on prolactin secretion and lactation. *Fertil Steril* 30:393, 1978

82. Lehtovirta P, Ranta T, Seppala M: Pyridoxine treatment of galactorrhea-amenorrhea syndromes. *Acta Endocrinol (Copenh)* 87:682, 1978

83. Abraham GE, Hargrove JT: Effect of vitamin B_6 on premenstrual symptomatology in women with premenstrual

tension syndrome; a double blind crossover study. *Infertility* 3:155, 1980

84. Morton JH, Addison H, Addison RG, et al: A clinical study of premenstrual tension. *Am J Obstet Gynecol* 65:1182, 1953

85. DePirro R, Fusco A, Bertoli A, et al: Insulin receptors during the menstrual cycle in normal women. *J Clin Endocrinol Metab* 47:1387, 1978

86. Heckel GP: Endogenous allergy to steroid hormones. *Surg Gynecol Obstet* 92:191, 1951

87. Kuchel O, Cuche JI, Buu NT, et al: Catecholamine excretion in "idiopathic" edema: decreased dopamine excretion. A pathogenic factor. *J Clin Endocrinol Metab* 44:639, 1977

88. Briggs M, Briggs M: Relationship between monoamine oxidase activity and sex hormone concentration in human blood plasma. *J Reprod Fertil* 29:447, 1972

89. Quigley ME, Yen SSC: The role of endogenous opiates on LH secretion during the menstrual cycle. *J Clin Endocrinol Metab* 51:179, 1980

90. Ropert JF, Quigley ME, Yen SSC: Endogenous opiates modulate pulsatile luteinizing hormone release in humans. *J Clin Endocrinol Metab* 52:583, 1981

91. Wardlaw SL, Wehrenberg WB, Ferin M, et al: Effect of sex steroids on β-endorphin in hypophyseal portal blood. *J Clin Endocrinol Metab* 55:877, 1982

92. Reid RL, Hoff JD, Yen SSC, et al: Effects of exogenous β-endorphin on pituitary secretion and its disappearance rate in normal human subjects. *J Clin Endocrinol Metab* 52:1179, 1981

93. Weitzman RE, Fisher DA, Minick S, et al: β-endorphin stimulates secretion of vasopressin in vivo. *Endocrinology* 101:1643, 1977

94. Lightman SI, Forsling ML: Evidence for endogenous opioid control of vasopressin release in man. *J Clin Endocrinol Metab* 50:569, 1980

95. Reid RL, Yen SSC: β-Endorphin stimulates the secretion of insulin and glucagon in humans. *J Clin Endocrinol Metab* 52:592, 1981

96. Wehrenberg WB, Wardlaw SI, Frantz AG, et al: β-endorphin in hypophyseal-portal blood: Variations throughout the menstrual cycle. *Endocrinology* 111:879, 1982

97. Cohen MR, Cohen RM, Pickar D, et al: Behavioral effects after high dose naloxone administration to normal volunteers. *Lancet* 2:1110, 1981

98. Collier HOJ, Roy AC: Morphine-like drugs inhibit the stimulation by E prostaglandins of cyclic AMP formation by rat brain homogenates. *Nature (Lond)* 248:24, 1974

99. Dawood MY: Dysmenorrhea. *Clin Obstet Gynecol* 26:719, 1983*

100. Budoff PW: Zomepirac sodium in the treatment of primary dysmenorrhea syndrome. *N Engl J Med* 307:714, 1982

101. Wood C, Jakubowicz D: The treatment of premenstrual symptoms with mefenamic acid. *Br J Obstet Gynecol* 87:627, 1980

102. Abraham GE, Lubran MM: Serum and red cell magnesium levels in patients with premenstrual tension, *Am J Clin Nutr* 34:2364, 1981

103. O'Brien PM: The premenstrual syndrome: A review of the present status of therapy. *Drugs* 24:140, 1982*

104. Day J: Danazol and the premenstrual syndrome. *Postgrad Med J* 55:87, 1979

105. Barbieri RL, Evans S, Kistner RW: Danazol in the treatment of endometriosis: Analysis of 100 cases with a 4-year follow up. *Fertil Steril* 37:737, 1982*

106. Meldrum DR, Chang RJ, Liu J, et al: "Medical oophorectomy" using a long-acting GnRH agonist—A possible new approach to the treatment of endometriosis. *J Clin Endocrinol Metab* 54:1081, 1982

107. Streeten DH: Idiopathic edema: Pathogenesis, clinical features, and treatment. *Metabolism* 27:353, 1978*

108. Edwards CRW, Besser G, Thorner MD: Bromocryptine-responsive form of idiopathic edema. *Lancet* 2:94, 1979

109. Ferris TF, Chonko AM, Williams JS, et al: Studies of the mechanism of sodium retention in idiopathic edema. *Trans Assoc Am Physicians* 86:310, 1973

110. Norbiato G, Bevilacqua M, Raggi U, et al: Effect of metoclopramide, a dopaminergic inhibitor, on renin and aldosterone in idiopathic edema: Possible therapeutic approach with levodopa and carbidopa. *J Clin Endocrinol Metab* 48:37, 1979

111. Sowers JR, Beck FW, Berg G: Altered dopaminergic modulation of 18-hydroxycorticosterone secretion in idiopathic edema: Therapeutic effects of bromocriptine. *J Clin Endocrinol Metab* 55:749, 1982

112. Thibonnier M, Marchetti J, Corvol P, et al: Abnormal regulation of antidiuretic hormone in idiopathic edema. *Am J Med* 67:67, 1979

113. Sowers J, Catania R, Paris J, et al: Effects of bromocriptine on renin, aldosterone, and prolactin responses to posture and metoclopramide in idiopathic edema: Possible therapeutic approach. *J Clin Endocrinol Metab* 54:510, 1982

114. MacGregor GA, Markandu ND, Roulston JE, et al: Is idiopathic edema idiopathic? *Lancet* 1:397, 1979

ANSWERS

1. d

2. e

3. a

4. e

5. c

23

Hirsutism and Virilism in Women

MARVIN A. KIRSCHNER

INTRODUCTION

Virilization represents a natural sequence of events occurring in boys at the time of puberty. This process follows the surge of endogenous testosterone secretion[1] and gradually transforms the child into an adult male. Virilization in women is an unnatural occurrence, frequently insidious in onset, usually associated with alarm and fear of societal rejection. The minor signs of virilization include coarse (terminal) body hair, acne, terminal facial hair, and menstrual disturbances (oligo- or amenorrhea). The more severe signs in the spectrum of events include clitorimegaly, shoulder muscle hypertrophy, temporal balding, deepening of the voice, and breast atrophy.[2-4] Virilization in women can in most cases be attributed to an overproduction of testosterone.[5,6] Figure 23-1 demonstrates a parallel increase in testosterone production rates with progressive signs of virilization. Fortunately, in most women with signs of virilization, testosterone production is only mildly elevated, and clinical symptoms remain in the "minor" categories.

MARVIN A. KIRSCHNER • Department of Medicine, New Jersey Medical School; and Newark Beth Israel Medical Center, Newark, New Jersey 07112.

HIRSUTISM

Hirsutism represents one of the early (minor) manifestations in the spectrum of virilism; it may be defined as the appearance of excessive coarse hair in facial and body regions, as demonstrated in Figure 23-2. The facial areas commonly involved include mustache, chin, sideburn, and beard areas, whereas the body regions frequently include chest, circumareolar areas, mid-line abdomen (linea alba), and thighs. In classifying the severity of hirsutism, Bardin and Lipsett[5] suggested assigning a plus sign (+) to each of the facial areas of involvement; thus 1–4+ hirsutism may be used. This method does not take into account either the density of terminal hairs in each of these areas or of other regions involved. Ferriman and Gallway[7] suggested that hirsutism be classified according to terminal hair density in many body sites, including facial regions. This method of classification places great emphasis on excessive growth of body hair with less emphasis on facial hair growth, when in fact it is the latter that is generally more disturbing to the patient.

Although the true incidence of hirsutism is unknown, excessive or unwanted hair growth is a common complaint in women seeking endocrinologic consultation.[3] It has been estimated that approximately one-third of women between the ages of 14 and 45 have excessive upper lip hair and

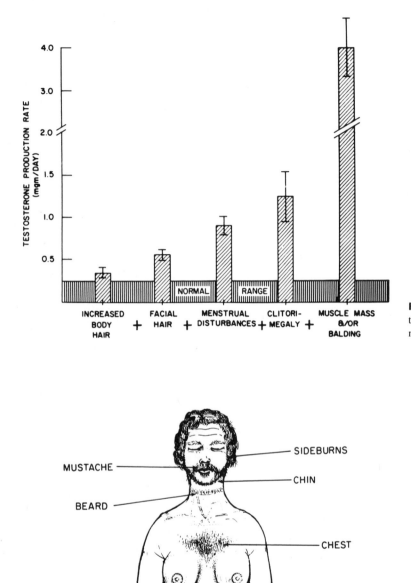

FIGURE 23-1. Testosterone production rates in women with increasing manifestations of virilization.

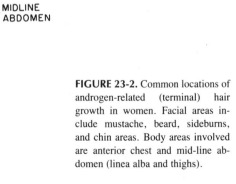

FIGURE 23-2. Common locations of androgen-related (terminal) hair growth in women. Facial areas include mustache, beard, sideburns, and chin areas. Body areas involved are anterior chest and mid-line abdomen (linea alba and thighs).

that 6–9% have unwanted hair on the chin and sides of the face.[3,8,9] Facial hair becomes more prevalent in postmenopausal women, and as many as 75% of women over the age of 60 have excessive facial hair.[10]

Excessive facial and body hair in women represents a dual problem: (1) the actual presence of excessive coarse hair as a clinical abnormality, and even more difficult, (2) the women's reaction to the problem. Women of Mediterranean or Semitic origin frequently accept the presence of dark facial and body hair as part of their genetic background, whereas in women of other ethnic origins, the presence even of small amounts of fine, downy upper lip hair causes alarm. Thus, hirsutism may be perceived as a severe threat by a particular woman, yet other women may be undisturbed by major amounts of hair growth and even other signs of virilism. In either case, appropriate physical evaluation and recommendations for treatment should be provided.

Classification of Hair

Hair may be classified into three basic types.

1. *Lanugo hair* is fine, short hair covering the entire body of the developing fetus. It usually completes its growth cycle before birth. It is lightly pigmented.
2. *Vellus hair* is similar to the fetal lanugo hair but makes its appearance in postnatal life. It is thin in caliber, soft, and generally unpigmented. Excessive accumulation of vellus hair may give a "peach fuzz" appearance, particularly when the hair is localized in the facial region. On rare occasions, vellus hair may grow excessively long, giving rise to hypertrichosis.
3. *Terminal hair* is coarse, dark-pigmented hair that is frequently curved or corkscrew in configuration. This hair type normally populates the pubic and axillary regions of both sexes at puberty and in men gives rise to the beard and general body hair. The presence of terminal hair on the face, chest, and/or abdominal regions (Fig. 23-2) usually causes women to seek medical or cosmetic relief. A given hair follicle can produce either vellus or terminal hair in response to appropriate stimuli, in most cases androgenic stimuli. Furthermore, the distinction between vellus and terminal hair may occasionally be difficult, since the

process of hair follicle stimulation is a gradual one. In view of the association of terminal hair growth with androgenic stimulation, consideration of androgen production and its influence on the hair follicle seems warranted.

ORIGIN OF TESTOSTERONE IN NORMAL WOMEN

In normal women, the daily production rate of testosterone averages 230 ± 30 µg, with little variation throughout the menstrual cycle.[11–13] The origin of testosterone is schematically represented in Figure 23-3. Testosterone is secreted directly by the ovaries[14–18] and adrenals[15,16,19–22] and also arises from the peripheral metabolism of prehormones.[5,15,16,23] On the basis of testosterone concentrations in ovarian and adrenal venous blood samples obtained from endocrinologically normal women, we previously suggested that approximately 25% of the daily testosterone production rate arises from direct adrenal secretion and 25% arises directly from ovarian secretion.[6,15] The remaining 50–60% arises from extragonadal metabolism of prehormones, chiefly androstenedione, and to a lesser extent, dehydroepiandrosterone

ORIGIN OF TESTOSTERONE IN WOMEN

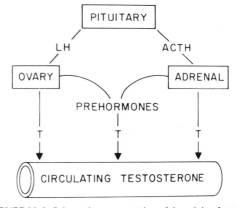

FIGURE 23-3. Schematic representation of the origin of testosterone in women. Testosterone is secreted both by the ovary and the adrenals. These sites also produce prehormones (chiefly androstenedione), which are transformed to testosterone *via* extragonadal metabolism, accounting for approximately 50% of the total daily testosterone production rate.

(DHEA). Androstenedione is similarly secreted by both adrenals and ovaries,[15,16] the latter being related to the phase of menstrual cycle.[11,14] Over the course of the menstrual cycle, approximately one-half the androstenedione arises from the ovaries, and one-half is of adrenal origin. DHEA is largely of adrenal origin, but its contribution to testosterone is minor.[4,24] These prehormones are transformed at several sites, including liver, fat, and skin, and then reenter the circulation as testosterone. Thus, in normal menstruating women, roughly one-half the total blood production rate of testosterone and its contributing prehormones is ovarian, and one-half is of adrenal origin.

ANDROGEN EXCESS IN HIRSUTISM

Although Figure 23-1 demonstrates a close correlation between increased production rates of testosterone and clinical signs of virilism, there is now evidence that most women with hirsutism and/or signs of virilism overproduce a variety of C_{19} androgens,[25] as listed in Table 23-1. In rare cases, virilism may be caused by an ovarian or adrenal tumor that produces a predominant androgen, i.e., testosterone or androstenedione.[26-30] In most hirsute women, however, hyperplasia of ovarian tissue and/or adrenal tissue is responsible for the increased androgens produced. In these cases, a variety of C_{19} compounds are produced in excessive amounts, either by direct secretion from the abnormal adrenals and/or ovaries or *via* extragonadal metabolism from secreted prehormones, as listed in Table 23-1. Evidence for direct secretion of a variety of androgens in hirsute women comes from many ovarian and adrenal venous catheterization studies.[14,17,26,31-34] The role of prehormonal contribution to active androgens has been determined by tracer kinetic studies.[5,16,23] The origin of excessive androgens in women with hirsutism is considered separately; however, it is apparent that the process of hair follicle stimulation and resultant terminal hair growth in women begins with increased production of androgens.

ANDROGEN METABOLISM IN THE SKIN

The skin and its appendages have an active role both in producing androgens from circulating prehormones and in serving as target organs for the action of androgens,[35] as shown in Figure 23-4.

Of the various secreted androgens, testosterone exhibits the greatest biologic activity in most test systems[36] and is capable of binding with androgen receptors at target tissue sites. Since stimulation of the sensitive hair follicle appears to be an androgen-receptor-mediated event, it seems most likely that the stimulus leading to hair follicle growth is excessive production of testosterone, which then binds to androgen receptors in the hair follicle, as shown in Figure 23-4A.

The next and critical step in the process of hair follicle stimulation is activation of the enzyme 5α-reductase, transforming receptor-bound testosterone to dihydrotestosterone (DHT) at the local hair follicle site,[37,38] as shown in Figure 23-4B. There is ample evidence, beginning with the pioneer work of Wilson and Gloyna[39,40] to the studies of Mauvais-Jarvis et al.[41-44] and the fascinating observations made by Imperato-McGinley and colleagues[45,46] that DHT is formed locally at many sites of androgen action and that it mediates androgen action in such tissues as prostate, seminal vesicles, and hair follicles.[37-40,47] Incubation of skin from hirsute women demonstrated active transformation of testosterone to DHT, compared with similar incubations from normal women.[42-44,48] Increased production rates of DHT in hirsute women (Table 23-1) are thus explained as arising almost entirely from precursor (prehormone) metabolism at androgen target organs rather than from increased secretion from the ovaries or adrenals.[49-51] Locally produced DHT is in turn metabolized to androstanediol, which has also been found at the local hair follicle sites. This latter C_{19} steroid is not only a metabolite of DHT but has inherent androgenic properties as well.[36,42,50,52]

The hair follicle that has been activated by testosterone to produce DHT and androstanediol begins to proliferate and grow terminal (thick) hair. The

TABLE 23-1. Androgen Overproduction in Hirsute/Virilized Women

Secreted androgens
    Testosterone
    Androstenedione
    Androstendiol
    Dihydroepiandrosterone sulfate
    Dehydroepiandrosterone
Nonsecreted androgens
    Dihydrotestosterone
    Androstanediol

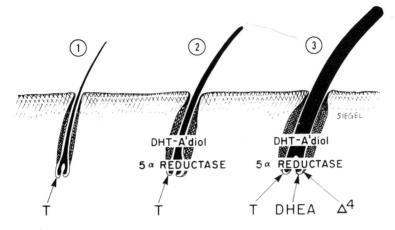

FIGURE 23-4. Proposed sequence of events demonstrating androgen-related hair follicle growth. (A) Increased plasma testosterone binds with androgen receptor at the hair follicle level. (B) Testosterone stimulates 5α-reductase, leading to local production of dihydrotestosterone and androstanediol, which stimulate hair follicle growth. (C) Increased hair follicle stimulation and increased 5α-reductase activity enables lesser prehormones such as DHEA and androstenedione to be metabolized directly to dihydrotestosterone (multiplier effect).

androgen-stimulated hair follicle with its increased 5α-reductase activity secondarily becomes capable of responding to circulating levels of lesser androgens, such as dehydroepiandrosterone (DHEA), dehydroepiandrosterone sulfate (DHEAS), and androstenedione, transforming them directly to DHT and androstanediol locally and leading to further hair follicle growth, as shown in Figure 23-4C. This represents the multiplier effect, as suggested by Mauvais-Jarvis et al.[44]

This sequence of events does not explain the predilection of terminal hair growth for certain anatomic regions of the body (e.g., face, pubic areas). It does, however, relate terminal hair growth to androgen overproduction and explains how the stimulated hair follicle may transform non-testosterone precursors to the potent androgens DHT and androstanediol for continued growth, even if the initiating testosterone source has been removed.

TESTOSTERONE CLEARANCE VERSUS HIRSUTISM

In normal women, the major site of testosterone metabolism (clearance) appears to be the liver.[15] In situations in which there is excessive production of testosterone, it appears that the liver cannot extend its clearance capabilities and is thus unable to meet the needs for increased androgen metabolism.[2,5,15] In these cases, extrahepatic or secondary sites of testosterone metabolism are developed. Although we had assumed that extrahepatic sites of testosterone clearance probably occurred in skin, hair follicles, and other androgen target tissues, the more recent demonstrations that testosterone is further converted to DHT and androstanediol at hair follicle sites makes this guess appear probable.

On the basis of patterns of plasma testosterone levels and metabolic clearance rate (MCR), we have suggested that an orderly sequence of events develops when testosterone production rates are increased, leading to hair follicle growth as a secondary means of testosterone metabolism. As shown in Figure 23-5, increased testosterone production rates (from whatever sources) results in elevated plasma testosterone levels as well as in increased free testosterone, since the sex hormone binding globulin (SHBG) is generally at its maximal capacity in normal women[3,9,13,19] and is thus easily exceeded. The increased free testosterone binds to androgen receptors in dormant hair follicles, resulting in local production of DHT, thus beginning the process of papillary hyperplasia and terminal hair growth. At a somewhat later stage, the stimulated hair follicle becomes capable of transforming sufficient amounts of testosterone to DHT and its metabolite androstanediol. This new secondary site of increased testosterone clearance normalizes the

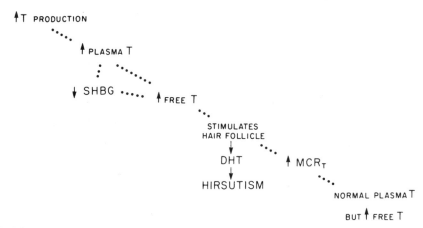

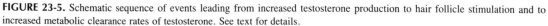

FIGURE 23-5. Schematic sequence of events leading from increased testosterone production to hair follicle stimulation and to increased metabolic clearance rates of testosterone. See text for details.

total plasma testosterone level. Indeed, approximately one-third of hirsute women have normal plasma testosterone levels despite elevated testosterone production rates. In such women, if only plasma testosterone were measured, one might mistakenly conclude that there was no abnormality of testosterone and that hirsutism in such cases might even be due to factors such as heightened skin sensitivity to "normal" circulating androgens.[4,43]

The apparent enigma of increased testosterone production rates associated with normal circulating testosterone levels can be explained by increased MCR probably from participation of skin and hair follicles in testosterone metabolism. Support for the above hypothesis is gained from recent findings of increased plasma androstanediol glucuronide levels in hirsute women. Increased blood levels of this androgen metabolite appear to reflect hair follicle participation in androgen metabolism and reflect increased testosterone production rates, despite apparently normal plasma testosterone levels.

At a still later (or more advanced) stage, testosterone production rate increases further and exceeds the clearance capabilities of both the liver as well as the secondary skin and hair follicle sites. At this advanced stage, there is increased plasma testosterone along with increased MCR. It should be pointed out that all three stages have been observed in hirsute women; however, the transition from one stage to another in a given patient remains theoretical.

To summarize, it appears that in normal women

the liver is the major site of testosterone metabolism. In states of excessive testosterone production, the liver cannot extend its clearance capabilities, and extra testosterone appears in the blood as biologically active androgen. The increased circulating free testosterone induces 5α-reductase in sensitive skin and hair follicles. Thus, the hair follicle becomes a secondary site of androgen metabolism, unfortunately at the expense of hair follicle stimulation and terminal hair growth.

CAUSES OF VIRILIZATION IN WOMEN

The common causes of virilization and hirsutism in women are listed in Table 23-2.

Exogenous Agents

In assessing possible causes of virilization in women, the physician must not overlook the possibility that exogenous androgens or other drugs may be the cause of hair growth.[53] The use of androgen-related anabolic agents, androgens used in the treatment of breast cancer, corticoids, and oral contraceptives must be ruled out as possible causes of hair growth.[53,54] Several drugs that have been associated with excessive hair growth, although not necessarily in the androgen-related areas, are diphenylhydantoin, minoxidil, and diazoxide.[53,55,56] These agents should be discontinued, if possible, if cosmetically disturbing hair growth results.

TABLE 23-2. Causes of Hirsutism and Virilism in Women

Exogenous agents
  Androgens
  Anabolic agents (androgen derivatives)
  Oral contraceptives
  Dilantin
  Minoxidil
  Diazoxide
Endogenous androgen overproduction
  Tumors
    Adrenocortical tumors
    Adenomas
    Carcinomas
    Ovarian tumors
      Arrhenoblastomas
      Hilar cell tumors
      Lipoid cell
      Kruckenberg
  Nontumor states
    Adrenal
      Congenital adrenal hyperplasia
        11-Hydroxylase deficiency
        21-Hydroxylase deficiency
        Late-onset CAH
      Cushing's syndrome
    Ovarian (androgenized ovary syndrome)
    Idiopathic hirsutism[a]
    Polycystic ovary syndrome[a]
    Hyperthecosis[a]

[a]Probably spectrum of common origin.

Endogenous Androgen Overproduction

In the nonpregnant woman, only the ovaries and adrenals are capable of secreting androgens, such as testosterone and its major prehormones, androstenedione, and DHEA. Thus, disease states that affect the adrenals and ovaries are responsible for the virilizing syndromes in women. Other tissues, such as skin, liver, lungs, and adipose cells, are capable of limited steroidal transformations. These tissues can activate adrenal and ovarian prehormones to biologically potent androgens.

Tumors

The major diagnostic concern in evaluating the hirsute or virilized women is to exclude the rare possibility that excessive androgens may be originating from an androgen-producing tumor of either the adrenals or the ovaries.

Adrenocortical Tumors. Virilization is a well-established manifestation of many adrenal neoplasms, both benign and malignant.

Benign adrenal tumors. Most benign adrenal neoplasms are discovered during the workup of the patient for Cushing's syndrome. In such cases, androgen overproduction is part of excessive adrenal secretion of a large number of hormones, chiefly cortisol.[31,57,58] On rare occasions, a benign androgen-secreting adenoma may be found in evaluating a woman for major elevations of androgen production. There have indeed been several reports of androgen-secreting adrenal adenomas responsive to human chorionic gonadotropin (hCG) and suppressed by exogenous estrogens.[27,30,58,59]

In most adrenal tumors, very high levels of other androgens, such as DHEA, DHEAS, and androstenedione are also found in adrenal venous effluents and in the peripheral circulation.[18,31,57,58] Successful removal of benign adenomas may normalize many of the virilizing signs, but subsequent quiescence of the stimulated hair follicle cannot be guaranteed with certainty. The physician is advised not to be overly optimistic in predicting total cessation of hirsutism in such cases.

Adrenal carcinoma. Virilization is fairly common in women with adrenocortical carcinoma and may be disproportionate to the signs of hypercortisolemia. In a study of women with metastatic adrenal carcinoma, testosterone production rates ranged from high normal to values greater than those seen in men. In some of these women, major amounts of the plasma testosterone were derived from androstenedione, and in others testosterone was either secreted or produced from some other plasma steroid precursor.[29,60] Women with virilization due to adrenocortical carcinoma will commonly produce massive amounts of a variety of androgen prehormones reflected by major increases in urinary 17-ketosteroids (17-KS) (30–150 mg/day)[28] as well as by massive increases in plasma DHEAS. Diagnosis of adrenal mass lesions has been greatly aided by abdominal computed tomography (CT) scans.[61] Although adrenal venous catheterizations showing increased androgen levels in one adrenal vein may be a useful diagnostic aid, at other times adrenal catheterization studies may not be very helpful, since adrenal blood flow may become so great that large adrenal androgen gradients may not be appreciated on the side of the tumor (MA Kirschner, unpublished observation).

Ovarian Tumors. Androgen-producing tumors of the ovary have been reported in association with several cell types, including arrhenoblastomas, hilar cell tumors, Kruckenberg tumors, and lipoid cell tumors. These tumors may be quite small and may secrete only testosterone or combinations of testosterone and prehormones. In general, ovarian tumors do not hypersecrete the profusion of prehormones seen in adrenal tumors. Thus, other androgenic parameters, such as urinary 17-ketosteroids and plasma DHEA or DHEAS, may not be elevated. In many reported cases of androgen-producing ovarian tumors, the diagnosis was suspected by finding signs of virilization in association with persistent elevations of plasma testosterone in excess of 200 ng/dl.[17,35,62] Evaluation of women with suspected virilizing ovarian tumors has been aided by ovarian vein catheterization with effluent analysis for testosterone and its immediate prehormones.[17,35,58] At medical centers lacking catheterization capabilities, the suspecting surgeon/gynecologist should be prepared to perform diagnostic laparotomy with ovarian bisection. As some of these tumors are quite small and deep seated, snip biopsy of the ovarian capsule *via* laparoscopy will often miss them and prove nondiagnostic.

As in the case of adrenal tumors, successful removal of the ovarian tumor will likely normalize the androgen abnormalities and lead to reversal of many signs of virilism over time. Nevertheless, the stimulated hair follicle may involute quite slowly; thus the physician is cautioned against being overly optimistic regarding reversal of the hirsutism.

Nontumor States

Adrenal Causes

Congenital adrenal hyperplasia. Children with congenital adrenal hyperplasia secondary to C_{21} hydroxylase or C_{11} hydroxylase deficiency have elevated plasma testosterone levels and corresponding degrees of virilism. Androstenedione and DHEA levels in plasma from these patients are often markedly increased and are generally higher than those of other virilized subjects.[63,64] These prehormones serve as a precursor for 50–90% of the testosterone produced in these syndromes. As a result of markedly elevated prehormone production, urinary 17-KS excretion is usually elevated, as are other chemical parameters of androgen overproduction. The major steroid excesses in these patients are 17-hydroxyprogesterone (17-HP) and 21-deoxycortisol

(in cases of C_{21} hydroxylase deficiency) and 11-deoxycortical or compound S in cases of C_{11} hydroxylase deficiency. The management of children with congenital adrenal hyperplasia has been aided by the use of testosterone measurements. ACTH suppression and corticoid replacement is monitored using testosterone suppression as an important treatment objective.

Adult-onset congenital adrenal hyperplasia. In recent years there have been numerous reports of women with peripubertal onset of hirsutism and menstrual disturbances; in these women excessive levels of 17-HP are found, either in "basal state" or in response to ACTH administration. Such women appear clinically identical to women with idiopathic hirsutism or polycystic ovary syndrome, but the hormonal profile demonstrating microgram amounts of 17-HP per deciliter in plasma suggests a mild form of C_{21} hydroxylase deficiency brought out by adrenarche and associated with mild elevations of testosterone.[65–71,118–124] HLA haplotypes have been similar to those reported in early-onset congenital adrenal hyperplasia (CAH).[66] In such cases, the excess androgens are generally easily suppressed by exogenous glucocorticoids. It has been estimated that 5% of women with idiopathic hirsutism may indeed have adult-onset CAH. A new diagnostic test, proposed by Milewicz and Vecsei, i.e., measurement of plasma 21-deoxycortisol levels, may serve to screen hirsute women for possible late onset C_{21} hydroxylase CAH.[72]

Recently New et al.[73] reported elevated DHEA and other Δ^5 steroids in some women with peripubertal onset of hirsutism. These and other studies[74] led to the suggestion that such women have a mild form of 3β-ol deficiency as the cause of their hirsutism. The frequency of this entity requires confirmation.

Cushing's hyperplasia. Although hirsutism is not a manifestation of cortisol excess *per se,* it is frequently part of the clinical picture of hyperadrenocorticism. Detailed studies of testosterone production in Cushing's hyperplasia have not been reported; however, plasma testosterone and prehormone concentrations are mildly elevated as part of the generalized increase in adrenal hormone production. The diagnosis of this cause of virilism is usually not difficult.

Ovarian Causes

Androgenized ovary syndrome. Most women in whom hirsutism develops in the second to fourth decades of life without other signs of virilism or

Cushing's syndrome can be divided into two large groups on the basis of ovarian histology: (1) those with normal ovaries, and (2) those with polycystic or sclerocystic ovaries. The findings in this latter group of women were described initially by Stein and Leventhal and bear their familiar eponym, Stein–Leventhal syndrome.[75,76] Although the initial description included such clinical features as obesity, hirsutism, amenorrhea, and sterility, there have since been many descriptions of women with enlarged polycystic ovaries in whom none of these clinical criteria is seen.[77-80] Hyperthecosis, a condition associated with the presence of isolated luteinized thecalike cells in the ovarian stroma, has sufficient histologic and hormonal similarity to be included as well in the spectrum of androgenized or polycystic ovary (PCO) syndrome.[79,81,82]

Idiopathic hirsutism. This designation is assigned to hirsute women in whom no specific etiologic diagnosis is apparent and in whom examination reveals normal-size ovaries. In general, women with idiopathic hirsutism have lesser degrees of hyperandrogenism than do those with polycystic ovarian disease or hyperthecosis.[5,31] Laboratory tests to assess virilization such as urinary 17-KS, plasma, or urinary testosterone are often normal in these women, leading some workers to suspect that the underlying abnormality in this condition is end-organ hypersensitivity to normal circulating androgens.[4,43] We have found androgen production rates elevated in 44 consecutive women with idiopathic hirsutism,[31] supporting the hypothesis that virilism is initiated by excessive testosterone production but that secondary adaptations of the hair follicles to metabolize testosterone may obscure these androgen measurements.[24]

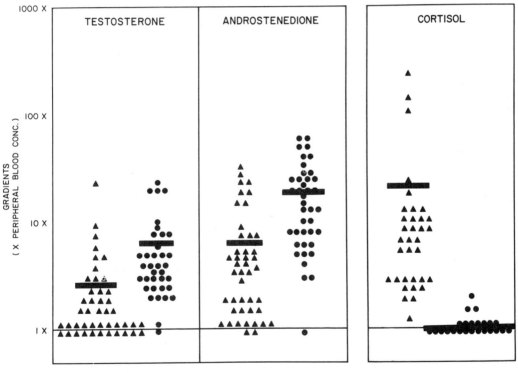

FIGURE 23-6. Gradients of testosterone, androstenedione, and cortisol observed in adrenal and ovarian venous blood of 44 women with idiopathic hirsutism. Approximately one-half the women have no gradient of testosterone in adrenal venous effluents, whereas 42 of 44 women had significant testosterone gradients. The mean gradient for testosterone was higher in ovarian versus adrenal vein effluents. Similar findings are observed for androstenedione. These data suggest that the ovaries are the major contributor to excessive androgens. (From Kirschner et al.[32])

The origin of excessive androgens in hirsute women with no known disease of the adrenals or ovaries has been investigated by direct adrenal and ovarian vein catheterization with effluent sampling for androgens (Fig. 23-6). Higher testosterone and androstenedione gradients were noted in ovarian venous effluents as compared with adrenal vein samplings.[16,32] Combining these venous gradients with kinetic studies of testosterone production and prehormone conversion to testosterone, it was possible to identify the source of excessive androgens to the ovaries in most women with idiopathic hirsutism. On the basis of these data, we believe that idiopathic hirsutism is an ovarian abnormality, probably a mild or early form of the polycystic or androgenized ovarian syndrome.

Polycystic ovarian disease. This abnormality represents a heterogeneous disorder with generally more severe manifestations than noted in women with idiopathic hirsutism.[5,32] There is evidence of an X-linked hereditary transmission in this or these disorders.[3] The size and histologic appearance of the polycystic ovaries are quite varied, ranging from nests of luteinized thecalike cells within the ovarian stroma to include the general phenomenon of hyperthecosis, a thick surface capsule, and numerous atretic follicles.[3] The ovarian stroma is often hyperplastic.

Laboratory tests have demonstrated that women with polycystic ovaries have higher production rates of androgens and higher levels of plasma testosterone and prehormones such as androstenedione and DHEA than do women with idiopathic hirsutism.[5,32] Increased extraglandular production of estrogens (chiefly estrone) results from the excessive androgens (chiefly androstenedione).[83] A fairly uniform finding in patients with PCO syndrome has been elevated plasma luteinizing hormone (LH) and lower-than-expected follicle-stimulation hormone (FSH), resulting in a high LH/FSH ratio.[3,18,65,80–87] Baird et al.,[65] Yen et al.,[86] and Rebar et al.[85] reported that elevated LH levels in this syndrome are largely due to increased amplitude of the pulsatile LH surge, probably related to increased sensitivity of the pituitary to luteinizing hormone releasing factor (LH-RF). By contrast, these workers noted that the decreased FSH levels were associated with absence or reduced pulsatile secretory pattern, little day-to-day variation, and decreased magnitude of FSH response to the releasing hormone.[65,80,83,85,86]

Studies performed by Rebar,[85] Yen,[80,83,86] and Baird [65,84] and their associates have all suggested that the hypothalamic–pituitary system is intact in patients with PCO syndrome. The changes observed merely exhibit (chronically) the heightened LH-RH sensitivity thought to be related to extraglandular production of estrogens. Yen and colleagues[80,83,86] proposed a mechanism to explain the persistent anovulation noted in patients with the

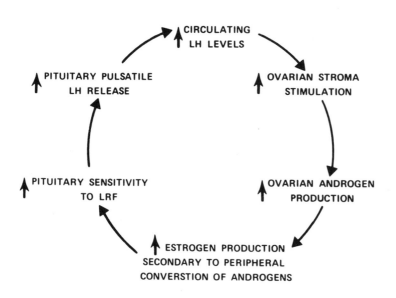

FIGURE 23-7. Proposed mechanism for persistent anovulation and ovarian stimulation in women with polycystic ovary syndrome. Increased LH levels lead to ovarian stromal stimulation and excessive androgen production. Increased androgen production results in hirsutism, follicular atresia within the ovary, and increased estrogens in the peripheral circulation. The increased estrogens increase pituitary sensitivity to LH-RH and perpetuation of the cycle. (From Yen.[80])

PCO syndrome (see Fig. 23-7). Circulating LH levels stimulate ovarian production of androgens. Increased androgens within the developing follicle may lead to atresia and subsequent anovulation. Furthermore, the increased ovarian androgens are secreted into the systemic circulation, where 2–4% are transformed to estrogens. Hyperestrogenemia leads to increased pituitary sensitivity to LH-RH, similar to that noted in the preovulatory phase of the normal menstrual cycle. Although the hypothesis proposed by Yen explains the self-perpetuating nature of the abnormalities of hormones and ovarian androgens noted in PCO syndrome, the pathogenesis of this cycle remains speculative. Certainly the associated findings of obesity, diabetes mellitus, hypertriglyceridemia, and so forth, which are noted in a greater-than-normal frequency in patients with this syndrome, are not readily explained, except possibly as an associated genetic abnormality.

Much interest in recent years has centered on whether the abnormalities observed in women with PCO syndrome represent a different pathologic entity from idiopathic hirsutism or indeed differing stages in a spectrum of a single pathologic process. There are several lines of evidence suggesting that idiopathic hirsutism is but an earlier stage in a single pathologic spectrum better termed "the androgenized ovary syndrome." These data are based on similarities of (1) steroid secretory profiles, (2) dynamic testing of androgen suppression and stimulation, and (3) therapeutic responses (or lack of responses) to various drug regimens.

Stromal hyperthecosis. Ovarian stromal hyperthecosis (thecomatosis, thecosis, or diffuse luteinization of ovarian stroma) is a condition of undetermined origin, characterized clinically by virilization and pathologically by diffuse hyperplasia and luteinization of the ovarian stroma. Plasma testosterone levels have been found to be elevated in this condition, mostly from direct ovarian secretion of testosterone,[26] although Givens et al.[88] described familial ovarian hyperthecosis with either increased androstenedione or testosterone, or both. The patients in this latter study were of interest because they presented a broad clinical spectrum, ranging from mild hirsutism and normal menses to marked virilization and amenorrhea. The likely relationship of this entity with PCO disease has led to the concept that this abnormality represents an end-stage or more severe form of polycystic ovary syndrome.[21,88]

CLINICAL CLUES IN EVALUATING HIRSUTISM

In evaluating a woman with either hirsutism or virilism, or both, the following clinical features may be of diagnostic value:

1. *Onset of hirsutism.* If virilizing signs occurred before puberty, diagnostic considerations include congenital adrenal hyperplasia, childhood Cushing's syndrome, and ovarian tumors. Such cases warrant more extensive diagnostic evaluation.
2. *Rapidity and severity of symptoms.* Hirsutism that is rapidly progressive and associated with menstrual disturbances and clitorimegaly should raise suspicion of a serious underlying process (e.g., tumor).
3. *Testosterone overproduction.* Whether benign or malignant, tumors generally produce large amounts of testosterone and thus are often associated with major signs of virilization and significant elevations of plasma testosterone or other parameters of androgen production. By contrast, ovarian or adrenal hyperplasia generally results in production of smaller amounts of testosterone. These abnormalities are usually associated only with hirsutism or the less severe symptoms.
4. *Menstrual pattern.* If normal cyclic menses persist despite excessive hair growth, androgen production is likely to be only minimally elevated, and the problem is most likely associated with minimally abnormal adrenal function and normal-appearing or polycystic ovaries. Limited screening of androgen values is worthwhile in order to rule out major androgen overproduction and will serve to provide baseline data for subsequent empiric treatment attempts. Most women with lesser degrees of virilism unexplained by definable adrenal or ovarian disease probably have a mild form of the androgenized ovary syndrome, a spectrum of abnormalities that includes idiopathic hirsutism, polycystic ovary disease, and, in its later stages, hyperthecosis.

LABORATORY TESTS FOR VIRILIZATION

Assuming that exogenous agents have been excluded as the cause of virilization, the major diag-

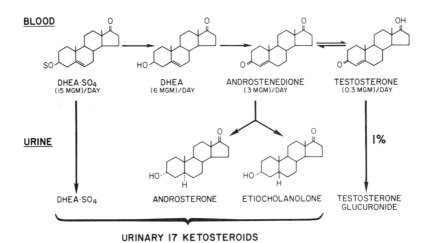

FIGURE 23-8. Origin or urinary 17-ketosteroids in women. The major contributory androgens are dehydroepiandrostenedione (DHEA) and dehydroepiandrostenedione sulfate (DHEAS), which are primarily adrenal secretory products. Testosterone is a minor contributor to urinary 17-ketosteroids in women.

nostic task is to rule out correctable etiologies that could be producing excessive amounts of testosterone, causing hirsutism or virilism in the patient. In this regard, several laboratory tests can serve as useful screens to help decide which patients should be evaluated further, to pursue possible tumor or other diagnoses. The tests are as follows:

1. *Urinary 17-ketosteroids.* This measurement is a bulk estimate of many C_{19} androgen metabolites containing a ketone group at position 17, as shown in Figure 23-8. Since the weak preandrogens DHEAS and DHEA, the major contributors to 17-KS, originate primarily in the adrenal cortex,[4,89] 17-KS excretion is usually a better reflection of adrenal androgen metabolites compared with ovarian androgens. 17-KS excretion is usually normal or slightly elevated in most hirsute women. Significant elevations of more than 30–35 mg/day should alert the clinician to the possibility of excessive androgen production, generally of adrenal origin (i.e., tumor or hyperplasia).

2. *Urinary 17-hydroxycorticoids.* Usually estimated along with the 17-KS, urinary 17-hydroxycorticoid (17-OHCS) can be of help when Cushing's syndrome or congenital adrenal hyperplasia is suspected. A less specific assay such as the 17-KS test may be more useful than the traditional Porter-Silber method, since it will include a wider spectrum of C_{21} steroids (such as might be found in congenital adrenal hyperplasia) in addition to the

traditional cortisol metabolites.[90] In cases in which congenital adrenal hyperplasia is suspected, more sensitive tests include measurement of 17-HP and/or 11-deoxycortisol (compound S) in plasma.

3. *Plasma testosterone.* In approximately 60% of women with hirsutism and virilization, plasma testosterone is elevated,[16,32] a feature that serves as a marker to determine the effectiveness of treatment programs. In the remaining 30–40% of patients, however, plasma testosterone is not elevated, and the clinician *may* overlook androgen overproduction as causative; in such cases, further evaluation should include free testosterone measurement. Plasma testosterone levels that are persistently elevated above 200 ng/dl should alert the clinician to the possibility of major pathology in the adrenals or ovaries; in such cases, further anatomic diagnostic attempts may be required.

4. *Free testosterone.* Since testosterone is transported in plasma bound to a β-globulin, SHBG, it is the unbound or free testosterone that appears to be the biologically active moiety.[91,92] This measurement considers the total testosterone level as well as the fraction that is dialyzable (free fraction)[92,93]:

$$\text{Free testosterone} = \text{total testosterone} \times \text{dialyzable fraction}$$

The measurement of free testosterone correlates extremely well with estimates of testosterone production rate and serves as a better guide of biologically

TABLE 23-3. Comparison of Plasma Testosterone, Dialyzable Fraction as Index of SHBG, and Free Testosterone Concentration in Women

Group	Plasma T (ng/dl)	Dialyzable T (%)	Free T (ng/dl)
Normal women			
Normal weight	38	1.3	0.49
Obese	35	2.4[a]	0.84[a]
Hirsute women			
Normal weight	68[b]	2.3[b]	1.56[b]
Obese	60[c]	2.8[c,d]	1.68[c,d]

[a] 1 vs. 2.
[b] 1 vs. 3.
[c] 2 vs. 4.
[d] 3 vs. 4.

active testosterone than the total testosterone measurement.

Free testosterone measurements may be particularly useful in assessing androgen overproduction in the obese woman.[24,25] Obesity leads to lowered levels of SHBG in both men and women[24,94]; increased testosterone clearance rates result, leading to lower total plasma testosterone levels.[24,51,95] Thus, a hirsute woman who is also obese will have lower plasma testosterone level than that found in her nonobese counterpart and may even exhibit false-normal values. In such cases, free testosterone measurement in the obese woman will be elevated and will assist in determining the degree of hyperandrogenism. Table 23-3 lists mean values for total and free testosterone levels in normal, obese, and hirsute women, demonstrating the usefulness of the free testosterone measurement.

5. *Plasma androstenedione.* Although this major precursor of testosterone usually is mildly elevated in most women with hirsutism and virilism, a two- to threefold elevation of androstenedione, in the range of 500 ng/dl or higher, may indicate serious underlying pathology.

6. *LH and FSH.* Women with PCO disease often have increased LH and lowered FSH levels. Thus, the finding of increased LH and an increased LH/FSH ratio may provide diagnostic insights.

7. *Serum prolactin.* In 20–30% of women with the clinical picture of PCO syndrome, serum prolactin levels have been found to be mildly elevated.[96] A relationship of plasma prolactin elevation with adrenal androgen production has been suggested by several studies, but the mechanism of prolactin stimulation of the adrenal is unclear. It is uncertain whether women with PCO syndrome and mild elevations of serum prolactin have early pituitary microadenomata or whether this association is a coincidental one.[96a] Measurement of prolactin is suggested in hirsute women as a screen for major elevations suggestive of a pituitary tumor. The potential use of dopamine suppressors in women with PCO syndrome, whether associated with increased prolactin or with normal prolactin levels, is currently being explored (J Vaitukaitis, personal communication, 1984).

8. *Androstanediol glucuronide.* This obscure androgen metabolite holds great promise as the most sensitive marker of androgen stimulation of the hair follicle.[95,97,98] Androgen-induced stimulation of the hair follicle leads to local dihydrotestosterone (DHT) production. Androstanediol and androstanediol glucuronide (3α-diol G) represent metabolites of this process.[97] Of great interest have been the studies reported by Horton et al.[97] and confirmed by our laboratory[95] that 3α-diol G levels are 10–12-fold elevated in women with hirsutism (Fig. 23-9). Values of 200–400 μg/dl in hirsute women make this a potentially easily measured metabolite to serve as a marker of hirsutism and a potential guide to effective therapy. In PCO patients without hirsutism, A–diol G levels have been reported to be normal. Similarly, in obese nonhirsute women, a variety of androgen production rates have been found elevated but A–diol G abnormalities are also minimal. Thus, A–diol G appears to be an excellent chemical marker of the stimulated hair follicle.

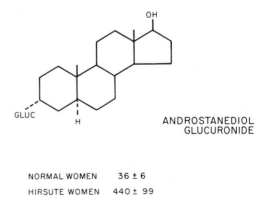

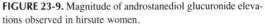

| NORMAL WOMEN | 36 ± 6 |
| HIRSUTE WOMEN | 440 ± 99 |

FIGURE 23-9. Magnitude of androstanediol glucuronide elevations observed in hirsute women.

In the clinical evaluation of the virilized woman, the above laboratory measurements can help decide whether a significant virilizing process exists or whether the problem is one of limited androgen overproduction to be treated by empiric means. If potentially serious underlying pathology is suspected from the androgen screening tests, confirmation of abnormal values is probably warranted, but further endocrine suppression or stimulation tests are only of limited use and entail many diagnostic pitfalls of false-positive and/or false-negative results.[59,81,99-102] At this point, anatomic investigation seems entirely in order. Adrenal and ovarian vein catheterization tests, abdominal CT scans, and ultrasound may be of help in localizing suspected tumors. Tedious and technically difficult venographic procedures should probably be performed only at centers at which expertise in this area exists. Laparoscopy and snip biopsy of the ovary are widely used in confirming the presence of PCO disease; however, this approach may miss a deep-seated interstitial tumor and is less useful than laparotomy with ovarian bisection in locating the small but potent androgen-secreting tumor.

TREATMENT

Treatment of excessive coarse (terminal) hair growth in facial regions, chest, breast, or other areas of the body is generally a difficult therapeutic task. Treatment schemes include (1) suppression of hyperandrogenism or use of antiandrogens in the hope of preventing new hair growth; (2) removal of existing unwanted hair (in most cases a combination of both approaches is necessary, with neither method, if used alone, being entirely effective; and (3) treatment of coexisting obesity, if this is an associated problem.

Suppression of Hyperandrogenism

Oral Contraceptives

These agents appear to have three actions useful in the treatment of hirsutism. Oral contraceptives act to suppress hyperandrogenism in women with idiopathic hirsutism or PCO syndrome, probably *via* suppression of pituitary LH secretion. These agents likely also serve as direct antiandrogens at the level of the hair follicle. Finally, the estrogens serve to elevate SHBG levels, increasing the fraction of circulating testosterone that is bound, and thus biologically inactive.[97,103-105] Givens et

al.[104] suggested use of Ortho-Novum 2 mg for 21-day cycles beginning on day 5 after the onset of menses. This regimen usually results in regularization of menstrual flow and promotes anovulatory cycles for those women desiring contraception. Measurement of basal plasma testosterone (or better still, free testosterone) and again, after approximately one to two cycles of therapy, will help confirm that hyperandrogenic parameters are suppressed by the therapy. Should these changes be noted during the first one or two cycles on oral contraceptives, the clinician can be encouraged to proceed for the lengthy time (12 months or more) generally needed to see clinical improvement. The patient may first observe no new areas of facial or body hair growth, followed by softening or thinning of the existing terminal hairs, and finally less frequent need to remove unwanted hair. This sequence of events will occur in approximately 50% of women treated; however, only one-third of women treated with oral contraceptives will eventually achieve sufficient improvement to enable them to discontinue their depilatory efforts.

Although androgen suppression by oral contraceptives or other means may occur within days,[97,102] the major effects of androgen suppression on terminal hair growth occurs slowly, and the patient should be told in advance not to expect significant results for approximately 9-12 months. Cyclic therapy may be carried for a 12-15-month period, followed by a 3-month rest period.

Oral contraceptives should not be offered as therapy for patients who have a family history of breast cancer or previous history of breast nodules, who are over 40 years of age, or who have major doubts or fears regarding their use. Patients for whom oral contraceptives are prescribed should be followed up periodically to be certain that oral contraceptives are not resulting in hypertension, diabetes mellitus, or other untoward effects.

Occasionally patients will claim that the 2-mg dosage of Ortho-Novum is "too strong," causing nausea or vomiting, or both. In these circumstances, it may be desirable to use a less potent agent such as Ovulin-21.

Glucocorticoids

Exogenous glucocorticoids may be useful in suppressing hyperandrogenism, particularly in the rare cases of late-onset CAH or in milder cases of PCO disease or idiopathic hirsutism. If a test regimen of dexamethasone given in a dose of 2-4 mg/day for

3–4 days results in either suppression of testosterone or free testosterone parameters into the "normal" range, this regimen may be tried on a long-term basis. Prednisone given in a dosage of 5–7.5 mg (at bedtime) to suppress endogenous nocturnal adrenal secretion has been widely recommended.[8,12,87,106,107] This dosage schedule rarely produces any of the undesirable side effects of high doses of steroids. In our clinical experience, glucocorticoid therapy often results in normalization of menses and improvement of androgen-related acne but in diminished hair growth in only approximately 25% of hirsute women.

In some cases, glucocorticoids may be coupled with oral contraceptives into a combined regimen, as suggested by Casey et al.[103]

Antiandrogens

Spironolactone This agent has been demonstrated to inhibit androgen action, probably at the peripheral (receptor) level.[108–110] Used in a dose of 50–200 mg/day, spironolactone has been reported to produce amelioration in 20–30% of women with excessive body or facial hair growth.

Cimetidine. The histamine blocker has been reported to reduce hair growth by acting as an inhibitor of androgen receptor activity. Cimetidine, in a dosage of 300 mg qid may produce a beneficial effect if given for a period of months.[111] There is no widespread experience with this agent for treatment of hirsutism.

Cyproterone Acetate. This antiandrogen has been used extensively in European clinics with favorable results in 60–90% of women, far better than those achieved by any of the above regimens.[111–113] Cyproterone has been used in dosages from 2.5 to 100 mg/day along with estrogens in a reverse sequential regimen. Unfortunately, this drug is not yet approved for use in the United States, pending further clinical trials.

Removal of Existing Hair

Most hirsute women have already explored various methods of treating unwanted hair by the time they seek medical advice. Nevertheless, it is useful to review these methods with the patient so that proper guidance can be offered and misconceptions or superstitions as to these various methods can be openly discussed at a professional level.

Bleaching

In some cases, excessive hair growth in the mustache and sideburn areas can be controlled cosmetically by bleaching.[114] Commercial preparations using a 6% hydrogen peroxide solution, along with ammonia and a few soap chips to form a simple paste, can be applied by dabbing with a swabstick for a period of 15–30 min, depending on skin tolerance. In women with sensitive skin, shorter exposure times are advised. This procedure can be repeated on a daily basis, provided that no extensive skin irritation is caused by the depilatory mixture. Should skin sensitivity develop, shorter exposure times or a weaker concentration of ammonia can also be tried. In patients with very sensitive skin, a mild steroid cream may also be used under physician guidance. Bleaching preparations using potassium persulfate are best avoided in view of the potential anaphylactoid reactions that have been reported.[105]

Tweezing

This seems to be the most commonly used and cosmetically acceptable method for removal of individual long terminal hairs on the chin, chest, and even breast area. Whereas infrequent tweezing is generally without risk, folliculitis may develop at the exposed pore. The patient should be advised to prepare the skin with a mild antiseptic in an attempt to prevent secondary folliculitis.

Hot Wax Epilation

This method represents a form of mass plucking. Carefully performed, hot wax epilation can be acceptable to some women; however, ingrown hairs can develop, as can acute and chronic folliculitis, which in turn may lead to chronic scarring. If inspection of such depilitated regions reveals evidence of multiple ingrown hairs or skin pitting, alternate methods of depilation should be recommended.

Chemical Depilatories

Chemical keratolytic agents have been available at cosmetic counters in the form of cream applications. Whereas such agents (e.g., Nair or Neet) are used widely for hair removal in body regions they are generally less successful in facial hair areas. The use of chemical depilatories is often time consuming and is associated with skin irritation in the more sensitive regions. In these regions, such keratolytic agents should be used only if they do not cause undue local skin irritation. Again, a low-potency topical corticosteroid may be required after each application to relieve undue skin irritation.

Shaving

Shaving is the safest of the mechanical methods of hair removal, since hairs are clipped at the skin with little or no damage to the hair follicle apparatus and little abrasion of the skin surface. Although this method has gained wide acceptance in removal of the leg and underarm hair, many women are fearful of shaving regions of the face. It is commonly believed that shaving of hair results in stimulation of the hair follicle and more rapid regrowth. Shaving does not accelerate the rate of hair regrowth, although the early "stubble" during the initial days after shaving appears thicker and unacceptable to many women. Women need to be reassured that shaving does not promote rapid hair regrowth and that shaving in combination with antiandrogen drug therapy may lessen the need for depilatation time.

Electrolysis

By far the most satisfactory method of permanent hair removal is electrolysis.[114,115] After careful antiseptic preparation of the skin, a thin electrified needle is inserted along the hair shaft to a point below the skin, presumably to the level of the hair follicle. An electric current of predetermined voltage is introduced, coagulating the hair root. Older methods using galvanic currents are time consuming and have largely been replaced by short-wave radiofrequency thermolysis units that generate local temperatures of 170–200°F and produce electrocoagulation of the hair root. When properly performed in the hands of a qualified electrologist, the procedure is safe and relatively painless. The treated hair is easily removed with no resistance or discomfort. The technique of electrolytic removal of the hair follicle at the root is largely an empiric one. The electrologist arrives at a decision to use a particular amplitude and duration of electrical current on the basis of such factors as skin sensitivity and thickness of the hair follicle to be electrocoagulated. After electrolysis, a temporary blanching of the hair follicle is generally followed by a mild erythemia lasting 15–20 min. Under optimal conditions, electrolysis is an effective procedure for hair

removal and probably the most effective method currently available. However, the field of electrolysis is largely an unlicensed and medically unsupervised activity in most states, and technical skills of electrologists vary greatly. Referral to a skilled electrologist (if available in your area) is frequently the most important advice that the physician can provide. In the absence of such direct information, an electrolysist who is licensed or who carries "degrees" by self-policing organizations should be sought.

In recent years, several products have been marketed that use the principle of an electrified tweezer. These have been widely advertised for home use. This approach seems unsound, since the hair shaft is a poor electrical conductor with little chance of transferring sufficient current to the hair roots for electrocoagulation. The use of such a do-it-yourself apparatus should be discouraged, since their effectiveness is probably that of simple plucking.

Treatment of Obesity

Although obesity may not be part of the patient's complaint, it is seen in 50–60% of women who present for evaluation and therapy of PCO syndrome.[77] Successful management of obesity in such women may have a beneficial effect on menstrual irregularities, on infertility, and on hirsutism. Certainly, PCO patients with morbid obesity (i.e., 50 or more lb above ideal body weight) can be expected to have more complications from a pregnancy, and it is likely that pharmacologic management of the hirsutism is made more difficult by coexisting obesity. Thus, in devising a treatment regimen for the woman with PCO syndrome, management of the obesity component becomes as important in the overall plan as treatment of any of the other complaints.

In women with lesser degrees of obesity (i.e., 40 lb or less), a program of calorie restriction can be offered. A well-balanced 1000-calorie diet offered by self-help groups such as Weight Watchers and Lean Line can be an effective method of weight control. Such approaches generally offer the possibility of 8–10 lb of weight loss per month for the not-too-obese woman.

In women whose hirsutism is complicated by major obesity, simple calorie-restriction methods are not very effective for normalization of body weight, since they take too long to accomplish their goals and have an unacceptable dropout rate. We have found a protein-sparing modified fast[116] an effective method of achieving major weight reduction.[2,117] Patients undergoing major weight loss are advised to defer any desires to become pregnant during the period of weight loss. Management of the hirsutism by means of pharmacologic agents or the use of local hair-removal agents, or both, can be started along with the weight-reduction program.

It is apparent that in the obese woman with hirsutism and/or PCO syndrome, major weight loss by itself will go a long way to improve self-image.

SUMMARY

Hirsutism or coarse thick (terminal) hair growth in facial and body regions is one of the signs of virilization and is caused by excessive production of either testosterone or other androgens, or both. The most common etiology of hirsutism in women is the nontumorous state, chiefly ovarian in origin. The androgenized ovary syndrome represents a spectrum of abnormalities ranging from idiopathic hirsutism to polycystic ovary syndrome to ovarian hyperthecosis. Of the various laboratory tests to evaluate hirsutism, simple measurements of plasma testosterone, free testosterone, and most recently androstanediol glucuronide seem to provide the best chemical evidence of androgen abnormalities. Treatment of hirsutism/virilism in women is difficult and is frequently unsatisfactory. Treatment schemes include suppression of androgens *via* glucocorticoids, oral contraceptives, and antiandrogens, as well as the use of local depilatory methods.

QUESTIONS

1. The spectrum known as virilization does *not* include
   a. anovulation.
   b. temporal balding.
   c. breast atrophy.
   d. abnormal patterns of sexual behavior.
   e. linea alba hair growth.

2. All the following hormonal changes have been observed in women with polycystic ovary syndrome except
   a. elevated prolactin.
   b. increased LH, decreased FSH.
   c. increased FSH, decreased LH.

   d. increased estrone production.
   e. increased androstenedione production.

3. It is most accurate to state that approximately one-third of hirsute women have
   a. elevated testosterone production rates.
   b. normal plasma testosterone levels, yet all have increased testosterone production rates.
   c. have normal plasma testosterone levels because of increased peripheral metabolism to estrogens.
   d. increased plasma testosterone levels because of elevated SHBG levels.
   e. no abnormalities of androgen production or plasma levels.

4. All the following treatment schemes have been reported with variable success in the treatment of hirsutism, except
   a. use of minoxidil.
   b. use of Ortho-Novum.
   c. use of Spironolactone.
   d. glucocorticoids + oral contraceptives.
   e. progestin only.

REFERENCES

1. Faiman C, Winter JSD: Gonadotropins and sex hormone patterns in puberty, clinical data, in Grumbach MM, Grave GD, Mayer FE (eds): *The Control of the Onset of Puberty*. New York, Dunn Witey & Sons, 1974, pp 32–61
2. Bardin CW, Kirschner MA: The clinical usefulness of testosterone measurements in virilizing syndromes, in Sunderman FW, Sundermann FW Jr, Green WH (eds): *Laboratory diagnosis of endocrine diseases*. St Louis, Mosby, 1971, pp 559–572
3. Givens JC: Hirsutism and hyperandrogenism. *Adv Intern Med* 21:221–247, 1976
4. Lipsett MB: Hirsutism, in DeGroot LJ, Cahill GF, Odell WD, et al (eds): *Endocrinology*, Vol. 3. New York, Grune & Stratton, 1979, pp 1451–1456
5. Bardin CW, Lipsett MB: Testosterone and androstenedione blood production rates in normal women with idiopathic hirsutism or polycystic ovaries. *J Clin Invest* 46:891–902, 1967
6. Kirschner MA: Virilism in women, in Gold JJ, Josimovich JB (eds): *Gynecologic Endocrinology*. Hagerstown, MD, Harper & Row, 1980, pp 594–609
7. Ferriman D, Gallway JD: Clinical assessment of body hair growth in women. *J Clin Endocrinol Metab* 21:1440–1447, 1961
8. Abraham GE, Maroulis GB, Buster JE, et al: Effect of dexamethasone on serum cortisol and androgen levels in hirsute patients. *Obstet Gynecol* 47:394–402, 1976
9. Vermeulen A, Verdonck L, Vander Straeten M, et al: Capacity of the testosterone-binding globulin in human plasma and influence of specific bindings of testosterone on

its metabolic clearance rate. *J Clin Endocrinol Metab* 29:1470–1480, 1969

10. Melick R, Taft HP: Observations on body hair in old people. *J Clin Endocrinol Metab* 19:1597–1599, 1959

11. Abraham GE: Ovarian and adrenal contribution to peripheral androgens during the menstrual cycle. *J Clin Endocrinol Metab* 39:340–346, 1974

12. Abraham GE: Evaluation and treatment of the hyperandrogenized woman, in Scholler R (ed): *Endocrinology of the Ovary*. Paris, Sepe, 1978, pp 395–422

13. Anderson DC: The role of sex hormone binding globulin in health and disease, in James VHT, Serio M, Giusti G (eds): *The Endocrine Function of the Human Ovary*. London, Academic, 1976, pp 141–158

14. Baird DT: Ovarian steroid secretion and metabolism in women, in James VHT, Serio M, Giusti G (eds): *The Endocrine Function of the Ovary*. New York, Academic, 1976, pp 125–133

15. Kirschner MA, Bardin CW: Androgen production and metabolism in normal and virilized women. *Metabolism* 21:667–687, 1972

16. Kirschner MA, Jacobs JB: Combined ovarian and adrenal vein catheterization to determine the site(s) of androgen overproduction in hirsute women. *J Clin Endocrinol Metab* 33:199–209, 1971

17. Moltz L, Schwartz U, Hammerstein J: Ovarian vein catheterizations in patients with virilizing ovarian neoplasma. *J Clin Endocrinol Metab* 1986 (in press)

18. Rivarola MA, Saez JM, Jones HW, et al: The secretion of androgens by the normal, polycystic and neoplastic ovaries. *Bull Johns Hopkins Hosp* 121:82–88, 1967

19. Baird DT, Uno A, Melby J: Adrenal secretion of androgens and oestrogens. *J Endocrinol* 45:135–136, 1969

20. Burger HG, Kent JR, Kellie AE: Determination of testosterone in human peripheral and adrenal venous blood. *J Clin Endocrinol Metab* 24:432–441, 1964

21. Gandy HM, Peterson RE: Measurement of testosterone and 17-ketosteroids in plasma by the double isotope dilution derivative technique. *J Clin Endocrinol Metab* 28:949–977, 1968

22. Wieland RB, DeCourey C, Levy RP, et al: $C_{19}O_2$ steroids and some of their precursors in blood from normal human adrenals. *J Clin Invest* 44:159–168, 1965

23. Horton R, Tait JF: Androstenedione production and interconversion rates measured in peripheral blood and studies on the possible site of its conversion to testosterone. *J Clin Invest* 45:301–312, 1966

24. Kirschner MA, Samojlik E, Silber D: A comparison of androgen production and clearance in hirsute and obese women. *J Steroid Biochem* 19:607–614, 1983

25. Kirschner MA, Samojlik E, Silber D: Obesity distorts androgen assessment in hirsute women. *Proceedings of Sixth International Congress on Hormonal Steroids, Jerusalem*, 1982

26. Bardin CW, Lipsett MB, Edgcomb JH, et al: Studies of testosterone metabolism in a patient with masculinization due to stromal hyperthecosis. *N Engl J Med* 277:399–402, 1967

27. Givens JR, Andersen RN, Wiser WL, et al: A gonadotropin responsive adrenocortical adenoma. *J Clin Endocrinol Metab* 38:126–133, 1974

28. Lipsett MB, Hertz R, Ross GT: Clinical and pathophysiologic aspects of adrenocortical carcinoma. *Amer J Medicine* 35:374–383, 1963

29. Saez JM, Loras B, Morera AM, et al: Studies of androgens and their precursors in adrenocortical virilizing carcinoma. *J Clin Endocrinol Metab* 32:462–469, 1971

30. Werk E, Sholiton LJ, Kalejs L: Testosterone secreting adrenal adenoma under gonadotropin control. *N Engl J Med* 289:767–769, 1973

31. Kirschner MA, Zucker IR, Jespersen DL: Ovarian and adrenal vein catheterization studies in women with idiopathic hirsutism, in James VHT, Serio M, Giusti G (eds): *Endocrine Function of the Human Ovary*. London, Academic, 1975, pp 443–456

32. Kirschner MA, Zucker IR, Jespersen D: Idiopathic hirsutism—An ovarian abnormality. *N Engl J Med* 294:637–640, 1976

33. Milewicz A, Silber D, Mielecki T: The origin of androgen synthesis in polycystic ovary syndrome. *Obstet Gynecol* 62:601–604, 1983

34. Serio M, Dell'Acqua S, Calabresi E, et al: Androgen secretion by the human ovary; measurement of androgens in ovarian venous blood, in James VHT, Serio M, Giusti G (eds): *The Endocrine Function of the Ovary*. London, Academic, 1976, pp 471–479

35. Meldrum DR, Abraham GE: Peripheral and ovarian venous concentrations of various steroid hormones in virilizing ovarian tumors. *Obstet Gynecol* 53:36–43, 1979

36. Hilgar AG, Hummel DJ: Androgenic and myogenic endocrine bioassay data, In: US Dept. of Health, Education and Welfare, Publication 1:1964

37. Takayasu, S, Adachi K: The conversion of testosterone to 17β-hydroxy-5α-androstane-3-one (dihydrotestosterone) by human hair follicles. *J Clin Endocrinol Metab* 34:1098–1101, 1972

38. Voigt W, Fernandez EG, Hsia SL: Transformation of testosterone into 17β-hydroxy-5α-androstan-3-one by microsomal preparations of human skin. *J Biol Chem* 245:5594–5599, 1970

39. Bruchovsky N, Wilson JD: The conversion of testosterone to 5α-androstan-17β-ol-3-one by rat prostate in vitro. *J Biol Chem* 243:2012–2021, 1968

40. Wilson JD, Gloyna RE: The intranuclear metabolism of testosterone in the accessory organs of reproduction. *Recent Prog Horm Res* 26:309–336, 1970

41. Mauvais-Jarvis P, Bercovici JP, Crepy O, et al: Studies on testosterone metabolism in subjects with testicular feminization syndrome. *J Clin Invest* 49:31–40, 1970

42. Mauvais-Jarvis P, Charransol G, Bobas-Masson F: Simultaneous determination of urinary androstanediol and testosterone as an evaluation of human androgenicity. *J Clin Endocrinol Metab* 36:452–459, 1973

43. Mauvais-Jarvis P, Kuttenn F: Idiopathic hirsutism: The respective roles of the hypersecretion of androgens and of their metabolism in the skin, in Scholler P (ed): *Endocrinology of the Ovary*. Paris, Sepe, 1978, pp 423–438

44. Mauvais-Jarvis P, Kuttenn F, Gauthier-Wright F: Testosterone 5α-reduction in human skin as an index of androgenicity, in James VHT, Serio M, Giusti G (eds): *The Endocrine Function of the Human Ovary*. London, Academic, 1976, pp 481–494

45. Imperato-McGinley J, Guerrero L, Gautier T, et al: Steroid 5α-reductase deficiency in man: An inherited form of male pseudohermaphroditism. *Science* 186:1213–1215, 1974

46. Peterson RE, Imperato-McGinley J, Gautier T, et al: Male pseudohermaphroditism due to steroid 5α-reductase deficiency. *Am J Med* 62:170–191, 1977

47. Bardin CW, Bullock LP, Sherins RJ, et al: Androgen metabolism and mechanism of action in male pseudoher-

maphroditism: A study of testicular feminization. *Recent Prog Horm Res* 29:65–109, 1973

48. Thomas PK, Ferriman DG: Variations in facial and pubic hair growth in white women. *Am J Phys Anthropol* 15:171, 1975

49. Ito T, Horton R: The source of plasma dihydrotestosterone in man. *J Clin Invest* 50:1621–1627, 1971

50. Mahoudeau, JA, Bardin CW, Lipsett MB: The metabolic clearance rate and origin of plasma dihydrotestosterone in man and its conversion to the 5α-androstanediols. *J Clin Invest* 50:1338–1344, 1971

51. Silber D, Samojlik E, Kirschner MA: Dihydrotestosterone production rates and metabolism in normal, hirsute and obese women (in preparation.)

52. Kinouchi T, Horton R: 3α-Androstanediol kinetics in man. *J Clin Invest* 54:646–653, 1974

53. Karpas AE: Introgenic hirsutism, in Mahesh VB, Greenblatt RB (eds): *Hirsutism and Virilism.* Boston, Wright PSG, 1983, pp 205–212

54. A.M.A.: *Drug Evaluation of Contraceptive Agents,* 4th ed. 1980, p 683

55. Arnold HL Jr, Odom RB: Diseases of the skin appendages, in: *Andrews' diseases of the Skin.* Philadelphia, Saunders, 1982, p 955

56. Snyder CH: Syndromes of gingival hyperplasia, hirsutism and convulsions. *J Pediatr* 67:499–502, 1965

57. Eisenberg H: Radiologic techniques in tumor localization, in DeGroot LJ, Cahill GF, Odell WD, et al (eds): *Endocrinology.* New York, Grune & Stratton, 1979, pp 2125–2143

58. Kirschner MA: Adrenal and gonadal venous catheterization studies in hirsute women, in Mahesh VB, Greenblatt RD (eds): *Hirsutism.* Boston, Wright PSG, 1983, pp 309–332

59. Blichert Toft M, Vijlsted H, Kehlet H, et al: Virilizing adrenocortical adenoma responsive to gonadotrophin. *Acta Endocrinol (Copenh)* 78:77–85, 1975

60. Bardin CW, Lipsett MB, French A: Testosterone and androstenedione production rates in patients with metastatic adrenal cortical carcinoma. *J Clin Endocrinol Metab* 28:215–220, 1968

61. Weyman PJ, Glazer H: The adrenal glands, in Lee JKT, Fagel S, Stanley S (eds): *Computed Body Tomography.* New York, Raven, 1981, pp 379–392

62. Osborn RH, Bradbury JT, Yannone ME: Androgen studies in a patient with lipoid-cell tumor of the ovary. *Obstet Gynecol* 33:666–672, 1969

63. Horton R, Frasier SD: Androstenedione and its conversion to plasma testosterone in congenital adrenal hyperplasia. *J Clin Invest* 46:1003–1008, 1967

64. Rivarola MA, Saez JM, Migeon CJ: Studies of androgens in patients with congenital adrenal hyperplasia. *J Clin Endocrinol Metab* 27:624–630, 1967

65. Baird DT, Corker, CS, Davidson DW, et al: Pituitary ovarian relationships in polycystic ovary syndrome. *J Clin Endocrinol Metab* 45:798–809, 1977

66. Chrousos GP, Loriaux DL, Mann DL, et al: Late-onset 21-hydroxylase deficiency mimicking idiopathic hirsutism or polycystic ovarian disease. *Ann Intern Med* 96:143, 1982

67. Fisher AA, Dooms-Goosens A: Persulfate bleach reactions. *Arch Dermatol* 112:1407, 1976

68. Gourmelen M, Pham-theun-Trung MT, Bredon MG, et al: 17-hydroxyprogesterone in the cosyntropin test: Results in normal and hirsute women and in mild congenital adrenal hyperplasia. *Acta Endocrinol (Copenh)* 90:481–489, 1979

69. Lobo, RA, Goebelsman U: Adult manifestation of congenital adrenal hyperplasia due to incomplete 21-hydroxylase deficiency mimicking polycystic ovarian disease. *Am J Obstet Gynecol* 138:720–726, 1980

70. Newmark S, Dluhy RS, Williams SH, et al: Partial 11- and 21-hydroxylase deficiencies in hirsute women. *Am J Obstet Gynecol* 127:494–598, 1977

71. Rosenwaks Z, Lee PA, Jones GS, et al: An attenuated form of congenital virilizing adrenal hyperplasia. *J Clin Endocrinol Metab* 49:335–339, 1979

72. Milewicz A, Vecsei P: 21-Deoxycortisol (21-DF) and 17-OH progesterone (17-OHP) responses to ACTH in hirsute women, in *Program of the Endocrine Society, San Antonio,* 1983

73. New MI, Kohn B, Lerner AJ, et al: Late onset attenuated 3β-hydroxy steroid dehydrogenase deficiency adrenal hyperplasia as a cause of hirsutism in peripubertal females, in *Proceedings of the Sixty-fifth Meeting of the Endocrine Society, San Antonio,* 1983 (no. 720)

74. Lobo RA, Goebelsmann U: Evidence for reduced 3β-ol-hydroxysteroid dehydrogenic activity in some hirsute women, thought to have polycystic ovary syndrome. *J Clin Endocrinol Metab* 53:394–400, 1981

75. Leventhal ML: The Stein–Leventhal syndrome. *Am J Obstet Gynecol* 76:825–838, 1958

76. Stein IF, Leventhal ML: Amenorrhea associated with bilateral polycystic ovaries. *Am J Obstet Gynecol* 29:181–191, 1935

77. Goldzieher JW, Green JA: The polycystic ovary 1: Clinical and histologic features. *J Clin Endocrinol Metab* 22:325–338, 1962

78. Jeffcoate TNA: The androgenic ovary, with special reference to the Stein-Leventhal syndrome. *Am J Obstet Gynecol* 88:143–156, 1964

79. Maury WP Jr: The multicystic ovary: The gray zone of the Stein-Leventhal syndrome. *South Med J* 57:868–877, 1964

80. Yen SSC: Chronic anovulation due to inappropriate feedback system, in Yen SSC, Jaffe RB (eds): *Reproductive Endocrinology.* Saunders, Philadelphia, 1978, pp 306–314.

81. Givens JR, Andersen RN, Umstot ES, et al: Clinical findings and hormonal responses in patients with polycystic ovarian disease with normal vs. elevated LH levels. *Obstet Gynecol* 47:388–395, 1976

82. Judd HL, Scully RE, Herbst AL, et al: Familial hyperthecosis: Comparison of endocrinologic and histologic findings with polycystic ovarian disease. *Am J Obstet Gynecol* 117:976–982, 1973

83. Yen SSC, Chaney C, Judd HL: Functional aberrations of the hypothalamic–pituitary system in polycystic ovary syndrome: A consideration of the pathogenesis, in James VHT, Serio M, Giusti G (eds): *The Endocrine Function of the Ovary.* London, Academic, 1976, pp 373–385

84. Baird DT: Pituitary ovarian relationships in disorders of menstruation, in James VHT, Serio M, Giusti G (eds): *The Endocrine Function of the Human Ovary.* London, Academic, 1976, pp 349–357

85. Rebar R, Judd HL, Yen SSC, et al: Characterization of the inappropriate gonadotropin secretion in polycystic ovary syndrome. *J Clin Invest* 57:1320–1329, 1976

86. Yen SSC, Vela P, Rankin J: Inappropriate secretion of follicle-stimulating hormone and luteinizing hormone in polycystic ovarian disease. *J Clin Endocrinol Metab* 30:435–442, 1970

87. Yen SSC, Vela P, Ryan KJ: Effect of clomiphene citrate in polycystic ovary syndrome: Relationship between serum gonadotropin and corpus luteum function. *J Clin Endocrinol Metab* 31:8–13, 1970

88. Givens JR, Wiser WL, Coleman SA, et al: Familial ovarian hyperthecosis: A study of two families. *Am J Obstet Gynecol* 110:959–972, 1971

89. Nieschlag E, Loriaux DL, Ruder HJ, et al: The secretion of dehydroepiandrosterone and dehydroepiandrosterone sulfate in man. *J Endocr* 57:123–134, 1973

90. Liddle G: The adrenal cortex, in William RFT (ed): *Textbook of Endocrinology*. Philadelphia, Saunders, 1981, pp 260–262

91. Rosenfield RL: Plasma testosterone binding globulin and indexes of the concentration of unbound plasma androgens in normal and hirsute subjects. *J Clin Endocrinol Metab* 32:717–728, 1971

92. Vermuelen A, Stoica A, Verdonck L: The apparent free testosterone concentration as an index of androgenicity. *J Clin Endocrinol Metab* 33:759–767, 1971

93. Chopra IJ, Abraham GE, Chopra U, et al: Circulating estradiol-17β in males with Graves' disease. *N Engl J Med* 286:124–126, 1972

94. Schneider G, Kirschner MA, Berkowitz R, et al: Increased estrogen production in obese men. *J Clin Endocrinol Metab* 48:633–638, 1979

95. Samojlik E, Silber D, Kirschner MA: Why aren't all obese women hirsute? *Proceedings of the Sixty-fifth Meeting of the Endocrine Society, San Antonio*, 1983 (no. 211)

96. Givens JR, Andersen RN, Wiser WL, et al: Dynamics of suppression and recovery of plasma FSH, LH, androstenedione and testosterone in polycystic ovarian disease using an oral contraceptive. *J Clin Endocrinol Metab* 38:727–737, 1974

96a. Besser GM, Thorner MO, Wass JAH: Prolactin and ovarian dysfunction, in Scholler R (ed): *Endocrinology of the Ovary*. Paris, Sepe, 1978, pp 359–376

97. Horton R, Hawks D, Lobo R: 3α-17β-Androstanediol glucuronide in plasma, a marker of androgen action in idiopathic hirsutism. *J Clin Invest* 69:1205, 1982

98. Lookingbill DP, Maries JG, Demers L, et al: Increased levels of plasma 3α-androstanediol glucuronide in women with acne, in *Proceedings of the Sixty-Fifth Meeting of the Endocrine Society, San Antonio*, 1983 (no. 727)

99. Bardin CW, Hembree WC, Lipsett MB: Suppression of testosterone and androstenedione production rates with dexamethasone in women with idiopathic hirsutism and polycystic ovaries. *J Clin Endocrinol Metab* 28:1300–1306, 1968

100. Ettinger B, Goldfield EB, Burrill RC, et al: Plasma testosterone stimulation-suppression dynamics in hirsute women. *Am J Med* 54:195–200, 1973

101. Givens JR, Andersen RN, Ragland JB, et al: Adrenal function in hirsutism. *J Clin Endocrinol Metab* 40:988–1000, 1975

102. Kirschner MA, Bardin CW, Hembree WC, et al: Effect of estrogen administration on androgen production and plasma luteinizing hormone in hirsute women. *J Clin Endocrinol Metab* 30:727–732, 1970

103. Casey JH, Burger HG, Kent JR, et al: Treatment of hirsutism by adrenal and ovarian suppression. *J Clin Endocrinol Metab* 26:1370–1374, 1966

104. Givens JR, Andersen RN, Wiser WL, et al: The effectiveness of two oral contraceptives in suppressing plasma androstenedione, testosterone, LH and FSH, and in stimulating plasma testosterone binding capacity in hirsute women. *Am J Obstet Gynecol* 124:333–339, 1976

105. Hancock KW, Levell MJ: The use of oestrogen/progtogen preparations in the treatment of hirsutism in the female. *J Obstet Gynaecol Br Commonw* 81:804, 1974

106. Casey JH: Chronic treatment regimen for hirsutism in women. Effect on blood production rates of testosterone and on hair growth. *Clin Endocrinol* 4:313–325, 1975

107. Nichols T, Nugent CA, Tyler FH: Glucocorticoid suppression of urinary steroids in patients with idiopathic hirsutism. *J Clin Endocrinol Metab* 26:79–86, 1966

108. Cumming DC, Yang JC, Rebar RW, et al: Treatment of hirsutism with spironolactone. *JAMA* 247:1295–1298, 1982

109. Milewicz A, Silber D, Kirschner MA: Therapeutic effects of spironolactone in polycystic ovary syndrome. *Obstet Gynecol* 61:429–432, 1983

110. Shapiro G, Evron S: A novel use of spironolactone: Treatment of hirsutism. *J Clin Endocrinol Metab* 51:429–432, 1980

111. Hammerstein J, Moltz L, Schwartz U: Antiandrogens in the treatment of acne and hirsutism. *J Steroid Biochem* 19:591–597, 1983

112. Hammerstein J, Mechies J, Leo-Rossberg I, et al: Use of cyproterone acetate (CPA) in treatment of acne, hirsutism and virilism. *J Steroid Biochem* 6:827–836, 1975

113. Kutten F, Rigand C, Wright F, et al: Treatment of hirsutism by oral cyproterone acetate and percutaneous estradiol. *J Clin Endocrinol Metab* 51:1107–1111, 1980

114. Castrow FF, Givens JR, Kirschner MA: Hirsutism: When a woman wants epilation. *Patient Care* Sept 1977, pp 1–12

115. Shapiro J: *Electrolysis*. New York, Dodd, Mead, 1981

116. Genuth SM, Castro JH, Vertes V: Weight reduction in obesity by outpatient semistarvation. *JAMA* 230:987–991, 1974

117. Kirschner MA, Schneider G, Ertel N, et al: Supplemental starvation: A successful method for control of major obesity. *J Med Soc NJ* 76:175–199, 1979

118. Blankstein J, Faiman C, Reyes FI, et al: Adult-onset familial adrenal 21-hydroxylase deficiency. *Am J Med* 68:441–448, 1980

119. Correade Oliveira RF, Novaes LP, Lima MB, et al: A new treatment for hirsutism. *Ann Intern Med* 83:817–819, 1975

120. Hamilton JB: Age, sex and genetic factors in the regulation of hair growth in man. A comparison of caucasian and Japanese populations, in Montagna W, Ellis RA (eds): *The Biology of Hair Growth*. New York, Academic, 1958.

121. Horton R, Romanoff E, Walker J: Androstenedione and testosterone in ovarian venous and peripheral plasma during ovariectomy for breast cancer. *J Clin Endocrinol Metab* 26:1267–1269, 1966

122. Judd HL, Spore WW, Talner LB, et al: Preoperative localization of a testosterone secreting ovarian tumor by retrograde venous catheterization and selective sampling. *Am J Obstet Gynecol* 120:91–96, 1974

123. Kirschner MA, Sinhamahapatra S, Zucker IR, et al: The production, origin and role of dehydroepiandrosterone and 5-androstenediol as androgen prehormones in hirsute women. *J Clin Endocrinol Metab* 37:183–189, 1973

124. Lipsett MB, Kirschner MA, Wilson H, et al: Malignant lipoid cell tumor of the ovary: Clinical, biochemical and etiologic considerations. *J Clin Endocrinol Metab* 30:336–344, 1970

125. Rivarola MA, Singleton RT, Migeon CJ: Splanchnic ex-

traction and interconversion of testosterone and androstenedione in man. *J Clin Invest* 46:2095–2100, 1967

126. Robyn C, Tukumbane M: Hyperprolactinemia and hir-
     sutism, in Mahesh VB, Greenblatt RB (eds): *Hirsutism
     and Virilism.* Boston, Wright PSG, 1983, pp 189–204

127. Schweikert HV, Wilson JD: Regulation of human hair
     growth by steroid hormones. II. Androstenedione metabo-
     lism in isolated hairs. *J Clin Endocrinol Metab* 39:1012–
     1019, 1974

128. Stahl NL, Teeslink CR, Greenblatt RB: Ovarian, adrenal
     and peripheral testosterone levels in the polycystic ovary
     syndrome. *Am J Obstet Gynecol* 117:194–200, 1973

129. Vigersky RA, Mehlmen I, Glass AR, et al: Treatment of
     hirsute women with cimetidine. *N Engl J Med* 303:1042,
     1980

ANSWERS

1. d

2. c

3. b

4. a

24

Lactation and Galactorrhea

DAVID L. KLEINBERG

INTRODUCTION

Mammary development in women is one of the earliest events of puberty. During breast development there is a gradual increase in circulating estrogens as well as an increase in prolactin,[1,2] most likely due to the rising titers of estrogen. Normal breast development (thelarche) occurs under the influence of a combination of hormones including estrogens, progesterone, adrenal steroids, growth hormone, and prolactin. Of these, prolactin and estrogen are thought to be the most important. The classic studies of Lyons, Li, and Johnson examining the combined and individual effects of these hormones on mammary development in hypophysectomized, oophorectomized, and adrenalectomized rats provided evidence that although development was optimal in the presence of the combination of hormones listed above, no mammary development occurred in the absence of prolactin, even when large doses of estrogen were employed.[3]

The individual and synergistic actions of estrogen and prolactin during mammary development are complex and have not been well worked out.

One might presume that estrogen may affect mammary growth, since in other systems (e.g., chick oviduct and MCF-7 human breast cancer cells[4]) estradiol increases cell division, DNA production, and new protein formation. The role of prolactin in the process of breast growth and development is also not well understood. A direct effect on thymidine incorporation into DNA has not been noted in careful studies carried out on mouse mammary tissue[5] but has been found in rabbit tissue.[6] Because of these discrepancies, some investigators have questioned the role of prolactin in mammary mitogenesis and have begun to reexamine the clearly vital role of the pituitary gland and the possibility that the pituitary gland contains mammary mitogens other than prolactin. Recent studies in monkeys provide evidence that the primate pituitary contains factors other than prolactin that participate in the process of normal mammary growth.[6a]

Whatever its effect on growth, prolactin has lactogenic effects on the mammary gland, even during the developmental stages.[7]

Hypothetically, once breast development has occurred, normal concentrations of circulating lactogenic hormones and steroids may act on mammary epithelial cells to maintain them in a state of readiness for eventual milk production. This speculation is suggested by studies in subhuman nulliparous and virgin primates in which mammary

DAVID L. KLEINBERG • Department of Medicine, New York University Medical Center; and Department of Endocrinology, Veterans Administration Medical Center, New York, New York 10016.

tissues, under basal conditions, were found to contain α-lactalbumin[8]; and these same tissues responded readily to prolactin in vitro with markedly increased α-lactalbumin production. During pregnancy, the breast undergoes further lobuloalveolar proliferation presumably under the influence of rising titers of prolactin, placental lactogen, estrogens, and progesterone.[9] In pregnant mice, histologic evidence of milk production becomes obvious at some point during the second half of pregnancy[10]; if tissues are removed shortly before milk production becomes microscopically visible, prolactin will stimulate milk formation in organ culture.[5,11] In humans, elevated mean levels of the milk protein α-lactalbumin can be detected during the second and third tremesters of pregnancy, providing evidence that some milk production is taking place during pregnancy.[12,13] The role of estrogens in alveolar development and preparation for lactation is a complicated one. Estrogen stimulates the normal pituitary to secrete prolactin[14,15] and is probably an important factor in the marked proliferation of pituitary lactotrophs during pregnancy.[16] It synergizes with prolactin or other pituitary substances to promote breast differentiation, but in high concentrations it inhibits milk production. In fact, estrogens are sometimes used to diminish postpartum lactation and breast engorgement. We have recently found that estradiol in physiologic concentrations or higher directly antagonizes the lactogenic effect of prolactin on the primate mammary gland in vitro,[17,18] which explains the clinical observation.

Active lactation begins shortly after parturition. A precipitous decrease in estrogen[19] and progesterone[20] after expulsion of the placenta is believed to be the stimulus. Continued milk production is maintained by episodic bursts of prolactin in response to each suckling episode,[21] even though baseline prolactin concentrations fall off postpartum and after a time may be indistinguishable from normal. The so-called milk letdown phenomenon, which can be triggered by psychic stimuli such as the cry of a hungry baby, does not seem to affect prolactin. This contraction of myoepithelial elements is probably an effect of oxytocin, as in animals. Recently careful studies have been started in humans.

A role for growth hormone in mammary mitogenesis and lactogenesis in humans has not been given adequate attention. In contrast to rodents, in which growth hormone is weakly lactogenic, the human material has been found to be as potent a lactogen as human prolactin in subhuman primates.[22] Thus, growth hormone, which acts ditectly on mammary epithelium cells, may have some importance in the process of mammary growth and development and in lactogenesis. It is unlikely that growth hormone secretion plays a major role in postpartum lactation, since growth hormone secretion is partially inhibited postpartum.

Several possible maneuvers may be considered to suppress lactation and breast engorgement in women who do not wish to nurse. High-dose long-acting estrogens, usually in combination with testosterone, have been effective,[23] but up to 20–40% of patients develop delayed engorgement.[24] Consideration of the side effects of estrogens, including an increase in the frequency of thromboembolism,[25,26] must be taken into account. Prolactin-lowering ergot derivatives (e.g., bromocriptine) have also been found to be effective suppressors of puerperal lactation, but rebound lactation may occasionally occur, requiring another course of treatment.[27] Simple measures consisting of ice packs, a tight binder or brassiere, and analgesics are usually sufficient.

The only well-established endocrine disease that makes nursing impossible is Sheehan's syndrome or other forms of pituitary insufficiency in which prolactin is deficient. One of the first indications that a patient has postpartum pituitary necrosis resulting from hemorrhage and subsequent hypotension is often inability to nurse because of the prolactin deficiency.[28] Other problems with lactation are generally thought to be of emotional origin but have not been well studied.

GALACTORRHEA

Since the original report of Chiari on inappropriate postpartum lactation and amenorrhea more than 100 years ago, a wide variety of causes of galactorrhea have been identified. Interest in this disorder was heightened because of the development of a sensitive bioassay[11] and subsequently a radioimmunoassay (RIA)[29] for human prolactin, the hormone largely responsible for most cases of galactorrhea. These developments have made physicians and lay people more aware of the significance of galactorrhea. It is now a very common disorder indeed.

In 1977 we published an analysis of 235 patients with galactorrhea, which enabled us to examine the relative frequency and underlying pathologic disorders that cause galactorrhea.[30] This chapter relies heavily on that experience and on our own subsequent experience and that of others.[31–33] Each major category or cause of galactorrhea is considered separately. Major findings in patients from our original series with each type of galactorrhea are listed in Table 24-1, and individual serum prolactin concentrations are presented in Figure 24-1.

In a study comparing prolactin levels in galactorrhea patients with those of normal individuals, prolactin levels in 102 normal men versus levels in women without galactorrhea are presented in Fig-

TABLE 24-1. Summary of Data in 235 Patients with Galactorrhea[a]

Diagnosis	No. of patients	Duration of galactorrhea (years)	Amenorrhea (%)	History of pregnancy (%)	Onset after childbirth (%)	Normal gonadotropins (%)	Mean prolactin (ng/ml)
Women							
Pituitary tumors	42	6.9 (0.4–23)[b]	81	51	31	58	376 (15–4000)
Idiopathic with menses	76	6.7 (0.1–30)	0	87	64	87	18.0 (1–120)
Idiopathic with amenorrhea	20	5.2 (0.5–11)	100	25	10	50	89.1 (4.6–285)
Chiari-Frommel syndrome	18	3.5 (1.0–13)	100	100	100	71	45.5 (3.2–230)
Postabortion	3	0.4 (0–1)	—	100	—	NA[c]	173 (9.9–300)
Postoophorectomy	1	(5 days)	100	100	0	NA[c]	85
Postlaparotomy	1	0.9	0	0	0	NA[c]	6.9
Oral contraceptive withdrawal	12	1.5 (0.1–4)	100	83	0	83	43.5 (6.6–170)
Oral contraceptive-induced	11	1.9 (0.5–4)	—	33	9	45	50.3 (4.8–180)
Phenothiazines	9	3.1 (0.6–12)	22	78	11	33	43.6 (12.4–110)
Benodiazepines	4	5.3 (0.5–10)	25	75	0	100	8.9 (4.5–14)
Isoniazid	1	0.1	100	100	0	100	3.0
Reserpine	1	1.5	0	100	100	100	23
Primary hypothyroidism	10	3.1 (0.2–17)	30	100	57	100	29.3 (12.1–55)
Hyperthyroidism	1	4	0	100	0	NA[c]	7.8
Cushing's disease	1	15	0	100	100	NA[c]	35
Empty-sella syndrome	5	1.95 (1–8)	40	80	40	80	10.4 (4.1–20)
Precocious puberty	1	0.3	0	0	0	—	7.9
Sarcoidosis	3	2.7 (1–5)	100	66	33	33	38.7 (21–58)
Schuller-Christian disease	1	0.5	100	100	0	—	97
Head trauma	1	0.5	100	0	0	NA[c]	67
Men							
Pituitary tumors	6	1.3 (1 day–3 years)	—	—	—	40	2630 (4.5–10,000)
Idiopathic	2	0.5	—	—	—	—	235 (220–250)
Klinefelter's syndrome thioridazine	1	1	—	—	—	100	8.2
Isoniazid	1	0.2	—	—	—	NA[c]	12.2
Orchiectomy and estrogen	1	1	—	—	—	100	30
Refeeding	1	2	—	—	—	100	9.4
Androgen therapy	1	0.25	—	—	—	—	9.4

[a]From Kleinberg et al.[30]
[b]Figures in parentheses denote ranges.
[c]Not available.

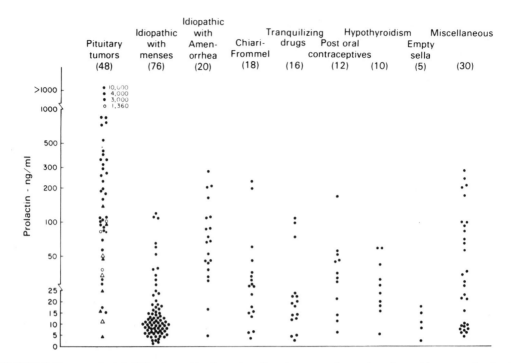

FIGURE 24-1. Plasma prolactin in 235 patients with galactorrhea of varying causes. Among the patients with tumors, triangles denote patients with acromegaly. Open circles or triangles denote patients studied only after radiotherapy or operation. (From Kleinberg et al.[30])

ure 24-2. As a group, women have slightly but significantly higher serum prolactin levels than men. The normal range in our laboratory is 1–25 ng/ml in women and 1–20 ng/ml in men. We view any consistent value over 15 ng/ml as suspiciously high. Because of considerable variability among prolactin preparations used for the RIA, normal levels may vary significantly from laboratory to laboratory.

DEFINITION AND DIAGNOSIS OF GALACTORRHEA

Galactorrhea can be defined as a unilateral or bilateral persistent discharge from the nipple that looks like milk and occurs in non-nursing individuals. Although usually white, the discharge may be yellowish or cream colored or may have a greenish hue. A black, brown, or reddish discoloration suggests the presence of blood. If a test for occult

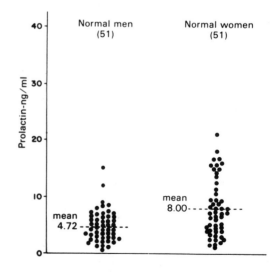

FIGURE 24-2. Plasma prolactin in 102 normal men and women 18–67 years of age. (From Kleinberg et al.[30])

blood is positive, an underlying breast tumor (often an intraductal papilloma) should be suspected.*

The amount of milk may range from a small drop which appears after manipulation to a profuse flow without stimulation. Sometimes even when galactorrhea is present it may not be obvious to the examiner or the patient, and careful attempts to express milk should be made by both. If the nature of the fluid is in doubt, the presence of milk can be confirmed by fat stains and measurement of milk proteins such as α-lactalbumin; α-lactalbumin has been found in concentrations ranging from 0.9–3.8 mg/ml of milk from galactorrhea patients.

CAUSES OF GALACTORRHEA

Pituitary Tumors

Forbes and colleagues brought to attention the relationship of pituitary tumors to galactorrhea. Since prolactin measurements in serum have been available, it has become obvious that this serious cause of galactorrhea is a relatively common one. In our series of 235 patients with galactorrhea, 20% of the 224 women had radiologically evident pituitary tumors. If only those patients with associated amenorrhea were counted, the frequency of pituitary tumors as a cause of galactorrhea rose to 34%. At the time this report was published the determination of a pituitary tumor was made by lateral skull films or in some cases polytomography. Therefore, the very large group of patients with microadenomas was missed. It is now clear that the great majority of patients with amenorrhea and galactorrhea with elevated prolactin concentrations have pituitary tumors. Most pituitary tumors that cause galactorrhea appear as chromophobe adenomas on sections stained with hematoxylin-eosin. Recent advances in immunocytochemical staining provide evidence that these tumors, once thought to be functionless, do indeed contain intracytoplasmic prolactin-laden granules.[36] These techniques permit functional classification of pituitary tumors making histologic identification of individual hormone-producing cytoplasmic granules within cells possible.

---

*Haagensen[34] reports that some women may develop bilateral bloody nipple discharge during pregnancy, but it disappears after delivery. The present author has seen two patients who had blood-tinged bilateral galactorrhea and in whom no underlying tumors were found, despite repeated physical examinations, mammographies, and cytology.

Signs and Symptoms

Hyperprolactinemia is found in the great majority of patients with pituitary tumor-associated galactorrhea (Fig. 24-1). The mean serum prolactin level in our series of 48 patients with pituitary tumors was 658 ng/ml (range: 4.5–10,000). As a group, patients with such tumors have the highest prolactin concentrations. Pituitary tumors were found in all patients whose prolactin concentrations were above 300 ng/ml and in 57% of those women whose serum prolactin concentrations were above 100 ng/ml. Although a very high level of serum prolactin (>300 ng/ml) is tantamount to the presence of a prolactin-secreting pituitary tumor, a large number of tumor patients have prolactin levels of under 100 ng/ml. In fact, most patients with microadenomas have prolactin concentrations in that range. Hypersecretion of growth hormone (GH) can itself cause galactorrhea, since human GH possesses intrinsic lactogenic activity that closely approximates the potency of human prolactin.[7,22] Although in this series it was rare to encounter normal concentrations of prolactin in patients with prolactin-secreting tumors, this author has since seen a number of patients with tumors in which prolactins were only intermittently elevated or consistently in the high normal range (i.e., >16 ng/ml). Several patients with acromegaly had galactorrhea. Prolactin is elevated in approximately 50% of acromegalics. In this disorder galactorrhea can occur with or without hyperprolacinemia.

In order for galactorrhea to occur, even in the presence of highly elevated prolactin concentrations, we assume that some degree of prior hormonal priming of the breast by steroid hormones is necessary. Not all patients with pituitary tumors develop galactorrhea. In an early study of patients with pituitary tumors, it was estimated that more than 60% were prolactin secreting. It was found that only 19 of 28 women (68%) with prolactin-producing tumors had galactorrhea, although highly elevated prolactin concentrations (in one case to 46,000 ng/ml) were found in the remaining nine patients. The concept that mammary epithelium must be primed in order for milk production to develop is further emphasized by the relatively infrequent occurrence of galactorrhea in men with prolactin-secreting pituitary tumors.[30,37]

Amenorrhea is present in most women with prolactin-secreting pituitary tumors (81% in our series, and higher in others).[30,31] In five of our patients, amenorrhea was primary. This unexpectedly high incidence of prolactin-producing pituitary tumors causing primary amenorrhea suggests that prolactin measurement be carried out in all patients with this disorder. Even though amenorrhea is so common in patients with prolactin-producing pituitary tumors, however, the presence of menses does not rule out a tumor. This is evidenced by the fact that 8 of 42 patients were having menstrual periods at the time their diagnoses were made; periods were regular in three and irregular in five of the eight patients. Since the completion of this study, it has become apparent that those patients with pituitary tumors and menses have lower prolactin as a group than do those with amenorrhea (usually <100 ng/ml). Even slight to moderate elevations of prolactin can cause shortened luteal phases that can be normalized by lowering prolactin with ergot drugs.[38] Often menses in patients with elevated prolactin are anovulatory. Galactorrhea and amenorrhea may be noted simultaneously, but one may precede the other by months or years. Gonadotropins are most often either within the normal range for menstruating women or low. Even normal levels of gonadotropins in the presence of amenorrhea and hypoestrogenism must be considered abnormal, since production of gonadotropins by the pituitary should increase markedly under these conditions. The mechanism by which prolactin interferes with normal menstrual function is still controversial, but the abnormality is thought to be either at the level of the hypothalamus or the ovary. Sauder and colleagues[41] found that the pattern of gonadotropin secretion over 24 hour periods was altered in hyperprolactinemic patients and that the secretory pattern was normalized during bromocriptine therapy. In contrast, Klibanski et al.[41a] found that patterns of gonadotropin secretion in tumor patients were heterogeneous. There is good evidence that elevated levels of prolactin inhibit ovarian steroid secretion.[40,40a] That the abnormality is not in the pituitary itself is suggested by the fact that gonadotropins respond normally to gonadotropin-releasing hormone (GnRH) in most patients with pituitary tumors. Patients with elevated prolactin frequently complain of decreased libido, vaginal dryness, and other symptoms associated with hypoestrogenism.

In addition to galactorrhea and amenorrhea, functioning pituitary tumors can result in other endocrine abnormalities, on one hand because of overproduction of prolactin and other hormones by the tumor itself and on the other because of hypopituitarism due to pressure necrosis of adjacent normal pituitary and hypothalamic tissue. GH-producing tumors were found in 14% of our tumor patients with galactorrhea who also had clinical acromegaly. Coexisting hyperprolactinemia, most often of minimal or moderate degree, occurs in up to 50% of acromegalic patients.[14] In addition, there have been rare reports of galactorrhea in patients with prolactinomas that also secrete thyroid-stimulating hormone (TSH)[42] or ACTH.[43]

Hypopituitarism caused by destruction of normal tissues may be present and can range from being asymptomatic to full blown, which when untreated may be incompatible with life. For this reason, patients with pituitary tumors should all be suspected of having possible hypopituitarism. The incidence of pituitary insufficiency affecting GH, TSH, ACTH, and other hormones with MSH activity increase with larger, more destructive tumors and especially after surgical or radiologic treatment of tumors. Of these, GH is the most frequently deficient. It produces few clinical sequelae, the major one being reduction of insulin requirements in diabetic patients. Secondary hypothyroidism, for which laboratory evidence consisting of low serum thyroxine concentrations together with normal or unmeasurable serum TSH, was found in 6 of our 48 patients (12.5%). Typical clinical signs and symptoms of hypothyroidism occur, ranging from mild sluggishness, intolerance to cold, and dryness of skin to profound myxedema. Symptoms of ACTH deficiency range from inability to handle major stress (e.g., surgery) to a picture resembling addisonian crisis, without the typical electrolyte disturbances, which may lead to collapse and death. This very severe disorder should be suspected often. Early and often vague symptoms including asthenia, malaise, nausea, anorexia, or hypopigmentation of the skin should alert the physician to the possibility of glucocorticoid insufficiency. Although aldosterone secretion may be slightly lower in ACTH-deficient individuals than in normal subjects, the hyponatremia and hypoosmolality in these patients resemble those of inappropriate secretion of antidiuretic hormone (SIADH). If due to hypocorticism, this inability to secrete a water load and tendency toward water intoxication can be reversed by physiologic replacement of steroids. It should be pointed out that the SIADH can be caused by hypothyroidism or by infiltration of or surgical trauma to the hypothalamus as well. Diabetes insipidus, when present, is generally a surgical side effect but may result from a large tumor extending into the hypothalamus.

Local manifestations of pituitary tumors include

loss of vision due to pressure on the optic nerves as the tumor extends above the sella turcica. Because of impingement on the inferior medial aspect of the optic nerves, the earliest visual-field losses are in the superior temporal quadrants, followed by bitemporal hemianopsia, nasal field losses, and eventual blindness if tumor growth continues.

Headaches are a frequent complaint of patients with pituitary tumors. Cranial nerve involvement of the third, fourth, and sixth nerves, or sometimes the first, occurs rarely. Infrequently interruption of the blood supply to the tumor may lead to thrombosis and hemorrhage, producing sudden severe headache, visual-field disturbance, and perhaps collapse. This so-called pituitary apoplexy must be recognized immediately and treated to avoid catastrophe.

Recent advances in computed tomography (CT) now permit the diagnosis of tumors ranging from several millimeters in diameter to large invasive ones. This technological advance has, for practical purposes, made routine skull films and polytomography almost obsolete in making the initial diagnosis of a pituitary tumor. By the time this book is published, the resolution of magnetic resonance imaging (MRI) may have been improved to the point of replacing the CT scan, but at present the CT scan is better for these purposes. The advantages of the MRI are that patients are exposed to lower doses of radiation and do not require injections of contrast material. High-dose radiation can theoretically result in cataract development. Nevertheless, the CT scan, taking proper precaution, is the procedure of choice.

Pharmacologic and Physiologic Tests in Pituitary Tumors

Stimulation or suppression of prolactin with pharmacologic agents has not been as helpful in the diagnosis of prolactin-secreting tumors as have their counterpart tests used in other endocrine disorders, like acromegaly and Cushing's disease. Stimulation by chlorpromazine did not double serum prolactin in any of the nine tumor patients tested. However, similar abnormalities may occur in nontumor patients with galactorrhea; the chlorpromazine stimulation test[44] was abnormal in 19 of 36 patients with galactorrhea of other causes.[30] Dopamine agonists, which lower prolactin in normals, also lower prolactin in patients with tumors. We found that L-dopa (500 mg p.o.) lowered serum prolactin by more than 50% in four of nine patients

with pituitary tumors. Although not used in tests of pituitary function, other dopamine agonists (e.g., bromocriptine) are much more effective than L-dopa in lowering serum prolactin. These drugs normalize prolactin in the large majority of patients with prolactin-secreting pituitary tumors.

When carefully interpreted, results of thyrotropin-releasing hormone (TRH) or metoclopramide stimulation tests may be helpful in making the diagnosis of pituitary tumor in selected instances. Although most tumor patients have had subnormal responses to TRH (less than a doubling of prolactin)[30] and metoclopramide,[45] normal responses to TRH have rarely been reported.[31] In the most difficult situation, that of a patient with a tumor on CT scan and a normal or high normal prolactin or that of a patient with an elevated prolactin and a normal CT scan in whom one suspects a tumor too small to see, a TRH or metoclopramide test may be helpful in making a diagnosis. In most instances, however, none of these tests appears to be more valuable than measurement of serum prolactin under basal conditions.

Treatment

Recent advances in transsphenoidal surgery, radiotherapy, and the development of prolactin-lowering ergot drugs provide a variety of therapeutic modalities for pituitary tumors. These can be employed singly or in combination, depending on the patient's endocrine status, expectation of fertility, and the size and degree of local invasion of the tumor.

MICROADENOMAS

Prolactin-secreting microadenomas (<10 mm diameter) are much more common than larger tumors and, when diagnosed, are most often found in women. Whether they occur with greater frequency in men, but remain undiagnosed, is yet to be determined. Unfortunately, no means has been developed to predict the growth characteristics of individual tumors. Most are either slow growing or remain stable for long periods of time.[46,47] Occasionally tumors may grow very rapidly and aggressively; therefore, all must be followed closely. Although patients with microadenomas tend to have lower prolactin concentrations than those with macroprolactinomas, prolactin levels vary widely from high normal to close to 1000 ng/ml.

There are a number of options that one may chose for treating these patients. Because microprolactinomas are generally slow growing, some endocrinologists have tended to choose a course of watchful waiting with periodic physical examinations, measurement of prolactin several times a year, and repeat CT scans every year or two. We have tended to reserve this approach for patients with regularly recurring ovulatory menses. For others, we have tended to recommend some form of therapy to lower prolactin because of the increased risk of osteoporosis in hyperprolactinemic amenorrheic patients[48] and because some tumors grow.

The only available means of curing patients with prolactin secreting tumors (i.e., normalizing prolactin and restoring ovulatory menses and fertility without disturbing other pituitary functions) is transsphenoidal surgery. Surgeons who are expert in this procedure can expect to cure 70–90% of patients with microprolactinomas.[49−55] With time, however, it has recently become evident that a significant minority of these patients develop recurrent hyperprolactinemia. Hardy,[56] who had initially reported a cure rate of approximately 90% has recently reported a recurrence rate of 40%.[56] Laws and colleagues[57] found hyperprolactinemia to recur in up to 25% of cases.[57] Side effects of surgery include, among others, hypopituitarism, diabetes insipidus, cerebrospinal fluid (CSF) leaks, visual deficits, and infections.

Although ergot drugs are highly effective in lowering prolactin and restoring normal menses and fertility in patients with prolactin-producing microadenomas, they do not, as far as we know, cure them.[51,58−65] Prolactin rises to pretreatment levels shortly after discontinuing medication and in most cases in which menses had been restored, amenorrhea reappears. Most microadenomas are objectively reduced in size during ergot therapy. In the series by Bonneville et al.[66] bromocriptine treatment was found to reduce tumor size in nearly 80% of those patients with microadenomas.[67] We found that pergolide, a long-acting synthetic ergot, reduced or altered tumor size in six of nine patients with microadenomas.[67] The major drawback of ergot therapy, as we see it, is committing patients to 30 or more years of drug treatment and the possibility of some still unidentified long term complications (e.g., adverse interaction with other medications). Side effect and suggestions on drug administration can be found below.

LARGE TUMORS

Because of actual or potential visual deficits or blindness in patients with large invasive tumors, some form of therapy is advised except under unusual circumstances. Classically, transsphenoidal surgery has been the treatment of choice for patients with tumors and visual impairment. The surgical cure rate of large tumors is very low (<28%).[49,52−55,68] The object of surgery is to reduce pressure on the optic nerves to improve vision. In a recent series, Wilson and Dempsey[55] found that vision was improved in 40 of 60 patients (66.7%) with large tumors causing visual defects. Most of these tumors were non-prolactin-secreting, however. In cases in which the entire tumor is not removed radiotherapy is then usually instituted. It is now possible and feasible to determine the degree of tumor removal using the high-resolution CT scanners together with prolactin determinations. If postoperative radiotherapy is not given to patients with large incompletely removed tumors, the recurrence rate is very high (up to 90%), suggesting that large tumors have a greater propensity for future regrowth than do smaller ones.[69,70] Radiotherapy alone has often been used in patients with tumors too large to completely remove surgically but not causing significant visual-field defects; radiotherapy can improve impaired visual fields in patients with visual defects. It has been estimated that tumor growth can be controlled for long periods of time in approximately 75% of patients treated with surgery and radiotherapy or radiotherapy alone.[70] Thus, these forms of therapy are highly effective in reversing or improving visual deficits and controlling further tumor growth. Unfortunately, they do not often lead to improved endocrine function. Prolactin is rarely reduced enough to permit restoration of menses.

Ergot drugs that lower prolactin are also highly effective in reducing the size of prolactin secreting pituitary tumors as judged by objective radiologic criteria. In eight recent prospective series designed to evaluate the effect of bromocriptine or lisuride on large pituitary tumor size in males and females, objective tumor shrinkage was noted in 78 of 112 patients with macroadenomas (69.6%).[51,63,71−76] These data are presented in Table 24-2. Thirty patients had visual field defects; in 19 or 63.3%, there was complete normalization or improvement in vision. Prolactin concentrations before and during therapy were reported in seven of the eight series. Prolactin was normalized to the equivalent of less

TABLE 24-2. Effects of Bromocriptine and Lisuride on Large Pituitary Tumors

Investigators	Drug	Daily dose (mg)	X-ray	No. of patients	No. with shrinkage	%
McGregor et al.[63]	Bromocriptine	20	CT + metrizamide	5	5	100
Chiodini et al.[119]	Bromocriptine or lisuride	7.5–20 0.6–2	CT	29	18	62
Sobrinho et al.[72]	Bromocriptine	7.5	Polytomography	11	8	73
Prescott et al.[75]	Bromocriptine	20 20	CT + metrizamide	6	6	100
Spark et al.[73]	Bromocriptine	7.5–25	CT	9	7	78
Wollesen et al.[71]	Bromocriptine	30–60	CT	15	13	87
Wass et al.[74]	Bromocriptine	7.5–60	CT + metrizamide	18	11	61
Weiss et al.[76]	Bromocriptine	7.5–10	CT	19	10	53
Total				112	78	69.6

than 25 ng/ml in 72 of 96 patients (75%). Tumor shrinkage occurred in some patients even though prolactin did not reach the normal range. Conversely tumor growth may occur in an occasional patient while taking bromocriptine despite normalization of prolactin. A precise estimate of the number of patients with large invasive tumors in whom menses were returned or libido and potency improved is not possible to ascertain from these studies. Improvement in sexual function occurred in a number of them and in our experience there is a greater chance of such improvement occurring in patients treated with ergots than with surgery or radiotherapy. The larger and more invasive the tumors, however, the less likely for sexual function to return despite normalization of prolactin. Sexual function is improved in patients in whom there are a sufficient number of gonadotrophs remaining in the pituitary gland; restoration of sexual function should not be expected in patients with panhypopituitarism. Those patients who respond to GnRH with increases in LH and FSH might be those who are more likely to experience return of sexual function during therapy with ergots. Occasionally disordered thyroid or adrenal function can be improved with ergot therapy.[74]

We have recently evaluated the efficacy of using pergolide for tumor shrinkage.[67] Of 13 patients with macroadenomas, tumor shrinkage was noted in 10 patients (77%) (eight men, two women). Decreased density of tumor was noted in an eleventh. Reduction in size was estimated at greater than 40% in seven of the ten patients. An example of tumor shrinkage in a patient who experienced marked tumor growth despite three craniotomies to remove a regrowing pituitary adenoma and radiotherapy can be seen in CT scans before and during therapy with pergolide in Figure 24-1. Thus, pergolide is at least as effective in shrinking tumors as bromocriptine and has the advantage of a much longer duration of action.

Macroadenomas vary in size from 1 cm in diameter to very large invasive tumors extending out of the sella turcica in all directions and may have significantly different rates of growth. Therefore, a tumor of just over 1 cm in diameter presents a different clinical problem than one that is larger and more destructive. The growth potential of intermediate-size tumors has not been studied. Such tumors in women present a greater risk of visual deficits if they become pregnant than smaller ones because of their proximity to the optic nerves. Because the cure rate of macroadenomas is significantly less than of microadenomas, potential visual problems during pregnancy would be avoided if the cure rate of surgery were improved. A recent report suggested that pretreatment with bromocriptine significantly improves the surgical cure rate of large tumors.[76] Ten of 19 patients with large (stage III–IV) prolactin-secreting tumors had reduction in tumor size. Of the 10 patients whose tumors had shrunk on bromocriptine, seven have had surgical "cures" (reduction of prolactin to 10 ng/ml or less). Only two of the nine nonresponders had normal prolactin levels postoperatively. Assuming further confirmation of these observations, medication followed by surgery may be preferable in selected patients with tumors.

The major drawback of ergot therapy is that it does not, as far as we know, lead to permanent cures. Tumor shrinkage may occur very rapidly in some patients with symptomatic improvement occuring within days after starting medication. Unfortunately, present evidence indicates that tumors reexpand if medication is discontinued.[77,78] Several groups have suggested that the reason for this rapid reduction and reexpansion is that bromocriptine acts by reducing cell volume rather than by tumor necrosis.[79,80]

Thus, treatment with ergot drugs is effective in the treatment of large pituitary tumors. It is probably as effective as surgery and/or radiotherapy in reducing tumor size; the possibility of restoration of normal sexual function is also an advantage.

PREGNANCY AND PITUITARY TUMORS

One of the major benefits of ergot therapy of pituitary tumors, restoration of fertility, is also a potential hazard. It has been suggested that the incidence of clinically significant tumor expansion during pregnancy is 35%[11] in patients with macroadenomas and 5% in the microadenoma group. We reviewed data from six reports of groups of 9 to 76 patients with tumors. Overall, complications during pregnancy occurred in 17 of 136 patients (12.5%). Complications included visual-field defects, ocular palsies, severe headaches, diabetes insipidus, and pituitary apoplexy.[52,81-86]

Although the great majority of pregnancies in patients with very small tumors proceed uneventfully, there is a small but definite risk of visual and other complications due to rapid tumor growth. That must be kept in mind and discussed with the patient before prescribing these drugs. In our view patients with large tumors ought to be advised against pregnancy because of the very high incidence of visual complications. In these patients, one might consider surgery, radiotherapy, or yttrium implantation prophylactically before pregnancy. A lower incidence of complications during pregnancy has been reported in patients who received radiotherapy[81] or yttrium-90 implantation.[85] Complete surgical removal of tumors transsphenoidally has permitted uneventful pregnancies in large numbers of patients. To our knowledge, no report on the effectiveness of partial tumor removal has appeared. It is important to keep in mind that a small number of tumors grow despite surgery or radiotherapy.

Regardless of the size of the tumor, we strongly suggest that patients have formal visual-field examinations before and periodically during pregnancy.

In the event that visual defects occur during pregnancy there are several steps that might be taken. High-dose corticosteroid therapy may reduce tumor volume by reducing edema, thereby improving vision. Transsphenoidal surgery during pregnancy has proved effective in relieving pressure on the optic nerves in some cases. Bromocriptine has recently been given to a few patients during pregnancy. Tumor shrinkage and improved visual fields were well documented in at least one of these.[88] The patient delivered twins with 1-min Apgar scores of 10; the body weight of one of the children was low. Although the incidence of birth defects is not increased in women taking bromocriptine,[89] the effects of long-term administration of ergots during pregnancy have not been adequately studied. We therefore advise against its use during pregnancy.

IDIOPATHIC GALACTORRHEA WITH MENSES

The largest single group of patients with galactorrhea are those in whom menstrual periods are present and who have no discernible cause for their galactorrhea. The great majority (87%) of our patients had been pregnant, and in most (64%) galactorrhea started postpartum and persisted in some cases for up to 30 years. In our experience, patients with this disorder account for about one-third of galactorrhea cases. The true prevalence of this condition is probably much higher than our figures indicate, since many women consider breast discharges in the absence of menstrual abnormalities normal. Furthermore, the presence of galactorrhea is not always looked for during a history and physical examination.

Serum Prolactin

In contrast to patients with pituitary tumors, serum prolactin levels in this group are generally within the normal range (1–25 ng/ml). We found prolactin to be normal in 65 of 76 patients (Fig. 24-1), the mean for these 65 being 9.9 ng/ml. In 11 others, prolactin was high, ranging from 28 to 120 ng/ml. The mean for the entire group, including the 11 patients with prolactin concentrations above 25 ng/ml, was 17.2 ng/ml (significantly higher than the mean for normal controls). Patients with higher prolactin concentrations probably represent a separate subgroup with a different prognosis.

Mechanisms

Whether or not idiopathic galactorrhea with regular menses is a disease or a normal or exaggeration of a normal physiologic event is uncertain. The only relatively firm evidence that this sort of galactorrhea may be pathologic is the fact that 57% of our patients had blunted prolactin responses to chlorpromazine stimulation. By contrast, several lines of experimental evidence that suggest that this type of galactorrhea may be normal or may reflect a greater sensitivity of some mammary glands to normal concentrations of prolactin. First, milk proteins are normally present in both subhuman primate and human mammary glands whether or not prolactin is high; concentrations of α-lactalbumin are expectedly higher in animals and humans with high prolactin levels who are either nursing or pregnant. That physiologic concentrations of prolactin are lactogenic in nonlactating nonpregnant primates is evidenced by our observation that long-term inhibition of prolactin by ergot drugs leads to reduced concentrations of α-lactalbumin in their mammary glands. Thus, assuming that our observations in normal primates are indicative of what occurs in humans, it may be normal for small amounts of milk to be produced by the mammary gland, particularly in patients previously exposed to high levels of prolactin and other mammary stimulants during a pregnancy. Why some individuals continue to lactate after a pregnancy and others do not is not immediately apparent, but it is possible that, among other explanations, some tissues are more sensitive than others to prolactin or that some forms of prolactin may be more biologically potent than others.

Workup and Treatment

In approaching a patient with galactorrhea, it is important to ascertain whether prolactin concentrations are elevated, a chore that may not be as simple as it first appears. Most laboratories arbitrarily set 25 ng/ml as the upper limit of normal for prolactin. Because of the extreme lability of human prolactin and because of variability in preparations used, incubation times, and other methodologic differences, prolactin assays vary widely from laboratory to laboratory. Thus, a level of 18 ng/ml of prolactin might be the mean for normal women of childbearing age in some laboratories; in our laboratory, we would view it as a suspicously high concentration and suggest that it be repeated and followed. Until better standardization of prolactin assays is available it is important that physicians be familiar with the characteristics and precision of the assays being employed and be particularly suspicious of repeatedly high normal prolactin concentrations as indicative of a possible underlying tumor or other disorder.

In patients with persistent postpartum galactorrhea in whom menses are perfectly regular, prolactin is at or close to our mean for normal age matched women without galactorrhea, and no underlying cause of galactorrhea can be found, we generally suggest no further workup except for yearly measurements of prolactin. If menses become irregular or if prolactin is high normal or becomes frankly high or if there is a fertility problem, we do more extensive workups. They might include high-resolution CT scans, more frequent prolactin determinations, measurements of growth hormone and parameters of thyroid, adrenal, and ovarian function, and other endocrine studies tailored to the specific problem. Only if galactorrhea is troublesome to patients do we suggest therapy with bromocriptine or other dopamine agonists.

IDIOPATHIC GALACTORRHEA WITH AMENORRHEA

Patients with galactorrhea and amenorrhea who do not have tumors on CT scan and in whom other known causes of galactorrhea have been ruled out are grouped together as "idiopathic." These patients are probably similar to those originally described by Argonz and del Castillo.[90] The incidence of this type of galactorrhea has not been ascertained. We initially included 9% of 235 patients with galactorrhea in this category. Many of them, however, would have been found to have pituitary tumors had CT scans been available at that time. There is, however, an increasingly large number of patients who have galactorrhea, amenorrhea, and hyperprolactinemia who do not have pituitary tumors. The mechanism of their galactorrhea has not been ascertained.

Treatment

Several modes of therapy are reasonable. In patients in whom immediate fertility is not the goal, one may choose to watch closely and suggest periodic X-ray studies of the sella turcica and serum prolactin measurements. In view of the correlation between the height of the serum prolactin level and tumor presence and size, a progressive or marked elevation of prolactin levels might stimulate earlier intervention.

Bromocriptine is highly effective in these patients and readily restores menstrual function. Because of an increased risk of osteoporosis in patients with hyperprolactinemia[48] bromocriptine may be the treatment of choice for idiopathic galactorrhea with amenorrhea.

CHIARI-FROMMEL SYNDROME

Postpartum galactorrhea and amenorrhea with uteroovarian atrophy constitute a syndrome originaly described by Chiari during the mid-1800s and by Frommel in 1882.[91] In our series, 18 patients (8%) had this sort of galactorrhea and amenorrhea for periods of 6 months to 11 years postpartum (mean: 3.5 years). Prolactin concentrations in these patients ranged widely from 4.6 to 285 ng/ml, with a mean of 45.5 ng/ml for the entire group. Prolactin levels were within the normal range of less than 25 ng/ml in seven patients and elevated in the remainder. Serum gonadotropins were normal in 71%, but again the absence of markedly elevated gonadotropin levels in a milieu of decreased concentrations of circulating estrogens indicates a primary abnormality at the level of the pituitary or hypothalamus.

No definite abnormality has been uncovered to explain persistent hyperprolactinemia. Whatever the mechanism, this disorder might be considered an exaggeration of normal, since menses frequently do not return immediately postpartum, even in women who do not nurse.

Not infrequently, patients with Chiari-Frommel syndrome have spontaneous resumption of menses with or without disappearance of galactorrhea. At times they may become pregnant without an intervening period.[30,92,93] Six of our patients became pregnant 8 months to 2 years after the onset of galactorrhea; only four had menstrual periods before conception. In patients who do not resume normal ovulatory function, treatment with ergot drugs should be considered.

By definition, patients with Chiari-Frommel syndrome do not have radiologically apparent pituitary tumors. It cannot be assumed, however, that patients who develop galactorrhea and amenorrhea postpartum do not have pituitary tumors. Among our previously reported patients with pituitary tumors, 31% noted galactorrhea postpartum. All patients presenting with amenorrhea and galactorrhea more than 6 months postpartum should have CT scans. Particular attention should be paid to thyroid function in these patients; hypothyroid patients may develop postpartum galactorrhea, sometimes with associated amenorrhea (see Hypothyroidism).

SURGERY AND TRAUMA

Galactorrhea occurring as a surgical side effect is uncommon, but it may appear several days to weeks postoperatively and may last for periods of from weeks to, in some cases, years. Although amenorrhea may acompany the galactorrhea, menses are most often unaffected. In addition to galactorrhea after pituitary stalk section[94] followed by moderate prolactin elevations,[14] inappropriate lactation has been reported after thoracoplasty,[95,96] hysterectomy,[97] and cholecystectomy.[98] Of the two patients in our series who had postsurgical galactorrhea, one had an elevated prolactin concentration 5 days postoophorectomy, and the other had normal prolactin levels 1 month postlaparotomy.

Although a number of mechanisms, including interruption of nerve supply, have been postulated as causes of this sort of galactorrhea, a major factor may be stress-induced hyperprolactinemia during surgery. In a group of women studied before, during, and after surgery, prolactin levels were generally found to be 100–200 ng/ml during surgery.[99] Speculatively a short-lived prolactin increase of this magnitude or stress-induced prolactin elevation that persists might be responsible.

In one patient galactorrhea and amenorrhea followed severe head trauma during an airplane accident. The elevated prolactin of 67 ng/ml could have been a result of stress. Other endocrine abnormalities, including amenorrhea alone, diabetes insipidus, and SIADH, have been noted after head trauma as well.

DRUGS

Various medications can cause galactorrhea. In our series, 17% of patients were believed to have drug-induced galactorrhea. Those drugs most often implicated are discussed below.

Oral Contraceptives

In patients taking oral contraceptives, galactorrhea has been noted to occur both after discontinuation of the drugs and during their administration. Precise assignment to one or the other of these categories is not always possible because of uncertainty about the exact time of onset of galactorrhea in relation to periods of starting and stopping the drug. It has been established that as many as 2.2% of women who stop taking birth control pills develop amenorrhea, but eventually most menstruate spontaneously[100]; a small number of these patients also have galactorrhea.[101,102] We have studied 12 patients with this sort of galactorrhea and amenorrhea. Serum prolactin was higher than normal in 8 of the 12 patients, the mean for the entire group being 43.5 ng/ml (range: 6.6–170 ng/ml).[30] The period of follow-up in our patients was not long enough to predict whether the height of the serum prolactin was in any way related to prognosis.

Because of the possibility of an underlying pituitary tumor, we recommend that CT scans of the sella turcica and serum prolactin measurements be carried out in all patients who develop galactorrhea and amenorrhea, even if they coincide with discontinuation of oral contraceptives. Spontaneous remissions have been observed in some patients with post-pill amenorrhea and galactorrhea, but in others signs and symptoms continue for years. In these cases periodic reexamination is advised.

Besser and Thorner[59] treated six patients with postpill galactorrhea and amenorrhea with bromocriptine. Prolactin was normal in two and elevated in four patients. The return to spontaneous menses occurred in all cases. Prolactin-lowering ergot drugs will probably be considered the treatment of choice for this disorder. Treatment with clomiphene has not been as reliable.[101]

Oral contraceptive administration may cause galactorrhea as well.[103] The mechanism is uncertain, but it may be related to the prolactin-stimulating property of estrogens or a direct effect on the breast, or both. We have 11 patients in whom galactorrhea was thought to be related to starting birth control pills. Although the mean serum prolactin level was elevated to 50.3 ng/ml, prolactin was in the normal range in seven patients in whom galactorrhea was thought to be related to starting birth control pills. The group was heterogeneous in that one of the patients had galactorrhea only during withdrawal bleeding, another had preexisting idiopathic galactorrhea with regular menses that worsened on taking the pills, and a third developed galactorrhea while taking the pills, followed by a 6-month period of amenorrhea and galactorrhea after stopping them; 7 of these 11 patients had preexisting men-

strual abnormalities. Treatment consists of discontinuing oral contraceptives and correcting underlying abnormalities if they exist.

Tranquilizing Drugs

Dopamine antagonist tranquilizing drugs, including all phenothiazines and butyrophenones, elevate prolactin. Galactorrhea associated with taking these drugs is most likely brought on by drug-induced prolactin increases. Estimates of the frequency of galactorrhea in hospitalized psychotic patients taking large doses of these drugs have been as high as 25%.[104] In our series, nine patients were classified as having galactorrhea resulting from phenothiazines. The mean prolactin level in these patients was 43.6 ng/ml, ranging from 12.4 to 110 ng/ml. Only two of nine patients taking phenothiazines had amenorrhea, but menses were irregular in most cases. Menstrual irregularity is common among untreated psychiatric patients with severe emotional disorders, but the irregularity may also be a side effect of major tranquilizers. It has not yet been established whether prolactin is in part responsible for these menstrual abnormalities.

In patients who develop galactorrhea and elevated serum prolactin levels while taking phenothiazines, a cause-and-effect relationship can be established if galactorrhea disappears and prolactin concentrations fall after discontinuing the drugs; however, underlying illness usually precludes such maneuvers. Clinical judgment, taking into account such variables as the presence or absence of amenorrhea and the degree of serum prolactin elevation, must be used to determine which patients should have more extensive periodic workups for possible underlying pituitary tumors.

Some patients have developed galactorrhea while taking minor tranquilizers of the benzodiazepine group. These drugs, which include chlordiazepoxide and diazepam, do not raise prolactin. A causal relationship between benzodiazepines and galactorrhea has not been firmly established.

Other Drugs

Antihypertensive medications, including reserpine and α-methyldopa, have been reported to cause galactorrhea. Although these drugs are thought to elevate prolactin, careful studies in humans are necessary to confirm this presumption.

Isoniazid, like some antihypertensive drugs, can cause both gynecomastia[105] and galactorrhea.[30]

Among our patients, one woman and one man developed galactorrhea shortly after starting isoniazid. Prolactin was within the normal range in both cases.

HYPOTHYROIDISM

Primary hypothyroidism as a cause of galactorrhea was first described in children with precocious menstruation and enlargement of the sella turcica.[106] Since that time, a number of patients with postpartum galactorrhea and amenorrhea who were initially diagnosed as having the Chiari-Frommel syndrome have been found to have hypothyroidism.[107-109] Treatment with thyroid hormone has resulted in the return of menses and the reduction of previously elevated levels of TSH and prolactin.[110,111] In our series, 10 patients with primary hypothyroidism had galactorrhea, but associated amenorrhea was only noted in three cases. There was a prior history of pregnancy in all patients, and galactorrhea clearly began after childbirth in four. Prolactin was elevated in five patients and was in the normal range in the remaining five. The mean for the entire group was 29.3 ng/ml (range: 12.1–55 ng/ml). Serum prolactin fell from a mean of 31.1 to 10 ng/ml in response to treatment with thyroid hormone in five patients who were so tested.[30]

For reasons that have not been elucidated, some patients with primary hypothyroidism (with or without galactorrhea) have moderate prolactin elevations.[14] In women in whom breast epithelial elements have been primed by the hormones of pregnancy, a slight elevation of prolactin, even to levels within the normal range, may be stimulus enough to cause galactorrhea. Thyroid replacement should result in the lowering of both prolactin and TSH and stimulate resumption of absent menses if caused by myxedema. Failure to respond to such therapeutic measures should alert the physician to the possibility of some other etiologic factor. Highly elevated prolactin levels (greater than 75 ng/ml) are not usual in patients with primary hypothyroidism. Their presence should also suggest a pituitary tumor or other cause of hyperprolactinemia. It should be pointed out that longstanding primary hypothyroidism may itself lead to pituitary hyperplasia or adenoma formation.[112]

EMPTY SELLA SYNDROME

Galactorrhea can occur in patients with the empty sella syndrome.[30,113] Five galactorrhea patients in our series had enlarged sella turcicae found to be empty by pneumoencephalography. Prolactin concentration was normal in all, the mean level being 10.4 ng/ml, but on repeated testing one of the patients was found to have one value of 23 ng/ml. In contrast to patients with tumors, response to TRH (Fig. 24-3) was normal in four of five patients tested, and all of five tested had normal response to L-dopa. The only abnormality besides the amenorrhea in two patients was failure to respond to chlorpromazine stimulation in three of four patients tested. In general, endocrine disturbances in the empty sella syndrome are infrequent and usually mild.[114,115]

Although several hypotheses have been suggested to explain the development of any empty sella, two attractive ones are (1) an anatomic defect in the diaphragma sellae leading to sella enlargement from increased CSF, and (2) necrosis and disappearance of a previously present tumor. We have recently seen a patient who had a pituitary tumor above an empty sella. Whether or not CSF gained access to the sella because of infarction of tumor tissue within the sella is unclear, but a progressive fall in prolactin has been noted in patients undergoing pituitary apoplexy.[116]

MISCELLANEOUS

In addition to the causes of galactorrhea discussed above, nonpuerperal lactation has occurred in patients who had disorders including primary hyperthyroidism, pregnancies interrupted by abortion, precocious puberty, sarcoidosis, and Hand-Schüller-Christian disease (Table 24-1).

In men,[30] who develop galactorrhea much less frequently than women, pituitary tumors were the most common cause of galactorrhea. In addition, drugs, including phenothiazines, isoniazid, estrogens, and androgens in the treatment of aplastic anemia, have been implicated. One prisoner of war developed galactorrhea after release and refeeding, while in two no cause could be found (Table 24-1).

TREATMENT OF GALACTORRHEA WITH PROLACTIN-LOWERING ERGOT DRUGS

Prolactin-lowering ergot drugs, including bromocriptine[59,61] and lergotrile mesylate,[30] have been extremely effective in the treatment of galactorrhea-amenorrhea syndromes. L-dopa, which lowers prolactin transiently, is only rarely effective

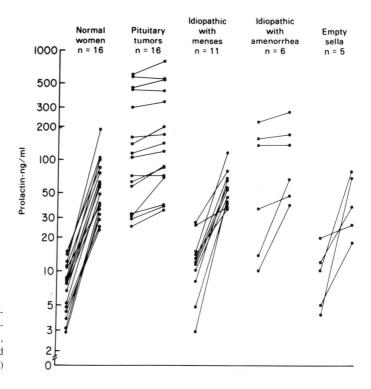

FIGURE 24-3. Serum prolactin concentrations before (left-hand dots) and after (right-hand dots) thyrotropin-releasing hormone, 500 μg IV, in patients with galactorrhea and in normal subjects. (From Kleinberg et al.[30])

and has not been generally used. Bromocriptine is the most widely used ergot drug. In patients with amenorrhea and galactorrhea who do not carry a definite diagnosis of pituitary tumors (see Pituitary Tumors), bromocriptine in doses of 2.5 mg bid or tid has resulted in prolactin inhibition to levels within the normal range in the vast majority of patients.[35,39,59,61,117] Disappearance of galactorrhea, return of menses, and fertility when desired are usual. As noted by Friesen and Tolis,[61] return of menses most often occurred within 3 months of starting medication, and pregnancy was noted generally within the first 6 months. Medication should be discontinued as soon as pregnancy has been diagnosed to avoid any adverse effects on the fetus, although no increase in the number of birth defects in humans had been noted. Our own experience and that of others indicates a high rate of recurrence of hyperprolactinemia with galactorrhea and amenorrhea when these drugs are withdrawn. The optimal duration of therapy has not been established, although some patients have received these drugs for more than 12 years.[59] Side effects are listed in Table 24-3. We routinely start patients with the smallest dose of medication in order to avoid side effects, which can be formidable. Bromocriptine (1.25 mg) or pergolide (25 μg) is administered just

before bedtime together with a small feeding. Daily contact is maintained with patients until they are stable. The dose of bromocriptine is then slowly increased to 1.25 mg bid and then tid. Medication is increased until prolactin is normalized or a daily dose of 7.5 mg is reached. Higher doses are occa-

TABLE 24-3. Side Effects of CB-154 in the Treatment of 78 Patients with Galactorrhea-Amenorrhoea[a,b]

Symptom	Acute		Chronic	
	Incidence	%	Incidence	%
Nausea	20[c]	25.3	6[d]	7.6
Nausea and vomiting	4[a]	5.1	3	3.8
Headache	4	5.1	2	2.5
Dizziness	3	3.8	2	2.5
Nasual congestion	2	2.5	1	1.3
Fatigue	4	5.1	—	—
Tinnitus	2	2.5	—	—
Heartburn	2	2.5	1	1.3
Tender breasts	—	—	3	3.8

[a]From Friesen and Tolis.[61] CB-154 was an earlier trade name for bromocriptine.
[b]Five patients discontinued because of side effects. If a symptom occurred in only one patient, it was not included in the above table.
[c]One patient had severe symptoms.
[d]Two patients had severe symptoms.

sionally necessary to shrink tumors, but a total daily dose of 7.5 mg is usually sufficient to reduce tumor size. Theoretically, too high a dose of bromocriptine or pergolide might inhibit gonadotropins and sexual function. Blood pressure should be taken with the patient in the supine and standing positions at every visit and visual fields should be evaluated frequently. If patients develop gastrointestinal discomfort, we keep them on the smallest dose of medication until they are comfortable and increase it very slowly. If tumors are present, we follow their size by CT scans taken in the coronal plane. We generally wait approximately 6 months to rescan patients, but in some cases we repeat scans more often. If tumor shrinkage is noted, scans are done less frequently so as to avoid exposure to radiation. If no tumor shrinkage is noted, we reevaluate our plans for therapy. It is important to remember that prolactin will likely increase and tumors regrow relatively rapidly after stopping medication.

Side effects of bromocriptine are similar to those of pergolide, but no transaminase elevations of major degree have been reported. Adverse reactions to bromocriptine are discussed elsewhere.[118] Sobrinho[72] reported two patients who suffered reversable loss of vision (partial in one case) while taking bromocriptine; we have also encountered such a patient.

SUMMARY

Lactation depends upon adequate preparation of the mammary gland during pregnancy. A number of known hormones (e.g., estrogen and prolactin) and possibly undiscovered hormones synergize to increase mammary gland mass and begin the process of milk production. Withdrawal of high levels of estrogen and probably progesterone, which inhibit the lactogenic action of prolactin on the mammary gland during pregnancy, permit the onset of active lactation. Milk release, which is stimulated by suckling, is mediated by oxytocin.

Most patients with galactorrhea and amenorrhea have prolactin-secreting pituitary adenomas. Many of the tumors are small and cause signs and symptoms such as amenorrhea or galactorrhea due to increased prolactin concentrations. Larger tumors may impinge upon neighboring anatomical structures and produce more serious problems (e.g., visual field defects). The most helpful and important tools in making the diagnosis of a prolactinoma are serum prolactin determinations, CT scans of the sella turcica, and visual field examinations.

Other causes of the galactorrhea–amenorrhea syndrome include acromegaly, hypothyroidism, pregnancy, trauma, and drugs, in addition to presumed abnormalities in the hypothalamus. Galactorrhea by itself may be caused by any of the above diseases or by rarer causes of the galactorrhea–amenorrhea symdrome. Galactorrhea also occurs in otherwise normal individuals. In those patients with so-called "idiopathic galactorrhea with menses," prolactin is normal, and diagnosis is made after ruling out other causes of galactorrhea.

Therapy is directed at reducing elevated prolactin levels with drugs such as bromocriptine in order to restore ovulatory menses and fertility and reduce tumor size in patients with prolactin-secreting tumors. Transsphenoidal adenomectomy without radiation for microadenomas, or with postoperative radiation or ergot therapy for larger tumors, is also an option. Occasionally radiation is used as the sole treatment. Treatment of other causes of galactorrhea should be individualized depending upon the cause. In many instances galactorrhea requires no therapy.

Pituitary tumors can enlarge during pregnancy and cause visual and other complications which may be serious. This problem occurs most often in patients who have macroadenomas or larger microadenomas.

QUESTIONS

1. Full lactation depends on

    a. the presence of prolactin.
    b. stimulation of the mammary gland by estrogen and progesterone.
    c. prior stimulation by estrogen, progesterone, prolactin, growth hormone, and adrenal corticosteroids.

2. In a 30-year-old women with 5 years of amenorrhea, galactorrhea, and infertility, found to have a prolactin level of 40 mg/ml, normal growth hormone and thyroid function studies, negative sella CT scan, and normal visual fields, the most suitable initial therapy of infertility is

    a. bromocriptine.
    b. sellar yttrium therapy.
    c. transsphenoidal surgery.

REFERENCES

1. Ehara Y, Yen S, Siler TM: Serum prolactin levels during puberty. *Am J Obstet Gynecol* 121:995, 1975
2. Jenner MR, Kelch RP, Kaplan SL, et al: Hormonal changes in puberty. IV. Plasma estradiol, LH, and FSH in prepubertal children, pubertal females, and in precocious puberty, premature thelarche, hypogonadism, and in a child with a feminizing ovarian tumor. *Clin Endocrinol* 34:521–530, 1972
3. Lyons WR, Li CH, Johnson RE: The hormonal control of mammary growth and lactation. *Recent Prog Horm Res* 14:219, 1958
4. Lippman ME, Bolan G: Oestrogen-responsive human breast cancer in long term tissue culture. *Nature (Lond)* 256:592–593, 1975
5. Topper YJ: Multiple hormone interactions in the development of mammary gland in vitro. *Recent Prog Horm Res* 26:287, 1970
6. Bourne RA, Bryant JA, Grierson D, et al: Prolactin-stimulated deoxyribonucleic acid syntheses in rabbit mammary tissue. *Biochem J* 130:10p, 1972
6a. Kleinberg DL, Niemann W, Flamm E, Cooper P, Babitsky G, Valensi Q: Primate mammary development: Effects of hypophysectomy, prolactin inhibition, and growth hormone administration. *J Clin Invest* 75:1943–1950, 1985
7. Kleinberg DL, Todd J, Niemann W: Evidence that prolactin stimulates α-lactalbumin production in mammary tissues from premenarcheal rhesus monkeys. *Endocrinology* 104(6):1569–1573, 1979
8. Kleinberg DL, Todd J, Niemann W: Prolactin stimulation of α-lactalbumin in normal primate mammary gland. *J Clin Endocrinol Metab* 47:435–441, 1978
9. Tyson JE, Hwang P, Guyda H, et al: Studies of prolactin secretion in human pregnancy. *Am J Obstet Gynecol* 113:14–20, 1972
10. Elias J: Cultivation of adult mouse mammary gland in hormone-enriched synthetic medium. *Science* 126:842, 1957
11. Kleinberg DL, Frantz AG: Human prolactin: Measurement in plasma by in vitro bioassay. *J Clin Invest* 50:1557–1568, 1971
12. Kleinberg DL, Todd J, Groves ML: Studies on human α-lactalbumin: Radioimmunoassay measurement in normal human breast and breast cancer. *J Clin Endocrinol Metab* 45:1238–1250, 1977
13. Kleinberg DL, Warren M: α-Lactalbumin production during human pregnancy, (submitted for publication)
14. Frantz AG, Kleinberg DL, Noel GL: Studies on prolactin in man. *Recent Prog Horm Res* 28:527–590, 1972
15. Yen SSC, Ehara Y, Siler TM: Augmentation of prolactin secretion by estrogen in hypogonadal women. *J Clin Invest* 53:652–655, 1974
16. Herbert DC, Hayashida T: Histological identification and immunochemical studies of prolactin and growth hormone in the primate pituitary gland. *Gen Comp Endocrinol* 24:381–397, 1974
17. Kleinberg DL, Todd J, Babitsky G, et al: Estradiol inhibits prolactin induced α-lactalbumin production in normal primate mammary *in vitro*. *Endocrinology* 110:279–281, 1982
18. Kleinberg DL, Todd J, Babitsky G: Inhibition by estradiol of the lactogenic effect of prolactin in primate mammary tissue: Reversal by antiestrogens LY 156758 and tamoxifen. *Proc Natl Acad Sci USA* 80:4144–4148, 1983
19. Meites J, Sgouris JT: Effects of altering the balance between prolactin and ovarian hormones on initation of lactation in rabbits. *Endocrinology* 55:530–534, 1954
20. Kuhn NJ: Progesterone withdrawal as the lactogenic trigger in the rat. *J Endocrinol* 44:39–54, 1969
21. Noel GL, Suh HK, Frantz AG: Prolactin release during nursing and breast stimulation in postpartum and non-postpartum subjects. *J Clin Endocrinol Metab* 38:413–423, 1974
22. Kleinberg DL, Todd J: Evidence that human growth hormone is a potent lacogen in primates. *J Clin Endocrinol Metab* 51:1009–1013, 1980
23. Womack WS, Smith SW, Allen GM, et al: A comparison of hormone therapies for suppression of lactation. *South Med J* 55:816, 1962
24. Markin KE, Wolst MD: A comparative controlled study of hormones used in the prevention of postpartum breast engorgement and lactation. *Am J Obstet Gynecol* 50:467, 1945
25. Tindall VR: Factors influencing puerperal thromboembolism. *Br J Obstet Gynaecol* 75:1324, 1968
26. Turnbull AC: Puerperal thromboembolism and the suppression of lactation. *Br J Obstet Gynaecol* 75:1321, 1968
27. Varga L, Lutterbeck PM, Pryor JS, et al: Suppression of puerperal lactation with an ergot alkaloid: A double-blind study. *Br Med J* 2:743–744, 1972
28. Sheehan HL: The incidence of postpartum hypopituitarism. *Am J Obstet Gynecol* 68:202–223, 1954
29. Hwang P, Guyda H, Friesen H: A radioimmunoassay for human prolactin. *Proc Natl Acad Sci USA* 68:1902–1906, 1971
30. Kleinberg DL, Noel GL, Frantz AG: Galactorrhea: A study of 235 cases, including 48 with pituitary tumors. *N Engl J Med* 296:589–600, 1977
31. Boyd AE III, Reichlin S, Turksov RN: Galactorrhea-amenorrhea syndrome: Diagnosis and therapy. *Ann Intern Med* 87:165–175, 1977
32. Tolis G, Somma M, Van Compenhout J, et al: Prolactin secretion in 65 patients with galactorrhea. *Am J Obstet Gynecol* 118:91–101, 1974
33. Gomez F, Reyes FI, Faiman C: Nonpuerperal galactorrhea and hyperprolactinemia. Clinical findings, endocrine features and therapeutic responses in 56 cases. *Am J Med* 62:648–660, 1977
34. Haagensen CD: *Diseases of the Breast*. Philadelphia, Saunders, 1971, p 778
35. Forbes AP, Henneman PH, Griswold GC, et al: Syndrome characterized by galactorrhea, amenorrhea and low urinary FSH: Comparison with acromegaly and normal lactation. *J Clin Endocrinol Metab* 14:265–271, 1954
36. Vacca LL, Rosario SL, Zimmerman EA, et al: Application of immunoperoxidase techniques to localize horseradish peroxidase-tracer in the central nervous system. *J Histochem Cytochem* 23:208–215, 1975
37. Antunes JL, Housepian EM, Frantz AG, et al: Prolactin-secreting pituitary tumors. *Ann Neurol* 2:148–153, 1977
38. Seppala M, Hirvonen E, Rauta T: Hyperprolactinemia and luteal insufficiency. *Lancet* 1:229, 1976
39. Dunaif AE, Zimmerman EA, Frantz AG, et al: Prolactin and its receptor: Intracellular localization in the ovary by immunoperoxidase technique. *Clin Res* 25:293A, 1977
40. McNatty KP, Sawres RS, McNeilly AS: A possible role

for prolactin in control of steroid secretion by the human graafian follicle. *Nature (Lond)* 250:653–655, 1974

40a. Demura R, Ono M, Demura H, Shizume K, Oouchi H: Prolactin directly inhibits basal as well as gonadotropin-stimulated secretion of progesterone and and 17 β-estradiol in the human ovary. *J Clin Endocrinol Metab* 54:1246–1250, 1982

41. Sauder SE, Frager M, Case GD, Kelch RP, Marshall JC: Abnormal patterns of pulsatile luteinizing hormone secretion in women with hyperprolactinemia and amenorrhea: responses to bromocriptine. *J Clin Endocrinol Metab* 59:941–948, 1984

41a. Klibanski A, Beitins IZ, Merriam GR, McArthur JW, Zervas NT, Ridgway EC: Gonadotropin and prolactin pulsations in hyperprolactinemic women before and during bromocriptine therapy. *J Clin Endocrinol Metab* 58:1141–1147, 1984

42. Horn K, Erhardt F, Fahlbusch R, et al: Recurrent goiter, hyperthyroidism, galactorrhea and amenorrhea due to a thyrotropin and prolactin-producing pituitary tumor. *J Clin Endocrinol Metab* 43:137, 1976

43. Levin ME, Daughaday WH, Levy I: Persistent lactation associated with pituitary tumor and hyperadrenal corticism. *Am J Med* 27:172–175, 1959

44. Kleinberg DL, Noel GL, Frantz AG: Chlorpromazine stimulation and L-dopa suppression of prolactin in man. *J Clin Endocrinol Metab* 33:873–876, 1971

45. Barbarino A, De Marinis L, Maira G, et al: Serum prolactin response to thyrotropin-releasing hormone and metoclopramide in patients with prolactin-secreting tumors before and after transsphenoidal surgery. *J Clin Endocrinol Metab* 47:1148–1151, 1978

46. Koppelman MCS, Jaffe MJ, Rieth KH, et al: Hyperprolactimenia, amenorrhea and galactorrhea. *Ann Intern Med* 100:115–121, 1984

47. March CM, Kletzky OA, Davajan V, et al: Longitudinal evaluation of patients with untreated prolactin-secreting pituitary adenomas. *Am J Obstet Gynecol* 139:835–844, 1981

48. Klibanski A, Neer RM, Beitins IZ, et al: Decreased bone density in hyperprolactinemic women. *N Engl J Med* 303:1511–1514, 1980

49. Hardy J: Transsphenoidal surgery of hypersecreting pituitary tumors, in Kohler PO, Ross GT (eds): *Diagnosis and Treatment of Pituitary Tumors.* New York, American Elsevier, 1973

50. Randall RV, Laws ER Jr, Abboud CF, et al: Transsphenoidal microsurgical treatment and prolactin producing pituitary adenomas: Results in 100 patients. *Mayo Clin Proc* 58:108–121, 1983

51. Corenblum B, Webster BR, Mortimer CS, et al: Possible antitumor effect of 2 bromo-ergocriptine (CB-154 Sandoz) in 2 patients with large prolactin secreting pituitary adenomas. *Clin Res* 23:614A, 1975

52. Lamberts SWJ, Klijn JGM, DeLange SA, et al: The incidence of complications during pregnancy after treatment of hyperprolactinemia with bromocriptine in patients with radiologically evident pituitary tumors. *Fertil Steril* 31(6):614–619, 1979

53. Post K, Biler B, Adelman L, et al: Selective transsphenoidal adenomectomy in women with galactorrhea-amenorrhea. *JAMA* 242:158–162, 1979

54. Tindall GT, McLanahan CS, Christy JH: Transsphenoidal microsurgery for pituitary tumors associated with hyperprolactinemia. *J Neurosurg* 48:849–860, 1978

55. Wilson CB, Dempsey LC: Transsphenoidal microsurgical removal of 250 pituitary adenomas. *J Neurosurg* 48:13–22, 1978

56. Serri O, Rasio E, Beauregard H, et al: Recurrence of hyperprolactinemia after selective transsphenoidal adenomectomy in women with prolactinoma. *N Engl J Med* 309:280–283, 1983

57. Laws ER: Role of surgery in the management of prolactin adenomas, in McCleod R (ed): *Fourth International Congress on Prolactin Proceedings.* New York, Raven, 1985

58. Besser GM, Parke L, Edwards CRW, et al: Galactorrhoea: Successful treatment with reduction of plasma prolactin levels by bromoergocriptine. *Br Med J* 3:669–672, 1972

59. Besser GM, Thorner MO: Bromocriptine in the treatment of the hyperprolactinemia-hypogonadism syndromes. *Postgrad Med J* 52:64–70, 1976

60. Del Pozo E, Brun Del Re R, Varga L, et al: The inhibition of prolactin secretion in man by CB-154 (2-Br-α-ergocriptine). *J Clin Endocrinol Metab* 35:768–771, 1972

61. Friesen HG, Tolis G: The use of bromocriptine in the galactorrhea-amenorrhea syndromes: The Canadian cooperative study. *Clin Endocrinol [Suppl]* 6:91s–99s, 1977

62. George SR, Burrow GN, Zinman B, et al: Regression of pituitary tumors, a possible effect of bromergocriptine. *Am J Med* 66:697–702, 1979

63. McGregor AM, Scanlon MF, Hall K, et al: *Reduction in size of a pituitary tumor by bromocriptine therapy.* N Engl J Med 300:291–293, 1979

64. Thorner MO, Gluckiger E, Calne DB (eds): *Bromocriptine—A Clinical and Pharmacological Review.* New York, Raven, 1980, pp 56–99

65. Von Werder K, Fahlbusch R, Rjosk H-K: Bromocriptine therapy of macroprolactinomas. *Neuroendocrinol Lett* 3:328, 1981 (abst)

66. Bonneville JF, Poulignot D, Cattin F, et al: Computed tomographic demonstration of the effects of bromocriptine on pituitary microadenoma size. *Radiology* 143:451–455, 1982

67. Kleinberg DL, Boyd AE III, Wardlaw S, Frantz AG, George A, Bryon H, Hilas S, Greising J, Hamilton D, Seltzer T and Sommers CJ: Treatment of prolactin and growth hormone secreting pituitary tumors with pergolide. *N Engl J Med* 309:704–709, 1983

68. Dominque JN, Richmond IL, Wilson CB: Results of surgery in 114 patients with prolactin secreting adenomas. *Am J Obstet Gynecol* 137:102–108, 1980

69. Emani B: Conventional radiotherapy and pituitary tumors, in Post KD, Jackson IMD, Reichlin S (eds): *The Pituitary Adenoma.* New York, Plenum, 1980, pp 437–458

70. Sheline GE: Treatment of chromophobe adenomas of the pituitary gland and acromegaly, in Kohler PO, Ross GT (eds): *Diagnosis and Treatment of Pituitary Tumors.* Amsterdam, Excerpta Medica, 1973, pp 201–216.

71. Wollesen F, Andersen T, Karle A: Size reduction of extrasellar pituitary tumors during bromocriptine treatment. *Ann Intern Med* 96:281–286, 1982

72. Sobrinho LG, Nunes MC, Calhaz-Jorge C, et al: Effect of treatment with bromocriptine on the size and activity of prolactin producing pituitary tumors. *Acta Endocrinol (Copenh)* 96:24–29, 1981

73. Spark RF, Baker R, Beinfang DC, et al: Bromocriptine

reduces pituitary tumor size and hypersecretion. Requiem for pituitary surgery? *JAMA* 247:311–316, 1982

74. Wass JAH, Williams J, Charlesworth M, et al: Bromocriptine in the management of large pituitary tumors. *Br Med J* 284:1908–1911, 1982

75. Prescott RWG, Johnston DG, Taylor P, et al: Hyperprolactinaemia men—Response to bromocriptine therapy. *Lancet* 1:245–248, 1982

76. Weiss MH, Wycott RN, Yardley R, et al: Bromocriptine treatment of prolactin-secreting tumors: Surgical implications. *Neurosurgery* 12:640–642, 1983

77. Thorner MO, Martin WH, Rogol AD, et al: Rapid regression of pituitary prolactinomas during bromocriptine treatment. *J Clin Endocrinol Metab* 51:438–445, 1980

78. Thorner MO, Perryman RL, Rogol AD, et al: Rapid changes of prolactinoma volume after withdrawal and re-institution of bromocriptine. *J Clin Endocrinol Metab* 53:480–483, 1981

79. Tindall GT, Kovacs K, Horvath E, et al: Human prolactin-producing adenomas and bromocriptine: A histological, immunocytochemical, ultrastructural, and morphometric study. *J Clin Endocrinol Metab* 55:1178–1183, 1982

80. Rengachary SS, Tomita T, Jefferies BF, et al: Structural changes in human pituitary tumor after bromocriptine therapy. *Neurosurgery* 10:242–251, 1982

81. Thorner MO, Edwards CRW, Charlesworth M, et al: Pregnancy in patients presenting with hyperprolactinaemia. *Br Med J* 2:771–774, 1979

82. Bergh T, Nillius SJ, Enoksson P, et al: Bromocriptine-induced pregnancies in women with large prolactinomas. *Clin Endocrin* 17:625–631, 1982

83. Bergh T, Nillius SJ, Wide L: Clinical course and outcome of pregnancies in amenorrhoeic women with hyperprolactinaemia and pituitary tumours. *Br Med J* 8:875–880, 1978

84. Child DF, Gordon H, Mashiter K, Joplin GF: Pregnancy, prolactin, and pituitary tumours. *Br Med J* 4:87–89, 1975

85. Kelly WF, Doyle FH, Mashiter K, et al: Pregnancies in women with hyperprolactinaemia: Clinical course obstetric complications of 41 pregnancies in 27 women. *Br J Obstet Gynecol* 86:698–705, 1979

86. Lamberts SWJ, Seldenrath HJ, Kwa HG, et al: Transient bitemporal hemianopsia during pregnancy after treatment of galactorrhea-amenorrhea syndrome with bromocriptine. *J Clin Endocrinol Metab* 44:180–184, 1977

87. Dommerholt HBR, Assies J, Van Der Werf AJM: Growth of a prolactinoma during pregnancy. *Obstet Gynecol* 61:117–120, 1983

88. Maeda T, Ushiroyama T, Okuda K, et al: Effective bromocriptine treatment of a pituitary macroadenoma during pregnancy. *Obstet Gynecol* 61:117–120, 1983

89. Turkatj I, Braun P, Krupp P: Surveillance of bromocriptine in pregnancy. *JAMA* 247(11):1589–1591, 1982

90. Argonz J, del Castillo EB: A syndrome characterized by estrogenic insufficiency, galactorrhea and decreased urinary gonadotropin. *J Clin Endocrinol Metab* 13:79–87, 1953

91. Sharp EA: Historical review of a syndrome embracing utero-ovarian atrophy with persistent lactation (Frommel's disease). *Am J Obstet Gynecol* 30:411–414, 1935

92. Lippard CH: The Chiari-Frommel syndrome. *Am J Obstet Gynecol* 82:724–726, 1961

93. Greenblatt RB, Carmona N, Hagler WS: Chiari- Frommel syndrome. A syndrome characterized by galactorrhea, amenorrhea and pituitary dysfunction: Report of two cases. *Obstet Gynecol* 7:165–170, 1956

94. Ehni G, Eckles NE: Interruption of pituitary stalk in the patient with mammary cancer. *J Neurosurg* 16:628–652, 1959

95. Grossman S, Buchberg AB, Brecher E, et al: Idiopathic lactation following thoracoplasty. *J Clin Endocrinol* 10:729–734, 1950

96. Salkin D, Davis EW: Lactation following thoracoplasty and pneumonectomy. *J Thorac Surg* 18:580–590, 1949

97. Sachs HB: Lactation after hysterectomy in a nulliparous woman. *Am J Obstet Gynecol* 78:204–207, 1959

98. Lavoie J: Lactation after surgery. *Can J Surg* 11:464–465, 1968

99. Noel GL, Suh HK, Stone JC, et al: Human prolactin and growth hormone release during surgery and other conditions of stress. *J Clin Endocrinol Metab* 35:66–77, 1972

100. Everard JR, Buxton BH, Erickson D: Amenorrhea following oral contraception. *Am J Obstet Gynecol* 124:88–91, 1976

101. Gambrell RD, Greenblatt RB, Mahesh VB: Post-pill and pill-related amenorrhea-galactorrhea. *Am J Obstet Gynecol* 110:838–848, 1971

102. Shearman RP: Prolonged secondary amenorrhea after oral contraceptive therapy. *Lancet* 1:64–66, 1971

103. Gregg WI: Galactorrhea after contraceptive hormones. *N Engl J Med* 273:1432, 1966

104. Hooper JH Jr, Welch VC, Shackelford RT: Abnormal lactation associated with tranquilizing drug therapy. *JAMA* 178:506–507, 1961

105. Koang NK, Tseng-Chi H, Chia-Lun J, et al: Endocrine function during treatment of pulmonary tuberculosis with INH. *China Med J* 75:100–109, 1957

106. Van Wyk JJ, Grumbach MM: Syndrome of precocious menstruation and galactorrhea in juvenile hypothyroidism: An example of hormonal overlap in pituitary feedback. *J Pediatr* 57:416–435, 1960

107. Jackson, WPU: Post-thyroidectomy hypothyroidism, hypoparathyroidism, exopthalmos and galactorrhea with normal menstruation. *J Clin Endocrinol Metab* 16:1245–1250, 1956

108. Kinch RAH, Plunkett ER, Devlin MC: Postpartum amenorrhea-galactorrhea of hypothyroidism. *Am J Obstet Gynecol* 105:766–773, 1969

109. Ross F, Nusynowitz ML: A syndrome of primary hypothyroidism, amenorrhea and galactorrhea. *J Clin Endocrinol Metab* 28:591–595, 1968

110. Boroditsky RS, Faiman C: Galactorrhea-amenorrhea due to primary hypothyroidism. *Am J Obstet Gynecol* 116:661–665, 1973

111. Edwards CRW, Forsyth IA, Besser GM: Amenorrhoea, galactorrhoea, and primary hypothyroidism with high circulating levels of prolactin. *Br Med J* 3:462–464, 1971

112. Kleinberg DL: Pituitary tumors and failure of endocrine target organs. *Arch Intern Med* 1979

113. Bar RS, Mazzaferri EL, Malarkey WB: Primary empty sella, galactorrhea, hyperprolactinemia and renal tubular acidosis. *Am J Med* 59:863–866, 1975

114. Brisman R, Hughes JEO, Holub DA: Endocrine function in 19 patients with empty sella syndrome. *J Clin Endocrinol Metab* 34:570–573, 1972

115. Neelon FA, Goree JA, Lebovitz HE: The primary empty

sella: Clinial and radiographic characteristics and endocrine function. *Medicine (Baltimore)* 52:73–92, 1973

116. Silverman VE, Boyd AE III, McCrary JA, et al: Pituitary apoplexy following chlorpromazine stimulation. *Arch Intern Med* 1978

117. Varga L, Wenner R, del Pozo E: Treatment of galactorrhea-amenorrhea syndrome with Br-ergocriptine (CB 154) restoration with ovulatory function and fertility. *Am J Obstet Gynecol* 117:75, 1973

118. Boyar RM, Kapen S, Finkelstein JW, et al: Hypothalamic-pituitary function in diverse hyperprolactinemic states. *J Clin Invest* 53:1588–1598, 1974

119. Chiodini P, Liuzzi A, Cozzi R, et al: Size reduction of macroprolactinomas by bromocriptine or lisuride treatment. *J Clin Endocrinol Metab* 53:737–743, 1981

ANSWERS

1. c

2. a

Hormone-Producing Tumors of the Ovary and Placenta

FRANK E. CHANG and MOON H. KIM

INTRODUCTION

As the ovary and placenta are endocrine organs, any neoplastic lesion arising from them may be active in hormone production. Although rare, they present interesting and challenging problems to clinicians. Hormone-producing ovarian tumors make up approximately 5% of all ovarian tumors. The histological diversity of these tumors is great and includes both primary and metastatic tumors of the ovary. Table 25-1 classifies these hormone-producing tumors into five major categories. Although androgens and estrogens are the most common hormones secreted by these tumors, human chorionic gonadotropin (hCG), thyroxine (T4), serotonin, and human placental lactogen (hPL) may be secreted as well. The clinical presentation is therefore extremely interesting in many of these cases. Although in vivo and in vitro studies of hormone production as well as ultrastructural studies have increased our understanding of these tumors, the histogenesis and pathophysiology of many of these tumors remains poorly understood. The trophoblastic diseases, hydatidiform mole and choriocar-

cinoma, are well known for their secretion of chorionic gonadotropin. With advanced chemotherapy, the treatment of these conditions has been successful. Although chorionic gonadotropin, particularly the β-subunit, serves as a biological marker, these trophoblastic neoplasms also produce other peptide hormones and steroid hormones.

OVARIAN TUMORS

Gonadal Stromal–Sex Cord Tumors of the Ovary

The embryological derivation of granulosa cells, theca cells, Sertoli-Leydig cells, and fibroblasts is unresolved. The classification of the ovarian tumors composed primarily of these cell types is therefore not uniform. Various investigators believe that granulosa cells and Sertoli cells are formed from the mesonephric and coelomic epithelial components of the sex cords.[1] Others dispute this epithelial derivation, citing the inability to demonstrate sex cord formation embryologically in the ovary. Instead, they believe that the granulosa and Sertoli cells are derived primarily from the mesenchymal anlages and should therefore be classified as gonadal–stromal tumors.[2] The World Health Organization (WHO) classification for this

FRANK E. CHANG and MOON H. KIM • Department of Obstetrics and Gynecology, Ohio State University Hospitals, Columbus, Ohio 43210.

501

TABLE 25-1. Classification of Hormone-Producing Tumors

Category	Hormones produced
1. Gonadal stromal–sex cord tumors	
Granulosa/thecal tumors	Estrogens, androgens
Sertoli–Leydig tumors	Androgens, estrogens
Gynandroblastomas	Estrogens, androgens
2. Functioning stromal tumors	Androgens, estrogens
Brenner tumor	
Fibroma	
Cystadenoma	
Metastatic carcinoma	
Gonadal dysgenesis	
3. Germ cell tumors	
Choriocarcinomas	hCH, hPL
Teratomas	Thyroxine, serotonin, hCG
Dysgerminomas	hCG, androgens, estrogens
4. Mixed germ cell and stromal tumor	Androgens, estrogens
Gonadoblastomas	
5. Hyperplasia	Androgens
Luteoma of pregnancy	
Hilus cell hyperplasia	

group of tumors (Table 25-2) does not resolve this issue, as it groups them under the combined heading of gonadal–stromal sex cord tumors of the ovary.

Granulosa Cell Tumor

Eighty percent of all gonadal–stromal sex cord tumors are granulosa cell tumors. They are classically associated with estrogen secretion, although certain granulosa cell tumors are virilizing.[3–6] The granulosa cell tumor is a low-grade malignancy; recurrences can occur as late as 20 years after the initial treatment.

Pathology. Frequently granulosa cell tumors are classified as granulosa–theca tumors because of the

TABLE 25-2. Classification of Gonadal Stromal–Sex Cord Tumors

Granulosa–stromal cell tumors
  Granulosa cell tumor
  Thecoma–fibroma
Sertoli–Leydig (androblastomas)
  Well differentiated
    Tubular adenoma of Pick
    Folliculome lipidique of Lecene (lipid filled)
    Sertoli–Leydig cell
Gynadroblastoma

common association of granulosa cells and theca cells in these tumors. Pure granulosa cell tumors or pure thecomas are not as frequently found as the mixed granulosa–theca tumors. Macroscopically, the granulosa cell tumors range from a few millimeters in size to extremely large tumors weighing more than 30 lb. They comprise 10% of all solid ovarian tumors, and 95% of them are unilateral. The larger granulosa cell tumors tend to be solid with cystic areas separated by friable, yellowish tissue, often with areas of necrosis.[7]

Microscopically, the pure granulosa cell tumors are highly differentiated. The typical microfollicular pattern, consisting of Call-Exner bodies, is often seen. These bodies consist of small cavities filled with eosinophilic fluid surrounded by granulosa cells that have "grooved" nuclei. Varying amounts of stromal tissue are found interspersed among the granulosa cells and luteinization of both granulosa and theca cells occasionally occurs.

Clinical and Endocrinological Aspects. These tumors are generally classified as feminizing tumors. They may occur at any age and because of the estrogen production by these tumors, may result in menstrual disorders. In very young girls, isosexual pseudoprecocity may be the first signs of an estrogen-producing tumor.[8] Thelarche and menarche are noted prematurely, and occasionally accelerated growth may occur. Regression of secondary sexual characteristics, however, occurs with the removal of these tumors in prepubertal girls. Women of reproductive age typically complain of irregular menses, dysfunctional uterine bleeding, and breast tenderness. Any postmenopausal woman who manifests signs of increased estrogen production, should be evaluated for the possibility of an estrogen-producing tumor. Because these tumors can reach very large sizes, patients may initially present with abdominal fullness and discomfort and occasionally even present with an acute abdomen due to rupture of the tumor.

Virilization occurs in 2–3% of patients with granulosa cell tumors,[3–6] occurring more often with the more cystic tumors.[5] Microscopically, these virilizing granulosa cell tumors have no Leydig cells nor are there any elements suggestive of it being a gynandroblastoma. The androgens are believed to be most likely produced by the luteinized stromal tissue rather than the granulosa cells. Estrogen production from the tumor was originally thought to be from the granulosa cells exclusively, but histochemical studies and ultrastructural studies have indicated that the theca cell in combination with the granulosa cell probably are the sources of estrogen production.[2,9] Tumors that consist almost entirely of granulosa cells with no theca cells, however, still have areas of stroma that are luteinized and able to produce estrogens.

Because of increased production of estrogen, women with estrogen-producing tumors are at risk of developing endometrial hyperplasia and adenocarcinoma of the endometrium. Fox et al.[10] noted that 6.5% of their series of patients with granulosa cell tumors had endometrial adenocarcinoma. McDonald et al.[11] reviewed 72 cases of endometrial adenocarcinoma associated with a feminizing tumor of the ovary. The endometrial cancer in these patients tended to be of a lower grade and stage, with a much higher 5-year survival rate than was found in patients whose endometrial cancers were not associated with a feminizing tumor.

Reported 10-year survival rates for patients with granulosa cell tumors range from 60 to 90%.[8,12] Initial treatment is dictated by the extent and spread of the tumor, the age of the patient and her wishes regarding future pregnancies. The degree of differentiation of the tumor does not correlate with the risk of recurrence or metastases, although the tumors showing capsular and lymphatic invasion tend to recur.[2] It is recommended that postmenopausal women or women with large tumors undergo total abdominal hysterectomy and bilateral salpingo-oophorectomy. Unilateral oophorectomy and long-term follow-up consisting of frequent pelvic examinations and monitoring of estrogen levels is a reasonable approach for younger women with unilateral involvement. Most recurrences are confined to the pelvis or abdominal cavity although occasionally distant metastases may be found. Response to chemotherapy and irradiation are unpredictable at best and should be reserved for the treatment of recurrences.[13] Monitoring of serum estradiol levels serves as a biological marker.

Thecomas

The pure thecomas, or fibrothecomas, do not have the typical Call-Exner bodies characteristic of the granulosa cell tumors. Thecomas tend to be more solid and firm in consistency. Microscopically, the cells are elongated with oval-shaped nuclei, so that these cells closely resemble fibroblasts. They can contain varying amounts of lipid within the cells and can even be confused with Sertoli–Leydig tumors. The pure thecoma is almost always benign. Occasionally, thecomas can be virilizing or associated with estrogen production although generally they are endocrinologically inert.[2,8,14] Treatment consists of a unilateral oophorectomy in younger patients, as most cases are unilateral.

Sertoli–Leydig Cell Tumors

Sertoli–Leydig cell tumors, also known as androblastomas or arrhenoblastomas, are generally considered virilizing ovarian tumors. They can be, however, endocrinologically inactive or even feminizing. They are considered of low-grade malignancy and are very rare tumors. Approximately 0.5% of all ovarian tumors fall within this category.[15]

Pathology. Grossly these tumors may be microscopic in size, although very large tumors may be encountered. They resemble granulosa–theca tumors grossly and are generally solid. Cystic and hemorrhagic areas are noted in the larger tumors. The solid tumors (unilateral in 95% of cases) are yellowish in color and rubbery in consistency, and there is rarely any extension of the tumor beyond its capsule.

It is simplest to think of these tumors as attempts to recapitulate an early stage of testicular differentiation. Microscopically, Sertoli-like cells make up immature seminiferouslike tubules that can vary greatly in their differentiation. The highly well-differentiated tumor that consists entirely of these cordlike patterns are considered pure Sertoli cell tumors, also known as tubular androblastomas, or Pick's adenoma. These highly differentiated tumors are generally inactive endocrinologically whereas the undifferentiated forms are usually virilizing, and occasionally feminizing.

The second type of cell found in other tumors of this group, except the pure Sertoli cell tumor, is the hilar, or Leydig cell. These cells are polygonal in shape, usually found in clusters near the hilar region of the ovary and contain varying amounts of lipid. They are homologous to the Leydig cell of the male gonad and are derived from the gonadal stroma. They are thought to be primarily responsible for the androgen production. The characteristic Reinke crystal, an eosinophilicprotein secretion, is a long rodlike structure found in the cytoplasm of the hilar or Leydig cell. The crystals are often surrounded by a clear halo when stained with hematoxylin and eosin. The Sertoli–Leydig tumor therefore is a combination of these two cell types in the same tumor. The degree of differentiation varies between these two cell types, so that at times it may be difficult to decide whether these tumors are sarcomas. Occasionally glandular tissue, muscle cells, neural tissue, and even cartilage may be found interspersed in this tumor.[15]

At the opposite end of the Sertoli–Leydig continuum is the pure Leydig cell or hilus cell tumor, which is unilateral in 95% of cases. Because they resemble adrenal cortex cells at times, they have also been classified as adrenal rest tumors or lipoid cell tumors. These tumors consist of lipid containing cells that usually contain the Reinke crystals resembling Leydig cells. Grossly these tumors may be small nodules in the hilar region of the ovary, or they may only be microscopic in size although the largest tumor reported is 15 cm.

Clinical Aspects. These tumors are most often found in women less than 40 years of age and are more common in women aged 20–30 years. Although classically thought of as masculinizing tumors, a significant proportion are nonsteroidogenic or even feminizing.[16,17] The patient with a virilizing tumor usually will present first with signs of defeminization, such as secondary amenorrhea, regression of breast development, and loss of typical female contours. Gradually the patient notices hirsutism and, in extreme cases, clitoromegaly and even temporal balding. These tumors can be quite small, and the diagnosis may be very difficult.

Evaluation should consist of baseline androgen studies, including serum testosterone, dehydroep-iandrosterone sulfate (DHEA-S), and androstenedione or urinary 17-ketosteroids (17-KS). Typically these patients will have very elevated testosterone and androstenedione levels with marginally elevated or normal serum DHEA-S or urinary 17-KS. The differential diagnosis should be entertained to exclude adrenal pathology such as virilizing adrenal adenoma or Cushing's syndrome. Generally there is poor suppression of the elevated serum androgens with dexamethasone or oral contraceptives. Occasionally pelvic ultrasounds or abdominal–pelvic computed tomograph (CT) scans may help in evaluating the size of the ovaries or adrenals, although with smaller tumors the scans may be normal. Selective catheterization angiographically may demonstrate an abnormal secretion of testosterone from one ovary in cases in which scans are not diagnostic,[18,19] but they are rarely indicated clinically.

Both in vivo studies in vitro studies of Leydig cell tumors have demonstrated that the major secretory products from these tumors are testosterone and androstenedione.[20,21] Even in patients with feminizing signs, there does not appear to be excessive estrogen secretion from the tumor suggesting that peripheral conversion of elevated serum androgens to estrogens may account for the feminization.

As most of these tumors are unilateral, therapy may consist of unilateral oophorectomy in younger women as long as there appears to be no metastasis or involvement of the contralateral ovary. In patients with large tumors or in older patients, total abdominal hysterectomy and bilateral salpingo-oophorectomy is recommended. Generally, virilization will regress, and feminization will return in women who preserve functioning ovarian tissue.

Gynandroblastoma

The gynandroblastoma is an extremely rare group of ovarian tumors, first described by Meyer in 1930.[22] This tumor consists histologically of both granulosa cell elements and arrhenoblastoma elements. Clinically the patient may be virilized and/or have signs of feminization, however the diagnosis can only be made histologically. Grossly the tumor is usually a few centimeters in size and often multilocular. Microscopically, cells similar to Sertoli cells and granulosa cells are intermixed. These tumors are almost always benign and unilateral oophorectomy or total abdominal hysterectomy and bilateral salpingo-oophorectomy is indicated, depending on the age of the paitent.

Tumors with Functioning Stroma

Primary ovarian tumors, which are considered endocrinologically inert, can be associated with ovarian hypersecretion of both estrogens and androgens. Similarly, metastatic lesions to the ovary can also be associated with feminization or virilization in certain patients.[2,23] Clearly these tumors or metastases are not the source of these hormones but there seems to be an undefined mechanism by which they stimulate the ovary to hypersecrete these hormones.

The types of tumors involved are varied, and include Brenner tumors, fibromas, cystadenomas, benign teratomas, and the Krukenberg tumors of the ovary.[2,23,24] Most cases are associated with feminization although virilization is occasionally seen. Apparently the luteinized stroma often found in these cases is responsible for the steroid production. The mechanism by which the stromal tissue is initially stimulated is unclear. Woodruff and others believe that mechanical stimulation of the stroma by the proliferating tissue is responsible.[23,25] Others have speculated that some undefined substance, perhaps hCG is secreted by the tumor which then stimulates the ovarian stroma.[2]

Patients with pure gonadal dysgenesis have been noted on occasion to have hirsutism as well.[26,27] These patients are phenotypically female but have streak gonads which lack ova. Karyotypically, these patients may be 46XX, 46XY, or 45X, and all three have been associated with virilism.[27-29] It may be that hilus cells, which are hyperplastic in some of these dysgenetic ovaries, may be responsible for the increased androgen production or that excessively stimulated luteinized stroma may be implicated.[26]

Germ Cell Tumors

Germ cell tumors are endocrinologically very interesting, as they may secrete a variety of hormones.[30,31] These tumors are derived from germ cells that migrate from the yolk sac to the gonadal ridge. The specific hormone-producing tumors listed in Table 25-1 are all grouped under germ cell tumors because of their presumed common histogenesis.

Dysgerminoma

Meyer[22] first described the dysgerminoma in 1931 as a tumor consisting of cells resembling earlier undifferentiated germ cells. While it is a malignant tumor, it has a comparatively higher 5-year survival rate in relationship to the other malignant germ cell tumors. The dysgerminoma occurs most frequently in women under 30 years of age and make up 3–5% of all ovarian malignancies.[32,33]

Pure dysgerminomas are solid tumors with areas of necrosis and hemorrhage. Usually they are unilateral, yellow or gray in color, ranging in diameter from a few centimeters to up to 50 cm.[34] Microscopically the cells are typically large, polygonal cells with a basophilic staining cytoplasm. These cells are grouped uniformly in islands or cords, separated by lymphocytic stroma. The nuclei are prominent and ovoid or round in shape.

The pure dysgerminomas are considered endocrinologically inert. However, several cases of precocious puberty, virilism, and elevated hCG titers have been associated with supposedly pure dysgerminomas.[34-36] Most commonly, dysgerminomas are associated with other germ cell elements, such as syncytiotrophoblastic or choriocarcinomatous cells.[37] These other cell types are responsible for hormonal secretion. Androgens can be secreted by luteinized stroma, occasionally found with dysgerminomas.

Treatment for most cases should consist of a total abdominal hysterectomy and bilateral salpingo-oophorectomy plus external radiation for cases where spread has been documented. It is sensitive to radiation therapy. In very young girls or women desiring to maintain their reproductive function, a conservative salpingo-oophorectomy for a localized dysgerminoma may be performed if bisection of the remaining ovary and node sampling prove negative. It is useful to follow hCG titers for those patients who present with elevated hCG titers.

Choriocarcinoma

Pure choriocarcinoma of the ovary is rare. Choriocarcinoma may be nongestational or gestational in nature, and it may be associated with other germ cell elements to form a mixed germ cell tumor. Gestational choriocarcinoma of the ovary may result from metastases from an intrauterine or ectopic gestation, or it may be associated with an ovarian pregnancy.

Prognostically, it is important to differentiate between nongestational and gestational choriocarcinoma of the ovary if possible. Gestational choriocarcinoma generally responds to single agent chemotherapy, either methotrexate or actinomycin

D.[38] By contrast, nongestational choriocarcinoma carries a poor prognosis and responds poorly even to a triple chemotherapeutic regimen.[39] Both types of tumors consist of hemorrhagic cystic masses, although the mixed germ cell tumors tend to have more solid components. Microscopically, both tumors contain syncytiotrophoblastic and cytotrophoblastic cells. hCG is produced by the syncytiotrophoblast in varying amounts. Quantification, although useful for follow-up, cannot differentiate between the gestational and nongestational ovarian choriocarcinoma.[40] hPL has recently been found in a large percentage of patients with ovarian choriocarcinoma.[41] It has not proved a clinically useful marker, however.

Treatment is initially surgical. In a young patient, unilateral adnexectomy may be performed if the tumor is small and confined to the ovary. More extensive involvement of the tumor dictates a more extensive surgical approach. Chemotherapy following surgical treatment is indicated.

Teratomas

Teratomas can be classified as either immature malignant teratomas or mature benign teratomas. The mature teratomas producing hormones can be further subclassified so as to include the predominantly monodermal tumors, the most common being the struma ovarii and carcinoid types.

Struma Ovarii. Boettlin was first to describe the presence of thyroid tissue in an ovarian dermoid in 1839. Thryoid tissue is found in anywhere from 7 to 20% of dermoid cysts; however, the term *struma ovarii* is reserved for tumors that consist of at least 50% thyroid tissue. The incidence of struma ovarii is approximately 2.7% of ovarian teratomas. Clinically only 5% of these patients have evidence of being hyperthyroid.[42] Thyrotoxicosis is extremely rare and most patients have no evidence of excessive thyroxine production.[43] Sixteen percent of patients will have an enlarged thyroid gland, and they typically regress with surgical removal of the struma ovarii.[42]

These tumors resemble thyroid glands especially when most of the tumor is found, on microscopic examination, to consist of thyroid tissue. Microscopically, the tumors resemble normal thyroid tissue with the typical eosinophilic acini lined by columnar or flat epithelial cells. Although most are benign, malignant changes have been reported.[44,45] Metastases can occur and usually involve intraperitoneal spread first. Ascites is found in 17% of cases but doesn't correlate with malignancy.[42]

Therapy consists of oophorectomy for benign struma ovarii. In cases of malignant degeneration, total abdominal hysterectomy and bilateral salpingo-oophorectomy with evaluation of the periaortic lymph nodes is indicated. This can be followed by radioactive[131] I or external radiation therapy.[46]

Carcinoid. A rare tumor, carcinoid of the ovary, is either primary or metastatic in origin. The primary ovarian carcinoid tumors consist of two types of tumors, islet carcinoid or trabecular carcinoid. These tumors are rarely malignant, but one-fourth to one-third of cases are associated with the characteristic carcinoid syndrome, which is due primarily to serotonin.

The tumor is usually solid and often resembles a solid teratoma. Microscopically, there are solid nests of polygonal cells with hyperchromatic nuclei also arranged in an acinar pattern. They are derived from enterochromaffin cells of the gastrointestinal or respiratory tract and produce serotonin.[47,48] Because the blood returned from the ovary to the systemic circulation bypasses the liver, inactivation of serotonin does not take place normally as it would with other intestinal carcinoids. Therefore, a higher percentage of patients may complain of flushing, diarrhea, or cardiovascular problems.

Treatment generally consists of excision of the ovary where local involvement only is found. Metastases of intestinal carcinoids to the ovary is rare but the prognosis in these cases is much poorer than localized primary carcinoid of the ovary.

Mixed Germ Cell and Stromal Tumor

Gonadoblastoma are tumors that consist of both germ cell elements and derivatives of sex cord stroma.[49] These tumors were first described by Scully in 1953 and are usually found in dysgenetic gonads. Typically, the patient is phenotypically female but chromatin negative in 90% of cases.[15] The karyotypes usually show Y chromosome or its fragment. More than 50% of these patients have some evidence of virilization and generally the patients have amenorrhea with poorly developed secondary sexual characteristics.

These tumors are of low malignancy potential, although when associated with other germ cell elements they may have a poorer prognosis. Grossly, these are solid tumors often with areas of calcification and hyalinization. Microscopically, they are composed of large germ cell elements surrounded by stroma. The germ cell elements are combined with cells resembling Sertoli or granulosa-type cells. The stroma usually contains luteinized stroma cells or Leydig cells, which are probably involved in androgen secretion.[50,51] Most likely, the gonadotropins are responsible for stimulating the stroma to increased androgen production, although the tumor may be autonomous in secreting hormones.[50]

Treatment consists of removing both ovaries as in most cases the ovaries are dysgenetic. Metastasis is uncommon unless associated with other germ cell elements. Unfortunately, virilization usually does not regress despite removal of the gonadoblastoma.

Luteoma of Pregnancy

An interesting and controversial entity is the luteoma of pregnancy first described by Sternberg[52] in 1963. It is characteristically a solid ovarian enlargement, either unilateral or bilateral, usually found incidentally at the time of cesarean sections or postpartum tubal ligations. It should not be considered a true neoplasm, as it almost always regresses after delivery. Its true incidence is difficult to assess, as it is associated with maternal or fetal virilization in approximately 14–40% of the documented cases.[53,54] Approximately 100 cases have been described in the literature since its initial description.[55]

Pathology. Morphologically, it is smooth, multinodular, and gray with reddish brown areas involving either one or both ovaries. Often these ovaries can be as large as 25 cm in diameter and can even lead to dystocia.[53] Microscopically, the cells are typically uniform in size and polyhedral in shape, with a slightly eosinophilic appearance. They resemble luteinized stromal tissue. Some believe that focal areas of preexisting luteinized stromal tissue become hyperplastic under the influence of chorionic gonadotropins to become luteomas.[52,56] Others believe that they are derived from luteinized theca tissue.[57] While its true origin is uncertain, it is agreed that these luteomas are separate from the corpus luteum and are not derived from them.

Clinical and Endocrinological Aspects. Unless extreme virilization occurs during pregnancy, the presence of a luteoma is rarely suspected. Although in most series, maternal and/or fetal virilization oc-

curs in only 25–30% of cases, these luteomas produce significant quantities of androgens.[54] Several in vivo and in vitro studies demonstrated that luteomas produce primarily testosterone, androstenedione, DHEA and DHEA-S.[55,58] Serum levels of estradiol and estrone (E_2 and E_1) and lower androgen concentration in cord blood (compared with maternal serum) suggest that the aromatization of androgens to estrogens in the placenta may prevent severe virilization of the fetus in many cases.[58]

Regression of these luteomas occurs spontaneously after delivery, obviating the need to remove the ovaries if a frozen section reveals a luteoma of pregnancy. However, the removal of luteoma may be considered if a female fetus is confirmed during pregnancy because of the possibility of virilization. Androgen concentrations decrease during the postpartum period, and signs of virilization eventually regress.[56]

PLACENTAL TUMORS (GESTATIONAL TROPHOBLASTIC DISEASE)

The term gestational trophoblastic disease, as its name implies, is preceded by a pregnancy. Commonly this category of placental tumors is subdivided into hydatidiform moles, invasive moles (chorioadenoma destruens) and choriocarcinoma. While the great majority of patients present with a hydatidiform mole, a significant proportion do not have regression of the disease following a dilatation and curettage (D & C) and require further evaluation and chemotherapy. Because of the great advances in chemotherapy, choriocarcinoma is no longer uniformly fatal and extremely high survival rates can be achieved even in patients with widely metastatic disease. Another great advance has been the ability to quantitate serum hCG concentrations by newer sophisticated radioimmunoassay (RIA) techniques that measure the β-subunit of the hCG molecule specifically. This has improved our ability to detect earlier choriocarcinoma as well as guide therapy.

Hydatidiform Mole and Invasive Mole

The hydatidiform mole is a pregnancy in which characteristic hydropic vesicles have replaced normal chorionic villi. They may be associated with no identifiable fetal tissue, abnormally developing embryos, or normally developing pregnancies. They are benign and regress spontaneously following a D

& C more than 80% of the time. In the remaining patients, persistently elevated hCG titers are found with persistent trophoblastic disease in the form of a locally invasive mole (chorioadenoma destruens), a persistent mole, or metastatic disease usually associated with choriocarcinoma.

Pathologically, there is a spectrum of hydatidiform changes associated with varying trophoblastic proliferation. Hydatidiform swelling of villi and the absence of normal villous blood vessels may involve only a part of the placental tissue or may be found throughout. The villi are surrounded by the proliferative trophoblastic tissue, and it is this tissue that is most helpful in determining prognosis. In general, the more proliferative anaplastic patterns are associated with persistently elevated titers later. The invasive mole is usually only locally invasive and diagnosed at the time of hysterectomy, although curettage specimens can demonstrate myometrial invasion.

The patient complains of vaginal bleeding in more than 80% of cases. The size of the uterus is greater than size for dates in 50% of cases and smaller than size for dates in 30% of cases.[59] Fetal heart tones are absent and ultrasound examination reveals the typical "snowstorm" appearance often seen with hydatidiform moles. Commonly, both ovaries are enlarged, and the typical multicystic theca–lutein cysts stimulated by very high hCG titers can be seen on ultrasound. After the initial diagnosis of a hydatidiform mole is made, a baseline chest roentgenogram should be obtained. Suction curettage followed by sharp curettage is the initial treatment of choice. Close follow-up is mandatory, as 3–5% of these patients will develop choriocarcinoma and 10–15% will have persistent trophoblastic disease or locally invasive trophoblastic disease. An enlarged uterus greater than size for dates and a very high initial hCG titer place the patient at higher risk. Initially, weekly serum β-hCG RIAs should be performed to quantitate serum hCG titers. In addition, frequent pelvic examinations are performed. hCG titers should continue to decrease and no longer be detectable after 12 weeks.[60] The patient should be on oral contraceptives, if not contraindicated, for 1 year, and titers should be followed during that time. Titers that plateau or rise mandate a thorough metastatic workup and placement on chemotherapy.

Patients with molar pregnancies can also present with signs of hyperthyroidism. hCG may be able to stimulate the thyroid in large concentrations. These patients may present in thyroid storm and have elevated free thyroxine and [131] I uptake.

Choriocarcinoma

Choriocarcinoma in the United States is relatively rare, occurring in approximately 1 of 40,000 pregnancies. With the introduction of methotrexate by Li and Hertz in 1956 for the treatment of choriocarcinoma, the survival rate for patients has increased dramatically.[61] Subsequent use of actinomycin D, chlorambucil, and other newer chemotherapeutic drugs and treatment regimens have further improved our ability to treat even widely metastatic disease successfully.

Choriocarcinoma is preceded by a hydatidiform mole in more than 50% of cases. The patient may present with abnormal vaginal bleeding and persistently elevated hCG titers or may present many months later with symptoms of metastatic disease. In more than 80% of women with metastases, the lung is involved. Thirty percent have vaginal involvement, and approximately 10% will have metastases to the brain or liver.

Grossly, the tumor appears hemorrhagic and resembles infarcted tissue. It may be very friable, and invasion deep into the myometrium is common. Microscopically, choriocarcinoma is composed of proliferating trophoblast; both syncitiotrophoblast and cytotrophoblast are found. The proliferating trophoblast is often surrounded by areas of necrosis and hemorrhage.

Treatment is based on clinical staging of the disease. The New England Trophoblastic Disease Center (NETDC) has developed a staging system that considers various factors, such as initial hCG titers, size of uterus, distant metastases, duration of disease, and previous history, which have been shown to have prognostic significance. These staging systems have proved helpful in guiding the choice of chemotherapeutic agents and regimens to obtain optimal results. Patients with initial hCG titers 100,000 mIU/ml, uterus greater than size for dates, prolonged (greater than 4 months) duration of disease prior to treatment, and distant metastases to brain and liver are placed in the high-risk category.

Methotrexate was used alone initially in the treatment of choriocarcinoma.[61] Goldstein et al.[62] introduced the use of citrovorum rescue factor in conjunction with methotrexate to reduce toxicity. Later Ross et al.[38] in 1965 added actinomycin D sequentially and achieved better results. In 1970 Hammond and Parker [63] introduced the triple chemotherapeutic regimen of methotrexate, actinomycin D and chlorambucil for the treatment of high-risk metastatic disease. Survival rates of 70–80% can be achieved in these high-risk patients.

More recently, Bagshawe[64] in 1976 introduced a seven-drug regimen that incorporated the use of very high doses of methotrexate that may be useful for patients with CNS involvement or resistance to triple chemotherapy regimens.

Surgical treatment may be performed along with adjunctive chemotherapy for certain patients no longer desiring reproductive function. Brewer et al.[28] demonstrated that hysterectomy alone for presumed localized choriocarcinoma was associated with only a 41.4% 5-year survival rate. Chemotherapy at the time of surgery is not associated with higher complication rates.

SUMMARY

Hormone-producing tumors of the ovary and placenta are very rare tumors. They often produce very interesting and diverse clinical pictures and become challenging clinical problems. Although some pure forms of tumors producing a single hormone have been found, most secrete more than one hormone. As techniques for measuring hormones have become more sophisticated, the ability to measure very small quantities of hormone has allowed for better and early diagnosis and treatment. The abnormally secreted hormones can serve as very useful markers in evaluating the effectiveness of treatment and prognosis of the diseases.

QUESTIONS

1. What is the incidence of endometrial andenocarcinoma in patients with granulosa cell tumors and what is the prognosis?

2. Describe the typical presentation of a patient with a Sertoli–Leydig tumor?

3. What factors place patients with choriocarcinoma in a high-risk category and decrease survival rates?

REFERENCES

1. Morris J, Scully RE: *Endocrine Pathology and the Ovary.* St. Louis, Mosby, 1958
2. Norris HJ, Chorlton I: Functioning tumors of the ovary. *Clin Obstet Gynecol* 17:189–228, 1974
3. Giuntoli RL, Celebre JA, Wu CH, et al: Androgenic function of a granulosa cell tumor. *Obstet Gynecol* 47:77–79, 1976
4. Ireland K, Woodruff JD: Masculinizing ovarian tumors. *Obstet Gynecol Surv* 37:603, 1982
5. Norris HJ, Taylor HB: Virilization associated with cystic granulosa tumors. *Obstet Gynecol* 34:629–635, 1969
6. Taylor HC, Velasco ME, Flores SG, et al: Amenorrhea and failure to virilize in a patient with a testosterone secreting granulosa cell tumor. *Clin Endocrinol* 16:557, 1982
7. Goldston WR, Johnston WW, Fetter BF, et al: Clinicopathologic studies in feminizing tumors of the ovary. *Am J Obstet Gynecol* 112:422–429, 1972
8. Busby T, Anderson GW: Feminizing mesenchymomas of the ovary. *Am J Obstet Gynecol* 68:1391–1420, 1954
9. Ryan KJ, Petro Z: Steroid biosynthesis by human ovarian granulosa and thecal cells. *J Clin Endocrinol Metab* 36:46–51, 1966
10. Fox H, Agrawal K, Langley F: A clinical pathological study of 92 cases of granulosa cell tumors of the ovary with specific reference to the factors influencing prognosis. *Cancer* 35:231, 1975
11. McDonald TW, Malkesian GD, Gaffey TA: Endometrial cancer associated with feminizing ovarian tumor and polycystic ovarian disease. *Obstet Gynecol* 49:654–658, 1977
12. Evans AT, Gaffey TA, Malkasian GD, et al: Clinico-pathological review of 118 granulosa and 82 theca cell tumors. *Obstet Gynecol* 55:231, 1980
13. Malkesian GD, Webb MJ, Jorsensen ED: Observations on chemotherapy of granulosa cell carcinomas and malignant ovarian teratomas. *Obstet Gynecol* 44:885, 1974
14. Nokes JM, Claiborne HA, Reingold WN: Thecoma with associated virilization. *Am J Obstet Gynecol* 78:722, 1959
15. Blaustein A (ed): *Pathology of the Female Genital Tract* 2nd ed. New York, Springer-Verlag, 1982
16. Teilum G: Classification of testicular and ovarian androblastoma and Sertoli cell tumors. *Cancer* 11:769, 1958
17. Mandel FP, Voet RL, Weiland AJ, et al: Steroid secretion by masculinizing and feminizing hilus cell tumors. *J Clin Endocrinol Metab* 52:779, 1981
18. Judd HL, Spore WW, Talner LB, et al: Preoperative localization of a testosterone-secreting ovarian tumor by retrograde venous catheterization and selective sampling. *Am J Obstet Gynecol* 120:91, 1974
19. Weiland AJ, Bookstein JJ, Cleary RE, et al: Pre-operative localization of virilizing tumors by selective venous sampling. *Am J Obstet Gynecol* 131:798, 1978
20. Lamberts SWJ, Timmers JM, Oosterom R, et al: Testosterone secretion by cultured adrenoblastoma cells: Suppression by a luteinizing hormone-releasing hormone agonist. *J Clin Endocrinol Metab* 54:450, 1982
21. Muremura M, Nakamura T, Matsuura K, et al: Endocrine profile of an ovarian androblastoma. *Obstet Gynecol* 59:100(S), 1982
22. Meyer R: Pathology of some special ovarian tumors and their relation to sex characteristics. *Am J Obstet Gynecol* 26:505, 1933

23. Ober WB, Pollak A, Gerstman KE, et al: Krukenberg tumor with androgenic and progestational activity. *Am J Obstet Gynecol* 84:739, 1962

24. Cotton DB, Hanson FW, et al: A mucinous cystadenoma associated with testosterone production. *J Reprod Med* 26:276, 1981

25. Woodruff JD, Williams TJ, Goldberg B: Hormone activity of the common ovarian neoplasm. *Am J Obstet Gynecol* 87:679, 1963

26. Judd HL, Scully RE, Atkins L, et al: Pure gonadal dysgenesis with progressive hirsutism. *N Engl J Med* 282:881, 1970

27. Swyer GIM: Male pseudo-hermaphroditism: A hitherto undescribed form. *Br Med J* 2:709, 1955

28. Brewer JI, Rhinehart JJ, Dunbar RW: Choriocarcinoma: Report of 5 or more years survival from Albert Matthieu Chorionepithelioma Registry. *Am J Obstet Gynecol* 81:574, 1961

29. Bardin DW, Rosen S, Lemaire WJ: In vivo and in vitro studies of androgen metabolism in a patient with pure gonadal dysgenesis and Leydig cell hyperplasia. *J Clin Endocrinol* 29:1429, 1969

30. Creasman WT, Fetter BF, Hammond CB: Germ cell malignancies of the ovary. *Obstet Gynecol* 53:226, 1979

31. Felmus LB, Pedowitz P: Clinical malignancy of endocrine tumors of the ovary and dysgerminoma. *Obstet Gynecol* 29:344, 1967

32. Mueller DW, Topkins P, Lapp WA: Dysgerminoma of the ovary. *Am J Obstet Gynecol* 60:153, 1950

33. Talerman A, Huyzinga WT, Kuiper T: Dysgerminoma: Clinicopathologic study of 22 cases. *Obstet Gynecol* 41:136, 1973

34. Asadourian LA, Taylor HB: Dysgerminoma: An analysis of 105 cases. *Obstet Gynecol* 33:370, 1969

35. Usizima H: Ovarian dysgerminoma associated with masculinization. *Cancer* 9:736, 1956

36. Hain AM: An unusual case of precocious puberty associated with ovarian dysgerminoma. *J Clin Endocrinol Metab* 9:1349, 1949

37. Neigus I: Ovarian dysgerminoma with chorioepithelioma. *Am J Obstet Gynecol* 69:838, 1955

38. Ross GT, Goldstein DP, Hertz R, et al: Sequential use of methotrexate and Actinomycin D in treatment of metastatic choriocarcinoma and related trophoblastic disease in women. *Am J Obstet Gynecol* 93:223–229, 1965

39. Smith JP, Rutledge F; Advances in chemotherapy for gynecologic cancer. *Cancer* 36:669, 1975

40. Jacobs AJ, Newland JR, Green RK: Pure choriocarcinoma of the ovary. *Obstet Gynecol Surv* 37:603, 1982

41. Van Nagell JR: Tumor markers in ovarian cancer. *Clin Obstet Gynecol* 10:197–212, 1983

42. Smith FG: Pathology and physiology of struma ovarii. *Arch Surg* 53:603, 1946

43. Woodruff JD, Markley RL: Struma ovarii: Demonstration of both pathologic change and physiologic activity; report of four cases. *Obstet Gynecol* 9:707, 1957

44. Gonzalez-Angulo A, Kaufman RH, Braungardt CD, et al: Adenocarcinoma of thyroid arising in struma ovarii. *Obstet Gynecol* 9:1349, 1949

45. Pardo-Mindau FJ, Vasquez JJ: Malignant struma ovarii: Light electron microscopic study. *Cancer* 51:337, 1983

46. Woodruff JD, Rauh JT, Markley RL: Ovarian struma. *Obstet Gynecol* 27:194, 1966

47. Robboy SJ, Norris HJ, Scully RE: Insular carcinoid primary in the ovary. *Cancer* 36:404, 1975

48. Serratoni FT, Robboy SJ: Ultrastructure of primary and metastatic ovarian carcinoids: Analysis of 11 cases. *Cancer* 36:157, 1975

49. Kurman RJ, Norris HJ: Malignant mixed germ cell tumors of the ovary. *Obstet Gynecol* 48:579, 1976

50. Kedzia H: Gonadoblastoma: Structures and background of development. *Am J Obstet Gynecol* 147:81, 1983

51. Scully RE: Gonadoblastoma: A review of 74 cases. *Cancer* 25:1340, 1970

52. Sternberg WH, Barclay DL: Luteoma of pregnancy. *Am J Obstet Gynecol* 95:165, 1966

53. Garcia-Bunuel R, Berek JS, Woodruff JD: Luteomas of pregnancy. *Obstet Gynecol* 45:407, 1975

54. Jewelewicz R, Perkins RP, Dyrenfurth I, Vande Wiele RL: Luteomas of pregnancy: A cause for maternal virilization. *Clin Obstet Gynecol* 17:229, 1974

55. Zander J, Mickan H, Holzman K, et al: Androluteoma syndrome of pregnancy. *Am J Obstet Gynecol* 130:170, 1978

56. Rice BF, Barclay DL, Sternberg WH: Luteoma of pregnancy: Steroidogenic and morphologic consideration. *Am J Obstet Gynecol* 104:871, 1969

57. Norris HJ, Taylor HB: Luteoma of pregnancy. *Am J Clin Pathol* 47:557, 1967

58. Verkauf BS, Reiter EO, Hernandez L, et al: Virilization of mother and fetus associated with luteoma of pregnancy: A case report with endocrinologic studies. *Am J Obstet Gynecol* 129:274, 1977

59. Goldstein DP, Berkowitz RS: *Gestational Trophoblastic Neoplasms.* Philadelphia, Saunders, 1982

60. Morrow CP, Kletzky OA, DiSaia PJ, et al: Clinical and laboratory correlates of molar pregnancy and trophoblastic disease. *Am J Obstet* 128:424, 1977

61. Li MC, Hertz R, Spencer DB: Effect of methotrexate therapy upon choriocarcinoma and chorioadenoma. *Proc Soc Exp Biol Med* 93:361, 1956

62. Goldstein DP, Goldstein PR, Bottomley P, et al: Methotrexate with citrovorum rescue factor for non-metastatic gestational trophoblastic neoplasms. *Obstet Gynecol* 48:321, 1976

63. Hammond CB, Parker RT: Diagnosis and treatment of trophoblastic disease. *Obstet Gynecol* 35:132, 1970

64. Bagshawe KD: Treatment of trophoblastic tumors. *Ann Acad Med* 5:273, 1976

ANSWERS

1. In the series of Fox and Langely, 6.5% of patients with granulosa cell tumors had associated endometrial adenocarcinoma. The endometrial cancer tends to be of a lower grade and stage; therefore, 5-year survival rates have been higher than in those patients with endometrial adenocarcinoma not associated with a granulosa cell tumor.

2. The patient is typically premenopausal and presents with complaints of hirsutism, deepening voice and decrease in breast size. Extreme virilization is not uncommon.

3. Patients who have very high initial hCG titers (>100,000 mIU/ml), duration of disease of more than 4 months, and metastases to the liver or brain have a poorer prognosis.

Steroid Receptors in Breast, Uterine, and Ovarian Malignancy
Diagnostic and Therapeutic Applications

EUGENE R. DESOMBRE, JOHN A. HOLT, and ARTHUR L. HERBST

INTRODUCTION

That certain human cancers might be hormone dependent was suggested in 1836, when Cooper reported a correlation between breast cancer growth and the menstrual cycle.[1] The first report of surgical endocrine ablation for breast cancer came in 1896, when Sir George Beatson[2] showed that oophorectomy in premenopausal women could effect regression of widespread breast cancer. These observations, predating the establishment of the discipline of endocrinology, lay dormant until after the major efforts to isolate and identify steroid hormones that led to studies demonstrating the effectiveness of hormone therapy for breast cancer with either estrogens[3] or androgens.[4] Since breast cancer occurs most frequently in postmenopausal women, the major impetus to endocrine therapy for breast cancer followed the important demonstration by Huggins

and Bergenstal[5] that adrenalectomy in postmenopausal patients with metastatic breast cancer could effect a striking remission. Subsequently, hypophysectomy was also shown to effect remission of metastatic breast cancer.[6,7]

Although dramatic histologic changes in the endometrium during the menstrual cycle and the dependence of the uterus on cyclic hormone levels for its maintenance and growth were demonstrated decades earlier, it was not until 1961 that the first report of responsiveness of some endometrial carcinomas to progestin treatment was published by Kelley and Baker.[8] The histologic effect of progesterone administration on hyperplasia and carcinoma in situ of the endometrium was reported several years earlier.[9] With both breast and endometrial carcinoma, it soon became evident that not all patients responded to hormone therapy. Thus the need arose to develop a method that would predict which cancers are hormone dependent in order to restrict treatment to those patients most likely to benefit. On the basis of current methodology to measure the steroid receptor content in a sample of the tumor, it is possible to predict the response to endocrine therapy for most breast cancers, and there are indications that

EUGENE R. DESOMBRE • Ben May Laboratory for Cancer Research, The University of Chicago, Chicago, Illinois 60637. JOHN A. HOLT and ARTHUR L. HERBST • Department of Obstetrics and Gynecology, The University of Chicago, Chicago, Illinois 60637.

similar success may be available for patients with endometrial carcinoma.

As compared with knowledge on sex steroid receptors in breast and endometrial tumors, information on ovarian cancers has developed primarily during the past 5 years and is more limited in scope, particularly with respect to understanding the biologic function of these receptors. An additional problem is the many histologic types of ovarian tumors. In the adult, epithelial adenocarcinomas are most common, particularly those of the serous and mucinous variety. This chapter limits consideration of sex steroid receptors to epithelial tumors of the ovary.

HORMONAL CONTROL OF GROWTH OF REPRODUCTIVE TISSUES

Studies during the past several decades have elucidated the general features of steroid hormone interaction with target tissues.[10–13] It is generally accepted (Fig. 26-1) that the action of the hormone is effected by the association of the hormone with the specific receptor protein, present in unique quantities in responsive cells. The principal action of the hormone receptor complex takes place in the cell nucleus, where the activated receptor complex, by an as yet not fully understood process, can in-

duce new nucleic acid synthesis characteristic of the particular hormone-dependent tissue. This leads to the response of the tissue, which in the case of estrogen often includes growth stimulation. The currently accepted model for the interaction of estrogen with its target tissues holds that the steroid enters the target cell by passive diffusion. The driving force for the retention of the estrogens by these cells however is the presence of the high-affinity receptor proteins for the steroid. While it has been widely believed that the receptors reside mainly in the cytoplasm of the unstimulated target cell (based on their presence in hypotonic extracts of such tissue, the so-called "cytosolic extracts"), recent data[14,15] indicate that a considerable portion of the free receptor may initially reside within the nucleus. Regardless of the initial localization of the free receptor, the association of estrogen with the receptor protein endows the complex with an important new property, the ability to undergo a steroid and temperature-dependent activation. This activation causes an increase in the affinity of the receptor for estrogens and also substantially enhances the ability of the receptor complex to bind to chromatin or DNA. The activated complex is not extractable from the cells or nuclei by hypotonic or physiologic salt concentrations but usually requires 0.4 M or a higher concentration of KCl to remove it from the chromatin. It is believed that this high-affinity association of the estrogen receptor complex with the chromatin is the basis for the biologic responses to estrogens. While increases in amounts of high-affinity nuclear estrogen receptor complex have been related to increases in biologic responses in model systems, the nature of the changes elicited by the binding of the receptor to chromatin and the details of how these changes enhance transcription are unknown.

BREAST CANCER

Early Studies of Hormone Dependence

The recognition that the female reproductive tract of experimental animals contains estrogen receptor or estrophilin was first shown by the unique ability of these tissues to take up and retain administered tritiated estrogens. Parallel studies with hormone-dependent rat mammary tumors[16,17] demonstrated the same avidity for estrogens. In 1961, Folca et al.[18] administered the tritiated synthetic estrogen, hexestrol, to several women with ad-

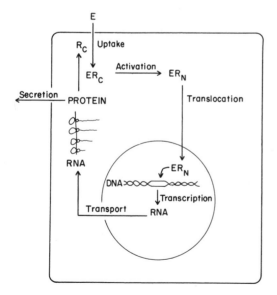

FIGURE 26-1. Schematic diagram for the interaction of estrogen (E) with the estrogen receptor (R) in a target cell.

vanced breast cancer and observed a higher retention of this estrogen by breast cancer tissue of women whose tumors responded to adrenalectomy than in tumors of nonresponding patients. In vitro methods were soon developed to study breast cancer tissue,[19] which showed promise as a means to identify hormone-responsive tumors.

As indicated in Figure 26-1, it is now evident that the specific uptake of tritiated estrogen by hormone-responsive normal and neoplastic tissues depends on the tissue content of specific estrogen receptors. Direct assay for these proteins is accomplished by solubilizing the major portion of the tissue complement of estrogen receptor as a cytosolic extract in hypotonic buffer and employing sedimentation analysis of the cytosols incubated with tritiated estradiol. The receptor was originally identified by the specific binding of estradiol in 4 S and 8 S regions of sucrose-density gradients. Using this method, studies at the University of Chicago correlated the clinical responses to endocrine therapy with the estrogen receptor (ER) status for 42 patients with metastatic breast cancer and reported that the patients experiencing remissions were almost exclusively from the patients with ER-containing cancers.[19] In 1974 the results of a workshop on estrogen receptors and breast cancer[20] confirmed that assay for cytosol estrogen receptor could predict the response of breast cancer patients to endocrine therapy.

Current Status of Estrogen Receptor Assays for Breast Cancer

In 1979 the National Cancer Institute (NCI) sponsored a conference to evaluate the current status of the usefulness of steroid receptor assays in breast cancer (the papers were published as a supplement to the December 1980 issue of *Cancer*). A Consensus Report[21] concluded that ''results of ER assays provide valuable information for making clinical decisions on the type of therapy to be employed'' for patients with metastatic breast cancer. Table 26-1 presents a tabulation of the meeting findings correlating endocrine-induced remissions of breast cancer with ER content of the tumor in nearly 2000 patients. About 55% of patients whose breast cancers contained estrogen receptor had an objective remission to endocrine therapy, while few patients whose cancers lacked receptor benefited.

Whereas an assay for estrogen receptor can identify a group of patients (ER lacking) who have little likelihood of responding to endocrine therapy, it

TABLE 26-1. Clinical Correlations of Breast Cancer Remissions to Endocrine Therapy and Estrogen Receptor Content

| Investigators | Remissions/cases[a] | | | |
	ER +	%	ER −	%
Blamey et al.[58]	13/30	(43)	5/27	(19)
Dao and Nemoto[38]	64/119	(54)	4/56	(7)
Degenshein et al.[178]	27/45	(60)	1/15	(7)
DeSombre and Jensen[36]	39/62	(63)	4/108	(4)
Lippman and Allegra[39]	77/139	(55)	6/105	(6)
Maass et al.[179]	64/93	(69)	3/76	(4)
Manni et al.[180]	68/105	(65)	2/21	(10)
McCarty et al.[170]	32/58	(55)	7/40	(17)
Nomura et al.[48]	29/45	(64)	0/36	(0)
Osborne et al.[40]	69/145	(48)	5/53	(9)
Paridaens et al.[37]	14/31	(45)	0/18	(0)
Rubens and Hayward[171]	46/136	(34)	5/55	(9)
Singhakowinta et al.[172]	20/30	(67)	2/23	(11)
Skinner et al.[173]	17/30	(57)	5/44	(11)
Wittliff[23]	37/67	(55)	0/44	(0)
Young et al.[174]	46/83	(55)	6/22	(27)
Total	662/1218	(54)	55/743	(7)

[a]Estrogen receptor positive and estrogen receptor negative.

would obviously be useful to be able to identify more specifically those patients who will respond. Before the advent of receptor assays, clinicians often used relevant clinical information to help in the choice of therapy. Parameters such as disease-free interval and site of visceral metastases seem to be associated with response to endocrine therapy. Indeed, Byar and co-workers[22] found that while ER status was the single most important parameter for predicting response to endocrine therapy, clinical information could also substantially improve the probability of response prediction.

While a number of investigators have suggested assay of additional characteristics of the ER as a means to improve predictability of response to endocrine therapy, none has received widespread confirmation or acceptance. Such assays include consideration of sedimentation coefficient,[23] ionic differences in receptor,[24] differences in ER size or shape,[25] as well as evaluation of the ability of breast cancer ER to bind to oligo(dT)-cellulose.[26] As yet, few correlations exist to confirm the initial results using these assays. Furthermore, it is evident that proteases present in breast cancers are able to change the size and apparent ionic form of the receptor, often during the tissue preparation.[27,28]

From our understanding of the interaction of estrogen with its target tissues, it would seem reasonable that the effective ER complex would be tightly bound to the nucleus of the cancer cells. It would therefore be reasonable to assay for this nuclear form of the receptor complex. Several preliminary reports suggest that consideration of the tumor content of both the cytoplasmic (i.e., low salt extractable) and nuclear (i.e., high salt extractable) estrogen receptor may be useful in predicting breast cancer response to therapy.[29-32] Nonetheless, the total number of patients whose response has been related to nuclear receptor content is small, and this procedure is subject to more analytic difficulty because of the more stringent conditions usually required for an exchange assay to measure receptor complex, which is already tightly bound to endogenous hormone. The recent availability of antibody to estrogen receptor holds the promise of simpler and more reliable assays for nuclear receptor, which should lead to more widespread evaluation of the usefulness of such assays for breast and other possibly hormone-dependent tissues.

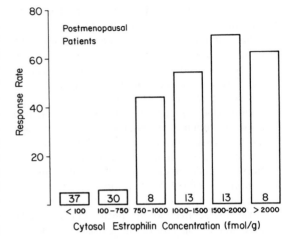

FIGURE 26-2. Relationship between the rate of response to endocrine therapies of postmenopausal breast cancer patients and the cytosol estrogen receptor (ER) content of their cancers. The number in each bar gives the number of patients in that group. The receptor content is derived from a cytosol ER assay be sedimentation analysis under nonsaturating conditions[36] and is expressed as femtomoles per gram wet weight of tissue.

Quantitative Estrogen Receptor and Endocrine Responses

Although original studies differentiated breast cancers on the basis of the presence or absence of estrogen receptors, it was evident that the amounts of estrogen receptor contained in human breast cancer tissue range from undetectable amounts to very high levels, similar to amounts found in normal tissues of the reproductive tract. Several laboratories[33-35] began relating the response of breast cancer patients to endocrine therapy with the quantity of receptor. As shown in Figure 26-2, our results from postmenopausal patients suggest that there is an increase in response rate to endocrine therapy as a function of the receptor content of the tumor. The data suggest that not only patients whose tumors lack detectable amounts of estrogen receptor but also those whose cancers contain small, but measurable, amounts of ER show little response to endocrine therapy. As has been noted in a number of laboratories, the levels of estrogen receptor present in breast cancers of premenopausal women tend to be lower than those found in postmenopausal women. Nonetheless, it appear that there is a relationship between the quantity of ER and the probability of response to endocrine therapy in premenopausal breast cancer patients as well.[36] On the basis of such quantitative considerations, we

have established empirical levels of receptor, derived from sedimentation assays at subsaturating levels of estrogen, which appear to separate tumors into clinically relevant categories referred to as "estrophilin-rich" and "estrophilin-poor." Using such quantitative considerations, the responses of the 170 patients (Table 26-2) show an overall response rate of 63% for ER-rich cancers, and possibly even a higher response in the group of patients treated by endocrine ablation alone. Other investigators have noted a similar relationship between response rate and quantity of estrogen receptors. Heuson and co-workers reported[37] increasing response rates with increasing ER concentration, which reached an 80% response in patients with the highest level of estrogen receptor. The work of Dao and Nemoto,[38] Lippman and Allegra,[39] and McGuire et al.[40] shows similar direct correlations between receptor content and probability of receiving objective benefit from endocrine therapy.

Progestin Receptors and Endocrine Response

Efforts to characterize more precisely the patients who would respond to endocrine therapy led a number of laboratories to search for other protein markers of hormone dependence. Recognizing that progesterone receptor (PR) is an estrogen-depen-

TABLE 26-2. Remissions to Endocrine Therapy for Patients with ER-Negative and ER-Positive Tumors[a]

Treatment	ER-rich[b]	ER-poor[b]
Ablation		
Adrenalectomy	4/6	0/20
Adrenalectomy + oophorectomy	14/19	1/17
Hypophysectomy	2/4	0/9
Oophorectomy	9/12	1/30
Total ablation	29/41 (71%)	2/76 (3%)
Hormone therapy		
Androgen	0/1	0/4
Estrogen	4/5	1/9
Estrogen + progestin	5/13	1/18
Antiestrogen	1/2	0/1
Total hormone therapy	10/21 (48%)	2/32 (6%)
Total endocrine therapies	39/62 (63%)	4/108 (4%)

[a]ER-positive correspond to lesions with >750 fmole/g tissue for postmenopausal patients and >300 fmole/g tissue for premenopausal patients.
[b]Objective remissions per total cases.

dent protein in the normal reproductive tract,[41–43] Horwitz and McGuire[44] suggested that progesterone receptor should be assayed as a second marker in human breast cancer tissue. Early results[43] showed that this additional information was helpful. Table 26-3 presents the clinical correlation of endocrine treatment responses related to the status of both estrogen and progestin receptors. Patients whose lesions contain both estrogen and progestin receptors have the highest probability of remission to endocrine therapy. Whereas 78% of patients whose lesion contained both receptors obtained remissions, about 57% (154 plus 58 divided by 202 plus 171) of the ER-positive patients responded. It appears that lesions containing only one of the two steroid receptor proteins have a lower yet significant remission rate. Therefore, on the basis of the apparent receptor phenotype, one finds a difference in response to endocrine therapies.

Because both quantitative ER levels and the combination of ER and PR positivity each appear to provide better predictability of endocrine response, it has been of interest to see whether both parameters could be related. Data from McGuire's laboratory[40] indicated that with increasing tumor content of estrogen receptor there is an increase in the percentage of tumors containing progestin receptor. It is not yet clear whether these parameters are equally useful or whether additional information may be obtained by consideration of the quantity of progestin receptor. Since progestin receptor is a labile tissue protein, it is crucial that stabilizing agents such as molybdate[45,46] be added to cytosols for assay of progestin receptor. There have been significant problems in establishing adequate quality-control procedures for estrogen and progestin receptors, but such efforts are important for the application of quantitative ER, and particularly PR, assays to multi-institution clinical protocols.[47]

Receptor Assays of the Primary Tumor—Prediction of Subsequent Response

Initial studies correlating endocrine response of breast cancer patients with steroid receptor assays

TABLE 26-3. Clinical Correlations of Breast Cancer Remissions to Endocrine Therapy and ER and PR Content

Investigators	Remissions/total cases			
	ER+PR+	ER+PR−	ER−PR+	ER−PR−
Allegra et al.[175]	11/14	8/14	0/4	0/12
Brooks et al.[176]	4/6	2/7	—	—
Dao and Nemoto[38]	10/13	18/31	—	2/28
Degenshein et al.[178]	26/33	3/14	1/1	0/14
King[177]	10/11	3/15	0/2	2/9
Manni et al.[180]	15/24	3/5	—	0/2
McCarty et al.[170]	33/40	2/20	1/3	—
Osborne et al.[40]	16/20	14/45	—	3/20
Skinner et al.[173]	9/12	2/6	2/3	3/30
Young et al.[174]	20/29	3/14	1/2	2/9
Total	154/202 (78%)	58/171 (34%)	5/15 (33%)	12/124 (10%)

were generally conducted on samples of metastatic disease. It then became important to determine whether later endocrine responses could be predicted from initial steroid receptor assays of the primary cancer. In a small patient series,[36] it appeared that an ER assay of the primary tumor would generally predict a subsequent response to endocrine therapy. Of the 13 patients with ER-rich cancers, nine had objective remissions to endocrine therapy 5–49 months after the initial receptor assay, while only one of the 21 receptor-poor patients responded. Nomura et al.[48] reported a 50% response rate to subsequent endocrine therapy in the 18 patients whose primary tumors were ER rich, a percentage similar to that obtained when the metastatic tumor was assayed.

The basic biologic question is how well the receptor phenotype of the metastasis reflects that of the primary tumor. It appears that a substantial proportion of breast cancers retain their receptor phenotype; nonetheless, a lower proportion of metastatic breast cancer is receptor positive in comparison with the primary lesions. Many investigators have found good agreement between the quantity of receptor in primary and metastatic lesions. Paridaens et al.[37] reported on two or more sequential ER assays in 46 patients; 88% of the samples showed qualitative agreement over a period of 1–63 months. Brennen et al.[49] found a 60–65% concordance of primary and metastatic tumors from the same patient, and Peetz et al.[50] reported 88% agreement when comparing multiple synchronous assays and 83.5% agreement for sequential assays with no intervening therapy. When the second receptor determination was preceded by chemotherapy or hormonal therapy, about one-third showed significant differences, and most commonly receptor-positive tumors became receptor negative. Mobbs[51] found similar concordance for synchronous and sequential tumor assays but also indicated that bilateral tumors, believed by many to arise from independent sites, appear to have independent receptor values.

An important basic question is whether endocrine therapies change the proportion of receptor-containing cells and thereby decrease the receptor content in such tumors. Allegra et al.[52] reported that sequential assays were generally concordant in patients who received no intervening therapy. However, patients given hormonal therapy between the times of two assays showed a distinct decrease in tumor receptor content, with the major decreases in all eight receptor-positive cancers. Since these investigators allowed 10–14 days between cessation of hormone therapy and excision of the tumor, the hormone therapy should not have affected the assay results. Data from the Ben May Laboratory[53] are not entirely consistent with this view. Several patients in our series who had remissions to endocrine therapy subsequently relapsed but still retained substantial amounts of estrogen receptor in their tumors. Taylor et al.[54] reported that the ER content in both responding and nonresponding patients decreased after endocrine therapy. In the group of responders, however, ER assay was performed at the time of relapse, and 10 of 14 tumors still had significant amounts of estrogen receptor after successful endocrine therapy. These results suggest that recurrence of disease after successful endocrine therapy does not necessarily lead to the emergence of receptor-negative tumor cells, nor does reduction in receptor content predict that endocrine therapy will be ineffective. Indeed, it has been known for some time that patients who have responded to initial endocrine therapy are good candidates for subsequent endocrine treatment.

Steroid Receptors—Prognosis and Survival

Knight et al.[55] were the first to observe that the presence of estrogen receptor appeared to relate to the time to recurrence of breast cancer. Soon thereafter, the Michigan Cancer Foundation[56] and the Tenovus Institute[57] presented confirmatory information on the prognostic value of ER content of breast cancer tissue. Subsequent results[40,58,59] indicated that the disease-free interval of patients with ER-positive breast cancers was significantly longer than that of patients with receptor-negative lesions, independent of lymph node status, menopausal status, or the size or location of the primary tumor.

Most results indicate that significant differences in disease-free interval are related to ER status in breast cancer patients with stage I and II disease. However, Hahnel et al.[60] observed that 5 years after mastectomy, the differences related to receptor status of the primary tumors were no longer evident, and subsequent differences correlated with regional lymph node involvement. Even if this were generally found, it would still be a distinct advantage to be able to identify patients who are most likely to have a recurrence within the first several years of primary therapy, based on the tumor ER content. Lippman and Allegra[39] confirmed that patients with ER-positive tumors tend to have a longer disease-free interval but noted that the duration was unrelated to the quantity of receptor.[61] Clark et al.[62] suggest that the PR concentration may provide a better correlation than ER concentration with the disease-free survival of patients with breast cancer. However, earlier Lippman and Allegra[39] were unable to find any additional prognostic value, over that provided by ER assay, by the assay of progestin, androgen, or glucocorticoid receptor in breast cancer. It should be noted that Nordenskjold et al.,[63] reported an increase in symptom-free survival related to increasing concentration of estrogen receptor in breast cancer. They also found that patients with low receptor content and those with receptor-negative tumors had similar short survival times. Godolphin et al.[64] reported a linear trend of survival and ER concentration, independent of adjustment for stage and menopausal status. In both studies, however, it is apparent that postrecurrence survival benefits related to receptor status were significant only in patients on hormone therapy. Therefore, data from a number of studies[62,64–67] suggest that the ER status of the lesion is a prognostic parameter that must be considered with lymph node status in order to assess the risk of recurrence.

NORMAL AND NEOPLASTIC UTERUS

Steroid Receptors in the Normal Uterus

Early studies at the University of Chicago[68] and the Imperial Cancer Research Fund[69] showed that the human uterus is also able to take up and retain unchanged tritiated estradiol administered in vivo. Since these observations, many investigators have documented changes in the level of cytoplasmic estrogen and progesterone receptors in the human uterus.[59,70–79] There is a general consensus that both ER and PR levels are higher during the proliferative than during the secretory phase of the menstrual cycle with the PR peak possibly occurring a few days later than the ER peak, near midcycle.

There is evidence from studies of patients receiving exogenous steroids that progesterone is actually responsible for the secretory phase decrease in ER and PR.[75] Pollow and co-workers[80] studied patients with gonadal dysgenesis who were treated with estrogen followed by estrogen and progesterone and who then underwent endometrial curettage. They found that both ER and PR levels in the endometrium were three- to sixfold higher during estrogen treatment than when estrogen was combined with progesterone. Interestingly, patients who were continued for 22 days on estrogen alone showed no decrease in receptor content at the time the lower receptor levels were seen in patients receiving progesterone along with estrogen.

A number of investigators have compared the steroid receptor content and receptor characteristics in the postmenopausal and premenopausal uterus. Strathy et al.[78] found the estrogen receptor of the postmenopausal endometrium to have a similar dissociation constant to that of ER of the uterus of cycling women; these workers also documented that changes in ER concentration were related to the location of the endometrium in the uterus. While the range of ER concentration in postmenopausal uteri may vary by 10-fold, it is clear that the postmenopausal uterus does contain substantial levels of estrogen receptor. It has been reported[81] that significant levels of PR occur in the postmenopausal uterus only after stimulation by estrogen.

Spelsberg's laboratory[79] reported that the estrogen receptor of the postmenopausal uterus had less affinity for chromatin than estrogen receptor extracted from premenopausal uteri. They also reported differences in the isoelectric focusing patterns of receptor from the premenopausal compared with the postmenopausal uterus, but Pellikka and co-workers[82] found that after addition of diisopropylfluorophosphate (DFP) and molybdate, which inhibit proteolysis and stabilize the receptor, the isoelectric focusing patterns were the same. It is possible that the degradation of the postmenopausal uterine estrogen receptor, obtained in the absence of DFP and molybdate, is also responsible for its altered affinity for chromatin.

Janne[83] studied endometriosis tissue largely from ovarian sites and found that the PR content was only about one-half that found in the endometrium, and the ER content was even lower. The hormonal regulation of the receptors in such tissue appeared to differ significantly from that of the normal cyclic endometrium as well.

Other steroid receptors have been identified in normal endometrium,[84,85] but neither the androgen nor glucocorticoid receptor content seems to vary in a consistent manner during the menstrual cycle, as judged from the limited data available.

Evidence from Tsibris et al.[86,87] and from Kauppila et al.[88] indicates that the concentration of ER and PR forms a gradient in the uterus, highest near the oviduct and lowest at the endocervix. Although the largest decrease in receptor content within a single uterus seems to occur between the corpus and cervical regions of the uterus, there may be significant differences in the fundus as well. These results may confound the interpretations of numerous studies of curettage samples, since the uterine location of such tissue would affect the results. Nonetheless, the Finnish investigators,[88] who also observed such topologic differences in receptor content of hyperplastic endometrium, contend that relative differences in the uterus are not sufficiently large to invalidate receptor assays performed on curettage tissue, especially in cases of hyperplasia or neoplasia, for which the data might have clinical value.

The classic nuclear or salt extractable forms of steroid receptors in the uterus would be expected to be present as a complex associated with endogenous hormone, requiring more complicated and less reliable exchange-assay procedures. As a result, fewer reports are available to document changes in the nuclear receptor in the normal human uterus. Bayard et al.[70] carried out extensive assays on endometrial samples from more than 300 patients and presented data on the salt extractable nuclear receptor complex as well as on the classic cytosolic estrogen and progestin receptors duing the menstrual cycle. These investigators reported a slight decrease in the cytosolic estrogen receptor from the early to late proliferative period and a substantial decrease with the onset of the secretory phase of the cycle. There was the expected increase in nuclear receptor from the early to late proliferative phase due to the increase in circulating estrogen levels. These nuclear ER levels continue into the early secretory phase but decrease by the late secretory phase. A similar pattern was seen for the progestin receptor, with a greater increase in cytosolic receptor from early to late proliferative endometrium and the somewhat later peak in the nuclear receptor complex, which occurred during the early secretory phase of the cycle. Interestingly, several laboratories have identified unoccupied receptor associated with nuclei[89-91] in normal, hyperplastic, and malignant human endometrium. Levels have been found to be highest in the mid-follicular period of the cycle.[88]

To understand the nature and function of constituents of the endometrium, recent studies have employed a variety of methods, including enzyme treatment, to separate glandular epithelium from the stromal tissue. Fleming et al.[92] confirmed that the changes in ER concentration measured in the endometrium during the menstrual cycle could be documented separately in the glands and stroma.

They also reported that the ER content tended to be higher in stroma than in glands. By contrast, Satyaswaroop et al.[93] reported as much as a 10-fold greater concentration of progestin receptor in epithelial cells in comparison to separted stroma. Both groups suggest that collagenase treatment of the tissue resulted in lower amounts of receptor. King et al.[94] confirmed a higher PR content in the epithelium in comparison with the stroma and suggested that the level of receptor measured in the collagenase-treated separated fractions could account for the levels measured in the intact tissue.

Studies of the receptor content of endometrial cells in primary monolayer or organ culture are complicated by the rapid changes that occur in vitro. Fleming et al.[71] reported that cyclic nucleotides can elicit rapid changes in the estrogen binding of both normal endometrium and the endometrial cancer cell line, HEC-1, in vitro. These workers found that molybdate, commonly used to stabilize receptor in hypotonic tissue extracts, can elevate specific estrogen binding. It is not clear whether this estradiol binding, measured with very high concentrations of tritiated estradiol, correlates directly to estrogen receptor measured by conventional means.

Receptors in Hyperplastic or Neoplastic Endometrium

Generally the level of progestin receptor in hyperplastic endometrium is higher than levels seen in either proliferative or secretory normal endometrium.[73,95] It is less clear whether the level of estrogen receptor is likewise elevated in hyperplasias. A major problem with such studies is that hyperplasias can be focal and provide insufficient uniform tissue for biochemical analysis. Unlike the normal breast, which has low receptor content, the normal endometrium, as we have seen, has usually substantial quantities of ER and PR, in both premenopausal and postmenopausal women. It will therefore be of considerable importance to use methods that identify the location of the receptor in tissue sections. Although numerous reports have appeared purporting to identify estrogen and progestin receptors by histochemical methods in human breast cancer tissue, it is clear that such methods are not capable of detecting the receptor proteins.[96] With the availability of antibodies to estrogen receptor, accurate immunocytochemical ER measurements are feasible. Preliminary reports indicate their usefulness to characterize the distribution of estrogen receptors in human breast cancer tissue[14,97] as well as in the normal human endometrium.[98]

Numerous workers have reported the concentration of estrogen and progestin receptors in endometrial carcinoma.[73,76,81,84,85,99,100] The percentage of endometrial carcinomas reported to contain receptors varies from 30 to 100%, but some of these series involve relatively small numbers of patients. In one of the largest series,[100] about 55% of the endometrial carcinomas were found to contain both estrogen and progestin receptor. A major reason for such discrepancies in receptor prevalence in endometrial carcinoma is the well-documented difference in occurrence of receptors with the histologic differentiation of the tumor and stage of the cancer. Generally the percentage of endometrial carcinomas that contain either ER or PR decreases with increasing stage, and few contain receptor when the cancer has progressed beyond stage II.[73,81,100] Creasman et al.[101] find a direct relationship between the receptor content and extent of disease. There seems to be general agreement that the well-differentiated endometrial carcinomas have higher levels of both ER and PR.[73,84,95,101,102] Some exceptions are from Pollow's group,[59] who found increases in ER concentration with decreasing degree of differentiation, and Martin et al.,[81] who found higher levels of progestin receptor, but lower levels of estrogen receptor, in well-differentiated tumors.

Steroid Receptors and Response to Endocrine Therapy

At least four groups have correlated steroid receptor content of endometrial carcinomas with response to progestin administration.[81,95,101,103] Generally, patients who have high levels of progestin receptor are most likely to respond to endocrine therapy. Since not all these investigators have assayed for both estrogen and progestin receptors, the relative status of each of these receptor proteins cannot be definitively assessed. Erlich et al.[95], the only investigators who employ a high PR cutoff (50 fmole/mg cytosol protein), report that seven of the eight patients with PR-positive lesions showed some objective response to progesterone therapy, while only one of the 16 PR-negative patients responded. Unfortunately, only two patients of this series of 24 obtained complete remissions, one classified as PR positive and one as PR negative.

Benraad et al.[103] reported that seven of eight patients who had cancers containing measurable estrogen receptor experienced some improvement on progestin therapy. Two lesions were found to be PR negative, and both patients responded to progestin therapy. Nonetheless, the accumulated data on tumor response and PR content[95] indicate that 88% of responders had PR-positive tumors, while only 6% of nonresponders contained progestin receptor. Considering the difficulty in reproducing PR results among laboratories[47] and the lability of the progestin receptor to degradation, these early clinical correlations suggest that steroid receptor assays may provide useful data for making therapeutic decisions in cases of endometrial carcinoma.

It is curious that different approaches to endocrine therapy have developed for breast and endometrial cancers. Antiestrogens, most frequently tamoxifen, are used commonly in cases of breast cancer. Progestin therapy has occasionally been shown effective for breast cancer, but it is most commonly used for endometrial carcinoma, and antiestrogens have seldom been used. However, Mortel et al.[104] have suggested that a tamoxifen challenge test may predict hormone responsiveness in endometrial carcinoma. These workers propose to assay endometrial carcinomas for cytosol and nuclear estrogen receptor before and after an 8-hr challenge treatment with tamoxifen. The effectiveness of tamoxifen would be indicated by increases in the nuclear ER content of the lesion, as well as an increase in the nuclear to cytosol ER ratio, before and after tamoxifen challenge. While such short-term tamoxifen treatment did not change the content of progestin receptors, tamoxifen administration to endometrial cancer patients for 5–7 days did produce a statistically significant increase in PR content of the cancers.[104]

Both Gurpide and Tseng[105] and Pollow et al.[106] proposed that patient responses to progestin therapy could be based on assays of the progestin-dependent endometrial enzyme, 17β-hydroxysteroid dehydrogenase (17-HSD). These investigators reported up to fourfold increases in enzyme activity, as well as a reduction of cytosol ER, in tumors responsive to progestins. Obviously both the tamoxifen challenge test and the above use of 17-HSD before and after progestin treatment would require the sequential excision of lesions, which is not always possible. However, such procedures can provide evidence for biologic effectiveness of hormone therapy early in the treatment course.

Effect of Progestin Therapy on Receptors

It has been speculated[81] that one of the problems with progestin therapy for endometrial carcinoma is the tendency of progestins to eliminate assayable cytosol progestin receptor. If the effectiveness of treatment depends on progestin receptor, one might expect only a short-term response. Janne et al.[73] reported that treatment with medroxyprogesterone acetate (MPA) for 4 weeks did reduce the level of estrogen and progestin receptor in both hyperplastic and neoplastic human endometrium. Prody et al.[85] also reported that MPA lowered progestin receptor but effected no change in ER. In an interesting study that may have considerable relevance to combination endocrine treatment, Kokko et al.[107] treated normal women with MPA alone or in combination with tamoxifen for 3 weeks. Treatment with MPA atrophied the endometrium, reduced 17-HSD activity, and decreased cytosol estrogen and progestin receptors. Tamoxifen alone had no effect on estrogen receptor, progestin receptor, 17-HSD (while increasing circulating sex steroid concentrations), and 3-week combination treatment with MPA and tamoxifen not only caused endometrial atrophy and a more dramatic drop in 17-HSD, but actually increased the level of cytosol ER. These workers conclude that the stimulatory effects of progestin treatment are short lived and by 3 weeks PR levels are depressed. It is possible that the addition of an antiestrogen, like tamoxifen, maintains levels of progestin receptor, thereby enhancing the effects of MPA and also taking advantage of the antiestrogenic effect of the tamoxifen.

STEROID RECEPTORS AND OVARIAN TUMORS

Steroid Sensitivity of Ovarian Tissues

Ninety percent of the carcinomas of ovarian origin arise from the surface epithelium.[108,109] This ovarian surface epithelium is derived from coelomic epithelium, which in the embryo is contiguous with the epithelium that gives rise to the steroid-sensitive epithelia of the female reproductive tract.[110] Because of this proximity, the surface epithelium of the ovary might be expected also to be hormone responsive. Indeed, the epithelia seen in ovarian neoplasia often closely resemble the epithelia of the endocervix, endometrium, and/or fallopian tubes.[111] Because it is now known that the morphologic characteristics of the epithelia of the

female reproductive tract and their responses to steroid hormones are in part dependent on their associated stroma,[112] the variety of histologic types of ovarian epithelial neoplasia suggests that the ovary is multipotent in its capacity to permit or induce mimicry of most types of reproductive tract epithelia. Observations on the normal ovarian surface epithelium in the rat in vitro[113,114] support the view that steroid hormone receptors, when present in ovarian tumors, may represent retention or expression of vestiges of differentiated steroid hormone receptor control systems.

A major problem has been to demonstrate the presence of steroid receptors in the normal ovarian epithelium. This is technically difficult because the epithelium consists of a single cell layer in vivo and because of the difficulty of retaining steroid responsiveness in cultured cells. This dilemma of having to explain an apparent dearth of receptors in the normal ovarian epithelium is analogous to that associated with the apparent lack of steroid receptors in normal breast tissue; however, breast tissue is more obviously responsive to steroid hormones. The presence of receptor proteins for estrogen, progestin, androgen, and glucocorticoid has been demonstrated in ovarian granulosa cells,[115–118] but this is the only cell compartment of the ovary in which there is strong evidence of the presence of these proteins in nonmalignant cells. Laboratories usually do not detect receptor proteins for the sex steroids in normal theca, corpus luteum, and stroma, although they may be present at low concentrations.[119–124] This contrasts with the readily demonstrated steroid receptors in the normal endometrium and myometrium and in the normal tissues of the fallopian tubes.

Characteristics of Steroid Receptor Proteins in Ovarian Cancers

The receptor proteins most frequently observed in ovarian tumors are those for estrogen and progestin,[114,119,121–135] glucocorticoid,[119] and androgens.[124,127,129,133] Based on physicochemical criteria, the receptor proteins for steroid hormones in ovarian carcinomas are, in most instances, indistinguishable from such proteins found in the classic steroid-sensitive target tissues, e.g., normal uterus and cancers of the breast. Thus, analytic procedures developed for the receptor proteins in other types of tissue can usually be expected to be applied directly, or with only slight modification, to ovarian tumors.[120–122,130] The estrogen and progestin receptors in ovarian adenocarcinomas can bind a variety of the estrogen and progesterone analogues, agonists, and antagonists, including tamoxifen[136] and its potent metabolite, monohydroxytamoxifen.[137]

As with breast carcinomas, it has not been possible to use fluorescein-tagged ligands for histochemical localization of estrogen receptor in ovarian adenocarcinomas.[126] However, because the ER protein in ovarian carcinomas is recognized by monoclonal antibodies raised against estrogen receptor derived from human breast cancer,[137,138] it is to be expected that immunocytochemical localization of estrogen receptor in ovarian cancers can be accomplished as has been reported for breast carcinomas[14,97] and endometrium.[98]

When present, the amounts of cytoplasmic estrogen receptor in tumors originating in the epithelium of the ovary are of the same order of magnitude (15–1500 fmoles/mg DNA, 50–7000 fmoles/g wet wt., or 3–200 fmoles/mg soluble protein) as the amounts observed in breast cancers and in cancerous or normal endometrial tissue.[122,128,139] The levels of estrogen and progestin receptors in a given patient may vary among various sites of metastatic disease.[125,134,139] However, ER levels in omental metastases were found not to be consistently higher or lower than those in the ovarian site.[134] Steroid receptor proteins are rarely found in metastases of ovarian cancers if they are absent from the primary.[120,122,125,134,139] As might be expected, the metastases to the ovaries from cancers of non-steroid-sensitive tissues, such as bowel, do not contain steroid receptors, whereas the metastases of receptor-rich breast and endometrial cancers can express steroid receptor activity in their metastases to the ovary.[120,125,136] There is some indication that the mean concentrations of receptors for sex steroid hormones in ovarian carcinomas are lower in premenopausal than in postmenopausal patients.[122,128] Chemotherapy, including combination chemotherapy, is reported to have little effect on the levels of sex steroid receptors in ovarian carcinomas.[140] In ovarian carcinoma, the effects of direct radiation therapy on its receptor content, character, and function are unknown. Nor is it known what effects prior irradiation of a site may have on receptor parameters in subsequent tumors growing in that site.

Although receptors for sex steroid hormones can be demonstrated in both cytoplasmic and nuclear extracts, a clear demonstration of cell-regulatory functions for these proteins in ovarian cancers has not yet been reported. Attempts to use plasminogen activator,[141] 17β-hydroxysteroid dehydrogenase,[123] or peroxidase[139] as postgenome markers of sex steroid action have not been successful in ovarian cancers. It has not been possible to show induction or regulation of one category of sex steroid receptor protein either by a steroid in its own class or by other categories of steroids or antisteroidal compounds. For example, tamoxifen regulation of estrogen and progestin receptors has not been shown in ovarian carcinomas. Regulation of receptor expression by sex steroids and antisteroidal compounds may be demonstrated in new cell lines of human ovarian carcinomas grown in immunodeficient mice.[142] The current hypothesis is that the receptor proteins for steroid hormones in ovarian cancers are physicochemically similar to those in tissues with steroid-sensitive growth and differentiation, but that the cellular responses are not the same.

Steroid Receptors in Ovarian Tumors According to Histologic Type, Grade, and Stage

All the principal types of epithelial (including clear cell, formerly called mesonephroid) and sex cord-stromal cancers of the human ovary have been reported to contain steroid receptors. In contrast, ovarian germ cell tumors rarely, if ever, contain sex steroid receptor proteins.[100,120,128,136,139,143–147] The serous tumors express steroid receptors more frequently than do mucinous tumors.[100,120,122,126,128,136,143] Most laboratories frequently detect sex steroid receptors in endometrioid tumors; in one reported series, incidence rates were 81% and 72% for estrogen and progestin receptor, respectively, with values taken as positive at >10 fmoles and >25 fmoles/mg protein, respectively.[145] In general, the amounts and the frequency of occurrence of receptors decrease with dedifferentiation of the endometrioid tumor.[100,120,122,126,143–145] Thus, the amounts and occurrence of receptor for progestin are usually low in anaplastic endometrioid tumors. Occasionally, however, PR or ER proteins, or both, are present in high concentrations (i.e., above 1600 fmoles/mg cytosol protein) in poorly differentiated endometrioid tumors. The high receptor content in some poorly differentiated tumors may be an indication of breakdown of the systems that regulate receptor expression. This concept may offer a partial explanation for the lack of inverse correlation between tumor grade and receptor content for most series of serous ovarian carcinomas. The presence of receptor for progestin is usually accompanied by the presence of receptor for estrogen in most ovarian carcinomas. The amounts of receptors for sex steroid hormones in ovarian adenocarcinomas are believed to be independent of disease stage,[100,120,126,134] but in recurrent disease, low receptor levels have been noted.[100,120] Most benign ovarian tumors have low or nondetectable levels of sex steroid receptors.[125,128,136]

Receptors in Ovarian Carcinomas and Patient Survival

Several investigators have reported longer survival in patients who had tumors with high levels of estrogen and/or progestin receptor,[120,126,135,148] whereas other investigators found no such relationship.[122,134,139,149] Because of the small number of patients studied to date, the prognostic significance of either estrogen receptor or progestin receptor content for ovarian carcinomas has not been established, in contrast to the findings for breast carcinoma.[96]

Endocrine Therapy against Ovarian Carcinoma

Several studies obtained encouraging results when progestins were used for the treatment of ovarian cancers,[125,150–158] with favorable responses estimated to be as high as 30–40%.[159] However, this early optimism for progestin as a possible active agent against ovarian carcinomas could not be substantiated in clinical trials on progestin for treatment of tumors that had failed to respond to conventional cytotoxic chemotherapy.[160–162] In these trials, progestin was well tolerated but was ineffective in most cases (less than 5% objective response rates). It has been speculated that progestin might be of benefit for some endometrioid ovarian tumors, particularly for those in which progestin receptors can be demonstrated.[161,162] In ovarian carcinomas, attempts have been made to induce progestin receptors by giving estrogens such as ethinyl-estradiol and subsequently medroxyprogesterone acetate.[163] Sufficient data for evaluation of the efficacy of such hormonal regimens are not yet available.

The use of antiestrogens, particularly tamoxifen, against ovarian carcinomas is being investigated actively, with attempts to correlate response with sex steroid receptor status, thus far with mixed success.[122,164,165] Tamoxifen[136] and one of its potent antiestrogenic metabolites, monohydroxytamoxifen, bind to the ER protein in ovarian carcinomas.[137] Like most antiestrogens, tamoxifen exhibits some estrogenic characteristics, e.g., it induces progestin receptor in endometrial cancer cells.[104,107] Whether tamoxifen displays similar activity in ovarian carcinomas is unknown. Because sex steroid receptors can persist even after intensive combination chemotherapy,[140,149] adjuvant use of progestins and antiestrogens might be effective. It remains unknown how extensively the regulation of cell growth and of differentiation in nonmalignant or malignant ovarian epithelial cells is affected by steroid hormones. For this reason, the future value of hormonal therapy against these tumors remains uncertain.

Novel Uses of Receptors in Ovarian Carcinoma

The presence of estrogen receptor in a large percentage of epithelial ovarian tumors, even after extensive chemotherapy,[140,149] offers the potential to use the receptors for imaging and possibly for treatment of some of these tumors. Recently, radiolabeled estrogen derivatives have been shown to localize in ER-rich tissues.[166] Their use could provide a method for imaging of ER-rich ovarian carcinomas. In addition, appropriate high-specific-activity radiopharmaceutical agents (e.g., ^{123}I, ^{80}Br and ^{80m}Br, and ^{77}Br) can now be attached to high-affinity ER ligands, such as R2858 (Moxestrol)-like analogues.[167,168] These agents could localize in the tumor cell nucleus to exert a cytotoxic effect, as has been reported for ER-rich models of human breast cancer.[169] It is known that a prototypical γ-emitting radiolabeled estrogen, 16α-[^{125}I]iodoestradiol, binds to the estrogen receptor found in specimens of metastatic epithelial ovarian carcinoma.[138] Such radiolabeled sex steroid receptor ligands could provide new modalities for the therapy of patients who have steroid-receptor-rich ovarian tumors. Current investigations are directed toward evaluation of these possibilities.

SUMMARY

The hormonal dependence of certain malignancies had been suspected for more than a century; in modern times they have provided an important basis for effective clinical therapy. Studies of the biochemical basis of the dependence of certain normal tissues, and their neoplastic counterparts, on steroid hormones have led to the identification of specific high-affinity soluble cellular proteins, or receptors, which have been implicated as mediators of the physiologic actions of the hormones. Results correlating the presence of estrogen receptors in human breast cancers with patient responses to various types of endocrine therapy, both ablative and additive, have shown that essentially only patients whose breast cancers contain estrogen receptor obtain remissions from endocrine therapy. While few ER-negative patients respond, one-half to two-thirds of ER-positive patients benefit. Knowledge of the quantity of estrogen receptor, or alternatively the presence of progestin receptors (PR), improves the accuracy of identifying patients most likely to respond to endocrine therapy. Furthermore, the steroid receptor content of the lesion is prognostic for the length of recurrence-free survival and overall survival. ER and PR levels in the normal human uterus have been shown to change during the menstrual cycle, with both found in highest concentrations during the proliferative phase. At least one-half of endometrial carcinomas contain receptors for sex steroid hormones, but with increasing stage or degree of dedifferentiation there is a concomitant decrease in receptor content, and fewer of the less differentiated cancers contain receptors. Correlations of response of the endometrial cancers to endocrine therapy, most frequently with progestins, have shown remissions generally associated with higher levels of receptors, especially progestin receptor. While less is known about the variation of steroid receptor content of the normal human ovary, estrogen and progestin receptors, indistinguishable by physical characteristics from the receptors of the normal reproductive tract, have been identified in epithelial malignancies of the ovaries. Primary and metastatic ovarian carcinomas have been shown to contain receptors, and their presence is independent of the stage of disease, while in endometrioid tumors the receptor concentration and frequency of receptor occurrence decrease with dedifferentiation. Mucinous carcinomas of the ovary less frequently contain estrogen and progestin receptors than do serous carcinomas. Despite some early encouraging reports, only a low proportion of ovarian cancers are found to respond to progestin therapy. The concentration of estrogen and progestin receptors in breast and endometrial cancers provides information about the likelihood of response to endocrine therapy and, in the case of breast cancer, relates to the length of disease-free survival of the patient.

ACKNOWLEDGMENTS. The laboratory and clinical studies from the University of Chicago described in this chapter were supported by National Cancer Institute grants CA 02897, CA 14599, and CA 27476, CB 14358, CB 43969, by Abbott Laboratories, by Mothers' Aid Research Fund for CLIH, and the Women's Board of the University of Chicago Cancer Research Foundation.

QUESTIONS*

1. Estrogen receptors

   a. are membrane constituents with high affinity for estrogens but not for other steroid hormones.
   b. are intracellular proteins with high affinity for estrogens but not for other steroid hormones.
   c. complex with estrogens resulting in nucleic acid synthesis.

2. Estrogen receptor levels in breast carcinomas

   a. are generally predictive of clinical outcome.
   b. indicate "endocrine-responsiveness" if the content is high.
   c. tend to be present in metastases if they are present in the primary tumor.

3. Progestin receptors in endometrial tissue

   a. increase in amount in response to estrogens.
   b. are markers for hormone-dependent endometrial carcinomas.
   c. are found in highest concentrations in the premenopausal uterus, in samples from the fundus, and in lowest concentrations near the endocervix.

4. Estrogen receptors in ovarian carcinomas

   a. appear to have the same physicochemical properties as those from breast carcinoma.
   b. affect cellular growth in tumors that are estrogen-receptor rich.
   c. are found in both primary ovarian carcinomas and metastases.

*More than one answer may be correct.

REFERENCES

1. Cooper AP: *The Principles and Practice of Surgery*. London, Cox, 1836, pp 333–335
2. Beatson GT: On the treatment of inoperable cases of carcinoma of the mamma. Suggestions for a new method of treatment with illustrative cases. *Lancet* 2:104–107, 1896
3. Haddow A, Watkinson JM, Patterson E: Influence of synthetic estrogens upon advanced malignant disease. *Br Med J* 2:393–398, 1944
4. Nathanson IT: Clinical investigative experience with steroid hormones in breast cancer. *Cancer* 5:754–762, 1952
5. Huggins C, Bergenstal DM: Inhibition of human mammary and prostatic cancer by adrenalectomy. *Cancer Res* 12:134–141, 1952
6. Luft R, Olivecrona H: Experiences with hypophysectomy in man. *J Neurosurg* 10:301–316, 1953
7. Pearson OH, Roy BS, Harrold CC: Hypophysectomy in treatment of advanced breast cancer. *JAMA* 161:17–21, 1956
8. Kelley RM, Baker WH: Progestational agents in the treatment of carcinoma of the endometrium. *N Engl J Med* 264:216–222, 1961
9. Kistner RW: Histologic effects of progesterone on hyperplasia and carcinoma in situ of the endometrium. *Cancer* 12:1106–1122, 1959
10. Gorski J, Gannon F: Current models of steroid hormone action: A critique. *Annu Rev Physiol* 38:425–450, 1976
11. Jensen EV, DeSombre ER: Estrogen–receptor interaction. *Science* 182:126–134, 1973
12. O'Malley BW, Means AR: Female steroid hormones and target cell nuclei. *Science* 183:610–620, 1974
13. Yamamoto KR, Alberts BM: Steroid receptors: Elements for modulation of eukaryotic transcription. *Annu Rev Biochem* 45:721–746, 1976
14. King WJ, Greene GL: Monoclonal antibodies localize oestrogen receptor in the nuclei of target cells. *Nature (Lond)* 307:745–747, 1984
15. Martin PM, Sheridan PJ: Towards a new model for the mechanism of action of steroids. *J Steroid Biochem* 16:215–229, 1982
16. King RJB, Cowan DM, Inman DR: The uptake of [6,7-3H]oestradiol by dimethylbenzanthracene-induced rat mammary tumours. *J Endocrinol* 32:83–90, 1965
17. Mobbs BG: The uptake of tritiated oestradiol by dimethylbenzanthracene-induced mammary tumours of the rat. *J Endocrinol* 36:409–414, 1966
18. Folca PJ, Glascock RF, Irvine WT: Studies with tritium labelled hexoestrol in advanced breast cancer. *Lancet* 2:796–798, 1961
19. Jensen EV, Block GE, Smith S, et al: Estrogen receptors and breast cancer response to adrenalectomy. *Natl Cancer Inst Monog* 34:55–70, 1971
20. McGuire WL, Carbone PP, Vollmer EP: *Estrogen Receptors in Human Breast Cancer*. New York, Raven, 1975
21. DeSombre, ER, Carbone PP, Jensen EV, et al: Special report: Steroid receptors in breast cancer. *N Engl J Med* 301:1011–1012, 1979
22. Byar DP, Sears ME, McGuire WL: Relationship between estrogen receptor values and clinical data in predicting the response to endocrine therapy for patients with advanced breast cancer. *Eur J Cancer* 15:299–310, 1979
23. Wittliff JL: Steroid–receptor interactions in human breast carcinoma. *Cancer* 46:2953–2960, 1980
24. Kute TE, Heidemann P, Wittliff JL: Molecular heterogeneity of cytosolic forms of estrogen receptors. *Cancer Res* 38:4307–4313, 1978
25. MacFarlane JK, Fleiszer D, Fazekas AG: Studies on estrogen receptors and regression in human breast cancer. *Cancer* 45:2998–3003, 1980
26. Myatt L, White JO, Fernandez MD, et al: Human breast tumor cytosol oestrogen receptor binding to oligo(dT)-cellulose. *Br J Cancer* 45:964–967, 1982
27. Miller LK, Tuazon FB, Niu E, et al: Human breast tumor estrogen receptor. Effects of molybdate and electrophoretic analyses. *Endocrinology* 108:1369–1378, 1981
28. Tilzer LL, McFarland RT, Plapp FV, et al: Different ionic forms of estrogen receptor in rat uterus and human breast carcinoma. *Cancer Res* 41:1058–1063, 1981
29. Laing L, Calman KC, Smith MG, et al: Nuclear oestrogen receptors and treatment of breast cancer. *Lancet* 2:168–169, 1977
30. Leake RE, Laing L, Calman KC, et al: Oestrogen-receptor status and endocrine therapy of breast cancer: Response rates and status stability. *Br J Cancer* 43:59–66, 1981
31. MacFarlane JK, Fazekas AG: Nuclear oestradiol receptors and regression of human breast cancers. *Lancet* 2:565, 1982
32. White JO, Fernandez MD, Burn JI, et al: Activated oestrogen receptors and clinical response in human breast cancer. *Lancet* 2:219, 1982
33. Jensen EV, Polley TZ, Smith S: Prediction of hormone dependency in human breast cancer, in McGuire WL, Carbone PP, Vollmer EP (eds): *Estrogen Receptors in Human Breast Cancer*. New York, Raven, 1975, pp 37–56
34. Jensen EV, Smith S, Moran EM, et al: Estrogen receptors and hormone dependency in human breast cancers, in Namer M (ed): *Hormones and Breast Cancer*. Paris, INSERM, 1975, pp 29–37
35. Leclercq G, Heuson JC, Deboel MC, et al: Oestrogen receptors in breast cancer: A changing concept. *Br Med J* 1:185–189, 1975
36. DeSombre ER, Jensen EV: Estrophilin assays in breast cancer: Quantitative features and application to the mastectomy specimen. *Cancer* 46:2783–2788, 1980
37. Paridaens R, Sylvester RJ, Ferrazzi E, et al: Clinical significance of the quantitative assessment of estrogen receptors in advanced breast cancer. *Cancer* 46:2889–2895, 1980
38. Dao TL, Nemoto T: Steroid receptors and response to endocrine ablations in women with metastatic cancer of the breast. *Cancer* 46:2779–2782, 1980
39. Lippman ME, Allegra JC: Quantitative estrogen receptor analyses: The response to endocrine and cytotoxic chemotherapy in human breast cancer and the disease free interval. *Cancer* 46:2829–2834, 1980
40. Osborne CK, Yochmowitz MG, Knight WA III, et al: The value of estrogen and progesterone receptors in the treatment of breast cancer. *Cancer* 46:2884–2888, 1980
41. Falk RJ, Bardin CW: Uptake of tritiated progesterone by the uterus of the ovariectomized guinea pig. *Endocrinology* 86:1059–1063, 1970
42. Milgrom E, Atger M, Baulieu E-E: Progesterone in uterus and plasma. IV. Progesterone receptor(s) in guinea pig uterus cytosol. *Steroids* 16:741–754, 1970
43. O'Malley BW, Sherman MR, Toft DO: Progesterone "receptors" in the cytoplasm and nucleus of chick oviduct target tissue. *Proc Natl Acad Sci USA* 67:501–508, 1970

44. Horwitz KB, McGuire WL, Pearson OH, et al: Predicting response to endocrine therapy in human breast cancer: An hypothesis. *Science* 189:726–727, 1975

45. Anderson KM, Marogil M, Bonomi PD, et al: Stabilization of human breast cancer progesterone (R5020) receptor by sodium molybdate. *Clin Chim Acta* 103:367–373, 1980

46. Anderson KM, Phelan J, Marogil M, et al: Sodium molybdate increases the amount of progesterone and estrogen receptor detected in certain human breast cancer cytosols. *Steroids* 35:273–280, 1980

47. Jordan VC, Zava DT, Uppenburger U, et al: Reliability of steroid hormone receptor assays: An international study. *Eur J Cancer Clin Oncol* 19:357–363, 1983

48. Nomura Y, Yamagata J, Takenaka K, et al: Steroid hormone receptors and clinical usefulness in human breast cancer. *Cancer* 46:2880–2883, 1980

49. Brennan MJ, Donegan WL, Appleby DE: The variability of estrogen receptors in metastatic breast cancer. *Am J Surg* 137:260–262, 1979

50. Peetz ME, Nunley DL, Moseley HS, et al: Multiple simultaneous and sequential estrogen receptor values in patients with breast cancer. *Am J Surg* 143:591–594, 1982

51. Mobbs BG: Effect of time and therapy on the hormone receptor status of breast carcinomas. *Can Med Assoc J* 127:217–221, 1982

52. Allegra JC, Lippman ME, Thompson EB, et al: Relationship between the progesterone, androgen and glucocorticoid receptor and response to endocrine therapy in metastatic breast cancer. *Cancer Res* 39:1973–1979

53. DeSombre ER, Jensen EV: Effect of endocrine ablative surgery on breast cancer cytosol estrogen receptor content. *Postgrad Med* 42:15–19, 1981

54. Taylor RE, Powles TJ, Humphreys J, et al: Effects of endocrine therapy on steroid-receptor content of breast cancer. *Br J Cancer* 45:80–85, 1982

55. Knight WA, Livingston RB, Gregory EJ, et al: Estrogen receptor is an independent prognostic factor for early recurrence in breast cancer. *Cancer Res* 37:4669–4671, 1977

56. Rich MA, Furmanski P, Brooks SC: Prognostic value of estrogen receptor determinations in patients with breast cancer. *Cancer Res* 38:4296–4298, 1978

57. Maynard PW, Blamey RW, Elston CW, et al: Estrogen receptor assay in primary breast cancer and early recurrence of disease. *Cancer Res* 38:4292–4295, 1978

58. Blamey RW, Bishop HM, Blake JRS, et al: Relationship between primary breast tumor receptor status and patient survival. *Cancer* 46:2765–2769, 1980

59. Pollow K, Lubbert H, Boquoi E, et al: Characterization and comparison of receptors for 17β-estradiol and progesterone in human proliferative endometrium and endometrial carcinoma. *Endocrinology* 96:319–328, 1975

60. Hahnel R, Woodings T, Vivian AB: Prognostic value of estrogen receptors in primary breast cancer. *Cancer* 44:671–675, 1979

61. Allegra JC, Lippman ME, Thompson EB, et al: Estrogen receptor status: An important variable in predicting response to endocrine therapy in metastatic breast cancer. *Cancer* 16:323–331, 1980

62. Clark GM, McGuire WL, Hubay CA, et al: Progesterone receptors as a prognostic factor in stage II breast cancer. *N Engl J Med* 309:1343–1347, 1983

63. Nordenskjold B, Wallgren A, Gustafsson S, et al: Steroid receptor levels and prophylactic endocrine therapy of mammary carcinoma. *Acta Obstet Gynecol Scand* 101:49–51, 1981

64. Godolphin W, Elwood JM, Spinelli JJ: Estrogen receptor quantitation and staging as complementary prognostic indicators in breast cancer: A study of 583 patients. *Int J Cancer* 28:677–683, 1981

65. Kinne DW, Ashikari R, Butler A, et al: Estrogen receptor protein in breast cancer as a predictor of recurrence. *Cancer* 47:2364–2367, 1981

66. Nicholson RI, Campbell FC, Blamey RW, et al: Steroid receptors in early breast cancer: Value in prognosis. *J Steroid Biochem* 15:193–199, 1981

67. Furmanski P, Saunders DE, Brooks SC, et al: The prognostic value of estrogen receptor determinations in patients with primary breast cancer: An update. *Cancer* 46:2794–2796, 1980

68. Davis ME, Wiener M, Jacobson HI, et al: Estradiol metabolism in pregnant and non-pregnant women. *J Obstet Gynecol* 87:979–990, 1963

69. Brush MG, Taylor RW, King RJB: The uptake of [6,7-3H]oestradiol by the normal human female reproductive tract. *J Endocrinol* 39:599–607, 1967

70. Bayard F, Damilano S, Robel P, et al: Cytoplasmic and nuclear estradiol and progesterone receptors in human endometrium. *J Clin Endocrinol Metab* 46:635–648, 1978

71. Fleming H, Blumenthal R, Gurpide E: Rapid changes in specific estrogen binding elicited by cGMP or cAMP in cytosol from human endometrial cells. *Proc Natl Acad Sci USA* 80:2486–2490, 1983

72. Fleming H, Gurpide E: Rapid fluctuations in the levels of specific estradiol-binding sites in endometrial cells in culture. *Endocrinology* 108:1744–1750, 1981

73. Janne O, Kauppila A, Kontula K, et al: Female sex steroid receptors in normal, hyperplastic and carcinomatous endometrium. The relationship to serum steroid hormones and gonadotropins and changes during medroxyprogesterone acetate administration. *Int J Cancer* 24:545–554, 1979

74. Kreitmann B, Bugat R, Bayard F: Estrogen and progestin regulation of the progesterone receptor concentration in human endometrium. *J Clin Endocrinol Metab* 49:926–929, 1979

75. Natrajan PK, Muldoon TG, Greenblatt RB, et al: The effect of progestins on estrogen and progesterone receptors in the human endometrium. *J Reprod Med* 27:227–230, 1982

76. Rodriquez J, Sen KK, Seski JC, et al: Progesterone binding by human endometrial tissue during the proliferative and secretory phases of the menstrual cycle and by hyperplastic and carcinomatous endometrium. *Am J Obstet Gynecol* 133:660–666, 1979

77. Rubin BL, Gusberg SB, Butterly J, et al: A screening test for estrogen dependence of endometrial carcinoma. *Am J Obstet Gynecol* 114:660–669, 1972

78. Sanborn BM, Kuo HS, Held B: Estrogen and progestogen binding site concentrations in human endometrium and cervix throughout the menstrual cycle and in tissue from women taking oral contraceptives. *J Steroid Biochem* 9:951–955, 1978

79. Strathy JH, Coulam CB, Spelsberg TC: Comparison of estrogen receptors in human premenopausal and postmenopausal uteri: Indication of biologically inactive receptor in postmenopausal uteri. *Am J Obstet Gynecol* 142:372–382, 1982

80. Lubber H, Pollow K, Rommler A, et al: Estradiol and progesterone receptor concentrations and 17β-hydroxy-

steroid-dehydrogenase activity in estrogen-progestin stimulated endometrium of women with gonadal dysgenesis. *J Steroid Biochem* 17:143–148, 1982

81. Martin PM, Rolland PH, Gammerre M, et al: Estradiol and progesterone receptors in normal and neoplastic endometrium: Correlations between receptors, histopathological examinations and clinical responses under progestin therapy. *Int J Cancer* 23:321–329, 1979

82. Pellikka PA, Sullivan WP, Coulam CB, et al: Comparison of estrogen receptors in human premenopausal and postmenopausal uteri using isoelectric focusing. *Obstet Gynecol* 62:430–434, 1983

83. Janne O, Kauppila A, Kokko E, et al: Estrogen and progestin receptors in endometriosis lesions: Comparison with endometrial tissue. *Am J Obstet Gynecol* 141:562–566, 1981

84. Prodi G, De Giovanni C, Galli MC, et al: 17β-estradiol, 5α-dihydrotestosterone, progesterone and cortisol receptors in normal and neoplastic human endometrium. *Tumori* 65:241–253, 1979

85. Prodi G, Nicolett G, De Giovanni C, et al: Multiple steroid hormone receptors in normal and abnormal human endometrium. *J Cancer Res Clin Oncol* 98:173–183, 1980

86. Tsibris JCM, Cazenave CR, Cantor B, et al: Distribution of cytoplasmic estrogen and progesterone receptors in human endometrium. *Am J Obstet Gynecol* 132:449–454, 1978

87. Tsibris JCM, Fort FL, Cazenave CR, et al: The uneven distribution of estrogen and progesterone receptors in human endometrium. *J Steroid Biochem* 14:997–1003, 1981

88. Kauppila A, Janne O, Stenback F, et al: Cytosolic estrogen and progestin receptors in human endometrium from different regions of the uterus. *Gynecol Oncol* 14:225–229, 1982

89. Fleming H, Gurpide E: Available estradiol receptors in nuclei from human endometrium. *J Steroid Biochem* 13:3–11, 1980

90. Geier A, Beery R, Levran D, et al: Unoccupied nuclear receptors for estrogen in human endometrial tissue. *J Clin Endocrinol Metab* 50:541–545, 1980

91. Levy C, Mortel R, Eychenne B, et al: Unoccupied nuclear oestradiol-receptor sites in normal human endometrium. *Biochem J* 185:733–738, 1980

92. Fleming H, Namit C, Gurpide E: Estrogen receptors in epithelial and stromal cells of human endometrium in culture. *J Steroid Biochem* 12:169–174, 1980

93. Satyaswaroop PG, Wartell DJ, Mortel R: Distribution of progesterone receptor, estradiol dehydrogenase, and 20alpha-dihydroprogesterone dehydrogenase activities in human endometrial glands and stroma: Progestin induction of steroid dehydrogenase activities in vitro is restricted to the glandular epithelium. *Endocrinology* 111:743–749, 1982

94. King RJB, Townsend PT, Siddle N, et al: Regulation of estrogen and progesterone receptor levels in epithelium and stroma from pre- and postmenopausal endometria. *J Steroid Biochem* 16:21–29, 1982

95. Ehrlich CE, Young PCM, Cleary RE: Cytoplasmic progesterone and estradiol receptors in normal, hyperplastic, and carcinomatous endometria: Therapeutic implications. *Am J Obstet Gynecol* 141:539–546, 1981

96. DeSombre ER: Steroid receptors in breast cancer, in McDivitt R, Oberman H, Ozello L (eds): *The Breast*. Baltimore, Williams & Wilkins, 1984, pp 149–174

97. Greene GL: Application of immunochemical techniques to the analysis of estrogen receptor structure and function, in Litwack G (ed): *Biochemical Actions of the Hormones*. New York, Academic, 1984, pp 207–239

98. Press MF, Greene GL: An immunocytochemical method for demonstrating estrogen receptor in human uterus using monoclonal antibodies to human estrophilin. *Lab Invest* 50:480–488, 1984

99. Neumannova M, Kauppila A, Vihko R: Cytosol and nuclear estrogen and progestin receptors and 17β-hydroxysteroid dehydrogenase activity in normal and carcinomatous endometrium. *Obstet Gynecol* 61:181–188, 1983

100. Vihko R, Isotalo H, Kauppila A, et al: Female sex steroid receptors in gynecological malignancies: Clinical correlates. *J Steroid Biochem* 19:827–832, 1983

101. Creasman WT, McCarty KS, Barton TK, et al: Clinical correlates of estrogen- and progesterone-binding proteins in human endometrial adenocarcinoma. *Obstet Gynecol* 55:363–370, 1980

102. McCarty KS Jr, Barton TK, Fetter BF, et al: Correlation of estrogen and progesterone receptors with histologic differentiation in endometrial adenocarcinoma. *Am J Pathol* 96:171–183, 1979

103. Benraad TH, Friberg LG, Koenders AJM, et al: Do estrogen and progesterone receptors (E2R and PR) in metastasizing endometrial cancers predict the response to gestagen therapy. *Acta Obstet Gynecol Scand* 59:155–159, 1980

104. Mortel R, Levy C, Wolff J, et al: Female sex steroid receptors in postmenopausal endometrial carcinoma and biochemical response to antiestrogen. *Cancer Res* 41:1140–1147, 1981

105. Gurpide E, Tseng L: Potentially useful tests for responsiveness of endometrial cancer to progestagen therapy, in Brush MG, King RJB, Taylor RW (eds): *Endometrial Cancer*. London, Bailliere Tindall, 1978, pp 252–257

106. Pollow K, Boquoi E, Lubbert H, et al: Effect of gestagen therapy on 17β-hydroxysteroid dehydrogenase in human endometrial carcinoma. *J Endocrinol* 67:131–132, 1975

107. Kokko E, Janne O, Kauppila A, et al: Effects of tamoxifen, medroxyprogesterone acetate, and their combination on human endometrial estrogen and progestin receptor concentrations, 17β-hydroxysteroid dehydrogenase activity, and serum hormone concentrations. *Am J Obstet Gynecol* 143:382–388, 1982

108. Czernobilsky B: Primary epithelial tumors of the ovary, in Blaustein A (ed): *Pathology of the Female Genital Tract*. New York, Springer-Verlag, 1977, pp 453–504

109. Lingeman CH: Etiology of cancers of the human ovary: A review. *J Natl Cancer Inst* 53:1603–1618, 1974

110. Langman J: Embryology and congenital malformations of the female genital tract, in: Blaustein A (ed): *Pathology of the Female Genital Tract*. New York, Springer-Verlag, 1977, pp 1–12

111. Julian CG: Germinal epithelial neoplasia of the ovary. *Clin Obstet Gynecol* 17:241–257, 1974

112. Cunha GR, Chung LWK, Shannon JM, et al: Stromal–epithelial interactions in sex differentiation. *Biol Reprod* 22:19–42, 1980

113. Hamilton TC, Davis P, Griffiths K: Oestrogen receptor-like binding in the surface germinal epithelium of the rat ovary. *J Endocrinol* 95:377–385, 1982

114. Hamilton TC, Davies P, Griffiths K: Steroid-hormone re-

ceptor status of the normal and neoplastic ovarian surface germinal epithelium, in Greenwald GS, Terranova PF (eds): *Factors Regulating Ovarian Function*. New York, Raven, 1983, pp 81–85

115. Jacobs BJ, Suchocki S, Smith RG: Evidence for a human ovarian progesterone receptor. *Am J Obstet Gynecol* 138:332–336, 1980

116. Richards JS: Hormonal control of ovarian follicular development: A 1978 perspective. *Recent Prog Horm Res* 35:343–373, 1979

117. Schreiber JR, Nakamura K, Erickson GF: Rat ovary glucocorticoid receptor: Identification and characterization. *Steroids* 39:569–584, 1982

118. Schreiber JR, Ross GT: Further characterization of a rat ovarian testosterone receptor with evidence for nuclear translocation. *Endocrinology* 99:590–596, 1976

119. Galli MC, DeGiovanni C, Nicolette G, et al: The occurrence of multiple steroid hormone receptors in disease-free and neoplastic human ovary. *Cancer* 47:1297–1302, 1981

120. Kauppila A, Vierikka P, Kivinen S, et al: Clinical significance of estrogen and progestin receptors in ovarian cancer. *Obstet Gynecol* 61:320–326, 1983

121. Lele SB, Piver MS, Barlow JJ, et al: Comparison of cytosol estrogen receptor status in ovarian carcinoma using different radiolabeled ligands and methods. *J Surg Oncol* 21:155–158, 1982

122. Pollow K, Schmidt-Matthiesen A, Hoffman G, et al: ³H-Estradiol and ³H-R5020 binding in cytosols of normal and neoplastic human ovarian tissue. *Int J Cancer* 31:603–608, 1983

123. Vierikko P, Kauppilla A, Vihko R: Cytosol and nuclear estrogen and progestin receptors and 17β-hydroxysteroid dehydrogenase activity in non-diseased tissue and in benign and malignant tumors of the human ovary. *Int J Cancer* 32:413–422, 1983

124. Wurz H, Wassner E, Citoler P, et al: Multiple cytoplasmic steroid hormone receptors in benign and malignant ovarian tumors and in disease-free ovaries. *Tumor Diagn Ther* 4:15–20, 1983

125. Bergqvist A, Kullander S, Thorell J: A study of estrogen and progesterone cytosol receptor concentration in benign and malignant ovarian tumor and a review of malignant ovarian tumors treated with medroxyprogesterone acetate. *Acta Obstet Gynecol Scand* 101:75–81, 1981

126. Creasman WT, Sasso RA, Weed JC, et al: Ovarian carcinoma: Histologic and clinical correlation of cytoplasmic estrogen and progesterone binding. *Gynecol Oncol* 12:319–327, 1981

127. Friberg LG, Kullander S, Persijin JP, et al: On receptors for estrogens (E2) and androgens (DHT) in human endometrial carcinoma and ovarian tumors. *Acta Obstet Gynecol Scand* 57:161–164, 1978

128. Hahnel R, Kelsali GR, Martine JD, et al: Estrogen and progesterone receptors in tumors of the human ovary. *Gynecol Oncol* 13:145–151, 1982

129. Hamilton TC, Davies P, Griffiths K: Androgen and oestrogen binding in cytosols of human ovarian tumours. *J Endocrinol* 90:421–431, 1981

130. Holt JA, Lorincz MA, Hospelhorn VD: Sulfhydryl sensitivity and [125-I]-16α-iodo-17β-estradiol binding of estrogen receptor in ovarian epithelial carcinomas. *J Steroid Biochem* 18:41–50, 1983

131. Janne O, Kauppila A, Syrjala P, et al: Comparison of cytosol estrogen and progestin receptor status in malignant and benign tumors and tumor-like lesions of human ovary. *Int J Cancer* 25:175–179, 1980

132. Jones LA, Edwards CL, Freedman RS, et al: Estrogen and progesterone receptor titers in primary epithelial ovarian carcinomas. *Int J Cancer* 32:567–571, 1983

133. Kusanishi H, Tamaya T, Wada K, et al: Characterization of steroid receptors in human ovarian cancer. *Asia Oceania J Obstet Gynecol* 8:427–432, 1982

134. Schwartz PE, LiVolsi VA, Hildreth N, et al: Estrogen receptors in ovarian epithelial carcinomas. *Obstet Gynecol* 59:229–238, 1982

135. Spona J, Gitsch E, Salzer H, et al: Estrogen- and gestagen-receptors in ovarian carcinomas. *Gynecol Obstet Invest* 16:189–198, 1983

136. Holt JA, Caputo TA, Kelly KM, et al: Estrogen and progestin binding in cytosols of ovarian adenocarcinomas. *Obstet Gynecol* 53:50–58, 1979

137. Holt JA, Jordan VC, Tate AC, et al: Binding of [³H]monohydroxytamoxifen in ovarian carcinoma. *Br J Obstet Gynecol* 90:751–758, 1983

138. Holt JA, Lorincz MA, King WJ: Antibody-recognized [125-I]-estradiol–receptor complex in ovarian epithelial carcinoma. *Obstet Gynecol* 62:231–235, 1983

139. Holt JA, Lyttle CR, Lorincz MA, et al: Estrogen receptor and peroxidase activity in epithelial ovarian carcinomas. *J Natl Cancer Inst* 67:307–318, 1981

140. Holt JA, Richman CM, Podczaski E, et al: Effect of chemotherapy on cytoplasmic estrogen receptors (ERc) in advanced epithelial ovarian carcinoma. *Gynecol Oncol* 17:266, 1984 (abst)

141. Isotalo H, Tryggvason K, Vierikko P, et al: Plasminogen activators and steroid receptor concentrations in normal, benign, and malignant breast and ovarian tissues. *Anticancer Res* 3:331–336, 1983

142. Hamilton TC, Young RC, McKoy WM, et al: Characterization of a human ovarian carcinoma cell line (NIH:OVCAR-3) with androgen and estrogen receptors. *Cancer Res* 43:5379–5389, 1983

143. Ford LC, Berek JS, Lagasse LD, et al: Estrogen and progesterone receptors in ovarian neoplasms. *Gynecol Oncol* 15:299–304, 1982

144. Quinn MA, Pearce P, Rome R, et al: Cytoplasmic steroid receptors in ovarian tumours. *Br J Obstet Gynecol* 89:754–759, 1982

145. Rendina GM, Donadio C, Giovannini M: Steroid receptors and progestinic therapy in ovarian endometrioid carcinoma. *Eur J Gynaecol Oncol* 3:241–224, 1982

146. Schwartz PE, MacLusky N, Sakamoto H, et al: Steroid-receptor proteins in nonepithelial malignancies of the ovary. *Gynecol Oncol* 15:305–315, 1983

147. Young PCM, Grosfeld JL, Ehrlich CE, et al: Progestin- and androgen-binding components in a human granulosa-theca cell tumor. *Gynecol Oncol* 13:309–317, 1982

148. Leibach S, Miller N, Slayton RE, et al: Hormone receptors in ovarian carcinoma. *Proc Am Assoc Cancer Res* 24:176, 1983 (abst)

149. Richman CM, Holt JA, Herbst AL: Persistence of estrogen receptor in advanced epithelial ovarian carcinoma after chemotherapy. *Obstet Gynecol* 65:257–263, 1985

150. Briggs MH, Caldwell ADS, Pitchford AG: The treatment of cancer by progestogens. *Hosp Med (Lond)* 2:63–69, 1967

151. Geisler HE: Megestrol acetate for the palliation of advanced ovarian carcinoma. *Obstet Gynecol* 61:95–98, 1983

152. Guthrie D: The treatment of advanced cystadenocarcinoma of the ovary with gestronol and continuous oral cyclophosphamide. *Br J Obstet Gynecol* 86:497–500, 1979

153. Jolles B: Progesterone in the treatment of advanced malignant tumors of breast, ovary and uterus. *Br J Cancer* 16:209–221, 1962

154. Malkasian GD Jr, Decker DG, Jorgensen ED, et al: 6-dehydro-6,17- and dimethylprogesterone (NSc-123018) for the treatment of metastatic and recurrent ovarian carcinoma. *Cancer Chemother Rep* 57:241–242, 1973

155. Mangioni C, Franceschi S, La Vecchia C, et al: High dose medroxyprogesterone acetate (MPA) in advanced epithelial ovarian cancer resistant to first or second-line chemotherapy. *Gynecol Oncol* 16:352–359, 1981

156. Varga A, Henriksen E: Effect of 17α-hydroxy-progesterone 17-n-caproate on various pelvic malignancies. *Obstet Gynecol* 23:51–62, 1964

157. Ward HWC: Progestogen therapy for ovarian carcinoma. *J Obstet Gynaecol Br Commonw* 79:555–559, 1972

158. Weeth JB: Large dose progestin palliation: Valuable in solid tumor patients. *Proc Am Soc Clin Oncol* 15:165, 1974 (abst)

159. Tobias JS, Griffiths CT: Management of ovarian carcinoma. *N Engl J Med* 294:818–823, 877–882, 1976

160. Aabo K, Pedersen AG, Hald I, et al: High-dose medroxyprogesterone acetate (MPA) in advanced chemotherapy-resistent ovarian carcinoma: A phase II study. *Cancer Treatm Rep* 66:407–408, 1982

161. Malkasian GD Jr, Decker DG, Jorgensen EO, et al: Medroxyprogesterone acetate for the treatment of metastatic and recurrent ovarian carcinoma. *Cancer Treatm Rep* 61:913–914, 1977

162. Slayton RE, Pagano M, Creech RH: Progestin therapy for advanced ovarian cancer: A phase II Eastern Cooperative Oncology Group Trial. *Cancer Treatm Rep* 65:895–896, 1981

163. Jolles CJ, Freedman RS, Jones L: Estrogen and progestogen therapy in advanced ovarian cancer: Preliminary report. *Gynecol Oncol* 16:352–359, 1983

164. Myers AD, Moore GE, Major FJ: Advanced ovarian carcinoma: Response to antiestrogen therapy. *Cancer* 48:2368–2370, 1981

165. Schwartz PE, Keating G, MacLusky N, et al: Tamoxifen therapy for advanced ovarian cancer. *Obstet Gynecol* 59:583–588, 1982

166. Toft DO, Wahner HW: Radiochemical probes for steroid hormone receptors. *J Nucl Med* 23:411–419, 1982

167. Gibson RE, Francis BE, Jagoda EL, et al: The properties of I-125-labeled 11β-methoxy-17alpha-iodovinyl-estradiol (IMOX). *J Nucl Med* 24:49, 1983

168. Katzenellenbogen JA, McElvany KD, Senderoff SG, et al: 16alpha-[77Br]bromo-11beta-methoxyestradiol-17beta; a gamma-emitting estrogen imaging agent with high uptake and retention by target organs. *J Nucl Med* 23:411–419, 1982

169. Bonzert DA, Hochberg RB, Lippman ME: Specific cytotoxicity of 16alpha-[125-I]iodoestradiol for estrogen receptor containing breast cancer cells. *Endocrinology* 110:2177–2179, 1982

170. McCarty KS Jr, Cox C, Silva JS, et al: Comparison of sex steroid receptor analyses and carcinoembryonic antigen with clinical response to hormone therapy. *Cancer* 46:2846–2850, 1980

171. Rubens RD, Hayward JL: Estrogen receptors and response to endocrine therapy and cytoxic chemotherapy in advanced breast cancer. *Cancer* 46:2922–2924, 1980

172. Singhakowinta A, Saunders DE, Brooks SC, et al: Clinical application of estrogen receptor in breast cancer. *Cancer* 46:2932–2938, 1980

173. Skinner LG, Barnes DM, Ribeiro GG: The clinical value of multiple steroid receptor assays in breast cancer management. *Cancer* 46:2939–2945, 1980

174. Young PCM, Ehrlich CE, Einhorn LH: Relationship between steroid receptors and response to endocrine therapy and cytotoxic chemotherapy in metastatic breast cancer. *Cancer* 46:2961–2963, 1980

175. Allegra JC, Barlock A, Huff KK, et al: Changes in multiple or sequential estrogen receptor determinations in breast cancer. *Cancer* 45:792–794, 1980

176. Brooks SC, Saunders DE, Singhakowinta A, et al: Relation of tumor content of estrogen and progesterone receptors with response of patient to endocrine therapy. *Cancer* 46:2775–2778, 1980

177. King RJB: Analysis of estrogen and progesterone receptors in early and advanced breast tumors. *Cancer* 46:2818–2821, 1980

178. Degenshein GA, Bloom N, Tobin E: The value of progesterone receptor assays in the management of advanced breast cancer. *Cancer* 46:2789–2793, 1980

179. Maass H, Jonat W, Stalzenbach G, et al: The problem of non-responding estrogen receptor-positive patients with advanced breast cancer. *Cancer* 46:2835–2837, 1980

180. Manni A, Arafah B, Pearson OH: Estrogen and progesterone receptors in the prediction of response of breast cancer to endocrine therapy. *Cancer* 46:2838–2841, 1980

ANSWERS

1. b, c

2. a, b, c

3. a, b, c

4. a, c

27

Understanding and Managing of Pregnancy in Women with Diabetes Mellitus

W. N. SPELLACY

INTRODUCTION

The woman with abnormal carbohydrate metabolism has a long history of problems with reproduction. Before the introduction of insulin, she would rarely live to puberty and, if she did, her poorly controlled hyperglycemia usually resulted in amenorrhea and infertility. Successful pregnancies were very unusual at that time. In 1924 the first successful pregnancy in an insulin-treated diabetic was reported by Graham.[1] During the next 25 years there were many reports demonstrating that insulin-treated women lived and that their fertility was normal. There was a high perinatal mortality rate, however; this was best predicted by the White classification, which related principally to the duration of the disease state.[2] The next 25 years saw advances in management leading to better glucose control and detailed fetal health and maturity assessment. These management changes produced not only a gradual fall in perinatal mortality to levels that are

not different now from those experienced by other women but a concomitant decrease in morbidity as well.[3] In addition, basic information about metabolism in pregnancy led to new insights about the disease and the value of mass screening, so that now the milder cases are also detected. Diabetes mellitus complicating pregnancy is common but manageable; furthermore, the risk of heredity to the offspring is 2–5%. This chapter discusses the metabolic changes that accompany pregnancy, describes detection procedures, outlines the potential maternal and infant problems for the diabetic, and describes a plan of management that can lead to a successful pregnancy outcome.

METABOLIC CHANGES IN PREGNANCY

Carbohydrate metabolism during pregnancy has been the central focus for many investigations for many years. Before 1960, the emphasis was on the measurement of blood glucose levels during pregnancy.[4] Pregnant women were shown to have a lower fasting glucose level and a prolonged glucose tolerance curve with higher values at the later times during the tolerance test than nonpregnant women.

W. N. SPELLACY • Department of Obstetrics and Gynecology, University of Illinois College of Medicine, Chicago, Illinois 60612.

The explanations for these findings were (1) a constant drain of glucose from the mother to the uterus, thereby decreasing the basal level; and (2) delayed gastrointestinal emptying time due to the smooth muscle relaxation effects of progesterone, thereby prolonging the tolerance curve. When insulin was injected into pregnant women, less hypoglycemic effect was seen demonstrating ''insulin resistance'' accompanying the gestation.[5]

Radioimmunoassay (RIA) techniques for measuring blood insulin levels were used to study the physiology of normal pregnancy.[6] It was demonstrated that hyperinsulinemia develops in normal women during their pregnancy; this is maximal at the end of the pregnancy where the insulin released during a glucose tolerance test is two to three times greater than when they are not pregnant.[7]

Since insulin does not cross the placenta and the hyperinsulinemia persists after fetal death, it is clear that these changes represent a placental–uterine rather than fetal effect. Many studies of insulin receptor activity in peripheral leukocytes have been performed because the cells are easy to obtain, but the importance of blood cells as target tissues for insulin activity appears limited. Nonetheless these studies show that progesterone lowers binding by reducing both the receptor numbers and their affinity. Pregnant women show lower binding than do women in the follicular phase of their cycle but similar binding to that seen during the luteal phase.[8] Studies of receptors in fat cells during pregnancy show some reduction as well.[9] The overall insulin receptor change is not as marked as that predicted from the studies of insulin levels or insulin resistance, thus suggesting that a ''postreceptor'' alteration may also be taking place.

A search for the mechanism causing this insulin resistance has been a primary focus of investigation over the past decade. Progesterone is markedly elevated during pregnancy and can cause some reduction in insulin receptor binding as seen in the luteal phase of the cycle.[8] Free cortisol is also elevated in pregnancy and could contribute to this receptor alteration.[7] While the placenta makes large quantities of human placental lactogen (hPL), few data support the role of hPL as a major factor in this change.[10] Since the metabolic clearance rate for insulin in pregnancy varies little from that found in nonpregnancy, the effect of placental insulin degradation (insulinase) seems minimal.[7] Glucagon secretion is little affected by pregnancy in the fasting state and seems to be more suppressed by hyperglycemia in pregnancy, so it is probably not contributing to the insulin resistance either.[11] Prolactin can cause insulin resistance and hyperinsulinemia.[12] Since pregnancy is associated with a marked elevation of blood prolactin levels coming from both the maternal pituitary gland and the uterine decidual area, it is probably a major factor in the process. In vitro studies show that prolactin can markedly reduce insulin binding to its receptors.[13] Other alterations such as those of chromium, pyridoxine, and xanthurenic acid may have some minor effects as well.[7] In general, however, it appears that the insulin resistance accompanying normal pregnancy occurs as a result of progesterone and or cortisol with prolactin acting at peripheral key target tissues.

DETECTION OF DIABETES

The characteristics of women who are susceptible to the development of diabetes during pregnancy have been well delineated; they include obesity, positive family history for diabetes, glucosuria, prior elevated blood glucose, and prior stillborn, anomalous, or macrosomic infants. While these characteristics assist in screening, they have now been replaced by a more sensitive blood screening test. The test that has been best evaluated is the measure of the blood glucose level 1 hr after the woman ingests 50 g glucose orally.[14] This blood value should normally be less than 130 mg/dl (plasma <150). Recent studies suggest that by lowering the plasma value to 135 mg%, one can even improve the sensitivity, yet more false-positive values would obviously result.[15] The screening test is usually done at the weeks 24–28 of pregnancy. Repeat screening may be done later in high-risk women. If the screening test exceeds that upper limit, the patient should then have a 3-hr oral glucose tolerance test performed using a 100-g glucose load. That test must be done after a 10-hr fast, and the patient does not need to collect urine samples during the test, as (1) they are almost always positive for glucose, (2) the patient's movement to and from the lavatory invalidates the blood test, and (3) a diagnosis of diabetes cannot be made from the urine values. The upper limits of normal for the glucose tolerance test in pregnancy are listed in Table 27-1.[16]

If two values exceed these upper limits, the patient has gestational diabetes mellitus, whereas if all levels are below these limits, the test is considered normal.[16] If only one value is abnormal, the test is considered borderline abnormal, and it should be

TABLE 27-1. Upper Limits for the Glucose Levels during an Oral Glucose Tolerance Test Using a 100-g Load

Value	Time			
	Fasting (mg/dl)	1 hr (mg/dl)	2 hr (mg/dl)	3 hr (mg/dl)
Blood	90	165	145	125
Plasma	105	190	165	145

[a]From O'Sullivan and Mahan.[16]

repeated in about 4 weeks. With the use of the routine blood glucose screen plus the glucose tolerance test on the abnormal screening results, very few women with carbohydrate abnormalities will go undetected during pregnancy. It is therefore recommended that every pregnant woman be screened in this manner.

INSULIN-DEPENDENT DIABETES MELLITUS

Maternal Problems

The risks of maternal death or significant long-term morbidity due to pregnancy are remote, but potential acute problems can occur in the pregnant diabetic patient. The seven problems most often encountered are listed in Table 27-2.

Hypoglycemia

During the first 20 weeks of gestation, the woman is susceptible to the development of hypoglycemia.[17] While there has been some slight increased sensitivity to insulin action described in that time period probably due to the effect of relaxin on receptors,[13] the most common reason for the problem is that the high chorionic gonadotropin levels affect appetite and cause anorexia, nausea, and/or vomiting. As a result, there is a decreased caloric intake and hypoglycemia ensues unless the insulin dosage is reduced. There are no good data to sug-

TABLE 27-2. Common Problems Experienced by the Pregnant Woman with Diabetes Mellitus

Hypoglycemia	Retinopathy
Hyperglycemia	Hypertension
Insulin shifts	Hydramnios
Urinary tract infections	

gest that transient periods of maternal hypoglycemia adversely affect the fetus. Indeed, during transient maternal hypoglycemic spells, the fetal glucose levels are maintained *via* glycolysis and gluconeogenesis, and there is a reversal of the placental gradient with fetal glucose going to the maternal side.

Hyperglycemia

Maternal hyperglycemia tends to occur during the last 20 weeks of pregnancy and is mainly related to the insulin resistance that develops at that time.[17] Hyperglycemia is the most serious of all the maternal problems during pregnancy, since glucose crosses the placenta by facilitated diffusion with ease; therefore, fetal hyperglycemia also occurs at that time. Since almost all the serious problems for the infant including death are highly associated with and are probably caused by maternal hyperglycemia, it must be avoided if possible; if hyperglycemia occurs, it must be treated aggressively.

Insulin Shifts

Since type 1 diabetic patients are dependent on exogenous insulin, pregnancy-induced insulin resistance will generally affect their insulin needs. If blood glucose levels are to be kept constant, the pregnant diabetic will have to increase her insulin dose two to three times during the pregnancy; most of this change will occur between the twentieth to thirtieth weeks of gestation. As soon as the placenta is removed, there is a return of insulin sensitivity when the insulin dose can be abruptly reduced by about one-half. This insulin need will gradually move toward the prepregnancy level by about 6–8 weeks postpartum; thereafter, the long-term needs will not be different because of the prior pregnancy.

Urinary Tract Infections

All pregnant women are at risk for urinary tract infection (UTI), and the diabetic has an even higher risk.[18] This results in part from the physiologic dilatation of the urinary tract that accompanies pregnancy, which results in poor emptying of urine and ureteralvesical reflux. In addition, there is normally glucosuria in all pregnancies; if there is any maternal hyperglycemia, it is more marked. This provides a substrate for bacterial growth. Most bacteria enter the urinary tract of women during intercourse when the bacteria colonized in the introitus and urethra are massaged into the bladder. Significant bacteriuria is found in about 30% of urine samples obtained after coitus.[19] The general pregnancy risk of UTI is about 10%; for the diabetic it increases to about 20%.[18] As a result, urine cultures are required at the first prenatal visit for all pregnant women and again at 30–32 weeks gestation for the diabetic. If the patient becomes symptomatic, they are again repeated. All positive cultures must be appropriately treated with antibiotics, and follow-up cultures are necessary to assure cure.

Retinopathy

The retina of diabetic patients goes through exacerbations and remissions in terms of their diabetic pathology and many studies have shown this to continue in pregnancy as well. The risk of background retinopathy becoming worse in pregnancy is about 15–20%.[20] This frequency does not seem to be related to the blood glucose control at that time but more to the duration of the disease state.[19-21] One type of lesion, proliferative retinopathy, has a much higher frequency of exacerbation in pregnancy, with rates as high as 80–90% being demonstrated.[20] Since this is a serious medical problem with long-term sequelae, proliferative retinopathy has been a medical indication for therapeutic abortion in the past. Newer retinal therapies, especially those of laser coagulation, have proved, however, to be an effective means of dealing with this lesion. Studies of laser-treated cases show a rate of progression in pregnancy of only about 15–20%, which is not different from that seen with background disease.[20] Thus, proliferative retinopathy is no longer considered a medical indication for therapeutic abortion, but all pregnant diabetics must have a complete retinal examination early in pregnancy and serially during the pregnancy, with appropriate treatment given to those with a proliferative lesion.

Hypertension

Hypertension occurs in about 7% of all pregnant women, but the diabetic, with her potential for vascular disease, is at increased risk for this problem. Most series of diabetic pregnancies show a frequency of hypertension complicating the pregnancy of about 25%.[7] The blood pressure change may be the only sign seen in pregnancy, for Clesley and associates[22] demonstrated that the later risk of the devel-

opment of diabetes is increased 2 and 3.8 times in women who had eclampsia during their first or later pregnancies, respectively.

Hydramnios

Increased accumulations of amniotic fluid are infrequent during pregnancy and are generally reported with an incidence of 0.4%.[23] The diabetic woman is more susceptible to this problem, for whom the frequency is generally considered to be about 20%. While the mechanism is not clearly understood, some cases are due to the increased fetal anomaly rate with associated poor fetal swallowing and some are due to fetal glucosuria and polyuria resulting from maternal hyperglycemia. This can also cause an osmotic pressure gradient that pulls water into the amniotic sac.

Infant Problems

The infant of the diabetic mother (IDM) is the major problem with diabetes complicating pregnancy, for the IDM can be affected with significant and permanent morbidity or mortality. There is no increase in the spontaneous abortion rate in diabetics unless they are poor in glucose control.[24] It is very important to consider some of the other potential IDM problems; seven of these are listed in Table 27-3.

Congenital Anomalies

It has been recognized for years that the IDM is at an increased risk for congenital anomalies, with the incidence being about three times the expected.[7,17] While any anomaly may occur, sacral agenesis is a unique anomaly for this group.[25] Women with infants having sacral agenesis should be carefully screened for diabetes mellitus. Studies of anomalous infants from diabetic mothers have shown that the insult probably occurs during the third to sixth weeks of pregnancy.[25] Additional studies using hemoglobin A_1C suggest that maternal hyperglycem-

TABLE 27-3. Common Problems Experienced by the Infant of the Diabetic Mother

Abortion	Macrosomia
Congenital anomalies	Hypocalcemia
Respiratory distress	Hyperbilirubinemia
Hypoglycemia	Death

ia may be the etiologic factor.[26] The hemoglobin A[1]C theoretically would screen the preceding month of pregnancy for hyperglycemia, for if the blood glucose rises above normal range, some of the glucose couples covalently with valine on the β-chain of hemoglobin and remains there for the life span of the red cell. This glucose-tagged hemoglobin moves faster in electrophoresis and is termed A[1]C.[27] Since circulating red cells have an average of about 4–5 weeks of remaining life, an episode of hyperglycemia can be retrospectively detected over the next month or two by measuring the level of blood hemoglobin A[1]C. The elevated test result strongly suggests prior hyperglycemia but does not tell precisely what level the glucose reached or how frequently it was elevated.

If the HbgA[1]C level is normal at the end of the first trimester, the anomaly rate is not increased, whereas if the HbgA[1]C level is elevated at that time, the anomaly rate is increased.[26] The importance of this observation in terms of understanding the mechanism for anomaly production (hyperglycemia) as well as counseling for it is now being tested in multiple centers by the National Institutes of Health (NIH).

Respiratory Distress Syndrome

The IDM is at an increased risk for the development of respiratory distress syndrome (RDS), and in some studies this risk has been increased five- to sixfold.[28] In animal systems, the cortisol induction of pulmonary surfactant synthesis can be inhibited with insulin. This may be important in the human, for if fetal hyperglycemia and hyperinsulinemia result when maternal hyperglycemia occurs, the lung maturation may be affected.[29] While the amniotic fluid lecithin/sphingomyelin (L/S) ratio can predict RDS in the neonate in most pregnancies, it does not seem to be as significant for the IDM.[30] Thus, for this group only, the amniotic fluid phosphatidylglycerol level is needed to determine the infant's ability to carry on normal respiration.[31]

Hypoglycemia

A normal fetus produces little insulin and, when challenged with a glucose load, it has a delayed release of insulin.[32] In the nursery, the normal neonate cannot handle glucose well and needs several days of eating in order to be able to release insulin promptly and control blood glucose.[7] If the fetus is exposed to chronic hyperglycemia as a result of poor maternal control, it begins to produce large amounts of insulin in utero. The result is that neonatal hypoglycemia is an expected sequela after the cord is clamped, as maternal glucose is no longer available, but the insulin secretion persists. Since the brain needs glucose as a substrate, neonatal hypoglycemia can cause significant brain damage and permanent cerebral palsy. Thus, we have a condition that could (1) be prevented (control maternal blood glucose levels), (2) be detected (measure blood glucose frequently in the early hours of life in the IDM), and (3) be treated (with parenteral glucose given to the hypoglycemic IDM). Therefore, brain damage from this cause in the IDM should no longer occur.

Macrosomia

The fetus uses principally three substances to grow: oxygen, which diffuses easily across the placenta; glucose, which moves by facilitated diffusion; and amino acids, which are actively transported to the fetus. The glucose is burned with oxygen to produce energy in the form of ATP, which is then used to produce proteins from the amino acids. The principal fetal hormones regulating this growth seem to be insulin and somatomedins, both of which are significantly correlated with birth weight.[33,34] If the maternal blood glucose level is elevated, a larger amount of glucose is transported to the fetus, and it grows larger. Macrosomia is defined as birth weight of more than 4500 g, which is commonly seen with maternal obesity and/or diabetes.

The two problems associated with infant macrosomia are immediate and delayed. The initial problem relates to dystocia in vaginal delivery and the possibility of injury to the fetus, especially brachial nerve injuries, clavicle fracture, and death. Thus, if the infant is known to be macrosomic, it is better to circumvent the vaginal delivery and avoid the possible birth trauma with an elective cesarean section. Detection of the macrosomic fetus can be done using ultrasound imaging. Since a major storage organ for the fetus is the liver, most of the techniques incorporate that measurement (abdominal circumference) into the formulas for fetal weight estimates.[35] The long-term problem of macrosomia is that these infants tend to remain obese as they grow up.[36] This carries other health hazards such as diabetes and hypertension.

Finally, the discovery of macrosomia should alert the obstetrician to the possibility that the mother has diabetes. Since all pregnant women should be screened for diabetes with a blood glucose test, the past history of macrosomic infants has less importance in the detection of diabetes today. The main screening is for the postpartum woman who has just delivered a macrosomic infant. Here a single fasting blood sample should be drawn before hospital discharge and a fasting glucose level determined. This glucose value assures the physician that the patient will not be sent home with uncontrolled diabetes. Studies with hemoglobin A_1C postpartum on women with macrosomic neonates have shown that this test has little clinical value.[37] Women with macrosomic infants should then have an oral glucose tolerance test performed some 6–8 weeks later in the postpartum period to screen for a more subtle glucose metabolic abnormality.

Hypocalcemia

Another common problem for the IDM is neonatal hypocalcemia with resultant tetany.[38,39] The pregnant diabetic woman tends to have normal free blood calcium levels but low magnesium levels.[40] This may be the cause of the problem or it may be related to the high growth hormone levels in the IDM.[41] Calcitonin levels are normal in the IDM, but parathyroid hormone concentrations are elevated.[42] While the precise mechanism for this problem is unknown, its frequent occurrence demands monitoring and treatment if indicated.

Hyperbilirubinemia

Jaundice of the newborn is much more common in the IDM.[38,39] This may be due to polycythemia secondary to fetal hypoxia or prematurity secondary to early delivery. While the precise cause is not clear, the neonatologist must monitor the bilirubin levels and treat the problem if needed.

Death

The IDM has been recognized as a high risk for perinatal mortality but with modern management this risk has decreased to a point where it is now similar to that for infants from normal women.[3] Previously all diabetics were classified according to the duration of the mother's disease and her blood vessel involvement (Whites' classification), which permitted prediction of the outcome of the pregnancy.[2] Today the IDM in most of the White classes do so well that there is little need to use the system to determine infant prognosis. It does permit determination of the severity of the disease in the population under study, however, and is therefore useful in research reporting. The perinatal deaths can occur in either the fetal or neonatal time period. The fetal deaths tend to occur either with significant maternal hyperglycemia or during the last weeks of the pregnancy. The mechanism for the death is incompletely understood but may relate to rapid movements of glucose, electrolytes, and water into cells causing dysfunction such as cardiac arrest. Another possible explanation is poor oxygenation due to an altered RBC oxygen-carrying capacity when the cells are labeled with glucose (high hemoglobin A_1C).[43] This increased risk for fetal death demands three principles in management: namely, good glucose control, serial fetal assessments, and early delivery, discussed in the section on Management.

Neonatal deaths generally occur from three causes: respiratory distress with resultant hyaline membrane disease, intravascular hemorrhage, or congenital anomalies. The first of these can be predicted from amniotic fluid studies of phosphatidylglycerol, thereby eliminating this problem with elective deliveries.[44] If the delivery can be postponed until after 32 weeks gestation and if birth trauma is avoided, intraventricular hemorrhage should rarely occur. Careful control of maternal blood glucose levels in the third to sixth weeks of pregnancy should reduce the risk of congenital anomalies.[26]

Management

The management of the diabetic during her pregnancy is difficult, time consuming, and expensive, but the results are rewarding, for one can expect a normal pregnancy outcome. Table 27-4 outlines some of the steps in the management of the diabetic expectant patient. Some of the management steps have already been discussed, such as the urine culture studies. Since the patient is at high risk for blood vessel disease, she needs cardiac (ECG), renal (creatinine clearance), and eye studies.

The two major goals of the management program are good glucose control and early timed delivery. Several steps must be taken in an effort to achieve these goals.

Good Glucose Control

In order to obtain a consistently good outcome, "pregnancy-type" glucose control must be

TABLE 27-4. Management of the Pregnant Diabetic

Usual diet plus 300 cal
Split insulin treatment
Home blood glucose monitoring
Frequent office visits
24-hr urine glucose tests
Hemoglobin A_1C measurements
Periodic amniotic fluid glucose assessments
Urine culture at first visit and at 30–32 weeks
Serial ultrasound examinations starting before 20 weeks
Serial fetal heart rate tests starting at 26–27 weeks
Amniotic fluid phosphatidylglycerol studies
Delivery in perinatal center
Serial retinal studies and laser treatment as needed
Cardiac (ECG) and renal (creatinine clearance) assessment

achieved; this means lower glucose levels than those of a nonpregnant population. The mother can go through the pregnancy with some hyperglycemia without increased morbidity, yet the fetus cannot tolerate hyperglycemia. The tight control is solely for the fetus. The three major steps needed to achieve tight control are diet, insulin treatment, and glucose monitoring.

Diet. There have been many diet descriptions for the diabetic pregnant woman, but little is really known about its composition or how it should differ from that for the low-risk pregnant woman. There is an increased caloric need during pregnancy and lactation and this is suggested to be an additional 300 and 500 cal/day, respectively. While the protein needs are also presumably increased and set between 1.3 and 1.5 g/kg per day, food supplement studies of malnourished populations suggest that the main need is for calories alone.[45] Thus, the diet should contain about 2300 cal/day or about 38 cal kg of ideal body weight. This can be distributed as 1.3 g protein per kilogram per day, 250 g carbohydrate per day, and the remainder in fat. The patient has a critical role in her own care, for she must learn her new diet and be extremely compulsive in taking the precise caloric load at the same times throughout the pregnancy. There is no way to control blood glucose if she consumes a widely varying daily caloric intake. A teaching session should be conducted at the first pregnancy encounter to help her understand her responsibilities and provide her with the information on diet. A nutritionist can greatly assist the health care team in this effort.

Insulin. Insulin does not cross the placenta but glucose does, so there is no fetal risk from insulin administration as long as the blood glucose levels are kept normal.[46] It is easier to control glucose if the insulin is given by continuous pump infusion, but there are still occasional mechanical problems with the ambulatory pumps. While these temporary breakdowns may not create much of a problem for the mother, the resultant hyperglycemia may be a serious problem for the fetus. Thus, while pumps are being included more and more in ambulatory diabetic management and will probably replace injections at some point for many patients, today most pregnant diabetics are still managed with injections in the ambulatory setting and by continuous intravenous infusions during labor or cesarean section.[47] The home injections give better control if they are split into two or three injections per day. In addition, mixtures of long- and short-acting insulin provide better control. One pattern administers two-thirds of the total dose of insulin in the morning as two-thirds long-acting and one-third short acting and the remaining one-third the total dose in the evening as one-half long acting and one-half short acting. Many variations of this program can be used. While in the hospital, blood glucose can be easily controlled by giving 120 ml 5% dextrose in water per hour intravenously plus 0.5 to 1 unit of regular insulin per hour intravenously, using an infusion pump. In most patients this will maintain the blood glucose value between 70 and 80 mg/dl.

Oral hypoglycemic agents are not used in pregnancy, for they have been associated with increased rates of congenital anomalies and prolonged hypoglycemia in the neonate. In addition, a significant number of women break away and develop severe hyperglycemia while taking them, and thus require supplementary insulin. A woman who is taking these drugs when she becomes pregnant should be switched to insulin injections for the duration of the pregnancy.

Glucose Monitoring. The only way to be certain that glucose control is adequate is to measure it, and the more measurements that are done the more certain one becomes about that level of control. The best measurements are blood studies, which can easily be done on an outpatient basis. In the past patients were instructed to record urine glucose values several times per day and to report these to the physician. However, since these are poorly correlated with blood values in pregnancy, that practice is no longer continued in obstetrics. Rather, the patient is instructed to do finger sticks several times per day and to measure the blood glucose concentration using paper enzyme systems with the assistance of simple home colorimeters.[48] This is done accurately and easily and allows for ambulatory management as opposed to hospital care, which greatly reduces the costs of care in this high-risk population. The patients need to check their bloods several times per day, e.g., fasting, before lunch, 1 hr after a meal to assess peak values, and before bedtime. The values should not exceed those used as criteria in the pregnancy glucose tolerance test listed in Table 27-1. Frequent office visits are necessary and, if high levels are measured, she can call her physician immediately.

Additional glucose monitoring should be done using tests that look at wider windows of time, since the blood values represent only the instant that the blood was drawn. Three other determinations are useful, namely: 24-hr urine total glucose levels, amniotic fluid glucose levels, and hemoglobin A_1C levels. The 24-hr urine collection can be done by the patient the day before the office visit and brought in with her. It reflects her daily glycemic profile and, usually with good control, contains only 1–2 g glucose. It can be quickly dipsticked before being sent to the laboratory to assess the control while the patient is still in the office. When the amniotic fluid is being sampled for fetal maturity studies, an aliquot can be obtained and sent for glucose measurements. Amniotic fluid glucose decreases as pregnancy advances and reflects maternal blood values for the previous week.[33] Normally

it is less than 25 mg/dl; high levels correlate well with poor condition of neonates, such as low Apgar scores.[49] The hemoglobin A_1C levels reflect the previous 4–5 weeks of glucose control and are useful long-term overall monitors. In general, in normal pregnancy, because blood glucose levels are reduced, the hemoglobin A_1C levels are lower than in nonpregnancy.[27] Since hemoglobin F (HbgF) migrates at about the same speed as $HbgA_1C$, and since HbgF is elevated to varying levels in pregnant women according to the chorionic gonadotropin levels, the methodology used to measure $HbgA_1C$ must exclude HbgF.

Timed Early Delivery

The timing of delivery in a high-risk pregnancy involves the assessment to two types of infant risk. These are illustrated in Figure 27-1.

Infant Death Risk. The first risk is that of staying in the uterus, and in general the longer one remains there the more likely that death will occur there. In the normal woman this risk begins to go up after the forty-second week, whereas in abnormal women with diabetes mellitus or hypertension, this risk may go up much earlier in the pregnancy (area B in Fig. 27-1). The specific risk must be assessed with serial fetoplacental function tests; these tests must be started at a time when there is an opportunity to save the infant with delivery. In most intensive care nurseries today, there are some normal survivors after 26–27 weeks gestation (650–700-g birth

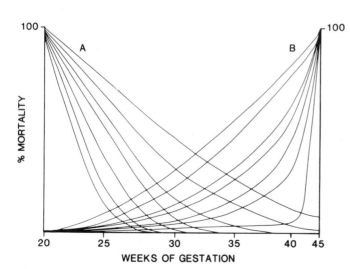

FIGURE 27-1. The two major risk factors for the fetus vary and include prematurity risks if delivered (area A) and stillbirth risks if they remain undelivered (area B).

weight), making it a logical time to begin the testing. A large number of these tests are used in perinatal medicine, and many have been tested in pregnant diabetic populations. Those that are predictive are estriol, nonstress tests, and contraction stress tests. Assessment of the IDM with estriol determinations can be done successfully, but these tests require daily sampling, and the measurements should be of plasma free estriol.[50] This is not practical at most perinatal centers. A more practical means of study is monitoring the fetal heart rate. Whereas many obstetricians moved to utilize the nonstress test (NST) because it was easy and convenient, several sources of data today suggest that it is not sensitive enough to use in diabetics on a weekly basis.[51-53] The test that provides the best assessment of fetal death risk is the weekly oxytocin contraction stress test (OCT). A negative test consisting of no fetal heart rate decelerations in a 10-min time period that includes three contractions suggests very little risk for fetal death during the next week, provided blood glucose control stays good.[51-53] Suspicious or positive tests suggest varying degrees of fetal jeopardy that need to be carefully evaluated in terms of the heart rate reactivity as well as other assessments of fetal and placental well-being. These could include breathing motions of the fetus and its cardiac preejection period measurements.

Fetal Maturity Tests. The risks for the prematurely delivered newborn involve two general problems: RDS and intraventricular hemorrhage (IVH) (area A in Fig. 27-1). The IVH results from disruption of immature blood vessels in the germinal plates within the ventricles and usually occurs in infants delivered before the thirty-second week of gestation or in infants with significant head trauma. There are no known perinatal tests that can predict that problem except fetal age assessment, which can best be done using serial ultrasound scans started before the twentieth week of gestation and measuring structures such as the gestational sac diameter, head biparietal diameter, femur length, and abdominal or chest circumference.[54] Assessment of the risk of neonatal RDS can be made from studies of the amniotic fluid surfactant levels, and for the IDM this means measurement of the amniotic fluid content of phosphatidylglycerol and the L/S ratio.[30,31] These tests are usually first done at about the thirty-seventh week of gestation if there are no problems up to that time, as determined by the fetal well-being risk assessments. Most IDMs

are mature and ready for delivery at about the thirty-eighth week of gestation.

Delivery

The delivery should be performed at a tertiary perinatal center where a team is available to manage all the potential problems for the mother and infant. Team members include maternal-fetal medicine subspecialty obstetricians, neonatologists, internal medicine diabetologists, obstetric anesthesiologist, nurses, nutritionists, and social workers. The management of premature labor can best be done using magnesium sulfate as the tocolytic drug, since the β-mimetic agents cause significant material hyperglycemia. The type of delivery is determined by obstetric factors, but fetal macrosomia must be assessed with ultrasound and, if found, that delivery should be by an elective cesarean section. During the labor-delivery time, the glucose level is most easily controlled using intravenous glucose and insulin treatment as noted earlier. Blood glucose and electrolytes must be measured frequently during this time. If labor is attempted then careful fetal assessment must be done using continuous electronic fetal heart rate monitoring with fetal scalp blood pH studies to assess any abnormal heart rate findings.

GESTATIONAL DIABETES

The woman with a mildly abnormal glucose tolerance test does not pose as serious a risk to the infant as one with insulin-dependent diabetes mellitus. Often these patients are obese. The goals of management are similar, however, and these are to keep blood glucose normal and to make serial assessments of fetal well-being. In general the glucose management relies first on dietary treatment; if this fails, the patient will then have to receive insulin therapy. If the fasting blood glucose levels are abnormal, diet treatment alone is less likely to succeed. Blood glucose (fasting and 1-hr percutaneous values) can be monitored at the office on a weekly basis, and both values need to be normal. The fetus can be assessed with frequent NST or weekly OCT; if these are normal, the pregnancy can be allowed to proceed to term gestation. Before induction of labor, ultrasound assessment for macrosomia should be performed. The need for cesarean section in this group is only slightly increased. After delivery, the abnormal glucose tolerance test usually reverts to normal, and the disease becomes subclinical for years. Regular glucose monitoring should be advised.

FAMILY PLANNING

Patients with diabetes mellitus pose a problem in terms of the family planning program.[55] These patients should understand that their reproductive problems increase with age; therefore, if possible, they should plan to have their children during the early years of their disease process. Once they have completed their family size they should be offered surgical sterilization, as this avoids the failures and problems of contraception. For the child-spacing time in their reproductive life plan, they have several safe choices.

First, the use of oral contraceptives is relatively contraindicated. When oral contraceptives (OC) were introduced into clinical medicine, the major concerns were the pregnancy rates and bleeding patterns. It was not until many years after their introduction into clinical use that reachers began to evaluate their effects on other body functions, including metabolism. The first report of their effects on blood glucose was in the early 1960s; later, many laboratories reported that the drugs were responsible for significant alterations in carbohydrate metabolism.[56–58] After many years of such reports, it became clear that several changes were common: few significant alterations in fasting blood glucose levels; significant elevations of the glucose tolerance test results, especially with the oral test as compared to the intravenous test; and elevations of plasma insulin levels during the glucose tolerance test.[56–58] It also became clear that women's responses varied with OCs for about 4% of "normal" women developed diabetic-type glucose tolerance tests when using the OCs, whereas about 44% of the gestational diabetic or subclinical diabetic women did so.[58] A major concern about these metabolic changes was that the OCs were also associated with an increased risk of myocardial infarction.[59] Whether the metabolic changes were responsible for the vessel wall changes remains unknown. It is clear that the synthetic steroids in the OC have a potentially detrimental effect on carbohydrate metabolism resulting in higher plasma insulin and blood glucose levels, especially in the high-risk subclinical gestational diabetic populations. This was clearly different from the normal menstrual cycle, where minimal changes in carbohydrate metabolism occur between the follicular and luteal phases. Thus, there are two major concerns. First, women with gestational subclinical diabetes may be made overt with the drugs and need medical treatment as a result. Second, women with diabetes mellitus are already at increased risk for accelerated atherogenesis and small vessel disease. Since oral contraceptives are also associated with accelerated atherogenesis, this may produce an additive adverse effect. The conclusion is that the OC is a poor choice for the diabetic.

Another contraceptive to be considered is the IUD. One major concern is that they are associated with increased risk of pelvic infections generally considered to be 1.5–2-fold elevated. The diabetic is characteristically susceptible to infections. Some studies have been published, however, showing that IUD use in diabetics is without any increased frequency of infections.[55] If this method is used, the patient should be informed of the potential complication.

The best method for these women is barrier forms of contraception as the diaphragm and contraceptive cream or condoms and contraceptive cream. There are no method risk factors, and the only problems are the higher pregnancy rates associated with the method and the nuisance factors of a coital act-associated method. They should be offered and encouraged, however.

SUMMARY

Diabetes mellitus complicating pregnancy is now a frequent problem that can be detected and managed. The insulin resistance accompanying normal pregnancy makes this an ideal time to detect subclinical disease. The problems for the mother are numerous but not serious. The problems for the infant are very serious and often permanent. All the infant problems seem to be due to hyperglycemia. The two goals of therapy are to keep maternal blood glucose "normal for pregnancy" throughout the entire gestation and to time the date of delivery by using serial biophysical and biochemical tests of fetal–placental health and maturity. Unique risks with contraceptives make a special family planning program important as well.

QUESTIONS

1. Type I IDDM is a disease whose heredity is based on susceptibility to autoimmune disease. The concor-

dance rate for identical twins is 50%. The risk to an offspring of a diabetic mother is

- a. 50%.
- b. 25%.
- c. 2–5%.
- d. none of the above.

2. In insulin-requiring diabetic pregnancy, the highest positive correlation has been noted between the size of the infant at birth and the maternal

- a. height and weight.
- b. weight gain in pounds per week.
- c. obesity greater than 115% of ideal body weight.
- d. fasting plasma glucose concentration.
- e. plasma triglyceride concentration.

3. In the pregnant woman, insulin

- a. has less biologic activity.
- b. freely passes the placenta.
- c. has normal secretory patterns in response to glucose stimuli.
- d. does not alter placental metabolism.

4. Studies of amniotic fluid glucose concentrations show

- a. a rise to 29–30 weeks of pregnancy and then a plateau until delivery.
- b. a good correlation between the levels before delivery and the neonates status immediately after birth.
- c. a short lag time, so that the concentrations poorly reflect the glucose profiles of the mother.
- d. a turnover rate half-life of 46 min.
- e. high levels with toxemia of pregnancy.

5. Patients with diabetes mellitus complicating pregnancy

- a. should not receive long-acting insulin immediately before delivery, as it will persist in the neonate for 24–26 hrs.
- b. require monitoring with blood insulinase studies to detect placental insufficiency.
- c. may produce neonates with respiratory problems secondary to insulin blockage of cortisol activity on the lungs.
- d. can be expected to require approximately 475 kcal more of food intake during the last half of their gestation.

REFERENCES

1. Graham G: A case of diabetes mellitus complicated by pregnancy, treated with insulin. *Proc R Soc Med* 17:102–104, 1924
2. White P: Diabetes mellitus in pregnancy. *Clin Perinatol* 1:331–347, 1974*
3. Jovanovic L, Peterson CM: Management of the pregnant Insulin-dependent diabetic woman. *Diabetes Care* 3:63–68, 1980
4. Burt RL: Carbohydrate metabolism in pregnancy. *Clin Obstet Gynecol* 3:310–325, 1960
5. Burt RL: Further observations on reactivity to insulin in normal pregnancy. *Obstet Gynecol* 13:433–436, 1959
6. Spellacy WN, Goetz FC: Plasma insulin in normal late pregnancy. *N Engl J Med* 268:988–991, 1963
7. Spellacy WN: Carbohydrate metabolism in pregnancy, in Fuchs F, Klopper A (eds): *Endocrinology of Pregnancy*, Philadelphia, Harper & Row, 1983, pp 161–175*
8. Tsibris JCM, Raynor LO, Buhi WC, et al: Insulin receptors in circulating erythrocytes and monocytes from women on oral contraceptives or pregnant women near term. *J Clin Endocr* 51:711–717, 1980
9. Pagano G, Cassader M, Massobrio M, et al: Insulin binding to human adipocytes during late pregnancy in healthy, obese and diabetic state. *Horm Metab Res* 12:177–181, 1980
10. Spellacy WN, Cohn JE: Human placental lactogen levels and daily insulin requirements in patients with diabetes mellitus complicating pregnancy. *Obstet Gynecol* 42:330–333, 1973
11. Kuhl C, Holst JJ: Plasma glucagon and the insulin: Glucagon ratio in gestational diabetes. *Diabetes* 25:16–23, 1976
12. Gustafson AB, Banasiak MF, Kalkhoff RK, et al: Correlation of hyperprolactinemia with altered plasma insulin and glucagon: Similarity to effects of late human pregnancy. *J Clin Endocr* 51:242–246, 1980
13. Jarrett JC II, Ballejo G, Saleem TH, et al: The effect of prolactin and relaxin on insulin binding by adipocytes from pregnant women. *Am J Obstet Gynecol* 149:250–255, 1984
14. O'Sullivan JB, Mahan CM, Charles D, et al: Screening criteria for high-risk gestational diabetic patients. *Am J Obstet Gynecol* 116:895–900, 1973
15. Carpenter MW, Couston DR: Criteria for screening tests for gestational diabetes. *Am J Obstet Gynecol* 144:768–773, 1982
16. O'Sullivan JB, Mahan CM: Criteria for the oral glucose tolerance test in pregnancy. *Diabetes* 13:278–285, 1964
17. Pedersen J: *The Pregnant Diabetic and Her Newborn*. 2nd ed. Baltimore, Williams & Wilkins, 1977
18. Vejlsgaard R: Studies on urinary infections in diabetics. III. Significant bacteriuria in pregnant diabetics and in matched controls. *Acta Med Scand* 193:337–341, 1973
19. Buckley RM Jr, McGuckin M, MacGregor RR: Urine bacterial counts after intercourse. *N Engl J Med* 298:321–324, 1978
20. Dibble CM, Kochenour NK, Worley RJ, et al: Effect of pregnancy on diabetic retinopathy. *Obstet Gynecol* 59:699–704, 1982
21. Moloney JBM, Drury MI: The effect of pregnancy on the natural course of diabetic retinopathy. *Am J Ophthalmol* 93:745–756, 1982

*Review article or chapter.

22. Chesley LC, Annitto JE, Cosgrove RA: The remote prognosis of eclamptic women. Sixth periodic report. *Am J Obstet Gynecol* 124:446–459, 1976
23. Queenan JT, Gadow EC: Polyhydramnios: Chronic versus acute. *Am J Obstet Gynecol* 108:349–355, 1970
24. Crane JP, Wahl N: The role of maternal diabetes in repetitive spontaneous abortion. *Fertil Steril* 36:477–479, 1981
25. Mills JL, Baker L, Goldman AS: Malformations in infants of diabetic mothers occur before the seventh gestational week—Implications for treatment. *Diabetes* 28:292–293, 1979
26. Miller E, Hare JW, Cloherty JP, et al: Elevated maternal hemoglobin A_1C in early pregnancy and major congenital anomalies in infants of diabetic mothers. *N Engl J Med* 304:1331–1334, 1981
27. Widness JA, Schwartz HC, Kahn CB, et al: Glycohemoglobin in diabetic pregnancy: A sequential study. *Am J Obstet Gynecol* 136:1024–1029, 1980
28. Robert MF, Neff RK, Hubbell JP, et al: Association between maternal diabetes and the respiratory-distress syndrome in the newborn. *N Engl J Med* 294:357–360, 1976
29. Smith BT, Giroud CJP, Robert M, et al: Insulin antagonism of cortisol action on lecithin synthesis by cultured fetal lung cells. *J Pediatr* 87:953–955, 1975
30. Cruz AC, Buhi WC, Birk SA, et al: Respiratory distress syndrome with mature lecithin/sphingomyelin ratios: Diabetes mellitus and low APGAR scores. *Am J Obstet Gynecol* 126:78–82, 1976
31. Hallman M, Teramo K: Amniotic fluid phospholipid profile as a predictor of fetal maturity in diabetic pregnancies. *Obstet Gynecol* 54:703–707, 1979
32. Spellacy WN, Gall SA, Carlson KL: Carbohydrate metabolism of the normal term newborn: Plasma insulin and blood glucose levels during an intravenous glucose tolerance test. *Obstet Gynecol* 30:580–583, 1967
33. Spellacy WN, Buhi WC, Bradley B, et al: Maternal, fetal and amniotic fluid levels of glucose, insulin and growth hormone. *Obstet Gynecol* 41:323–331, 1973
34. Bennett A, Wilson DM, Liu F, et al: Levels of Insulin-like growth factors I and II in human cord blood. *J Clin Endocrinol* 57:609–612, 1983
35. Ogata ES, Sabbagha R, Metzger B, et al: Serial ultrasonography to assess evolving fetal macrosomia—Studies in 23 diabetic women. *JAMA* 243:2405–2408, 1980
36. Pettitt DJ, Baird HR, Aleck KA, et al: Excessive obesity in offspring of Pima Indian women with diabetes during pregnancy. *N Engl J Med* 308:242–245, 1983
37. Coen RW, Porreco R, Cousins L, et al: Postpartum glycosylated hemoglobin levels in mothers of large-for-gestational age infants. *Am J Obstet Gynecol* 136:380–382, 1980
38. Pildes RS: Infants of diabetic mothers. *N Engl J Med* 289:902–904, 1973*
39. Tsang RC, Ballard J, Braun C: The infant of the diabetic mother: Today and tomorrow. *Clin Obstet Gynecol* 24:125–147, 1981*
40. Cruikshank DP, Pitkin RM, Reynolds WA, et al: Altered maternal calcium homeostasis in diabetic pregnancy. *J Clin Endocrinol* 50:264–267, 1980
41. Bergman L, Westerberg B, Lindstedt G, et al: Possible involvement of growth hormone in the pathogenesis of early neonatal hypocalcemia in infants of diabetic mothers. *Biol Neonate* 34:72–79, 1978
42. Bergman L, Kjellmer I, Selstam U: Calcitonin and parathyroid hormone-relation to early neonatal hypocalcemia in infants of diabetic mothers. *Biol Neonate* 24:151–160, 1974

43. Madsen H, Ditzel J: Changes in red blood cell oxygen transport in diabetic pregnancy. *Am J Obstet Gynecol* 143:421–424, 1982
44. Cunningham MD, Desai NS, Thompson SA, et al: Amniotic fluid phosphatidylglycerol in diabetic pregnancies. *Am J Obstet Gynecol* 131:719–724, 1978
45. Lechtig A, Habicht JP, Delgado H, et al: Effect of food supplementation during pregnancy on birth weight. *Pediatrics* 56:508–520, 1975
46. Spellacy WN, Goetz FC, Greenberg BZ, et al: The human placental gradient for plasma insulin and blood glucose. *Am J Obstet Gynecol* 90:753–757, 1964
47. Rudolf MCJ, Couston DR, Sherwin RS, et al: Efficacy of the insulin pump in the home treatment of pregnant diabetics. *Diabetes* 30:891–895, 1981
48. Jovanovic L, Peterson CM, Saxena BB, et al: Feasibility of maintaining normal glucose profiles in insulin-dependent pregnant diabetic women. *Am J Med* 68:105–112, 1980
49. Archimaut G, Belizán JM, Ross NA, et al: Glucose concentration in amniotic fluid: Its possible significance in diabetic pregnancy. *Am J Obstet Gynecol* 119:596–602, 1974
50. Distler W, Gabbe SG, Freeman RK, et al: Estriol in pregnancy. V. Unconjugated and total plasma estriol in the management of pregnant diabetic patients. *Am J Obstet Gynecol* 130:424–431, 1978
51. Freeman RK, Anderson G, Dorchester W: A prospective multi-institutional study of antepartum fetal heart rate monitoring. I. Risk of perinatal mortality and morbidity according to antepartum fetal heart rate test results. *Am J Obstet Gynecol* 143:771–777, 1982
52. Freeman RK, Anderson G, Dorchester W: A prospective multi-institutional study of antepartum fetal heart rate monitoring. II. Contraction stress test versus nonstress test for primary surveillance. *Am J Obstet Gynecol* 143:778–781, 1982
53. Barrett JM, Salyer SL, Boehm FH: The nonstress test: An evaluation of 1,000 patients. *Am J Obstet Gynecol* 141:153–157, 1981
54. Seeds JW, Cefalo RC: Relationship of fetal limb lengths to both biparietal diameter and gestational age. *Obstet Gynecol* 60:680–685, 1982
55. Spellacy WN: Family planning and the diabetic mother. *Semin Perinatol* 2:395–399, 1978*
56. Spellacy WN: A review of carbohydrate metabolism and the oral contraceptives. *Am J Obstet Gynecol* 104:448–460, 1969*
57. Spellacy WN: Carbohydrate metabolism in male infertility and female fertility—Control patients. *Fertil Steril* 27:1132–1141, 1976
58. Kalkhoff RK: Effects of oral contraceptive agents on carbohydrate metabolism. *J Steroid Biochem* 6:949–956, 1975*
59. Mann JI, Vessey MP, Thorogood M, et al: Myocardial infarction in young women with special reference to oral contraceptive practice. *Br Med J* 2:241–245, 1975

ANSWERS

1. c

2. d

3. a

4. b

5. c

V

Infertility and Its Future

28

Investigation of the Infertile Couple

WILLIAM C. ANDREWS

INTRODUCTION

Infertility is defined as a failure to achieve conception during 1 or more years of intercourse of adequate frequency without the use of contraception. Primary infertility indicates those patients who have never conceived. Secondary infertility indicates previous pregnancy but failure to conceive subsequently during one or more years of unprotected intercourse. Absolute infertility or sterility indicates those individuals who have an absolute factor preventing conception. Relative infertility involves conditions that are potentially correctable after diagnosis.

Eighty percent of couples attempting pregnancy achieve a conception within 1 year with regular intercourse of reasonable frequency. An additional 10% achieve conception by the end of the second year. Ten percent will remain infertile at the end of 2 years.

The 1976 National Survey of Family Growth, classified 6,954,000 (25.3%) of all married couples with the wife of childbearing age as having a fecun-

dity impairment. Many of these couples, however, did not desire children or additional children.

The increased incidence of pelvic inflammatory disease (PID) with the use of intrauterine devices (IUDs) may increase the number of infertile women, but the decrease in PID found with the use of oral contraceptives may counterbalance this trend.

Female factors in infertility account for approximately 40–50% of cases. Forty percent involve male factors, and the remainder involve problems in both members of the couple. Approximately 20–30% of the problems are tubal or peritoneal in origin, 25% are ovulatory problems, and 5–10% are cervical.

Problems of ovulation may be anovulation or oligo-ovulation. In addition, some patients may have inadequate production of progesterone, resulting in inadequate development of the endometrium for implantation of a fertilized egg. Defects of ovulation can occur at any of the three levels of the hypothalamic–pituitary–ovarian axis: (1) hypothalamic or higher CNS factors, including drug related or psychogenic factors; (2) pituitary factors, including tumors or destructive vascular lesions; and (3) gonadal factors, including premature ovarian failure, ovarian tumors, or ovarian dysgenesis. Additional factors such as significant deviations from normal weight, chronic illness, meta-

WILLIAM C. ANDREWS • Department of Obstetrics and Gynecology, Eastern Virginia Medical School, Norfolk, Virginia 23507.

bolic disease, including hypothyroidism and diabetes, and the adrenogenital syndrome or other disturbances of the adrenal gland may be involved in the etiology of ovulation defects.

Mechanical obstruction or unfavorable environment at any of the four levels of the female reproductive tract can prevent conception. Cervical mucus of adequate quantity and quality must be present. The endometrium must be adequately prepared and free of synechia or significant adhesions. Cervical problems may be the result of chronic infection, inadequate hormonal stimulation or immunologic factors. The intrauterine environment may be rendered hostile by hormonal inadequacy, infection, scarring, or tumors. Tubal problems range from complete obstruction to limitation of tubal motility by peritubal adhesions. Peritoneal factors in infertility in addition to peritubal adhesions include endometriosis, a common disease and frequent cause of infertility. Approximately 35% of infertile women, where no other cause for infertility is found in the couple, will be found to have endometriosis. It is estimated that 6–15% of infertile patients have endometriosis as a sole cause of their infertility.

On the male side, infertility may be produced in absolute fashion by azospermia or in a relative manner by oligospermia of varying degrees. Orchitis, in particular mumps orchitis, is a common cause of azospermia. It is estimated that 15% of men who have mumps after puberty will become sterile. General state of health, drug intake, and chronic use of alcohol and marihuana all may affect spermatogenesis. Infections such as prostatitis or seminal vesiculitis may lower fertility. Obstructive disorders of the male genital tract are a less common cause of infertility if infections are treated promptly with antibiotics. Ejaculatory disturbances such as retrograde or absent ejaculation may be associated with long-term diabetes mellitus, which can also interfere with spermatogenesis. Retrograde ejaculation may also be produced secondary to retroperitoneal or pelvic surgery that interrupt sympathetic nerve passways.

INVESTIGATION OF INFERTILITY

Any couple desiring children who do not achieve a pregnancy within 2 years of adequate exposure should have a systematic evaluation of their reproductive function. The investigation should be performed for women 30 years of age or older after one year of exposure. Earlier investigation may be recommended in young women because of their own concerns or because of factors in their history or physical examination suggesting the presence of an abnormality in reproductive function. The success rate for treatment of infertility declines with length of infertility and increasing age; if indicated adequate investigation and treatment should not be unnecessarily postponed.

Steps in the investigation should be outlined to the couple together if possible. The investigation should, in most cases, be completed within 3–6 months, and prolonged investigation or basal temperature determinations should be avoided if possible to avoid undue psychic stress.

INVESTIGATION OF THE FEMALE

History

The history should include duration of infertility, previous contraceptive history, fertility in other marriages, sexual exposure of patient and previous consort(s), previous obstetric history (if any, which should include number of pregnancies and abortions, length of time required to initiate each pregnancy, complications of any pregnancy), a detailed menstrual history, and a history of any previous infections. The general medical history should include chronic and hereditary disease. The surgical history should be directed especially toward abdominal or pelvic surgery. The sexual history should include particularly frequency of intercourse and postcoital practices. The psychosomatic evaluation should focus on general and infertility problems. A history of any previous tests or therapy for infertility should be obtained.

Physical Examination

The general physical examination should be performed to rule out any disease affecting general health, with special attention to normality of weight, any abnormal distribution of hair. Examination of the genital tract should include adequacy of hymeneal opening; evidence of vaginal infections; cervical tears or infection; uterine size, shape, and mobility; presence of adnexal masses or fixation; and tenderness or nodularity in the uterosacral ligaments.

Laboratory Investigation

Laboratory data should include at least a routine urine and CBC. Additional studies should be performed as indicated by history, physical, or subsequent findings. The sequence in which infertility tests should be performed may be determined by history or physical findings, which suggests looking at one or another factor first. In the absence of such clues, the following suggested sequence is a logical approach. The semen analysis should be obtained early in the investigation (details to be discussed later), as a major defect on this one test may obviate doing any further testing on the female.

Ovulatory Factors

Abnormalities of ovulation are a frequent cause of infertility and, since the adequacy of ovulatory function may be determined noninvasively, this should be one of the first factors studied in the female. Problems of ovulation include a range from luteal phase dysfunction to anovulation to amenorrhea.

Basal Body Temperature Charting

This is the simplest, least expensive method of assessing presumptive ovulation; it should be the initial test in the female. It should not be the only test of ovulatory function. The patient should be instructed to take her temperature with a basal body thermometer on first awakening in the morning. The temperature may be taken orally or rectally, but the oral route is perfectly adequate and less stressful. The thermometer should be shaken down in advance, the temperature should be recorded on a chart with adequate scope to portray changes. A sustained rise of over 0.6°F maintained for at least 10 days represents presumptive ovulation. A monophasic level throughout the cycle suggests anovulation. Presumptive ovulation is at the nadir of the curve and not at the rise. Temperature taking should not be used to determine the time for conception in a given cycle, but only in retrospect. Continuation of the chart during the investigation is of help in determining timing of postcoital tests and endometrial biopsies but should not be continued for more than 3–4 months, except when necessary for management of ovulation induction. Prolonged use of temperature charting may result in sexual dysfunction, particularly in the male partner.

Endometrial Biopsy

Properly timed endometrial biopsy is not only helpful in establishing presumptive ovulation but also in determining the adequacy of endometrial development and indirectly luteal function and is also of value in ruling out endometritis, particularly of tubercular origin. The biopsy should be performed one to two days prior to an expected period. (Use of the basal temperature chart helps in planning the timing of the biopsy.) A Novak suction currette or the equivalent may be employed, using a single lateral wall sweep of the endometrial cavity. Studies suggest that this does not interrupt a conception in that cycle but, if of concern to the patient, barrier contraception may be employed during that cycle. Premedication with a prostaglandin synthetase inhibitor 1 hr before the procedure or the use of narcotics reduces discomfort, but in an occasional case a paracervical block may be necessary in the very sensitive patient. Cramping is usually brief, and premedication alone is adequate. Endometrial slides should be read and dated according to the criteria of Noyes, Hertig, and Rock by an individual interested and experienced in the interpretation. Dating should be from the subsequent not the preceding period. Absence of secretory change confirms anovulation or the rare progesterone receptor defect, where proliferative endometrium is found in a cycle at the same time as luteal-phase serum progesterone levels.

When the endometrium is found to be 2 or more days behind in development, a diagnosis of luteal-phase defect is suggested; this must be confirmed by a repeated biopsy or serum progesterone determinations at the mid-luteal phase in a subsequent cycle.

Serum Progesterone

Serum progesterone levels follow a parabolic curve during the luteal phase of the menstrual cycle. Serial daily progesterone determinations throughout the luteal phase provide the most accurate determination of luteal function, but expense and inconvenience preclude this for clinical use. A single serum progesterone obtained 7 days after the nadir of the basal temperature chart is reasonable presumptive evidence of ovulation and is useful in confirming or refuting a luteal-phase defect suggested on endometrial biopsy. A level of ≥3 ng/ml suggests ovulation; 3–10 ng/ml is indicative of inadequate luteal function; ≥ 15 ng/ml suggests good luteal function; and 10–15 ng/ml is a borderline range the significance of which is unclear. Additional laboratory studies are indicated in several situations.

Amenorrhea

When amenorrhea is present the following tests are indicated

1. Rule out pregnancy by a serum test for human chorionic gonadotropin (hCG). Pregnancy is the most common cause of amenorrhea in the reproductive years.
2. Test serum follicle stimulating hormone (FSH) to exclude primary ovarian failure.
3. Perform thyroid studies for thyroid-stimulating hormone (TSH), triiodothyronine (T3), and thyroxine (T4).
4. Test the prolactin level, which may be elevated with or without galactorrhea. Serum should be obtained from patient in morning in a fasting state. If elevated, ascertain whether the patient is taking any medication such as phenothiazide, α-methyldopa, or reserpine, which could iatrogenically elevate prolactin. If prolactin is elevated above 100 ng/ml, the patient should be checked radiographically for macro- or micropituitary tumors by roentgenograms of the sella turcica or by tomograms or computed tomography (CT) scans. Third-generation CT scans have proved most effective in detecting microadenomas.
5. In cases of primary amenorrhea, karyotyping should also be performed.

Oligomenorrhea or Anovulatory Cycles

For patients with oligomenorrhea or anovulatory cycles

1. Obtain serum prolactin levels.
2. Perform thyroid studies.
3. Test FSH and LH levels to identify polycystic ovarian disease (Stein-Leventhal syndrome). Absent or infrequent ovulation, normal FSH and relatively elevated LH establishes the diagnosis.
5. Evaluate androgen levels. Dehydroepiandrosterone sulfate (DHEA-S) is a good screen for excessive androgen production by adrenal glands. Serum testosterone is indicated to detect excess androgen of ovarian origin. If elevated, morning and evening cortisol studies should be performed and corticosteroid suppression tests performed to differentiate adrenal hyperplasia from adrenal tumors in cases of elevated DHEA-S levels.

Determination of Tubal Patency

Uterotubal Insufflation

Insufflation of carbon dioxide gas, or Rubin's test, is employed less frequently today than in previous years but may be useful as a screening test for tubal patency. There is also a clinical impression that this may at times be therapeutic. The test should be performed after the end of menstruation and before ovulation and should be performed with equipment that controls the pressure of CO_2, with the pressure not exceeding 200 mm Hg. Apparatus should also measure and record the pressures and variations in pressures during the tests, with kymographic tracing of changes in pressures during the tests. The kymographic tracing of falls in pressure indicating passage of the gas. Patency is confirmed by the presence of shoulder pain when the patient sits up following the test.

Hysterosalpingography

This test should be performed at some point in every couple's evaluation of fertility unless an absolute cause of sterility has been found. This test is not only of value in demonstrating the presence or absence of tubal patency and the point of occlusion, if present, but is also of value in demonstrating structural abnormalities of the uterine cavity. This test should be performed between the end of menses and prior to ovulation. There is debate as to whether oil- or water-based media should be used for hysterosalpingography, with advantages and disadvantages to each. Increased viscosity and slow dissipation and absorption of oil-based media provides more distinct radiographic shadows. The water-based medium is believed to have a wider margin of safety. Seven of the nine deaths from hysterosalpingography reported in the literature occurred with oil-based media. The oil-based media also carries a greater risk of granuloma formation, foreign body reaction, and chemical peritonitis.

Insufflation at Laparoscopy

This procedure is discussed in the section on laparoscopy.

Evaluation of Cervical Factor

A postcoital test is performed to determine the quality and quantity of cervical mucus and the ability of the sperm to penetrate the mucus. Cervical mucus is only favorable for sperm penetration at the time of ovulation or immediately before it; thus, the timing of the test requires the use of the basal temperature chart to estimate time of expected ovulation, performing the test on that day or 1 or 2 days before. In the event of an unfavorable test, the timing should be rechecked as to when ovulation apparently did occur in that cycle; the test should be repeated at a more appropriate time if inappropriately timed initially. Couples should be instructed to avoid intercourse for 2 days before the day of the test and to avoid any intravaginal medication or douching on the days preceding the test.

There is debate as to the appropriate interval between normal intercourse and the performance of

the test. For logistical reasons, an interval of 2–4 hr has proved practical in my experience.

In performing the test, the cervix should be cleansed, using saline-moistened sponges. Cervical mucus is aspirated with a polyethylene suction catheter attached to a syringe to provide suction. As the catheter is withdrawn from the cervix, a string of mucus usually trails behind and should be measured for *spinbarkeit*. This may need to be cut with scissors near the cervical os to prevent pulling the specimen out of the catheter. A scoring system for cervical mucus has been devised by Insler (Table 28-1). Attention should be paid to the abundance, clarity, lack of viscosity, and *spinbarkeit* ($\geq$5 cm); on microscopic examination, the mucus should be checked for white blood cells (WBC). If WBC are present, the mucus should be cultured.

There is also debate as to the number of motile sperm necessary to define a normal test. Some investigators believe that there should be 20 or more motile sperm per high-power field (hpf), while others consider it as normal if five or more are found. In general, the shorter the interval between intercourse and the test, the higher number of motile sperm that will be found in the cervical mucus.

Table 28-1. Cervical Scoring System[a,b]

Parameter	0	1	2	3
Amount of mucus	None	Scant; a small amount of mucus can be drawn from the cervical canal	Dribble; a glistening drop of mucus seen in the external os; mucus easily drawn	Cascading; abundant mucus pouring out of the external os
Spinnbarkeit	None	Slight; uninterrupted mucus thread may be drawn approx. one-fourth the distance between the external os and vulva	Moderate; uninterrupted mucus thread may be drawn approx. one-half the distance between the external os and vulva	Pronounced; uninterrupted mucus thread may be drawn the whole distance between the external os and vulva
Ferning	None: amorphous mucus	Linear; fine linear ferning seen in a few spots; no side branching	Partial; good ferning with side branches in parts of the slide; linear ferning or amorphous mucus in other parts	Complete; full ferning in the whole preparation
Cervix	Closed; mucosa pale pink; the external os hardly admits a thin applicator		Partially open; mucosa pink; the cervical canal easily penetrable by an applicator	Gaping; mucosa hyperemic, the external os patulous

[a]A score of 10–12 just before ovulation is considered adequate.
[b]Insler et al.[13]

Shaking sperm are considered an abnormal finding. The postcoital test should not be performed in lieu of semen analysis but rather as an adjunct providing additional information about the mucus and the sperm ability to penetrate the mucus.

The finding of immotile sperm in good-quality cervical mucus in a properly timed test in which the consort has a normal semen analysis, suggests the presence of an immunologic factor. This may be diagnosed by (1) serum agglutination tests (Kibrick), (2) immobilization tests (Isojima), or (3) clinical tests cross-matching the wife's cervical mucus against donor semen and the husband's semen against donor preovulatory cervical mucus.

Laparoscopy

Laparoscopy should be performed in all infertility workups, except where an absolute cause of sterility has already been determined, or a significant contraindication to laparoscopy exists. Laparoscopy may be performed in the proliferative or luteal phase of the cycle but preferably should be performed in the luteal phase shortly after ovulation to observe for stigma of ovulation or a corpus luteum as further confirmation of ovulation and to help rule out the luteinized unruptured follicle syndrome (LUF). The couple should be advised to use double-barrier contraception, (e.g., foam and condoms) during the cycle in which the procedure is to be performed. General anesthesia provides better relaxation, hence better visualization of the pelvic organs. Adequate visualization is further enhanced by the use of the two puncture technique, employing a wand to permit visualization of the posterior surfaces of the ovaries, where at times endometriosis may be found in the absence of any other visible disease in the pelvis. In addition to visualizing both sides of the ovaries, the whole length of both tubes should be visualized, as well as the anterior and posterior walls of the uterus, anterior pelvis, and the cul-de-sac. The appendix can also often be visualized and at times is a site of endometriosis. A dilute solution of indigo carmen dye should be injected into the endometrial cavity for tubal perturbation. Indigo carmen is preferable to methylene blue, as it is rapidly absorbed. If a dilatation and curettage (D & C) is to be performed, it should be done after the laparoscopy rather than before, to decrease the chance of endometrial tissue being introduced into the peritoneal cavity.

The American Fertility Society Endometriosis Classification Form is a convenient tool for accurately and quickly documenting the findings at laparoscopy, if endometriosis or adhesions are found (Fig. 28-1).

Laparoscopy, although usually without sequelae, should be considered major surgery. The risks should be recognized and explained to the patient and the procedure performed with all safeguards to minimize complications.

Hysteroscopy

This procedure should be employed for patients showing filling defects on hysterosalpingography or where submucus myoma or synechia are suspected on clinical grounds.

INVESTIGATION OF THE MALE

History

A history of previous fertility or lack thereof should be elicited. A general medical history should be taken with particular reference to sexually transmitted diseases, epididymitis, mumps orchitis, chronic disease (particularly diabetes), and the use of prescription or recreational drugs (e.g., marihuana) or alcohol. The surgical history should be directed particularly toward herniorrhaphy, operations on the testes, or other surgery in the genital area. The occupational history should be directed toward exposure to chemicals, x-rays, radar, or extreme heat or to the use of "jockey" shorts. A sexual history should be obtained, and information regarding any previous fertility testing should be elicited.

Physical Examination

A general physical examination should be performed to determine the general state of health and the condition of the reproductive system, which should exclude hypospadias as well as a check for testicular size (excluding epididymis: normal 3.6–5.5 (average 4.6) × 3.1–3.2 cm (average 2.6)), testicular and epididymal consistency, presence of vas deferens, prostate size and consistency. A careful search for varicocele should be performed in the upright position. In small varicoceles, reflux of blood flow during the Valsalva manuever may be the only physical sign.

Laboratory Investigation

A routine urinalysis and complete blood count (CBC) should be performed. In men over age 30,

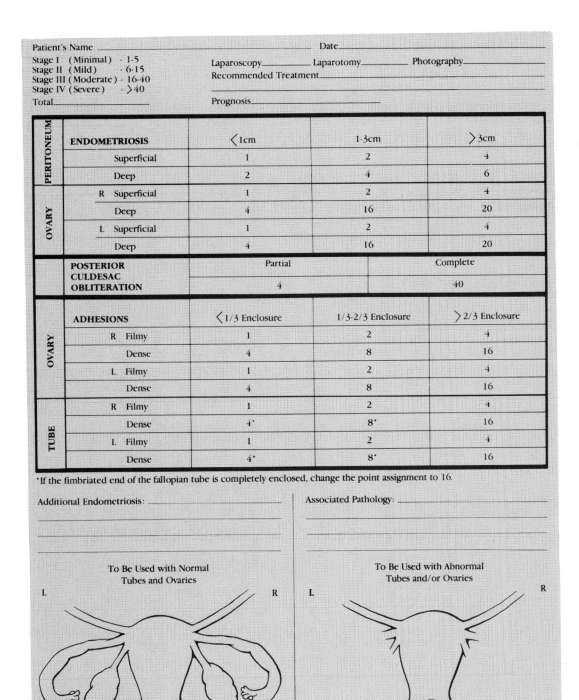

Patient's Name _____ Date_____

Stage I (Minimal) - 1-5
Stage II (Mild) - 6-15
Stage III (Moderate) - 16-40
Stage IV (Severe) - >40
Total_____

Laparoscopy_____ Laparotomy_____ Photography_____
Recommended Treatment_____

Prognosis_____

PERITONEUM	**ENDOMETRIOSIS**	<1cm	1-3cm	>3cm
	Superficial	1	2	4
	Deep	2	4	6
OVARY	R Superficial	1	2	4
	Deep	4	16	20
	L Superficial	1	2	4
	Deep	4	16	20

	POSTERIOR CULDESAC OBLITERATION	Partial	Complete
		4	40

	ADHESIONS	<1/3 Enclosure	1/3-2/3 Enclosure	>2/3 Enclosure
OVARY	R Filmy	1	2	4
	Dense	4	8	16
	L Filmy	1	2	4
	Dense	4	8	16
TUBE	R Filmy	1	2	4
	Dense	4*	8*	16
	L Filmy	1	2	4
	Dense	4*	8*	16

*If the fimbriated end of the fallopian tube is completely enclosed, change the point assignment to 16.

Additional Endometriosis: _____   Associated Pathology: _____
_____   _____
_____   _____

To Be Used with Normal Tubes and Ovaries
L   R

To Be Used with Abnormal Tubes and/or Ovaries
L   R

FIGURE 28-1. American Fertility Society revised classification of endometriosis. (Courtesy of the American Fertility Society.)

fasting multiphasic serum chemistries should be obtained. If a family history of diabetes is present, a 2-hr postprandial blood sugar should be performed. A complete seminal fluid examination should be performed by an experienced technician trained in semen analysis or by a physician experienced in this analysis.

In men with azoospermia, oligospermia, or low-volume ejaculate, or in those with problems of sexual potency, serum FSH, LH, and testosterone levels should be obtained, as well as prolactin. Seminal fluid fructose should be assayed in the presence of azospermia and testes of normal size. Absence of fructose suggests congenital absence of seminal vesicles or of portions of the ductal system, or both.

Semen Analysis

Findings on semen analysis may vary widely from time to time for the same individual; conclusions as to fertility of a man should not be made on the basis of a single unfavorable specimen. The specimen should be collected by masturbation after a 2-day interval of abstinence, collected in a dry, clean glass or plastic jar, and delivered to the laboratory within 2 hr. It should be kept at ambient temperature in transit if not collected at the laboratory.

Criteria of Evaluation

Seminal Fluid Volume. The normal adult range is between 2–6 ml; volume above 6 ml has been suggested as a cause of infertility, but this is not well established. A volume of less than 1 ml has been demonstrated to be a factor in infertility.

Sperm Concentration. The normal adult range is between 60 and 200 million sperm/ml; 20–60 million/ml should be considered a borderline range, although many pregnancies occur within this range. Motility is a major factor in determining the significance of these levels. Below 20 million is considered oligospermic, and pregnancies very rarely occur below the 10-million/ml range. It should again be emphasized that repetitive tests are necessary to establish this diagnosis. Polyspermia or concentration above 200 million/ml is associated with infertility for reasons undetermined.

Sperm Morphology. Careful assessment of morphology with the use of properly stained slides and

interpretation by well-trained individuals is an essential part of the analysis. If a varicocele is present, there is usually an increase in numbers of tapered sperm forms, An increase in the percentages of immature germ cells suggests the presence of D/D 13, 14 translocation, or asymptomatic genital tract infections.

The average normal percentages for various sperm forms and immature germ cells are as follows: oval, 73%; large 2.7%, small, 8.6%; tapered, 6.1%; amorphous, 8.6%, Dup., 1%; and immature, 0.5%. More than 50% of the sperm should have normal morphology.

Sperm Motility. Sperm motility is probably the most significant factor in assaying the ability of a given specimen to fertilize oocytes. Motility should be reported as progressively motile, sluggishly motile, and immotile. More than 50% should be progressively motile.

Agglutination. The specimen should be checked for sperm agglutination. Agglutination of more than 50% of the sperm may result in infertility.

Leukocytes. The presence of WBC in the ejaculate suggests prostatitis or seminal vasiculitis and requires further investigation.

FURTHER STUDIES FOR UNEXPLAINED INFERTILITY

In cases where a cause of the infertility has not been identified, the following procedures should be performed.

Serial Sonography

Serial ultrasound observations of the developing follicle may be performed to detect ovulation and diagnose or exclude LUF syndrome.

Cultures

Semen may be checked for *Ureaplasma,* or the cervix may be cultured for *Ureaplasma* or *Chlamydia.* There is still uncertainty as to the significance of these organisms in infertility, but pregnancies have been reported after the use of doxycycline or tetracycline treatment of these infections or even on an empirical basis.

Hamster Oocyte Penetration Test

The significance of the findings of this test are not totally established but may identify males who, in spite of apparently normal semen analysis, are unable to fertilize a spouse. For this test, hamsters are superovulated; the oocytes are collected and denuded of the zona pellucida. Semen to be tested is incubated with the denuded ova and the percentage of ova penetrated compared with a control. Generally a normal specimen will penetrate from 16–100% of the ova, while in cases of "established" infertility 9% or less of the ova will be penetrated.

SUMMARY

Various common causes of female and male infertility are described. The importance of continued counseling during the gradual evaluation and treatment of a couple is emphasized. The steps to be taken in the workup of female and male partners in cases of infertility are outlined in terms of initial evaluation of history, physical examination, laboratory tests, and special investigative technique.

QUESTIONS

1. List three tests or special investigations that will assist in the diagnosis of a condition preventing passage of eggs or sperm through the female reproductive tract.

2. Name two endocrine disorders that may prevent normal ovulation.

BIBLIOGRAPHY

1. Abraham GE, Moroulis BG, Marshall JR: Evaluation of ovulation and corpus luteum function using measurement of plasma progesterone. *Obstet Gynecol* 44:522–525, 1974
2. Andrews WC: Luteal phase defects. *Fertil Steril* 32:501–509, 1979
3. Ansari AH: Diagnostic procedures for assessment of tubal patency. *Fertil Steril* 31:469–480, 1979
4. Behrman SJ, Kistner RS: *Progress in Infertility.* Boston, Little, Brown, 1976
5. Belsey M, et al: *Laboratory Manual for the Examination of Human Semen and Semen–Cervical Mucus Interaction,* Singapore, Press Concern, 1980
6. Corson SL: Use of the laparoscopy in the infertile patient. *Fertil Steril* 32:359–369, 1979
7. Moghissi KS: The function of the cervix in human reproduction. *Curr Probl Obstet Gynecol* 7:1–58, 1984
8. Moghissi KS, Wallach EE: Unexplained infertility. *Fertil Steril* 39:5–21, 1983
9. Noyes RW, Hertig AT, Rock J: Dating the endometrial biopsy. *Fertil Steril* 1:3, 1950
10. Siegler AM: Hysterosalpingography. *Fertil Steril* 40:139–158, 1983
11. Vallee RF, Sciarra JJ: Current status of hysteroscopy in gynecologic practice. *Fertil Steril* 32:619–632, 1979
12. Wallach EE, Kempers RD: *Modern Trends in Infertility and Conception Control,* Vol. II, Hagerstown, MD, Harper & Row, 1982
13. Insler V, Melmed H, Eichenbrenner I, et al: The cervical score: A simple semiquantitative method for monitoring of the menstrual cycle. *Int J Gynec Obstet* 10:223–228, 1972

ANSWERS

1. Hysterosalpingography, tubal insufflation, and laparoscopic chromo perturbation.

2. Polycystic ovarian disease and hyperprolactinemia.

29

Male Infertility

EMIL STEINBERGER

INTRODUCTION

The incidence of infertility is difficult to establish. This is true not only because detailed epidemiological studies are lacking, but also because the definition of the infertile state is subjective. It depends on the couple's and the physician's perception of the time interval necessary for a conception to occur. Some couples may wait years before consulting a physician, others will see a physician several months after lack of success. Possibly if they would wait longer conception would occur and the couple would not become a statistic. The available information suggests that between 0.4 and 15% of marriages in the United States are involuntarily childless.

As recently as the 1950s, the female was frequently considered the principal cause of a couple's infertility. Textbooks dealing with infertility problems focused primarily on the female, by and large ignoring the male contribution to this problem. As it became apparent that abnormalities in the male might significantly contribute to the couple's infertility problem, more and more attention was paid to the "male" factor. The incidence of "male infer-

tility" as the cause of barren marriages has been variously quoted to be in the range of 30–50%.[1]

Along with the realization that an abnormality of the reproductive system could be detected in the male partner of a substantial number of infertile couples, the focus of the evaluation shifted from the female to the "responsible partner," whether female or male. Since the two partners of a couple were commonly seen by two different physicians practicing different specialties (gynecology or urology), communication problems have rendered management of an infertile couple difficult, and frequently produced less than optimal results. During the past 15 years, physicians became aware of the shortcomings of the concept of a "partner-directed" approach, and a "couples-directed" approach was proposed.[2] This concept was supported by various investigators and practitioners dealing with disorders of the reproductive system.[3-5]

When evaluating a couple's fertility potential, the physician must not be unduly concerned with the "absolute" fertility potential of either partner but rather with the potential of the *couple* to produce offspring. In some instances, the male partner may indeed be the primary cause of a couple's infertility although his fertility potential might be adequate for fathering a child with a different, more fertile female partner. In such a case, although a definite defect in the male partner's reproductive system may be present, one may elect to treat the female

EMIL STEINBERGER • Texas Institute for Reproductive Medicine and Endocrinology; and Department of Internal Medicine, University of Texas Medical School at Houston, Houston, Texas 77002.

partner vigorously instead of focusing on the male, particularly if treatment of the male would involve lengthy and difficult procedures. The converse may also be the case. Consequently the investigation and treatment of infertility must involve the couple rather than each partner separately. The couple should ideally be seen by a physician, or by a team of physicians, conversant with the various medical and surgical disciplines related to the disorders of the reproductive system in both sexes. Both partners should undergo the initial evaluation simultaneously. It should be stressed that examination of the male involves evaluation of specific functions of the male reproductive system rather than determination of an "absolute" fertility potential. The only direct and reliable approach to the assessment of an absolute fertility potential would be to mate the male partner with an "absolute fertile" female. That is obviously impractical even if it were possible to determine the absolute fertility of the female.

This chapter deals with diagnosis and therapy of reproductive system disorders in the male partner of the infertile couple. The material discussed touches briefly on current concepts dealing with the physiology, pathology, and etiology of the male reproductive system disorders associated with fertility disturbances. Sophisticated diagnostic techniques, made possible by recently acquired understanding of the basic aspects of reproductive system function, are outlined. Therapeutic modalities for the management of the male infertility unfortunately still lag seriously behind those for the female in their sophistication; nevertheless, an attempt is made to discuss therapy critically where applicable.

MALE PHYSIOLOGY

Structural Considerations

General

The male reproductive system consists of gonads, their excretory ducts, and several exocrine glands (sex accessory glands) which provide the bulk of the secretions composing the ejaculate. The testis is suspended in the scrotum by the spermatic cord (funiculus spermaticus), which contains the vas deferens, blood vessels, nerves, and the cremasteric muscle. The scrotum, in addition to housing the gonads, serves also as a specialized organ aiding in heat regulation and protection of the testes against physical injury. It is a complicated structure composed of a thin layer of skin lacking subcutaneous adipose tissue, the dartos muscle, the superficial perineal fascia, the external spermatic fascia, the internal spermatic fascia, and the parietal leaf of the tunica vaginalis (Fig. 29-1). The testis is an oblongoid, approximately 4.5 cm in its longest diameter and 2.8 cm in width, weighing 30–45 g.

The parenchyma of the testis is surrounded by a capsule composed of three layers; the visceral layer of the tunica vaginalis, the tunica albuginea, a dense fibrous membrane resting on a thin layer of areolar connective tissue rich in blood vessels, and the tunica vasculosa (Fig. 29-1). Appropriately functioning scrotal structures are essential for normal testicular function. Even small elevations in intratesticular temperature lead to testicular dysfunction. The involvement of testicular envelopes in the production of testicular lesions by mechanisms other than temperature elevation (e.g., hydrocele, vascular changes, increase in intratesticular pressure, impairment of free movement of the testis within the scrotum) is still not clearly understood. It has been demonstrated that the testicular capsule contracts spontaneously and that these contractions can be influenced by acetylcholine (ACh). The role of the contractions is not clear at this time, although it has been suggested that they may be involved in the transport of spermatozoa through the seminiferous tubules.[6] If this function is confirmed, abnormalities in the contractile capacity or pattern of contraction of the testicular capsule may indeed be involved in abnormalities leading to fertility disturbances.

The testicular parenchyma consists of seminiferous tubules, which exhibit a highly complex pattern of convolutions. The tubules are embedded in a connective tissue matrix containing interstitial cells of Leydig, blood vessels, lymphatics, nerves, and a large number of macrophages. Although the seminiferous tubules of human testes show an extremely complicated and irregular pattern of convolutions, anastomoses, and blind pouches, they basically form closed loops terminating in the tubuli recti. The tubuli recti empty into the rete testis, which is connected by a number of small ducts, the ductuli efferentes, with the epididymal duct at the caput epididymis.

The Seminiferous Tubules

The seminiferous tubules occupy approximately 75% of the volume of the parenchyma. Consequently, damage to the seminiferous tubules result-

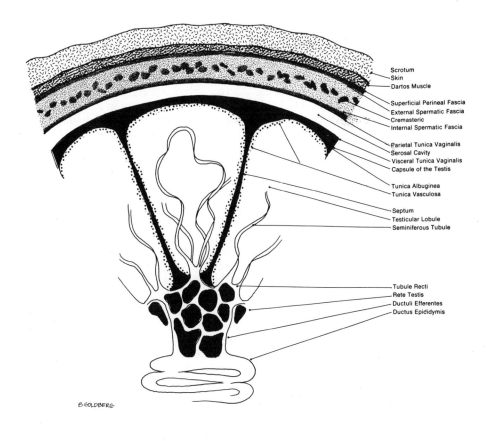

Scrotum
Skin
Dartos Muscle

Superficial Perineal Fascia
External Spermatic Fascia
Cremasteric
Internal Spermatic Fascia

Parietal Tunica Vaginalis
Serosal Cavity
Visceral Tunica Vaginalis
Capsule of the Testis

Tunica Albuginea
Tunica Vasculosa

Septum
Testicular Lobule
Seminiferous Tubule

Tubule Recti
Rete Testis
Ductuli Efferentes
Ductus Epididymis

B GOLDBERG

FIGURE 29-1. Diagrammatic section of the testis and its envelopes.

ing in atrophy of the seminiferous epithelium produces an overall decrease in the size of the testes and softening of the organ. The tubules are surrounded by a complex membrane (tunica propria, or limiting membrane), which consists of peritubular cells (fibroblasts), myoid cells (contractile elements), several layers of collagen fibrils, and a basement membrane composed of an acellular mucopolysaccharide matrix on which surface rests the seminiferous epithelium. The limiting membrane is extremely sensitive to pathological processes and responds to them with characteristic proliferative changes, such as fibrosis (overproduction of fibroblasts) and/or "hyalinization" (excessive deposition of the acellular mucopolysaccharide layer).

The Seminiferous Epithelium

Formation of spermatozoa, or the process of spermatogenesis, takes place in the seminiferous epithelium within the seminiferous tubules. The newly formed spermatozoa are shed from the surface of the epithelium into the lumen of the seminiferous tubules and are transported through the excretory system of the testes (tubuli recti, rete testis, and ductuli efferentes) into the epididymis. During the transit through the epididymis, they undergo physiological maturation and are stored in the cauda (the tail of the epididymis).

The spermatogenic or seminiferous epithelium is composed of somatic cells, the Sertoli cells, and germ cells in various stages of development. The germ cells exhibit a variety of morphological characteristics depending on the stage of their development. The microscopic appearance of germ cells had already been described in the nineteenth century, when they were classified into the various morphological types and their developmental pattern was partly clarified.[7] It has been suggested that the cells residing at the periphery of the epithelium near the basement membrane, the spermatogonia, are the least differentiated germ cells, which divide to form spermatocytes. The spermatocytes are unique cells which, immediately after formation, enter the S phase of meiosis, acquire a 4n complement of DNA, and enter the lengthy meiotic prophase which terminates in reduction division resulting in formation of haploid cells, the spermatids, which contain a 1n DNA complement. The spermatids do not further divide but undergo a complicated process of metamorphosis (spermiogenesis) culminating in formation of flagellate, motile cells, the spermatozoa (Fig. 29-2).

Investigation of the details of the sperm cell development in the animals led to the discovery of the "cycle of the seminiferous epithelium."[7,8] It has been observed that the various germ cells form a number of precisely defined cellular associations, each occupying a segment of the seminiferous tubule and succeeding one another cyclically. Each complete sequence of changes of the cellular associations in a given segment of the seminiferous tubule was coined "the cycle of the seminiferous epithelium." The concept of the "wave of the seminiferous epithelium" defines the spatial relationships of the various cellular associations along the length of the seminiferous tubule. Thus the

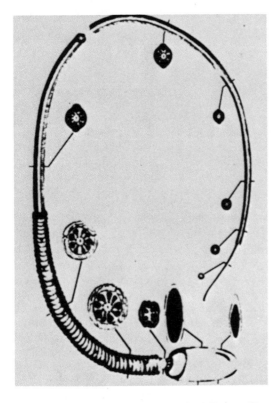

FIGURE 29-2. Human spermatozoon. (From Fawcett.[17])

"wave is in space what the cycle is in time."[9] In all mammals, including a number of primates, the spermatogenic process is orderly and follows the principles described above (for review, see Steinberger and Steinberger[10]). In man (Fig. 29-3), although the cycle of seminiferous epithelium is present,[11] the "wave" is irregular, so that the numerical relationships are poorly defined.[12] The spermatogenic process in human testes has been described as "clonal" in nature rather than a "wave."[13] Nevertheless, the kinetics governing the divisions of the individual germ cell and its progeny or a small group of cells (a "clone") are probably fairly precise. The characteristically well-defined temporal relationships of cellular divisions found in lower species are also found in human testes. This regularity permitted relatively accurate timing of the human spermatogenic process. Heller and Clermont[14] determined that human spermatogenesis requires approximately 64 days. The precision of cell divisions permitted the development of quantitative techniques of evaluation of the numerical relationships in the seminiferous epithelium of human testes. These techniques, although relatively precise, are time consuming and difficult to adopt for routine studies of the testes.[15] Recently, a relatively simply and rapid morphological technique has been developed to quantitate with precision the yield of spermatozoa from a testicular biopsy specimen.[16]

Since spermatozoa are continuously produced in adult testes, a constant supply of germ cells is essential. The mechanism governing this process is still unclear. The evidence points toward a concept of a "self-renewing" stem cell (for review, see Steinberger and Steinberger[10]). In man, however, the stem cell-renewing process has not been studied in sufficient detail to permit any generalizations. This is unfortunate because an understanding of this process is of utmost importance from diagnostic, prognostic, and therapeutic points of view in interpretation of testicular biopsies from men with spermatogenic disturbances.

The only somatic elements within the seminiferous epithelium are the Sertoli cells. They line the basement membrane, and their cytoplasm forms extensive processes which envelop germ cells and form specialized junctions with cytoplasm of neighboring Sertoli cells (Fig. 29-4). For details of Sertoli cell structure, see the recent review by Fawcett.[17]

A wide variety of substances present in peripheral circulation are excluded from the semi-

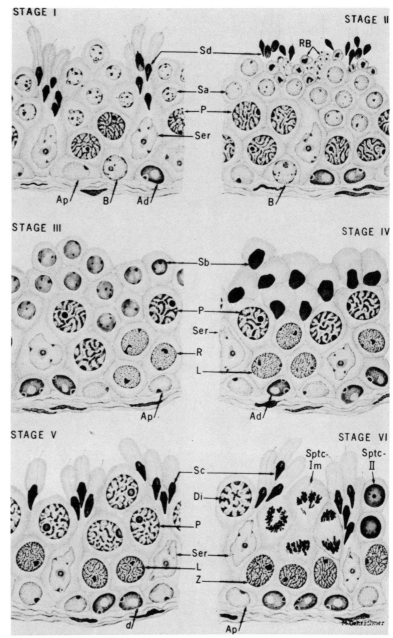

FIGURE 29-3. Cellular composition and topography of the six typical cellular associations found repeatedly in human seminiferous tubules. These cell associations, corresponding to stages of the cycle of the seminiferous epithelium, are numbered stages I–VI. Ser, Sertoli nuclei; Ap and Ad, pale and dark type A spermatogonia; B, type B spermatogonia; R, resting primary spermatocytes; L, leptotene primary spermatocytes; Z, zygotene primary spermatocytes; P, pachytene primary spermatocytes; Di, diplotene primary spermatocytes; Sptc-II, secondary spermatocytes in interphase; Sa, Sb, Sc, and Sd, spermatids at various steps of spermiogenesis; RB, residual bodies. (From Clermont:[135] Physiol Rev 52:198, 1972.)

niferous tubule fluid. This finding suggests the presence of a blood–testis barrier similar to the blood–brain barrier. The Sertoli–Sertoli junctional complexes (tight junctions), which divide the germinal epithelium into basal and adluminal compartments, form the ultrastructural basis for the blood–testis barrier. The basal compartment contains the spermatogonia, and the adluminal compartment contains the remaining complement of germinal epithelium cells. Although the presence of a blood–testis barrier has been demonstrated in human testes, its physiological importance is unclear.[17]

Sertoli cells do not proliferate in adult testes; the only divisions occur in fetal and early postnatal

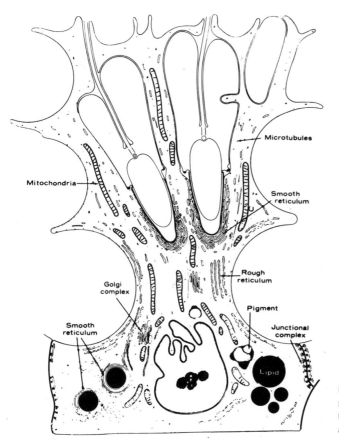

Mitochondria

Microtubules

Smooth reticulum

Golgi complex

Rough reticulum

Pigment

Smooth reticulum

Junctional complex

Lipid

FIGURE 29-4. Typical Sertoli cell, showing its shape and relationships to the germ cells as well as the form and distribution of its principal organelles and inclusions. (From Fawcett.[17])

life.[18] This amitotic state of adult Sertoli cells is not influenced in vivo by hormones or other physiological alterations.

Interstitial Tissue

The interstitial tissue is composed of fibroblasts, collagen and elastic fibrils, blood vessels, lymphatics, nerves, macrophages, and Leydig cells. Many features of the interstitial tissue are common to most mammalian species. However, human interstitial tissue exhibits several distinguishing characteristics: a relative paucity of lymphatics, the presence of crystalloids of Reinke in Leydig cells, the presence of large numbers of macrophages, and the characteristic clumping of Leydig cells.

In adult testes and under normal physiological conditions, Leydig cells do not divide. They are primarily concerned with synthesis of androgens and exhibit the characteristic ultrastructure of steroid-producing cells (Fig. 29-5).

The Sex Accessories

Seminal Vesicles. The seminal vesicles and the ejaculatory ducts develop in the embryo from the lower portion of the wolffian duct and differentiate functionally at puberty under the influence of androgens. In man the seminal vesicles are paired tubular structures 10–20 cm long, with numerous outpouchings of the alveolar glands. The glandular tissue is surrounded by muscle and connective tissue layers. The lumen is filled with mucoid secretions that provide the major contribution toward the total volume of the ejaculate. The vesicles empty into the ejaculatory duct. It should be emphasized that seminal vesicles do not serve as the storage site for the spermatozoa; the few sperm cells occasion-

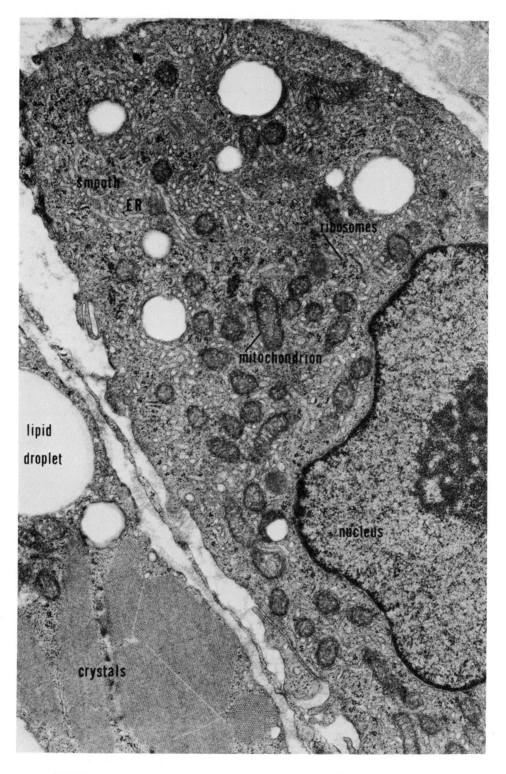

FIGURE 29-5. Ultrastructure of a human Leydig cell. (Courtesy of Dr. A. K. Christensen.)

ally found in the seminal vesicles are thought to be there as a result of reflux action.

The growth and secretory activity of the seminal vesicles are under the influence of androgens.

Prostate. The human prostate begins to develop in the 12-week-old fetus from a number of epithelial buds originating from the proximal urethra. The buds ultimately develop into posterior, middle, and lateral lobes. The gland remains in a fetal state of development until puberty, when it begins to develop in response to androgens. In an adult man, the prostate consists of 30–50 branches of tubuloalveolar glands, which, together with their ducts, form lobules embedded in fibromuscular stroma. The ducts empty into the prostatic urethra in the area of the verumontanum. The gland is surrounded by a multilayered capsule consisting of an inner muscle layer, a heavy connective tissue layer, and an outer layer of loose areolar connective tissue. The glandular epithelium of the prostate is highly responsive to androgens and rich in acid phosphatase. The prostatic secretions form part of the ejaculate.

Vas Deferens. The 50-cm (20-inch)-long tubular structure connects the tail of the epididymis with the ejaculatory duct and serves as the conduit and storage site for the spermatozoa. The wall of the vas is composed of adventitia, vasculosa, muscularis, and mucosa. The latter is composed of cylindrical epithelium. The ampulla is the specialized portion of the vas prior to its entrance into the ejaculatory duct. The ampulla forms a dilated portion of the vas with marked folding of the mucosa and is also a site of spermatozoan storage.

The ejaculatory duct traverses the prostate to enter the posterior urethra. Its mucosa is lined by simple cylindrical epithelium and is thrown into numerous folds.

ANDROGEN PRODUCTION BY THE TESTIS

The testis is the primary site of androgen production in the male. The major circulating androgen is testosterone. By definition, androgens are steroid hormones capable of stimulating the development and of maintaining the normal function of male sex accessory organs. A number of steroids other than testosterone also exhibit the biological action of androgens, such as androstenedione and dehydroepiandrosterone, which are weak androgens, and

5α-dihydrotestosterone (DHT), which is a potent androgen. In addition to androgens, the testis secretes a number of other steroids, including estradiol and 17-hydroxyprogesterone, the latter being the second major secretory product of the testes.

The Steroid Biosynthetic Pathways

The ultimate precursor of all steroid hormones is acetate, from which cholesterol is synthesized. Cholesterol can be synthesized de novo from acetate in the Leydig cells, or it can be derived from systemic circulation.

The conversion of cholesterol (a C_{27} steroid) to androgens (C_{19} steroids) is depicted in Figure 29-6. The first step in the biosynthetic pathway involves cleavage of the cholesterol side chain, resulting in formation of C_{21} steroids. The first C_{21} steroid produced is pregnenolone, which is thought to be a nonhormonal steroid. Pregnenolone is then converted through a series of intermediates to testosterone. The pathway through progesterone is called the $\triangle^4$ pathway, and the one through dehydroepiandrosterone the $\triangle^5$ pathway. The biosynthetic process involves basically a series of cleaving reactions (the side chain of cholesterol, a C_{27} steroid, is cleaved to form pregnenolone, a C_{21} steroid, cleavage of the side chain of C_{21} steroids results in formation of C_{19} steroids) and a series of reduction reactions. In the androgen target tissues, e.g., the prostate, testosterone is further reduced to DHT (dihydrotestosterone or androstanolone and androstanediol).

The biosynthetic process involves sequential participation of several subcellular organelles of the Leydig cell. The cholesterol is delivered to the mitochondria, where it is converted to pregnenolone; pregnenolone is transported from the mitochondria to the microsomes, where it is converted to testosterone (for review, see Steinberger[19]).

The available evidence suggests that in the human testis the $\triangle^4$ pathway predominates. Although the various intermediates formed in the process of androgen biogenesis should theoretically remain in the cell, this is not the case. The pathway apparently "leaks" a number of the intermediates, particularly 17-hydroxyprogesterone, which is secreted by the testes and appears in the testicular venous effluent in rather large quantities.

The plasma and the urine of adult men also contain estrogens. There is considerable evidence that

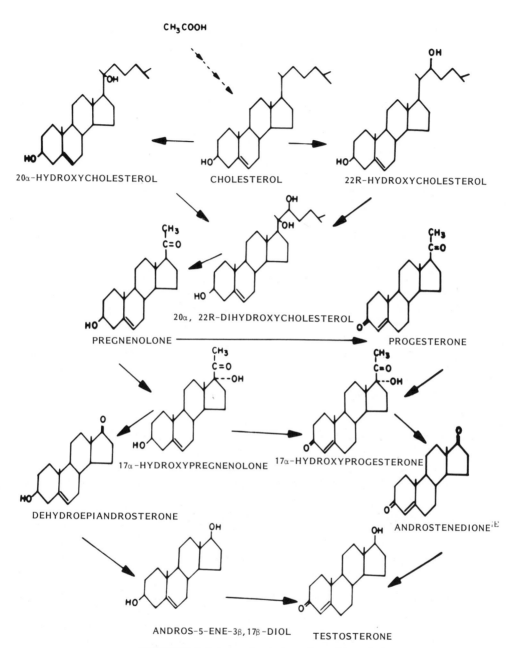

CH₃COOH

20α-HYDROXYCHOLESTEROL   CHOLESTEROL   22R-HYDROXYCHOLESTEROL

20α, 22R-DIHYDROXYCHOLESTEROL

PREGNENOLONE ————————————————→ PROGESTERONE

17α-HYDROXYPREGNENOLONE   17α-HYDROXYPROGESTERONE

DEHYDROEPIANDROSTERONE

ANDROSTENEDIONE

ANDROS-5-ENE-3β,17β-DIOL   TESTOSTERONE

FIGURE 29-6. Pathway of testicular androgen biosynthesis.

the testes are capable of synthesizing and secreting estradiol.

Regulation of Steroidogenesis

Numerous studies demonstrated that in the testes luteinizing hormone (LH) stimulates androgen pro-duction by facilitating the conversion of cholesterol to pregnenolone. Thus the major site of LH action on steroidogenesis is stimulation of the side chain cleavage of cholesterol (for review, see Hall[20]). Recent evidence suggests that LH may also influence the side chain cleavage of pregnenolone and/or progesterone.[21]

The molecular mechanisms concerned with LH stimulation of steroidogenesis involve specific binding of LH to Leydig cell membrane receptors; this triggers a series of biochemical events, including stimulation of adenyl cyclase activity, formation of cAMP, and ultimately synthesis of specific proteins. Although this is the basic mechanism for the induction and maintenance of androgen synthesis, a number of other regulatory mechanisms enter into the picture as well. These involve product inhibition and substrate competition. For example, 20α-hydroxysteroid dehydrogenase competes with C_{17}–C_{20} lyase for 17-hydroxyprogesterone. This competition may divert the substrate from the androgen pathway and limit production of testosterone. Recent investigations of biogenesis of androgens in testes of men with oligospermia demonstrated defects in androgen biosynthesis associated with abnormalities in the biogenetic pathway characterized by this defect.[22]

Secretion of Steroids by the Testis: Transport and Metabolism

The major androgens secreted by the testis are testosterone and dihydrotestosterone. The testis secretes approximately 6 mg testosterone in 24 hr. The liver is the major site of testosterone metabolism. The hormone levels in the blood are kept relatively constant because the ratio between secretion and disposal rates is fixed. The disposal rate can be determined by computing the metabolic clearance rate (MCR), defined as the apparent volume of whole blood or plasma from which a substance is completely and irreversibly removed per unit of time. The MCR is usually expressed in liters per day.[23] In man the MCR for testosterone is approximately 1000 liters/day.[24]

Important insights into various in vivo metabolic processes can be derived or inferred from the MCR, since it is the sum of splanchnic and extrahepatic clearance. A variety of physiological and pathological factors, such as degree of binding of testosterone to plasma proteins, the hepatic function, the posture, aging, drugs, and hypo- or hypermetabolic states, can alter the MCR. Consequently, a "normal" plasma concentration of testosterone can be associated with an altered production rate owing to the variety of factors related to the metabolic clearance or the metabolism of testosterone. Furthermore the plasma testosterone levels vary widely from 0.25 to 1.2 µg/dl. This variation can be caused in part by variations in binding protein con-

centration as well as by the rapid oscillatory pattern in plasma testosterone levels. These variations prompt to question the diagnostic validity of measurements of testosterone in a single blood sample. Recently it has been demonstrated that when three samples are taken 30 min apart and pooled and the determination is performed on the pooled sample, one can obtain 95% probability of the mean value.[25] Furthermore, stress, whether emotional or secondary to surgery, can reduce testosterone values.

A number of steroids which are the intermediates in the biosynthetic pathway of androgens are also secreted by the testis. These include pregnenolone, progesterone, 17α-hydroxypregnenolone, dehydroepiandrosterone, and androstenedione. The adult testis also secretes estradiol (10–15 µg/day), but this accounts for only 20–25% of the total estradiol in the circulation of man, the remainder being the product of peripheral aromatization of both testicular and adrenal androgens.[24] The testis secretes approximately 50–100 µg dihydrotestosterone, as well as 1–2 mg 17αOH-progesterone, a steroid whose biologic role in the male is not known.

Sex Steroid Binding

Testosterone is transported in plasma bound to proteins. A fraction of testosterone is weakly bound to albumin, but this fraction is considered to be similar dynamically to unbound testosterone. The testosterone-binding protein is a β-globulin that has a high affinity and limited capacity for testosterone. All 17β-hydroxysteroids, including estradiol and dihydrotestosterone but not conjugated steroids, bind to this protein, which also called the sex hormone binding globulin (SHBG) or testosterone-estradiol binding globulin (TeBG). As described previously for corticosteroid-binding globulin (CGB), TeBG is also synthesized in the liver and it increases during pregnancy, after estrogen administration, and in hyperthyroidism. It is generally accepted that "free" or albumin-bound androgens are hormonally active. Methods are available to determine free testosterone.

It should be noted that intratesticular concentration of testosterone is approximately 100 times higher than blood concentration. This high intratesticular concentration of testosterone is considered necessary for completion of meiotic division; consequently a drop in intratesticular levels will interfere with the spermatogenic function.[26]

Androgen Metabolism

Testosterone is metabolized essentially by two pathways. The predominant pathway involves oxidation at the 17-position, leading to formation of weak androgens, e.g., androsterone, and the other to formation of 5α-reduced androgens. In the former, the 17-keto pathway, the liver is the major organ of metabolism; in the latter, a relatively minor but important pathway, production of dihydrotestosterone (DHT) and androstanediol occurs predominantly in androgen target tissues.

The major 17-ketosteroid metabolites of testosterone are androsterone and etiocholanolone, which are conjugated in the liver as glucuronides and sulfates to make them water soluble so that they can be excreted in the urine. These C_{19} steroids are measured in the urine as ketosteroids. It is now well established that the measure of urinary ketosteroids is not an appropriate reflection of testicular function and biological androgenicity, since the ketosteroid metabolites are derived not only from testosterone but primarily from metabolism of adrenal steroids, e.g., dehydroepiandrosterone and androstenediol. Only about 20% of ketosteroids found in the urine are derived from testicular androgens. Actually castrated men excrete ketosteroids within the normal range for intact individuals. Because of this consideration, the determination of the levels of ketosteroids or their fractions in the urine for evaluation of androgen production by the testis is not valid.

Biochemical Features of Androgen Physiology

During the past 20 years, considerable information has accumulated concerning the biochemical mechanisms of androgen action (for review, see Mainwaring[27]). It appears that the primary effect of androgens on the target cell is the end result of changes in mechanisms of gene expression, particularly in nuclear transcription of specific RNA molecules which in turn regulate the biogenesis of specific proteins in the cytoplasm. This is accomplished with the aid of specific intracellular androgen receptor proteins, which bind with the steroid and translocate it from the cytoplasm to the nucleus, where it can associate with nuclear chromatin that regulates RNA transcription (Fig. 29-7).

Most of the biological effects of androgens seem to depend on the regulation of the synthesis of the various enzymes and other proteins in responsive tissues. In these tissues (e.g., the prostate), testosterone enters the cell where, in the cytoplasm, its A ring is reduced by 5α-reductase to form dihydrotestosterone, which is bound to a specific receptor. The androgen–receptor complex is translocated into the nucleus, where intranuclear proteins, the "acceptors," facilitate the association of the androgen–receptor complex with nuclear chromatin. This induces transcription of an appropriate message and intranuclear processing of this transcript. As a result, de novo synthesis of a pertinent messenger RNA (mRNA) and its subsequent accumulation in association with cytoplasmic poly-

Target cell

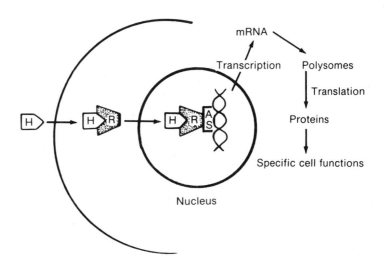

FIGURE 29-7. Molecular mechanisms of steroid hormone action. H, hormone; R, receptor; AS, nuclear acceptor.

ribosomes take place, as well as appropriate changes in rates of synthesis of specific proteins.

Hormonal Control of Spermatogenesis

The observation in the nineteenth century that patients with intracranial lesions failed to develop sexually led clinicians and pathologists to suggest that the controlling center for gonadal development and function must be located within the brain. The modern concepts of the endocrine basis of testicular control evolved from Smith's[28] studies, which demonstrated that the pituitary gland secretes substances (gonadotropins) responsible for stimulation of gonadal growth and maintenance. Subsequently it was shown that two pituitary hormones, luteinizing hormone (LH) or interstitial cell-stimulating hormone (ICSH) and the follicle-stimulating hormone (FSH), play a role in the regulation of testicular function, ICSH being responsible primarily for stimulation of androgen production and FSH being involved in the process of spermatogenesis. During the 1960s, a hypothesis was proposed that the spermatogenic process can be maintained qualitatively by testosterone alone, but in immature testes the induction of complete spermatogenesis is more complicated, requiring the interaction of several hormones. It has been suggested that testosterone is probably essential for the initiation of spermatogonial divisions but primarily for allowing completion of meiotic division of the spermatocytes. FSH was thought to be involved in and responsible for creating conditions favorable for spermatid maturation and thus formation of spermatozoa (for review, see Steinberger and Steinberger[29]).

These concepts were derived primarily from experiments in lower species, particularly the rat. Studies in man were difficult to carry out because it is almost impossible to create in man an appropriate experimental model in which various endocrine and physiological parameters can be manipulated in a precise fashion. Nevertheless, it appears that in man gonadotropins of human origin will initiate spermatogenesis in a hypogonadotropic or hypophysectomized male. Human menopausal gonadotropins (hMG, Pergonal), which exhibit both LH and FSH activity, will induce spermatogenesis in these patients. Since all studies dealing with the initiation of spermatogenesis in man used gonadotropin preparations containing LH, the question of the role of androgens in the initiation of spermatogenesis and in the completion of the

meiotic division remained unclear. It would be reasonable to assume that LH in the gonadotropin preparations stimulated androgen production by the Leydig cells and thus was responsible for the initiation of the spermatogenesis and completion of the meiotic division. However, this assumption is debated by many investigators, beginning with Hotchkiss,[30] who showed that administration of testosterone to normal men results in suppression of spermatogenesis and that, in men with gonadotropin deficiency, spermatogenesis cannot be induced by the administration of testosterone. This is in disagreement with findings in lower species where testosterone was shown to be capable of both initiating spermatogenesis and allowing the meiotic division to be completed.

Clinical evidence is available to clarify this issue, and an explanation for this discrepancy has been offered. A rat requires approximately 1–2 mg/day testosterone for maintenance of spermatogenesis. If this dose is extrapolated to man, a daily dose of 4–8 mg/kg or 300–600 mg per individual would have to be administered to obtain similar results. Since no preparations of testosterone are available that would permit administration of such a high dose, and since such a high dose was never attempted in man, it is possible to assume that the reason for the inability to influence spermatogenesis with testosterone in man is the inability to administer a sufficiently high dose. Furthermore, in the rat the intratesticular concentration of testosterone is approximately 10-fold that of blood, whereas in man it appears to be 50- to 100-fold; thus possibly even higher peripheral circulating levels of testosterone would have to be produced before an intratesticular concentration of testosterone adequate for maintenance of spermatogenesis could be obtained.

The demonstration in the testes of the various components of the biochemical system involved in polypeptide–hormone action and the demonstration of responsiveness of the system to FSH established the role of FSH in spermatogenesis. Subsequently, the Sertoli cells were shown to be the primary site of FSH action in the testes. On the basis of the most recent biochemical information, the following hypothesis has been proposed (Fig. 29-8).

FSH, delivered to the interstitial area of the testes *via* the arterial system, diffuses through the seminiferous tubule basement membrane and binds to specific receptors on the Sertoli cell membranes. There it activates adenyl cyclase and stimulates production of cAMP, which promotes DNA-dependent RNA synthesis resulting in synthesis of specif-

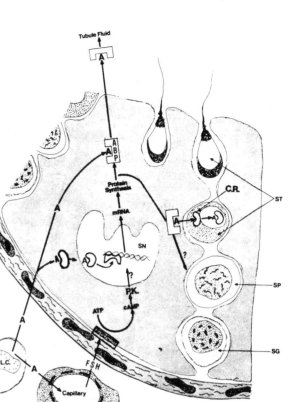

FIGURE 29-8. Sertoli and germ cells and the biochemical mechanisms concerned with their function. SN, Sertoli cell nucleus; SG, spermatogonium; SP, spermatocyte; ST, spermatid; LC, Leydig cell; PK, cAMP-dependent phosphokinase; A, testosterone; FSH, follicle-stimulating hormone; CR, cytoplasmic receptor; ABP, androgen-binding protein; receptor; chromatin acceptor.

ic proteins, including a specific androgen-binding protein (ABP).

Androgens diffuse from the interstitial area into the seminiferous epithelium, where they are bound and concentrated by a specific FSH-induced androgen binding protein (ABP). This creates a high androgen concentration in the vicinity of germ cells. The ABP–androgen complex facilitates transfer of androgens to specific types of germ cells. In the germ cell cytoplasm the androgens are bound to a specific cytoplasm receptor. The androgen–receptor complex is then translocated into the nucleus, where it binds to an acceptor site on the chromatin and induces changes necessary for germ cell maturation. The biochemical details of the latter steps are still unclear (for review, see Steinberger[31]).

DISORDERS OF TESTICULAR FUNCTION ASSOCIATED WITH INFERTILITY

Various approaches were used to classify the numerous testicular abnormalities that interfere with gametogenesis. The most commonly proposed classification divides all testicular disorders into three groups: (1) those associated with high gonadotropin levels, (2) those with normal gonadotropins, and (3) those with low gonadotropins. The gonadotropin levels, however, do not necessarily reflect the primary abnormality, and although the gonadotropin levels provide a convenient "handle" in diagnostic evaluation of the patient, they frequently do not reflect the etiology or pathophysiology of the disorder. Information has accumulated that now permits more precise categorization of the various testicular disorders; this time-honored and previously highly useful classification is not used in the present discussion. Instead, an attempt is made to classify the disorders of testicular function on the basis of etiology.

Testicular Disorders Secondary to Hypothalamic–Pituitary Dysfunction

This group of testicular abnormalities comprises several diagnostic categories:

1. Complete selective prepubertal gonadotropic failure (hypogonadotropic eunuchoidism)
2. Selective postpubertal gonadotropin failure (hypogonadotropic hypogonadism)
3. Postpubertal panhypopituitarism
4. "Fertile eunuch" syndrome (isolated LH deficiency or Pasqualini syndrome)

In all these disorders, the pathophysiology is based on inadequate secretion of gonadotropin by the pituitary gland, resulting in lack of testicular development or in testicular atrophy if the condition commences after puberty. These disorders can usually be diagnosed clinically. They represent a small fraction of patients with infertility, but they can easily be diagnosed, and in most instances specific and effective therapy is available.

Complete Selective Prepubertal Gonadotropin Failure (Hypogonadotropic Eunuchoidism)

Upon physical examination, the characteristic clinical features of "eunuchoidism"—eunuchoid skeleton, high-pitched voice, small prepubertal-sized testes of normal consistency, lack of bitemporal scalp hair recession, sparse or absent pubic hair, and diminished body hair growth are noted. If anosmia is present, the condition is classified as Kallman's syndrome.

The diagnosis can usually be made on the basis of history and physical examination and confirmed by appropriate laboratory studies. The etiology of this condition is not entirely clear. The disorder probably is the final expression of a spectrum of disorders with a common denominator of diminished or absent gonadotropin production. It probably is not caused by primary pituitary disease, since the gonadotropin levels rise in response to LHRH administration. Although optimistic reports suggesting efficacy of LHRH therapy have been published, many variations in the responses were reported. It was not until the pulsatile nature of LHRH release was demonstrated to be essential for normal physiological responses that LHRH therapy could be used effectively. The development of small, portable computerized infusion pumps permitted evaluation of clinically effective methods for delivery of LHRH in precise pulsatile fashion. Using this delivery system, a number of workers reported successful initiation or reinitiation of androgen biosynthesis and spermatogenesis with hypergonadotropic hypogonadism.[32,33] Before the introduction of pulsatile LHRH therapy, the most effective form of therapy was the combination of human chorionic gonadotropin (hCG) and human postmenopausal gonadotropins (hMG). Numerous therapeutic regimens have been suggested. We prefer a 6–8-week treatment with 2500 IU hCG twice a week followed by HMG 1 vial (75 IU FSH and 75 IU LH) twice weekly in addition to the hCG. Since completion of the spermatogenic process requires 2–3 months, therapy must be continued for several months before spermatozoa can be expected to appear in the ejaculate. The patient with normal olfactory acuity and selective gonadotropin failure, normal karyotype, and no evidence of organic lesions in the brain or the pituitary gland may respond to treatment with 25 mg clomiphene citrate (Clomid) administered daily for several months.

Selective Postpubertal Gonadotropin Failure (Hypogonadotropic Hypogonadism)

Although this is considered a rare condition, partial failures may occur more commonly among males with diminished sperm production than was previously considered. When complete failure is present, the patient may complain of diminished libido and potency, a decrease in the rate of beard growth, and a decrease in body hair. There is a decrease in gonadotropin and testosterone levels; however, there is no clinical picture of eunuchoidism, because the skeletomuscular and sexual development was complete prior to the onset of gonadotropic deficiency. Therapy with hCG and hMG is usually effective in reinitiating spermatogenesis; similarly, pulsatile LHRH therapy may be also attempted.

Postpubertal Panhypopituitarism

This condition may be idiopathic, secondary to a pituitary tumor, or iatrogenic, secondary to hypophysectomy. Regardless of etiology, the testicular deficiency associated with this disorder can be treated successfully with gonadotropins or LHRH in the same fashion as the other hypogonadotropic states.

The "Fertile Eunuch" (Isolated LH Deficiency or Pasqualini Syndrome)

In this condition, the serum FSH level is usually within normal range, but LH is decreased or undetectable and testosterone levels are markedly depressed. The spermatogenic activity is depressed, and the sperm output may vary from several million spermatozoa per milliliter to azoospermia. Most likely, isolated deficiency of LH is the underlying etiologic factor. Therapy with hCG is usually effective in stimulating additional androgen production and improving the sperm production.

Congenital or Developmental Testicular Disorders

Testicular Dystopia

Lack of testicular descent (cryptorchidism) or inadequate or inappropriate descent induces pathological changes in the testes which result in either azoospermia or severe oligospermia. The etiological factors responsible for the failure or inappropriate descent are unclear. In some instances, particularly in unilateral cryptorchidism, anatomical abnormalities that prevent normal descent have been demonstrated. A genetic etiology for seminiferous epithelium failure in cryptorchid testes has also been suggested. If the latter were the case in all instances, therapy directed toward placement of testes into the scrotum whether surgical or hormonal would ameliorate the spermatogenic defect, but this is not always the case. The possibility should be considered that testicular dystopia has multiple etiologic factors, including a genetic factor. It is of particular importance to note that the incidence of testicular dystopia in Klinefelter's syndrome, Sertoli cell-only syndrome, and hypogonadotropic eunuchoidism, is relatively high. This emphasizes the importance of a complete workup, including cytogenetic evaluation, endocrine studies, and testicular biopsy of patients with testicular dystopia.

The question of medical versus surgical therapy in testicular dystopia has been the topic of controversy. In patients with unilateral cryptorchidism the chances of an anatomic defect are higher, and frequently a primary surgical approach is utilized. It should be stressed, however, that even in cases of unilateral cryptorchidism, the patient may respond to hormonal therapy. Fundamentally it is the end result of therapy that must be considered in evaluating its efficacy. If fertility is used as the primary criterion, opinions in the literature vary greatly. Charny[34] is pessimistic. Others, however, have published data demonstrating a relatively high frequency of fertility after orchidopexy.

The usual hormonal therapeutic approach involves a trial of therapy, usually the administration of 2000 IU hCG 2 or 3 times weekly for 6–8 weeks. If no definite response is observed, an additional course of therapy is instituted after a rest period of several months. Failure of medical therapy calls for surgical intervention. The age when therapeutic intervention is to be commenced (whether surgical, medical, or a combination of both) has also been a point of controversy. Most of the authorities suggest ages 5–7 years as optimal.

Congenital Anorchia, The Vanishing Testis, or Functional Castrate Syndrome

Relatively few cases of this disorder have been reported.[35] They are phenotypic males with a 46, XY karyotype presenting with eunuchoid characteristics and lack of pubertal development. The development of the derivatives of wolffian ducts is perfectly normal and there is an absence of derivatives of the mullerian ducts. The testes are not palpable, the penis is small, and there is a lack of beard growth and absence of pubic hair. The etiology of this condition is unclear. Because of the normal development of the wolffian duct derivatives and regression of the mullerian derivatives, some degree of testicular function must have been present in these males during fetal life. Possibly an intrauterine infection, testicular torsion, or other intrauterine catastrophy resulted in complete destruction of the gonadal tissues. A finding of extremely high LH and FSH levels associated with lack of response to a hCG test is almost diagnostic for this disorder. In questionable cases, exploratory surgery in search of an undescended testes may be required. While obviously no therapy to restore fertility is available, a successful testicular transplant from an identical twin was recently reported;[36] thus a possibility to restore fertility in selected cases indeed exists.

Sertoli Cell-Only Syndrome (Del Castillo's Syndrome)

Sertoli cell-only syndrome has been considered to be a genetic abnormality, however no direct evidence for this etiology has been provided. The disorder is characterized by azoospermia associated with a total absence of germ cells in the testes, elevated gonadotropic levels, and normal androgen levels. There are no other associated congenital abnormalities. No therapy is available to induce spermatogenesis.

Ullrich–Turner Syndrome or Male Turner Syndrome

In this rare condition, there are phenotypic characteristics of Turner's syndrome, including short stature, low-set ears, webbed neck, "shield" chest, cardiovascular anomalies, cubitus valgus, cryptorchidism, spermatogenic defects, and clinical signs of diminished androgen function. However, in most instances no chromosomal abnormalities are noted. No therapy for the spermatogenic defect is available.

Congenital Syndromes Associated with Hypogonadism

Several syndromes are associated with hypogonadism, each characterized by a variety of systemic abnormalities:

Prader Willi Syndrome: Characterized by mental retardation, neonatal muscular hypotonia, and hypogonadism frequently associated with cryptorchidism and massive obesity. The patients suffer uncontrollable hyperphagia and impaired temperature regulation. Because of these symptoms, hypothalamic dysfunction has been suspected.

Laurence–Moon–Biedl Syndrome: Characterized by growth retardation, mental deficiency, polydactyly, obesity, retinitis pigmentosa, and hypogonadism.

Familial Cerebellar Ataxia: Associated with nerve deafness and hypogonadism.

Alström Syndrome: Resembles the Laurence–Moon–Biedl syndrome. No mental retardation or polydactyly is present, but patients exhibit a variety of metabolic disorders including hypertriglyceridemia, hyperuricemia, and acanthosis nigricans.

No adequate therapy for hypogonadism is available for this group of syndromes.

Chromosomal Abnormalities

Chromosomal abnormalities are detected in a relatively small number of men seeking help for infertility. The incidence has been reported to vary between 2 and 21%, depending on the composition of the population studied. In studies containing large numbers of men with severe oligospermia or azoospermia the incidence is higher.[37,38] Hendry et al.[39] reported a 3.5% incidence of somatic chromosomal abnormality and a 10.5% incidence of ' chromosome in a group of subfertile men. Despite relatively low incidence of chromosomal abnormalities, and the fact that some, particularly somatic chromosomal abnormalities, may be unrelated to the fertility impairment, chromosomal analysis in patients with severe oligospermia or azoospermia is probably indicated.

Specific Syndromes Associated with Chromosomal Abnormalities

Klinefelter's Syndrome. The clinical picture of this syndrome was first described by Klinefelter et al.[40] Patients exhibit eunuchoid habitus, very firm pea-size testes and azoospermia. A relatively high percentage exhibit gynecomastia, light beard growth, and female hair distribution. There is an increased incidence of other system disorders (e.g., diabetes mellitus, mental disorders). Microscopic examination of the testes reveals a characteristic pattern of severe hyalinization of seminiferous tubules, aspermatogenesis and formation of large clumps of Leydig cells in the interstitial spaces. Endocrine evaluation demonstrates markedly elevated FSH and LH levels, normal or decreased testosterone levels and blunted response to hCG. Cytogenetic evaluation indicates the presence of an extra X chromosome; thus, the number of chromosomes is 47 rather than the normal 46, and the karyotype is 47,XXY. The high incidence of poly-X and poly-Y complements results in even higher than 47 chromosomes in some cases, as well as variety of deletions and mozaicisms. No therapy for restoration of spermatogenesis is available. Some of these men produce inadequate amounts of testosterone; others do not or may develop testosterone deficiency in the future. Proper monitoring of the androgen status is necessary and testosterone therapy is appropriate where indicated.

XYY Syndrome. Although this condition affects approximately 0.2% of the male population, its relation to gonadal dysfunction is poorly defined and highly variable.[41] Spermatogenesis may vary from perfectly normal to azoospermia. Men with XYY chromosome complement are tall and frequently have acne; most are found in correctional facilities for antisocial behavior. Hormonal levels vary from normal to elevated gonadotropins and depressed androgens.

The XX or Sex-Reversal Syndrome. These patients clinically resemble men with Klinefelter's syndrome. They exhibit male phenotype, male psychosexual identification, and relatively normal male body habitus. In most cases, pubic hair growth is diminished, the penis and scrotum are normal, and the testes are small, showing microscopic characteristics similar to those found in Klinefelter's syndrome. Until recently, no explanation for the 46-XX karyotype in patients with testes was available. Wachtel et al.[42] provided immunological evidence for the presence of H-Y antigen in patients with 46,XX karyotype. This finding suggests the presence of Y-chromosome-associated, testis-determining genetic material. These patients, however, lack normal physiological expression of gonadal maleness, as evidenced by defective spermatogenesis. A possibility exists that these patients are examples of another variant of Klinefelter's syndrome expressed by the presence of two X chromosomes and a part of the Y chromosome.

Spermatogenic Dysfunction Associated with Defects in Activity of Steroidogenic Enzymes

During the past several years, specific deficiencies in steroidogenic enzymes resulting in abnormal androgen production have been described. The disturbed androgen production results in somatic and reproductive tract abnormalities. The disorders can be subdivided into three groups: (1) systemic deficiencies involving the adrenal glands and the testes, (2) deficiencies involving only the adrenal glands, and (3) specific deficiencies in testicular steroidogenesis activity.

Various forms of congenital adrenal hyperplasia belong to the first category. They can be characterized by deficiencies in the 3β-hydroxysteroid dehydrogenase and $\triangle^4$-isomerase system, 17α-hydroxylase,[17–21] lyase, or deficiencies of the cholesterol sidechain cleaving enzymes. The end result of these enzymic deficiencies is a hypoandrogenic state resulting in spermatogenic arrest. The customary therapy for congenital adrenal hyperplasia calls for administration of corticosteroids. This results in correction of the adrenal deficiency, but produces no improvement in testicular function. No testis-directed therapy is yet available for patients with congenital adrenal hyperplasia. These forms of congenital adrenal hyperplasia must be differentiated from hyperandrogenic disorders of the adrenal glands (group 2) associated with normal intratesticular steroidogenic enzymes. In this condition, the adrenal-derived high androgen levels suppress pituitary gonadotropins and induce secondary hypogonadotropic hypogonadism. Corticoid therapy to suppress adrenal androgens restores normal gonadotropin secretion and leads to the reestablishment of normal pituitary–gonadal interaction and normal spermatogenic function.

In the third category of steroid enzyme disorders, the abnormality resides in the steroidogenic tissue of the testis, while the adrenal function remains intact. One of these abnormalities described recently is excessive 5α-reduction of early steroidal precursors in the biogenetic pathway of androgens. This abnormality reduces the capacity of the testis to produce testosterone. It can be treated successfully with high doses of human gonadotropins.[43] Deficiencies in other enzymes have also been demonstrated in some patients with unexplained oligospermia.[22] Careful evaluation of patients with idiopathic oligospermia will most likely uncover more instances of specific enzyme deficiencies. The ability to uncover specific biochemical lesions in this group of patients should aid substantially in our ability to manage the difficult problem of idiopathic oligospermia.

Spermatogenic Dysfunction Associated with Genetic Defect in the Mechanism of Androgen Action on Target Cells

Abnormalities in the molecular mechanisms leading to expression of androgen action in the target cell may lead to severe systemic and gonadal consequences. Four types of gonadal abnormalities have been described: (1) complete testicular feminization; (2) incomplete testicular feminization; (3) familial complete male pseudohermaphroditism, type 2; and (4) familial complete male pseudohermaphroditism, type 1. (In conditions 1, 2, and 3, the individual exhibits female phenotype and is usually reared as a female; these conditions are not discussed here.) The familial incomplete male pseudohermaphroditism, type 1, however, is associated with a male phenotype characterized by hypospadias, incomplete virilization at puberty, gynecomastia, and azoospermia. The term, familial incomplete male pseudohermaphroditism, type 1, has been coined by Wilson et al.[44] who also demonstrated an X-linked inheritance for this syndrome. Similar to syndromes listed under 1, 2, and 3, the underlying biochemical lesion is a defect in androgen receptors in the target cell. The condition encompasses a spectrum of clinical phenotypes. They vary from patients with diminished sperm counts, hypospadias, and gynecomastia, to patients with a total lack of virilization.

Because of the varying nature of the clinical picture, a number of syndromes were coined to characterize specific constellations of clinical signs and symptoms. All these syndromes probably have the same underlying etiology related to defective androgen receptors. They are discussed in a descending order of clinical severity.

Lubs Syndrome: Characterized by masculine skeletal development, normal pubic and axillary hair, partial labioscrotal fusion, and partial wolffian duct development.[45]

Gilbert-Dreyfus Syndrome: Characterized by a phenotypic male presenting with a small phallus, hypospadias, incomplete wolffian duct structure development and gynecomastia.

Reifeinstein Syndrome: Clinically similar to Klinefelter's syndrome but with normal 46,XY karyotype, patients usually exhibit male phenotype, perineal hypospadias, bifid scrotum, gynecomastia, high gonadotropin levels, and azoospermia. The testes show a striking microscopic resemblance to Klinefelter's syndrome.[46]

Rosewater Syndrome: Characterized by gynecomastia and infertility,[47] this is probably the mildest form of familial, incomplete male pseudohermaphroditism, type 1. Members of the same family may exhibit phenotypes corresponding to either the mildest (Rosewater syndrome) or most severe (Lubs syndrome) form. They all may be the expression of a single gene mutation resulting in defective androgen receptors.

As a group, these patients will have high plasma testosterone levels and high LH levels. The latter suggest defective feedback control by testosterone secondary to defective testosterone receptors. No therapy is available for these patients.

Infectious Causes of Testicular Dysfunction

Testicular damage can occur as a result of an infectious process involving primarily the testicle, in response to a systemic infection (e.g., upper respiratory or oral), or as a result of infection involving the sex accessory glands.[48]

The best-documented cause of spermatogenic damage secondary to infection is that of mumps orchitis. Diagnosis is usually made on the basis of history and appearance of the testicular biopsy. Unilateral involvement in most instances does not cause infertility, although a diminished sperm count may be present. Bilateral involvement results in severe oligospermia or azoospermia. No therapy is available once the damage has occurred.

Systemic infections, whether bacterial or viral, and infections of the seminal vesicles or the prostate may cause depression of sperm production. Frequently the depression is temporary in nature. The abnormality in sperm count may occur some months after a relatively minor infection, and spontaneous recovery may not occur for an additional several months. Consequently, a careful history of systemic infections is essential before any extensive diagnostic procedures such as testicular biopsies are contemplated, because in these patients the abnormality may correct itself spontaneously.

Evidence has been provided suggesting T-mycoplasma infections of the reproductive tract may be one of the causative factors of male infertility.[49] Because a number of investigators have been unable to confirm this suggestion,[50,51] the question of the role of T-mycoplasma infections in male infertility remains uncertain.

Nonspecific or gonorrheal epididymitis may cause permanent, partial, or complete epididymal block associated with severe oligospermia or azoospermia. History and physical examination frequently provide important clues pointing toward this etiology of oligospermia or azoospermia. On physical examination of the scrotal content, thickening and irregularity of epididymal structures can be detected; however, a definitive diagnosis can be made most effectively during scrotal exploration. The block produces whitish areas or small fluid-filled cysts in the epididymis that are easily detected by the naked eye.

Immunological Factors

Ever since the reports of Wilson[52] and Rümke[53] suggesting the presence of immunological factors in some infertile men, numerous studies have been reported on this topic (for reviews, see refs. 54–56). Two types of antibodies, sperm agglutinating and sperm immobilizing, have been demonstrated. Although both were shown to occur more frequently in partners of infertile couples, the relationship of the antibodies to infertility is still not entirely clear.[54,56] The most commonly utilized tests for immunological studies are the Kibrik sperm agglutination test,[57] the Franklin-Dukes sperm agglutination test,[58] and the Isojima sperm immobilizing test.[59]

Neurological Causes

Extensive lesions of the spinal cord are frequently associated with testicular dysfunction. In paraplegia, varying degrees of impotence, ejaculatory disturbances, and azoospermia or severe oligospermia are present. Whether the neurological deficit produces the spermatogenic damage or whether the damage is secondary to the associated disturbances in testicular temperature regulatory mechanism is unclear.

Myotonia Dystrophica

Testicular damage occurs in approximately 80% of all cases. Whereas pubertal development is normal, testicular atrophy occurs at varying times after puberty and is usually associated with infertility. The microscopic appearance of the testis is frequently similar to that observed in Klinefelter's syndrome, but no cytogenetic abnormalities have been detected. The spermatogenic damage varies in degree and sometimes can be associated with limited sperm production. There is no associated androgen deficiency, but substantially elevated levels of LH and FSH have been demonstrated, suggesting that it is a primary testicular disorder. The etiology of the testicular lesion is unknown. There is no known therapy for this condition.

Physical and Chemical Agents—Ionizing Radiation

The information concerning the response of the human testis to radiation is still only fragmentary in spite of the fact that a considerable body of information has accumulated. In man microscopic studies of the testis suggest that the germinal elements are the most sensitive to radiation, while the Sertoli cells and Leydig cells are relatively radioresistant. Although basic characteristics of the response of germinal epithelium to ionizing radiation are similar in all mammals, specific quantitative differences exist, particularly in the timing of postregression recovery and details of the effect on specific types of spermatogonia. In man a dose as low as 15 rad causes a reduction in sperm count, and 100 rad causes rapid morphological damage to germ cells. There is an increased number of both stable and unstable chromosome aberrations in the testicular cells following exposure to 100 rad.[60,61]

In man testicular damage is caused, in most instances, by accidental exposure to radiation or exposure secondary to treatment of neoplasias. No reliable form of medical therapy has been found to prevent, protect, or treat germinal epithelium damage resulting from exposure to ionizing radiation. In some instances spontaneous recovery of spermatogenesis takes place. The degree of recovery depends on the dose and length of exposure; however, no reliable information is available whether or not the sperm formed after the recovery are genetically intact. It is probably advisable to inform individuals who have experienced severe damage to the germinal epithelium that in spite of recovery the possibility of genetic lesions in offspring is real.

Thermal Effects

Extensive literature in animals clearly demonstrates the sensitivity of the germinal epithelium to temperature elevations as little as 1° or 2°F above that of normal intratesticular environment. In man the normal intratesticular temperature is 2°–3°F lower than body temperature. Reports of testicular damage following febrile illness or artificially induced elevation of intratesticular temperature provided direct evidence for the detrimental effects of heat on the human testis. Since only a slight increase in temperature is sufficient to damage the testis, suggestions have been made that wearing tight clothing, jockey-type shorts, or athletic supporters may be implicated in the induction of intratesticular hyperthermia with resulting oligospermia. Similarly postsurgical or postinflammatory conditions requiring tight bandages that bring the testicles close to the body may induce a hyperthermic condition in the testes, resulting in damage. The heat-induced damage is reversible if the exposure is brief. After chronic exposure, the lesion is irreversible, and there is no medical treatment available.

Chemical Agents

A variety of chemical agents have been shown to produce testicular damage. The patient may be exposed to these agents either in the course of his normal employment or as therapy for a variety of diseases (e.g., cancer, nephrotic syndrome). In many instances a spontaneous complete or at least partial recovery may take place following exposure to various therapeutic agents (e.g., mercaptopurines, cyclophosphamide, methotrexate, chlorambucil, nitrogen mustard, vincristine, procarbazine, triethylenemelamine, or nitrofurans). Although the return of fertility would seem to be a positive sign, the occurrence of recovery must be viewed with caution. Animal experiments provide evidence that these agents induce mutations in the stem cells of the germinal epithelium, and these mutations may then be transferred through the spermatozoa to the offspring.[62,63] Consequently it is possible to see a return of fertility in human males treated with these agents, but the possibility that, under these conditions, mutant genes will be introduced into the human genetic pool with entirely unknown consequences both for the offspring and particularly for future generations must be considered.

Exposure to a variety of industrial toxics and pollutants that are, or may potentially be, hazardous to the male reproductive system, has become of serious medical concern, particularly since a relatively large segment of population may be chronically exposed to these chemicals. For example, boron found in such diverse sites as artesian drinking water and in factories producing boric acid or dibromochloropropene (DBCP, a soil fumigant) has been shown to induce severe testicular damage and infertility in a large segment of workers and farmers who were exposed to these chemicals while engaged in their production or application.[64] Unfortunately, none of these chemicals produces a sufficiently characteristic pathological or clinical picture to allow the physician who may be investigating a patient with infertility to make a specific diagnosis. Thus one depends totally on a careful history obtained from the patient concerning the exposure. No specific therapy to reverse the pathological picture is available. Varying degrees of spontaneous recovery of spermatogenesis have been reported following cessation of the exposure. In utero exposure of the male fetus to certain substances has also been shown to be damaging to the reproductive system after the individual reaches maturity. Specifically, in utero exposure to DES administered to the mother during pregnancy has been shown to induce epididymal pathology and spermatogenic damage in the offspring.[65]

A number of reports appeared in the literature suggesting that a variety of narcotic and psychedelic drugs may interfere with normal male reproductive function and may cause damage to germ cells expressed by congenital anomalies in offspring. The information on this topic is, however, even more limited than information concerning the cytotoxic and alkylating agents, and it is even more controversial. At this moment it is difficult to state whether these agents do indeed produce a serious effect on the germinal epithelium.

Vascular Abnormalities

Interference with the Normal Blood Supply. Unfortunately only limited information is available on the effect of interruption of blood supply on the human testis (for review, see Steinberger[66]). In experimental animals, extensive studies have been conducted on this topic. Most data suggest that temporary interruption, up to 90 min, produces no damage to spermatogenesis. After 120 min of ischemia, severe generalized damage to all germ cells in the seminiferous tubules is produced. Extrapolation of these observations to man is difficult. Clinical studies suggest that 360 degree torsion of the testis of less than 12 hr duration may not produce necrosis of the testis. However, the degree of spermatogenic impairment after such an episode varies greatly. Furthermore, it should be noted that in the case of torsion, not only is the testicle deprived of the blood supply, but there is interference with venous drainage as well. Limited experimental studies in man where the internal spermatic artery at the external inguinal canal has been interrupted suggest that within 24 hr of interruption morphological changes occur in the seminiferous epithelium. After 5 days of blood flow interruption, necrosis of the testis takes place.[67]

Varicocele. Varicocele is a condition in which the veins draining the testicle became dilated and the venous drainage impaired. The first mention of this condition was made over 400 years ago when "a compact pack of vessels filled with melancholic blood" was described. It was not until the second half of this century that Tulloch[68] reported beneficial effects of varicocelectomy in infertile males. Charny[34] introduced and Dubin and Amelar[69] popularized this operation in the United States.

A varicocele occurring exclusively on the right side is suggestive of a pathological lesion involving the right retroperitoneal space or an intraperitoneal lesion in the vicinity of the drainage of the right internal spermatic vein into the vena cava. This condition will not be discussed here. A varicocele occurring on the left side or bilaterally appears "to be related either to the congenital absence or incompetency of valves in the left spermatic vein. The unusually long length, erect posture of man, and the right-angle termination of the gonadal vein poorly enable the vein to resist incompetency and consequently retrograde flow."[70]

Unfortunately only scanty information is available for the incidence of varicocele in the normal fertile male population. The available reports suggest that in the normal population it varies from 8%[71] to 14%.[72] There is no information available on the incidence of varicocele in men who recently fathered children. Although considerable evidence has accumulated suggesting a cause–effect relationship between varicocele and male infertility and an increased incidence of varicocele in infertile males, the statistics are difficult to interpret because of great variation in the type of patient population seen by different investigators. The estimates range from 4.6% in the study of a group of 5000 patients[73] to 39% in a group of 1294 patients.[74] Similarly, there is no agreement as to the type of testicular abnormality associated with varicocele.

MacLeod[75] suggested that infertile patients with varicocele exhibit a characteristic pattern of sperm morphology: an increased incidence of tapered, amorphous, and immature sperm; however, he later reported that 50% of men with varicocele do not demonstrate any abnormalities in their seminal fluid.[76] Other authorities in more recent studies suggested that most infertile patients with varicocele exhibit morphological abnormalities of spermatozoa, but many show sperm counts within normal range.[23] It appears that varicocele indeed may have an etiologic relationship to testicular abnormalities, although a clear and specific relationship has not yet been established. Similarly, a definite cause–effect relationship between correction of varicocele, improvement in seminal fluid characteristics, and increased incidence of pregnancy remains to be demonstrated. Since changes in sperm count and morphology occur only in 50–80% of patients after ligation of varicocele,[75] the parameter frequently utilized in assessment of therapeutic success has been the pregnancy rate. Some authors report no changes in seminal fluid characteristics subsequent to varicocele ligation but an increase in the conception rate.[77] Many reports on the effects of varicocelectomy provide either no information concerning the female partner or only a statement that "no abnormality was present in the female." Recently a report was published on a group of infertile patients, with both partners followed by the same team of physicians. The males were divided into two groups, those left untreated and those whose varicocele was ligated. The wives in both groups were carefully evaluated and treated. The incidence of pregnancy in the wives of men who had varicocelectomy did not differ from those whose husbands were not operated[78] and were the same as those reported in literature for operated patients.

The mechanism by which varicocele produces testicular damage is still unclear. The early suggestions that it interferes with the cooling mechanism of the testis has been discarded, although the final proof to warrant this conclusion has not been provided.[79] A toxic effect on the testes of adrenal steroids draining to the vascular bed of the testis because of the reflux from the adrenal vein has been suggested.[80] Recently a suggestion was made that an increased concentration of catecholamines in the spermatic vein may be the causative factor of spermatic damage in men with varicocele.[81] Evidence for the possibility of compromised Leydig cell function has also been presented recently.[82]

Although a considerable body of data has accumulated implicating the varicocele in male infertility, a review of critical analysis of these data clearly indicates that a great deal of work will still be necessary to clarify the relationship between varicocele and testicular function, the mechanism by which varicocele possibly produces testicular damage, and the role played by varicocele ligation in therapy.

DIAGNOSTIC EVALUATION OF THE INFERTILE MALE

The evaluation of the infertile male can be divided into two major phases: (1) the initial evaluation, and (2) extensive diagnostic investigation.

The initial evaluation is designed to define the following parameters: (1) the ability on the part of the male to produce a satisfactory ejaculate, (2) the ability to deliver the ejaculate at the appropriate time to the appropriate area of the female reproductive tract, and (3) the capacity of the spermatozoa to penetrate ovulatory cervical mucus and retain adequate motility in it.

A thorough history and physical examination may by themselves provide sufficient clues to allow the examiner to detect the presence of a well-defined disorder that may affect testicular function: an endocrine disorder, genetic or developmental disorder, neurologic disorder, sexual dysfunction, anatomic abnormality, or gonadal damage secondary to exposure to toxic substances or various forms of irradiation. Physical examination frequently yields information that is directly supportive of diagnostic clues found in the course of obtaining the history.

During physical examination of the genitalia, special attention is paid to the position of the testes in the scrotum, as well as their size and consistency; the epididymis is examined for structural irregularities, indurations, and cysts. To detect a possible varicocele, the pampiniform plexus is examined with the patient standing and executing the Valsalva maneuver. A rectal examination is conducted to exclude the possibility of prostatic or seminal vesicle disease.

It must be stressed, however, that perfectly normal history and physical examination may still be associated with severe abnormalities of sperm production. Consequently, careful and extensive evaluation of the seminal fluid is the second essential step. Although the technical aspects of seminal fluid examination are relatively simple, in order to make this examination meaningful considerable attention to this procedure is essential. The patient must be instructed in the collection of the specimen and in the pitfalls that may cause erroneous results. For adequate evaluation of sperm output, the specimen must be collected by masturbation and the patient appropriately instructed in order to prevent loss of a portion of the ejaculate. The physician must become aware of the customary frequency of the patient's ejaculatory activity. Some practice frequent ejaculations, daily or even several times each day; this may seriously influence the sperm count. In view of the documented variability in the quality of the ejaculate, particularly pronounced in patients with oligospermia, it is necessary to examine several (four to six) specimens obtained after a 2- or 3-day period of abstinence and at varying intervals.

It is difficult, and at times impractical, during the course of evaluating the male fertility potential, to follow a rigid outline. However, general guidelines can be suggested.

The initial steps of evaluation of male fertility are summarized in Figure 29-9. It will be noted that even if the complete history and physical examination as well as the examination of six seminal fluid specimens are normal, further steps are essential. The postcoital tests evaluate penetration and survival of spermatozoa in the cervical mucus. If that also is normal, one can go one step further and conduct the sperm freezing test. It has been shown that spermatozoa of men with fertility problems do not survive freezing as well as spermatozoa from highly fertile men; thus this test may provide a clue for spermatozoan inadequacy. An abnormal postcoital test may indicate an immunological problem or "cervical hostility" of unknown etiology. An in vitro sperm penetration test is then performed in a crossover fashion (between husband's sperm and wife's mucus, wife's mucus and donor sperm, and husband's sperm and donor mucus) in an attempt to pinpoint the abnormality. Obviously, when the history and the physical examination provide a clue for the presence of an abnormal condition, a workup for that suspected condition needs to be conducted in addition to the evaluation of the six seminal fluid specimens. When the history and physical examination are normal and the seminal fluid is abnormal, the abnormality of the seminal fluid may be one of the abnormalities mentioned in Figure 29-9.

The analysis of the seminal fluid may provide information useful for diagnosis of pathology in the various segments of the reproductive tract. Abnormal volume (high or low) suggests a disturbance in the secretory function of the seminal vesicles, whereas absence of fructose suggests either a block of the ejaculatory ducts or congenital absence of the seminal vesicles or the ejaculatory duct. This finding requires further studies, including a vesiculogram and vasograms. White blood cells and bacteria in seminal fluid are most frequently associated with prostatis or seminal vesiculitis. Teratospermia points toward an intratesticular abnormality. Severe oligospermia may be associated not only with testicular disease but also with partial obstruction of the epididymal duct.

When severe oligospermia or azoospermia is detected, endocrine evaluation is in order (Fig. 29-10). Normal findings on endocrine evaluation in patients with azoospermia suggest a complete block of the testicular excretory system. However, a par-

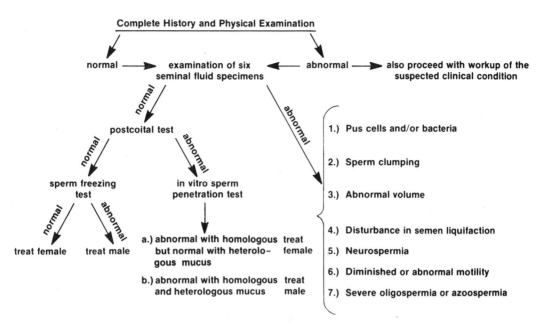

FIGURE 29-9. Initial evaluation of the male reproductive system.

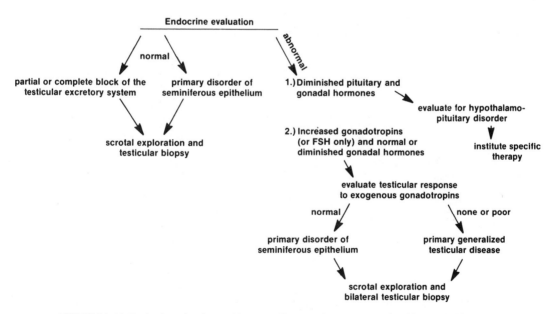

FIGURE 29-10. Evaluation of patients with severe oligospermia or azoospermia with normal Hx and Px.

tial epididymal and/or vasal block, primary testicular disease due to enzyme defects in androgen biosynthetic pathway, or a primary testicular defect may also be associated with normal endocrine findings.

If endocrine evaluation suggests diminished pituitary and gonadal hormone production, a hypothalamic–pituitary disorder is most likely present, and its careful evaluation may permit specific therapy. When increased gonadotropins are detected or if only FSH levels are increased while the gonadal hormones are within normal levels or slightly diminished, severe seminiferous epithelium damage for which no therapy is available is the most likely diagnosis and no further workup is usually indicated.

When scrotal exploration is conducted, several procedures can be carried out during the course of this surgery. First, inspection of the scrotal contents allows one to ascertain whether the epididymis and vas are normal. An abnormality in the epididymis, congenital absence of the vas associated with a partial or complete block as well as the presence of a varicocele can usually be detected at this point. Appropriate corrective procedures can be undertaken. A biopsy is obtained from both testicles. The fragments of testicular tissue can be used for morphological, cytogenetic, and biochemical investigations.

We feel that exploration of the scrotum should replace simple biopsy because it permits adequate visualization of the testis, the epididymis, and a portion of the vas. It should be emphasized again that an epididymal block may exist not only in the presence of azoospermia but also in patients with oligospermia. An epididymal block can be diagnosed by visual inspection because of the characteristic appearance of the epididymis with areas of dilated epididymal ductal system or even formation of a small cyst (Fig. 29-11). Evaluation of testicular biopsy is only useful if appropriate techniques for procurement of the tissue are utilized and the tissue is adequately processed; otherwise this procedure becomes a useless exercise. Microscopic examination of the tissue should be conducted only by an experienced individual who can not only properly interpret the findings but also determine whether the tissue was properly obtained and processed. Artifacts of inappropriate surgical or laboratory techniques are extremely common and lead to erroneous conclusions when interpreted by inexperienced observers.

The recently developed techniques for evaluation of steroid biosynthetic pathways, although they re-

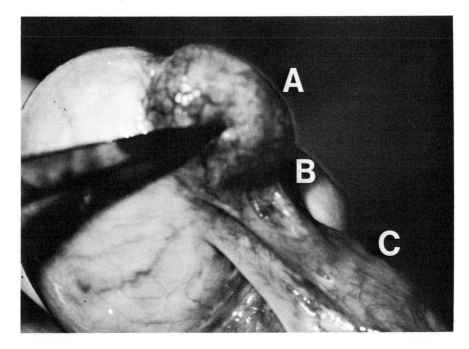

FIGURE 29-11. Epididymal block. A, caput epididymis; B, block; C, corpus epididymis. (Courtesy of Dr. R. Schoysman.)

quire relatively sophisticated laboratory facilities, are helpful not only in the diagnosis of specific enzymic abnormalities of the androgen biogenetic pathways but also in the choice of successful therapy.

Obviously not all diagnostic procedures need to be carried out in each case. The selection of an appropriate plan of diagnostic investigation depends on each diagnostic step, including scrotal exploration and biopsy and the findings during surgery.

LABORATORY EVALUATION OF TESTICULAR FUNCTION

Tests available for evaluation of testicular function can be divided into two principal categories: those dealing with evaluation of the spermatogenic process and those dealing with evaluation of the endocrine aspects of gonadal function.

Some of the procedures described here are utilized as part of a routine workup for all patients. Others are employed only when there is a clear indication. The third group of techniques described here are available primarily in research laboratories. It is important to emphasize that one cannot make rigid suggestions concerning the precise role of the various tests and the sequence of their employment during diagnostic workup. Each patient has to be considered as an individual case, and depending on the indications and available facilities, the diagnostic investigation has to be appropriately designed. It is of primary importance for the physician who embarks upon evaluation of male reproductive function to become thoroughly familiar not only with the relevance, sensitivity, precision, and normal values for each of the diagnostic techniques but also with the limitations and reliability of the laboratory that he or she utilizes.

Evaluation of Endocrine Factors

Plasma Hormone Levels

The endocrine evaluation of the infertile male is based principally on the ability to measure the various hormones in body fluids and tissues. Three different techniques have been used to measure hormones: bioassays, chemical techniques, and competitive binding assays. While all three methods are still useful, the competitive binding assays (including RIAs) have come to the forefront in the past several years. The RIA offers superior precision

and sensitivity. However, these qualities are achieved only when the procedure is performed by experienced personnel under well-supervised conditions. Although the RIA has become a routine method and is available in many clinical laboratories, and although a variety of commercial kits have been developed that greatly simplify the assay procedure, in many instances, unfortunately, this very simplicity has resulted in serious drawbacks. Materials which do not provide adequate specificity and precision are sometimes utilized. The relative simplicity of the technique lulls the laboratory supervisors and technicians into a false sense of security, resulting in the production of data that are not only of little use to the clinician but at times detrimental to precise diagnosis. Consequently, physicians must make themselves aware of the various shortcomings and must request from the laboratory information concerning the methodology used, including specificity of the antibody, precision of the assay, the accuracy and reproducibility of the technique and the details of the quality controls employed. Since the normal range for each hormone varies among different laboratories, it is important to know how the normal range was established in the laboratory. Frequently laboratories use blood samples from their own employees to establish a "normal" range. Since these employees are usually not really investigated for "normalcy," the "normal" range may not be accurately represented, leading to misinterpretation of the data by the physician.

The interpretation of the laboratory data must be also tempered with some knowledge of physiologic factors that may influence the results. First, both the gonadotropins and the plasma steroids, particularly testosterone, show rapid and wide fluctuation with time. Plasma testosterone values may vary in excess of 100% in blood samples obtained at intervals of several minutes. Consequently a single value should be interpreted cautiously, and accuracy can be improved by utilizing either integrated blood sampling techniques[83] or pooled aliquots of three blood samples taken at 20-min intervals.[25]

In evaluating testosterone values, an additional parameter must be taken into consideration. Steroids, including testosterone, circulate largely bound to a plasma protein and, in the case of testosterone, to a testosterone-binding globulin (TBG). Variations in the levels of the carrier protein affect circulating testosterone levels. Since only free (unbound) testosterone is metabolically active, total testosterone levels may not provide adequate information, and the determination of TBG may become necessary. TBG determination involves the quantitation of the saturation capacity of serum for androgens (testosterone or dihydrotestosterone). The normal range for an adult man is 5–11 μg/dl. Furthermore, it should be kept in mind that the circulating steroid levels represent the integrated end result of testicular production, peripheral metabolism, renal clearance, and extragonadal production. Techniques for the determination of both the production and metabolic clearance rate are available.[84] However, for the routine evaluation of a male with infertility problems, they may not be important.

Owing to the differences in methodology, normal ranges for plasma hormone levels vary among laboratories, and the normal range for each laboratory is usually wide. For example, the range for normal LH level may range from undetectable to 5 mIU/ml in some laboratories,[85] while in others the normal range may be from 5–20 mIU/ml.[86] Similar variations in normal ranges have been reported for FSH. Consequently, diagnosis of low gonadotropin production based solely on circulating levels may be misleading, since in many instances very low or undetectable levels are reported to be within normal range. To overcome this difficulty, a variety of function tests can be used. Similarly, the normal range for testosterone levels in adult male plasma varies greatly among different laboratories. In general it has been reported to range between 200 and 1200 ng/dl. Difficulty in diagnosing a hypoandrogenic state may arise when a low normal level is observed, since it is impossible to conclude whether the low level is normal or whether this individual would normally produce considerably higher amounts of testosterone. A variety of function tests are available to establish normalcy in patients who show low values that are still within normal ranges.

Evaluation of the Hypothalamic–Pituitary Axis

The first step in evaluating the hypothalamic–pituitary axis is the measurement of plasma gonadotropin levels. If the gonadotropin levels are suspiciously low, function tests can be conducted. Clomiphene citrate and GnRH stimulation tests are usually utilized for this purpose.

Clomiphene Citrate Test. Clomiphene citrate is thought to stimulate secretion of GnRH, which in turn results in the release of gonadotropins by the pituitary gland. Usually the release of LH is greater than that of FSH. The test is conducted in the following fashion. Clomiphene citrate, 100–200 mg/day, is administered for 5 days. Baseline gonadotropin levels are obtained on the day before administration of the drug and the day after the last dose. The response is considered normal if the LH shows doubling of the pretreatment levels.[87]

GnRH Stimulation Test. GnRH stimulates the anterior pituitary to release both LH and FSH. The LH release is usually considerably greater than that of FSH. The test is conducted in the following fashion. A baseline blood sample of FSH and LH is obtained; 100–500 μg GnRH is administered intramuscularly, and subsequently blood samples are obtained every 30 min for 3 hr. Both LH and FSH are measured in each blood sample. A normal response is characterized by a severalfold increase in LH levels and a smaller increase in FSH. Recently it has been suggested that intravenous administration of GnRH may provide more precise results.[88]

Interpretation of Results

Elevated levels of both LH and FSH: Primary testicular failure is associated with elevation of both gonadotropins. Testicular disease associated with failure of the germinal epithelium will also produce elevation of FSH with relatively normal LH levels. Where failure of both Leydig cells and germinal epithelium is present both LH and FSH are elevated. Patients with high FSH levels do not require further testing since neither clomiphene citrate nor GnRH stimulation will provide additional information.

Low or normal LH and FSH levels: In these patients, further testing may permit more precise localization of the lesion.

Absence of response to GnRH strongly suggests a pituitary dysfunction, and studies of other pituitary tropic hormones as well as radiographic evaluation of the pituitary fossa and other studies directed toward detection of intracranial lesions are indicated. Normal gonadotropin responses to GnRH associated with absence of response to clomiphene citrate is suggestive of hypothalamic disease and indicates further studies directed towards detection of an intracranial lesion.

Suppressed plasma gonadotropin levels may also be found in patients with hormone-producing gonadal tumors and in patients previously treated with gonadal hormones (estrogens or androgens).

Determination of Androgen Production by the Testis

Determination of plasma testosterone and "free" testosterone levels as described above is the basic form of evaluation of androgen production by the testis. An hCG stimulation test can be used for more precise evaluation of disturbed androgen production. Usually the hCG stimulation test involves daily administration of 1500–5000 IU hCG for 5 days.[87,89] We use the dose of 5000 IU for 4 days for adults and the lower dose for children. The plasma testosterone levels are measured 1 day before the first injection and the day after the last injection. The determinations are performed on pools of equal aliquots of several blood samples (three samples of 20-min intervals). A normal response produces at least doubling of the plasma testosterone levels. An abnormal response to hCG stimulation suggests local disturbance of Leydig cell function.

A more precise evaluation of Leydig cell function can be obtained by in vitro investigation of the androgen biosynthetic pathways in testicular tissue obtained at the routine testicular biopsy.[90,91] This technique permits detection of defects in specific enzymes involved in androgen biosynthesis and provides important diagnostic, therapeutic, and prognostic information.[22,43] These procedures are still expensive, complicated, and time consuming, hence not applicable for routine clinical use. It is hoped that simplification of these techniques will provide an approach to clinical diagnosis of specific Leydig cell deficiencies associated with testicular dysfunction.

Interpretation of Results. A subnormal plasma testosterone level may be the result of a hypothalamic–pituitary disorder or a primary dysfunction of the Leydig cell. The hypothalamic–pituitary basis for diminished androgen production can be iatrogenic in origin (secondary to administration of sex steroids or corticoids).[92] Depression of testosterone levels has been observed after physiological and surgical stresses,[93,94] possibly owing to an increase in corticosteroid levels in the stressed individuals. A careful history before measurement of androgens is necessary for appropriate interpretation of the results.

Failure of response to hCG suggests either absence of functional Leydig cells or severe disease of the Leydig cells. Diminution in the response is found in patients with Klinefelter's syndrome or other chromosomal abnormalities. The diminution in response may be associated with relatively normal baseline testosterone levels. In individuals with hypogonadotropic hypogonadism, hCG stimulation induces a brisk testosterone response.

Analysis of Seminal Fluid

Probably the most important single laboratory examination performed on a male patient with infertility is evaluation of the seminal fluid. The techniques are relatively simple procedures. Although very few changes have been introduced in the past 24 years, there is a need to apply highly standardized and precise methodology to obtain reliable results.

The collection of the specimen is as important as the analytical technique itself. The patient must be appropriately informed as to the method for proper collection and transport of the sample. The most precise and reliable method for obtaining the specimen is masturbation. Collection into a rubber condom produces misleading data on spermatozoan motility and inaccurate sperm counts and volume measurements. Coitus interruptus may result in incomplete collection and a biased sampling, since, if part of the ejaculate is lost, it is usually the first part, which contains the highest density of spermatozoa.

The patient should be provided with an appropriate container for collection of the specimen; otherwise the physician may expect the greatest variety of inappropriately sized and shaped containers and, most importantly, containers that may not be sufficiently free of traces of substances which may be detrimental to spermatozoan motility. The patient must be apprised of the need for a continence period of a minimum of 2 and a maximum of 5 days duration. The specimen should be delivered to the laboratory within 1 hour of collection and should be kept at room temperature (70°–80°F) rather than body temperature.[95] The seminal fluid is then examined macroscopically, microscopically, chemically, and immunologically. Macroscopic evaluation involves measuring the volume and the viscosity of the specimen; observation on the rapidity of liquefaction must also be made. Unusual color and/or odor should be noted.

Microscopic Examination. The specimen must be fully liquefied and adequately mixed before microscopic examination is performed. The most frequent cause of an erroneous sperm analysis is probably inadequate mixing of the sample. The spermatozoa have the tendency to settle, particularly those with poor motility. This introduces a bias in estimates of both count and motility. If no spermatozoa are observed during the initial examination, the specimen should be centrifuged and the sediment examined for the presence of spermatozoa.

Evaluation of motility. In most instances, motility is determined by subjective examination of the seminal fluid specimen. A drop of semen is placed on a clean glass slide and covered with a glass coverslip of standard size. The preparation is then examined by a trained observer at magnification of 400–600X, preferably with phase-contrast optics. Only spermatozoa with directional motility should be considered motile, and a minimum of 20 microscopic fields should be examined. The motility is expressed as percent of spermatozoa exhibiting directional motility. Some laboratories also report the estimate of viability, which is that fraction of sperm demonstrating any motion. Supervital stains can also be utilized to make the distinction between live and dead spermatozoa.[96] Recently an attempt has been made to develop objective techniques for evaluation of sperm motility; these include utilization of highly sophisticated laser techniques, computerized video techniques, and relatively simple stroboscopic techniques. It is the later technology, namely, utilization of simple stroboscopic apparatus,[97] possibly coupled with relatively simple computerization that may become applicable for both clinical and research directed objective analysis of sperm motility. Most laboratories still use subjective methods of evaluating sperm motilities. The physician must be familiar with the specific technique used in the laboratory employed as well as the range of error before using the data for making the final diagnostic conclusion.

Sperm count. The sperm count is performed in a fashion similar to that used for a blood count. The specimen is diluted 1 : 10 or 1 : 20, depending on sperm density, and counted in a hemocytometer. The sperm count is then reported as millions of spermatozoa per milliliter of seminal fluid or as a total sperm count, which means millions of spermatozoa per total ejaculate.

Some laboratories employ an electronic particle counter (Coulter counter), which is quicker and less subjective than a hemocytometer; however, particularly where low counts are present or where there is debris, a considerable amount of interference is encountered, resulting in erroneous results.[98]

Sperm morphology. This is usually assessed by microscopic examination of stained smears of seminal fluid. Most laboratories evaluate and classify 200 cells according to standardized criteria.[99–101] Morphological abnormalities are usually classified as those of sperm head (e.g., large, small, tapered, amorphous, duplicated, round, pearshaped, midpiece, or tail defects). The presence of immature germ cells is noted, and recognition of white cells or epithelial cells is of particular importance in differentiating between sloughed germinal epithelium cells and inflammatory cells derived from the sex accessory organs. Special staining techniques have been developed to differentiate between round spermatids and leukocytes.[102]

Chemical analysis. Chemical analysis of the seminal fluid is a point of controversy. Although a variety of tests have been suggested, only the test for the presence of fructose and the determination of pH are of value for clinical purposes.

Immunology. A number of reports in the literature suggest that the presence of antibodies against spermatozoa and/or constituents of the seminal plasma may interfere with fertility.[103] The mechanism by which the antibodies are produced is not entirely clear. Most likely the pathophysiology of this process involves injury to the male reproductive system resulting in exposure of the immunological system to the constituents of the spermatozoa as it may occur subsequent to vasectomy or following orchitis.

Two types of antibodies have been described: sperm agglutinating and sperm immobilizing. Sperm-immobilizing antibodies are probably associated with infertility. These antibodies can be detected in serum by the sperm-immobilizing test of Isojima.[59] Sperm-agglutinating antibodies can be detected either by the macroscopic test of Kibrick et al.[57] or the microscopic technique of Franklin and Dukes.[58] The prognostic value of these tests is still not entirely clear. No direct relationship between the type of the antibody and the degree of infertility has been established. Nevertheless a screening test for antibodies is useful as an additional parameter in defining the fertility state of the male.

Fertilizing Capacity. While determination of sperm density, motility, and morphology provides fundamental diagnostic and prognostic information about semen quality, none of these parameters addresses the issue of fertilizing capacity of the spermatozoa. The only way to assess the parameter would be to determine the capacity of the spermatozoa to fertilize human ova in vitro, an impractical approach because of a variety of ethical, legal, and technical issues. An alternative approach has been suggested by the pioneering work of Yanagimachi,[104] who demonstrated that spermatozoa of all eutherian species will penetrate zona pellucida-free hamster eggs and subsequently suggested that the ability of human spermatozoa to penetrate the denuded hamster egg may serve as a test for their fertilizing capacity.[105] There are still numerous basic problems with the sperm penetrate assay (SPA) as far as its clinical usefulness is concerned. Even disregarding the problem of extremely high cost and necessity for highly trained personnel to carry out the SPA, a number of fundamental problems will have to be solved before its clinical use could be fully justified. First, the interpretation of the results (''normal range'') varies significantly among various research laboratories.[106,107] It is still unclear what the SPA actually measures.[108] Nevertheless, the SPA definitely shows potential as an important adjunct in diagnostic evaluation of the male fertility potential. It is of interest to note that a definite positive correlation has been demonstrated between the results of SPA and the proportion of progressively motile spermatozoa showing a small amplitude of lateral head displacement.[109] On the other hand, successful penetration of zona free hamster eggs has been observed despite the presence of functional and/or structural abnormalities of the spermatozoa, abnormalities that preclude the fertilization of human eggs in vitro.[109]

Interpretation of Results. The analysis of the seminal fluid is the most important parameter for defining the fertility potential of the male. However, the definition of ''normal'' or ''fertile'' ejaculate has been changing considerably in the past decade. Recently it has been suggested that the fertility of a couple is a relative state which depends on the interaction of the fertility potentials of both the male and the female partners of the infertile couple.[2,110] Thus, a male with certain seminal fluid pictures could be defined as infertile or subfertile when mated with a specific female, but he could be quite fertile when mated with a female of much higher fertility. Nevertheless, despite all its shortcomings, the seminal fluid analysis still provides one of the most important objective parameters for evaluating male fertility.

The number of samples that have to be analyzed to obtain a clear picture of the average sperm output is still a matter of controversy and conjecture. A marked oscillation in sperm density has been observed when ejaculates of the same individual are examined at different times.[111] There is no controversy concerning the fact that a number of seminal fluid specimens should be examined. Investigators do not agree, however, on the number and time interval between examinations. Smith et al.[5,110] suggest examination of a minimum of six ejaculates. Sherins et al.[112] suggest a minimum of nine ejaculates over a period of 6 months.

Although there is a great variation in the normal sperm density, most authorities accept 20 million/ml as the dividing line between optimal fertility potential and subfertility. Recently a number of reports appeared in the literature suggesting that even this may be too high and that subfertility in a male should not be considered unless the sperm count drops below 10 million or possibly below 5 million/ml.[5,110,113] Similarly, there is no consensus concerning the dividing line between fertile and infertile man as far as the percentage of motile spermatozoa is concerned. Reports of pregnancies following insemination with semen showing motility of 25–30% are not uncommon.[114]

Although sperm morphology would appear to be a highly objective measure of sperm quality, the general criteria are not clearly defined. The American Fertility Society suggests that fertility is compromised when the percentage of abnormal sperm is above 40.[115] Others believe that an even higher percentage of abnormal sperm is still compatible with fertility.[116]

Testicular Biopsy. The surgical procedure involved in obtaining testicular biopsy is simple and relatively safe. The procedure can be conducted on an outpatient basis or when associated with testicular exploration as a minor inpatient procedure. It is of utmost importance that the surgical procedure, the processing of the tissue, and the microscopic interpretation are properly performed (Figs. 29-12A and 29-13A).

Although appropriate surgical techniques for testicular biopsy have been described in detail in the literature,[117] many surgeons are still using techniques that are inappropriate, resulting in mutilated tissue unsuitable for appropriate histological studies (Fig. 29-12B). The tissue is frequently removed with forceps and scissors or, even worse, by needle biopsy. Similarly, many laboratories still utilize formalin as the fixative. The resulting histological preparation is frequently worthless (Fig. 29-13B). The appropriate technique for biopsy involves making a small incision in the tunica albuginea, through

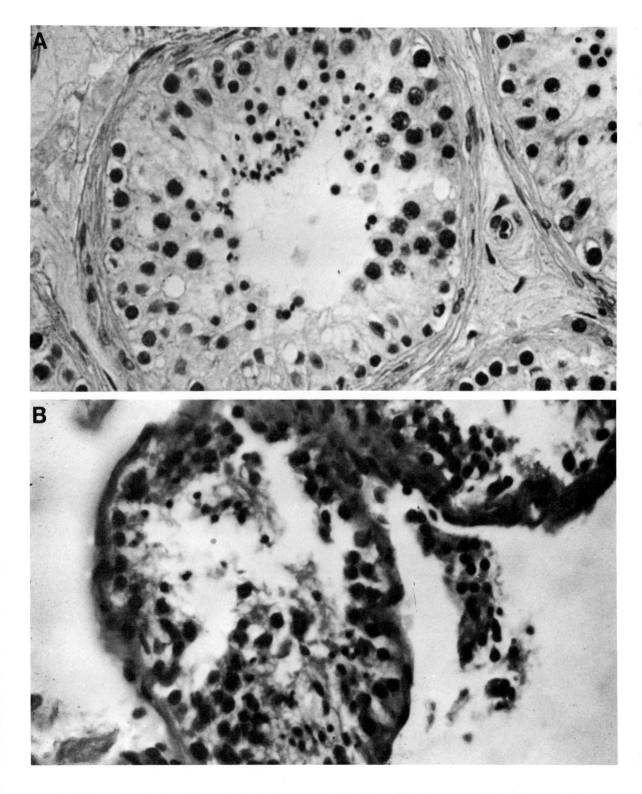

FIGURE 29-12. (A) Testicular biopsy obtained with proper surgical technique. (B) Inadequate surgical technique, resulting in distorted testicular biopsy.

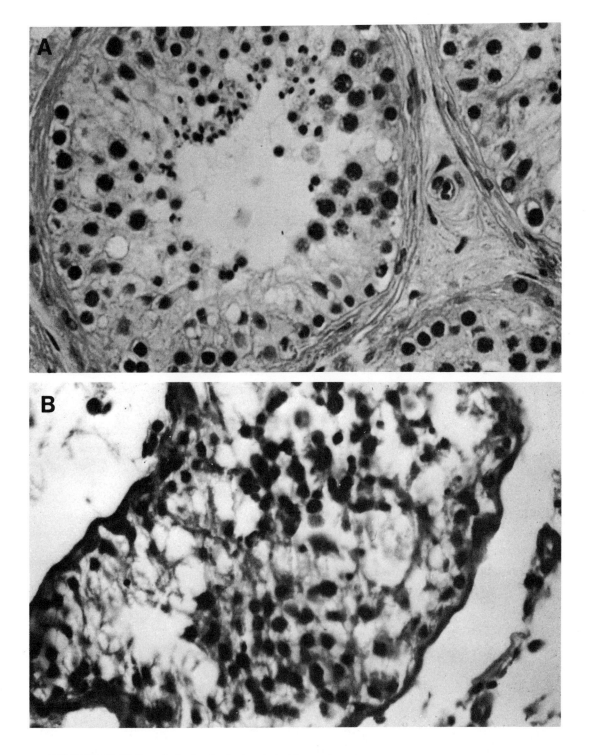

FIGURE 29-13. (A) Properly fixed and stained testicular biopsy. (B) Inadequate fixation of testicular biopsy (formalin).

which testicular tissue will bulge if the testicle is held firmly; the bulge is shaved off with a razor blade. Once the tissue is free, both razor blade and tissue are dropped into the fixative (Bouin's or Clelland's solution) so that no mechanical manipulation or pressure is applied to the specimen during the surgical procedure and before fixation. If these precautions are not observed, sloughing and distortion of the germinal epithelium will result in misinterpretation of the microscopic picture of the biopsy. The interpretation of the biopsy should be performed by an individual familiar with spermatogenesis, to avoid erroneous interpretations.

Frequently the indication for biopsy is severe oligospermia or azoospermia. Under these circumstances the possibility should be kept in mind that not only total but also partial obstruction of the epididymal duct may exist. Under these circumstances, a scrotal exploration should be performed in conjunction with the testicular biopsy. Visual examination of the epididymis will reveal an epididymal block.

Although a qualitative examination of the germinal epithelium is all that is necessary for routine evaluation of testicular biopsy, a number of quantitative techniques for evaluating spermatogenesis are available.[15] While most are still primary research tests some have been simplified to allow routine hospital application.[16] The application of these techniques is of particular importance as the assessment of testicular function needs to be made before the decision to perform microsurgery for epididymal block.

As mentioned in previous sections, testicular biopsy can also be used for in vitro evaluation of the androgen biosynthetic pathways. For this purpose, a small fraction of the biopsy (10–15 mg) is incubated with appropriate radiolabeled steroid precursors and the steroid metabolites formed are then separated, purified, and quantitated. From these data, defects in the various enzymes involved in androgen biogenesis can be diagnosed. Although still a research procedure, it is rapidly being simplified and will be available in the near future for routine evaluation of androgen biosynthesis in small portions of testicular biopsy.

SUMMARY OF THERAPEUTIC INTERVENTION

Male infertility results most frequently from inadequate sperm production. The inadequate sperm production can be caused by one of several conditions, including an endocrine disorder of the hypothalamic–pituitary axis; a specific but unexplained lesion of the seminiferous epithelium (e.g., the Sertoli cell-only syndrome); genetic abnormalities (e.g., Klinefelter's syndrome); seminiferous epithelium failure due to infections (e.g., mumps); idiopathic failure of the seminiferous epithelium; abnormalities of Leydig cell androgen biosynthesis; and a block of the excretory duct.

The therapy of a well-defined hypothalamic–pituitary problem is relatively simple. It requires administration of the appropriate amount of gonadotropic hormones. The dosage and the details of this form of therapy are described in the section on disorders of testicular function associated with infertility. Blocks of the excretory ducts, particularly a block of the epididymis or the vas deferens, can be corrected surgically with varying degrees of success. The success of epididymovasostomy is relatively low (10–30%) even in the hands of highly experienced reproductive systems surgeons. This procedure probably should not be undertaken except by appropriately trained surgeons. Nevertheless, it is a worthwhile approach in properly selected patients.[118] In cases of Sertoli cell-only syndrome, genetic abnormalities, or destruction of the germinal epithelium secondary to infection or vascular accidents, no therapy is available. However, the largest number of patients with diminished sperm production do not fall into these etiological categories. In most instances, the diagnosis of seminiferous epithelium failure of unknown etiology is made, and in a substantial percentage of these cases a varicocele can be detected.

Numerous reports in the literature suggest that high ligation of the spermatic vein is an effective form of therapy in patients with unexplained abnormalities of sperm production and varicocele.[69] Although this form of therapy appears to show promise, there is considerable evidence that, at least in patients with sperm counts of less than 10 million, no improvement in sperm output is observed.[78] Consequently, the efficacy of varicocelectomy or ligation of the spermatic vein in patients with varicocele as therapy for infertility still awaits confirmation. Furthermore, since only a fraction of patients with varicocele respond to surgery, it would be of great benefit to be able to select responders, although this has not proved successful.[119]

The medical therapy for patients with idiopathic seminiferous tubule failure has been the topic of numerous publications.[120] Numerous hormonal and nonhormonal agents have been claimed at one time or another to effect improvement. One of the more common forms of hormonal therapy has been thyroid hormone, specifically Cytomel. Although the initial reports suggested a beneficial response, no solid evidence could be marshalled subsequently in support of the effectiveness of this form of therapy in patients with oligospermia of unknown etiology.

Similarly, therapy with adrenal corticoids showed great promise.[121] There were a number of proponents as well as numerous opponents.[122] A review of the literature leads this author to the conclusion that this form of therapy is not warranted in patients who do not exhibit adrenal insufficiency.

In recent years, therapy with clomiphene citrate (Clomid) has led to the publication of a number of controversial papers. Clomiphene citrate has been demonstrated to stimulate gonadotropin production by the pituitary gland *via* its effect on the hypothalamus.[123] Significant improvements in sperm production in large numbers of patients treated with clomiphene have been reported by a number of investigators[124,125]; however, a number of other workers failed to support or confirm this observation.[126,127] As a matter of fact, suppression of spermatogenesis in normal man has been reported after administration of high doses of Clomid.[128] The possibility exists some patients with idiopathic oligospermia have (1) a subtle abnormality or deficiency in gonadotropin production, (2) a form of "insensitivity" of the Leydig cell to normal levels of gonadotropins, or (3) an abnormality requiring higher-than-normal circulating levels of gonadotropins. Under these circumstances, Clomid-induced elevation of circulating levels of gonadotropins may be beneficial. However, one must be able to select appropriate patients for the therapy. Thus an appropriate diagnosis has to be made in order to select the responder. This selection process has not yet been defined. Furthermore, even if we were able to select such patients, the question of the appropriate dose of Clomid would still have to be settled. Consequently, it appears that Clomid should be still considered an experimental drug with the potential to become part of an effective therapeutic regimen for patients with idiopathic oligospermia.

The effectiveness of gonadotropin therapy in patients with idiopathic seminiferous epithelium failure is difficult to evaluate for similar reasons. Again, as in the case of Clomid, some investigators reported a degree of success in a segment of the patient population after treatment with gonadotropins. However, as the patient population in these reports was randomly selected, analysis of the results is difficult. Nevertheless, even under these circumstances, it appears that a small segment of a random population of patients treated with gonadotropins shows a positive response. Further studies again will be essential to select the responders for this form of therapy.[120]

The use of testosterone treatment of idiopathic seminiferous epithelium failure also had a stormy history. One must differentiate between two forms of testosterone therapy. In one, testosterone is administered with the idea of replacing an inadequate level of testosterone in the patient. In the other, testosterone is administered in a sufficiently high dose to suppress the patient's own gonadotropins, hence to suppress his own testosterone production, induce arrest of spermatogenesis, and upon termination of the treatment induce a "rebound." Proponents of the latter form of therapy believe that, subsequent to the arrest of the germinal epithelium induced by testosterone treatment, regeneration with greater vigor occurs and the germinal epithelium is capable of producing spermatozoa at a higher rate than pretreatment levels. The rebound form of therapy involves administration of large doses of testosterone.[129] Improvement has been claimed by a number of investigators, and this form of therapy has been employed with varying degrees of success in the past 25 years.[130,131] Unfortunately, even in reports where successful outcome has been reported, again only a small segment of the patient population responded. This prompts the question, "Is there a group of responders which needs to be selected?" No adequate guidelines are available for the selection of such responders.

The administration of testosterone for the purpose of "stimulating" spermatogenesis[132] has not been documented to be effective. The suggested dose range is such that it probably does not elevate intratesticular levels of testosterone.

A variety of synthetic steroids have been reported to produce beneficial effects in patients with oligospermia. An orally active synthetic androgen allegedly showing little if any toxicity[133] has been suggested to be effective in stimulating sperm production in patients with oligospermia.[134] Reports of the beneficial effect of this agent have not been clearly documented, and its effectiveness as well as its safety must await further study.

Similarly, a number of nonhormonal agents have been periodically hailed for therapy of oligospermia. Among these are arginine, vitamin C, vitamin E, phenelzine sulfate, and pentoxifylline (methylxanthine derivative). To the best knowledge of this author, no adequately documented evidence has been provided in support of effectiveness of these agents.

SUMMARY

It appears that both medical and surgical forms of therapy in patients with undiagnosed oligo- or azoospermia are basically empirical, difficult and unrewarding. In patients amenable to surgical therapy, a definite group may respond beneficially. In patients for whom no surgical therapy is available, the response is even more difficult to evaluate. Unquestionably the ''shotgun'' form of medical therapy with a variety of agents, particularly Cytomel, vitamin E, and arginine, should not be accepted as appropriate. On the other hand, therapy with Clomid and appropriate gonadotropin preparations holds definite promise. The major problem is the ability of the physician to select responders, which in turn depends on the ability of the physician to make a highly precise diagnosis. The latter may require the availability of sophisticated laboratory facilities and properly trained personnel for both performance of the test and its interpretation.

Undoubtedly, the rapid advances in the understanding of the physiology and biochemistry of the male reproductive system will lead to clear understanding of the underlying causes of spermatogenic failure and to the development of simpler, more definite, more precise diagnostic techniques, which will result in improvement of our therapeutic efforts.

QUESTIONS

1. A genetic defect in the mechanism of androgen action on target cells (lack or deficiency of androgen receptors) is caused by

    a. Lubs' syndrome.
    b. Klinefelter's syndrome.
    c. Reinfeinstein's syndrome.
    d. Kallmann's syndrome.
    e. Alström's syndrome.

2. The testes synthesize and secrete

    a. androstenedione.
    b. Progesterone.
    c. Testosterone.
    d. Estradiol.
    e. Dihydrotestosterone.

3. In hypogonadotropic hypogonadism, spermatogenesis can be initiated and maintained by

    a. testosterone.
    b. LH.
    c. FSH.
    d. FSH and testosterone.
    e. LH and FSH.

4. The initial evaluation of a patient referred because of oligospermia requires

    a. complete history and physical examination.
    b. determination of fructose in the semen.
    c. determination of plasma LH, FSH, and testosterone.
    d. repeat semen analysis.
    e. complete thyroid function test.
    f. plasma ''androgen panel.''
    g. testicular biopsy.

5. In a patient with hypogonadotropic hypogonadism, therapy may result in appearance of spermatozoa in the ejaculate after a minimum of

    a. 2 weeks.
    b. 4 weeks.
    c. 12 weeks.
    d. 24 weeks.
    e. 32 weeks.

REFERENCES

1. Murphy DP, Torrano EF: Male fertility in 3620 childless couples. *Fertil Steril* 16:337, 1965
2. Steinberger E, Steinberger A: Testis: Basic and clinical aspects, in Balin H Glasser S (eds): *Reproductive Biology.* Amsterdam, Excerpta Medica, 1972, pp 144–267*
3. Newton J, Craig S, Joyce D: The changing pattern of a comprehensive infertility clinic. *J Biosoc Sci* 6:477, 1974
4. Sherins RJ: Clinical aspects of treatment of male infertility with gonadotropins: Testicular response of some men given HCG with and without pergonal, in Mancini RE, Martini L (eds): *Male Fertility and Sterility, Proceedings of Serono Symposia,* Vol 5. New York, Academic, 1974, p 545
5. Smith KD, Rodriguez-Rigau LJ, Steinberger E: The infertile couple, working with them as a couple, in Cockett ATK, Urry RL (eds): *Male Infertility. Workup, Treatment and Research.* New York, Grune & Stratton, 1977, pp 211–214
6. Davis JR, Langford GA, Kirby RJ: The testicular capsule,

*Review article or chapter.

in Johnson AD, Gomes WR, VanDemark NL (eds): *The Testis*, Vol 1. New York, Academic, 1970, p 282

7. von Ebner V: Untersuchungen uber den Bau der Samelkanalchen und die Entwicklung der Spermatozoiden bei den Säugentieren und beim Menschen, in *Rollet's Untersuchungen aus dem institut für Physiologie und Histologie in Graz*. Leipzig, 1871, p 200

8. Benda C: Untersuchungen uber den Bau des funktionierenden Samelkanalchens einiger Saugetiere und Folgerungen fur die Spermatogenase dieser Wirbeltierklasse. *Arch Mikrosk Anat* 30:49, 1887

9. Regaud C: Etude sur la structure des tubes séiminifères et sur la spermatogenèse chez les mammifères. *Arch Anat Microsc Morphol Exp* 4:101, 231, 1901

10. Steinberger E, Steinberger A: The spermatogenic function of the testis, in Greep R, Astwood E (eds): *Handbook of Physiology. Endocrinology*, Sect 7, Vol V: *Reproductive System–Male*. Baltimore, American Physiological Society—Williams & Wilkins, 1975, p 1*

11. Clermont Y: The cycle of the seminiferous epithelium in man. *Am J Anat* 112:35, 1963

12. Steinberger E, Tjioe DY: Kinetics and quantitative analysis of human spermatogenesis. *Proceedings of All-India Conference on Research in Reproduction and Fertility*. Indian Council of Medical Research. Technical Report Series No. 21:99, 1973*

13. Chowdhury AK, Steinberger A, Steinberger E: A quantitative study of spermatogonial population in organ culture of human testis. *Andrologia* 7(4):297, 1975

14. Heller CG, Clermont Y: Spermatogenesis in man and estimate of its duration. *Science* 140:184, 1963*

15. Steinberger E, Tjioe DY: A method for quantitative analysis of human seminiferous epithelium. *Fertil Steril* 19:960, 1968*

16. Rodriguez-Rigau LJ, Smith KD, Steinberger E: Correlation between sperm output and number of mature spermatids in human testicular biopsies. Sixth Annual Meeting, American Society of Andrology. New Orleans, LA, 1981. *J Androl* 2:24, 1981

17. Fawcett DW: Ultrastructure and function of the Sertoli cell, in Greep R, Astwood E (eds): *Handbook of Physiology. Endocrinology*, Sect 7, Vol V: *Reproductive System–Male*. Baltimore, American Physiological Society—Williams & Wilkins, 1975, p 21*

18. Steinberger A, Steinberger E: Replication pattern of Sertoli cells in maturing rat testis *in vivo* and in organ culture. *Biol Reprod* 4:84, 1971

19. Steinberger E: Biogenesis of androgens, in Giabian H, Plotz EJ (eds): *Mammalian Reproduction*. Heidelberg, Springer-Verlag, 1970, p 112*

20. Hall PF: Gonadotrophic regulation of testicular function, in Eik-Nes KB (ed): *The Androgens of the Testis*. New York, Marcel Dekker 1970, p 73*

21. Rodriguez-Rigau LJ, Tcholakian RK, Smith KD, et al: *In vitro* steroid metabolic studies in human testis. II. Metabolism of cholesterol, pregnenolone, progesterone, androstenedione and testosterone by testes of an estrogen-treated man. *Steroids* 30:729, 1977

22. Rodriguez-Rigau LJ, Weiss DB, Smith KD, et al: Suggestion of abnormal testicular steroidogenesis in some oligospermic men. *Acta Endocrinol (Copenh)* 87:400, 1978

23. Amelar RD, Dubin L: Male infertility. Current diagnosis and treatment. *Urology* 1:1, 1973*

24. Horton R: Sex steroid production and secretion in the male. *Andrologia* 10(3):183, 1978

25. Goldzieher JW, Dozier TS, Smith KD, et al: Improving the diagnostic reliability of rapidly fluctuating plasma hormone levels by optimized multiple-sampling techniques. *J Clin Endocrinol Metab* 43(4):824, 1976

26. Steinberger E, Smith KD, Tcholakian RK, et al: Steroidogenesis in human testis, in Mancini RE, Martini L (eds): *Male Fertility and Sterility*. New York, Academic, 1974, p 149*

27. Mainwaring WIP: *The Mechanism of Action of Androgens*. New York, Springer-Verlag, 1977, p 1

28. Smith PE: The disabilities caused by hypophysectomy and their repair. *JAMA* 88:158, 1927

29. Steinberger E, Steinberger A: Hormonal control of testicular function in mammals, in Knobil E, Sawyer WH (eds): *Handbook of Physiology. Endocrinology*, Sect 7, Vol V, Part 2: *Reproductive System–Male*. Baltimore, American Physiological Society—Williams & Wilkins, 1974, p 325

30. Hotchkiss RS: Effects of massive doses of testosterone propionate upon spermatogenesis. *J Clin Endocrinol Metab* 4:114, 1944*

31. Steinberger E: Hormonal regulation of the seminiferous tubule function, in French FS, Hansson V, Ritzen EM, Nayfeh SN (eds): *Hormonal Regulation of Spermatogenesis*. New York, Plenum, 1975, pp 337–352*

32. Mortimer CH, McNeilly AS, Fisher RA, et al: Gonadotrophin-releasing hormone therapy in hypogonadal males with hypothalamic or pituitary dysfunction. *Br Med J* 4:617, 1974

33. Nillius SJ: The therapeutic uses of gonadotrophin-releasing hormone and its analogues, in Beardwell C, Robertsson GL (eds): *BIMR Clinical Endocrinology. The Pituitary*. London, Butterworths, 1982, p 211

34. Charny CW: Effect of varicocele on fertility. *Fertil Steril* 13:47, 1962

35. Glenn JF, McPherson HT: Anorchism: Definition of a clinical entity. *J Urol* 105:265, 1971

36. Silber SJ, Rodriguez-Rigau LJ: Pregnancy after testicle transplant. The importance of treating the couple. *Fertil Steril* 33:454–455, 1980

37. Kjessler G: Fracteurs génétiques dans la subfertilé male humaine, in *Frécondité et stérilité du male. Acquisitions recéntes*. Paris, Masson, 1972

38. Smith KD, Steinberger E, Steinberger A, et al: Recent advances in human cytogenetics. *J Albert Einstein Med Ctr* 11:134–158, 1963*

39. Hendry WF, Polani PE, Pugh RCB, et al: 200 infertile males: Correlation of chromosome, histological, endocrine, and clinical studies. *Br J Urol* 47:899, 1976

40. Klinefelter JF Jr, Reifenstein EC Jr, Albright F: Syndrome characterized by gynecomastia, aspermatogenesis without A-Leydigism and increased excretion of follicle-stimulating hormone. *J Clin Endocrinol* 2:615, 1942

41. Baghdassarian A, Bayard F, Borgaonkar DS, et al: Testicular function in XYY men. *Johns Hopkins Med J* 136:15, 1975

42. Wachtel SS, Koo GC, Greg WR, et al: Serologic detection of a Y-linked gene in XX males and XX true hermaphrodites. *N Engl J Med* 295:750, 1976

43. Steinberger E, Ficher M, Smith KD: An enzymatic defect in androgen biosynthesis in human testis: A case report and response to therapy. *Andrologia* 6:59, 1974

44. Wilson JD, Harrod MJ, Goldstein JL, et al: Familial incomplete male pseudohermaphroditism, type 1. Evidence for androgen resistance and variable clinical manifestations in a family with the Reifenstein's syndrome. *N Engl J Med* 290:1097, 1974

45. Lubs HA, Jr, Vilar O, Bergenstal DM: Familial male pseudohermaphroditism with labial testes and partial feminization: Endocrine studies and genetic aspects. *J Clin Endocrinol Metab* 19:1110, 1959

46. Reifenstein EC Jr: Hereditary familial hypogonadism. *Clin Res* 3:86, 1947

47. Rosewater S, Gwinup G, Hamwi GJ: Familial gynecomastia. *Ann Intern Med* 63:377, 1965

48. Eliasson R: Parameters of male fertility, in Hafez ESE, Evans TN (eds): *Human Reproduction*. Hagerstown, MD, Harper & Row, 1973, p 39

49. Fowlkes DM, MacLeod J, O'Leary WM: T-mycoplasmas and human infertility: Correlation of infection with alterations in seminal parameters. *Fertil Steril* 26:1212, 1975

50. Delouvois J, Harrison RF, Blades M, et al: Frequency of mycoplasma in fertile and infertile couples. *Lancet* 1:1074, 1974

51. Taylor-Robinson D, Manchee RJ: *Mycoplasma Diseases of Man*. Jena, Fisher Verlag, 1969, p 113

52. Wilson L: Sperm agglutination due to autoantibodies. A new cause for sterility. *Fertil Steril* 7:262, 1956

53. Rümke P: The presence of sperm antibodies in the serum of two patients with oligospermia. *Vox Sang* 4:135, 1954

54. Ansbacher R, Yeung KK, Behrman SJ: Clinical significance of sperm antibodies in infertile couples. *Fertil Steril* 24:305, 1973

55. Rümke P: Autoantibodies against spermatozoa in infertile men. *J Reprod Fertil (Suppl)* 21:19, 1974

56. Shulman S: Immunity and infertility; A review. *Contraception* 4:135, 1971*

57. Kibrick S, Belding DL, Merrill B: Methods for the detection of antibodies against mammalian spermatozoa. II. A gelatin agglutination test. *Fertil Steril* 3:430, 1952

58. Franklin RR, Dukes CD: Antispermatozoal antibody and unexplained infertility. *Am J Obstet Gynecol* 89:6, 1964

59. Isojima S, Li, TS, Ashitaka Y: Immunologic analyses of sperm-immobilizing factor found in sera of women with unexplained sterility. *Am J Obstet Gynecol* 101:677, 1968

60. Paulsen CA: The study of irradiation effects on the human testis, including histologic, chromosomal and hormonal aspects. Progress Report to Atomic Energy Commission Contract AT (45-1):1781, 1966

61. Rowley M, Leach DR, Warner GA, et al: Effect of graded doses of ionizing radiation on the human testis. *Radiat Res* 59:665, 1974

62. Fox BW, Fox M: Biochemical aspects of the actions of drugs on spermatogenesis. *Pharmacol Rev* 19:21, 1967

63. Jackson H, Schnieden H: Pharmacology of reproduction and fertility. *Annu Rev Pharmacol* 8:467, 1968

64. Steinberger E, Lloyd, JA: Adverse effects of environmental exposure to pollutants on the male reproductive system, in Tarcher AB (ed): *The Principles and Practice of Environmental Medicine*. Plenum, 1986, (in press)

65. Steinberger E, Lloyd JA: Chemicals affecting the development of reproductive capacity, in Dixon RL (ed): *Reproductive Toxicology*. Target Organ Toxicology Series. New York, Raven, 1985, 1–20

66. Steinberger E: Effect of altered blood flow on the testes, in Johnson AD, Gomes WR, VanDemark NL (eds): *The Testis*, Vol III. New York, Academic, 1970, p 363

67. Iwasita K: Ortliche Blutzirkulationsstorung des Hodens. III. Mitteilung: Klinisch-experimentelle Beitrage zur Kenntnis des Einflusses der Samelstanggefass-Absperrung auf den Hoden. *Z Zellforsch* 45:126, 1939

68. Tulloch WS: Consideration of sterility factors in light of subsequent pregnancies: Subfertility in male. *Edinb Med J* 59:29, 1952

69. Dubin L, Amelar, RD: Varicocelectomy as therapy in male infertility: A study of 504 cases. *Fertil Steril* 26:217, 1975*

70. Brown JS, Dubin L, Becker M, et al: Venography in the subfertile man with varicocele. *J Urol* 98:388, 1967

71. Clarke BG: Incidence of varicocele in normal men and among men of different ages. *JAMA* 198:1121, 1966

72. Steeno O, Knops J, Declerck L, et al: Prevention of fertility disorders by detection and treatment of varicocele at school and college age. *Andrologia* 8:47, 1976

73. Klosterhalfen H, Schirren C: Uber die operative Wiederherstellung der Zengungsfahigkeit des Mannes. *Dtsch Med Wochenschr* 89:2234, 1964

74. Dubin L, Amelar RD: Etiologic factors in 1294 consecutive cases of male infertility. *Fertil Steril* 22:469, 1971*

75. MacLeod J: Seminal cytology in the presence of varicocele. *Fertil Steril* 16:735, 1965

76. MacLeod J: Further observations on the role of varicocele in human male infertility. *Fertil Steril* 20:545, 1969

77. Lindholmer C, Thulin L, Eliasson R: Semen characteristics before and after ligation of the left internal spermatic veins in men with varicocele. *Scand J Urol Nephrol* 9:177, 1975

78. Rodriguez-Rigau LJ, Smith KD, Steinberger E: Relation of varicocele to sperm output and fertility of male partners in infertile couples. *J Urol* 120:691, 1978

79. Stephenson JD, O'Shaughnessy EJ: Hypospermia and its relationship to varicocele and intrascrotal temperatures. *Fertil Steril* 19:110, 1968

80. Lindholmer C, Thulin L, Eliasson R: Concentrations of cortisol and renin in the internal spermatic vein of men with varicocele. *Andrologia* 5:21, 1973

81. Cohen MS, Plaine L, Brown JS: The role of internal spermatic vein plasma catecholamine determinations in subfertile men with varicoceles. *Fertil Steril* 26:1243, 1975

82. Rodriguez-Rigau LJ, Weiss DB, Zukerman Z, et al: A possible mechanism for the detrimental effect of varicocele on testicular function in man. *Fertil Steril* 30:577, 1978

83. Santen RJ, Bardin CW: Episodic luteinizing hormone secretion in man. Pulse analysis, clinical interpretation, physiologic mechanisms. *J Clin Invest* 52:2617, 1973

84. Persky H, Smith KD, Basu GK: Relation of psychologic measures of aggression and hostility to testosterone production in man. *Psychosom Med* 33:265, 1971

85. Smith KD, Tcholakian RK, Chowdhury M, et al: Rapid oscillations in plasma levels of testosterone, LH and FSH in men. *Fertil Steril* 25:965, 1974

86. Goebelsmann U, Horton R, Mestman JH, et al: Male pseudohermaphroditism due to testicular 17β-hydroxysteroid dehydrogenase deficiency. *J Clin Endocrinol Metab* 36:867, 1973

87. DeKretser DM, Deough EJ, Burger MG, et al: The response of infertile men to clomiphene and chorionic gonadotrophin stimulation, abst 20. Endocrine Society of Australia, August, 1973

88. Yen SSC, Vandenberg G, Siler TM: Modulation of pituitary responsiveness to LRF by estrogen. *J Clin Endocrinol Metab* 39:170, 1974

89. Lipsett MB, Migeon CJ, Kirschner MA, et al: Physiologic basis of disorders of androgen metabolism. *Ann Intern Med* 68:1327, 1968*

90. Danezis JM: Steroidogenesis in mammalian gonads as related to fertility and infertility. *Fertil Steril* 17:488, 1966
91. Rodriguez-Rigau LJ, Tcholakian RK, Smith KD, et al: *In vitro* steroid metabolic studies in human testis. I. Effect of estrogen on progesterone metabolism. *Steroids* 29: 771, 1977
92. Doerr P, Pirke KM: Cortisol-induced suppression of plasma testosterone in normal adult males. *J Clin Endocrinol Metab* 43:622, 1976
93. Kreuz LE, Rose RM, Jennings JR: Suppression of plasma testosterone levels and psychological stress. *Arch Gen Psychol* 26:479, 1972
94. Matsumoto K, Takeyasu K, Mizutani S, et al: Plasma testosterone levels following surgical stress in male patients. *Acta Endocrinol (Copenh)* 65:11, 1970
95. Harvey C, Jackson MH: Assessment of male fertility by semen analysis. *Lancet* 11:99, 1945
96. Eliasson R, Treichl L: Supravital staining of human spermatozoa. *Fertil Steril* 22:134, 1971
97. Makler A: A new multiple exposure photography method for objective human spermatozoal motility determination. *Fertil Steril* 30:192, 1978
98. Gordon DL, Herrigel JE, Moore DJ, et al: Efficacy of Coulter counter in determining low sperm concentrations. *Am J Clin Pathol* 47:226, 1967
99. Eliasson R: Correlation between the sperm density, morphology and motility and the secretory function of the accessory genital glands. *Andrologia* 2:165, 1970
100. Eliasson R: Analysis of semen, in Behrman SJ, Kistner RW (eds): *Progress in Infertility,* 2nd ed. New York, Little, Brown, 1975, p 691
101. MacLeod J: Human seminal cytology as a sensitive indicator of the germinal epithelium. *Int J Fertil* 9:281, 1964
102. Couture M, Ulstein M., Leonard J, et al: Improved staining method for differentiating immature germ cells from white blood cells in human seminal fluid. *Andrologia* 8:61, 1976
103. Alexander NJ: Sperm antibodies and infertility, in Cockett ATK, Urry RL (eds): *Male Infertility. Workup, Treatment and Research.* New York, Grune & Stratton, 1977, p 123
104. Yanagimachi R: Mechanisms of fertilization in mammals, in Mastroianni L Jr, Biggers JD (eds): *Fertilization and Embryonic Development in Vitro.* New York, Plenum, 1981, p 81
105. Yanagimachi R, Yanagimachi H, Rogers BJ: The use of zona-free animal ova as a test-system for the assessment of the fertilizing capacity of human spermatozoa. *Biol Reprod* 15:471, 1976
106. Paulsen CA: Another look at the sperm penetration assay. *Fertil Steril* 40:302, 1983
107. Aitken RJ, Best FSM, Templeton AA, et al: Fertilizing capacity of human spermatozoa: A study of oligozoospermia and unexplained infertility, in D'Agata R, Lipsett MB, Polosa P, van der Molen HJ (eds): *Recent Advances in Male Reproduction: Molecular Basis and Clinical Implications.* New York, Raven, 1983, p 13*
108. Gould JE, Overstreet JW, Yanagimachi H, et al: What functions of the sperm cell are measured by in vitro fertilization of zona-free hamster eggs? *Fertil Steril* 40:344, 1983
109. Aitken RJ, Best FSM, Richardson DW, et al: The correlates of fertilizing capacity in normal fertile men. *Fertil Steril* 38:68, 1982
110. Smith KD, Rodriguez-Rigau LJ, Steinberger E: Relation between indices of semen analysis and pregnancy rate in infertile couples. *Fertil Steril* 28:1314, 1977
111. Van Zyl JA, Menkveld R, Van W Kotze TJ, et al: Oligozoospermia: A seven year survey of the incidence, chromosomal aberrations, treatment and pregnancy rate. *Int J Fertil* 20:129, 1975
112. Sherins RJ, Brightwell D, Sternthal PM: Longitudinal analysis of semen of fertile and infertile men, in Troen P, Nankin HR (eds): *The Testis in Normal and Infertile Men.* New York, Raven, 1977, p 473
113. Zukerman Z, Rodriguez-Rigau LJ, Smith KD, et al: Frequency distribution of sperm counts in fertile and infertile males. *Fertil Steril* 28:1310, 1977
114. Steinberger E, Smith KD: Artificial insemination with fresh or frozen semen. *JAMA* 223:778, 1973
115. American Fertility Society: *How to Organize a Basic Study of the Infertile Couple.* Birmingham, AL, American Fertility Society, 1971
116. Freund M: Standards for the rating of human sperm morphology. *Int J Fertil* 11:97, 1966
117. Rowley MJ, Heller CG: The testicular biopsy: surgical procedure, fixation and staining techniques. *Fertil Steril* 17:177, 1966
118. Schoysman R: *Proceedings of the Ninth World Congress on Fertility and Sterility. Miami, FL,* April, 1977
119. Fernando N, Leonard JM, Paulsen, CA: The role of varicocele in male fertility. *Andrologia* 8:1, 1976
120. Steinberger E: Medical treatment of male infertility. *Andrologia (Suppl)* 8(1):77, 1976
121. Stewart BH, Montie JE: Male infertility: An optimistic report. *J Urol* 110:216, 1973
122. Mancini RE, Lavieri JC, Muller F, et al: Effect of prednisolone upon normal and pathologic human spermatogenesis. *Fertil Steril* 17:500, 1966
123. Bardin CW, Ross GT, Lipsett MB: Site of action of clomiphene citrate in men: A study of the pituitary–Leydig cell axis. *J Clin Endocrinol Metab* 27:1559, 1969
124. Paulsen DF, Wacksman J, Hammond CB, et al: Hypofertility and clomiphene citrate therapy. *Fertil Steril* 26:982, 1975
125. Reyes FI, Faiman C: Long-term therapy with low-dose Cisclomiphene in male infertility: Effects of semen, serum FSH, LH, testosterone and estradiol, and carbonhydrate tolerance. *Int J Fertil* 19:49, 1974
126. Dedes M, Da Rugna D: Erfahrungen mit Clomiphenzitrat bei Fertilitatstorungen des Mannes. *Praxis* 63:704, 1974
127. Foss GL, Tindall VR, Birkett JP: The treatment of subfertile men with clomiphene citrate. *J Reprod Fertil* 32:167, 1973
128. Heller CG, Rowley MJ, Heller GV: Clomiphene citrate: A correlation of its effect on sperm concentration and morphology, total gonadotropins, ICSH, estrogen and testosterone excretion, and testicular cytology in normal men. *J Clin Endocrinol Metab* 29:638, 1969*
129. Heller CG, Nelson WO, Hill IB, et al: Improvement in spermatogenesis following depression of the human testis with testosterone. *Fertil Steril* 1:415, 1950
130. Heckel NJ, Rosso WA, Kestel L: Spermatogenic rebound phenomenon after testosterone therapy. *J Clin Endocrinol Metab* 11:235, 1951
131. Rowley MJ, Heller CG: The testosterone rebound phenomenon in the treatment of male infertility. *Fertil Steril* 23:498, 1972
132. *Physicians' Desk Reference:* Oradell, NJ, Litton, 1977, pp 1417, 1512

133. Giarola A: Effect of Mesterolone on the spermatogenesis of infertile patients, in Mancini RE, Martini L (eds): *Male Fertility and Sterility. Proceedings of Serono Symposia,* Vol 5, New York, Academic, 1974, p 479

134. Mauss J: Ergebnisse der Behandlung von Fertilitat-storungen des Mannes mit Mesterolon oder einem Plazebo. *Arzneim Forsch* 24:1338, 1974

135. Clermont Y: Kinetics of spermatogenesis in mammals: Seminiferous epithelium cycle and spermatogonial renewal. *Physiol Rev* 52:198, 1972

ANSWERS

1. a, c

2. All

3. e

4. a, b, c, d

5. c

Surgical Treatment of Infertility

CELSO-RAMON GARCIA

INTRODUCTION

During the past decades, society has had an increasing awareness of the importance of the problems affecting reproduction.[1] Significant efforts have been devoted to improving our understanding at the basic level of the physiology of reproduction as well as its clinical applications in curbing or regulating fertility for the benefit of the very fertile segment of the population. Moreover, extension of such efforts also has been directed toward restoring or enhancing the anatomy and the physiology of those afflicted with misfortunate barrenness. Thus, such efforts have been equated to a double-edged sword—one edge aimed at increasing and the other at decreasing the fertility potential.

The special attention paid at the level of the physiology of the fallopian tube indeed has led to improved understanding of the physiologic events that have allowed for a series of applications culminating in in vitro fertilization. Thus, those who elect to manage tubal problems should be thoroughly familiar with normal adnexal anatomy and the physiology of tubal function. Such knowledge serves as

CELSO-RAMON GARCIA • Division of Human Reproduction, Department of Obstetrics and Gynecology, Hospital and Medical School of the University of Pennsylvania, Philadelphia, Pennsylvania 19104.

a basis for selecting patients who are to undergo treatment as well as for selecting and executing the appropriate procedures.

The uterine tube is a seromuscular organ whose contractile and secretory functions, while still poorly understood, are vitally concerned not only with supporting gamete well-being and transport, but with the fertilization of the gametes and in the subsequent development of the zygote as well. It is generally agreed that under normal conditions, the fallopian tube is the site of fertilization and early development. Thus, conception is necessarily preceded by efficient transport of the spermatozoa, transfer of the ovulated ovum from the follicle, and delivery of the morula into the uterus. The timing of the transport and changes in tubal environment are both critical factors during the initial phases of the embryonic development. This oviduct, some 10 cm in length, presents an intramural or interstitial, an isthmic, and an ampullary portion that ends in the infundibulum encompassing the fimbriated end and the tubal ostium. The prominence of the muscular layers in relationship to the secretory elements varies from one site to another. As one progresses from the less muscular distal segment, the secretory elements predominate, while at the proximal segment, the reverse is the case.[2] It is generally agreed that after ovulation, transport of the ovum requires a normal ovum pickup mechanism that implies freedom of the oviduct in its special structural relationship between the fimbria and the ovary.[3] While the precise relationship may vary from one species to another, either the ovisac or the fimbria appears to encompass or embrace the ovary at or near the site of the ovulation. Motility of the oviduct also appears to vary with the ovarian cyclic pattern, with estrogen influences appearing to enhance the motility as well as the secretion, while progesterone diminishes both.[4-6] By isolating segments of the oviduct while preserving the vascularity of each of the individual segments as well as that of the entire oviduct, the tubal fluid content of each of the segments has been evaluated. There is a diminution in fluid secretion as one proceeds from the ampulla toward the interstitial portion of the tube.[7]

In those mammals that have been studied, the cilia of the infundibulum beat in the direction of the tubal ostium toward the uterus.[8,9] The ovum, surrounded by an entourage of cumulus cells, provides a sticky matrix that enables the cilia to transport it with great efficiency. During the ovulatory process, the smooth muscle elements in the fimbria ovarica (the tubal-attracting muscles) are thought to contract and align the tubal ostium with the ovarian surface to establish an anatomic proximity between the oviduct and the ovary to enhance the ovum pickup ability.[10,11]

The infundibulum constitutes the most delicate segment of the oviduct with its complex vascularity. Large vascular plexuses, accompanied by muscular elements, are present in the fimbriated end of the tube. The functions of these vascular and muscular arrangements are not totally understood. Function aside, this vascularity signals to the surgeon the need for meticulous delicate handling of the fimbria ovarica, to avoid the distressing bleeding, which may be difficult to control. It is well to avoid the need for such hemostatic efforts, since they can lead to serious compromise of future function of this important structure.

During the past decade, such care has been improved enormously through the application of microsurgical techniques. Magnification permits easier recognition of tissue planes and anatomic landmarks. Magnification also allows for identification of the avascular planes as well as the sources of bleeding. Such anatomic precision has facilitated more accurate, less traumatic dissection with meticulous hemostasis. Every effort should be made to identify the appropriate planes to avoid and reduce bleeding and damage to the structures.

During the course of reconstruction of the damaged distal end of the tube, the surgeon should

approach this compromised or occluded oviduct and delineate these remaining elements of the fimbria ovarica whenever possible. They should be restored and preserved during the reconstruction. Teasing the tissues apart and dissecting through the scarred cleavage planes with the most delicate dissecting instruments after the initial incision through the point of conglutination is an appropriate approach afforded by microsurgical techniques. Such dissections will do more for accurate restoration of the anatomy than the sharp dissections through these tissues that prevent careful attention to the specific anatomic landmarks of this important organ. Resection and excision of tissues should be avoided until their usefulness has been assessed during the course of dissection and reconstruction.

In addition to the anatomic features, another mechanism of equal importance to that of the ovum pickup involves the fluid currents, which normally course through the oviduct lumen. While the cilia beat in the direction of the uterus, with transport being directed toward the uterus, the currents created appear to transport spermatozoa at greater speeds than their own propulsive forces would provide. These currents may be created by both ciliary activity as well as tubal motility, but the spermatozoa are transported in a direction opposite that of the ovum. It has been well established that particles placed in the cul-de-sac can be transported into the uterus and recovered at the cervix. Such mechanisms may explain the occasional ovum that may have been deposited in the cul-de-sac and picked up from the peritoneal cavity.

Understanding of the oviductal fluid that provides a suitable environment for the spermatozoa, the ovum and of the fertilization process, was incomplete until the introduction of in vitro fertilization, which has shed much light on these mechanisms. Nonetheless, the precise steps occurring in this tubal environment remain to be elucidated. The precise mechanism by which spermatozoa are capacitated, or rendered capable of ovum penetration, is still somewhat nebulous; it has been challenged by the finding that fertilization of human ova with freshly ejaculated spermatozoa has been accomplished in defined media. Nonetheless, changes in the outer layers of the acrosomal cap that are believed to occur permit the trypsinlike acrosomal enzyme to facilitate the penetration of the ovum. The ability to fertilize an egg varies with the maturity of the egg and sperm. Moreover, the fertilizable age of the mammalian ovum is quite limited.[12] In vitro fertilization studies also support this.

PATHOPHYSIOLOGY

Severe inflammatory changes can adversely affect the anatomy and the physiology of the oviduct. Distortion of the ostium, inadequate ovum pickup, intraluminal adhesions, or any number of anatomic alterations in the mucosal folds can seriously affect the normal function of the oviduct. Such alterations and anatomic distortions offer reasonable explanations for the increased incidence in ectopic pregnancies recorded in association with their presence.

Intraluminal adhesions have been documented through scanning electromicrographs of previously damaged oviducts. However, their presence at surgery may often present difficulties in documentation. Exploration of the tubal lumen with miniature intraluminal endoscopes may at best offer exploration of only the larger luminal diameters of the oviduct. The longitudinal rugae observed through radiocontrast salpingography are viewed as supporting a more favorable prognosis, while the absence of rugae, suggesting extensive fibrous replacement of the serociliary components, offers a poorer prognosis. It should be mentioned, however, that the distention of the lumen often flattens out these components, which can be seen to realign into the mucosal folds after decompression. Extensive damage of the oviducts presents evidence of severe fibrous replacement of the muscularis. No reliable objective means has been found by which to evaluate the ability of the tubal musculature to regenerate after restoration or for it to retain function even after long periods of distention.

The status of the tubal musculature cannot be assessed accurately by gross evaluation, even in the hands of the most experienced surgeon. Histologic sampling may not be adequate without further compromising the future tubal function. There is consensus that the fallopian tube, which presents a thick, rigid wall, offers a much poorer prognosis than the tube with a supple consistency. The variety, severity, and multiplicity of the arrangements of the oviduct can be infinite. The variations in pathology in one oviduct may be totally different from those in the other, present a totally different anatomic distortion.

Besides the variations in pathology, the location and severity may be variable from one site to the next. Such numerous permutations and combinations notoriously compound the assessment of the numerous different approaches used for the correction of the compromise of the hampered adnexa. What can be said about the oviduct similarly applies

to the ovary.[13] The causes of tubal dysfunction are generally secondary to inflammatory disease, even though the etiology may be multiple. When infectious in origin, the process may migrate along the surface, through the tubal lumen, through vascular transmission, through the peritoneal cavity *via* bowel contamination, or through a parametritis. On rare occasions, iatrogenically induced alterations may be produced by trauma, contamination, or diethylstilbestrol (DES) exposure of the intrauterine fetus. Endometriosis may also distort the adnexa, while embryologic distortions may be additive.

The disease process that has caused the tubal distortion or occlusion must be considered in the overall picture. Even when viewed through the operative microscope, only the end result of the effect of a variety of pathologic entities can be appreciated. Current methods of assessing the degree of distortion are really not adequate to permit a precise prognosis. Nevertheless, it is well recognized that the prognosis following surgical correction is greatly influenced by the disease processes responsible for the distal distortion. Moreover, there is no effective nonsurgical approach for the restoration of anatomic barrier distortions or abnormalities in the fallopian tube or in periadnexal structures, which may interfere with mechanisms of ovum capture and transport.

At the extreme end of the spectrum is the oviduct, which has been damaged by repeated or prolonged bouts of salpingitis. Most treacherous is that caused by *Mycobacterium tuberculosis,* which reaches the oviduct by hematogenous spread. Accordingly, it can be harbored asymptomatically until a stage of utter destruction with fibrosis and calcification occurs before it is detected. In these instances of tubercular tubal involvement, the prognosis after reparative surgery is utterly grim. Second only to *Mycobacterium tuberculosis, Gonococcus* is the most potent damaging organism. It reaches the oviduct by ascending surface spread, followed by secondary invaders. *Gonococcus* can produce severe endosalpingeal damage and eventually tubal occlusion. Clinically, *Gonococcus* produces the symptoms that more often lead to earlier antibiotic therapy, which may forestall severe damage unless the patient is exposed to repeated bouts. By contrast, *Chlamydia trachomata* is more insidious, since its symptoms are mild and treatment is often delayed, allowing for more severe pathologic damage. These ascending infections produce more damage to the endosalpinx than to the muscularis. *Streptococcus* and other organisms affect the adnexa from the peritoneal route and tend to lead to disease processes that exert their efforts in the peritubular and periovarian areas, often affording a more optimistic prognosis than had the endosalpinx been involved.

Periadnexal involvement, which interferes with tubal motility and ovum pickup, affords easier access to surgical restitution unless adhesions are very dense. The classic finding following moderately severe healed salpingitis is that of the occluded bilateral hydrosalpinx with extensive damage and loss of fimbria and spotty endosalpingeal and intraluminal adhesions with or without varying degrees of peritubal and periovarian adhesions. When periovarian adhesions are severe, extensive, and dense, the prognosis is very guarded in spite of demonstrable tubal patency. Such patients, presenting with massive ovarian involvement, should probably be discouraged from having reconstructive surgery. Among those with very severe or repeated bouts of pelvic infection, the tubes may be blocked at both extremities or at multiple sites. There is a general consensus that the prognosis for successful surgical correction of such oviducts is extremely guarded.

Pathology of extratubal origin secondarily affecting the tube and ovary, leading to adhesions involving these structures, does not cause marked endosalpingeal alteration. Classically, this occurs with the adnexal involvement occurring secondary to rupture of the appendix, which produces peritubal and periovarian adhesions after the initial inflammatory activity has subsided. More prolonged or severe infections of this kind of course can involve the endosalpinx unless the infection is aggressively treated early. Endometriosis is also a very common cause of periadnexal adhesions. Prior pelvic surgery, particularly ovarian wedge resection, often contributes to adnexal involvement with periovarian adhesions. This is particularly true when proper attention has not been paid to meticulous hemostasis or when devascularization with subsequent necrosis occurs.

In general, when peritubal and periovarian adhesions are observed, their distribution often suggests an altered mobility of the ovary and the tube; it is reasonable to conclude that they probably interfere with ovum pickup, thus contributing to decreased fertility. In many instances of periadnexal disease, the distal area of the tube, or the infundibulum, may actually be encased in adhesions and is occluded extrinsically. Such individuals as a group probably offer a better prognosis than those with a great endosalpingeal involvement.

CLASSIFICATION OF TUBAL DISEASE

A standard classification of tubal disease has been proposed in the hope of providing more objective means for comparison of reported results of reconstructive techniques. In the management of infertility in general, the physician should be mindful that the ultimate goal is not solely that of a successful pregnancy. Of equal importance is the ability to establish a prognosis and, among couples who are finally judged hopelessly sterile, to counsel them appropriately and provide early opportunity to plan their lives realistically. The development of standard classifications of tubally induced infertility presents a complicated, and perhaps insoluble, problem. On the surface, it would seem reasonable to classify along the lines of etiology. It is often difficult and sometimes impossible because one is viewing the end result of an insult to the pelvic structures which occurred much earlier in time. Various attempts at classification of periadnexal disease have been attempted. One presented by Hulka et al[14] is as follows:

Stage I   Minimal adhesions, most of ovary visible; patent tube
Stage II   More than 50% of ovarian surface free; distal tubal occlusion with rugae on hysterosalpingography
Stage III   Less than 50% of ovarian surface free; distal tubal occlusion with no rugae on hysterosalpingography
Stage IV   No ovarian surface visible, bilateral hydrosalpinx

The cobweblike adhesions (filmy and avascular) are rated type A and the scarifying (dense and vascular) type B. While each adnexa is rated individually, the score of the best side is the one used. Gomel[15] proposed the following classification of pathologic findings, which is more encompassing of the varied pathology:

Nature of adhesions
   Velamentous
   Vascular
   Fibrous
   Dense (gluing organs one to another)
Caliber of the oviduct (especially in cases of hydrosalpinx)
   <15 mm in diameter
   15–30 mm in diameter
   >30 mm in diameter
Status of the mucosa

Lush, with mucosal folds present
Mucosal folds moderately well preserved
Flat, with paucity of folds
Flat, with paucity of folds; also contains large areas of scarring or fatty infiltration (or both)
Status of the tubal wall
Normal
Thin
Edematous, thick, rigid
Intratubal adhesions
None
Occasional adhesions
Moderate adhesions involving distal oviduct
Extensive adhesions requiring excision of the distal segment
Intratubal adhesions at other sites
Length of tubal segment affected (especially important in cases of proximal and midtubal occlusion)
Additional pathology and its extent; i.e., the presence of endometriosis or uterine fibroids or other disorders that may affect the prognosis
Histologic diagnosis of the excised tubal segment or lesion (e.g., endometriosis, polyps, salpingitis isthmica nodosa, fibrosis, inflammation, tuberculosis, ectopic pregnancy, neoplasia, parasites)
Results of electron microscopic studies on microbiopsy
Chlamydia cultures on tubal fluid and microbiopsies

For endometriosis, the standard classification proposed by Acosta et al.,[16] with modifications, has served a useful purpose in evaluating the end results of surgical treatment. The American Fertility Society classification,[17] which represents a modification of the Acosta and the Kistner–Siegler–Behrman classifications, is now more uniformly used.

Problems in classification are often compounded by the marked variability in the involvement of one patient to the next. Even in the same patient, one side may be minimally involved while the other may be so massively compromised as to justify extirpation. One tube may have been removed previously, perhaps as a result of an ectopic pregnancy. The tube may be obliterated at multiple sites or involved at a single site, usually the proximal or distal portion. Nonetheless, it is generally agreed that the best prognosis following surgery is noted where there is minimal adnexal involvement by peritubal and periovarian adhesions and where the integrity of the tube has otherwise been preserved. At

the other extreme is the ovary surrounded by very dense occlusive adhesions rendering a guarded prognosis. Filmy and periadnexal adhesions that are easily dissected offer a significantly better prognosis.

While the peritubal and periadnexal tissues in general can be assessed and their variable compromise rated, our inability to evaluate the status of the endosalpinx with accuracy remains a significant obstacle. The observation of longitudinal rugae observed at hysterosalpingography is generally believed to support a more favorable prognosis. The absence of this endosalpingeal pattern is interpreted as severe endosalpingeal damage. Unfortunately, such patterns are not always discernible, making interpretation difficult.

It is generally agreed that observations at laparoscopy serve as the best basis for assessing the extent of pelvic pathology and establishing a prognosis. This represents a subjective evaluation, however, based largely on clinical judgment and requires extensive prior experience.

CLASSIFICATION OF OPERATIVE PROCEDURES

The 1980 classification recommended by the International Federation of Fertility Societies is probably the most useful. This classification is as follows:

Lysis of periadnexal adhesions (salpingolysis ovariolysis), classified according to adnexa with least pathology
Minimal: 1 cm of tube or ovary involved
Moderate: partially surrounding tube or ovary
Severe: encapsulating peritubal or periovarian adhesions (or both)
Lysis of extra-adnexal adhesion
Minimal
Moderate
Severe
Tubouterine implantation
Isthmic: implantation of isthmic segment
Ampullary: implantation of ampullary segment
Combination: different type of implantation on right and left sides
Tubotubal anastomosis
Interstitial (intramural)-isthmic
Interstitial (intramural)-ampullary
Isthmic-isthmic
Isthmic-ampullary

Ampullary-ampullary
Ampullary-infundibular (fimbrial)
Combination: different type of anastomosis on right and left tubes
Salpingostomy (salpingoneostomy); surgical creation of a new tubal ostium
Terminal
Ampullary
Isthmic
Combination: different type of salpingostomy on right and left tubes
Fimbrioplasty (reconstruction of existent fimbria)
By deagglutination and dilatation
With serosal incision (for completely occluded tube)
Combination: different type of fimbrioplasty on right and left tubes
Other reconstructive tubal operations (specific procedure should be stated)
Combination of different types of operations
Bipolar: for occlusion at both proximal and terminal end of tube (specific procedure should be stated)
Bilateral: different operations on the right and left sides (specific procedures should be stated)

REPARATIVE TUBAL SURGERY

The successful reconstructive surgery of the fallopian tubes includes not only the background related to the physiopathology but an appreciation of other factors that can modify tissue response to the surgery as well. These factors include patient selection, cycle timing of the surgery, the surgery adjuvants, and of paramount importance, the surgical techniques themselves.

Patient Selection

It is incumbent on the surgeon to review with the patient and the husband the status of the fallopian tubes as well as all the other factors involved in the reproductive process in the most objective manner. A realistic summation must be provided not only of possible alternatives but of the level of reasonable outcome that can be expected as well. The decision to proceed with an operative procedure solely to enhance fertility must be considered carefully by the couple to accept the risks and the discomforts of such a procedure. The barren couple should be af-

forded every opportunity to make this decision knowledgeably. Both husband and wife should be aware that results following tuboplasty vary considerably but that the rate of success is influenced by proper selection of the patient as well as the skill of the surgical team. Any given technique in the hands of a skillful dedicated surgeon will inevitably produce results superior to those obtained by a less caring and less technically skilled operator using a similar approach. The couple should be given a realistic appraisal of the prognosis in the hands of the surgeon who is responsible for the procedure expressed not only in the probability of success but in the probability of failure as well.

Since patients facing infertility are often desperate, this counseling is particularly essential. Every effort should be made in a most humane manner to discourage the couple from seeking surgery when it is clear that the extent of the disease is beyond the ability to treat it. The risks should be carefully reviewed. The couple should be impressed that failure to accept surgical treatment will not affect the patient's general health. The overall health status and the ability to sustain a subsequent pregnancy should be carefully reviewed. Medical conditions that would make a pregnancy hazardous, such as cardiac compromise, severe hypertension, or uncontrolled diabetes, must be ruled out. Moreover, all other factors contributing to infertility should be eliminated or measures taken that can correct them.

Among the factors that should be excluded are those of the inflammatory states. Before agreeing to perform a surgical procedure, it is encumbent on the surgeon to be sure that an active, ongoing inflammatory process is not extant. White blood count (WBC), differential, and sedimentation time, although nonspecific, should be included in the screening in addition to that of an endometrial biopsy obtained during the luteal phase early on in the patient's evaluation. Any suspicion of a chronic inflammatory process should signal the concern to rule out tuberculosis as the etiology. Cultures of the endometrium or of the menstrual effluvium should be carried out. At laparoscopy, any granulomatous lesions should be biopsied and intraperitoneal cultures performed.

Preoperative evaluation of the patient by laparoscopy represents the most reliable basis for arriving at a pertinent assessment of the status of the adnexa and with few exceptions should be performed routinely. It allows for the most effective assessment of adnexal function and its usefulness is enhanced when carried out by the surgeon who will eventually perform the definitive procedure. It will also form the firm basis for objective counseling. Proceeding directly to the operative procedure immediately after laparoscopy is probably unwise because of the small, but additional, risk of potential peritoneal contamination, weighted also by what might prove a lengthy operative procedure with its additional incumbent potential contamination. Moreover, this approach precludes meaningful counseling and assumes that the surgeon knows best what the patient's desires are. Moreover, since the results following adnexal surgery at this point are not completely satisfactory, every effort should be made to offer the patient the best possible chance of success by uncompromising adherence to the principles herein outlined.

Age

In the preoperative evaluation of the adnexa, a number of factors must be considered that materially affect prognosis, including the age of the patient. Surgery plays a limited role, at best, in the treatment of what has been referred to as geriatric infertility. In my personal experience of some 200 infertile women with ages 39–46, no pregnancies have occurred among women after the age of 42 who have undergone infertility surgery and, with few exceptions, this is also the case after the age of 40. It should be recalled that the age-specific fertility rates in all societies decreases appreciably after the age of 35, and more notably, after the age of 40.[17]

Pelvic Adhesions

The culpability of pelvic adhesions as the cause of infertility depends on their location and their relationship to the tubes and the ovaries. This is particularly true when the tubes are patent. A long-standing history of infertility in a patient whose ovaries are bound by adhesions to the lateral pelvic sidewalls, with a veil of adhesions between the ovaries and the fimbria, clearly represents an anatomic basis for the infertility. Selection of patients with adhesions for surgical treatment is judgmental and is based on visual evaluation of the adhesions in relationship to the tubal function. The problem can be compounded by the variance between the two adnexa. Certainly bilateral severe pelvic adhesions, densely involving the tubes or the ovaries or both, carry an unfavorable prognosis.

Cyclic Timing of Surgery

Whereas timing of surgery in the cycle may not be essential in general gynecologic procedures, the achievement of optimal results in infertility surgery depends on this factor. Surgical intervention should be scheduled in the preovulatory phase of the cycle. This preovulatory phase is generally viewed as the anabolic, regenerative phase. Moreover, the ovary is more vulnerable to periovarian adhesion dissection in the luteal phase of the cycle, when the possibility of damaging a recently formed corpus luteum is enhanced. Thus, scheduling the surgery in the proliferative phase of the cycle will simplify the dissection.

Surgical Adjuvants

Atraumatic Technique

The most fundamental underlying surgical approach requires that an atraumatic technique be supported with meticulous use of atraumatic instruments, fine nonreactive suture material, and proper attention to the anatomic reconstructions, including peritonealization of the tissues. A deep Trendelenburg positioning of the patient offers the advantage of allowing the bowel to be displaced into the upper abdomen with the least amount of trauma. A properly executed modified Pfannenstiel incision with a U-shaped dissection of the anterior sheath of the rectus from one lateral border of the rectus to the other permits ease of access to the lower abdomen and pelvis. The skin incision need not be large, since this tissue is more pliable than the underlying anterior sheath of the rectus. Nonetheless, this abdominal incision should provide adequate exposure. All laparotomy pads and sponges should be thoroughly soaked and rinsed well in warm physiologic saline before they are placed in the abdominal cavity. Such rinsing is particularly important to reduce the possibility of lint granuloma. The tissues should be irrigated and possibly dabbed, but not rubbed, to avoid tissue trauma. Saline irrigation should be used throughout, and there appears to be considerable advantage to adding 5000 units of heparin to each liter of physiologic saline. In primates, Ringer's lactated solution and the like offer no greater advantage in protecting the epithelium, despite advantages reported in rodent studies. Irrigation offers the best possibility for identifying small bleeding points and preventing the atmospheric air from drying the pelvic tissues under the heat of the operating room lights. Moreover, saline used for such irrigation should be drawn as needed from a sterile saline container through a sterile infusion set and should not be obtained through a syringe from a pan that may have been exposed to debris or lint from the operating room. Certainly it should not be obtained from a pan that contains abdominal lap pads and sponges, which give off a fair amount of lint.

Hemostasis

Various approaches are used to attain meticulous hemostasis. Larger bleeders may be controlled with pressure and clamped and appropriately ligated. For smaller bleeders, however, hemostasis can be ensured by laser techniques, bipolar microforcep coagulation, or by dissection with the thermal probe.

The laser is a more recent technique applied to gynecology, and the technology of the laser is still developing. This technique has little tissue reaction while affording fairly consistent hemostasis and rapid dissections. Bipolar microforcep coagulation likewise affords hemostasis of the smaller vessels and also affords the advantage of minimal tissue reaction.

Bipolar Techniques. Two point coagulation techniques have been initiated using the Bovie as its electrosurgical unit early in the 1930s. Two-point coagulation isolated circuitry soon followed. Continued improvement of the energy sources include damped-wave solid-state spark units, which provide a completely isolated current output along with the energy generator itself being grounded. The transformer impedances have been integrated with the rest of the circuitry to provide a waveform output causing minimal muscle stimulation for the amount of coagulation achieved. This requires a continuous wave cycle with a consistent degree of reliability. In the completely isolated circuitry bipolar coagulation system, the current flows between the two electrode tips. Neither tip has any significant current flow to the ground or to the patient. Moreover, using these electrode forceps, the tips must not be allowed to touch each other and be short-circuited since, under these circumstances, they will not provide coagulation. It is essential that the vessel or the tissue to be coagulated be held loosely between the tips of the forceps or the electrode tips.

It is preferable to use irrigation, since coagulation can be accomplished under saline while avoiding significant tissue heating and sticking to the forceps. When bipolar coagulation is used in a dry field without irrigation or in a collection of blood, the forceps tips become coated with the baked, charred blood insulating the electrodes and reducing or preventing effective coagulation. With continuous irrigation and suction, the minute bleeding points can be detected and coagulation accomplished with the fine points of the microbipolar forceps. Applying the completely isolated current source in short bursts permits hemostasis of the vessels generally encountered in the gynecologic microsurgical dissections. Bipolar coagulating techniques using very low currents under saline irrigation can also approximate and seal the edges of tiny peritoneal surface defects. Such welding techniques have been used by researchers accomplishing vascular anastomosis necessary to carry out renal transplants in mice.

Unipolar Techniques. Unlike the bipolar techniques that offer the most isolated current coagulation, the unipolar generator provides the current flow from the point of the electrode contact to the grounding plate attached to the patient.[18a] This point of contact represents only the tip of the iceberg, since the longer the length of application and the greater the current and current setting, the deeper and more pronounced are the effects of the conical spread of the induced currents from the point of contact to the underlying tissues. Coagulation of the small branch or vessel carried out using the unipolar technique may permit coagulation extending on to the parent vessel, which may unintentionally disrupt a few days later. Such disruptions may produce hemorrhagic accumulations and provide disquieting sequellae. When using the unipolar coagulating current, such as the case of the thermal probe, glass probes, or plastic rods must be used since contact with the thermal probe needle will extend the electric charge along the metal with which it comes in contact. The thermal probe does offer greater speed, but it has not been our experience that it offers enough to overcome the protective benefits of bipolar coagulation. The monopolar fine electrode technique, using the thermal probe (Siemmens) or the electrosurgical microelectrode (Martin), permits rapid dissection of adhesions. Even with meticulous care, the increased speed often leads to either incomplete resection or denudation of the viscera. The Malis CMC II electrosurgical unit provides both a coagulating and cutting current mode across the bipolar forceps tips. It uses a computer-generated current that simulates the aperiodic waveform of the spark gap generators.

Laser Techniques. The laser, which is the product of light amplification by stimulated emissions of radiation, uses various sources of energy. The most frequently used is the CO_2 laser, although the argon and neodynium–YAG are also available. The CO_2 laser can be beamed through a system of mirrors or passed through the lenses of a colposcope or microscope. A micromanipulator can be used to direct the beam by aid of a second helium–neon laser, providing a visible red aiming beam. The beam can also be brought into the field through an articulating arm and with a hand-held laser scalpel for free hand use. It permits dissection through adhesions or dissection through tissue with minimal extension of damage laterally into the healthy tissue and will allow for meticulous hemostasis. The laser potentially offers hemostasis, decreased tissue destruction, precision of dissection, and rapid operating time.

It must be stressed that proper instrumentation, assistance, and particularly extensive experience with this technique are essential.[18,19,20] Safety precautions with strict adherence to safety guidelines and techniques are also required. Laser techniques have been applied to salpingostomy, tubal anastomosis, lysis of adhesions, tubal coagulation, myomectomies, endometriosis, and so forth.[4,21–24] Cost and availability are disadvantages, with down time an annoying encumbrance.

Other Adjuvants

Good exposure is a sine qua non to assure meticulous surgical technique. The uterus and adnexa can be conveniently exposed in the operative field by well-moistened pads or forms placed in the cul-de-sac. This approach is far more effective than packing the vagina to accomplish a similar elevation of these structures since the latter tends to limit mobility.

For manipulation and exposure of the adnexa, a Williams clamp grasping the uterine ligament can be helpful in elevating these tissues into the field. Often a vein retractor can be utilized similarily to elevate the structures with traction on the ligament. The Williams clamp is a relatively atraumatic instrument that is preferable to the use of the standard Babcock clamp, the jaws of which can produce lacerations when compressing and elevating these delicate tissues.

A Buxton clamp or a Hellman-Siegler clamp placed at the cervicouterine junction is also useful not only in elevating the uterus but in affording better exposure of the posterior leaf of the broad ligament in addition to occluding the cervicouterine junction. When thus occluded, instilled tinted saline introduced by injection through the anterior uterine wall into the uterine cavity by hypodermic syringe can test for tubal patency or stain the mucosa when necessary.

Certainly, tenaculae, towel, clamps, and traction sutures should be avoided and not be placed on the fundus for elevation of the structures. Their use promotes tissue trauma and necrosis with increased likelihood of adhesions resulting from such damage. Every effort should be made to minimize any manipulation and to avoid those that could result in the formation of postoperative adhesions. In order to decrease tissue reaction, one should avoid creation of raw surfaces which expose tissue that has been traumatized. Meticulous hemostasis should be assured, and the delicate approximation of tissues should be substituted for brusk handling and erratic placement of large sutures compromising blood supply and providing tissue reaction. Foreign body contamination should likewise be avoided.

Magnification. The introduction of suitable magnification, either through the operative microscope or through improved loupes with wide-field vision has markedly benefited operative techniques by facilitating better dissections and restoration of the anatomic integrity and reducing tissue trauma. While the use of the operative microscope as well as the loupes does increase operative time, the former is more formidable because it produces a greater encumbrance. Loupes of 5–10-power magnification on lightweight eyeglass frames or head mounts ensure a more adequate working field. The operative microscope is often reserved for those instances requiring greater magnification for tissue repair or when using the laser. Good illumination and experience using the operative microscope can accommodate the surgeon working at lower powers of magnification similar to that of an experienced pathologist who reverts to high-power magnification only on infrequent occasions for histologic reviews. The achievement of competence in performing microsurgical manipulations should be learned not in the operating room while working on patients but in the laboratory on prepared tissues and subsequently on experimental animals. Only when proficient at this level is the surgeon prepared to carry out operative microscope dissections in patients.

The operating microscope and the loupes both afford a more accurate identification of pathologic tissues in addition to decreasing tissue dissection trauma. Greater appreciation of vascular bleeders with increased ability to achieve meticulous hemostasis and a notable increase in the precision of tissue approximation are also a consequence. Along with magnification, special fine instrumentation and tissue handling is essential.

During the course of reconstructive procedures, the use of magnification with the aid of loupes offers considerable advantage. The presence of the operative microscope, and indeed higher powers of magnification, can actually impede the efficient progress of the procedure and considerably increase the operative time.

Techniques to Prevent Pelvic Adhesion Formation. Postoperative adhesion formation is one of the principal causes of tuboplastic failure. No foolproof method has yet been devised to prevent adhesions consistently. One popular approach involves the use of dexamethasone combined with promethazine as first advocated by Replogle et al.[25] The standard regimen includes separate administration of dexamethasone, 20 mg, and promethazine, 25 mg, 6 and 3 hr before laparotomy, again at laparotomy dissolved in 250 ml physiologic saline, and instilled into the peritoneal cavity. Postoperatively, the dosage technique used is the same as that used preoperatively but at 4-hr intervals for a total of nine doses. More recently, smaller oral doses of 4 mg dexamethasone have been substituted in place of the 20-mg dosage preoperatively and postoperatively; they seem to have an adequate effect as judged over the past 5 years. The dexamethasone/promethazine approach appears to have been clinically useful, although its effectiveness has not been confirmed in the rhesus monkey.[26,27,28]

High doses of steroids are associated with general postoperative euphoria and a sense of patient well-being. The need for postoperative analgesics is considerably diminished, making the initial postoperative period more comfortable. The concomitant use of prophylactic antibiotics is usually recommended. The regimen should not be used if there is systemic contraindication to the use of steroids, such as healed pulmonary tuberculosis or a history of peptic ulcer.

Mild transient postoperative adrenal suppression has been reported in some patients following the 48-hr postoperative administration of this regimen.[6] Such has not been observed by the present author with the shorter 36-hr regimen when the dosage is at the 4-mg oral administration of dexamethasone.

High-molecular-weight dextran instillation has been advocated to prevent postoperative adhesions.[28] The data in the literature are still inconclusive. My experience noted the finding of a marked fibroblastic coating of the Silastic hood in three consecutive cases in which the high-molecular-weight dextran was used. Since such a repeated occurrence has never been seen by me with silicone prostheses, I have discontinued the use of high-molecular-weight dextran in my surgical armamentarium and have returned to the use of dexamethasone and promethazine.

Numerous other adjuvants to prevent adhesions have and continue to be advocated. Heparin exerts a beneficial effect on fibrin deposition. Systemically administered ibuprofen has also been advocated. In all instances, meticulous technique is probably the overriding factor.

Uterine Suspension. Particularly after ovariosalpingolysis or dissections with endometriosis, uterine suspension is usually recommended. The procedure for uterine suspension should be one that requires the simplist manner of fixation of the round ligament to the anterior abdominal wall. This produces a temporary forward displacement of the uterus and, it is hoped, prevents readherence of the old adhesion sites in the cul-de-sac and lateral pelvic walls.

Hydrotubation. The use of postoperative hydrotubation has been widely advocated. It is difficult to evaluate the efficacy of this approach from the literature inasmuch as most reports fail to document adequately the initial status of the tubes. More recent, Rock and Siegler et al.[29] have shown in their review, the value of this technique could not be demonstrated. It should be remembered, however, that hydrotubation is not without risk and in their large series, Ascenzo-Cabello et al.[30] reported a diagnosed posthydrotubation infection rate of 3.3%. It is not unreasonable to expect that the passage of fluid through the cervix into the adnexa on through the adnexa could be associated with a significant introduction of some bacteria that, despite broad antibiotic coverage, can occasionally find a favorable environment in the recently manipulated post-tuboplasty blood vessels and tissues. Although I have used postoperative hydrotubation early in my infertility surgical experience, I have come to discontinue this technique because of the above reasons and the lack of notable advantage in its use.

Prostheses. The use of prostheses in tuboplastic repair has been advocated for many years. More recently, it has fallen into less favor. It has been my practice, as well as others here at the University of Pennsylvania, to use the silicone prosthesis, the so-called Mulligan Hood (Dow-Corning Corporation, Midland, MI), in those cases in which the distal extremity has been completely occluded but not in instances of tubal patency, such as when dilatation is apparent with a restricted distal phimosis. Moreover, the occluded oviduct, which does not disclose edema and inflammatory changes, but in dissections discloses an anatomy that supports the fact that the newly opened distal end of the tube is unlikely to close over when the prosthesis is not used. During the past 5–6 years, I have advocated its use only in the more severe distortions and dissections where persistent patency appears tenuous. Significant differences of opinion exist concerning its use. These silicone prostheses, the Mulligan Hoods, are effective but only when special precautions to avoid contamination with lint or debris are observed. Reluctance to use them is due to the need to remove them some 6 months later. The second surgical procedure does afford an opportunity, however, for tidying up the pelvis. Careful teasing of any fibroblastic tissue on the hood or the oviduct must be totally removed.

Other stents, such as solid nylon rods and tubules, are of transient value. Strong opinions have been expressed about their advantages and disadvantages, with references made to their use in rodents. Earlier work done in primates indicated substantial value. I limit their use to the interstitial isthmic anastomoses, coiling the nylon #1 stents in the uterine cavity and removing them postoperatively on the third day.

Suture Material. Nonabsorbable sutures of fine caliber with special fine wires or needles have been widely used, with nylon being the material with the greatest usage. Polyglactin and polyglycolic sutures are also very useful and in many respects probably superior. Certainly catgut should be avoided. The size range of microsurgical suture material for gynecologic procedures can be limited to #6–#8-0 in caliber, while for vascular work, #8–#11-0 is more desirable. The caliber of the wires vary between 175 and 30 μm, with the size wire to be used dependent on the surgeon's experience and the desired needs related to the specific tissues. Because of their caliber and their electrostatic properties, the finer sutures are difficult to work with.

Instrument tying reduces some of these difficulties. They should be kept short and the needle kept in view at all times.

Surgical Reconstructive Procedures

The Paradoxical Oophorectomy

The surgeon is often confronted with a problem wherein a salpingectomy is contemplated that will leave the patient with a single oviduct and two ovaries. The relative infertility associated with transmigration of the ovum from the contralateral ovary raises the question of whether a paradoxical oophorectomy (removal of the ovary ipsilateral to the site of salpingectomy) of the isolated ovary is not in the patient's best interest. This has been advocated by several investigators.[31,32] The interval of time[32] between pregnancies is greater when there is an isolated ovary. Nonetheless, with present attitudes concerning in vitro fertilization and the need for having multiple retrieval of ova in preparation for the in vitro fertilization and embryo transfer, fewer paradoxical oophorectomies are being performed.

Management of the Peritoneal Factor—Pelvic Adhesions—Salpingo-ovariolysis

Pelvic adhesions, or the peritoneal infertility factor, have been observed in animal colonies with sterility as well as in humans where the mobility of adnexal structures is altered by adhesions fixing the ovaries and/or the oviducts to the lateral wall of the pelvis or to the posterior leaf of the broad ligament. Moreover, veils of adhesions interspersed between the ovary and the infundibulum are an apparent clear-cut anatomic explanation for the longstanding infertility of such individuals. The excision of adhesions, using atraumatic tissue handling, such as sharp dissection along the natural cleavage planes or through vaporization with the laser, aim to achieve a more normal anatomic restoration directed towards improvement of the tubo-ovarian relationships.

The role of pelvic adhesions causing infertility is dependent on the location of these adhesions and their relation to the activity of the adnexal structures. Under normal circumstances, a special relationship exists between the tube and ovary through separate and distinct projections of fimbriae originating at the tubal ostium and extending to the ovarian surface. This structure between the tube and ovary has often been referred as the fimbria ovarica, the tubal-attracting muscle, or the tuboovarian ligament. It contains smooth muscle and is believed to act as a fulcrum that facilitates the alignment of the tube and the ovary during ovulation, presumably to enhance the ovum pickup. Relieving the presence of adhesions that could compromise these activities has been noted to follow with an notable increase in the promptness with which pregnancy occurs.

Conglutinated Fimbria

A variance of the peritoneal factor is the coaptation or conglutination of fimbria that simulates a partial occlusion of the distal ostium of the oviduct interfering with the function of the ovum pickup by the infundibulum. These may result either from either congenital embryologic arrest of the fenestration of the distal end of the tube or from inflammatory activity, causing a fusion of these tissues. These are simply treated by bipolar coagulation dividing the conglutinated edges using the microforceps low-voltage bipolar coagulating current. The laser can likewise be used but requires having the backup protection for the tissue posterior or inferior to the beam of the laser. If the bipolar cutting current is used, the coagulated portion need not be incised with the use of the iris or Strulli scissors.

Preservation of the infundibulum structures should be the key effort. A probe or a fine instrument separating the tissues without damaging them is helpful in appreciating the cleavage planes among the scars and detection of the coaptation of fimbrial tissues. The hemostasis provided by the bipolar cutting current or the laser affords meticulous hemostasis, which does not require the ligation of the bleeding points.

Ovariolysis

The meticulous resection of adhesions from the surface of the ovary using bipolar cutting current facilitates this dissection with meticulous hemostasis of the surface. This meticulous hemostasis can be more easily achieved by irrigation with heparin in physiologic saline ensuring that all bleeding points are adequately controlled. Denuded or disrupted areas of the ovarian capsule should be plicated with interrupted sutures and by burying the knots. This should be carried out using a #6-0 caliber polyglactin or polyglycolic acid suture with a fine wire. Moreover, the dissected areas of the pos-

terior leaf of the broad ligament should likewise be plicated, bringing the healthy tissues together and burying the areas of the dissection after adequate hemostasis has been achieved. This reduces the probability of having the ovary become readherent to its old bed. It should be borne in mind that dense periovarian adhesions encasing the ovary to the lateral pelvic wall present the poorest prognosis.

CO_2 laser vaporization of adhesions shows considerable promise. With continuing improved technology, many cases may be eligible for the laparoscopic laser approach to salpingolysis and ovariolysis. Extensive experience and sound judgment are essential ingredients.

Proximal Tubal Occlusion

The uterotubal junction always requires a certain degree of concentration in trying to ensure that an occlusion is present. This requires that the attempt to demonstrate patency be assessed repeatedly. Once again, during the intraoperative procedure, the uterotubal junction should be reassessed. The reconstruction of the oviduct occluded at its proximal segment requires that this obstruction be resected and that the patent segments be reapproximated. If the obstruction is located at a superficial level of the myometrium, a reanastomosis to the uterine interstitial portion with the distal segment is feasible. In carrying out this anastomosis, the uterine cavity and the oviduct should be lavaged after occluding the cervicouterine junction with saline tinted with methylene blue under mild pressure, which allows for staining the endometrium and the endosalpinx. The methylene blue tinted saline is introduced into the uterine cavity transfundally by going through the anterior uterine wall until a sense of resistance is lost. In the case of tubal obstruction, obviously the staining will only be noted to the point at which patency ends. The distal segments of the oviduct, if they are to be stained, must be injected in a retrograde fashion. Care must be taken not to exert too much pressure, which would disrupt that delicate structure.

The excision of the occluded segment can be accomplished by incising the oviduct and extending the serial section type of resection of the occluded portion toward the uterotubal junction. On reaching the portion of the lumen where patency can be observed and the staining of the endosalpinx apparent, confirmation can be obtained through the use of magnification. A nylon #1 suture can be used as a stent that can be introduced through the proximal tubal lumen through the uterotubal junction into the uterine cavity. Cannulation of the oviduct from the proximal to the distal portion of the oviduct using a thin, blunt probe permits threading of a fine Teflon tubing through the oviduct onto the probe, which allows it to pull the tubing through the lumen. A nylon suture can then be threaded through the tubing to bring the nylon stent through the distal end of the tube[34] (Fig. 30-1). The stent permits the tubal segments to be carefully aligned. Some 12 in. of the stent should be introduced into the uterine cavity. This facilitates postoperative retrieval of the stent transcervically after an appropriate time interval. Fine suture material is used to approximate the muscularis. These are placed at four equidistant symmetrically located points[35] (Fig. 30-2). This approximation of the muscularis should be done with precision, with proper placement of either #8-0 or a #7-0 polygylcollic acid or polyglactin sutures using a fine-wire needle of about 100-μm caliber. The serosal surfaces are then repaired subsequently, using a #7-0 or a #6-0 polyglycolic or polyglactin suture. The stents used in these implantations can be removed either immediately postop-

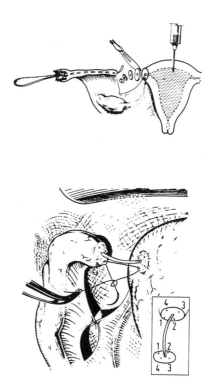

FIGURE 30-2. Tubocornual anastomoses. (From Winston.[35])

eratively or left in for some days. In the latter case, they are removed transvaginally.

Occlusions deep into the myometrium require an implantation technique with resection of the occluded segment being carried out by free hand scalpel, laser, or resection using a razor sharp trephine. A corneal trephine attached to a mandrel is functional for this procedure; it permits a most precise resection of the occluded portion of the oviduct leaving a smooth, clean incision. In fact, the trephine is truly a circular scalpel. Cork borers give poor results. The endosalpinx of the distal end of the oviduct is then brought in close approximation to the endometrium using two #4-0 polyglactin or polyglycollic acid suture. Additional sutures are brought through the serosa of the oviduct to affix it to the more superficial areas of the myometrium. The myometrial defects are then approximated, ensuring a better fixation of the oviduct within the uterine wall. The implantation is carried out using a stent similarly placed in the uterine cavity and retrieved some 72 hr later.

An alternate approach is favored by some workers. This entails implanting the oviduct in the posterior aspect of the uterus (Fig. 30-3). A transverse

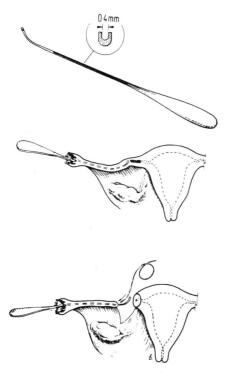

FIGURE 30-1. Threading the nylon #1 stent. (From Winston.[34])

TABLE 30-1. Results of Cornual Anastomosis (Microsurgical)

Surgeon	Winston[35]	Gomel[66]	Diamond[67]	Winston[68]	McComb and Gomel[69]	Meldrum[70]
Year	1977	1977	1979	1980	1980	1981
Number of cases	16	13	28	43	38	7
% Patent	—	78.6	82.1	—	—	100
Pregnancies						
% Intrauterine	68.6	53.8	75.0	60.5	52.6	57
% Extrauterine	6.3	7.7	0	2.3	5.3	14.3

incision is made along the posterior uterine wall and the oviduct implanted in the uterine cavity, facilitating visual approximation of endosalpinx to endometrium. The myometrial defect is loosely approximated. In the initial 14 patients with adequate follow-up, Peterson et al.[91] reported a 57% pregnancy rate with a 2% ectopic pregnancy rate and a 36% live-birth rate. This success is counterbalanced by the observation that 57% of the patients showed a myometrial defect in the implantation site of the transverse uterine incision. A 77% total patency rate of the oviducts indeed is a commendable achievement. Subsequent experience (Table 30-1) perhaps reflects a less successful approach and tempers one's attitude towards using this approach over the previous uterine tubal implantations in the cornual region.

Tubouterine implantations usually encompass isthmnic interstitial or uterine implantations or ampullary segment implantations. There may be a combination of an isthmic tubouterine implantation on one side or an ampullary tubouterine implantation on the other. The interstitial-isthmic tubal uterine implantation or anastomosis offers a better outlook than the interstitial-ampullary anastomosis.

Distal Tubal Occlusion

The salpingostomy, the neosalpingostomy, the neoampullostomy, or the ampulloplasty illustrates considerable diverse opinions on how to manage the distal occluded oviduct or the hydrosalpinx. This has been a perplexing problem from the earliest of times. A review of the historical perspec-

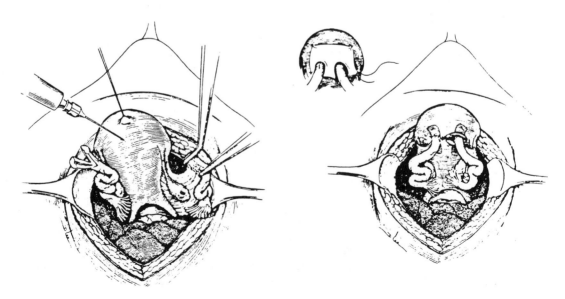

FIGURE 30-3. Posterior wall tubouterine implantation. (From Peterson et al.[91])

tives indicates that various techniques have been offered. Hydrotubation or the use of pertubation with consistent increasing pressures has been offered as a medical approach to the problem. However, since successes have been few and far between, this approach has not been widely accepted. Initially, amputation and eversion of a cuff of the ampulla was widely used. The linear incision of Chalier has been advocated by some, being reserved for those cases of hydrosalpinx observed during an acute inflammatory phase.

Historical perspectives disclose repeated attempts to treat the salpingostomy without having to use some means of maintaining the patency after the surgical salpingostomy has been created. In the earlier reports, allantoic membranes or some other sort of coating or covering was used, perceived as necessary to sustain the patency of the newly created ostium. A variety of devices have been used for the same purpose. In the experiences of the late John Rock of Boston and his followers, initially hydrotubation was applied followed by the use of gold or platinum wires, either in straight or spiral formation. This was subsequently followed by the use of a Teflon conical prosthesis and later by the use of a polyethylene prosthesis, and finally reaching the presently known Mulligan hood. This silicone prosthesis represents the product of all these prior experiences. It is of interest that most of the antagonists do not know how to use the Mulligan hood. The greatest resentment of the prosthesis is the need for a second laparotomy. Cognat[4] of Lyons, France, offered an approach that attempted to bypass a second procedure. Such approaches overlook the benefit of the pelvic toilet which the Mulligan prosthesis approach offers at the time of the second laparotomy when the prosthesis is removed. Indeed, some recommend the use of the laparoscopy some 6–8 weeks after the salpingostomy in order to perform a lysis of adhesions through the laparoscope. My personal experience has shown that the tissues are not healed any sooner than about 5–6 months. To be assured that all patients have their tissues healed adequately, it is best to wait 6 months following the salpingostomy. Lysis of adhesions, when not healed, have a high rate of recurrence.

Meticulous dissection of adhesions with the aid of bipolar microforceps coagulation assuring meticulous hemostasis is essential. Alternately, the use of laser vaporization of the adhesions is an approach advocated by those with experience with this technique.

The meticulous preparation of the entire pelvis prior to the salpingostomy and possible application of the Mulligan hood is also an essential ingredient. The second operation to retrieve the prosthesis should be carried not any sooner than six months following the initial procedure. Not only will this serve for the removal of the prosthesis, but it also affords the opportunity for a further meticulous reconstruction of whatever may appear to be necessary at that time. All fibroblastic tissue on the tube and on the hood must be gently teased away. Meticulous care to avoid foreign body contamination during the handling of the prosthesis in its initial application is utterly essential to avoid foreign body reactions. The silicone hood is a very nonreactive substance but is easily contaminated and should therefore not be touched with either the gloved hand or allowed to come into contact with cotton towels or any other objects. The use of the Claw hood retractor and holder (Automated Medical Products Corporation), is recommended for this purpose (Fig. 30-4).

The vascular network to the distal extremity of the oviduct makes this area especially vulnerable to trauma. Unnecessary manipulation can lead to bleeding, which would require hemostatic techniques through either suturing, bipolar coagulation, or laser. Every effort should be made to preserve as much of the tissues that remains in trying to recreate an infundibulum. In those instances in which the tube is completely sealed, there is considerable advantage to dissect the tissues apart along the scarred cleavage planes using fine dissecting instruments with the aid of either the operative microscope or the loupes. Table 30-2 demonstrates the advantages of microsurgical techniques. The point of conglutination should be identified as this more often makes the ideal location for the initial incision. This point of conglutination can be identified as a scarred dimple at the distal tubal extremity. After the oviduct is opened along the avascular planes, a fine clamp can be used to spread the tissues further, helping identify the appropriate tissue planes through which the dissection can be carried out and avoiding the unnecessary bleeding with its tissue damage that can be encountered if the incisions are made through the normal tissue, which is most vascular. Once the endosalpingeal lumen is identified and the adhesions in these areas dissected under magnification, the tube is then everted. A fine skin hook is indeed most useful for this purpose. The skin hook is passed along the inner tubal wall to a point some 5 cm from the newly created ostium. The skin hook is turned and the point of the skin

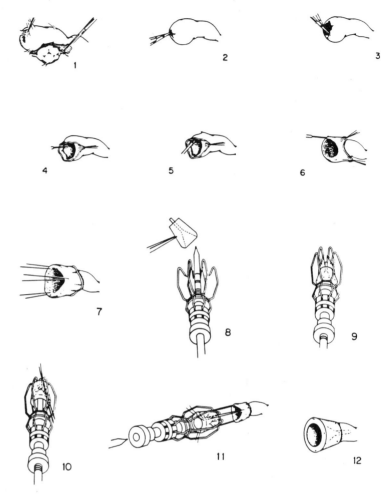

FIGURE 30-4. Salpingostomy. Application of the Silastic hood with the use of the Garcia claw. (1) Microsurgical dissection of adhesions. (2,3) Microsurgical dissection of scarred planes of hydrosalpinx. (4–6) Introduction of fine skin hook to evert cuff. (7) Equidistant placed mattress sutures through distal fold of cuff. (8) Picking up silastic hood with central rod of the Garcia tuboplasty claw. (9) Hood retracted, claw closed to be fitted onto Silastic hood. (10) Sutures brought through dome of hood using two Keith needles simultaneously traversing the hood to reduce likelihood of lacerating the Silastic hood. (11) Drawing oviduct into open Silastic hood. (12) Claw closed and removed and sutures tied after placing three additional sutures at base of hood.

hook insinuated through the tubal wall. Hence, the skin hook serves as a fulcrum over which the distal extremity of the tube can be easily everted. When the prior damage to the endosalpinx has been modest, this maneuver results in the exposure of endosalpinx which has a fimbrialike appearance. The extension of this tissue towards the ovary often allows for the identification of the remains of the fimbrio ovarica. The attachment of the fimbria ovarica to the ovary should be left undisturbed. The reconstruction is carried out with #6-0 or #7-0 polyglactin or polyglycolic acid sutures. A vertical mattress suture is applied at the mid-portion of the everted tube at the antimesosalpingeal wall to maintain the everted cuff of the newly created ostium. Similar management is carried out in the other oviduct. After finishing the second creation of the salpingostomy, the first repaired tube should be in-

spected to see if it shows signs of edema with a tendency for it to close. If this is the case, the silicone prosthesis should be applied. The silicone prosthesis is placed in the claw hood retractor and holder to avoid contamination and to apply it to the newly opened oviduct. The silicone prosthesis is held in place by prolene sutures; three at the dome and three at the base of the hood. If, however, the oviduct gives the appearance of staying open, there is little point in using the prosthesis. Patients who exhibit preservation of the patent fimbriated extremity after the perifimbrial adhesions are lysed or those presenting only distal phimosis are also not candidates for the use of the silicone prosthesis.

The second procedure is scheduled some 5–6 months after the application of the Silastic hood. The effectiveness of the silicone hood has been the subject of lengthy debate. I reserve the use of the

TABLE 30-2. Salpingostomy: Macrosurgical vs Microsurgical Results

Surgeon	Macrosurgical					Microsurgical						
	Siegler and Kontopoulos[71]	DeCherney and Kase[72]	Fayez and Suliman[73]	Garcia[74]	Swolin[75]	Siegler and Kontopoulos[71]	Gomel[76]	Winston[77]	DeCherney and Kase[72]	Fayez and Suliman[73]	Lassen[78]	Lauritsen et al.[79]
Number of cases	15	9	42	32	33	23	72	241	54	20	54	39
Pregnancies												
Total	33.3	22.2	26.2	37.5	45.4	39.1	38.8	34.4	44.4	40.0	38.9	43.5
% Term	13.3	22.2	16.7	18.1	24.2	21.7	29.2	17.5	25.9	35.0	31.5	23.1
% Ectopics	20.0	0	4.8	6.3	18.1	12.1	9.7	9.5	17.0	5.0	0	7.7

silicone hood only for those cases of true hydro-salpinx in which, upon opening the hydrosalpinx, the probability of maintaining patency is limited and in those cases where prior microsurgery failed to correct the hydrosalpinx. The prosthesis is applied only after careful reconstruction of the distal extremity by the methods described above. Indeed, in women who accepted the two stage procedure after the prior simple microsurgical approach failed, 7 of 10 cases to date have been rewarded with term pregnancies.

Difficulties associated with the use of the hood have occurred because of improper handling during its application. The Silastic prosthesis is electrostatic and easily picks up particles of lint and foreign material when inappropriately handled. The use of the Claw hood retractor and holder is essential in avoiding the contamination of the silicone hood. The hood offers the advantage of allowing healing of the newly reconstructed tubal ostrium under its protection. Perifimbrial adhesions can occur when the prosthesis is not used. These can frequently result in postoperative distal occlusion even after the most carefully meticulous dissections. The use of the silicone hood avoids these perifimbrial adhesions.

Removal of the silicone hood at the second laparotomy six months later requires that great care exercised in teasing away any fibroblastic material that may have accumulated beneath the hood. This fibroblastic tissue should be completely removed.

The second operation provides the additional opportunity to manage any pelvic adhesions which may have formed in the interim or to revise the distal ostium of the prior salpingostomy.

Mid-tubal Occlusion (Table 30-3 and Fig. 30-5)

The rise in frequency and popularity of tubal sterilization has been considerable in the United States. This seems to be related in part to the purported hazards of the oral contraceptive, which have minimized the appreciation of the benefits of the utter efficacy of the oral contraceptive. Equally devastating has been the despair faced by those selecting surgical contraception who, for various reasons, aspire to restore their procreative capabilities. Indeed, this change in attitude occurs all too soon after the surgical interruption of the oviduct, particularly when the sterilization is elected in association with pregnancy termination. The loss of a child or the loss of a mate with a subsequent acquisition of another mate may provide motivation toward wanting to restore their fertility. When the new mate has not exhibited proven fertility, restoration may not reach quite the same levels as when the mate has had proven fertility. Careful counseling of the patient—or the couple—is essential, since the success of the reversal of sterilization cannot be assured for all patients. Moreover, when disease processes affect the oviduct, these obstructions may be very vexing

TABLE 30-3. Results of Tubal Anastomosis

	Conventional			
Surgeon	Umezaki[80]	Siegler[81]	Rock[82]	Diamond[83]
Year	1974	1975	1981	1981
Number of cases	6	17	19	12
% Patent	80	—	—	50
Pregnancies				
% Intrauterine	50	50	47.4	41.6
% Extrauterine	0	0	0	0

	Microsurgical						
Surgeon	Garcia[84]	Gomel[85]	Winston[77]	Coronado[86]	Riggall[87]	Rock[82]	Diamond[83]
Year	1972	1980	1980	1981	1981	1981	1981
Number of cases	16	118	126	163	16	30	28
% Patent	87.5	—	—	—	81.2	—	92.9
Pregnancies							
% Intrauterine	50	64.4	57.9	75.5	31.3	66.7	76.9
% Extrauterine	0	0.8	2.4	3.7	6.3	3.3	—

when considering the restoration of fertility. By contrast, the reversal of sterilization offers more superior results, since more often they are not affected by disease processes and the microsurgical techniques, as currently used, yield pregnancy outcomes far superior than by macrosurgical approaches and also, far and beyond better than that which can be expected from in vitro fertilization and embryo transfer. Of course, when a bilateral salpingectomy has been performed as the surgical approach to contraception, in vitro fertilization and embryo transfer, if the ovaries are accessible, are probably the only option's available to the couple other than adoption.

Requests for reversal of tubal sterilization when performed for health or eugenic reasons require justification that must be most compelling, while still ensuring the protection of the rights of the individual. The past medical status that may have led to tubal interruption may have been overcome by medical or surgical means but might not substantiate physiologic competence to maintain a healthy course during a subsequent pregnancy. Often one encounters such situations following cardiac valvular surgery. Caution should be urged, and each contemplated pregnancy should be considered only after a careful review of the cardiac status lest a decline in the cardiac reserve be menacing while unappreciated by the patient herself.

Prior experience with various approaches to tubal sterilization reaffirm that tubal amputation, although effective in preventing pregnancy, is far too drastic to justify it as a routine approach. Resection of a small isthmic portion through cauterization or occlusion through compression with a clip or Silastic ring, or even tissue vaporization through the use of a YAG laser, is equally protective as the amputation. Although there are failures, these are low enough to be acceptable and do not vary greatly among the various techniques used when carried out properly.

In assessing future prognosis of restoration of fertility following an anastomosis, the length of the residual tube following sterilization plays an important role. Preservation of the distal segment to include the ampullary isthmic junction is essential. Moreover, a combined length of proximal and distal segments of 6 cm or more supports better pregnancy occurrence and outcome rates. Certainly when the combined total length is less than 3 cm, the prognosis for reversal is less justifiable under any but the most compelling reasons despite the fact that pregnancies have been reported with reconstructed oviducts of less than 2.5 cm total length.

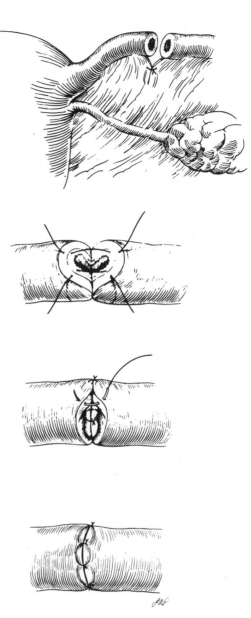

FIGURE 30-5. Tubal anastomosis. (From Reyniak.[38])

Further perplexing is the attitude towards reversal of sterilization presented by the third-party payers. Many insurance carriers exclude the reversal of sterilization and health care coverage of the individual for such procedures is also not covered in many states. Moreover, many surgeons will not perform a reversal of sterilization in single women. In this latter situation, each case needs to be assessed individually according to the needs of the patient and the judgment of the surgeon.

Preoperative evaluation should encompass a general health screening including a complete infertility review to detect possible medical contraindications. The restoration of tubal patency should be approached only after the medical or infertility deficits have been eliminated or acceptably corrected. Although Novy[37] reported the successful reversal of a Kroener distal tubal fimbriectomy, it should be emphasized that the success following the tubal fimbriectomy depends on how much distal tube has been resected; the probability of success being low if the entire ampulla has been excised. In these circumstances, surgical restitution is not advisable.

The mid-segmental isthmic–isthmic anastomosis is the most frequently performed. The technique for the restitution of patency of the oviduct for a prior tubal sterilization requires that one reconstruct or develop luminal compatibility of the segments that are to be anastomosed. The approximation is similar to that of a vascular anastomosis. The layers of the oviduct must be approximated to restore the anatomic integrity.[38] Various techniques are offered. Fine suture material is featured by all and, as time has progressed, most surgeons have no longer continued to use the #12-0–#10-0 nylon monofilament but are now using the #8-0 and #7-0 polyglactin or polyglycolic acid sutures which offer equally satisfying results. The approximation is initiated by placing a simple interrupted suture approximating the mesosalpinx. Simple interrupted sutures or interrupted mattress sutures are used to approximate opposite segments of the tube. The sutures are placed in the muscularis and can include the serosa where the lumen is patulous, as in the ampulla. The lateral mattress sutures evert the edges. Again, it should be emphasized that both of these approaches are used in the vascular anastomoses with equal success. Careful suture placement under direct microsurgical observation while monitoring the tension of the suture when tying these is essential. With proximal interstitial anastomoses, and particularly when the lumen is exceedingly narrow, the mucosa is approximated without the suture penetrating this layer. The sutures are placed simply in the muscularis.

Reports in the literature indicate pregnancy occurrence rates which are offered as corrected figures. While presenting gross rates may not give a fair picture, corrected values do tend to place the better foot forward, which also can be misleading. A new mate, particularly when the fertility has not been previously proven, may allow for wide vari-

ance. In my series of reversal of sterilizations, those women with new mates achieved a pregnancy less frequently than those who had reversal of sterilization and did not have a new mate. This was the case despite successful patency and careful attention to the male factor. The patency rate is agreed by all to be in the vicinity of 90–95%. The corrected pregnancy rates vary from 60 to 90% and reflect more than tubal status and technical competence of the individual surgeon.

Ectopic Pregnancy (Table 30-4)

The incidence of ectopic pregnancy appears to be increasing.[39] While the exact cause for ectopic pregnancy is unknown, it is agreed to be related to tubal disease or to follow repair of a damaged tube. Ectopic pregnancies are seen more frequently following the repair of a hydrosalpinx than with reversal of sterilization. When an ectopic pregnancy occurs in the posttubal repair, it represents a catastrophic situation for the patient. The patient, elated by the pregnancy, is then devastated by the grief of her view of this ectopic pregnancy and the need for further "unproductive" surgery.

The diagnosis of ectopic pregnancy requires a high index of suspicion. The prompt diagnosis not only allows for wide options of therapy, but also contributes significantly to lower morbidity and mortality. To make an early diagnosis, the classic triad of abdominal pain, amenorrhea, and vaginal bleeding more often are late signs. Anyone with a prior history of salpingitis, IUD use, progestagen use (particularly if used alone), oral contraceptive use, prior sterilization, prior ectopic pregnancy, endometriosis, in utero diethylstilbestrol exposure, or prior tubal surgery should be suspected of having an ectopic pregnancy. A negative β-subunit of hCG makes an ectopic pregnancy unlikely. β-hCG quantification titers should give normal values for normal intrauterine pregnancy with the corresponding doubling of the titer every 2 or 3 days during the first 6–8 weeks. Ultrasonography identifying an intrauterine pregnancy with a titer above 6500 mIU/ml also can safely exclude an ectopic pregnancy. There is probably less than a 2% chance of an ectopic pregnancy under these circumstances. However, if an intrauterine sac is not observed, an ectopic pregnancy is likely. This is particularly the case if the titer remains below 6000 mIU/ml but does not exclude the possibility of a missed abortion. A gestational sac and particularly identification of a fetal pole, or better that of a heartbeat, in

TABLE 30-4. Subsequent Outcome Following Surgery for Tubal Pregnancy: Random Comparison of Reports by Authors Reporting Both Conservational and Extirpative Management

	After Extirpative Surgery			
Surgeon	Skulj[33]	Ploman[88]	Timonen[89]	DeCherney[90]
Year	1960	1960	1967	1979
Number of cases	114	61	558	50
Pregnancies				
Intrauterine	32 (28%)	30 (49%)	—	—
Term Deliveries	22 (19%)	29 (48%)	— (29%)	21 (42%)
Ectopic Pregnancies	10 (9%)	5 (8%)	— (12%)	6 (12%)

	After Conservational Surgery			
Surgeon	Skulj[33]	Ploman[88]	Timonen[89]	DeCherney[90]
Year	1960	1960	1967	1979
Number of cases	92	88	185	48
Pregnancies				
Intrauterine	23 (25%)	14 (56%)	—	—
Term Deliveries	—	4 (47%)	— (27%)	19 (40%)
Ectopic Pregnancies	1 (1%)	11 (13%)	— (16%)	4 (8%)

the adnexa confirms an ectopic pregnacy. A gestational sac with a fetus with an in utero heartbeat strongly discounts the ectopic pregnancy.

When ultrasonography is questionable, laparoscopy can be most helpful. In the extremes, the above may not be so easy. Titers may be hedging, ultrasonography may show a questionable sac, or may be suggestive of a possible decidual sac and may lead to the frustrations through laparoscopy where adhesions may preclude seeing the adnexa effectively. Under these circumstances, a D & C and a frozen section of the tissue obtained could be helpful. The absence of chorionic villi with decidua or decidual reactions with signs of an Arias-Stella reaction is suggestive of an ectopic pregnancy. When a patient begins to have the disruption of the ectopic pregnancy, the classic triad becomes apparent. Nonetheless, ectopic pregnancies can mimic many abdominal syndromes. The patient with complaints of amenorrhea, abdominal pain, vaginal bleeding, dizziness, shoulder pain, fainting, nausea, rectal pain, or the passage of tissue should raise suspicion of an ectopic pregnancy. Patients should be warned that all tissue passed should be brought in for examination. The tissue, be it a decidual cast or the products of conception, can be most helpful in settling the differential diagnosis.

The physical findings of an adnexal tenderness or a mass with abdominal tenderness is highly suspect. Rebound tenderness usually suggests hematoperitoneum. Here the diagnosis should be obvious. Culdocentesis in such instances may give a false-negative result in up to 20% of cases. False-positive results occur in about 15–20% of cases because of the blood obtained coming from other sources. In my experience, culdocentesis has not been crucial in influencing the management of the ectopic pregnancy. Nonetheless, others advocate its use widely.

Laparoscopy is probably the most effective way to define the problem and detect the ectopic pregnancy. In many series, only 2–5% have been missed. Laparoscopy should not be done when the patient is in shock or the findings clearly indicate an ectopic pregnancy. The high index of suspicion, together with the rest of the clinical picture, is essential. Careful attention should be paid to the history and particularly to the menstrual pattern, the physical findings, the β-hCG titers, ultrasonography, and laparoscopy for this will best define the problem effectively.

When confronted with a patient with an ectopic pregnancy, if the diagnosis is made early enough, before the pregnancy has disrupted through the tube, all the options are available. These would be influenced by the desires of the patient and the propriety of the clinical situation. The management may vary depending on the patient's age, her desire for future fertility, and other gynecologic determinants, such as a history of abnormal cytology, menstrual dysfunction, or pelvic infections, in addition to location and severity of the ectopic pregnancy and the condition of the patient. It is essential that these be discussed with the patient or the couple as soon as ectopic pregnancy is suspected. Together with the couple, one can plan whether conservative tubal surgery or extirpative surgery, which might include salpingectomy, salpingo-oophorectomy, salpingectomy with tubal ligation of the other tube, and in rare instances, even hysterectomy, should be considered. Through such discussions, the patient can assume a more active role in her management. She must also be aware that conservational surgery might still offer an elevated risk of ectopic pregnancy. However, the latter does offer the best opportunity to preserve reproductive functions. With a ruptured ectopic, the procedures employed include teasing or extracting the products of conception through linear salpingotomy or tubal resection, depending on where the pregnancy is located. Expression of the products of conception should be avoided since such compressions produce further tissue disruptions and destruction. Mid-tubal ruptures may require partial resection of the tube. While the patient's condition may permit it, the tissue distortion more often suggests that subsequent scheduled anastomosis is preferable to proceeding with an anastomosis that has been suggested by others. Those that are done may be less likely to be successful because of the luminal disparity and the tissue fragility. In the ruptured ectopic pregnancy, other infertility surgery should be delayed, particularly in those instances where the hypovolemia is a factor. It is also not wise to operate on an occluded contralateral tube, since tubal surgery performed as an emergency yields poorer results than when scheduled appropriately.

In the unruptured tubal pregnancy, the tubal distortion is truly nowhere near that of the ruptured tube. Implantations in the ampulla may be gently extracted or teased with removal of the pregnancy through the ostium of the infundibulum. If this is not feasible, one may resort to a linear salpingotomy or ampullotomy. The mid-segmental site may be managed by a linear salpingotomy and the pregnancy extracted. It has been suggested that in the treatment of the interstitial pregnancy, the continuity of the oviduct might be established by performing a tubouterine implantation after resection of the damaged area. This more extensive procedure might better be delayed to a more opportune time. Interstitial pregnancies may not be diagnosed until uterine rupture, in which case the extent of damage may dictate hysterectomy as the more conservative approach for the protection of the patient.

Ectopic pregnancies that are unruptured have been treated through a laparoscopic approach. The application of this technique requires that the surgeon have experience and be an able laparoscopist armed with special instrumentation and equipment including the availability of a significant irrigation, suction, and pneumoperitoneal sustaining techniques in addition to coagulation and cutting cautery. It should be apparent that often there may be the need for laparotomy where the compressing fingers can easily control the bleeding and avoid the anxieties and the prospect of unintended damage to the adnexa. Elective surgery, such as incidental appendectomy, is controversial but is probably not advisable. This is particularly the case in the medically unstable patient as well as in those interested in conserving fertility.

ASSESSMENT OF TUBAL SURGICAL SUCCESS

The various factors to be considered in assessing the successes of tubal surgery include the initial selection of the patient population based on the variety, extent, and classification of the pathology observed, together with the size and length of follow-up of the series. Moreover, the results of a single surgeon's experience are probably more meaningful than those obtained through a series that combine operations by many surgeons within the same, or even multiple, institutions. It should be recalled that the technical variations of individual surgeons as well as the varied pathologies of the patients provides a mathematical exercise which cannot offer realistic or valid data. The literature provides much confusion for this reason. Moreover, successes may be measured according to the numbers of successes relative to patency, but it should be emphasized that assessing patency gives us nothing to indicate restoration of physiologic function. Although pregnancy is the acme of success, this may be confused by the elusive, enigmatic male contribution or other similar subtle difficulties responsible for the variability in pregnancy rates from one couple to another and which distort the results of series according to the promptness or lateness of their occurrence. Moreover, liberties are taken when reporting pregnancy; they may be based strictly on a positive pregnancy test or on the basis of term pregnancy or may include pregnancy losses even when they may not be documented histologically. Such confusions further complicate the interpretation of many figures. Crude gross rates are probably the ones that are less frequently presented. More often, the rates presented are adjusted or corrected figures. Life table analysis can better afford an opportunity for comparing time intervals, judging one series with another more effectively. It should also be stipulated that in those series in which patients are lost to follow-up and which are discarded rather than considered as a failure, the results may be unduly enhanced. As with any technically detailed surgical exercise, assessment of the role of the surgical dexterity of the individual surgeon is difficult, and perhaps impossible, to quantify. Nonetheless, it is probably the most significant ingredient.

PELVIC ENDOMETRIOSIS

There appears to be a concensus regarding the relationship between endometriosis and infertility. Although medical approaches to the management of endometriosis have been offered, opinions vary on their effectiveness when there is associated infertility.[40-43] Management of the surgery has also engendered some controversy.[41,44-47] Expectancy in the patient with limited disease has also been supported.[47] Surgical resection has some advantage in that it allows for more prompt expectancy of pregnancy than the medical modalities that suppress ovulation and menstruation. Little advantage is seen in combining these efforts. Indeed, preoperative use of danazol or the like may facilitate the surgery only to offer the disadvantage of incomplete resection of endometriosis, since the medical management may repress and obscure the lesions.

In those instances in which adnexal distortion is extensive, a pelvic restoration has been suggested. Adhesions are carefully dissected with meticulous attention directed toward hemostasis. Endometriomas are not electrocoagulated but are surgically excised with en bloc resection except when deep involvement of the bowel is encountered. Dissection of the broad ligament and uterosacrals demand careful attention to the broad ligamental vasculature and particularly the ureter. The latter should be identified as the dissection progresses to avoid unintended damage.

Ovaries are incised and the endometrioma excised by sharp resection and blunt dissection. Re-construction of the ovary should ensure meticulous hemostasis and obliteration of dead space; #3-0 or #4-0 polyglycolic acid or polyglactin sutures are used. The deeper layers are closed with a continuous spiralling circular or pursestring suture starting at the base. The capsule edges are approximated with a continuous baseball stitch, inverting the edges slightly, leaving a smooth surface.

Presacral neurectomy is often offered as an adjuvant to those women with severe dysmenorrhea or dyspareunia, or both. A uterine suspension, temporary in nature, such as the modified Olshausen, is performed to better assure anterior and superior pelvic positioning of the uterus and adnexa during the postoperative healing phase.

The application of the classification for endometriosis detailing the severity and the extent of the disease appears to be helpful in projecting the expectant outcome of this reproductive surgery. The American Fertility Society endometriosis scoring form is the simplest and most effective.

LEIOMYOMATA UTERI

Leiomyomata uteri are the most prevalent benign tumors found in the pelvic viscera, with an incidence of about 20% in women of reproductive age. In women desirous of preserving reproduction, the conservational surgical approach is desirable despite hysterectomy being touted as the treatment of choice in women who may have completed their childbearing. This is particularly supported by the potential of recurrence of myomas of 4%–30%[48,49] and of 3–32% requiring subsequent hysterectomy.[36,48-57]

The relationship of myomata to infertility has been debated.[49,51,52,54,56,57] The frequency of recurrent spontaneous abortion is dramatically reduced after myomectomy.[58,59] Nonetheless, the absolute association between myomata uteri and infertility is low, and many women conceive without difficulty despite the pressure of myomata. My experience supports that women with infertility associated with myomata uteri, and particularly those with a submucus locus, are promptly benefited by myomectomy.[60]

Myomectomies generally are performed *via* the abdominal route, with an incision appropriate to mass size, under general anesthesia. An adaptation of the Rubin hemostatic tourniquet technique reduces blood loss significantly. Laser also has been offered, but the capsule incision and traction for enucleation of the myoma affords the dissection allowing to clamp the principle vessels at the base. All defects produced by the enucleation of the myomata are closed to afford hemostasis and eliminate dead space. This is best done by using concentric spiraling pursestring stitches using #3-0 polyglycolic acid or polyglactin sutures. The surface area is approximated using #4-0 polyglactin suture with a baseball stitch imbricating the edge and leaving a smooth surface. Bipolar microcoagulation controls miniscule bleeding at the suture sites.

METROPLASTY

Uterine anomalies are infrequent and are often associated with pregnancy loss. The classification of mullerian anomalies of Buttram is recommended.[61] Resection of the uterine septum has been advocated by Jones,[62] while Straussman,[63] and later Tompkins,[64] use techniques that do not excise any tissue. I favor the Tompkins technique in the septate uterus, although the Straussman may have advantage in the arcuate uterus.

As in most all infertility surgery, the Pfannenstiel incision is used. Similarly as for myomectomy, a modified Rubin tourniquet may be applied for hemostasis. The uterus is evaluated seeking out the sulcus of the midline through which the incision is made in the anteroposterior orientation. Sutures of #3-0 vicryl are applied to the anterior and posterior walls of each side of the bivalved uterus. This allows for traction for extension of the incision as well as for hemostasis if the tourniquet is not used. The incision is extended downward along the midline until the common cavity is reached. The wall of the septum can easily be identified and incised on each side toward the uterine fundus. A metroplasty hook facilitates the direction of this incision. The anterior halves are then repaired in layers using interrupted #3-0 vicryl sutures; similarly, the posterior halves are united. The serosa is approximated with a #4-0 vicryl subserosal continuous approximation or with a baseball-type stitch approximating the edges. Before closing the fundal sutures in the approximation, a $\frac{1}{4}$-in. iodoform gauze pack is inserted into the uterine cavity dissecting the first portion toward the endocervical canal. This separates the two walls and prevents the possibility of adhesion formation. The pack is removed some 72–84 hr postoperatively. Significant improvement in fetal salvage is seen following septum revision.

Factors affecting fertility can be eliminated or improved to achieve the desired effect through properly selected surgical corrections.[65] Judgment, experience, and surgical dexterity are the key ingredients to such success.

SUMMARY

Selection of surgical procedure appropriate for correction of infertility has improved greatly during the last decade because of advances in our knowledge of physiology of the reproductive tract; the development of less traumatic instruments, suture materials, and electrical and laser cutting modes; and finally, the use of modern biostatistical methods for comparison of results.

In the area of physiology, operative and laboratory observations, including those adopted in in vitro fertilization programs, have afforded improved understanding of tubal propulsive forces for egg, sperm, and zygote, both physical and biochemical. The importance of the blood supply to the distal tube and fimbria ovarica are especially noteworthy.

The use of magnification by loupe or microscope, taken in conjunction with the development of a variety of synthetic fine suture materials, has invested the surgeon with the capability of coping differently with the four major processes of infertility amenable to surgery—those caused by infectious disease, prior surgery, endometriosis, and ectopic pregnancy. These new techniques now strongly affect the type of primary surgery chosen, e.g., surgical sterilization techniques and procedures used for extirpation of ectopic pregnancies.

Further comparative studies, and further understanding of the chemical interactions among the tube, gametes, and zygote, will undoubtedly lead to further improvements in surgical results.

REFERENCES

1. Aral SO, Cates W Jr: The increasing concern with infertility. Why now? *JAMA* 250:2327–2331, 1983
2. Mastroianni L Jr, Shah U, Abdul-Karim R: Prolonged volumetric collection of oviductal fluid in the rhesus monkey. *Fertil Steril* 12:417–424, 1961
3. Nalbondov AV: Comparative morphology and anatomy of the oviduct, in Hafez ESE, and Blandau, RJ (eds): *The Mammalian Oviduct.* University of Chicago Press, 1969, p. 47–55
4. Cognat M, Rochet Y: Notre experience de la salpingoplastie. *J Gynecol Obstet Biol Reprod (Paris)* 6:839–850, 1977
5. Fromm E, Garcia CR, Jeutter DC: Physiologic assessment of tubal motility—Extraluminal telemetric subject evaluation, ovum transport and fertility regulation. A World

Health Organization Symposium. Copenhagen, Scriptor, 1975, p. 107–125

6. Magyar DM: Hypothalamic–pituitary adrenocortical function after dexamethasone-promethazine adhesion regimen. *Obstet Gynecol* 63:182–185, 1984

7. David A, Brackett BG, Garcia CR, et al: Composition of rabbit oviductal fluid in ligated segments of the fallopian tube. *J Reprod Fertil* 19:285–289, 1969

8. Coutinho EM: Physiologic and pharmacologic studies of the human oviduct. *Fertil Steril* 22:807–815, 1971

9. Cristoph FN, Dennis KJ: The cellular composition of the human oviduct epithelium. *Br J Obstet Gynaecol* 84:219–221, 1977

10. Blandau RJ: Gamete transport—Comparative aspects, in Hafez ESE, Blandau RJ *The Mammalian Oviduct.* Chicago, University of Chicago Press, 1969, p. 129–162

11. Westman AD: A contribution to the question of the transit of the ovum from ovary to uterus in rabbits. *Obstet Gynecol Scand* 5:1–5, 1926

12. Garcia CR, Mastroianni L Jr: Microsurgery for treatment of adnexal disease. *Fertil Steril* 34:413–424, 1980

13. Hulka J, Omran K, Berger C: Classification of adnexal adhesions: A proposal and evaluation of its prognostic value. *Fertil Steril* 30:661–665, 1978

14. Gomel V: Classification of operations for tubal and peritoneal factors causing infertility. *Clin Obstet Cynecol* 23:1259–1260, 1980

15. Acosta AA, Buttram VC, Besch PK, et al: A proposed classification of pelvic endometriosis. *Obstet Gynecol* 42:19–25, 1973

16. *Classification of Endometriosis,* Special Contribution, American Fertility Society, December 1979, #32, p 633–664

17. DeCherney AH, Berkowitz G: Female fecundity and age. *N Engl J Med* 306:424–426, 1982

18. Daniell JF, Brow DH: CO_2 laser laparoscopy. *Obstet Gynecol* 59:761–764, 1982

18a. Fayez JA, McComb JS, Harper HA: Comparison of tubal surgery with CO_2 laser and the unipolar microelectrode. *Fertil Steril* 40:476–480, 1983

19. Daniell JF, Christianson C: Combined laparoscopic surgery and Danazol therapy for pelvic endometriosis. *Fertil Steril* 35:521–524, 1981

20. Danielle JF, Pittaway DE, Maxson NS: The role of laparoscopic adhesolysis in an in vitro fertilization program. *Fertil Steril* 40:49–52, 1983

21. Baggish MS, Chong AP: CO_2 laser microsurgery of the uterine tube. *Obstet Gynecol* 58:111–116, 1981

22. Fayez JA, Jobson VW, Lentz SS, et al: Tubal microsurgery with CO_2 laser. *Am J Obstet Gynecol* 146:371–373, 1983

23. Grunert GM, Franklin RR: What's new: The CO_2 laser in gynecologic fertility surgery. *Tex Med* 79:43–47, 1983

24. Kelly RW, Roberts DK: Experience with CO_2 laser in gynecologic microsurgery. *Am J Obstet Gynecol* 146:585–588, 1983

25. Replogle RL, Johnson R, Gross R: Prevention of postoperative adhesions with combined promethazine and dexamethasone therapy. *Ann Surg* 163:580–588, 1966

26. diZerega GS, Hodgen GD: Prevention of postoperative tubal adhesions: Comparative study of commonly used agents. *Am J Obstet Gynecol* 136:173–176, 1980

27. Seitz HM Jr, Schenker JG, Epstein S, et al: Postoperative intraperitoneal adhesions: A double-blind assessment of their prevention in the monkey. *Fertil Steril* 24:935–940, 1973

28. Holtz G, Baker ER: Inhibitors of peritoneal adhesions after lysis with 32% Dextran 70. *Fertil Steril* 34:394–395, 1980

29. Rock JA, Siegler AM, Meisel MB, et al: The efficacy of postoperative hydrotubation: A randomized prospective multicenter clinical trial. *Fertil Steril* 42:373–376, 1984

30. Ascenzo-Cabello J, De la Puente-Lanfranco R, Ascenzo AE: RLcent advances in human reproduction, in Compos dePaz A, Drill V, Hayashi M, et al (eds): *Proceedings of the First International Congress of Human Reproduction, Brazil, November 1974.* New York, American Elsevier, 1976, p 42–46

31. Jeffcoate TNA: Salpingectomy or salpingo-oophorectomy? *J Obstet Gynaecol Br Emp* 62:214–215, 1955

32. Scott JS, Lynch EM, Anderson JA: Surgical treatment of female infertility: Value of paradoxical oophorectomy. *Br Med J* 1:631–634, 1976

33. Skulj V, Pavlic Z, Stoiljkovic C, et al: Conservative operative treatment of tubal pregnancy. *Fertil Steril* 15:634–639, 1964

34. Winston RML: Tuboplasty, in Roberts DWT (ed): *Operative Surgery (Gynecology & Obstetrics).* London, Butterworth, 1977, p 152–164

35. Winston RML: Microsurgical tubo-cornual anastomosis for reversal of sterilization. *Lancet* 1:284–285, 1977

36. Loeffler FE, Noble AD: Myomectomy at the Chelsea Hospital for Women. *J Obstet Gynaecol Br Commonw* 77:167–170, 1970

37. Novy M: Reversal of Kroener fimbriectomy sterilization. *Am J Obstet Gynecol* 137:198–206, 1980

38. Reyniak JV: Reversal of female sterilization, in Reyniak JV, Lauersen NH (eds): *Principles of Microsurgical Techniques in Infertility.* New York, Plenum, 1982, p 139–159

39. Ectopic Pregnancies—United States, 1970–1980. Morbidity Mortality 33:201–202, 1984

40. Chalmers JA: *Endometriosis.* London, Butterworth, 1975

41. Greenblatt RG (ed): *Recent Advances in Endometriosis. Proceedings of Symposium, August, Georgia, March 5–6, 1975; Amsterdam, 1976.* Amsterdam, Excerpta Medica, 1975/1976

42. Reid D, Christian D, (eds): Medical versus surgical management of endometriosis, in *Controversy in Obstetrics and Gynecology.* II. Philadelphia, Saunders, 1974, p 631

43. Gray LA: Surgical treatment of endometriosis. *Clin Obstet Gynecol* 3:472–491, 1960

44. Hammond CB, Rock JA, Parker RT: Conservative treatment of endometriosis: The effects of limited surgery and hormonal pseudopregnancy. *Fertil Steril* 27:756–776, 1976

45. Rogers SF, Jacobs WM: Infertility and endometriosis: Conservative surgery approach. *Fertil Steril* 19:529–536, 1968

46. Williams TJ: The role of surgery in the management of endometriosis. *Mayo Clin Proc* 50:198–203, 1975

47. Garcia CR, David SS: Pelvic endometriosis: Infertility and pelvic pain. *Fertil Steril* 129:740–747, 1977

48. Bonney V: The technique and result of myomectomy. *Lancet* 220:171–177, 1931

49. Mussey RD, Randall LM, Doyle LW: Pregnancy following myomectomy. *Am J Obstet Gynecol* 49:508–513, 1945

50. Brown AB, Chamberlain R, TeLinde RW: Myomectomy. *Am J Obstet Gynecol* 71:159–163, 1956

51. Brown JM, Maklasian GD, Symmonds RE: Abdominal myomectomy. *Am J Obstet Gynecol* 90:126–12ᶜ, 1967

52. Buttram VC Jr, Reiter RC: Uterine leiomyomata: etiology, symptomatology, and management. *Fertil Steril* 36:433–445, 1981

53. Finn WF, Muller PF: Abdominal myomectomy: Special

reference to subsequent pregnancy and to the reappearance of fibromyomas of the uterus. *Am J Obstet Gynecol* 60:109–116, 1950

54. Malone LJ, Ingersoll FM: Myomectomy in infertility, in Behrman, SJ, Kistner RW *Progress in Infertility*. Boston, Little, Brown, 1975, p 85–90

55. Munnell EW, Martin FW: Abdominal myomectomy: Advantages and disadvantages. *Am J Obstet Gynecol* 62:109–120, 1951

56. Raney B, Frederick I: The occasional need for myomectomy. *Obstet Gynecol* 53:437–441, 1979

57. Israel SL, Mutch JC: Myomectomy. *Clin Obstet Gynecol* 455–466, 1958

58. Babaknia A, Rock JA, Jones HW Jr: Pregnancy success following abdominal myomectomy for infertility. *Fertil Steril* 30:644–647, 1978

59. Stevenson CS: Myomectomy for improvement of fertility. *Fertil Steril* 15:367–384, 1964

60. Garcia CR, Tureck RW: Submucosal leiomyomas and infertility. *Fertil Steril* 42:16–19, 1984

61. Buttram VC Jr, Gibbons WE: Mullerian anomalies: A proposed classification. *Fertil Steril* 32:40–46, 1979

62. Jones HW Jr, Rock JA: Surgical correction of the double uterus, in Jones W, Rock JA: *Reparative and Constructive Surgery of the Female Generative Tract*. Baltimore, Williams & Wilkins, 1983, p 182–183

63. Straussman EO: Operations for double uterus and endometrial atresia. *Clin Obstet Gynecol* 4:240–255, 1961

64. Tompkins P: Comments on the bicornuate uterus and twinning. *Surg Clin North Am* 42:1049–1062, 1962

65. Buttram VC Jr, Zanotti L, Acosta AA, et al: Surgical correction of the septate uterus. *Fertil Steril* 25:373–379, 1974

66. Gomel V: Tubal reanastomosis by microsurgery. *Fertil Steril* 28:59–65, 1977

67. Diamond E: A comparison of gross and microsurgical techniques for repair of cornual occlusion in infertility: A retrospective study, 1968–1978. *Fertil Steril* 32:370–376, 1979

68. Winston RML: Reversal of tubal sterilization. *Clin Obstet Gynecol* 23: 1261–1268, 1980

69. McComb P, Gomel V: Cornual occlusion and its microsurgical reconstruction. *Clin Obstet Gynecol* 23:1229–1241, 1980

70. Meldrum DA: Microsurgical tubal reanastomosis—the role of splints. *Obstet Gynecol* 57:613–619, 1981

71. Siegler AM, Kontopoulos V: An analysis of macrosurgical and microsurgical techniques in the management of the tuboperitoneal factors in infertility. *Fertil Steril* 32:377–383, 1979

72. DeCherney AH, Kase N: A comparison of treatment for bilateral fimbrial occlusion. *Fertil Steril* 35:162–166, 1981

73. Fayez JA, Suliman SU: Infertility surgery of the oviduct: Comparison between macrosurgery and microsurgery. *Fertil Steril* 37:73–78, 1982

74. Garcia CR: Surgical reconstruction of the oviduct in the infertile patient, in Behrman SJ, Kistner RW (eds): *Progress in Infertility*. Boston, Little, Brown, 1968, pp 223–262

75. Swolin K: Electromicrosurgery and salpingostomy: Long-term results. *Am J Obstet Gynecol* 121:418–419, 1975

76. Gomel V: Salpingostomy by microsurgery. *Fertil Steril* 29:380–387, 1978

77. Winston RML: Microsurgery of the fallopian tube: From fantasy to reality. *Fertil Steril* 34:521–530, 1980

78. Lassen B: Late results of salpingostomy combined with salpingolysis and ovariolysis by electromicrosurgery in 54 women. *Fertil Steril* 37:156–160, 1982

79. Lauritsen JG, Pagel JD, Vangsted P, et al: Results of repeated tuboplasties. *Fertil Steril* 37:68–72, 1982

80. Umezaki C, Katayama P, Jones HW Jr: Pregnancy rates after reconstructive surgery on the fallopian tube. *Obstet Gynecol* 43:418–424, 1974

81. Siegler AM, Perez RJ: Reconstruction of fallopian tubes in previously sterilized patients. *Fertil Steril* 26: 383–392, 1975

82. Rock JA, Katayama KP, Jones HW: Tubal reanastomosis: A comparison of Hellman's approach and a microsurgical technique, in Phillips JM (ed): *Microsurgery in Gynecology*. II. Downey, CA, A.A.G.L., 1981, p 176–183

83. Diamond E: A microsurgical study of the blood supply to the uterine tube and ovary, in Phillips JM (ed): *Microsurgery in Gynecology*. II. Downey, CA, A.A.G.L., 1981, p 228–240

84. Garcia CR: Oviductal anastomosis procedures, in Richart RM, Prager DJ (eds): *Human Sterilization*. Springfield, IL, Thomas, 1972, p 116–128

85. Gomel V: Microsurgical reversal of female sterilization. A reappraisal. *Fertil Steril* 33:587–597, 1980

86. Coronado JL: Reversal of tubal sterilization: A prospective study of 254 cases, in Phillips JM (ed): *Microsurgery in Gynecology*. II. Downey, CA, A.A.G.L., 1981, p 135–140

87. Riggall FC, Cantor B: Relationship of microsurgical reanastomosis to the type of previous sterilization, in Phillips JM (ed): *Microsurgery in Gynecology*. II, Downey, CA, A.A.G.L., 1981, p 172–175

88. Ploman L, Wicksell F: Fertility after conservative surgery in tubal pregnancy. *Acta Obstet Gynecol Scand* 39:143–152, 1960

89. Timonen S, Nieminen U: Tubal pregnancy, choice of operative method of treatment. *Acta Obstet Gynecol Scand* 46:327–339, 1967

90. DeCherney AH, Kase N: A conservative surgical management of unruptured ectopic pregnancy. *Obstet Gynecol* 54:451–455, 1979

91. Peterson EP, Musich JR, Behrman SJ: Uterotubal implantation and obstetric outcome after previous sterilization. *Am J Obstet Gynecol* 128:662–667, 1977

31

Medical Treatment of Infertility

WAYNE DECKER

INTRODUCTION

Ovulation defects are a major cause of infertility. It was not until about 20 years ago that pharmacologic means became available to induce ovulation consistently in the anovulatory woman. The first of these drugs to become available for general clinical use was clomiphene citrate, which remains the safest, the most broadly effective, and the most widely used of several agents now available.

Next in sequence of availability for practical clinical use was human menopausal gonadotropin (hMG), capable of stimulating ovulation under selected circumstances but sometimes responsible for serious and unexpected side effects.

The realization that excessive prolactin secretion has an adverse effect on ovulation followed the capability to detect and measure plasma levels of this endocrine hormone with accuracy.

Most recently, tentative use is being made of gonadotropin-releasing hormone and its analogues for more readily regulated effect and safer ovulatory response by the anovulatory woman. Although not yet practical for routine utilization, it deserves some detailed consideration in a chapter on the medical treatment of infertility. This chapter deals with those agents capable of inducing ovulation. Each has its precise place in the therapeutic scheme and each requires an understanding of its indications, mode of action, means of monitoring responses of its effects, and a clear understanding of its side effects and management.

CLOMIPHENE CITRATE

The development of pharmaceutical agents to induce ovulation in the nonovulating or oligo-ovulating woman constitutes the most significant advance in infertility therapy in this generation. Before these agents became available, little could be done to increase the ovulatory capability of these women.

Pharmacology

Clomiphene citrate is a nonsteroidal substance the structure of which bears a close resemblance to diethystilbestrol (DES); its steric structure has some similarities to estradiol. Although the precise mechanism of action of clomiphene is not totally understood, it is assumed that the essence of its ability to exert an antiestrogenic effect depends on the structural similarities to these compounds and is responsible for its affinity to estrogen binding sites in a variety of target organs. These include the uterus and vagina as well as the anterior pituitary and most

WAYNE DECKER • Fertility Research Foundation, New York, New York 10021.

importantly the hypothalamus, which appears to be not only the site of its activity but the area essential to ovulation induction as well. The influence of clomiphene on other target organs, most notably the anterior pituitary and possibly the ovaries themselves, may have a role in the mode of action.[1] By occupying estrogen-binding sites, clomiphene leads indirectly to the luteinizing hormone (LH) surge needed for ovulation.

Therapeutically administered doses of clomiphene from cycle days 5–9 result in a rise in serum LH and follicle-stimulating hormone (FSH) within a few days. On the sixteenth or seventeenth day of the clomiphene-treated cycle, estradiol rises to a level higher than that seen with spontaneous ovulation. Higher levels of estradiol seem to be needed in the induced cycle to affect an adequate LH surge needed for follicle rupture and ovum extrusion.

Clomiphene is an extremely safe drug. It has few significant side effects, can be taken orally, and requires only simple monitoring during its administration.

Indications

The major indications for the use of clomiphene are (1) oligomenorrhea, (2) hypothalamic amenorrhea, (3) secondary amenorrhea such as occurs with post-pill amenorrhea, (4) polycystic ovarian disease, and (5) luteal-phase deficiency.

Criteria for patient selection is important, but clinical trial in borderline cases is often justified. Patients must have an intact hypothalamic–pituitary–ovarian axis and should be producing suffi-

cient endogenous estrogen in order to bleed after the intramuscular administration of 100 mg progesterone in oil. If such a response fails to occur, serum levels of FSH and LH should be determined. If these are excessively high in amenorrheic woman, premature ovarian failure is indicated, and further attempts at ovulation induction will be unsuccessful.

Dosage

No clear correlation has been established between clomiphene dosage, its schedule of administration and the ultimate results. The usual dose of clomiphene is 50–200 mg/day for 5 days starting on the fifth day of cycle. Treatment is usually begun with the smallest dose (50 mg) (Fig. 31-1) and is increased in subsequent cycles, as indicated by responses shown on the basal body temperature (BBT) curve and the occurrence of adequate cervical mucus and the presence or absence of side effects. It has been our usual practice to initiate treatment with 100 mg/day, as experience indicates that this is generally found to be the most effective dose level (Fig. 31-2). If unpleasant or undesirable side effects result, such as visual disturbances or hostile mucous changes, the dose can be reduced to 50 mg/day to seek an effective ovulatory response. Doses above 200 mg/day do not appear to be effective in the absence of responses at lower levels.

There have been many variations in these schedules. Treatment has been started as early as the second or third day and continued for 7–10 days. These variations generally have not been found beneficial.

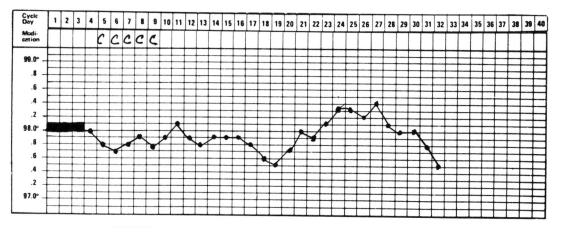

FIGURE 31-1. Poor response to clomiphene stimulation. c, clomiphene 50 mg.

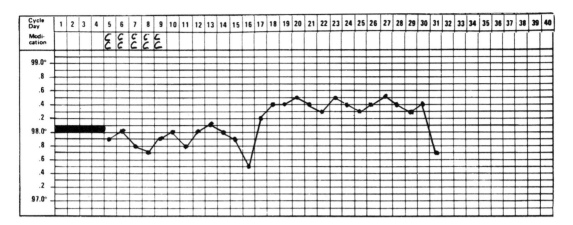

FIGURE 31-2. Clomiphene induction of ovulation. c, clomiphene 50 mg.

Monitoring

Cycles should be monitored with daily BBT recordings, midcycle evaluations of cervical mucus and pelvic examinations. Cervical mucus can best be evaluated with the postcoital test, which gives a clear indication of the character of the mucus in relationship to its compatibility with healthy sperm cells. Frequent postcoital testing on patients during clomiphene therapy may be justified as Clomid may induce thickening of cervical mucus.

Failure of Response

Failure to respond to ovulation indicators (i.e., BBT, cervical mucus) after adequate doses of clomiphene alone can often be corrected by the addition of human chorionic gonadotropin (hCG) 10,000 U IM 7–8 days after the last dose of clomiphene. It appears to enhance the LH surge (Fig. 31-3). Garcia et al.[2] reported a 55.8% pregnancy rate in a series of selected patients using this regimen. It is recommended that the timing of the injection coincide with the development of cervical mucus. An additional injection of hCG 10,000 U given 1 week later has been found helpful when the BBT level is not maintained in the luteal phase.

Some clomiphene failures associated with hirsutism and increased androgen levels may produce ovulatory responses with the addition of dexamethasone.[3] A reduction of nighttime ACTH can sometimes be achieved with the use of a daily dose of dexamethasone 0.5 mg at bedtime. The recommended initial dose of clomiphene is 50 mg D 5-9

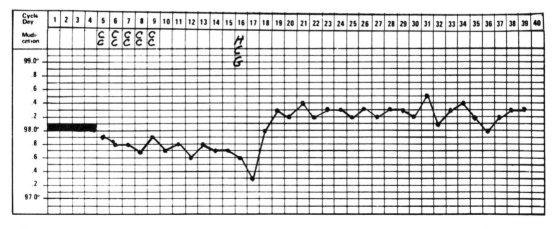

FIGURE 31-3. Clomiphene, hCG response, and pregnancy. hCG 10,000 μm.

but should be quickly increased to 100 mg, then 150 mg until the desired response is noted. We tend to discontinue this combination if a favorable response is not apparent in 3–4 cycles.

Cervical Mucus Changes

Because of its antiestrogen properties, clomiphene sometimes causes the cervical mucus to become thick and tenacious. This unfavorable occurrence can be perplexing. Efforts are sometimes made to counter this change by adding small doses of estrogen during the proliferative stage of the cycle. This is not always satisfactory, and it appears illogical to reverse the desired antiestrogen effect by the addition of estrogen. The added estrogen may result in delayed or erratic menstruation. Often the character of the mucus will show favorable changes under the influence of potassium iodide, a time-honored expectorant and the ingredient of some of the older cough remedies. Ten drops of a saturated solution of potassium iodide added to a half-glass of water or fruit juice and taken once or twice a day from days 9–18 will produce clear mucus of the desired consistency. Similar results have been observed with the use of cough preparations containing guaifenesin, an effective mucolytic agent.

Where either of these measures fail, the use of small doses of hMG may be unusually effective. Following the usual course of clomiphene from days 5–9, one ampule of hMG is injected on day 11 and again on day 13. This will usually produce a strong mucogenic response. The dose of hMG is not large enough to require the usual monitoring procedures. Patients on this dosage schedule of clomiphene tend to ovulate between the fifteenth and seventeenth days, and the addition of hMG does not appear to alter this response.

Side Effects

Other side effects of clomiphene include the following:

1. *Ovarian enlargement:* This results from follicular stimulation and rarely poses a significant problem. When enlargement is detected, ovarian size should be evaluated by pelvic examinations at about 2-week intervals. Pelvic sonography may be indicated if an anticipated decrease in size is not detected promptly. If enlargement persists after the next menstrual period, further clomiphene should be deferred. When normal ovarian size is reestablished, however, treatment can be safely resumed.
2. *Vasomotor disturbances:* A response to suppression of estrogen levels, the resultant flushes are of short duration. Patients can be assured they are of no serious significance.
3. *Partial alopecia:* This rare side effect indicates the need for discontinuation of the medication.
4. *Visual disturbances:* The cause of such symptoms as blurred vision, scotoma, and abnormal perception is unknown, but they disappear when medication is stopped. They may be dose related. Because of our lack of knowledge of this phenomenon, these symptoms are a contraindication to continued use of the drug.

Breast discomfort, painful ovulation, and abdominal bloating are the sequelae of desired ovulation and, although patients sometimes complain of these problems, they can be confidently reassured that they are not abnormal.

Luteal-Phase Deficiency

For oligo-ovulating women or for those with luteal-phase deficiencies, clomiphene is helpful. Luteal-phase deficiency diagnosed by endometrial biopsy (out of phase) and confirmed by subsequent BBT's (poor diphasic) and serum progesterone levels (low) respond to conventional clomiphene doses. Its use for the woman who ovulates irregularly will ensure consistent ovulation and will therefore enhance fertility.

Clomiphene is particularly useful in creating regularly predictable ovulation patterns in women who are undergoing artificial insemination with either their husband's semen or a donor's. This will reduce the required number of inseminations and increase pregnancy rates.

Certain orthodox Jewish couples must defer intercourse for specified intervals after the last bleeding. For women with short cycles, this may effectively avoid the time of ovulation. Conventional clomiphene treatment will delay ovulation until the days 15–17. There is no evidence to indicate that clomiphene enhances fertility in normally ovulating women, and there is probably no justification for its empiric use.

Duration of Treatment

Clomiphene therapy may be continued for as long as it is required to manage or correct all faulty fertility factors. There are innumerable instances of women who have repeated clomiphene during successive cycles for a year or longer. As long as an adequate response is noted and there are no unusual side effects, there is really no arbitrary limit to the duration of treatment.

Results

The pregnancy outcome from clomiphene was once thought to show an increase in multiple (twin) pregnancies and to result in a greater number of spontaneous abortions than pregnancies from spontaneous ovulations. Extensive experience now indicates that the results of these two groups of pregnancies is really very similar, with twin pregnancy and abortion rates about the same. Seventy to 80% of properly selected anovulatory women will be made to ovulate with effective doses of clomiphene. From this group, pregnancy rates will be essentially the same as those found in a normally ovulatory group of women.[4]

HUMAN MENOPAUSAL GONADOTROPIN

Human menopausal gonadotropins (hMG) available for the induction of ovulation in this country consist of ampules of equal parts of FSH and LH (75 IU each) extracted from the urine of postmenopausal women.

Selection of Patients

Treatment with these substances is effective in women with hypopituitarism, FSH and LH deficiency. In general, the same criteria for patient selection are used as for clomiphene. Almost without exception, however, hMG should be used only when the patient has failed to ovulate with clomiphene stimulation. There are rarely justifications for proceeding with hMG without first trying to induce ovulation with clomiphene. The reasons for this are obvious: hMG is expensive, it requires daily injections for an undetermined number of days, it requires careful clinical and laboratory monitoring, and it has the potential for sudden and serious side effects. For these reasons also, it should not be used as a therapeutic trial as may be done with clomiphene. Candidates for hMG therapy should be carefully worked up to rule out any other possible cause of their infertility. If other causes are found, it may be necessary to correct them before hMG treatment is instituted.

Pretreatment levels of FSH and LH should not be excessive. High levels of these gonadotropins in the anovulatory woman indicate ovarian failure; any treatment directed toward ovulation stimulation will be futile in this patient.

Treatment Schedules

Amenorrheic patients may be made to bleed with a single injection of 100 mg progesterone in oil or 5 days of oral Provera, 10 mg bid and thus demonstrate an intact hypothalamic–pituitary–ovarian axis with adequate endogenous estrogen priming.

With the cessation of bleeding, hMG injections can begin. In the hypopituitary patient with infertility, injections may be started directly but will require a greater dosage of hMG. Initial dosage is arbitrary. It is our practice during the first course of treatment to give a single ampule daily (Fig. 31-4). Monitoring consists of daily BBT, pelvic examination, and serum estradiol levels at least every other day. By the fourth day of treatment, there should be evidence of beginning production of clear cervical mucus, with rising estradiol levels reaching 300–500 pg/ml. If these levels are not reached, the dose of hMG is increased to 2 ampules/day from the sixth to eighth day of treatment. There should be a profuse flow of clear cervical mucus, and the serum estradiol should have reached a level of 1000 pg/ml or more. If not, continued hMG at the same or increased doses will be required. It is important that frequent evaluation of ovarian size be made. This is usually done by bimanual pelvic examination, but findings should be confirmed by sonography, if possible. This will also define the developing follicle. Some use sonography alone to determine the effect of hMG stimulation and use as its end-point follicular size without reference to estradiol levels. Generally, estradiol levels in conjunction with sonographic monitoring give the best assurance of proper dose levels.

When there is a profuse clear cervical mucus and estradiol levels have reached 1000–2000 pg/ml, ovulation is initiated by an injection of 10,000 U of human chorionic gonadotropin (hCG) given 24–48 hr after the last hMG injection. This may have to be repeated 48 hr later. Ovulation can be determined to

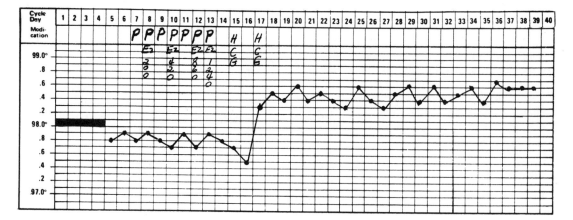

FIGURE 31-4. Typical hMG response and pregnancy. P, hMG; hCG 10,000 μm.

have occurred by a shift in BBT and a cessation of the flow of cervical mucus. Although ovulation will usually not occur until hCG has been given, about 10% of patients will ovulate without hCG after the estradiol level has reached 600 pg/ml or more. Patients should be advised of this and reminded to keep a regular schedule of intercourse.

If pregnancy fails to occur during the first course of treatment it should be repeated. Some knowledge will have been gained as to approximately how much hMG will be required to induce ovulation, and the dosage schedule can be adjusted more effectively to achieve this end. It must be remembered, however, that careful and precise monitoring must be continued because patients will not necessarily respond consistently during successive cycles of treatment. To lessen the burden of visits, the patient or her husband can be instructed in the preparation of the medication and the giving of the injection in the early stages of therapy.

Ovarian Hyperstimulation Syndrome

If the estradiol level rises above 2000 pg/ml or there is appreciable ovarian enlargement, hCG should be withheld. This will prevent excessive ovarian stimulation and the woman usually will not ovulate.

In spite of careful monitoring, ovarian hyperstimulation may occasionally occur. In its milder forms, abdominal pain with ovarian enlargement and abdominal distention may occur. These women need only be placed on limited physical activity, and in time the symptoms will subside and the ovarian enlargement will regress. Frequent and vigorous pelvic examinations should be avoided. Patients who undergo minimal hyperstimulation have a higher pregnancy rate than do those who are less symptomatic.

Ovarian hyperstimulation can be more severe with physical and physiologic changes that can be life threatening. Ovarian enlargement can be enormous, filling the abdomen with exquisitely tender masses. Ascites and pleural effusion occur. This shift of fluid from the intravascular space results in hemoconcentration hyperkalemia and circulatory disturbances. There may be hypotension and a fall in central venous pressure (CVP). The hematocrit will show evidence of hemoconcentration, which eliminates the concern that the symptom complex is the result of acute blood loss. Decreased renal perfusion results in increased water and salt reabsorption and low sodium excretion. Hyperkalemia and acidosis result.

Patients who experience severe ovarian hyperstimulation syndrome should be hospitalized and placed on bed rest and a strict monitoring program should be instituted. Pelvic and abdominal examinations are contraindicated. Serial determinations of hematocrit coagulation factors, urinary sodium and potassium, total protein and A/G ratio, BUN, creatinine, electrolytes, and electrocardiograms (ECGs) may be helpful. Diuretics should be avoided. Treatment should be geared to the expectation that the condition will resolve itself over a period of time; supportive measures are needed until that occurs.

Surgery is strictly contraindicated unless ovarian rupture and hemorrhage, a rare complication, occurs. In that event, the most conservative approach aimed at securing hemostasis should be undertaken.

At the onset of treatment, patients should be

made aware of the possibility of hyperstimulation occurring in the event they seek help from someone other than the physician who undertook the hMG therapy. A physician unfamiliar with this medication and its complications might interpret the sudden onset of symptoms and pelvic masses as an acute surgical emergency and act accordingly.

Repeat Treatment Courses

The question always arises how often hMG treatments can be repeated. Many authorities state categorically that after three ovulatory cycles have been achieved without pregnancy, further treatment with hMG should be discontinued. Others see no justification for this conservative approach. Many tend to continue treatment for six to eight cycles at which time, with the patient's approval and understanding, treatment is suspended for 2–3 months during which time the basic fertility factors are reviewed. If found normal, treatment can be resumed. Treatment may be continued as long as the patient is able to withstand it both emotionally and financially, unless there is a definite reason to indicate that pregnancy is unlikely or impossible. A number of pregnancies have resulted after 12–18 months of hMG-induced ovulation.

Results

Ninety percent of properly selected anovulatory women can be made to ovulate with hMG. Of these, 50–70% will achieve pregnancies. The abortion rate is probably slightly higher than that seen in other pregnancies. Significant fetal wastage results from multiple pregnancies, which occur at a rate of about 20%, of which 15% will be twins and 5% triplets or more. It is desirable to make the diagnosis of multiple pregnancies as early as possible which is best achieved by sonography.

COMBINED CLOMIPHENE AND hMG

The combined use of clomiphene and hMG offers several advantages over the use of either of these substances alone.[5] The combination is a considerably more potent ovulating stimulant than clomiphene alone. Comparable results for hMG alone can be anticipated, but with the use of smaller amounts of the latter drug this can materially reduce the cost of treatment. Although monitoring of the effects of the combined drugs must be just as stringent as with hMG, there seems to be less evidence of excessive stimulation.

Dose Schedule

The initial treatment cycle usually consists of clomiphene 150 mg/day from day 5 to 8 and single ampules of hMG from day 10 until the level of estradiol has reached 1000–2000 pg/ml (Fig. 31-5). hCG 10,000 U is then given 24 hr after the last injection of hMG and repeated at 48-hr intervals, if necessary, until evidence of ovulation is achieved. It is not unusual to find that hMG may be required for as few as 3–4 days with only a single ampule given each day.

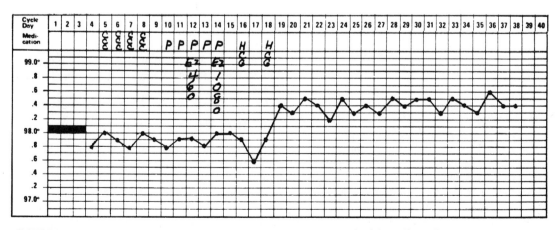

FIGURE 31-5. Combined clomiphene–hMG–hCG response and pregnancy. c, clomiphene 50 mg; P, hMG; hCG 10,000 μm.

GONADOTROPIN-RELEASING HORMONE

Historical Background

In 1960 Campbell et al.[6] and McCann et al.[7] independently demonstrated that a crude extract of the hypothalamus was capable of causing the release of LH from the anterior pituitary. Thus, hormone rather than a neuron link between these two structures was established. There was no practical therapeutic application for this discovery until 1971, when Schally et al.[8] and Guillemin et al.[9] isolated and characterized luteinizing hormone-releasing hormone (LHRH) from porcine hypothalamus. This enabled them to synthesize quantities that permitted its use in significant clinical trials. It was determined that not only did the injection of this substance cause the release of LH, but FSH as well, to a lesser degree. Because no specific FSH-releasing hormone has been identified, many investigators have chosen to refer to it as a gonadotropic hormone-releasing hormone (GnRH), a designation we prefer until its true nature is further clarified.

With the availability of larger amounts of GnRH, two early expectations for its use were apparent. It was hoped that with the use of this substance a provocative test would be available to distinguish a hypothalamic from a hypogonadotropic cause of hypogonadism. Its use for this purpose has not been entirely satisfactory because of a significant number of deceptive results. About 15% of patients with pituitary tumors have shown normal responses.[10]

For the anovulatory woman with infertility, the effectiveness of treatment with GnRH proved to have little advantage, if any, over more conventional means of ovulation induction. Lack of greater success appears to have resulted from a failure to appreciate the normal pulsatile nature of GnRH secretion. Equally disconcerting is its apparent short duration of action. GnRH has been stated to have a metabolic half-life of 2–8 min.

Advantages

GnRH administration for the induction of ovulation was assumed to have significant potential advantages over other forms of treatment. There should be a built-in safety factor against multiple ovulation and hyperstimulation not present with hMG. One could assume that ovarian estradiol production would control the GnRH, mediate gonadotropin release, and prevent multiple follicular development and ovarian hyperstimulation. However, despite the fact that Liu et al.[11] were consistently able to produce a single follicle in hypogonadotropic women with the administration of 1–5-μg doses of pulsatile GnRH, the administration of 10-μg pulses at 60-min intervals produced two to six follicles in six different patients. Apparently E_2 modulation can be overridden by larger doses of GnRH.

Analogues

Alteration of the molecular structure of GnRH results in the formation of a variety of analogues. The complexity of the molecular structure of GnRH permits construction of a wide variety of analogues that may act as agonists or antagonists. Agonists cause downregulation of GnRH receptors, while antagonists competively bind with these receptors. Antagonists are of relatively low potency, but a group of high-potency agonists referred to as superagonists have been developed. Those from this group are the most clinically effective. As many as 1000 analogues have been developed, and more will come. Among the hoped-for improvements in these altered molecular structures is an analogue displaying an effectively longer metabolic half-life.

BROMOCRIPTINE (See Chapter 23)

It is our practice to include in the routine fertility evaluation an endometrial biopsy and, at the same visit, serum progesterone and prolactin levels. In the event that the biopsy shows evidence of anovulation or luteal-phase deficiency, a relationship with hyperprolactinemia will immediately be apparent. Ten to 15% of anovulatory women will be found to have excessive levels of prolactin; less than one-half may have galactorrhea. Suppression of pulsatile GnRH secretion by prolactin is recognized as a cause of ovulation defects that range from hypoestrogenic amenorrhea to minimal luteal-phase abnormalities.

Etiology of Hyperprolactinemia

Prolactin levels in the lower elevated ranges (35–100 ng/ml) are usually due to vaguely recognized causes, which are of little clinical significance; however, these levels may be responsible for ovulatory dysfunction in these women. Care should be taken in assigning a causal relationship on the basis of minimal elevations of prolactin in a single instance. The pulsatile nature of prolactin secretion makes it possible to obtain apparently higher than normal levels in isolated blood samples. In instances of marginally elevated values, assays should be repeated so that the level of repetitive values can be determined. Morning fasting levels are more reliable than those found later in the day.

When the prolactin concentration rises above 100 ng/ml (normal <25 ng/ml), the possibility of prolactin secretion of micro- (smaller than 10 mm) or macroadenomata must be considered.

Evaluation of the Hyperprolactinemic Patient

Patients who show a lesser elevation of prolactin associated with infertility and ovulation defects must be evaluated to eliminate the possibility of premature ovarian failure.

When higher values (>100 ng/ml) are present, scans of the sella turcica are indicated to detect the possible presence of pituitary adenomas. Study of visual fields will help determine optic nerve compression from larger tumors. Patients with elevated prolactin levels may or may not show concomitant galactorrhea.

Treatment of Hyperprolactinemia and Pituitary Adenoma

In those patients who show only modest elevations of prolactin levels and in whom there are no indices of pituitary tumors, treatment with bromocriptine is as follows. When there is evidence of tumor, either micro- or macroadenoma, other considerations must be taken into account. Beginning in the early 1970s,[12-14] transphenoidal removal of the tumor became an effective means of treatment for many cases. Larger tumors had lower cure rates, and the infertile woman often failed to achieve normal prolactin levels or restored fertility. It soon became apparent that treatment with bromocriptine was capable of reducing prolactin synthesis as well as tumor growth and size in these patients. Bromocriptine has become the treatment of choice in women with ovulatory defects associated with hyperprolactinemia with or without pituitary adenomata.[15-17]

Treatment Method and Schedules

To accommodate for the short half-life and the physiologic pulsatile nature of its secretion, GnRH is best administered by pulsatile infusion pumps. These computerized, programmable pumps deliver desired doses at predetermined intervals. Effective induction of ovulation results when pulses vary between 2.5 and 20 μg GnRH with a frequency of 60–120 min. *Via* the pulsatile pump, the GnRH is delivered through a small subcutaneous needle fixed in place for the duration of the treatment.

This method of delivering medication is cumbersome and awkward but to date appears to be the best method for utilizing GnRH. Until pharmacologic improvements are made, it will have to do.

Other Uses

Other potential uses of GnRH and its analogues include male and female contraception, control of endometriosis and other gonadal steroid-responsive neoplasias, and the treatment of precocious puberty.

Pharmacology

Bromocriptine is a dopamine receptor agonist capable of activating postsynaptic dopamine reactors. It effectively reduces serum prolactin levels in hyperprolactinemic patients. Bromocriptine suppresses lactation in physiologically lactating women. This nonhormonal, nonestrogenic substance has little or no effect on pituitary hormones other than prolactin except for patients with acromegaly, in whom it lowers levels of growth hormone.

In patients with galactorrhea and amenorrhea, menses usually resume when lactation ceases and prolactin levels return to normal. Bromocriptine is effective when taken orally.

Treatment Schedules

Patients with ovulatory defects and infertility are treated essentially the same whether or not they exhibit galactorrhea. In the amenorrheic woman, bromocriptine 2.5 mg/day is given for the first week. This low dose is given initially to reduce the possibility of unpleasant side effects. These may be further reduced if the medication is taken at bedtime. After the first week and if side effects are not encountered, the dose is increased to 2.5 mg bid and continued daily until prolactin levels return to normal and menses resume. Occasionally the dose may need to be increased to 2.5 mg tid. After the resumption of menses, medication is continued until pregnancy results, as long as appropriate indices demonstrate that ovulation has occurred.

In some instances, ovulation may not return, even though prolactin levels have become normal. If this is the case, the administration of clomiphene in the usual dosage will generally be effective. If necessary, hCG can be supplemented as when clomiphene is given without bromocriptine.

Some women are reluctant to take bromocriptine, or for that matter any medication, if there is any possibility of pregnancy. After ovulation has been reestablished, bromocriptine can be given from the first day of the cycle and then interrupted after ovulation has occurred and resumed with the onset of the next menstrual period.

Whether given continuously or cyclically, the dose of bromocriptine can often be reduced to as little as 1.25 mg/day once ovulation has been reestablished and prolactin levels have returned to normal.

Side Effects

The dopamine effect of bromocriptine may be evident in side effects related to the cardiovascular and gastrointestinal systems. These may include headache and dizziness as well as nausea and diarrhea. Symptomatic hypotension can occur.

Management during Pregnancy

When pregnancy occurs, the medication should be discontinued. Particular attention during pregnancy must be given to those patients with pituitary adenomas. Recurrences of symptom-producing pituitary tumors during pregnancy have been reported,[16] and appropriate treatment may be required. This may consist of resumption of bromocriptine[18] or, in unusual circumstances, surgery.

Results

Almost all women who are anovulatory as a result of hyperprolactinemia will be made to ovulate with proper bromocriptine treatment. Pregnancies will therefore occur at a rate comparable to any group of ovulating women, taking into account the possibility of other factors (i.e., seminal, tubal) unrelated to hyperprolactinemia.

Of greater concern are the changes occurring in the associated pituitary tumors during the course of treatment. Bromocriptine reduces or arrests mitotic activity in adenomatous tissue; therefore, most pituitary tumors show a reduction in size during

treatment. Other symptoms such as visual-field disturbances are promptly relieved. Prolactin levels may begin to fall within 24 hr. Even large macroadenomas become smaller. Those that do not may be overhanging the edges of the sella turcica and are thus prevented from retracting.

The long-range effect of treatment of pituitary adenomas and its influence on their subsequent recurrence have not yet been fully evaluated.

SUMMARY

Effective therapeutic measures are available to induce ovulation in anovulatory women with physiologically responsive ovaries. Physicians undertaking these methods of treatment should be familiar with both the physiology of the deficiencies responsible for the ovulation defects and the pharmacology of the agents used for their correction. In addition to this specialized knowledge, some sophisticated laboratory and other diagnostic tools may be essential to the proper conduct of that treatment. Failure to use these adjuvant modalities may subject patients to unnecessary and serious complications. This is particularly true when undertaking the administration of hMG.

Clomiphene is an unusually effective drug for the induction of ovulation in a wide variety of anovulatory situations. It has the added benefit of being an extremely safe drug. Its use as a "fertility drug" to enhance the fecundity of patients without regard to the cause for their failure to conceive is unwarranted and unjustified. Such practice will seldom lead to pregnancy except by random chance. When used for properly selected patients, however, it represents probably the most valuable therapeutic tool available to the infertile, anovulatory woman.

Bromocriptine is a more recently accepted drug that offers a specific solution to a formerly poorly recognized and insoluble problem in hyperprolactinemic women. Careful diagnosis is again essential, and empiric prescriptions for undefined conditions represents a disservice.

GnRH is at the threshold of the therapeutic arena and only awaits significant refinements to make clinical application more acceptable and practical.

QUESTIONS

1. What is the major side effect of clomiphene citrate that may make it an undesirable agent for use in the "normal infertile" woman?

2. With excessively elevated estradiol levels during hMG induction of ovulation, how can hyperstimulation syndrome be prevented?

3. What are the effects of bromocryptine on pituitary microadenomas with hyperprolactinemia?

REFERENCES

1. Stahler E, Strum G, Dawme E: Direktwirkung von Clomiphen auf das Ovar. Untersucht am In Vitro Perfundierten Menschlichen Ovar. *Arch Gynak* 219:585, 1975
2. Garcia J, Jones GS, Wentz AC: The use of clomiphene citrate. *Fertil Steril* 28:707, 1977*
3. Lobo RA, Gysler M, March CM, et al: Clinical and laboratory predictors of clomiphene response. *Fertil Steril* 37:168, 1982*
4. Gorlitsky G, Kase NG, Speroff L: Ovulation and pregnancy rate with clomiphene citrate. *Obstet Gynecol* 51:265, 1978
5. March CM, Tredway DR, Mishel, DR Jr: Effect of clomiphene citrate upon amount and duration of human menopausal gonadotropin therapy. *Am J Obstet Gynecol* 125:699, 1976
6. Campbell HJ, Feurer G, Garcia J, et al: The infusion of brain extracts into the anterior pituitary gland and the secretion of gonadotrophic hormone. *J Physiol (Lond)* 157:1661, 1960
7. McCann SM, Talesnik S, Friedman H: LH releasing activity in hypothalamic extracts. *Proc Soc Exp Biol Med* 104:432, 1960
8. Matsuao H, Baba Y, Nair RMG, et al: Structure of the porcine LH and FSH releasing factor. *Biochem Biophys Res Commun* 43:1334, 1971
9. Birgus R, Butcher M, Ling N, et al: Structure du moléculaire du facteur hypothalamique (LRF) et l'origine ovine controlant la secretion de l'hormone gonadotrope hypophysaire de luteinisation (LH). *CR Acad Sci (D) (Paris)* 273:1611, 1971

*Review article or chapter.

10. Taymor ML: The use of luteinizing hormone-releasing hormone in Gynecology. *Obstet Gynecol Ann* 7:285, 1978*
11. Liu JH, Durfee R, Muse K, et al: Induction of multiple ovulation by pulsatile administration of gonadotropin-releasing hormone. *Fertil Steril* 40:18, 1983
12. Keye WR Jr, Chang RJ, Monroe SE, et al: Prolactin secreting adenomas in women II. Menstrual function, pituitary reserve and prolactin production following micro surgical removal. *Am J Obstet Gynecol* 134:360, 1979
13. Wiebe RH, Kramer RS, Hammond CB: Surgical treatment of prolactin-secreting micro adenomas. *Am J Obstet Gynecol* 134:49, 1979
14. Domingue JN, Richmond IL, Wilson CB: Results of surgery in 114 patients with prolactin-secreting pituitary adenomas. *Am J Obstet Gynecol* 137:102, 1980
15. McGregor AM, Scanlon MF, Hall R, et al: Effects of bromocriptine on pituitary size. *Br Med J* 2:700, 1979
16. Corenblum B: Successful outcome of ergocriptine-induced pregnancies in twenty-one women with prolactin-secreting pituitary adenomas. *Fertil Steril* 32:183, 1979
17. Hancock KW, Lamb JT, Gibson RM, et al: Conservative management of pituitary prolactinomas: Evidence of bromocriptine-induced regression. *Br J Obstet Gynaecol* 87:523, 1980*
18. Bergh T, Nillius SJ, Wide L: Clinical course and outcome of pregnancies in amenorrhoeic women with hyperprolactinaemia and pituitary tumours. *Br Med J* 1:875, 1978*

ANSWERS

1. The antiestrogen effect of clomiphene tends to make otherwise normal cervical mucus thick and tenacious and prevents its penetration by sperm.

2. Withhold hCG when estradiol levels appear too high.

3. Return to normal levels of prolactin, reduction in size of the microadenoma and restoration of fertility.

In Vitro Fertilization

A. A. ACOSTA, Z. ROSENWAKS, S. J. MUASHER, and J. GARCIA

INTRODUCTION AND OVERVIEW

In vitro fertilization (IVF) and pre-embryo replacement in the donor is one of several techniques now available or under consideration from a large therapeutic armamentarium for the treatment of the infertile couple. Other related techniques include (1) in vivo fertilization of oocytes obtained by superovulation, followed by pre-embryo transfer into synchronized recipients; (2) IVF followed by transfer of fresh or cryopreserved pre-embryos into another recipient (synchronization is necessary when a fresh pre-embryo is transferred); and (3) oocyte replacement into the uterine cavity, accompanied by previous or subsequent insemination (natural or artificial).

Because of the complexity of IVF programs in medical, legal, bioethical, technical, and other aspects, they should be considered and made available only by professionals who possess formal and extensive training and experience in the whole field of reproductive endocrinology and who have high-level laboratory facilities adequate for such complex therapeutic methods.

A. A. ACOSTA, Z. ROSENWAKS, and S. J. MUASHER • Department of Obstetrics and Gynecology, Eastern Virginia Medical School, Norfolk, Virginia 23507. J. GARCIA • Women's Hospital Fertility Center and IVF Program, Greater Baltimore Medical Center, Towson, Maryland 21204.

In every IVF program, there are several aspects to be considered: development of new clinical laboratory techniques, use of the tremendous potential for research that this kind of project generates, and provision for the high quality of training for reproductive endocrinologists.

The population requesting IVF services in every clinic is rapidly increasing, with applications from new patients and recycling of former patients, who had failures in previous attempts. New patients require careful screening from a medical point of view as well as for establishing the availability of the ovaries for translaparoscopic oocyte retrieval. With the possibility of new techniques for retrieval (ultrasonically guided transabdominal–transvesical, transurethral–transvesical, and transvaginal procedures), however, ovaries that are not available through the laparoscope can also be reached.

Different categories of patients are now being accepted into IVF programs: (1) patients with severe nonreparable tubal damage, absence of gonads and germ cells, or normal ovaries but absent uterus; and (2) patients who have not responded to conventional therapy for endometriosis, idiopathic fertility, intractable cervical mucus abnormalities, or the male factor.

The assisted recruitment of oocytes for fertilization requires careful stimulation and cycle monitoring in order to maximize the number of oocytes obtained without deterioration of quality. It has been our experience that standard, routine protocols cannot be used without paying the price in lower success and higher cancellation rates.

Different types of ovarian stimulation have been proposed, including the use of clomiphene citrate (CC), alone or in different combinations with human menopausal gondotropin (hMG) and pure follicle-stimulating hormone (FSH), followed by the ovulatory-triggering dose of human chorionic gonadotropin (hCG), a surrogate luteinizing hormone (LH) surge.

Monitoring these stimulated cycles requires the use of rapid hormonal assays to follow the endocrine ovarian response; daily examination of the estrogen target organs, such as cervical mucus (score) and vaginal epithelium (karyopyknotic index), to check on the biologic response of the patient; and finally ultrasonographic assessment of follicle growth to check on the morphologic response of the ovaries. After ovarian stimulation has been successfully performed, oocyte retrieval is carried out by any of the approaches mentioned above.

After insemination, successful fertilization and cleavage, pre-embryo transfer is carried out in the same surgical environment in which retrieval was performed. If pregnancy is achieved, careful monitoring of the early stages is required until a normal gestation is demonstrated. Routine obstetric care is then used in the follow-up of these patients.

Babies born by the IVF procedure, at least at present, are given a careful pediatric follow-up, including tests of physical and psychological development. A registry of babies born through IVF and pre-embryo transfer, or any of the variants mentioned, is being organized. Patients who fail at one of the steps described above (ovarian stimulation, oocyte retrieval, pre-embryo transfer) or who do not achieve a pregnancy are recycled into the program.

The different stages of this therapeutic method require a well-equipped endocrine laboratory to perform the rapid hormone assays, expert nursing care in the clinical and surgical fields, and an able embryology laboratory, which is a key part of the process. In the Norfolk program, the andrology laboratory also plays a major role, not only in investigating the male factor but also in performing support studies of quality control, which should be done routinely and meticulously to enhance the success rates.

The amount of information collected through IVF programs, including clinical and basic research data on the menstrual cycle, ovulation induction,

gamete physiology and interaction, and the early stages of embryo development and implantation, is overwhelming; a tremendous amount of literature has been published, based on these data. Information accumulated during the performance of these procedures should be carefully stored for future clinical use and research purposes. A special computerized program has been designed for this purpose in Norfolk. Worldwide interest in these programs is clearly demonstrated by the increasing demand for training in both the clinical and research aspects.

The constant development of new techniques, the need for pre-embryo manipulation, and the rapidly changing conditions in the fields of reproductive physiology and treatment of infertility have created ethical problems that need careful research and scrutiny before any modifications are introduced into the therapeutic modalities. It is important to emphasize the complexity of these programs, as well as their multidisciplinary nature, so that physicians and scientists introduced to these therapeutic procedures will not be surprised or discouraged by the multiple requirements and difficulties.

As a result of the availability of IVF and other modalities of assisted reproduction, several approaches to therapy in obstetrics and gynecology have changed. Every effort should be made to preserve the ovaries and uterus in women with benign pelvic pathology in order to preserve reproductive capabilities using the new procedures.

HISTORICAL BACKGROUND

Efforts to fertilize laboratory animal oocytes in vitro apparently began during the latter half of the nineteenth century, when Schenk reported fertilization and cleavage in culture of rabbit and guinea pig oocytes. No effort was made to establish a pregnancy at that time, however. The first documented in vivo fertilization followed by pre-embryo transfer and successful pregnancy was published by Heape[1] in 1890, but there is evidence that efforts had been made as early as 50 years before that successful experiment was conducted.

Austin,[2] in 1951, published some observations on the penetration of sperm into the mammalian egg, almost at the same time that Chang[3] described the need for "sperm capacitation" to achieve fertilization in vitro.

After all this information had become available, McLaren and Biggers,[4] in 1959, and Chang,[5] in

1959, were successful in accomplishing fertilization in vivo—followed by pre-embryo transfer and pregnancy—of mouse ova and fertilization in vitro of rabbit ova.

Brinster and Biggers,[6] in 1965, succeeded in fertilizing oocytes in vitro in explanted oviducts of mice; Whittingham,[7] in 1968, developed a culture medium in which IVF of mouse oocytes could be successfully accomplished.

Veterinarians, through the use of superovulation, in vivo fertilization, and surgical or nonsurgical pre-embryo transfer, have accumulated extensive experience in this field.

The first efforts in human subjects were made by Edwards et al. in 1965 and 1966,[8,9] followed by successful experiences during the 1970s.[10] When pre-embryo transfer was accomplished in humans, the same inefficiency of the natural reproductive cycle in animals was observed. It was not until July 25, 1978, that the first successful term pregnancy was delivered in England, followed by a second one in 1979.[11] A third baby was born in Australia on June 3, 1980.[12] The first program in the United States was officially started at the Eastern Virginia Medical School in March 1980, after 2 years of preparation and planning. The first term baby was delivered by cesarean section in Norfolk General Hospital on December 28, 1981.

Inability to retrieve oocytes through laparoscopy because of pelvic adhesions and the availability of percutaneous ultrasonically guided needle puncture, as well as the tranvaginal and transurethral–transvesical approaches, has prompted groups in Europe to use these techniques for oocyte retrieval. Several centers are now using these procedures routinely,[13–16] and some of them are trying to abandon laparoscopy as the routine technique.

It was believed that cryopreservation, extensively used in the past for semen samples, could be useful for pre-embryos. Pierre Soupart, among others, began working in the cryopreservation of pre-embryos with the idea of transferring them to the donor in subsequent cycles. The group at Monash University in Melbourne made extensive use of this technique to achieve successful pregnancies in the donor and in a surrogate mother. A recent symposium in Vienna (April, 1986) was organized to update this technique and to report the initial results.[17]

Other procedures have been proposed to overcome infertility in women with tubal problems or unable to produce oocytes. Fresh oocyte donation, followed by IVF and pre-embryo transfer to the patient/recipient, has also been used successfully by the Monash group. Uterine lavage, an alternate technique of pre-embryo donation, was developed at the Los Angeles County Harbor General Hospital (UCLA Medical School), with pregnancies resulting. In this method, donor eggs are artificially fertilized with the sperm of the patient's husband, flushed from the donor's uterus, and transferred to the patient's uterus. The Norfolk program established a successful donor oocyte project in 1985.

These new techniques have created medical, legal, and ethical problems that must be carefully studied and resolved before the techniques are widely adopted. The Ethics Committee of the American Fertility Society is preparing a full report on these ethical issues in reproductive medicine; the report will be released in September 1986.

PHYSIOLOGIC PRINCIPLES EMPLOYED

Fertilization of a natural oocyte by a spermatozoon occurs at the ampulla of the fallopian tube. This phenomenon is preceded by several physiologic events: (1) selection and development of dominant follicle, (2) triggering of the ovulatory LH and FSH mid-cycle peak through an intact hypothalamic–pituitary axis, (3) oocyte pickup by the fallopian tube, (4) sperm transport through normal endocervical–endometrial endosalpinx and tubal cavities, followed by (5) the presence of an adequate number of spermatozoa, with adequate ability to penetrate and fertilize the oocyte.

Abnormalities in any one of these physiologic events may cause fertilization to fail. The therapeutic method to be applied depends on the etiologic diagnosis of infertility. IVF can be used in the treatment of several abnormalities. This chapter refers primarily to the classic type of IVF with pre-embryo transfer, as used in the Norfolk program.

The indications for IVF have enlarged to include many factors not responding to routine treatment: male and female immunologic problems; intractable cervical mucus hostility; endometriosis; anomalies of the female genital tract, especially those due to exposure to diethylstilbestrol (DES); unexplained infertility (normal infertile couples); and the initial indication of irreparable tubal damage.

CLINICAL METHODS AND PROCEDURES

Patient Selection

Candidates for IVF should be patients in good general health. In our program the age of 40 has been set as a limit for admission.[18] Since it has been demonstrated that although these patients may respond well to stimulation, and fertilization may occur in an adequate number of oocytes, the obstetric outcome shows a very high number of pregnancy losses which, in our program, has reached 66%. Advanced age also carries an increased risk of chromosomal abnormalities.

At the beginning of the IVF procedure, the natural cycle was used and recommended for oocyte retrieval; normality of the menstrual cycle was originally a requirement for patient admission into programs, including the Norfolk program. As experience increased, it became obvious that the pregnancy rate with the natural cycle was very low, and therefore most programs began using stimulated cycles. Since then, minor menstrual irregularities have been found not to modify results, because ovulation stimulation, as used in most programs, can overcome these problems. However, patients with an abnormal pituitary–ovarian axis function (polycystic ovarian disease and variants) have proved to be very difficult to stimulate with any of the current protocols.

A hysterogram is requested of all patients in order to ascertain the presence of a normal endometrial cavity capable of carrying a pregnancy to term. Evaluation of the patient also includes a general physical and pelvic examination. Special laboratory tests are obtained only when indicated by the medical history. A screening laparoscopy is performed on patients with a history of pelvic inflammatory disease (PID) and/or several surgical procedures, in whom there is a strong suspicion of the ovaries being covered by adhesions, hence unavailable. The presence or absence of the fallopian tubes, the presence and extent of adhesions or endometriosis, the existence of any other type of pathology that might interfere with aspiration of the follicles, and the anatomy of the pelvic organs should be recorded. This information is useful not only at the time of retrieval and transfer but also during the ultrasonic monitoring of ovulation stimulation; it helps interpret the structures that are visualized with ultrasonography. It is also useful to determine, once the follicles develop, whether they are present predominantly in the ovary which is available, in patients with asymmetric pathology. In the Norfolk program, 5% of applicants show adhesions, precluding translaparoscopic access to the ovaries.

In some of those cases, before the availability of techniques now used for ovaries inaccessible by laparoscopy, a laparotomy with pelvic recon-

structive surgery was performed with good success. During the procedure, lysis of adhesions, removal of the fallopian tubes if present and nonfunctional, mobilization of the ovaries with uterine cornual or round ligament suspension, and uterine suspension were performed. The procedure had to be done meticulously and was helpful in 90% of cases.[19]

A detailed semen analysis of the husband is essential before patients are admitted into the program. Bacteriologic investigation of the seminal plasma, determination of acrosin and adenosine triphosphate (ATP) levels, and immunologic studies are carried out. In infertility due to the male factor, the male patient has a complete physical and urologic evaluation, and further testing is added to the routine protocol, namely, a separation of the motile fraction and a hamster zona-free oocyte penetration test.

Patient Monitoring

The final goal of patient monitoring is to maximize the number of mature (preovulatory) oocytes obtained, while minimizing the risk of impairing their quality.

THE NATURAL CYCLE

The first successful IVF attempt ending in the delivery of the first baby born through this procedure was the result of using the natural cycle.[11] As a consequence, Steptoe et al. recommended the natural cycle as the ideal source of oocytes, since stimulated cycles used before had produced no pregnancies. Similar results were reported by the Australian group. The cycle was monitored by daily urinary determinations to identify the mid-cycle LH surge, utilizing the commercially available Hi-Gonavis test. Laparoscopy was carried out 26 hr later to aspirate the single preovulatory follicle. The Norfolk program used the natural cycle in 1980. To predict ovulation, the patient was monitored daily by (1) determination of the karyopyknotic index in a fresh vaginal smear, (2) evaluation of the cervical mucus until changes were obtained that were considered indicative of adequate estrogen levels (clinical shift); the criteria used to consider the cervical mucus adequate were a volume >0.2 ml, a spinnbarkeit > 10 cm, and ferning of 4 +, (3) pelvic ultrasound to measure the diameter of the dominant follicle, and (4) serum estradiol (E_2) and LH levels. The frequency of LH determinations was

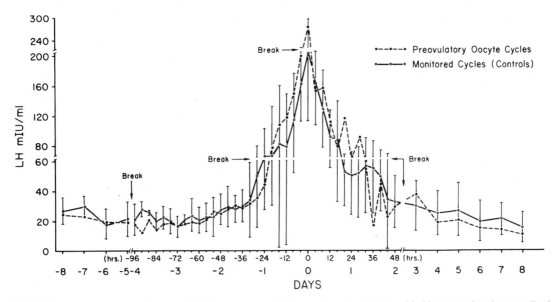

FIGURE 32-1. Daily and every 4 hr serum luteinizing hormone (LH) levels from day -8 to day +8 in 50 menstrual cycles normalized to the day of the LH peak. Solid bar: (—) cycles before retrieval cycle (controls); (---) cycles in which preovulatory eggs were retrieved. (From Garcia.[28])

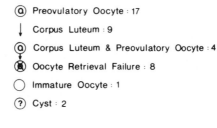

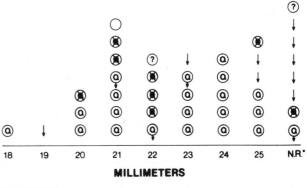

FIGURE 32-2. Follicle diameter by ultrasound in 41 natural cycles aspirated for in vitro fertilization. (From Garcia.[28])

*Not Reliable.

increased by taking blood samples every 4 hr when ovulation was considered imminent, in order to detect the ascending limb of the LH surge (Fig. 32-1). Laparoscopy and oocyte aspiration were performed at 28.5 hr from the ascending limb of the LH surge. It was determined that a true ascending limb was detected when levels were >50 mIU/ml. Preovulatory oocytes were obtained from follicles with a diameter varying from 18 to 25 mm (Fig. 32-2).

STIMULATION OF OVULATION

The term *stimulation of ovulation* is used in this chapter to indicate that treatment is given to normally ovulating and menstruating women to enhance the number of follicles produced during the cycle, as opposed to ovulation induction, in which treatment is given to anovulatory patients. Ovulation stimulation for IVF was attempted unsuccessfully during the 1970s; it was therefore abandoned and was not recommended. It was not until 1981 that different ovulation stimulation protocols were developed and adopted by various IVF groups.

Clomiphene Citrate and Spontaneous LH Surge

This is one of the most widely used protocols for stimulation of ovulation in IVF. The patient receives CC 50–150 mg/day for 5 days, beginning on day 2, 3, or 5 of the spontaneous menstrual cycle.[20-22] Follicular development is monitored by ultrasound alone or in combination with urinary or serum E_2 determinations and with urinary or serum LH assays, in order to detect the spontaneous LH surge. Laparoscopy for oocyte retrieval is usually scheduled 24–26 hr after the beginning of the LH surge (ascending limb). An average of 2.1 preovulatory oocytes are recovered per cycle with this procedure. Some disadvantages are the uncertainty of patient response, the need for monitoring every 4 hr in order to detect the LH surge (since in many instances it is triggered unexpectedly), and cancellation of 25–40% of cycles because of inadequate response or premature LH surge.

Clomiphene Citrate plus hCG as LH Surge Surrogate

CC is administered as indicated above. In addition, human chorionic gonadotropin (hCG) is administered when the ultrasound shows that the

diameter of the largest follicle is 18–20 mm or when the serum E_2 levels plateau.[22-26] The exogenous gonadotropins replace the endogenous LH surge. Laparoscopy is carried out 34–38 hr later.[27] A spontaneous LH surge may still occur, anticipating the hCG injection: If it is detected, laparoscopy should be scheduled 24–26 hr from the beginning of the surge; otherwise, the cycle must be cancelled.

Clomiphene Citrate plus hMG/hCG

Edwards adopted and modified Kistner's ovulation induction protocol[28] to be used in ovulation induction for IVF. CC (100 mg) is administered for 5–7 days, beginning on day 2 of the menstrual cycle, along with human menopausal gonadotropin (hMG). hMG is continued for three or four doses after the last CC administration. Patients are monitored by ultrasound or daily urinary or serum E_2 and/or LH determinations.[29] Lopata[30] reported better success with an individualized regimen based on the E_2 profile, and an expected LH surge still occurred. Therefore, early laparoscopy or cancellation has to be considered.

hMG/hCG

This protocol was designed by the Norfolk program in 1981. Two ampules of hMG (75 IU of LH/75 IU of FSH per ampule) are administered IM daily, starting on day 3 or 5 of the cycle, according to the length of the natural menstrual cycle (28 or 35 days).[31,32] Patients are monitored by (1) daily serum E_2 determinations, (2) daily ultrasound to estimate follicular development, and (3) daily pelvic examinations to obtain a karyopyknotic index at the vaginal level and an evaluation of the cervical mucus, beginning on day 3 of stimulation.

Three types of response to hMG have been described according to the serum E_2 level at the time hMG is discontinued. In the low responders, the E_2 levels are below 300 pg/ml; in the normal responders, the levels are usually 300–600 pg/ml; in the high responders, the levels are above 601 pg/ml.

The response of the target organs is considered adequate when changes at the karyopyknotic index level and at the cervical mucus level indicate a clinical shift, respresented by (1) a karyopyknotic index of 30% or more, (2) cervical mucus in an amount above 0.15 ml, (3) spinnbarkeit above 10 cm, (4) ferning of 4+, (5) clear and acellular microscopic appearance of the cervical mucus, and (6) dilation of the external cervical os.

hMG is administered in an individualized regimen rather than in a fixed protocol in order to tailor the dose to each patient's E_2 response. In the low responders, hMG administration is discontinued when a clinical shift has occurred over 3 consecutive days; in the normal responders, it is discontinued on the first day of a clinical shift. In the high responders, it is discontinued as soon as the 600 pg/ml level is obtained, regardless of the biologic parameters, except when ultrasound reveals ovarian follicles smaller than 11 mm in diameter. Usually on the day hMG is discontinued, ultrasound shows follicles with an average diameter of 14 mm.

hCG (10,000 IU) is administered IM 50 hr after the last hMG injection (long interval). Patients with specific indications may receive hCG 29–33 hr after the last hMG injection (short interval). Laparoscopy is carried out 34–36 hr later. Jones et al.[33] described several E_2 patterns at the end of ovulation stimulation, each one carrying a difference in pregnancy rate (Fig. 32-3).

Pure FSH/hCG

Pure FSH (Metrodin, Serono) contains 75 units of FSH per ampule, with less than 1 IU of LH. The Norfolk Program began using pure FSH for ovulation stimulation in 1981.[34] The rationale for using it at the beginning of the cycle, either alone or in combination with hMG, is to improve the recruitment phase of stimulation and consequently to retrieve more oocytes. When pure FSH is used alone, the follicular phase seems to be slightly longer and therefore could indicate patients with a rapid response and consequently a very short follicular phase. It seems that patients stimulated in this fashion have less tendency to trigger a spontaneous LH surge. Patients with a polycystic ovary (PCO) type of hypothalamic–pituitary–ovarian axis may benefit from the use of pure FSH stimulation. It can also be used when the patient has failed to respond to other protocols.

Combination of FSH–hMG/hCG

Using the same rationale, the FSH/LH ratio is increased using this type of stimulation, in which 2 ampules of pure FSH plus 2 ampules of hMG are given during days 3 and 4 of the menstrual cycle in the typical protocol. Once the recruitment phase

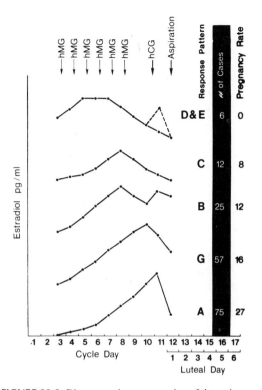

FIGURE 32-3. Diagrammatic representation of the various estradiol (E_2) patterns of response together with the number of cases in each pattern and the pregnancy rate by pattern. hcG, human chorionic gonadotropin; hMG, human menopausal gonadotropin; D&C; dilatation and curettage. (From Jones.[57])

terminates, stimulation is continued with 2 ampules of hMG alone. A long interval is usually used for the administration of hCG. The use of the combination protocol has several advantages: The mean number of preovulatory oocytes retrieved increases to 2.9–3.3; the fertilization rate is similar; the number of pre-embryos transferred is also increased; the cancellation rate is lower, and the number of low responders is also less. This protocol is now the routine stimulation used in the Norfolk program for new and repeat patients.

GnRH

Multiple follicular development has been reported after pulsatile administration of several doses of GnRH.[35] The experience with this stimulation in IVF is not extensive. Patients who failed to respond to the other protocols have occasionally responded to GnRH administered by pulsatile infusion. It has also been used for patients with a history of PCO or with hormonal evidence of impending ovarian failure (perimenopause) due to age or surgical trauma to the ovaries. The results are still preliminary, and no conclusions can be drawn.

OOCYTE RETRIEVAL AND ASPIRATION DEVICE

Several aspiration devices are described in the literature.[36–38] Minor differences can be seen in the type of trap and connecting tubes, needle length and gauge, and source of negative pressure. The trap is connected to a suction system set to generate a negative pressure of 100 mm Hg. In the Norfolk program a double-puncture laparoscopic technique has been used since the beginning, using an offset laparoscope with a 5-mm operating channel, through which the aspirating needle is passed. A Semm-type atraumatic grasping forceps is used for the intrapelvic maneuvers, especially to stabilize the ovary at the time of follicular puncture.

The Norfolk aspiration device consists of a 12-gauge needle (2.16 mm internal diameter) 43 cm in length, with a 45° blunt bevel. A small ring is placed 5 mm behind the tip of the needle to indicate the depth of penetration into the follicle and to seal the puncture site at the time of aspiration. The needle hub has one flat surface that indicates the direction in which the bevel is pointing. The needle attaches to one of the plastic tubes of the DeLee suction trap, which has a 20-ml capacity and is connected to 60-ml syringe by a second plastic tube, also provided by the manufacturer.[39] This device is capable of generating enough negative pressure for aspiration of the follicular fluid and oocyte (Fig. 32-4A,B).

Laparoscopy for follicular aspiration is done as an outpatient procedure under general endotracheal anesthesia.[40] The laparoscopy is performed in a routine fashion without vaginal, cervical, or intrauterine manipulation. Carbon dioxide (CO_2) is insufflated to create a pneumoperitoneum. The theoretical objection to the use of CO_2 is the potential change of follicular fluid pH; however, very little if any CO_2 gets into the device and therefore any change in pH is negligible. Two ml of Dulbecco's phophate-buffered saline is placed into the trap before follicular aspiration and an additional 2 ml is used to flush the system after aspiration. This technique tends to stabilize the pH even when CO_2 accidentally enters the trap. The aspiration procedure is monitored by a television camera attached to the laparoscope; this permits all members of the team to coordinate the procedure.

A routine inspection of the pelvic cavity is carried out during laparoscopy; special attention is given to the amount and characteristics of the peritoneal fluid. If it is hemorrhagic, it may indicate that ovulation has already occurred, and prompt aspiration of the cul-de-sac fluid is necessary to retrieve the extruded oocyte and to prevent its exposure to the CO_2 present in the abdominal cavity. The ovaries should then be inspected carefully, with a search for the presence of a fresh corpus luteum. If ovulation has occurred, the corpus luteum is irrigated immediately, since in many instances the oocyte is still inside the follicle. If a functional fallopian tube is present, the ampullary portion should be irrigated as well, in case the oocyte has already been picked up by the tube. Early ovulation occurs in about 10% of patients after administration of hMG/hCG.

Follicular aspiration is carried out, ideally starting with the largest follicle. After each aspiration, the follicle is immediately irrigated with 4 ml Dulbecco's buffer solution at pH 7.4. In 92% of aspirations, the oocyte is obtained in the original fluid, but in approximately 8%, it is recovered in the first or second follicular wash. All the follicles should be aspirated, since preovulatory oocytes have been recovered from small follicles (9–10 mm in diameter). Immature oocytes that are recovered have an 83% chance of in vitro maturation.[41] By contrast, in some IVF programs, only follicles that measure more than 15 mm in diameter are aspirated.[25]

Oocytes can be recovered in laparotomy.[42] Lately, different approaches to oocyte retrieval have been described in the literature (transabdominal–transvesical, transvaginal, and transurethral–transvesical).[13,14,43] The Norfolk program has utilized only the transabdominal–transvesical procedure to retrieve oocytes from ovaries that are not available for the translaparoscopic approach. Although the number of oocytes retrieved is smaller, the final results have been quite similar (Table I).

FOLLICULAR FLUID AND OOCYTE CHARACTERISTICS AT ASPIRATION

The follicular fluid volume correlates very well with the diameter of the follicle.[44] Normally, the fluid is straw colored with a pH of 7.2–7.4. The fluid hormonal milieu depends on the degree of

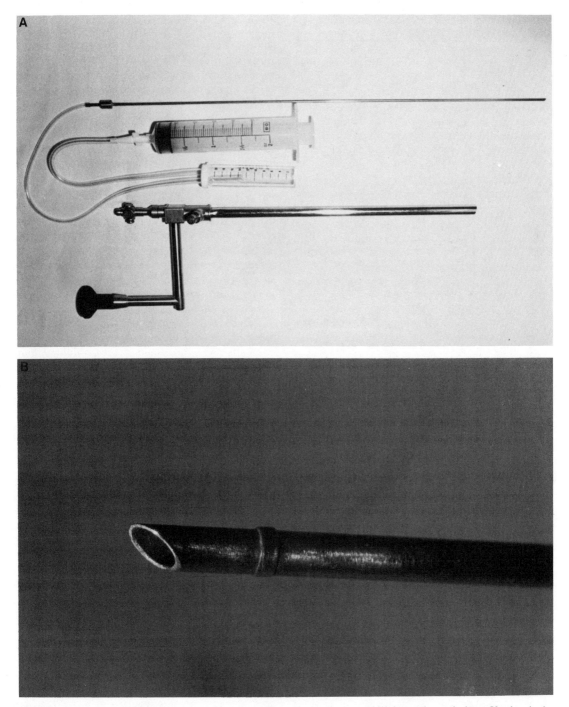

FIGURE 32-4. (A) Upper, photograph of an aspirating needle attached to the trap, which in turn is attached to a 50-ml aspirating syringe. Lower, offset laparoscope through which the aspirating needle can be passed. (B) Photograph of the tip of the aspirating needle showing the 45° bevel with a relatively blunt point and a band 5 mm from the distal tip of the needle. (From Jones.[34])

TABLE 32-1. Norfolk Program Transabdominal-Transvesical Oocyte Retrieval Results: Series 17–21 (November 1984–December 1985)

Patients	25		
One treatment cycle	17		
More than one treatment cycle	8	6	2 attempts
		2	4 attempts
Transvesical approach only	23		
Transvesical and laparoscopy combined	2		
Cycles (transvesical approach only)	35		
Follicles punctured	131		
Follicles punctured/cycle	3.74		
Oocytes retrived	95		
Oocytes/cycle	2.71		
Oocytes/follicle	0.72		
Fertilization rate (P.O. oocytes)	85%		
Transfers	29		
Transfer rate/cycle	82%		
Pregnancies	6	1 singleton (born)	
		1 set twins (born)	
		1 ectopic	
		3 ongoing	
Pregnancy rate/cycle	17%		
Pregnancy rate/transfer	20.68%		

follicular maturation. A high concentration of E_2 characterizes the mature follicle; progesterone (P) is on the rise and 17-hydroxyprogesterone, FSH, and LH are also present. By contrast, these follicles have a low concentration of Δ^4-androstenedione, oocyte maturation inhibitor (OMI), luteinization inhibitor (LI), and inhibin.[45–52] High levels of androstenedione and OMI are present in follicular fluid from immature or degenerating follicles.

The stage of follicular oocyte maturation is determined by microscopic scanning at the time of retrieval, using either a dissecting or an inverted microscope. The oocyte is usually found in a matter of seconds after the fluid arrives at the laboratory, although occasionally it may take longer.

The morphologic characteristics of the cumulus and the corona cell layers, the appearance of the ooplasm, the presence of a germinal vesicle or polar body, and the appearance of the membrana granulosa cells are the criteria by which the stage of oocyte maturation is classified.[53] Mature or preovulatory oocytes present expanded cumulus and corona radiata, a clear and regular ooplasm, a first polar body visible under the cell mass, and mature,

round, and loose membrana granulosa cells (Fig. 32-5). The presence of a polar body is a good indicator to classify an oocyte as preovulatory, metaphase II (M II). Some other kinds of preovulatory-appearing oocytes do not show the presence of a polar body and are still in metaphase I (MI), since the germinal vesicle has already disappeared. Some M II oocytes extrude the first polar body within 15 hr of retrieval and are considered mature; others take a longer period of time to extrude the first polar body and are considered as M I (immature) oocytes. Immature oocytes may or may not lack cumulus, the corona cells are almost always compact, and a germinal vesicle is present (Fig. 32-6). An atretic or degenerated oocyte displays a contracted, misshapen, dark (brown-black) ooplasm (Fig. 32-7). Postmature oocytes sometimes present with very well-expanded cumulus or corona radiata but with a defective, ruptured zona pellucida, through which the oocyte can be partially or totally extruded (ghost zona). Our program has named those oocytes "fractured zona" (Fig. 32-8).[54]

Mature granulosa cells are large and loosely aggregated; they exhibit some degree of luteinization. The cells are well dispersed in the fluid of preovulatory follicles. By contrast, immature granulosa cells are compact and shed in sheets and have a rather scanty cytoplasm.

A semen sample is obtained, after a 3–5-day period of sexual abstinence, immediately after laparoscopy is performed or 2–4 hr thereafter, depending on the stage of maturation of the oocytes retrieved. Semen is allowed to liquify at room temperature, and in the normal male only 1 ml is diluted with 2 ml insemination medium, Ham's F–10 with 7.5% fetal cord serum (FCS). It is mixed and centrifuged for 10 min. The supernatant is then discarded and the pellet resuspended and centrifuged as before. The procedure is repeated twice. The sperm are then incubated for 60 min in an atmosphere of 5% CO_2 in air. Finally, the supernatant containing the motile fraction of sperm is removed. Sperm concentration and motility are determined. A final concentration of 50,000 motile sperm/ml of insemination fluid (total of 3 ml) is added to the oocyte.

The preovulatory oocytes are inseminated after a period of in vitro preincubation. The preincubation time depends upon the maturity of the ooytes, established at aspiration.[55,56] Immature oocytes undergo in vitro maturation after a long preincubation of 22–36 hr.[41]

Several culture media have been used for IVF,

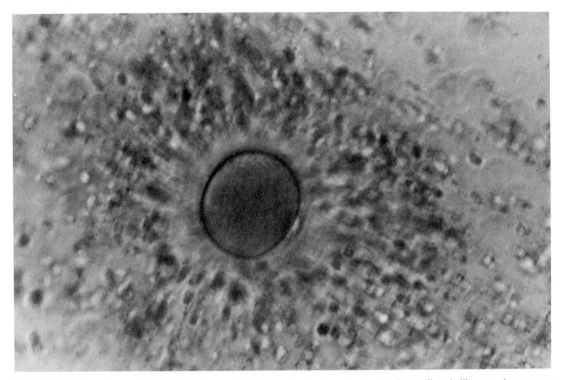

FIGURE 32-5. Preovulatory oocyte. Photomicrograph showing the corona radiata, granulosa cells, vitelline membrane, zona pellucida, and first polar body. (x100)

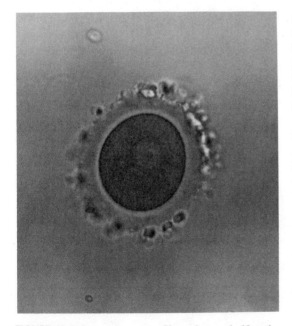

FIGURE 32-6. Immature oocytes. Photomicrograph. Note the presence of the germinal vesicle and compactness of the corona around the zona pellucida. (X100)

most of them supplemented with inactivated maternal blood serum. The insemination medium used in the Norfolk program consists of Ham's F-10 supplemented by 7.5% heat-inactivated FCS; 3 ml of medium/oocyte is used in the organ culture dish. Incubation is always carried out in an atmosphere of 5% CO_2 in air with 98% humidity.

A total of 150,000 spermatozoa are put into contact with each oocyte for an interval of 12–18 hr. After fertilization, the oocytes are transported to fresh culture medium, supplemented with a higher concentration of human FCS (15%), now referred to as growth medium.

The presence of two pronuclei or the extrusion of a second polar body is the parameter required to ascertain fertilization (Fig. 32-9).[57] The presence of three or more pronuclei (polyspermia) occurs in 9.3% of all fertilized oocytes in our program (Fig. 32-10). Mechanical dispersion of the cumulus is therefore carefully carried out when the oocyte is still heavily covered by the cumulus, so that the number of pronuclei can be seen.

The fertilized oocytes are then replaced in the incubator. No further evaluation is done for 24 hr.

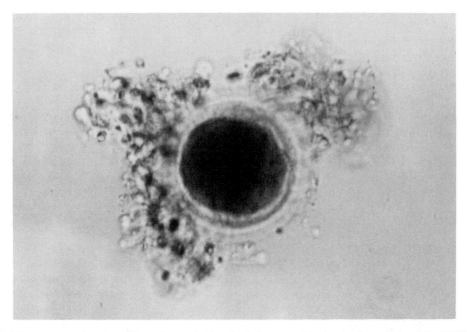

FIGURE 32-7. Atretic oocyte. Photomicrograph. Note the dark, retracted ooplasm and germinal vesicle. (X100)

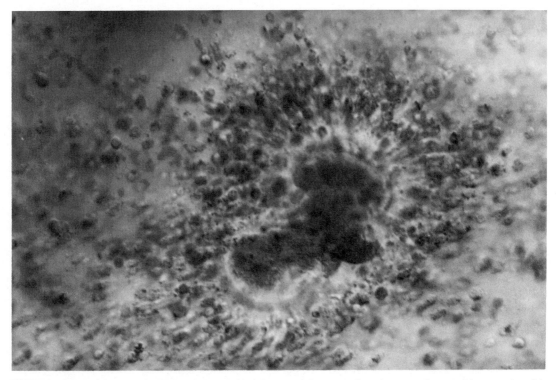

FIGURE 32-8. Fracture zona oocyte. Photomicrograph. Note the expanded corona radiata, the ruptured zona and the protrusion of the ooplasm. (X100)

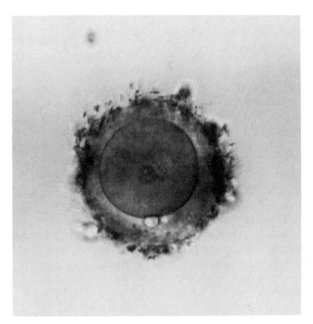

FIGURE 32-9. Two-pronuclei stage fertilized oocyte. Photomicrograph. Note the male and female pronuclei. The cumulus had been dispersed and several spermotozoa are still attached to the zona. (X100)

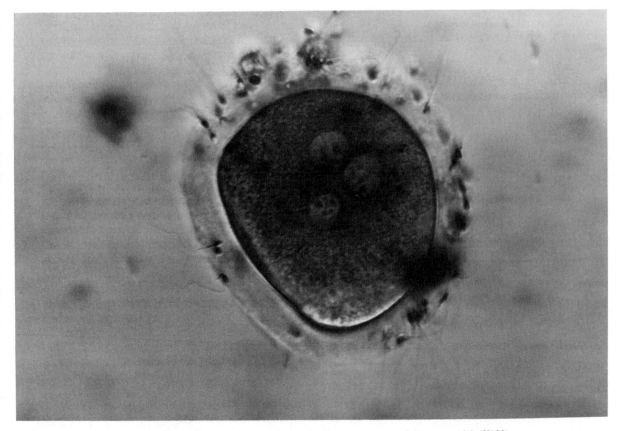

FIGURE 32-10. Polyspermia. Photomicrograph. Note the presence of three pronuclei. (X100)

A 4–8-cell pre-embryo is observed approximately 36–48 hr after insemination, and a 10–16-cell pre-embryo is observed at 48–72 hr (Figs. 32-11 and 32-12). Although it is desirable to observe pre-embryos that have cleaved as described, pregnancy has been obtained from concepti with slow or delayed cleavage. Pre-embryos with some degree of asymmetry and granular-appearing blastomeres are also capable of implanting and originating a viable pregnancy.

TRANSFER

Transcervical transfer is the only method used for pre-embryo transfer in humans. The procedure is usually performed 42–72 hr after insemination. However, pregnancies have been reported after transfers performed as early as 24 hr after insemination.

Pre-embryos are transferred to the endometrial cavity at any stage of cleavage, most commonly at the 4–8-cell stage. The pregnancy rate increases with the number of pre-embryos transferred, up to three or four and then reaches a plateau. Therefore, in the Norfolk program the maximum number of pre-embryos derived from preovulatory oocytes and transferred is 5. By limiting the number of concepti transferred, we try to compromise between increasing the pregnancy rate and decreasing the

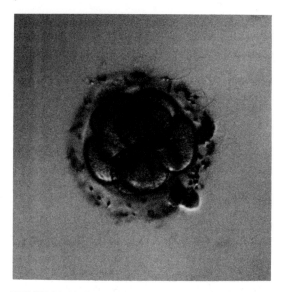

FIGURE 32-12. Seven- to eight-cell conceptus. Photomicrograph. Note that some spermotozoa are still attached to the zona. The cumulus is still attached to one side of the conceptus. (X100)

possibility of multiple pregnancies. The results in the Norfolk program from series 1–21 (1981–1985) are show in Table II. The total pregnancy rate ranges from 18% with a single pre-embryo transferred to 39% with five or more pre-embryos transferred.[58]

Several transfer devices have been described in the literature. The Norfolk program designed its own device, which consists of a Teflon catheter 46 cm in length and an inner diameter of 1.2 mm.[59] The tip of the catheter is solid and round, with a notch on one side, through which the pre-embryos are aspirated and ejected. The catheter is carried within a metal cannula that serves as a guide (Figs. 32-13 and 32-14).

During tranfer, the patient is placed in the knee–chest position. In a few cases when the uterus is retroverted and fixed, the transfer is performed in the dorsal-lithotomy position. The cervix may be grasped with a single-toothed tenaculum. The tip of the cannula is introduced approximately 1 cm into the endocervical canal, and the catheter is then advanced up to the fundus. When the top of the fundus is reached, it is withdrawn slightly and the pre-embryos are ejected in a small amount (50–90 μl) of growth medium.

The patient is requested to remain in bed in the prone position for approximately 4 hr after transfer; she is then released from the hospital with instruc-

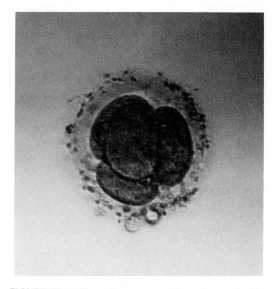

FIGURE 32-11. Four-cell conceptus. Photomicrograph. Note the regularity and symmetry of the blastomeres. (X100)

TABLE 32-2. Norfolk Series 1–21: Continuing Pregnancies by Number of Concepti Transferred

Number of concepti transferred	Number of transfer cycles	Transfers				% Continuing pregnancies
		% Total pregnancies (>6 weeks)	% Pregnancies (>8 weeks)	% Pregnancies (>12 weeks)	% Pregnancies (>26 weeks)	Total pregnancies
1	384	18	13	12	12	67
2	343	29	23	18	16	57
3	158	34	32	29	28	82
4	97	32	28	24	23	71
5+	96	39	35	21	21	54
Total	1078	27	22	18	17	65

tions to rest in bed until the next morning, when she resumes normal activities.

Blood samples to determine E_2 and P levels are drawn every other day during the luteal phase. Occasionally, luteal phase deficiencies occur after follicular aspiration, mainly when mild degrees of hyperstimulation have been induced during the follicular phase. Therefore, we empirically supplement the luteal phase in all patients, using a daily injection of P (25 mg IM), beginning on the day after laparoscopy and thus 1 day before transfer.

An hCG β-subunit determination is performed on day 11 after transfer (13 days after laparoscopy) and, if it is positive, the patient is instructed to start

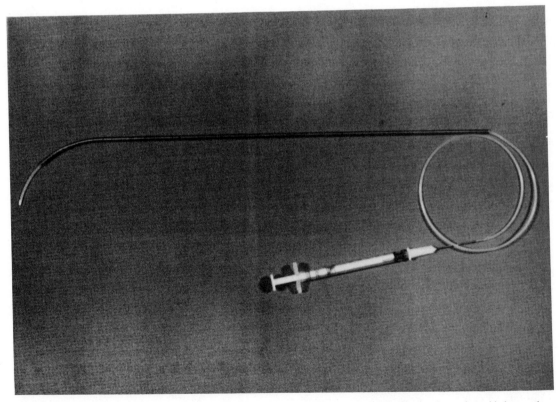

FIGURE 32-13. Photograph of the nylon transfer catheter and the 1-ml syringe attached to the distal end, together with the carrying cannula, the tip of which is placed just within the endocervical canal for the transfer. (From Jones.[34])

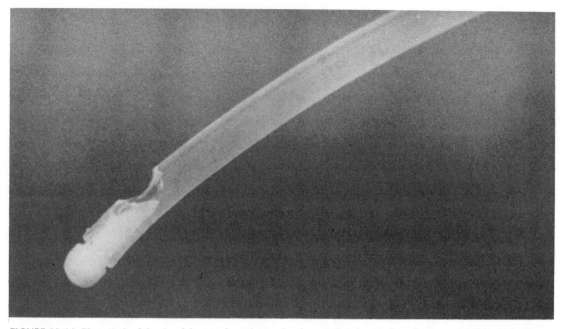

FIGURE 32-14. Photograph of the tip of the transfer catheter, showing a bullet-shaped plug of nylon and a side notch. (From Jones.[34])

17-hydroxyprogesterone caproate (Delalutin), 250 mg once a week, until week 16–18 of pregnancy. At approximately 8 weeks of pregnancy, an ultrasound is performed to determine pregnancy location and the number of fetal sacs and embryos present.

The rest of the obstetrical care is done on a routine basis, usually by the patient's own obstetrician.

RESULTS

Natural Cycle

A total of 41 laparoscopies were performed during 1980, when the natural cycle was used as the only method of oocyte retrieval. Preovulatory eggs were retrieved in 24 instances. Fresh corpora lutea were observed in nine patients and functional cysts in two others; technical failures impaired oocyte retrieval in nine patients. Although 19 patients went through IVF and pre-embryo transfer, no pregnancy was achieved.

Stimulated Cycle

A normal term pregnancy is the final goal of IVF with pre-embryo transfer. Pregnancy rate is there-

fore, the best indicator for evaluation of a program. Its efficiency can also be determined, however, at several stages: (1) the number of patients canceled because of deficient response to stimulation or a premature LH surge, (2) the number of follicles obtained and aspirated, (3) the number and quality of ooctyes retrieved, (4) the number of oocytes that fertilized and cleaved normally, and (5) the number of pre-embryos transferred.

In the Norfolk program from 1981–1985 (Table III), a total of 1,400 cycles were processed. The first treatment period (cycle) using hMG/hCG for ovulation stimulation established the criteria that were utilized, with minor modifications according to the type of stimulation protocol used in the rest of the program. Two pregnancies occurred out of 31 cycles in this initial experience. An average of 4.1 oocytes/cycle were retrieved; 40% were classified as preovulatory, 31.5% as immature, and 28% as atretic.

As shown in Table III, a total of 1,209 transfers were performed; in 1078 transfers, at least one pre-embryo, derived from a preovulatory oocyte, was replaced. A total of 298 pregnancies were obtained for a total pregnancy rate/transfer of 24.34%. When the outcome of pregnancy was reviewed from series 1–20 (1981–August 1985), 100 patients delivered, 23 had a clinical miscarriage, 30

TABLE 32-3. Norfolk Study: 1981–1985

Year	Cycles	Transfer all	Transfer at least 1 preovulatory	Pregnancies all	Pregnancies at least 1 preovulatory	% All pregnancies/cycle	% All pregnancies/all transfer	% Preovulatory pregnancies at least 1 preovulatory transfer
1981	55	31	28	7	6	12.7	22.6	21.4
1982	207	155	130	34	30	16.5	21.9	23.1
1983	298	243	204	64	62	21.3	26.3	30.4
1984	372	355	310	87	87	23.4	26.0	28.1
1985	468	425	401	106	104	22.6	24.9	25.9

had a preclinical abortion, and 2 presented ectopic tubal pregnancies.[60] Twelve sets of twins and one set of triplets were delivered. When ultrasounds performed near week 8 of pregnancy are taken into account, 23 sets of twins and 3 sets of triplets were diagnosed.

When the results of the procedure are studied by original diagnosis (Table IV), the tubal category represented most of our patient population, followed by endometriosis, male factor, and idiopathic infertility. The pregnancy rate/transfer was quite similar except for the group with idiopathic infertility, who showed a 36.7% pregnancy rate. When the clinical pregnancy rate/transfer was obtained, the results tended to be quite similar in all categories. Pregnancy was also established in patients with other factors, such as hostile cervical mucus, sperm antibody problems, pelvic tuberculosis, and DES exposure.[61]

SUMMARY

IVF with pre-embryo transfer is now a well-established procedure in the therapeutic armamentarium of the infertility specialist. The results obtained in most of the experienced centers are approaching figures comparable to the success rate of the natural reproductive process, and in some centers the results are even better. Developments in the future may be slow, and a tremendous amount of research is needed to improve present results.

The fear that IVF could cause an increased number of chromosomal abnormalities, a great concern of scientists originally involved in the procedure, has been disspelled. In the collective experience of IVF groups worldwide, such a risk is no greater than in the general population.

General guidelines have been established for the startup of programs. The demand for training is overwhelming, and the number of groups active in the field is insufficient to provide it.

The possibility of overcoming infertility in patients who had no chances before the IVF procedure was developed, as well as the possibility of using variations of the classic method, have opened new avenues and has pushed the frontiers of infertility and human reproduction. The changes have been so substantial that the impact has reached the whole field of obstetrics and gynecology.

It is of utmost importance for all reproductive endocrinologists and fertility specialists to understand the complexity of these programs and to give serious consideration to all potential and theoretical

TABLE 32-4. Norfolk Series 1–21 by Diagnosis

Diagnosis	Transfer	Pregnancies	% Pregnancy/transfer	Pregnancy >12 weeks	% Pregnancy transfer >12 weeks transfer
All	1078	289	26.8	200	18.6
Tubal	724	192	26.7	139	19.2
Endometriosis	143	36	25.2	27	18.9
Male	50	12	26.1	10	21.7
Idiopathic	63	22	36.7	14	23.3
Transvesicle	26	7	26.9	6	23.0

problems before establishing these therapeutic modalities in their centers.

REFERENCES

1. Heape W: Preliminary note on the transplantation and growth of mammalian ova within a uterine foster mother. *Proc Royal Soc Lond [Biol]*, 48:457–458, 1890
2. Austin CR: Observations on the penetration of the sperm into the mammalian egg. *Aust J Sci Res B* 4:581–596, 1951
3. Chang MC: Fertilizing capacity of sperm deposited in the fallopian tube. *Nature (Lond)* 168:697–698, 1951
4. McLaren A, Biggers JD: Successful development and birth of mice cultivated *in vitro* as early embryos. *Nature (Lond)* 182:877–878, 1959
5. Chang MC: Fertilization of rabbit ova *in vitro*. *Nature (Lond)* 184:466–467, 1959
6. Brinster RL, Biggers JD: In vitro fertilization of mouse ova within the expanded fallopian tube. *J Reprod Fertil* 10:277–279, 1965
7. Whittingham DG. Fertilization of mouse eggs in vitro. *Nature (Lond)* 220:592–593, 1968
8. Edwards RG. Maturation "in vitro" of human ovarian oocytes. *Lancet* 2:926–929, 1965
9. Edwards RG, Donahue RP, Baramki TA, et al: Preliminary attempts to fertilize human oocytes matured *in vitro*. *Am J Obstet Gynecol* 96:192–200, 1966
10. Edwards RG, Steptoe PC, Purdy JM: Fertilization and cleavage *in vitro* of preovulatory human oocytes. *Nature (Lond)* 227:1307–1309, 1970
11. Steptoe PC, Edwards RG, Purdy JM: Clinical aspects of pregnancies established with cleaving embryos grown *in vitro*. *Br J Obstet Gynaecol* 87:757–768, 1980
12. Lopata A, Johnston IWH, Hoult IJ, et al: Pregnancy following intrauterine implantation of an embryo obtained by *in vitro* fertilization of a preovulatory egg. *Fertil Steril* 33:117–121, 1980
13. Lenz S, Lauritzen JG: Ultrasonically guided percutaneous aspiration of human follicles under local anesthesia: a new method of collecting oocytes for *in vitro* fertilization. *Fertil Steril* 38:673–677, 1982
14. Wikland M, Nilsson L, Hansson R, et al: Collection of human oocytes by the use of sonography. *Fertil Steril* 39:603–608, 1983
15. Feichtinger W, Kemeter P: Laparoscopic or ultrasonically guided follicle aspiration for in vitro fertilization. *IVF ET* 1:244, 1984
16. Parsons J, Riddle A, Booker M, et al: Oocyte retrieval for in vitro fertilization by ultrasonically guided needle aspiration via the urethra. *Lancet* 1:1076, 1985
17. Jones HW Jr: Improvement in IVF results. In Feichtinger W, Kemeter P (eds): *Future Aspects in Human In Vitro Fertilization*. Berlin: Springer-Verlag (in press)
18. Romeu A, Muasher SJ, Acosta AA, et al: Results of in vitro fertilization attempts in women forty years of age and older: The Norfolk experience. (Submitted to *Fertil Steril*, 1986)
19. Garcia JE, Jones HW Jr, Acosta AA, et al: Reconstructive pelvic operations for in vitro fertilization. *Am J Obstet Synecol* 153:172, 1985
20. Queenan J, O'Brien GD, Bains LM, et al: Ultrasound scanning of ovaries to detect ovulation in women. *Fertil Steril* 34:99–105, 1980
21. Wood C, Trounson AD, Leeton JF, et al: Clinical features of eight pregnancies resulting from *in vitro* fertilization and embryo transfer. *Fertil Steril* 38:92–96, 1982
22. Quigley MM, Maklad NF, Wolf DP: Comparison of two Clomiphene Citrate dosage regimens for follicular recruitment in an *in vitro* fertilization program. *Fertil Steril* 40:178–182, 1983
23. Vargas JM, Marrs RP, Kletzky DA, et al: Correlation of ultrasonic measurement of ovarian follicle size and serum estradiol levels in ovulatory patients following clomiphene citrate for *in vitro* fertilization. *Am J Obstet Gynecol* 144:569–573, 1982
24. De Crespigny LJ, O'Herlihy C, Hoult IJ, et al: Ultrasound in an *in vitro* fertilization program. *Fertil Steril* 35:25–28, 1981
25. Quigley MM, Wolf DP, Maklad NF, et al: Follicule size and number in human *in vitro* fertilization. *Fertil Steril* 38:678–687, 1982
26. Hoult IJ, De Crespigny LJ, O'Herlihy C, et al: Ultrasound control of clomiphene/human chorionic gonadotropin stimulated cycle for oocyte recovery and *in vitro* fertilization. *Fertil Steril* 36:316–319, 1981
27. Testart J, Frydman R: Minimum time lapse between luteinizing hormone surge on human chorionic gonadotropin administration and follicular rupture. *Fertil Steril* 37:50–53, 1982
28. Kistner RW: Sequential use of clomiphene citrate and human menopause gonadotropin in ovulation induction. *Fertil Steril* 26:192, 1976
29. Edwards RG, Steptoe PC: Current status of *in vitro* fertilization and implantation of human embryos. *Lancet* 2:1265–1269, 1983
30. Lopata A: Concepts in human *in vitro* fertilization and embryo transfer. *Fertil Steril* 40:289–301, 1983
31. Garcia JE, Jones GS, Acosta AA, et al: Human menopause gonadotropin/human chorionic gonadotropin follicular maturation for oocyte aspiration: Phase I, 1981, *Fertil Steril* 39:167–173, 1983
32. Garcia JE, Jones GS, Acosta AA, Wright G Jr. Human menopause gonadotropin/human chorionic gonadotropin follicular maturation for oocyte maturation: Phase II, 1981. *Fertil Steril* 39:174–179, 1983
33. Jones JW Jr, Acosta AA, Andrews MC, et al: The importance of the follicular phase to success and failure in *in vitro* fertilization. *Fertil Steril* 40:317–321, 1983
34. Jones GS, Garcia JE, Rosenwaks Z: The role of pituitary gonadotropins in follicular stimulation and oocyte maturation in the human. *J Clin Endocrinal Metab* 59:178, 1984
35. Liu JH, Durfee R, Muse K, et al: Induction of multiple ovulation by pulsatile administration of gonadotropin-releasing hormone. *Fertil Steril* 40:18–22, 1983
36. Renou P, Trounson AD, Wood C, et al: The collection of human oocytes for *in vitro* fertilization. An instrument for maximizing oocyte recovery rate. *Fertil Steril* 35:409–412, 1981
37. Mettler L, Seki M, Baukloh V, et al: Human ovum recovery via operative laparoscopy and *in vitro* fertilization. *Fertil Steril* 38:30–37, 1982
38. Lopata A, Johnston IWH, Leeton JF, et al: Collection of human oocytes at laparoscopy. *Fertil Steril* 25:1030, 1974
39. Jones HW Jr, Acosta AA, Garcia J: A technique for the aspiration of oocytes from human ovarian follicles. *Fertil Steril* 37:26–29, 1982
40. Evans JM: Anesthesia for *in vitro* fertilization oocyte retrieval. *Infertility* 6:97, 1983
41. Veeck L, Wortham JWE, Witmyer J, et al: Maturation and

fertilization of morphologically immature human oocytes in a program of *in vitro* fertilization. *Fertil Steril* 39:594–602, 1983

42. Mastroianni LJ, Turek RW, Blasco L, et al: Intrauterine pregnancy following ovum recovery at laparotomy and subsequent *in vitro* fertilization. *Fertil Steril* 40:536–538, 1983

43. Hamberger L, Wikland M. Clinical experience with ultrasound-guided follicle aspiration. *Arch Androl* 11:179, 1983

44. Mantzabinos T, Garcia J, Jones JW Jr: Ultrasound measurement of ovarian follicles stimulated by human gonadotropin for oocyte recovery and in vitro fertilization. *Fertil Steril* 40:461–465, 1983

45. Brailly S, Gougen A, Milgrom E, et al: Androgen and progestins in the human ovarian follicle. Differences in the evaluation of preovulatory, healthy nonovulatory, and atretic follicles. *J Clin Endocrinol Metab* 53:128–134, 1981

46. Carlson RS, Trounson AD, Findlay JK: Successful fertilization of human oocytes *in vitro:* Concentration of estradiol 17-Beta, Progesterone and androstenedione in the antral fluid of donor follicles. *J Clin Endocrinol Metab* 55:798–800, 1982

47. McNatty KP, Moore-Smith D, Makris A, et al: The microenvironment of the human antral follicle: Interrelationships among the steroid levels in antral fluid, the population of granulosa cells, Endocrinol Metab 49:851–860, 1979

48. Wrambly H, Kullander S, Liedholm P, et al: The success rate of *in vitro* fertilization of human oocytes in relation to the concentration of different hormones in follicular fluid and peripheral plasma. *Fertil Steril* 36:448–454, 1981

49. Channing CP, Liu CQ, Jones GS, et al: Decline of follicular oocyte maturation inhibitor coincident with maturation and achievement of fertilizability of oocytes recovered at midcycle of gonadotropin-treated women. *Proc Natl Acad Sci USA* 80:4184–4188, 1983

50. Sangal MK, Berger MJ, Thompson IE, et al: Development of graafian follicles in adult human ovary. I. Correlation of estrogen and progesterone concentration in antral fluid with growth of follicles. *J Clin Endocrinol Metab* 38:828–835, 1974

51. Channing CP: Follicular fluid survey and possible role of follicular fluid inhibit activity in the human. *Infertility* 6:251, 1983

52. Channing CP. Follicular fluid oocyte maturation and follicular control of granulosa cell maturation. *Infertility* 6:265, 1983

53. Sandow BA: Characteristics of human oocytes aspirated for in vitro fertilization. *Infertility* 6:143, 1983

54. Acosta AA, Jones GS, Garcia JE, et al: Correlation of human menopausal gonadotropin/human chorionic gonadotropin stimulation and oocyte quality in an *in vitro* fertilization program. *Fertil Steril* 41:196–201, 1984

55. Trounson AD, Mohr LH, Wood C, et al: Effect of delayed insemination on *in vitro* fertilization and transfer of human embryos. *J Reprod Fertil* 64:285–294, 1982

56. Testart J, Grydman E, DeMouzon J, et al: A study of factors affecting the success of human fertilization *in vitro*. I. influence of ovarian stimulation upon the number and conditions of oocytes collected. *Biol Reprod* 28:415–424, 1983

57. Veeck LL: Fertilization and development. *Infertility* 6:155, 1983

58. Garcia JE: *In vitro* fertilization. *Obstet Gynecol Annu* 14:45–72, 1985

59. Jones HW Jr, Acosta AA, Garcia JE, et al: On the transfer of concepti from oocytes fertilized *in vitro*. *Fertil Steril* 39:241–243, 1983

60. Andrews MC, Muasher SJ, Levy DL, et al: An analysis of the obstetric outcome of 125 consecutive pregnancies conceived in vitro and resulting in 100 deliveries. *Am J Obstet Gynecol* 154:848, 1986

61. Muasher SJ, Garcia JE, Jones HW Jr: Experience with diethylstilbesterol exposed infertile women in a program of *in vitro* fertilization. *Fertil Steril* (in press)

VI

New Frontiers in Gynecologic Endocrinology

Endocrine Control of the Secretory Immune System in the Reproductive Tract of the Female

Response of IgA, IgG, and Secretory Component in the Uterus to Sex Hormones

CHARLES R. WIRA and JOHN B. JOSIMOVICH

INTRODUCTION

The immunology of the female reproductive tract is of fundamental importance, particularly at the level of the mucosal surfaces. The mucosa serves a dual purpose, protecting the host against infectious agents as well as providing a safe environment for the successful growth of the allogeneic conceptus.[1,2] Protective mechanisms at these surfaces are of particular importance in the human, since the genital tract is essentially an open connection between the external environment and the peritoneal cavity. It is within the secretions bathing these surfaces that immunoglobulins A (IgA) and G (IgG),[3,4] along with other nonspecific agents,[5-7]

protect against both bacterial and viral invasion. The alterations that occur in the immune system during pregnancy and the close interrelationship of the maternal host with the antigenically different conceptus, demonstrate the intricate complexity and control exerted on genital tract and systemic immune mechanisms that result in species perpetuation and maternal protection.

THE IMMUNE SYSTEM IN THE FEMALE REPRODUCTIVE TRACT

The secretory immune system present in the female reproductive tract resembles that present at other mucosal sites in the body.[8,9] Cervical and vaginal secretions contain primarily secretory IgA (IgA bound to secretory component) and, to a lesser extent, IgG.[3,10,11] What remains to be established, however, is to determine the contributions of local synthesis versus serum transfer to the IgA and IgG pools in genital tract secretions. The relative contri-

CHARLES R. WIRA • Department of Physiology, Dartmouth Medical School, Hanover, New Hampshire 03756.
JOHN B. JOSIMOVICH • Department of Obstetrics and Gynecology and Department of Pathology, UMDNJ–New Jersey Medical School, Newark, New Jersey 07103.

bution of these sources is in part reflected by the region of the genital tract examined and the number of lymphocytes and/or plasma cells present. In human uteri, for example, plasma cells are either absent or found very infrequently during the menstrual cycle. Diffuse noncellular staining of IgA and IgG is found in the endometrium and in the epithelial regions of the uterus.[12-15] Secretory component, a glycoprotein synthesized by epithelial cells, which functions to transport IgA into mucosal secretions, is also present in uterine and oviductal epithelial cells.[12,15] By contrast, the cervix has significant numbers of IgA, IgG, and IgM lymphocytes.[12,13] IgA and IgG are present along cervical basement membranes and between columnar epithelial cells. Secretory component is also localized in these cells, but not in the squamous epithelium of the vagina.[12,13,16] The vagina of the human exhibits diffuse staining of IgA and IgG, but, as based on several studies, has very few if any lymphocytes or plasma cells.[12,13]

Local antibody synthesis has been demonstrated when antigens are introduced into the female genital tract. For example, *Brucella abortus* introduction into the uteri of cattle results in antibody titers in the vagina that are higher than in serum.[17] After acute infection with gonorrhea, trichomoniads, or *Candida albicans* in young women, cervical biopsies exhibit an increased number and predominance of IgA-plasma cells.[18] That cervicovaginal secretions represent an admixture of local and systemic origin was demonstrated when rhesus monkeys were immunized intravaginally with lipopolysaccharide (LPS) or T-4 coliphage.[19] Under these conditions, specific agglutinating and neutralizing antibodies were found in both serum and cervical secretions. After systemic immunization, high antibody titers were measured in serum with lesser activity measured in cervical aspirates. Aspirates had titers higher than those measured following vaginal application and correlated with serum levels.

In addition to serum contributions, antibodies may appear within the genital tract as a result of local synthesis by lymphocytes. After antigen sensitization at distant sites, lymphocytes migrate to the reproductive tissues.[20,21] Using an adoptive lymphocyte transfer system for injecting mesenteric node cells labled with [3H]thymidine into syngeneic mice, lymphocytes were demonstrated to migrate into intestinal, respiratory, mammary, and genital tissues. In other studies, oral immunization of mice with live herpes simplex virus (HSV-1) led to a reduced incidence and milder form of infection after vaginal challenge with cross-reacting HSV-II. Immunized mice had an accelerated pattern of vaginal viral elimination with a decreased rate of lethality as compared with unimmunized controls.[22]

HORMONAL INFLUENCE ON THE SECRETORY IMMUNE SYSTEM OF THE FEMALE REPRODUCTIVE TRACT

A number of studies have shown that variations occur in the uterine immune system during the menstrual and estrous cycle. During the luteal phase of the menstrual cycle, IgA and IgG in stromal and epithelial spaces were shown to reach maximal levels.[12,15] IgA increased during this time in parallel with the synthesis and accumulation of secretory component and then declined during the premenstrual period as measured by staining intensity.[12-15] These observations led to speculation

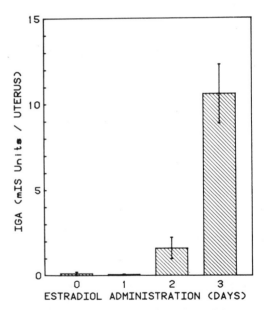

FIGURE 33-1. Time course of the effect of estradiol treatment on IgA accumulation in the uterine lumen of ovariectomized rats. Estradiol, $1.0 \mu g/0.1$ ml, in ethyl laurate was administered for 1, 2, and 3 days. Controls received only ethyl laurate. Animals (5/group) were sacrificed 24 hr after the last injection. Bars represent the mean per group and vertical lines on the bars indicate the SE. IgA results are reported as immunocytoma serum (IS) units; 1.0 IS unit is defined as the concentration of IgA in 1.0 mg lyophilized immunocytoma serum per milliliter distilled water. Day 2 and 3 IgA levels are, significantly ($p < 0.01$) greater than control. (Adapted from Wira and Sandoe.[26])

that progesterone regulates secretory component in the uterus, which in turn, transfers IgA into the uterine lumen. With regard to the presence of immunoglobulins in uterine secretions, our studies in the rat have demonstrated that IgA, IgG, and secretory component change during the estrous cycle.[23,24] At proestrus, which correlates with elevated serum estradiol levels,[24] all three were higher than at any other stage of the cycle. This cyclic pattern of immunoglobulin accumulation coincided well with the marked inhibition of *Escherichia coli* colony formation, which was highest at proestrus.[25]

In light of the information available suggesting that sex hormones might influence the immune system, we undertook to use the uterus of the rat as a model to study the interactions of estrogen and progesterone with the secretory immune system. The results of these studies, some of which are presented here, indicate that the sex hormones control several parameters of the immune system. Evidence is provided indicating that (1) estradiol stimulates both IgA and IgG accumulation within the uterine secretions, (2) the mechanisms involved in the movement of IgA and IgG into the uterine lumen are different, (3) IgA-positive cells migrate into the uterine tissues in response to hormone treatment, (4) secretory component is under hormonal control, and (5) expression of the uterine IgA and IgG response to estradiol requires the presence of an intact thymus. More recently, we have extended these studies to the human by measuring secretory components levels in uterine washes at various stages of the menstrual cycle.

EFFECT OF ESTRADIOL ON IgA AND IgG LEVELS IN THE UTERUS OF THE RAT

In order to measure IgA and IgG in uterine secretions, radioimmunoassays (RIAs) were developed using either solid phase[26] or double antibody precipitation.[27] Briefly, in the solid-phase RIA, rabbit anti-rat IgG (Miles Laboratories, Elkhart, Ind.) and goat anti-rat IgA (Dr. H. Bazin, Belgium) prepared against IgA-rich serum from rats with IR-22 immunocytomas were coupled to microcrystalline celluose or Sepharose-4B. Rat IgG and rat IgA-rich serum were radiolabeled with $Na^{125}I$. In the double-antibody assay, rabbit anti-goat IgG and goat anti-rabbit IgG (Miles Laboratories) were used as second antibodies. In each assay system, displacement of [^{125}I]immunoglobulin permitted direct calculation of the amount of immunoglobulin in each unknown. Our procedure for recovering uterine samples and for the measurement of lumen and tissue levels of IgA and IgG has been described previously.[26,17]

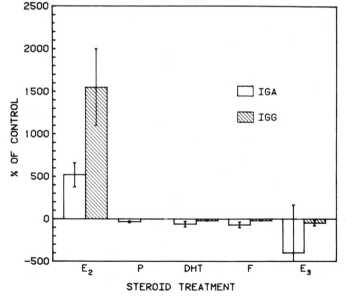

FIGURE 33-2. Influence of hormones on IgA and IgG levels in rat uteri. Ovariectomized rats were injected daily with 0.1 ml either ethyl laurate or 0.9% saline solution with either 1.0 μg estradiol (E_2) or estriol (E_3), 2 mg progesterone (P), 1.0 mg cortisol (F), or 1.0 mg of dihydrotestosterone (DHT). Twenty-four hours after the third injection, uterine luminal content was recovered and immunoglobulins measured. Results are expressed as percentage of control ±SE (six rats per group) that received only ethyl laurate or saline. E_2 value differs ($p < 0.01$) significantly from controls. (From Wira and Sandoe.[26])

Figure 33-1 shows the levels of IgA that accumulate in the uteri of ovariectomized rats following daily injection of estradiol 1 μg/day for 3 days. When secretions were collected 24 hr after each injection, a gradual increase was observed in IgA and IgG after 2 and 3 days of hormone exposure. In an earlier study, we had observed similar increases in intact rats at the proestrous stage of the estrous cycle.[23,26] These findings suggested that uterine IgA and IgG are regulated in the intact rat by estradiol. This conclusion was further supported by our observation that progesterone, cortisol, dihydrotestosterone, and estriol when administered at doses known to elicit physiologic effects in their respective target tissues, had no observable action in IgA and IgG levels on uterine target tissues (Fig. 33-2). We have observed in other studies, however, that progesterone given along with estradiol blocks the increase in both IgA and IgG that occurs after estradiol treatment alone.[28]

In light of the increases in IgA and IgG that resulted following estradiol treatment, we examined the time course of immunoglobulin appearance both within the tissues of the uterus (cytosol) as well as in the uterine lumen. As shown in Figure 33-3a, both IgA and IgG levels in uterine tissues increased rapidly within hours (3–6 hr) after two or three injections of estradiol. Tissue levels then declined between 6 and 24 hr after each injection. A similar increase (not shown) was found after a single treatment of estradiol. We have found that estradiol induces this rapid transfer of IgA and IgG from blood to tissue through serum transudation.[27] IgG and IgA also enter the uterine lumen (Fig. 33-3B), but their peaks of accumulation occur at different times. The time course for IgG paralleled that seen in the tissues with elevations observed at 3 hr postinjection. By contrast, IgA content did not change after the first (not shown) injection and did not begin to increase until 25 hr after the second injection of estradiol. With the third injection, IgA levels continued to rise and were maintained for the next 24-hour period. These results indicate that whereas estradiol has a stimulatory effect on IgA and IgG movement, the mechanisms controlling each immunoglobulin are distinctly different.

To determine whether IgA and IgG movement into the uterus was selective, the concentrations of both immunoglobulins were measured in blood, tissue and uterine fluid following estradiol treatment of ovariectomized rats. As shown in Figure 33-4, the concentrations of immunoglobulins var-

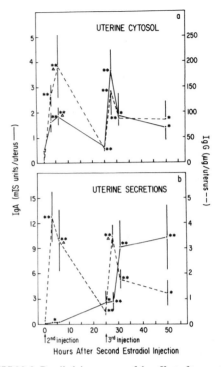

FIGURE 33-3. Detailed time course of the effect of two or three estradiol injections on the levels of IgA and IgG in uterine cytosol (A) and secretions (B) from ovariectomized rats. Arrows indicate the time of either the second or third injection. Immunoglobulin levels were measured at 3, 6, and 24 hr after each injection. Animals received either estradiol (1 μg/day) or saline (controls, indicated at 0 time point). Each point represents the mean ±SE of four to eight values. *, significantly ($p < 0.05$) greater than control; **, significantly ($p < 0.005$) greater than control; Δ, significantly ($p < 0.05$) greater than level at next time point. (From Sullivan and Wira.[30])

ied markedly. For IgG, the mean concentration was greatest in plasma, reduced in tissue and lowest in uterine fluid. By contrast, the concentration of IgA in uterine fluid was greater than that measured in blood or tissue. These findings indicate that whereas IgG, in response to estradiol, moves down a gradient from blood to lumen, IgA movement from tissue to lumen is against an apparent concentration gradient. The forms (monomer vs. polymer) of IgA vary from compartment to compartment.[29,30] Elution profiles of uterine tissue cytosol and plasma indicated that both monomeric and polymeric IgA were present. By contrast, when uterine fluid was passed over a Sepharose-6B column, only the polymeric form of IgA was present.

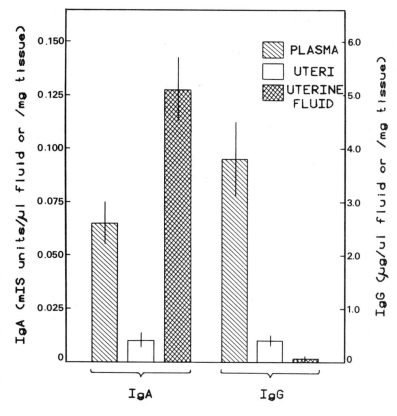

FIGURE 33-4. Concentrations of IgA and IgG in plasma, uterus, and uterine fluid of ovariectomized rats injected daily with estradiol (1 µg/day) in saline for 3 days. Bars represent the mean ±SE values of four to eight animals per group. IgA values in plasma are significantly different from those measured in the uterus ($p < 0.01$) and in the uterine fluid ($p < 0.05$). The IgG value in the uterus is significantly different from that in the plasma ($p < 0.01$) and in the uterine fluid ($p < 0.05$). (From Wira et al.[31])

CELLULAR ASPECTS OF THE IMMUNOGLOBULIN RESPONSE TO ESTRADIOL

To determine whether estradiol had any immunoglobulin-related effects on uterine epithelial cells and/or the migration of lymphocytes into the uterus of the rat, we evaluated the appearance and changes in these cell types both before and following hormone treatment by fluorescent microscopy. Fluorescinated anti-rat IgA was prepared and incubated with uterine sections before microscopic evaluation. As seen in Figure 33-5A, in the absence of estradiol very little IgA is associated with the epithelial cells lining the uterine lumen.[28] When the same stain is applied to uteri from rats treated with estradiol for 3 days, a marked accumulation of IgA is associated with the epithelial cells. The presence of IgA, as shown in Figure 33-5B, appears to be distributed throughout the cells, with increasing amounts present at the apical end. As a part of the stimulatory effect of estradiol, the morphology of

the epithelial cells changed from cuboidal (Fig. 33-5A) to columnar (Fig. 33-5B).

Estradiol also plays a central role in the migration of lymphocytes into the uterine tissues.[29] In the absence of estradiol, uteri from ovariectomized rats had no IgA-positive cells present. With estradiol, IgA-positive cells, as shown in Figure 33-5C, accumulated in the endometrial and myometrial regions at a time that coincided with the disappearance of lymphocytes from the blood[28] and the accumulation of IgA within the uterine lumen. Further studies, however, are necessary to distinguish between that portion of IgA which accumulates in uterine secretions as a result of local synthesis versus that which is derived from the transfer of IgA from blood to uterus.

More recently, a study was undertaken to determine whether the thymus plays a role in the endocrine control of the immune system in the uterus.[30] As shown in Table 33-1, when estradiol (1 µg/day) was given for 3 days to neonatally thymectomized rats, the luminal accumulation of IgA and IgG (not

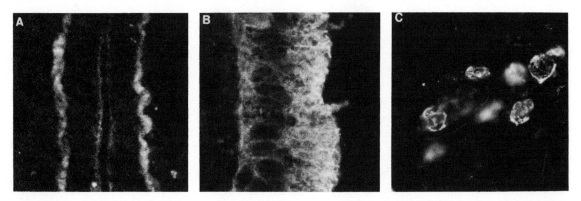

FIGURE 33-5. Fluorescent microscopic localization of IgA in uteri from rats after three daily injections of estradiol. Ovariectomized rats were injected with 1.0 μg estradiol in 0.1 ml saline (B,C). Controls (A) received only saline. Uteri were frozen and sectioned in a cryostat (−20°C) and cut into 8-μm sections. The IgG fraction of fluoresceinated goat anti-rat IgA was applied to tissue sections and indubated in a humid chamber for 24 hr at room temperature prior to saline-buffered washing and microscopic analysis. (From Wira et al.[28] and Wira et al.[9])

shown) was significantly lower than that measured in either the sham operated or intact ovariectomized rats. These findings suggest that estradiol control of the uterine immune response is in part regulated through hormone effects on the thymus. Whether the action of T cells is expressed systemically or directly at the level of the uterus remains to be established.

EFFECT OF ESTRADIOL AND PROGESTERONE ON SECRETORY COMPONENT

Secretory component (SC) is a glycoprotein that is synthesized and secreted by mucosal epithelial cells.[8,9] After binding to SC, IgA is transferred

from tissue to mucosal surfaces where it exerts its protective effect as secretory IgA (IgA bound to SC). In light of the central role played by SC in the secretory immune system, an RIA that measures free SC was developed to obtain direct evidence that SC is under the control of the female sex hormones. As seen in Figure 33-6, when estradiol was administered to ovariectomized rats in amounts known to exert physiologic effects, SC levels in uterine secretions increased significantly as compared with ovariectomized controls. As a part of these studies, SC and IgA accumulation in uterine secretions in response to estradiol were determined to see whether both followed the same time course of appearance.[31] As illustrated in Figure 33-7, IgA and SC increases were detected initially at 18 hr after the second injection of estradiol. This parallel

TABLE 33-1. Effect of Estradiol on IgA Levels in Uterine Secretions of Neonatally Thymectomized, Sham-Operated, and Thymus-Intact Ovariectomized Rats[a]

	Control	Estradiol-treated groups		
		Intact	Sham operated	Thymectomized
IgA (mIS units/uterus)	0.16	12.6[b]	19.2[b]	0.99[b,c]
	± 0.06	± 4.9	± 5.9	±0.51
Animals/group	10	8	8	5

[a]Adapted from Sullivan and Wira (30).
[b]Significantly ($p < 0.05$) greater than control. Animals were ovariectomized 7–10 days before receiving either estradiol (1.0 μg/day in saline or saline (control). Twenty-four hours after the last injection, rats were killed and uterine fluid was collected. All IgA values represent the mean ±SE of the animals indicated in each group.
[c]Significantly ($p < 0.05$) less than other estradiol-treated groups.

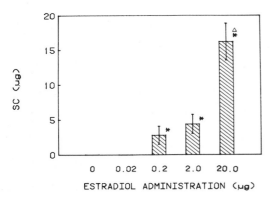

FIGURE 33-6. The effect of increasing doses of estradiol on secretory component (SC) levels in the uterine lumen. Ovariectomized rats were administered three daily injections of estradiol or saline and killed 23 hr later. Bars equal the mean ±SE of five values. *, significantly ($p < 0.005$) greater than control; Δ, significantly ($p < 0.005$) greater than other estradiol-treated groups. (From Sullivan et al.[33])

increase continued after the third injection of estradiol. The nearly identical patterns of accumulation are consistent with our hypothesis that IgA movement from tissue to lumen is mediated by estradiol regulation of uterine SC.

To test whether the stimulation of SC by estradiol involves both protein and RNA synthesis, uteri were incubated in culture media either in the presence or absence of RNA and protein inhibitors. The effect of actinomycin D, a known inhibitor of RNA synthesis, is shown in Figure 33-8. When uteri from ovariectomized rats injected with estradiol for 3 days were placed in media containing actinomycin D, SC release was markedly reduced relative to that of control-estradiol uteri. In other experiments, α-amanitin, a potent inhibitor of eukaryotic RNA polymerase II and messenger RNA (mRNA) synthesis, also significantly decreased the release of SC into the incubation media.[32] To determine whether estradiol control of SC production in-

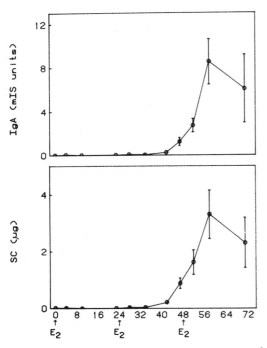

TIME AFTER ESTRADIOL ADMINISTRATION(hours)

FIGURE 33-7. Time course of the effect of one, two, or three estradiol treatments on SC and IgA content in uterine secretions of ovariectomized rats. Animals were injected with either estradiol (E_2, 2 μg/day) or saline controls, indicated as 0 time point. Each value is equal to the mean ±SE of 4 (E_2) or 12 (saline) determinations. (From Sullivan et al.[28])

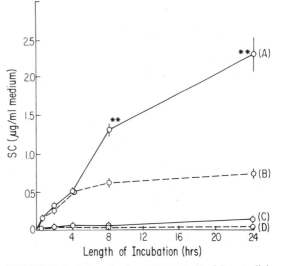

FIGURE 33-8. Antagonism by actinomycin D of the estradiol induced increase in uterine SC in vitro. After 3 days of in vivo estradiol (1.0 μg/day) or saline to ovariectomized rats, uterine horns were divided, slit lengthwise, and washed in saline before placement in incubation media (RPMI-1640, Gibco) or in media containing actinomycin D (20 μg/ml; Sigma). The curves shown are as follows: (A) estradiol; (B) estradiol/actinomycin D; (C) saline; (D) saline/actinomycin D. Each point on the curves indicates the mean ±SE of four determinations per time point. **, significantly greater ($p < 0.01$) than the value obtained from estradiol-treated uteri in actinomycin D containing media. (From Wira et al.[32])

volved protein synthesis, cycloheximide was added under similar incubation conditions.[33] The significant decrease in SC accumulation observed suggested that estradiol regulation of uterine SC production, in addition to involving RNA synthesis, also involves the stimulation of its synthesis.

LEVELS OF SECRETORY COMPONENT IN HUMAN UTERINE FLUID DURING THE MENSTRUAL CYCLE

In light of the evidence that steroid hormones regulate the humoral immune system in the reproductive tract of the rat, a study was undertaken to determine whether similar changes might be occurring in the uteri of women during the menstrual cycle. To measure the levels of SC in uterine secretions, uterine washes from women (aged 18–49) with histologically normal endometria were collected by lavage with a Gravlee jet wash device using isotonic glycine.[34] Levels of SC were measured by an RIA that recognized primarily free SC. As seen in Figure 33-9, the levels of SC in uterine secretions varied significantly with the stage of the menstrual cycle. When expressed as percentage of total wash protein, the amount of SC recovered was

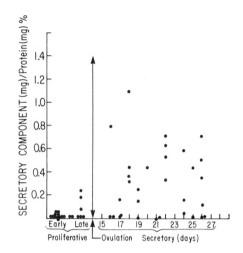

FIGURE 33-10. Content of secretory component in uterine washes during specific stages or days of the menstrual cycle. Only those values that could be accurately dated by the Pathology Department of the Massachusetts General Hospital are included in this graph. (From Sullivan et al.[34])

highest during the secretory phase, reduced during the proliferative phase and lowest during menstruation. Figure 33-10 shows the SC levels in washes taken on specific days of the menstrual cycle. Only those samples that could be dated by the examination of endometrial biopsies were included. The results presented indicate that post-ovulatory levels of SC throughout the secretory phase are higher than levels measured during the early and late proliferative phase of the menstrual cycle. These results are consistent with the finding of others indicating that intraepithelial IgA content in human uteri also increases during the secretory phase of the menstrual cycle.[12-15] Changing levels of SC are most likely due to changes in the endocrine balance that occurs during the menstrual cycle. Less clear, however, is the specific hormone or combination of hormones that controls the human secretory immune system in the uterus. One important observation made by Holinka and Gurpide[35] is that the endocrine signal for increasing some proteins in the uteri of women is different from that which stimulates the same proteins in the rat uterus. For example, glycogen synthetase is increased by estradiol in the rat but is regulated by progesterone in the human. Whether SC and other elements of the immune system are similarly regulated remains to be established.

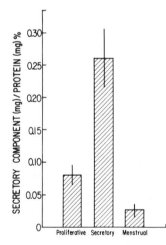

FIGURE 33-9. Secretory component levels in uterine luminal washes during the menstrual cycle. Bars represent the mean ±SE of 41 proliferative, 39 secretory, and 5 menstrual samples. SC levels, expressed as percentage of total wash protein and measured during the secretory phase of the menstrual cycle were significantly ($p < 0.001$) greater than those measured during the proliferative phase. (From Sullivan et al.[34])

EFFECTS OF STEROID HORMONES ON SYSTEMIC CELLULAR AND HUMORAL IMMUNE RESPONSES

Effects in the Fetus or Neonate

In newborn animals, Ahlquist[36] and Blair[37] showed that treatment with both male and female sex steroids, progestogens, and other steroids caused changes in lymphocyte counts and proliferative responses of splenic lymphocytes to mitogens, as well as alterations in spleen and thymus size. T- and B-cell function could, in certain instances, be long lasting. Furthermore, Shapiro and Slone[38] showed that children whose mothers were treated with diethylstilbestrol (DES) during pregnancy displayed changes in immune responses.

Effects in the Adult

Mathur et al.[39] showed that low doses of estradiol or progesterone enhanced antibody production to *C. albicans* but that higher doses of estradiol suppressed antibody production to this organism which causes afflication with greater frequency to women during pregnancy or who take estrogen-containing oral contraceptives. Furthermore, Halgason and Von-Schoultz[40] found a dose-related estrogen suppression of lymphocyte reactivity, as well as a synthetic ethinyl estradiol of 450–500 times greater effectiveness than estrone sulfate or estradiol-17β.

Progesterone, in contrast to estradiol, has been found to inhibit (and account for 80% of the inhibiting effect of pregnancy serum) lymphocyte cytoxicity;[41] while synthetic progestogen[42] can greatly increase the lymphocyte response to phytohemagglutinin (PHA) and allogeneic cells, with an increase in T-rosettes.

Earlier studies on the effects of combined estrogen–progestogen oral contraceptives (OC) by Keller et al.[43] showed depression of PHA mitogen responses of lymphocytes in 217 women, with effects lasting 1 year after stopping OC use, a finding confirmed by Bray.[44] Zane[45] noted disagreement among several groups as to the systemic immunoreactivity of women taking OCs, although Gerretsen et al.[46] confirmed increased sensitivity to cutaneous antigens. Zane further noted that these earlier and sometimes inconsistent studies were due to use of less specific lymphocyte function tests (e.g., proliferation), except for the skin allergy response. In studies requiring confirmation, using monoclonal antibody against total T, and T-cell subpopulations, Zane found that OCs lowered T helper to T suppressor cell ratio, accompanied by a reduced T-helper population coincidental with or attributable in part to increased T-suppressor activity. Zane's studies demonstrated OCs to lower serum concentrations of IgA, IgG, and IgM, although earlier studies had reported increased levels of IgG.[47,48] A recent study,[49] using low-estrogen-dose (35-μg) OCs, has shown enhanced pokeweed mitogen (PWM) (a B-cell mitogen) and Concanavalin A (ConA) (a T-cell mitogen) lymphocyte proliferation, suggesting that the inconsistencies in results cited above may in part be due to suppressive effects of higher pharmacologic doses of estrogen used in earlier studies.

CONCLUSIONS

The results presented indicate that the secretory immune system in the female reproductive tract of the rat is under the control of the female sex hormones. The nature of this control, as measured by changes in levels of IgA, IgG, and SC, indicates in our animal model that estradiol has a stimulatory effect and that progesterone antagonizes this action. Our understanding of the multiple levels at which estradiol interacts with the secretory immune system are presented schematically in Figure 33-11. In response to estradiol, IgA and IgG move rapidly from blood into the tissue space. This rapid influx, which occurs within 3–6 hr, is paralleled by the movement of IgG into the uterine lumen. Movement is most likely due to the stimulatory effect of

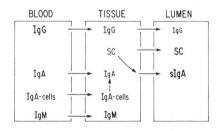

FIGURE 33-11. Summary design of the possible sites of action at which estradiol exerts an influence on the secretory immune system in the uterus of the rat. Changes in the sizes of the lettering among blood, tissue, and luminal compartments of the uterus depict apparent concentration gradients for each immunoglobulin and secretory component. (From Wira et al.[50])

estradiol on uterine fluid imbibition, characterized by serum transudation and the accumulation of fluid within the uterine lumen. The transfer of IgG is down a concentration gradient.

When IgA begins to accumulate, its presence coincides with a gradual increase in SC levels within the uterine lumen. The appearance of both follows a more gradual time course that involves 2–3 days of hormone treatment of the ovariectomized rat. When IgA moves from tissue to lumen in response to estradiol, it is against an apparent concentration gradient and is present as secretory IgA. The stimulatory effect of estradiol on SC as well as its time course of appearance are consistent with our working hypothesis that IgA movement is most likely controlled by estradiol regulation of uterine SC. Also shown in Figure 33-11 is the estradiol-induced accumulation of IgA-positive cells in the uterus. The hatched arrow from these cells to IgA suggests that local synthesis, in addition to serum transudation, may contribute to the pool of IgA that appears in the uterine lumen following hormone treatment. Also shown is a recent finding that IgM moves from blood to tissue as a part of the water imbibition step.[30] To date, however, no evidence has been obtained to suggest that this immunoglobulin enters the uterine lumen. Not included in this scheme is our finding that in the absence of an intact thymus, the response of the secretory immune system in the uterus to estradiol is markedly diminished. The mechanism(s) by which this effect is altered, however, remain(s) to be identified.

The studies of secretory component levels measured in uterine washes of women during the menstrual cycle indicate, as in the animal model, that the secretory immune system is under hormonal control. Based on our observations that SC levels are highest during the secretory phase, further studies need to be undertaken to identify the hormone(s) and mechanism(s) controlling SC levels.

Clearly, assessment of the importance of the changes brought about by estrogen, progesterone, or varying formulations of oral contraceptives on extragenital humoral and cellular immune function await careful studies like those under way in the reproductive tract.

Now that the effects of estrogen and progesterone on the humoral and cellular immune system have been demonstrated in the reproductive tract of the rat, and are becoming clearer in the human, further studies need to be carried out to investigate several questions:

1. Do differing estrogen : progesterone combinations in oral contraceptives affect genital tract resistance to infection?
2. What is the best site for immunization, and under what hormonal conditions should antigens be presented to protect against bacterial and viral pathogens?
3. How do these hormones alter resistance of the uterus to ascending infection after insertion of intrauterine contraceptive devices or after gonococcal salpingitis?
4. How is the immune system altered during pregnancy, and what role do the female sex hormones, as they regulate IgA, IgG, and SC, have in the survival of the fetus?

ACKNOWLEDGMENTS. The authors express their grateful appreciation to Dr. Brian Underdown at the University of Toronto, Canada, for his generous gifts of secretory component and antisera used in both the human and animal studies. We also express our appreciation to Dr. Herve Bazin for his kind gifts of goat anti-rat IgA and IgA-rich serum from rats with IR-22 immunocytomas. The research presented in this chapter was supported by research grants AI-13541 from the National Institutes of Health and CA-23108

QUESTIONS

1. In the ovariectomized rat, administration of estradiol

   a. increases movement of IgG into the uterine tissue.
   b. increases movement of IgG into the uterine luminal fluid.
   c. stimulates production of secretory component, which appears to aid IgA passage into the uterine lumen.
   d. all of the above.

2. Simultaneous administration of progesterone in the same preparation

   a. enhances the effects of estradiol noted in question 1.
   b. inhibits the effects of estradiol.
   c. has no effect.

3. In the human, estradiol

   a. enhances antibody production to *Candida albicans*.
   b. inhibits antibody production.

c. enhances antibody production at low doses but suppresses production at higher doses.

REFERENCES

1. Beer AE, Billingham RE: Immunobiology of mammalian reproduction. *Adv Immunol* 14:1–24, 1971
2. Edwards RG, Coombs RRA: Immunological interactions between mother and fetus, in Gell, PGH, Coombs RRA, Lachman PS, eds: *Clinical Aspects of Immunology.* London, Blackwell, 1975, pp 561–598
3. Labib RS, Tomasi TB Jr: Secretory immunoglobulin A, in Seligson D, ed: *C.R.C. Handbook Series in Clinical Laboratory Science Section F—Immunology.* Cleveland, CRC, 1978, pp 137–155
4. Ganguly R, Waldman RH: Local immunity and local immune responses. *Prog Allergy* 27:1–68, 1980
5. Klebanoff SJ, Smith DC: Peroxidase-mediated antimicrobial activity of rat uterine fluid. *Gynecol Invest* 1:21–30, 1970
6. Galask RP, Snyder IS: Antimicrobial factors in amniotic fluid. *Am J Obstet Gynecol* 106:59–65, 1970
7. Brownlee J, Hibbitt KG: Antimicrobial proteins isolated from bovine cervical mucus. *J Reprod Fertil* 29:337–347, 1972
8. Bienenstock J, Befus AD: Mucosal Immunology. *Immunology* 41:249–270, 1980
9. Brandzaeg P: Transport models for secretory IgA and IgM. *Clin Exp Immunol* 44:221–232, 1981
10. Chandra RK, Malkani PK, Bhasin K: Levels of immunoglobulins and uterine fluid in women using an intrauterine contraceptive device. *J Reprod Fertil* 37:1–16, 1974
11. Schumacher GFB: Humoral immune factors in the female reproductive tract and their changes during the cycle, in Dindsa D, Schumacher G, eds: *Immunological Aspects of Infertility, and Fertility Regulation.* New York, Elsevier/North-Holland, 1980, pp 93–141
12. Tourville DR, Ogra SS, Lippes J, et al: The human female reproductive tract: Immunohistological localization of γA, γG, γM, "secretory piece" and lactoferrin. *Am J Obstet Gynecol* 108:1102–1108, 1970
13. Rebello R, Green FHY, Fox H: A study of the secretory immune system of the female genital tract. *J Obstet Gynecol* 82:812–816, 1975
14. Hurliman J, Dayal R, Gloor E: Immunoglobulins and secretory component in endometrium and cervix. Influence of inflammation and carcinoma. *Virchows Arch* [Pathol Anat] 377:211–223, 1978
15. Kelley JK, Fox H: The local immunological defense system of the human endometrium. *J Reprod Immunol* 1:39–47, 1979
16. Hulka JF, Omran KF: The ut●ine cervix as a potential local antibody secretor. *Am J Obstet Gynecol* 104:440–442, 1969
17. Kerr WR: Vaginal and uterine antibodies in cattle with particular reference to *Br. abortus. Br Vet J* 111:169, 1955
18. Chipperfield EJ, Evans BA: The influence of local infection on immunoglobulin formation in the human endocervix. *Clin Exp Immunol* 11:219–223, 1972
19. Yang S-L, Schumacher GFB: Immune response after vaginal application of antigens in the rhesus monkey. *Fertil Steril* 32:588–598, 1979

20. McDermott MR, Bienenstock J: Evidence for a common mucosal immunologic system. I. Migration of B immunoblasts into intestinal, respiratory and genital tissues. *J Immunol* 122:1892–1898, 1979
21. McDermott MR, Clark DA, Bienenstock J: Evidence for a common mucosal immunologic system. II. Influence of the estrous cycle on B immunoblast migration into genital and intestinal tissues. *J Immunol* 124:2536–2539, 1980
22. Sturn B, Schneweis K-E: Protective effect of an oral infection with Herpes simplex virus type 1 against subsequent genital infection with Herpes simplex virus type 2. *Med Microbiol Immunol* 165:119–127, 1978
23. Wira CR, Sandoe CP: Sex steroid hormone regulation of IgA and IgG in rat uterine secretions. *Nature (Lond)* 268:534–536, 1977
24. Sullivan DA, Wira CR: Variations in free secretory component levels in mucosal secretions of the rat. *J Immunol* 130:1330–1335, 1983
25. Wira CR, Merritt K: Effects of the estrous cycle, castration and pseudopregnancy on E. coli in the uterus and uterine secretions of the rat. *Biol Reprod* 17:519–522, 1977
26. Wira CR, Sandoe CP: Hormonal regulation of immunoglobulins: Influence of estradiol on immunoglobulins A and G in the rat uterus. *Endocrinology* 106:1020–1026, 1980
27. Sullivan DA, Wira CR: Mechanisms involved in hormone regulation of immunoglobulins in the rat uterus. I. Uterine immunoglobulin response to a single estradiol treatment. *Endocrinology* 112:260–268, 1983
28. Wira CR, Sullivan DA, Sandoe CP: The role of estradiol in the accumulation of IgA and IgG in the rat uterine lumen. *J Steroid Biochem* 19:469–474, 1983
29. Wira CR, Hyde E, Sandoe CP, et al: Cellular aspects of the rat uterine IgA response to estradiol and progesterone. *J Steroid Biochem* 12:451–459, 1980
30. Sullivan DA, Wira CR: Hormonal regulation of immunoglobulins in the rat uterus. II. Uterine response to multiple estradiol treatments. *Endocrinology* 114:650–658, 1984
31. Sullivan DA, Wira CR: Estradiol regulation of secretory component in the female reproductive tract. *J Steroid Biochem* 15:439–444, 1981
32. Wira CR, Stern JE, Colby E: Estradiol regulation of secretory component in the uterus of the rat: Evidence for involvement of RNA synthesis. *J Immunol* 133:2624, 1984
33. Sullivan DA, Underdown BJ, Wira CR: Steroid hormone regulation of free secretory component in the rat uterus. *Immunology* 49:379–386, 1983
34. Sullivan DA, Richardson GS, MacLaughlin DT, et al: Variations in the levels of secretory component in human uterine fluid during the menstrual cycle. *J Steroid Biochem* 20:509, 1984
35. Holinka CF, Gurpide E: Hormone-related enzymatic activities in normal and cancer cells of human endometrium. *J Steroid Biochem* 15:183–192, 1981
36. Ahlquist J: Endocrine influences on lymphatic organs, immune responses, inflammation and autoimmunity. *Acta Endocrinol (Copenh)* 83 (suppl 206):5–131, 1976
37. Blair PB: Immunological consequences of early exposure of experimental animals to diethylstilbestrol and steroid hormones, in Herbst AL, Bern HA, eds: *Developmental Effects of Diethylstilbestrol (DES) in Pregnancy.* New York, Thieme–Stratton, 1981, pp 167–193

38. Shapiro S, Slone D. The effects of exogenous female sex hormones in the fetus. *Epidemiol Rev* 1:110–123, 1979

39. Mathur S, Mathur RS, Dawda H, et al: Sex steroids, hormones and antibodies to Candida albicans. *Clin Exp Immunol* 33:79–87, 1978

40. Helgason S, Von-Schoultz B: Estrogen replacement therapy and the mixed lymphocyte reaction. *Am J Obstet Gynecol* 141:395–399, 1981

41. Szekeres J, Scernus V, Pejtsic S, et al: Progesterone as an immunologic blocking factor in human pregnancy serum. *J Reprod Immunol* 3:333–339, 1981

42. Wybran J: Lynestrenol: A progesterone-like agent with immunostimulatory properties. *Cancer Res* 75:180–185, 1980

43. Keller AJ, Irvine WJ, Jordan J, et al: Phytohemagglutinin-induced lymphocyte transformation in oral contraceptive users. *Obstet Gynecol* 49:83–89, 1977

44. Bray RS: Some immune responses of Gambian women taking the combined oral contraceptive pill. *Contraception* 13:417–422, 1976

45. Zane HD: Immune reactivity among women on oral contraceptives. Doctoral thesis, Rutgers University, Newark, NJ, 1983

46. Gerretsen G, Krener J, Bleuminlt E, et al: Immune reactivity of women on hormonal contraceptives. Phytohemagglutin and concanavalin-A induced lymphocyte response. *Contraception* 11:25–28, 1980

47. Horne CHW, Howie PW, Weir RJ, et al: Effect of combined estrogen–progestogen oral contraceptives on serum levels of macroglobulin, transferrin, albumin and IgG. *Lancet* 1:49–50, 1970

48. Chandra RK: Serum levels of IgG and α_2-macroglobulin and incidence of cryo-fibrinogenemia in women taking oral contraceptives. *J Reprod Fertil* 28:463–467, 1972

49. Baker DA, Milch P. Immune alterations in women on low dose oral contraceptives. Abstract 291P in Abstracts, *Thirty-Second Annual Meeting Society of Gynecologic Investigators, Phoenix, March 1985*

50. Wira CR, Sullivan DA, Sandoe CP: Estrogen-mediated control of the secretory immune system in the uterus of the rat. *Ann NY Acad Sci* 409:534–551, 1983

ANSWERS

1. d

2. b

3. c

Epidermal Growth Factor and Its Receptor and Their Possible Relationships to Gynecologic Endocrinology

JOHN C. M. TSIBRIS

INTRODUCTION

Recent research in endocrinology is beginning to show that paracrine chemical substances such as epidermal growth factor may play important roles in fostering differentiation of epithelia, including tissues in the reproductive tract, raising implications for the understanding of hormone responsiveness and oncogenesis. The current enthusiasm for the study of peptide growth factors,[1] e.g., epidermal growth factor (EGF), and their cell-surface receptors, is based on the realization that most of them have mitogenic properties and regulate a cascade of events (pleiotropic response) in normally dividing cells. On the other hand, cells that are transformed (e.g., after exposure to retroviruses) produce proteins that have extensive primary sequence homology with these peptide growth fac-

tors, thus becoming independent of an exogenous supply of mitogens required for their growth. EGF and other peptide growth factors exert their biologic effect through specific receptor proteins located at the plasma membrane. An exciting discovery was made when the primary structure of the EGF receptor was determined and was compared with a data base of all known protein sequences.[2-4] Extensive homology was found between the EGF receptor and the protein encoded by a viral oncogene (*erbB*); oncogenes are genomic sequences in the cellular or viral genome that are considered responsible for the induction of neoplasia.

Since the discovery of EGF by Stanley Cohen in 1960, a great deal of progress has been made in understanding the structure of novel peptide growth factors, such as EGF, their receptors, and the mechanisms of their biologic action.[5] This account of recent findings about EGF and its receptor is aimed to describe some new exciting concepts which do not fall within the classic framework of endocrinology. It is hoped that the information gained from the study of EGF, its receptor, and the newly

JOHN C. M. TSIBRIS • Department of Obstetrics and Gynecology, and Department of Physiology and Biophysics, University of Illinois at Chicago, Chicago, Illinois 60612.

found families of peptide growth factors will broaden our perspective and clarify our understanding of how they and sex hormones/receptors interact to control normal and abnormal (neoplastic) growth of gynecologic tissues.

EPIDERMAL GROWTH FACTOR

Mouse EGF[5-7] is an energetically stable, acidic (pI = 4.6) polypeptide hormone with a molecular weight of 6045 (53 amino acids) and three disulfide (cystine) bonds, which are required for activity; EGF has no alanine, phenylalanine, or lysine residues (Fig. 34-1). EGF was discovered by S. Cohen during an attempt to isolate nerve growth factor from male mouse submaxillary glands. Extracts from these glands were injected into newborn mice and caused a precocious eyelid opening and eruption of the incisors; these observations became a bioassay and assisted in isolating EGF.

Under neutral pH, EGF can be isolated from male mouse submaxillary glands as a 74,000-M_r complex composed of two molecules of EGF and two molecules of a 30,000-M_r EGF-binding protein, which displays arginine esteropeptidase activity. Nerve growth factor (NGF) isolated from the same source is also bound to a homologous binding protein with arginine esteropeptidase activity. Since both EGF and NGF have arginine residues at their carboxy terminal, it is possible that EGF and NGF are produced from their precursor proteins by the action of these arginine esteropeptidases.

An unexpected discovery about the biologic activity of mouse EGF was made when the primary structure of human urogastrone, a urinary peptide that inhibits gastric secretion of HCl, was determined. Comparison revealed that human EGF and human urogastrone were identical molecules with a molecular weight of 5400. The primary sequence of urogastrone is similar to 70% of the mouse EGF sequence, and the latter is being used routinely (because of its easy accessibility) in all studies of EGF in human tissues and cell cultures. It is believed that EGF and its receptor, both of which are found in vertebrates (from sharks to human) and which seem to be conserved through evolution, must play a rudimentary role in metabolism and development.

Among the numerous biologic effects of EGF on epithelial tissues[6,7] are (1) induction of cell proliferation in the pericardium, kidney capsule, and bile duct; (2) control of the palate closure; (3) epithelial hyperplasia of the conducting airways in fetal lambs and rabbits and prevention of the development of hyaline membrane disease; (4) induction of tracheal budding in chick lung rudiments; (5) a direct hyperplastic effect on corneal cells in organ culture; and (6) promotion of healing of stomach ulcers. EGF induces increased synthesis of DNA, RNA, cyclic nucleotides, ornithine decarboxylase, and the synthesis/secretion of specialized proteins and complex carbohydrates (e.g., prolactin, collagen, hyaluronic acid).[7,8]

The mitogenic effects of EGF seen in vivo can also be demonstrated in organ or tissue cultures.[6] For example, EGF is mitogenic to human keratinocytes, granulosa cells, and rabbit endometrial cells. In human choriocarcinoma cells, EGF stimulates the secretion of chorionic gonadotropin (hCG). EGF regulates the number of gonadotropin receptors in testicular Leydig tumor and granulosa cells in culture. EGF also inhibits the ability of hCG

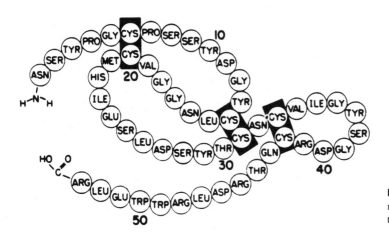

FIGURE 34-1. Amino acid sequence of mouse EGF showing the position of the three disulfide bonds. (From Cohen.[5])

to transform undifferentiated theca-interstitial cells into active androgen-producing cells,[9] indicating that the salivary gland, the main known producer of EGF, may influence the development of the follicle system (theca and granulosa cells).

Mouse EGF is synthesized in the submaxillary glands and is under androgen control; female mice apparently have a similar gland structure but less than 10% of the male EGF levels. Other sites of EGF synthesis must exist, since the removal of the submaxillary glands does not affect the blood EGF levels. Human EGF (urogastrone) is enriched in the submaxillary glands and in the Brunner's gland of the duodenum. EGF (urogastrone) is present in human milk, plasma (men and women have equal levels, 140–160 pg/ml), urine (men secrete approx. 800 ng/kg body weight per 24 hr and women 600 ng/kg per 24 hr),[7] cerebrospinal fluid (CSF), maternal and fetal blood, and amniotic fluid.

Infusion of EGF to sheep reversibly weakened, the attachment of the fleece, which then could be removed easily by hand.[10] Since EGF is androgen dependent in mice, this information may suggest a cause-and-effect relationship in baldness, perpetuating the myth that bald men have high testosterone levels. EGF and nerve growth factor are synthesized, stored, and secreted by the glandular epithelial cells of the prostate. EGF-like activity has also been detected in human testes, seminal vesicles, and epididymis.[11]

Since there is no single site of EGF synthesis, such "classic" endocrinologic studies as removal of the source of EGF and observation of the results of EGF deprivation cannot be done. Despite two decades of EGF study we still do not know the precise function of EGF in development and metabolism; perhaps recent insights into the interaction of EGF with its receptor and neighboring growth factors/receptors will point to new types of hormone interactions (paracrine and autocrine[12]) and will lead to more extensive applications of EGF to clinical problems such as the treatment of severe burns, corneal wounds, and ulcers.[6]

THE EGF RECEPTOR

Cells responsive to EGF have receptors for EGF on their surface membrane. Iodine-125-labeled EGF prepared by reacting EGF with chloramine-T + $^{125}I^-$ or with lactoperoxidase + H_2O_2 + $^{125}I^-$, has been used to determine EGF receptors in a variety of cultured cells (e.g., vulval car-

cinoma cells A431) or plasma membrane preparation from many tissues (e.g., placenta, liver, lung, endometrium). The specificity and high-affinity (dissociation constants are $10^{-9}–10^{-10}$ M) of $[^{125}I]$-EGF binding has also been used to set up radioreceptor assays for EGF.

It has been amply documented that after the initial binding of $[^{125}I]$-EGF to specific plasma membrane receptors, which are diffusely distributed and laterally mobile, the EGF–receptor complexes are clustered in clathrin-coated regions of the plasma membrane, and enter the cell by the temperature-dependent process of receptor-mediated endocytosis (for review, see Wileman et al.[13]). The process of endocytosis is common to many peptide hormone receptors (e.g., for insulin and platelet-derived growth factor) and a few other proteins, such as α_2-macroglobulin and low-density lipoproteins. Following internalization, the ligand (EGF) is degraded by lysosomal enzymes (this degradation is not a prerequisite for the stimulation of cell division). In hepatocytes it was shown that the EGF receptor is recycled back to the cell surface. This pathway of receptor movement as well as the structure and orientation of the EGF receptor have been studied extensively using ^{125}I-labeled, fluorescent, and ferritin-conjugated EGF[6] and polyclonal or monoclonal antibodies to the EGF receptor. Most studies have been done with placental receptors (because of readily available normal tissue) and with numerous cells in culture, especially the epidermoid carcinoma cell line A431, which expresses 50 times more receptors (2 million receptor sites per cell) than the majority of other cells. These studies have demonstrated the importance of the receptor, and not EGF itself, as the active "carrier" of the signals leading to EGF-specific pleiotropic responses and cell proliferation. However, the precise nature of these "signals" is unknown.

In 1978, Carpenter et al.[3] studied in A431 cells the effect of EGF on phosphorylation/dephosphorylation reactions, which are known to regulate many metabolic pathways; cell membranes were found to contain endogenous protein kinases, which phosphorylated serine and threonine residues. Carpenter et al.[3] found an EGF-specific protein kinase independent of cAMP, cGMP, and Ca^{2+}, which in the presence of ATP, Mn^{2+}, or Mg^{2+} phosphorylated endogenous membrane proteins (most prominently a 170,000-dalton protein) and added proteins such as casein, histones, and a variety of peptides. What was unusual, however, was that in all cases a tyrosine residue was phosphorylated. It has since been determined that this EGF-stimulated protein-tyrosine kinase (PTK) activity is intrinsic to the receptor, that the 170,000-dalton protein represents the intact receptor, and therefore the EGF receptor could phosphorylate itself (autophosphorylation). Purified EGF receptor from A431 cells could phosphorylate at tyrosine residues both the α- and β-subunits of the progesterone receptor from hen oviduct,[3] but the biologic significance of this or all other tyrosine phosphorylations is not yet clear.

Interestingly, receptor–PTK activity and autophosphorylation is a ligand-stimulated property common to other growth factor receptors, i.e., for insulin, insulinlike growth factor 1 (IGF-1) and platelet-derived growth factor (PDGF). Like the EGF receptor, these receptors can phosphorylate other endogenous or exogenous substrates in vitro. There are, however, growth factor receptors, for example, for interleukin 2, nerve growth factor, or IGF-2, which do not exhibit PTK activity.[3,14]

Primary Structure of the EGF Receptor

The complete amino acid sequence of the human EGF receptor has been deduced from the nucleotide sequence of complementary DNA (cDNA) clones (for review, see Hunter and Cooper[3]). This sequence does not contain information about post-translational modifications (e.g., phosphorylations) or secondary structure (e.g., position of disulfide bonds) but represents a giant step forward in integrating information from the myriad of experiments done with EGF-binding sites during the past 20 years. It gives unprecedented insight into structural features that seem to be repeated in the structures of other peptide growth factor receptors, such as the receptor for insulin.

The main features of the EGF receptor are as follows:

1. The receptor is a glycoprotein and consists of a single long stretch of 1186 amino acids with a 170,000–180,000 M_r. There is some uncertainty about the precise amount of carbohydrate present. Another receptor, the PDGF receptor is also a monomer whereas the insulin receptor is made of two α- and two β-subunits held together by disulfide bonds as a β.α.α.β. tetramer.
2. The NH$_2$-terminal is outside the cell, whereas the COOH-terminal is inside the cytoplasm (Fig. 34-2). On the basis of infor-

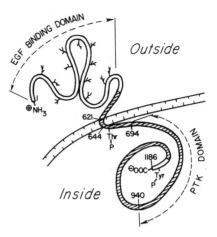

FIGURE 34-2. Schematic representation of the human EGF receptor at the cell surface. The EGF-binding site, located in the extracellular side, is cysteine rich and has 12 carbohydrate chains important in EGF binding (the exact size of the polypeptide chain, which folds to form the ligand-binding site, is unknown at this time). The 23-residue hydrophobic section spanning the plasma membrane is followed by a cytoplasmic 15-residue basic section containing threonine-654, which is phosphorylated by kinase C. The PTK (protein-tyrosine kinase) active site is made of residues 694–940 but, unlike PTK domains of other receptors, the main autophosphorylated tyrosine (residue 1173) is outside that polypeptide segment. The hatched segment represents a 600-residue section of the receptor, which shows significant homology with a glycoprotein encoded by the v-erb-B oncogene from the avian erythroblastosis retrovirus.

mation from the primary structure and numerous previous experiments with partial proteolysis of native EGF receptor, [^{125}I]-EGF binding, and antibodies, the EGF receptor can be divided in three domains:

a. An extracellular domain, consisting of 621 amino acids (approx. 80,000 M_r) and containing the binding site for EGF
b. A transmembrane domain, made up of 23, mainly hydrophobic, amino acids
c. An intracellular C-terminal domain, made up of 542 amino acids (approx. 65,000 daltons) and containing the protein-tyrosine kinase (PTK) active site. At the tail end of this domain, and outside the catalytic site, is the main tyrosine reside, position 1173, which becomes self-phosphorylated by the PTK activity of the receptor.

3. The NH_2-terminal region is rich in cysteine residues; it is assumed that disulfide bonds would be formed to stabilize the conformation of the extracellular domain. Twelve potential N-linked glycosylation sites (approx. 30,000 daltons)[15] are located in this domain and are probably important in EGF binding.

4. As is common among cytoplasmic sequences across transmembrane domains, there is a preponderance of basic amino acids in a 15-amino acid stretch following the putative 23-amino acid transmembrane domain. This basic section may interact with the plasma membrane phospholipid head groups and better anchor the receptor across the cell surface. Some important changes must occur in this region when EGF binds to the receptor to cause an allosteric activation of the PTK activity and during the endocytosis of the whole receptor.

5. An amazing story unfolded when the EGF receptor sequence was determined and revealed that an approximate 600 amino acid stretch (Fig. 34-2) has an 85% overall homology with a 74,000-dalton glycoprotein encoded by the virus-erb-B oncogene from an RNA tumor virus (avian erythroblastosis virus, AEV)[3]. The degree of identity is very high, considering the evolutionary distance between birds and humans and suggests that the cellular-erb-B locus encodes the EGF receptor in humans and birds. The human EGF receptor and a human v-erb-B-related sequence have been mapped on chromosome 7. The EGF receptor gene is amplified 15–20 times in the human epidermoid carcinoma A431 cells compared with DNA from normal diploid cells and could account for the increased EGF receptor production in these cells. Equally important is the fact that the v-erb-B sequence is missing the extracellular EGF-binding site (Fig. 34-2) but contains the PTK active site. Thus, the absence of the ligand binding domain signifies the removal of a control mechanism generated by ligand (EGF) binding and a possible continuous PTK activation leading to rapid proliferation, abnormal growth, and neoplasia.

Additional information reveals that the A431 cells secrete a 105,000-dalton protein[15] that is not derived from the membrane-bound EGF receptor and lacks PTK activity but that is homologous to the NH_2-terminal cell surface domain of the EGF receptor. Thus, the carcinoma A431 cells can produce one EGF receptor protein to be embedded in the plasma membrane and a separate, truncated, EGF receptor destined for secretion. The function of this secreted EGF-binding protein in terms of the paracrine or autocrine[12] cell regulation is unknown.

EGF Receptor, C-Kinase, and Phorbol Ester Tumor Promoters

Tyrosine phosphorylation is a relatively rare occurrence in the cell, since less than 1% of all phosphorylated amino acid residues are tyrosines; however, it appears to be an important regulatory modification. Serine and threonine phosphorylations can be catalyzed by kinase C, a membrane-associated, Ca^{2+}- and phospholipid-dependent enzyme. A special threonine residue seems important in signal transmission; it is located in position 654, among the basic amino acid stretch on the cytoplasmic side near the transmembrane domain of the EGF receptor (Fig. 34-2). Thr654 is probably phosphorylated in vivo by C-kinase, bringing about a significant modulation of the EGF receptor, i.e., a decrease in the affinity for EGF.

C-kinase is activated by and probably is the cell receptor for phorbol esters.[16] Phorbol esters are the most extensively studied and most potent tumor promoters and are diterpenes of plant origin. TPA (12-O-tetradecanoylphorbol-13-acetate), the most frequently used phorbol ester, has a diacylglycerol-like structure. Tumor promoters are a class of compounds that are not carcinogenic by themselves, but that can markedly increase tumorigenesis when given after a suboptimal dose of a tumor initiator, such as the chemical carcinogen benzo(a)pyrene.

Tumor promoters, like TPA, decrease the affinity or the number of EGF receptors in many cells by activating the C-kinase, which in turn phosphorylates Thr654 and several other serine residues.

Physiologic activators of C-kinase are Ca^{2+} and diacylglycerol. A unique effect of EGF on A431 cells is to stimulate the turnover of phosphatidylinositol and to increase the production of diacylglycerol, thereby activating membrane-bound C-kinase. This series of experiments[3,17,18] gives a better insight into the downregulation of EGF receptors in A431 by EGF. Until now, the literature was filled with "phenomenological" observations that compounds X,Y,Z could change the affinity or receptor number (usually estimated by

Scatchard plots of EGF binding data), but an understanding of the molecular mechanism of these changes was lacking. *Thr654* and other phosphorylation sites are likely points of such a signal transmission control.

A first step in phosphatidylinositol metabolism is its phosphorylation, followed by its breakdown to diacylglycerol and inositol triphosphate. It is not yet known whether the EGF receptor can catalyze the phosphorylation of phosphatidylinositol.

EGF and Transforming Growth Factor Receptors

Transforming growth factors (TGFs) are a family of polypeptides[4,19] that are produced by many tumor cells and can confer to normal cells anchorage-independent growth and a transformed phenotype. Unlike genetic cell transformation, the ''transformation'' of these cells is reversible upon removal of TGFs from the medium.[19] There are two types of TGFs.

α-TGF. This type has a molecular weight of 5600 and a 30–40% sequence homology with human and mouse EGF. α-TGF is produced only in tumor-derived cells or cells transformed by retroviruses, although it was recently isolated from normal human platelets. EGF and α-TGF are products of separate genes. α-TGF and EGF interact with equal potency with the EGF receptor in human placenta and A431 cells. α-TGF can mimic EGF and induce PTK activity and EGF receptor downregulation. The autocrine secretion of TGFs, especially α-TGF, may be an important mechanism in the malignant transformation of cells.[12]

β-TGF. This type is much more abundant than α-TGF and is present in both normal and tranformed cells. Neither α- or β-TGF alone can cause anchorage-independent growth of cells. β-TGF is thought to have a normal function in wound healing.[19] β-TGF, which does not bind to the EGF receptor, consists of two (probably identical) basic polypeptide subunits of 12,000 daltons, linked by disulfide bonds to form a 23,000–25,000-M_r dimer. Affinity labeling experiments with [^{125}I]-TGF-β have indicated that the β-TGF receptor is made of two subunits of 280,000–300,000 daltons; giving rise to a disulfide-linked glycosylated dimer of 565,000–615,000 daltons.

There is no cross-interaction among α-TGF, β-TGF, and their receptors, although the demonstration of the β-TGF/β-TGF receptor's transforming

activity requires the presence of other growth factors and their receptors, i.e., PDGF, EGF/α-TGF, and insulinlike growth factors (for review, see Massagué[19]).

EGF and Estrogen Receptors

In immature rats, administration of 17β-estradiol produced a threefold increase in the binding of [^{125}I]-EGF to uterine membranes.[20] However, we found no change in EGF binding to plasma membranes from nonmalignant human endometrium during the menstrual cycle (Fig. 34-3), refuting any apparent correlation between EGF receptors and sex hormones.[21] On the contrary, an apparent negative correlation may exist between EGF and estrogen receptors along the longitudinal uterine axis, since the endocervical region showed higher EGF binding than the fundal region of the endometrium; previous experiments[21] had shown that the fundus has significantly higher estrogen receptor levels than are found in the endocervix.

A significant inverse relationship between estrogen receptors and EGF receptors was found in primary breast tumors[22]; EGF receptors were found in a greater proportion of metastases than in primary tumors. Therefore, the presence of EGF receptors may be associated with metastatic potential, and the growth of estrogen receptor-negative tumors may

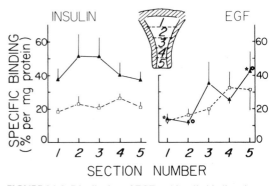

FIGURE 34-3. Distribution of EGF and insulin binding sites to plasma membrane preparations from the outlined five sections of the human uterine cavity (inset sketch). Each point is the mean value of EGF or insulin binding from 10–15 uterine specimens; the bars indicate the standard error. Squares and triangles indicate, respectively, data from the proliferative and secretory phases of the menstrual cycle. Whereas in each section there is no difference in EGF binding during the two phases of the cycle, there is significantly ($p < 0.02$) higher EGF binding in the endocervical than in the fundal regions. (From Sheets et al.[21])

be regulated by peptide growth factors (EGF, α-TGF) interacting with the EGF receptor.

SUMMARY

Growth factors like epidermal growth factor (EGF) and their receptors are involved in the regulation of cell proliferation; recent evidence suggests that they also have a key function in oncogenesis. EGF, a polypeptide originally isolated from male mice, has 53 amino acids and three disulfide bridges. It is secreted by many tissues but in largest concentration by the submaxillary gland and duodenum; it exhibits mitogenic and many other activities. Human EGF, smaller than mouse EGF, was formerly known as urogastrone (a urinary peptide that inhibits gastric secretion of HCl) and has 70% sequence homology with mouse EGF. Both EGFs bind to the EGF cell-surface receptor.

The recent determination of the primary structure of the human EGF receptor was a great accomplishment of recombinant DNA technology and protein chemistry revealing that the receptor consists of three sections or domains: (1) the N-terminal section, made up of 621 amino acids, is rich in carbohydrate and cysteine residues and extends into the extracellular side of the plasma membrane; (2) the transmembrane section, made up of 23 mostly hydrophobic amino acids; and (3) the C-terminal section, which is made up of 542 amino acids and extends into the cytoplasm. The EGF-binding site is located in the ''outside'' domain, whereas the intracellular domain contains the EGF-receptor's protein-tyrosine kinase (PTK) active site; the main tyrosine residue autophosphorylated (*via* an interior or intramolecular mechanism) by the PTK is located near the C-terminal. When EGF binds to its receptor the PTK activity is induced by some interchain allosteric signal. EGF receptor PTK can also phosphorylate histones and other cytoplasmic proteins in vitro.

In an unprecedented convergence of endocrinologic and viral oncogenesis research, it was found that among the 20 identified viral oncogens three encode proteins related to either a growth factor or a growth factor receptor. A close sequence similarity was found between the human EGF receptor and a protein encoded by the avian erythroblastosis virus-transforming gene, *v-erb-B*. However, the viral gene product is missing the EGF-binding site but maintains the PTK activity site, implying the loss of a regulatory control mechanism provided by the availability/binding of EGF. Thus, the potential continuous PTK activation could lead to rapid proliferation and eventually to neoplasia. It becomes clear that retroviruses employ cellular genes for growth factor receptors as part of their transforming strategy.

To date only α-transforming growth factor (α-TGF), a 6000-dalton peptide bearing 30–40% homology with EGF, can mimic EGF in terms of its binding to the EGF receptor, PTK activation, or receptor downregulation.

Research on EGF and its receptor provides new clues into the mechanism of action of peptide hormones. Further studies will certainly reveal important interactions between the classic sex steroid and peptide hormones and the new regulators of normal and neoplastic cell growth exemplified by epidermal growth factor.

QUESTIONS

1. A calcium-activated neutral protease can cleave off a 150–180-residue (20,000-dalton) polypeptide from the C-terminal of the EGF receptor.[23] How would that cleavage change the receptor's auto- and heterophosphorylation (PTK) activity? Explain your answer.

2. Which peptide growth factor, besides EGF, would bind to the EGF receptor?

3. What is the connection between EGF and viral oncogenesis?

REFERENCES

1. James R, Bradshaw RA: Polypeptide growth factors. *Ann Rev Biochem* 53:259–292, 1984*
2. Weinberg RA: Cellular oncogenes. *Trends Biochem Sci* 9:131–133, 1984*
3. Hunter T, Cooper JA: Protein-tyrosine kinases. *Ann Rev Biochem* 54:897–930, 1985*
4. Paul D: Growth factors, oncogenes and transformation. Part I: Growth factors and cell cycle control. *Arzneimittelforschung* 35:772–779, 1985*
5. Cohen S: The epidermal growth factor (EGF). *Cancer* 51:1787–1791, 1983*
6. Haigler HT: Epidermal growth factor: Cellular binding and consequences, in Guroff G (ed): *Growth and Maturation Factors*, Vol. 1. New York, Wiley, 1983, pp 119–153*
7. Daughaday WH, Heath E: Physiological and possible clinical significance of epidermal and nerve growth factors. *Clin Endocrinol Metab* 13:207–226, 1984*
8. Castor CW, Cabral AR: Growth factors in human disease:

The realities, pitfalls and promise. *Semin Arthritis Rheumatism* 15:33–44, 1985*

9. Erickson GF, Case E: Epidermal growth factor antagonizes ovarian theca-interstitial cytodifferentiation. *Mol Cell Endocrinol* 31:71–76, 1983

10. Moore GPM, Panaretto BA, Wallace ALC: Treatment of ewes at different stages of pregnancy with epidermal growth factor: Effects on wool growth and plasma concentration of growth hormone, prolactin, placental lactogen and thyroxin and on foetal development. *Acta Endocrinol (Copenh)* 105:558–566, 1984

11. Elson SD, Browne CA, Thorburn GD: Identification of epidermal growth factor-like activity in human male reproductive tissues and fluids. *J Clin Endocrinol Metab* 58:589–594, 1984

12. Sporn MB, Todaro GJ: Autocrine secretion and malignant transformation of cells. *N Engl J Med* 303:878–880, 1980

13. Wileman T, Harding C, Stahl P: Receptor-mediated endocytosis. *Biochem J* 232:1–14, 1985

14. Schlessinger J, Schreiber AB, Levi A, et al: Regulation of cell proliferation by epidermal growth factor. *CRC Crit Rev Biochem* 14:93–111, 1983

15. Weber W, Gill GN, Spiess J: Production of an epidermal growth factor receptor-related protein. *Science* 224:294–297, 1984

16. Horowitz AD, Weinstein IB: Tumor promoters and their relevance to endogenous growth factors, in Guroff G(ed): *Growth and Maturation Factors*, Vol. 1. New York, Wiley, 1983, pp 155–191*

17. Fearn JC, King AC: EGF receptor affinity is regulated by intracellular calcium and protein kinase C. *Cell* 40:991–1000, 1985

18. Wolf M, Levine H III, May WM Jr, et al: A model for intracellular translocation of protein kinase C involving synergism between Ca^{++} and phorbol esters. *Nature (Lond)* 317:546–549, 1985

19. Massagué J: The transforming growth factors. *Trends Biochem Sci* 10:237–240, 1985*

20. Mukku VR, Stancel GM: Regulation of epidermal growth factor receptors by estrogens. *J Biol Chem* 260:9820–9824, 1985

21. Sheets EE, Tsibris JCM, Cook NI, et al: In vitro binding of insulin and epidermal growth factor to human endometrium and endocervix. *Am J Obstet Gynecol* 153:60–65, 1985

22. Sainsbury JRC, Sherbet GV, Farndon JR, et al: Epidermal-growth-factor receptors and oestrogen receptors in human breast cancer. *Lancet* 1:364–366, 1985

23. King LE, Gates RE: Calcium-activated neutral protease purified from beef lung: Properties and use in defining structure of epidermal growth factor receptors. *Arch Biochem Biophys* 242:146–156, 1985

ANSWERS

1. Most likely, the degraded EGF receptor form (150,000 daltons) would retain some activity toward exogenous substrates, since the PTK active site (Fig. 34-2, residues 694–940) would not be affected. King and Gates[23] found that the 150,000-M_r and 170,000-M_r forms had comparable PTK activity toward exogenous substrates (heterophosphorylation). The autophosphorylation rate may go down because the protease would remove the main tyrosine residue (at position 1173) phosphorylated by the receptor PTK. Some autophosphorylation may remain, however, since there are other tyrosine residues, some within the PTK active site (Fig. 34-2), which are also phosphorylated. King and Gates[23] found that the 150,000-M_r form was autophosphorylated 10% as well as the native 170,000-M_r form.

2. The α-transforming growth factor, which is produced (almost exclusively) by transformed cells.

3. A retrovirus oncogene (*v-erb-B*) encodes for a polypeptide that has an 85% overall homology with the PTK domain of the EGF receptor. The retroviruses must use, in some yet unknown way, cellular oncogenes (proto-oncogenes) to cause cell transformation.

GLOSSARY OF ABBREVIATIONS

ADH   antidiuretic hormone

17-AHP   17α-hydroxyprogesterone

AID   artificial insemination by a donor

AIH   artificial insemination by the husband

ACTH   adrenocorticotropic hormone; adreno-corticotropin

AMP   adenosine monophosphate

APL   anterior pituitarylike hormone

ATP   adenosine triphosphate

BBT   basal body temperature

BEI   butanol-extractable iodine

BMR   basal metabolic rate

BSP   Bromsulphthalein

BTB   breakthrough bleeding

BUN   blood urea nitrogen

CAGS   congenital adrenogenital syndrome

CAH   congenital adrenal hyperplasia

C-21 compounds   21-carbon compounds

CBC   complete blood count

CCI   crowded cell index

CDGD   constitutional delay of growth and development

Clomid   clomiphene

CL   confidence limit

CNS   central nervous system

CNS–H-P   central nervous system–hypothalamus-pituitary

CRF   corticotropin-releasing factor; ACTH-releasing factor

CT   computed tomography

D & C   dilatation and curettage

DHEA   dehydroepiandrosterone

DHEAS   dehydroepiandrosterone sulfate

DHT   dihydrotestosterone

DIT   diiodotyrosine

DNA   deoxyribonucleic acid

E_2 17β-estradiol

EE   ethynyl estradiol

EI   eosinophilic index

ER   estrogen receptor

FCI   folded cell index

FELR   follicular estrogen with luteal replacement

FPLR   follicular progestin with luteal replacement

FSH   follicle-stimulating hormone

FSH-RF   follicle-stimulating hormone-releasing factor

GH   growth hormone

GN-RF   gonadotropin-releasing factor

hCG   human chorionic gonadotropin

hGH   human growth hormone

hCS   human chorionic somatomammotropin (known also as hPL)

5-HIAA   5-hydroxyindoleacetic acid

hMG   human menopausal urinary gonadotropin

17-HP   17-hydroxyprogesterone

hPG   human pituitary gonadotropin; human pituitary FSH

hPL   human placental lactogen (known also as hCS)

HPO axis   hypothalamus-pituitary-ovarian axis

ICSH   interstitial cell-stimulating hormone (same as LH)

IHP syndrome   immature hypothalamic-pituitary syndrome

ILA   insulinlike activity

IUD   intrauterine device

IVP   intravenous pyelogram

KPI   karyopyknotic index

17-KS   17-ketosteroid(s)

17-KGS   17-ketogenic steroid(s)

LATS   long-acting thyroid stimulator

LH   luteinizing hormone

LH-RF   luteinizing hormone releasing factor

LTH   luteotropic hormone (known also as PRL)

MCR   metabolic clearance rate

MI   maturation index

MIT   monoiodotyrosine

MSH   melanocyte-stimulating hormone

NAD   nicotinamide adenine dinucleotide

NADPH   reduced nicotinamide adenine dinucleotide phosphate (TPNH)

OAAD   ovarian ascorbic acid depletion

OC   oral contraceptive

17-OH   17-hydroxylated steroids

17-OHCS   17-hydroxycorticosteroid(s)

17-OH Progest-caproate   17α-hydroxyprogesterone-caproate

PAPS   3′-phosphoadenylylphosphosulfate

PBI   protein-bound iodine

PCO   polycystic ovarian disease

PID   pelvic inflammatory disease

PIF   prolactin-inhibiting factor

PMP   postmenstrual phase

PMS   pregnant mare serum; equine gonadotropin

PMSG   pregnant mare serum gonadotropin

PPA   postpill amenorrhea

PPAG   postpill amenorrhea galactorrhea

PR   progesterone receptor

PRL   prolactin (known also as LTH)

RAI   radioactive iodine

RF   releasing factors

RIA   radioimmunoassay

RNA   ribonucleic acid

SHBG   sex hormone binding globulin

T   testosterone

T3   triiodothyronine

T4   circulating thyroxine; tetraiodothyronine; L-thyroxine

T4I   thyroxine iodide

TBG   thyroxine-binding globulin

TBP   thyroxine-binding protein

TBPA   thyroxine-binding prealbumin

TeBG   testosterone-estradiol-binding globulin

TPNH   reduced triphosphopyridine nucleotide hormone (NADPH)

TRH   thyrotropin-releasing hormone

TSH   thyroid-stimulating hormone (or thyrotropic-stimulating hormone); thyrotropin

MISCELLANEOUS ABBREVIATIONS

MU   mouse units

IM   intramuscular

IU   international units

IV   intravenous

R   roentgen

μU   microunit

bid   two times a day

tid   three times a day

qid   four times a day

Index